DRUG	USE	DOSAGE	ROUTE	SIDE EFFECTS	OTHER MEDICAL ISSUES
Anticonvulsants—cont'd					
Lamotrigine (Lamictal)	Partial seizures	200 to 500 mg/day	PO	Leukopenia, anemia, disseminated intravascular coagulation, hepatitis, Stevens-Johnson syndrome	Must stop immediately in presence of rash
Levetiracetam (Keppra)	Grand mal, partial, psychomotor seizures	Maximum daily dose of 3000 ng	PO	Somnolence, asthenia, infection, dizziness	
Phenobarbital (Luminal)	CNS depressant	50 to 100 mg tid serum 15-40 mcg/ml	PO, IV	HA, vertigo, confusion, N/V, respiratory depression; respiratory arrest with IV	15 mg/kg IV in status epilepticus
Phenytoin (Dilantin)	Grand mal, psychomotor seizures; neuropathic pain	100 mg tid	PO, IV	Ataxia, sedation, HA, N/V, cardiac dysrhythmias	Level: 10 to 20 mcg/ml
Primidone (Mysoline)	Barbiturate; grand mal, focal, psychomotor seizures	250 mg tid to 500 mg qid	PO	Ataxia, sedation, HA, N/V, irritability	Level: 5 to 12 mcg/ml
Valproic acid (Depakote/Depakene)	Absence seizures; neuropathic pain	1000 to 3000 mg/day	PO	Ataxia, sedation, HA, N/V, aggression	Avoid in pregnancy
Antihypertensives					
ACE inhibitors	Antihypertensive		PO, IV	Nephrotic syndrome	
Alpha-blockers (Minipress, etc.)	Antihypertensive, control of sympathetic dystrophy		PO, IV	Syncope, sedation, HA, urinary retention	
Beta-blockers	Antihypertensive		PO, IV	Congestive heart failure, bradycardia, hypotension, peripheral vascular disease (PVD)	
Calcium channel blockers	Antihypertensive		PO, IV	Dizziness, HA, hypotension	
Direct vasodilators	Antihypertensive		PO, IV	Tachycardia, hypotension, HA	
Diuretics	Antihypertensive		PO, IV	Metabolic/electrolytes, cramps, hypotension, renal failure	
Postganglionic neuron inhibitors	Antihypertensive		PO, IV	Diarrhea, hypotension, depression	
Antidepressants					
Fluoxetine (Prozac)	Antidepressant	20 to 80 mg qd-bid	PO	Anxiety, tremor, insomnia, nausea, diarrhea	
MAO inhibitors	Antidepressant		PO	Dizziness, vertigo, HA, constipation, HTN	Patient must avoid tyramine/tryptophan
Sertraline (Zoloft)	Antidepressant	50 to 200 mg qd-bid	PO	Anxiety, tremor, insomnia, nausea, diarrhea	
Tricyclics (e.g., amitriptyline)	Antidepressant, pain control adjuvant		PO	Myocardial infarction (MI), hypotension, seizures, confusion, leukopenia, parathesias, N/V, coma, constipation, hepatitis	Best for continuous neuropathic pain

Continued on back endsheets

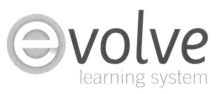 **evolve**
learning system

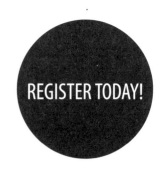 REGISTER TODAY!

To access your free Evolve Resources, visit:

http://evolve.elsevier.com/Gillen/stroke

Evolve Student Learning Resources for Gillen: Stroke Rehabilitation, *3E, offers the following features:*

- Activities for students to test their application and clinical thinking skills

- References linked to PubMed

- Glossary

Third Edition

STROKE REHABILITATION
A Function-Based Approach

Glen Gillen, EdD, OTR, FAOTA
Associate Professor of Clinical Occupational Therapy
Programs in Occupational Therapy
Columbia University
College of Physicians and Surgeons;
Honorary Adjunct Associate Professor
of Movement Sciences and Education
Teachers College
New York, New York

ELSEVIER
MOSBY

3251 Riverport Lane
St. Louis, Missouri 63043

STROKE REHABILITATION: A FUNCTION-BASED APPROACH,
THIRD EDITION

ISBN: 978-0-323-05911-4

Copyright © 2011, 2004, 1998 by Mosby, Inc., an affiliate of Elsevier Inc.

Notices

Knowledge and best practice in this field are constantly changing. As new research and experience broaden our understanding, changes in research methods, professional practices, or medical treatment may become necessary.

Practitioners and researchers must always rely on their own experience and knowledge in evaluating and using any information, methods, compounds, or experiments described herein. In using such information or methods they should be mindful of their own safety and the safety of others, including parties for whom they have a professional responsibility.

With respect to any drug or pharmaceutical products identified, readers are advised to check the most current information provided (i) on procedures featured or (ii) by the manufacturer of each product to be administered, to verify the recommended dose or formula, the method and duration of administration, and contraindications. It is the responsibility of practitioners, relying on their own experience and knowledge of their patients, to make diagnoses, to determine dosages and the best treatment for each individual patient, and to take all appropriate safety precautions.

To the fullest extent of the law, neither the Publisher nor the authors, contributors, or editors, assume any liability for any injury and/or damage to persons or property as a matter of products liability, negligence or otherwise, or from any use or operation of any methods, products, instructions, or ideas contained in the material herein.

Library of Congress Cataloging-in-Publication Data

Stroke rehabilitation : a function-based approach / Glen Gillen. -- 3rd ed.
    p. cm.
Includes bibliographical references and index.
ISBN 978-0-323-05911-4 (hardcover : alk. paper)
  1. Cerebrovascular disease--Patients--Rehabilitation. I. Gillen, Glen.
RC388.5.S85625 2011
616.8'1--dc22
                                    2010026437

Vice President and Publisher: Linda Duncan
Executive Editor: Kathy Falk
Managing Editor: Jolynn Gower
Publishing Services Manager: Anitha Rajarathnam
Project Manager: Mahalakshmi Nithyanand
Book Designer: Maggie Reid

Printed in the United States of America

Last digit is the print number: 9   8   7   6   5   4   3   2   1

Contributors

Guðrún Árnadóttir, PhD, MA, BOT
Private Practitioner, Associate Professor
Division of Occupational Therapy, Faculty of Health
University of Akureyri, Iceland;
Coordinator of Occupational Therapy Research and
    Development Projects, Occupational Therapy
Grensás, Landspítali, University Hospital
Reykjavík, Iceland

Sandra M. Artzberger, MS, OTR, CHT, CLT
Lecturer, Consultant, Hand Therapist
Rocky Mountain Physical Therapy
Pagosa Springs, Colorado

Wendy Avery, MS, OTR/L
Occupational Therapist
Amedisys Home Health
Bluffton, South Carolina

Matthew N. Bartels, MD, MPH
Assistant Professor of Clinical Rehabilitation Medicine
Columbia University
New York, New York

Clare C. Bassile, EdD, PT
Assistant Professor of Clinical Physical Therapy
Physical Therapy Program
Columbia University
New York, New York

Carolyn M. Baum, PhD, OTR, FAOTA
Associate Professor of Occupational Therapy and
    Neurology
Washington University School of Medicine
St. Louis, Missouri

Heather Edgar Beland, MS, OTR/L
Staff Therapist
Englewood Hospital and Medical Center
Englewood, New Jersey

Birgitta Bernspång, PhD, OT
Professor of Occupational Therapy
Department of Community Medicine and Rehabilitation
Umeå University
Umeå, Sweden

Karen A. Buckley, MA, OT/L
Clinical Assistant Professor
Department of Occupational Therapy
New York University
New York, New York

Helen S. Cohen, EdD, OTR, FAOTA
Associate Professor
Bobby R. Alford Department of Otorhinolaryngology
    and Communicative Sciences
Baylor College of Medicine
Houston, Texas

Salvatore DiMauro, MD
Lucy G. Moses Professor of Neurology
College of Physicians and Surgeons
Columbia University
New York, New York

Susan M. Donato, OTR/L
Occupational Therapist
Merrimack Special Education Collaborative
Chelmsford, Massachusetts

Catherine A. Duffy, OTR/L
Advanced Clinician, Occupational Therapy Department
New York-Presbyterian Hospital
Columbia University Medical Center;
Instructor in Clinical Occupational Therapy,
    Programs in Occupational Therapy
Columbia University
New York, New York

Janet Falk-Kessler, EdD, OTR, FAOTA
Associate Professor of Clinical Occupational Therapy
Director, Programs in Occupational Therapy
Columbia University
New York, New York

Jessica Farman, MS, OTR/L
Director of Rehabilitation
Belmont Manor Nursing Center
Belmont, Massachusetts

Susan E. Fasoli, ScD, OTR/L
Clinical Instructor
Physical Medicine and Rehabilitation
Harvard Medical School
Cambridge, Massachusetts;
Rehabilitation Manager
Rehabilitation Services
Newton Wellesley Hospital
Newton, Massachusetts

Glen Gillen, EdD, OTR, FAOTA
Associate Professor of Clinical Occupational Therapy
Programs in Occupational Therapy
Columbia University
College of Physicians and Surgeons;
Honorary Adjunct Associate Professor of Movement
    Sciences and Education
Teachers College
New York, New York

Sheila M. Hayes, BSN, MS, PT
Convent of Mary the Queen
Yonkers, New York

Leslie A. Kane, MA, OTR/L
Manager of Occupational Therapy
New York-Presbyterian Hospital and Columbia
    University Medical Center;
Instructor in Clinical Occupational Therapy
Programs in Occupational Therapy
Columbia University
New York, New York

Megan Kirshbaum, PhD
Founder and Executive Director
Through the Looking Glass;
Co-Director
The National Center for Parents with Disabilities
    and their Families
Berkeley, California

Josefine Lampinen, MSc
Council Certified Specialist in Occupational Therapy
Norrlands University Hosptial
Umeå, Sweden

Virgil Mathiowetz, PhD, OTR, FAOTA
Associate Professor
Program in Occupational Therapy
University of Minnesota
Minneapolis, Minnesota

Stephanie Milazzo, MA, OTR, CHT
Director of Rehabilitation
Rehab Resources Unlimited
Ossining, New York

Barbara E. Neuhaus, EdD, OTR
Adjunct Associate Professor (Retired)
Programs in Occupational Therapy
Columbia University
New York, New York

Susan L. Pierce, OTR, CDRS
Certified Driver Rehabilitation Specialist
Adaptive Mobility Services, Inc.
Orlando, Florida

Karen Halliday Pulaski, MS, OTR/L
Trauma Team Supervisor
Inpatient Rehabilitation
Moses Cone Health Systems
Greensboro, North Carolina

Ashwini K. Rao, EdD, OTR/L
Assistant Professor of Clinical Physical Therapy
Physical Therapy Program
Department of Rehabilitation Medicine
Columbia University
New York, New York

Karen Riedel, PhD, CCC-SLP
Director Speech-Language Pathology Department
Rusk Institute of Rehabilitation Medicine
New York University Medical Centers
New York, New York

Judith Rogers, OTR/L
Pregnancy and Birthing Specialist
Parenting Equipment Specialist
Through the Looking Glass
Berkeley, California

Kerry Brockmann Rubio, MHS, OTR/L
Lead Occupational Therapist
Maria Parham Hospital
Henderson, North Carolina

Patricia A. Ryan, MA, OTR/L
Senior Occupational Therapist
Department of Occupational Therapy
New York-Presbyterian Hospital
Columbia University Medical Center;
Instructor in Clinical Occupational Therapy
Programs in Occupational Therapy
Columbia University
New York, New York

Joyce S. Sabari, PhD, OTR, FAOTA
Associate Professor and Chair
Occupational Therapy Program
State University of New York—Downstate Medical
    Center
Brooklyn, New York

Mary Shea, MA, OTR, ATP
Clinical Manager, Wheelchair Clinic
Kessler Institute for Rehabilitation
West Orange, New Jersey

Celia Stewart, PhD, MS, CCC-SLP
Department Chair
Associate Professor
Communicative Sciences and Disorders
Steinhardt School of Culture, Education, and Human
    Development
New York University
New York, New York

Jennie W. Sullivan, OTR/L
Occupational Therapist
East Tennessee Children's Hospital
Knoxville, Tennessee

**Carolyn A. Unsworth, PhD, BAppSc (OccTher),
    AccOT, OTR**
Associate Professor
School of Occupational Therapy
La Trobe University
Bundoora, Victoria, Australia

Jocelyn White, BSc (OT)
Senior Occupational Therapist
Royal Perth Hospital
Shenton Park Campus
Perth, Western Australia

Timothy J. Wolf, OTD, MSCI, OTR/L
Instructor in Occupational Therapy and Neurology
Program in Occupational Therapy
Washingon University
St. Louis, Missouri

CONTRIBUTORS TO PREVIOUS EDITIONS

Lorraine Aloisio
Beverly K. Bain
Ann Burkhardt
Judith Dicker Friedman
Michele G. Hahn
Lauren Joachim
Christine M. Johann
Steve Park
Denise A. Supon
Jeffery L. Tomlinson
Nancy C. Whyte

To: Peg & Ed

Preface

The third edition of *Stroke Rehabiliation: A Function-Based Approach* strives to be the most up-to-date text on this topic, incorporating state of the art tools and techniques to maximize function and quality of life for those living with stroke. This edition's contributors include expert clinicians, researchers, and scientists from across the United States of America, Australia, Iceland, and Sweden. Contibutors are experts in various disciplines, including neurology, occupational therapy, physiatry, physical therapy, psychology, and speech and language pathology.

The current text combines aspects of background medical information, a comprehensive review of standardized and nonstandardized evaluation procedures and assessments, treatment techniques, and evidence-based interventions. It contains the most up-to-date research on stroke rehabilitation from a variety of rehabilitation settings and professions without losing its holistic perspective on the overall care of the people whose lives we as clinicians touch.

This text has overarching themes. First and foremost, clinicians are provided with specific suggestions to maintain a client-centered approach when working with stroke survivors. Furthermore, clinicians are challenged to use the most up-to-date treatment approaches (including both remediation and adaptation approaches) to decrease impairments, prevent secondary complications, improve the client's ability to perform meaningful activities, and, most important, decrease participation restrictions and improve quality of life.

Although this book is written primarily by occupational therapists, it is an appropriate reference for a variety of rehabilitation professionals, including physiatrists, physical therapists, speech and language pathologists, rehabilitation nurses, social workers, vocational counselors, and therapeutic recreation specialists. The immense value of an interdisciplinary team approach when working with the stroke survivor population cannot be overestimated. This text may also be beneficial to therapists who practice virtually alone in the community or as a case manager because its research on the specific topic of stroke rehabilitation is comprehensive. The terms *patient* and *client* have been used interchangeably; it is recognized that stroke rehabilitation can take place in multiple settings.

Educators and students can use this text in the classroom setting. Key terms, chapter objectives, review questions, and case studies have been provided as learning tools. A text that can appeal to the basic learner and the specialist alike, this book is a good investment for any clinician who plans to work with neurologically impaired persons—specifically, adults who have had a stroke. This text spans the continuum of care—from acute to long-term management—in a variety of roles and settings.

The first five chapters provide the necessary medical and therapeutic foundations that should be the basis of any intervention plan. Chapter 1 has been expanded to not only include medical management but also a comprehensive approach to acute stroke rehabilitation because current practice dictates that rehabilitation services begin within 24 hours of stroke in many cases. Acute care evaluations and interventions are clearly delineated for those working in intensive care units, step down units, and the acute hospital settings. The information in Chapter 2, Psychological Aspects of Stroke Rehabilitation, as well as in Chapter 3, Improving Participation and Quality of Life Through Occupation, should be implicit in any therapeutic interaction with this population. Chapters 4, Task-Oriented Approach to Stroke Rehabilitation, and 5, Activity-Based Intervention in Stroke Rehabilitation, provide readers with an overall view of current therapeutic approaches and should be understood before the chapters on specialized topics are read.

Chapters 6 through 15 focus on the motor control aspects of stroke rehabilitation. Chapter 6, Approaches to Motor Control Dysfunction: An Evidence-Based Review, provides the reader with critical information to evaluate traditional and current practice approaches. Specific topics related to motor control that are covered include trunk control (Chapter 7), balance (Chapter 8), vestibular dysfunction (Chapter 9), comprehensive approaches to upper extremity function and management (Chapter 10), use of cutting-edge technology to improve limb function after stroke (Chapter 11), acute and subacute edema control (Chapter 12), splinting of the neurological upper extremity (Chapter 13), functional mobility (Chapter 14), and gait (Chapter 15).

The following five chapters provide readers with insight into managing simple and complex visual, perceptual, cognitive, and speech/language impairments that interfere with daily function. Chapters focus on assessment and interventions related to visual and spatial skills

(Chapter 16), clinical reasoning during assessment and treatment planning for those with cognitive and perceptual deficits (Chapter 17), standardized assessment of the impact of cognitive-perceptual impairments on meaningful tasks (Chapter 18), function-based approaches to managing and evaluating cognitive and perceptual deficits (Chapter 19), and management of speech and language deficits (Chapter 20).

This text contains comprehensive chapters on specific aspects of daily living after a stroke, such as driving, sexuality, leisure, instrumental activities of daily living, resumption of parenting roles after stroke, mobility, and self-care. Specific interventions highlighted include dysphagia management, home adaptation, and wheeled mobility and seating prescription. Finally, two stroke survivors who share their thoughts, frustrations, and experiences provide readers with invaluable insights to the stroke recovery process.

It is my hope that this text will challenge practicing clinicians to consider their present approaches to stroke rehabilitation and serve as a foundation on which students can build their philosophies for intervention with the stroke population.

ACKNOWLEDGMENTS

I am grateful for all I have learned from the hundreds of stroke survivors I have interacted with over the past 21 years. It is my hope that this text will make a positive impact on improving the quality of life of those living with stroke. I am grateful to all of the professionals from my own community, across the country, and internationally for their contributions to this book. They accepted my challenge to put their knowledge and skill base into words. Their dedication to this project will inspire future generations of clinicians and researchers

I continue to appreciate the dedication and persistence of the staff at Elsevier for supporting my work for over a decade, specifically Kathy Falk, Megan Fennell, Jolynn Gower, and Melissa Kuster.

Glen Gillen

Contents

Pathophysiology, Medical Management, and Acute Rehabilitation of Stroke Survivors

key terms

acute management	hemorrhagic stroke	stroke diagnosis
decubitus ulcer	intensive care unit (ICU)	stroke management
early mobilization	ischemic stroke	stroke prevention

chapter objectives

After completing this chapter, the reader will be able to accomplish the following:

1. Describe the pathophysiology of stroke.
2. Explain the diagnostic workup of stroke survivors.
3. Understand the medical management of various stroke syndromes.
4. Describe interventions to prevent the recurrence of stroke and its complications.
5. Understand normal and abnormal responses to acute stroke rehabilitation.
6. Be familiar with standardized assessments used during acute stroke rehabilitation.
7. Implement a comprehensive treatment that is safe for the acute and ICU settings.
8. Write appropriate goals for the acute and ICU settings.
9. Be able to prevent secondary complications such as skin breakdown and contracture after stroke.

Pathophysiology and Medical Management of Stroke

Matthew N. Bartels

PREVALENCE AND IMPACT OF STROKE

Stroke remains the third leading cause of mortality in the United States after cardiovascular disease and cancer, accounting for 10% to 12% of all deaths.[15,127] Globally, stroke is the second leading cause of mortality in developed nations with 4.5 million deaths every year.[109] An estimated 550,000 strokes occur each year, resulting in 150,000 deaths and more than 300,000 individuals with significant disability.[119] The United States has an estimated 3 million stroke survivors today, which is double the number of survivors 25 years ago.[54] The economic impact of stroke in 2007 was estimated at $62.7 billion, markedly increased from the estimate in 2001 of $30 billion, of which $17 billion were direct medical costs and $13 billion were indirect costs from lost productivity.[119] Fortunately, modern medical interventions (mostly risk factor modifications) have decreased stroke mortality by approximately 7% per year in industrialized nations since 1970.[15] The advances continue, but with increased cost of care for more advanced treatments.

EPIDEMIOLOGY OF STROKE

Stroke is essentially a preventable disease with known, manageable risk factors.[16] The established risk factors for stroke include hypertension, cigarette smoking, obesity, elevated serum fibrinogen levels, diabetes, a sedentary lifestyle, and the use of contraceptives with high doses of estrogen.[101] The most important and easily treated of these risk factors is systolic hypertension. In the Multiple Risk Factor Intervention Trial, 40% of strokes were attributed to systolic blood pressures greater than 140 mm Hg.[130] Stroke incidence also increases exponentially with aging, with an increase in stroke from three in 100,000 individuals per year in the third and fourth decades of age to 300 in 100,000 individuals per year in the eighth and ninth decades of life.[16] Eighty-eight percent of stroke deaths occur among persons aged 65 years or older[15] Table 1-1 outlines modifiable and nonmodifiable risks.

Stroke prevention interventions have reduced mortality in industrialized nations primarily through treating hypertension in the elderly. Another cause of decreased mortality has been the establishment of dedicated stroke units that can prevent acute death and later development of life-threatening complications.

PATHOGENESIS AND PATHOLOGY OF STROKE

Definition and Description of Stroke Syndromes

Stroke. Stroke is essentially a disease of the cerebral vasculature in which a failure to supply oxygen to brain cells, which are the most susceptible to ischemic damage, leads to their death. The syndromes that lead to stroke compose two broad categories: ischemic and hemorrhagic stroke. Ischemic strokes account for approximately 80% of strokes, whereas hemorrhagic strokes account for the remaining 20%.[128]

Transient Ischemic Attack. Symptoms of a transient ischemic attack (TIA) include the focal deficits of an ischemic stroke within a clearly vascular distribution, but TIAs are reversible defects because no cerebral infarction ensues. The causes of TIAs can be thrombotic and embolic and could result from a cerebral vasospasm. By definition, the effects of TIAs must resolve in less than 24 hours. Since 35% of patients who have had a TIA will have a stroke within five years, they should have a complete evaluation for cerebrovascular disease and sources of embolism.[167] The treatment of TIAs depends on the source of the emboli or thrombi and can include anticoagulation therapy and/or surgery.

Ischemic Stroke

An ischemic stroke is the most common form of stroke with various causes. The one common endpoint among all the different subtypes of ischemic strokes is that injury results from tissue anoxia caused by an interruption of cerebral blood flow.

Table 1-1

Modifiable and Nonmodifiable Risks

TYPE OF RISK	RELATIVE RISK (PER 1000 PERSONS)
Modifiable risks	
Hypertension	4.0 to 5.0
Cardiac disease	2.0 to 4.0
Atrial fibrillation	5.6 to 17.6
Diabetes mellitus	1.5 to 3.0
Cigarette smoking	1.5 to 2.9
Alcohol abuse	1.0 to 4.0
Hyperlipidemia	1.0 to 2.0
Nonmodifiable risks	
Age	1 to 2/1000 at age 45– to 54–years-old to 20/1000 at age 75– to 84–years-old
Gender	1.2 to 2.1
Race (black or Hispanic)	2.0
Heredity	1.8 to 3.1

Embolic Stroke. Cerebral embolic strokes are the most common subtype of ischemic stroke. Embolic strokes usually are characterized by an abrupt onset, although they also can be associated with stuttering symptoms. Usually no heralding events occur, such as TIAs or previous small strokes evolving into larger strokes.[83] A warning with microemboli that cause smaller events are uncommon, and the usual clue to a possible embolic source is a completed stroke.[128] The source of approximately 40% of embolic strokes is unknown, even after the common sources have been evaluated extensively. Most embolic strokes of known cause occur after emboli that are cardiac in origin.[27] The second most common sources of emboli are atherothrombotic lesions that result in artery-to-artery embolisms. These lesions can be in the aorta, the carotid and vertebrobasilar systems, and, less frequently, smaller arteries.

Sources of Emboli

Cardiac Sources. Cardiac emboli can develop from numerous areas in the heart. Cardiac dysrhythmias, structural anomalies, and acute infarctions are the usual sources of emboli. The most common source of an embolism is the classical pattern of thrombosis in the left atrium of patients with atrial fibrillation. The usual mechanism of thrombus formation in atrial fibrillation is by clot formation in the left atrial appendage. This then breaks off and creates an embolus that can move through the arterial system. Patients older than 60 years are particularly prone to this type of embolization. Embolism is not limited to the brain, and infarction can occur in the kidneys, peripheral tissues, or any other location.

The most common cardiac structural cause of a cerebral embolism is due to a myocardial infarction.[83] In patients with left ventricular infarcts, particularly anterior wall and apical infarctions, the endocardial damage associated with a subendocardial or transmural infarction is an excellent nidus (a focal point where bacteria or other infectious agents thrive) for thrombus formation. The emboli most often develop during the first several weeks after the infarction, although the risk for developing them can persist for much longer.

Valvular heart disease also can result in thrombi, but they more frequently develop after valve replacement rather than result directly from the native valve. More commonly the native valvular heart disease causes the patient to be in atrial fibrillation and then to develop an embolus. Mechanical heart valves (e.g., St. Jude valves) are much more likely to cause emboli than porcine (tissue) valves, so patients with the mechanical type always continue to receive anticoagulation therapy.

Much less common sources of cardiac emboli are the vegetations resulting from bacterial endocarditis. These emboli cause small septic infarcts called mycotic aneurysms, which are at high risk of conversion to hemorrhagic infarcts. Other rare causes of cardiac emboli are atrial myxomas,

which are tumors of the heart endocardium. In addition, embolic infarctions also may result from cardiac and thoracic surgery.[83]

Cardiac emboli usually (80% of the time) occlude the middle cerebral artery, 10% of cardiac emboli occlude the posterior cerebral artery, and the rest occlude the vertebral artery or its branches.[83] Anterior cerebral artery embolization from the heart is rare. The severity of the clinical syndrome is related to the size of the embolus. An embolus of 3 to 4 mm can cause a large stroke by occluding the larger brain arteries. Blood clots undergo lysis over a few days with the establishment of recanalization through the clot. Because clots naturally lyse, a stroke can convert from ischemic to hemorrhagic when reperfusion distal to the occlusion is present, because the blood vessels in the ischemic distribution may no longer be intact. This can lead to leakage from these damaged arteries, arterioles, and capillaries, leading to a phenomenon called hemorrhagic conversion. The possibility of hemorrhagic conversion contraindicates the use of anticoagulation therapy as initial treatment for large embolic strokes.

Vascular Sources. Strokes vascular in origin are far less common than cardiac strokes but are still one major type of embolic stroke. The sources of vascular emboli are usually atheromatous plaques in the walls of the aorta, carotid arteries, or smaller vessels in the cerebral circulation. Platelet activation and the formation of a fibrin clot can occur rapidly. The most common areas affected by the emboli of the vascular system are the same as those affected by cardiac sources of emboli. The most common areas for ulcerated plaques in the cerebral blood supply are the aorta and the proximal internal carotid artery. The plaques in the carotid artery can be visualized by Doppler sonography of the carotid artery system.[128]

Paradoxical Sources. Congenital atrial septal defects can create the opportunity for emboli to cross from the right-sided (venous) circulation to the left-sided (arterial) circulation, a rare source of cerebral emboli. A common source of paradoxical embolic material is deep venous thrombosis (DVT). The modern techniques of transesophageal echocardiography with a "bubble study" help identify patients at risk for this condition. One performs a bubble study by injecting a small bolus of air into the venous circulation while the echocardiographer observes the heart. If the air bolus, which is seen easily, has no portion cross over to the left-sided circulation, then no shunt is present. If the bubbles cross into the left-sided circulation, then a shunt is possible. One of the most common atrial shunting abnormalities is a patent foramen ovale. In young patients or patients who have had TIAs or strokes, the treatment of choice is surgical repair of the lesion.

Unknown Sources. Thrombi of unknown source often occur in patients with known hypercoagulability syndromes. These syndromes can result from acquired diseases (e.g., lupus anticoagulant and metastatic tumors) or inborn errors of the coagulation system (e.g., protein S and C deficiencies).

Surgery or medication therapies such as estrogen replacement can induce iatrogenic causes of hypercoagulable states. Even when the patient is known to be in a hypercoagulable state, the source of the emboli may remain unknown. In many patients the entire workup is unrevealing.

Thrombotic Stroke

A thrombotic stroke can result from a variety of causes, but most causes are related to the development of abnormalities in the arterial vessel wall. Atherosclerosis, arteritis, dissections, and external compression of the vessels are causes. In addition, some patients with hematological disorders develop thrombosis. The spectrum of disease includes stroke and TIA, and often the difference between a thrombotic and an embolic stroke may be difficult to determine. Thrombosis and embolism are often both present, especially in patients with atherosclerotic disease. The exact mechanism of infarction from thrombosis is still being debated, but atherosclerosis does play a significant role. Hypertension with associated microtrauma of the arterial intima is thought to play a role, as is hypercholesterolemia.[104,128] TIAs may result from the formation of microthrombi and their embolization. Large vessel thrombosis can also occur in extracranial vessels, such as the vertebral and carotid arteries, leading to devastating strokes.[117]

Pathophysiology. Atherosclerotic plaque formation is greatest at the branching points of major vessels and forms in areas of turbulent flow. Chronic hypertension is a common precursor, and damage to the intimal wall may be followed by lymphocyte infiltration. Foam cells then develop, and the first stage of atherosclerosis is formed. Calcification and narrowing with resultant turbulent flow follow. In this setting of turbulent flow, plaque ulceration can become a site for thrombus formation. If the thrombus forms and is degraded rapidly, a transient ischemic phenomenon can occur, which is the setting of a TIA. Classically, the symptoms of internal carotid disease include amaurosis fugax and monocular blindness. If the clot does not break up or lyse, a cerebral infarction can occur. The size and severity of the infarction depends on available collateral circulation and the size of the occluded vessel. In patients with extensive atherosclerotic disease, however, a limited amount of collateral circulation is available, and the sparing from collateral circulation may be limited.

Atherothrombotic Disease. The most common site for the development of atherosclerosis and the subsequent development of atherothrombosis that leads to TIAs and stroke in the anterior circulation is the origin of the carotid artery and in the posterior circulation is the top of the basilar artery. Other sites of atherosclerosis include the carotid siphon and the stems (bases) of the middle cerebral artery, anterior cerebral artery, and origin of the basilar artery.[51] The atheromatous plaques are sources of emboli that can cause distal symptoms in a TIA or stroke. These embolic events are similar events from other embolic sources. Table 1-2 lists common stroke syndromes, and Figs. 1-1 to 1-3 explain the anatomy of these strokes. Atherosclerotic disease is screened most readily by carotid Doppler ultrasonography and transcranial Doppler imaging. Magnetic

Table 1-2

Common Stroke Syndromes

ANATOMICAL DISTRIBUTION	STROKE SYNDROME
Common carotid artery	Often resembles middle cerebral artery (MCA) but can be asymptomatic if circle of Willis is competent
Internal carotid artery	Often resembles MCA but can be asymptomatic if circle of Willis is competent
Middle cerebral artery	

Main stem	Contralateral hemiplegia
	Contralateral hemianopia
	Contralateral hemianesthesia
	Head/eye turning toward the lesion
	Dysphagia
	Uninhibited neurogenic bladder
	Dominant hemisphere
	  Global aphasia
	  Apraxia
	Nondominant hemisphere
	  Aprosody and affective agnosia
	  Visuospatial deficit
	  Neglect syndrome

Table 1-2

Common Stroke Syndromes—cont'd

ANATOMICAL DISTRIBUTION	STROKE SYNDROME
Upper division	Contralateral hemiplegia; leg more spared
	Contralateral hemianopia
	Contralateral hemianesthesia
	Head/eye turning toward the lesion
	Dysphagia
	Uninhibited neurogenic bladder
	Dominant hemisphere
	Broca (motor) aphasia
	Apraxia
	Nondominant hemisphere
	Aprosody and affective agnosia
	Visuospatial deficit
	Neglect syndrome
Lower division	Contralateral hemianopia
	Dominant hemisphere
	Wernicke aphasia
	Nondominant hemisphere
	Affective agnosia
Anterior cerebral artery (ACA)	
Proximal (precommunal) segment (A1)	Can be asymptomatic if circle of Willis is competent, but if both ACAs arise from the same stem, then:
	Profound abulia (akinetic mutism)
	Bilateral pyramidal signs
	Paraplegia
Postcommunal segment (A2)	Contralateral hemiplegia; arm more spared
	Contralateral hemianesthesia
	Head/eye turning toward the lesion
	Grasp reflex, sucking reflex, gegenhalten
	Disconnection apraxia
	Abulia
	Gait apraxia
	Urinary incontinence
	Anterior choroidal artery
	Contralateral hemiplegia
	Hemianesthesia
	Homonymous hemianopsia
Posterior cerebral artery	
Proximal (precommunal) segment (P1)	Thalamic syndrome:
	Choreoathetosis
	Spontaneous pain and dysesthesias
	Sensory loss (all modalities)
	Intention tremor
	Mild hemiparesis
	Thalamoperforate syndrome:
	Crossed cerebellar ataxia
	Ipsilateral third nerve palsy
	Weber syndrome:
	Contralateral hemiplegia
	Ipsilateral third nerve palsy
	Contralateral hemiplegia
	Paralysis of vertical eye movement
	Contralateral action tremor

Continued

Table 1-2

Common Stroke Syndromes—cont'd

ANATOMICAL DISTRIBUTION	STROKE SYNDROME
Postcommunal segment (P2)	Homonymous hemianopsia
	Cortical blindness
	Visual agnosia
	Prosopagnosia
	Dyschromatopsia
	Alexia without agraphia
	Memory deficits
	Complex hallucinations
Vertebrobasilar syndromes	
Superior cerebellar artery	Ipsilateral cerebellar ataxia
	Nausea/vomiting
	Dysarthria
	Contralateral loss of pain and temperature sensation
	Partial deafness
	Horner syndrome
	Ipsilateral ataxic tremor
Anterior inferior cerebellar artery	Ipsilateral deafness
	Ipsilateral facial weakness
	Nausea/vomiting
	Vertigo
	Nystagmus
	Tinnitus
	Cerebellar ataxia
	Paresis of conjugate lateral gaze
	Contralateral loss of pain and temperature sensation
Medial basal midbrain (Weber syndrome)	Contralateral hemiplegia
	Ipsilateral third nerve palsy
Tegmentum of midbrain (Benedikt syndrome)	Ipsilateral third nerve palsy
	Contralateral loss of pain and temperature sensation
	Contralateral loss of joint position sensation
	Contralateral ataxia
	Contralateral chorea
Bilateral basal pons (locked-in syndrome)	Bilateral hemiplegia
	Bilateral cranial nerve palsy (upward gaze spared)
Lateral pons (Millard-Gubler syndrome)	Ipsilateral sixth nerve palsy
	Ipsilateral facial weakness
	Contralateral hemiplegia
Lateral medulla (Wallenberg syndrome)	Ipsilateral hemiataxia
	Ipsilateral loss of facial pain and sensation
	Contralateral loss of body pain and temperature sensation
	Nystagmus
	Ipsilateral Horner syndrome
	Dysphagia and dysphonia

resonance angiography (MRA) and carotid and cerebral angiography can further elucidate lesions, which can be treated surgically or medically.

Lacunar Syndrome. A lacunar stroke occurs in one of the perforating branches of the circle of Willis, the middle cerebral artery stem, or the vertebral or basilar arteries. The occlusion of these vessels results from the atherothrombotic or lipohyalinotic blockage of one of these arteries. The development of disease in these arteries correlates closely with the presence of chronic hypertension and diabetic microvascular disease.[107,128] These are small vessels, 100 to 300 μm in diameter, that branch off the main artery and penetrate into the deep gray or white matter of the cerebrum.[107] The resulting infarcts are from 2 mm to 3 cm in size and account for

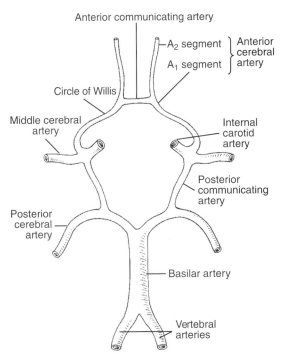

Figure 1-1 Circle of Willis and cerebral circulation.

roughly 20% of all strokes. These types of strokes usually evolve over a few hours and sometimes can be heralded by transient symptoms in lacunar TIAs. Lacunar strokes can cause recognizable syndromes (Table 1-3). The basic lacunar syndromes are (1) pure motor hemiparesis from an infarct in the posterior limb of the interior capsule or pons, (2) pure sensory stroke from an infarct in the ventrolateral thalamus, (3) ataxic hemiparesis from an infarct in the base of the pons or the genu of the internal capsule, and (4) pure motor hemiparesis with motor apraxia resulting from an infarct in the genu of the anterior limb of the internal capsule and the adjacent white matter in the corona radiata. Recovery from a lacunar stroke often can be dramatic, and in some individuals, near complete or complete resolution of deficits can occur in several weeks or months. In patients who have had multiple lacunar infarcts, a syndrome characterized by emotional instability, slow abulia (impairment in or loss of volition), and bilateral pyramidal signs known as pseudobulbar palsy will develop. This diagnosis is based on the symptoms and the use of computerized tomography (CT) or magnetic resonance imaging (MRI). MRI is especially useful in this situation for detecting small lesions in the deep brain structures or brainstem; the ability of CT to see lesions clearly in these areas is limited.[29]

Hemorrhagic Conversion. As a sequela of an embolic or ischemic infarction, a purely ischemic infarct may convert into a hemorrhagic lesion. Thrombi can migrate, lyse, and reperfuse into an ischemic area, leading to small hemorrhages (petechial hemorrhages) because the damaged capillaries and small blood vessels no longer maintain their integrity. These damaged areas then can coalesce (combine) and form a hemorrhage into ischemia.[83] These conversions are more common in large infarcts, such as an occluded middle cerebral artery, or in a large

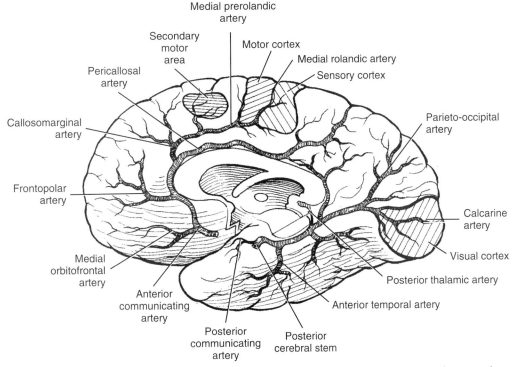

Figure 1-2 Medial view of brain with anterior and posterior cerebral artery circulation and areas of cortical function.

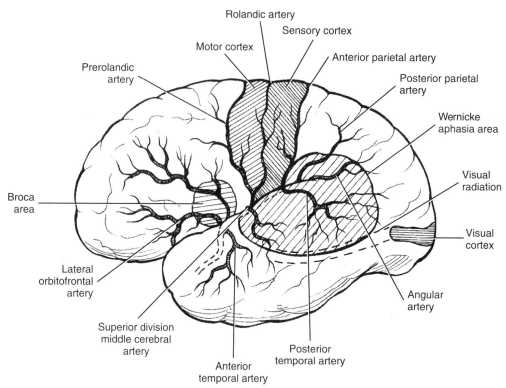

Figure 1-3 Lateral view of brain with middle cerebral artery and its branches and areas of cortical function.

Table 1-3

Lacunar Stroke Syndromes and Their Anatomical Sites

LACUNAR SYNDROME	ANATOMICAL SITES
Pure motor	Posterior limb of internal capsule
	Basis pontis
	Pyramids
Pure sensory	Ventrolateral thalamus
	Thalamocortical projections
Ataxic hemiparesis	Pons
	Genu of internal capsule
	Corona radiata
	Cerebellum
Motor hemiparesis with apraxia	Genu of the anterior limb of the internal capsule
	Corona radiata
Hemiballismus	Head of caudate
	Thalamus
	Subthalamic nucleus
Dysarthria/clumsy hand	Base of pons
	Genu of anterior limb of the internal capsule
Sensory/motor	Junction of the internal capsule and thalamus
Anarthric pseudobulbar	Bilateral internal capsule

infarction in the distribution of a lenticulostriate artery. In patients who have large infarcts with possibility of hemorrhage, anticoagulation therapy is not used because of the risk of hemorrhagic conversion. These types of hemorrhages have characteristics in common with hemorrhagic strokes.

Hemorrhagic Stroke

Hemorrhagic strokes have numerous causes. The four most common types are deep hypertensive intracerebral hemorrhages (ICHs), ruptured saccular aneurysms, bleeding from an arteriovenous malformation (AVM), and spontaneous lobar hemorrhages.[83]

Hypertensive Bleed. Hypertensive cerebral hemorrhages usually occur in four sites: the putamen and internal capsule, the pons, the thalamus, and the cerebellum. Usually these hemorrhages develop from small penetrating arteries in the deep brain that have had damage from hypertension. The pathological features of hypertension include lipohyalinosis (fat infiltration of pathologically degenerated tissue) and Charcot-Bouchard aneurysms.[50] The usual hypertensive ICH develops over the span of a few minutes but occasionally can take as long as 60 minutes. Unlike ischemic infarcts, hemorrhagic bleeds do not follow the anatomical distribution of blood vessels but dissect through tissue planes spherically. This commonly leads to severe damage and complications, such as hydrocephalus and mass shift (movement of brain tissues to one side to accommodate the volume of the hemorrhage).[83,128] Within 48 hours of the hemorrhage, macrophages begin to phagocytize the hemorrhage at its outer margins. Patients with a cerebral hemorrhage often experience a rapid recovery within the first two to three months after the hemorrhage. ICHs usually occur while patients are awake and often while they are under emotional stress. Vomiting and headache are associated commonly with ICH and are unique features that differentiate ICHs from ischemic strokes. Table 1-4 outlines the four major hypertensive ICH syndromes.

Lobar Intracerebral Bleed. Lobar hemorrhages are ICHs that occur outside the basal ganglia and thalamus in the white matter of the cerebral cortex. These types of hemorrhages and hypertension are not correlated clearly; the most common underlying condition in patients with this type of ICH is the presence of AVMs.[83] Other associated conditions include bleeding diatheses, tumors (e.g., melanoma or glioma), aneurysms in the circle of Willis, and a large number of idiopathic cases.[49] Patients with lobar ICH initially have acute onset of symptoms, and most lobar ICHs are small enough to cause discrete clinical syndromes that may resemble focal ischemic events. Because lobar bleeds occur far from the thalamus and the brainstem, coma and stupor are much less common than they are in patients with hypertensive ICHs. Headaches are also common and can help differentiate lobar bleeds from ischemic strokes, which they can resemble so closely.[126] Detection of a hemorrhage on a CT scan or MRI is the best way to distinguish these two entities.

Saccular Aneurysm and Subarachnoid Bleed. A saccular aneurysm rupture is the most common cause of a subarachnoid hemorrhage (SAH).[150] Saccular aneurysms occur at the bifurcation (branching) points of the large arteries in the brain and are most commonly found in the anterior portion of the circle of Willis.[83] An estimated 0.5% to 1% of normal individuals harbor saccular aneurysms.[158] Despite the high number, bleeding from them is rare (6 to 16 per 100,000). Unlike other stroke syndromes, however, the incidence of SAH has not declined since 1970.[102] The rupture risk correlates best with the size of the aneurysm. Aneurysms smaller than 3 mm have little chance of hemorrhage, whereas aneurysms 10 mm or larger have the greatest chance of rupture.[95] SAH usually is characterized by acute, abrupt onset of a severe headache of atypical quality.[102] These headaches are often the most severe that patients have ever experienced.

Table 1-4

The Four Major Hypertension Intracerebral Hemorrhage Syndromes

TYPE	STRUCTURES INVOLVED	CLINICAL SYNDROME	COMMENTS
Putamenal	Internal capsule Basal ganglia	Contralateral hemiplegia Coma in large infarcts Eyes deviate away from lesion Can have stupor/coma with brainstem compression Decerebrate rigidity	Most common
Thalamic	Thalamus Internal capsule	Contralateral hemiplegia Prominent contralateral sensory deficit for all modalities Aphasia if dominant (left) thalamus involved Homonymous visual field defect Gaze palsies Horner syndrome Eyes deviate downward	
Pontine	Pons Brainstem Midbrain	Coma Quadriparesis Decerebrate rigidity Severe acute hypertension Death	Can lead to a locked-in syndrome
Cerebellar	Cerebellum	Nausea and vomiting Ataxia Vertigo/dizziness Occipital headache Gaze toward the lesion Occasional dysarthria and dysphagia	Nystagmus and limb ataxia are rare

A brief loss of consciousness, nausea and vomiting, focal neurological deficits, and a stiff neck at the onset of symptoms also may occur. The diagnosis is based on clinical suspicion, subarachnoid blood found on the CT scan, or blood found in the cerebrospinal fluid from a spinal tap. One determines the definitive location of the aneurysm by cerebral angiography.

The development of further delayed neurological deficits results from three major events: rerupture, hydrocephalus, and cerebral vasospasm. Rerupture occurs in 20% to 30% of cases within one month if treatment is not aggressive, and rebleeding has an associated mortality rate of up to 70%.[102] Hydrocephalus occurs in up to 20% of cases, and aggressive management often is required. Chronic hydrocephalus is also common and often requires permanent cerebrospinal fluid drainage (shunting). Vasospasm also is a common problem after SAHs, occurring in approximately 30% of cases.[102] The normal time course for vasospasm is an onset in three to five days, peak narrowing in five to 14 days, and resolution in two to four weeks. In half of cases, the vasospasm is severe enough to cause a cerebral infarction with resulting stroke or death. Even with modern management, 15% to 20% of patients who develop vasospasms still suffer strokes or die.[96] A permanent ischemic deficit develops in approximately 50% of patients with symptomatic vasospasms after SAHs.[69] Vasospasm therefore must be treated rapidly and as aggressively as possible to prevent permanent ischemic damage.

Arteriovenous Malformation. AVMs are found throughout the body and can occur in any part of the brain. They are usually congenital and consist of an abnormal tangle of blood vessels between the arterial and venous systems. They range from a few millimeters in size to large masses that can increase cardiac output because of the amount of their blood flow. The larger AVMs in the brain tend to be found in the posterior portions of the cerebral hemispheres.[50] AVMs occur more frequently in men, and if found in one family member, they have a tendency to be found in other members. AVMs are present from birth, but bleeding most often occurs in the second and third decades of life. Headaches and seizures are common symptoms, as is hemiplegia. Half of AVMs initially occur as ICHs. Although rebleeding in the first month is rare, rebleeding is common in larger lesions as more time passes. Contrast CT, MRA, and MRI are useful noninvasive tests, whereas cerebral angiography is the best test for delineating the nature of the lesion. The management of these lesions is accomplished best by a team approach, a combination of surgical treatment and interventional angiography for definitive management. Treatment of hydrocephalus and increased intracranial pressure is the same as treatment for SAH and ICH.

Posttraumatic Hemorrhagic Stroke. A traumatic brain injury commonly results in hemorrhagic damage to the brain in addition to ischemic and other injuries. The four major types of injury caused by traumatic brain injury include SAH and ICH, diffuse axonal injury, contusions, and anoxic injury from hypoperfusion (decreased flow in the vessels) and hypoxemia (decreased oxygen level). This combination of injuries leads to a constellation of findings that mixes the features of a number of individual ischemic and hemorrhagic injuries.

Other Causes of Stroke and Strokelike Syndromes

Arterial and Medical Disease. Numerous medical conditions can result in arterial system diseases and lead to thrombosis and thromboembolism. Some conditions may cause disease in the cerebral vasculature (Table 1-5).

Strokelike Syndromes. A number of conditions in addition to TIAs and cerebral infarctions can cause transient paralysis. These conditions generally resolve spontaneously with no long-term sequelae. The most common cause of transient hemiparesis is Todd paralysis, which develops postictally (after a seizure). Todd paralysis results from neurotransmitter depletion and neuronal fatigue in focal areas of the brain caused by the extremely high neuronal firing rate during a seizure.[37] Patients usually regain function within 24 hours. Another common cause of focal neurological deficits is migraine headaches. These headaches are actually thought to result from cerebral vasospasms, but an actual ischemic infarct rarely if ever occurs. The deficits resolve with the resolution of the migraine and are not permanent.

Cerebral Neoplasm. Obviously, cerebral neoplasms (whether primary or metastatic) can lead to focal neurological deficits that resemble a stroke. The treatment of the sequelae and the long-term management of the deficits are the same as they are in stroke patients. Treating the primary lesions is the focus of the acute care. Often the initial symptoms are seizures and ICHs.

STROKE DIAGNOSIS

The diagnosis of stroke and differentiation of stroke from strokelike syndromes is based on the clinical presentation and physical examination of the patient. The examiner needs to differentiate a true stroke from syndromes that can mimic a stroke, such as Todd paralysis, seizures, multiple sclerosis, tumors, and metabolic syndromes. Most often, the patient's symptoms in the emergency room include an acute onset of weakness or other neurological deficits. The patient history can help identify the risk factors for stroke and the nature of the lesion. The physical examination includes a general medical examination and a neurological examination. Only after a diagnosis of stroke

Table 1-5

Medical Conditions That Cause Arterial System Disease

CONDITION	FEATURES*	TREATMENT
Vasculitic/inflammatory		
Systemic lupus erythematosus	Most commonly associated vasculitis with stroke	Treat lupus
	Vasculitic, thrombotic, and embolic events occur	Anticoagulation with warfarin
	Greater than 50% recurrence rate	
	Antiphospholipid antibody may play a role	
Binswanger disease	Rare condition	No clear treatment
	Diffuse subcortical infarction	Anticoagulation
	Diffuse lipohyalinosis of small arteries	
Scleroderma	Stroke in 6% of patients	No clear treatment
	Antiphospholipid antibody may play a role	Anticoagulation
Periarteritis nodosa	Can cause a CNS vasculitis	Treat underlying condition
	Can cause embolic stroke	
Temporal arteritis	Can cause a CNS vasculitis	Treat underlying condition
	Can cause embolic stroke	
Wegener granulomatosis	Can cause a CNS necrotizing vasculitis	Treat underlying condition
	Can cause thrombotic stroke	
Takayasu arteritis	Can cause embolic stroke	Treat underlying condition
		Anticoagulation
Isolated angiitis of the CNS	Rare primary CNS vasculitis	Treat underlying condition
	Headache, multiinfarct dementia, lethargy	
Fibromuscular dysplasia	Mostly in young women	Anticoagulation
	Often asymptotic	Surgical dilation of the carotid arteries (if necessary)
	Can be associated with TIA and stroke	
Moyamoya disease	Vasooclusive disease of the large intracranial arteries	Role of anticoagulation controversial because of risk of hemorrhage
	Mainly in Asian population	Role of surgery controversial
	Cause of strokes in children and young adults	
Hypercoagulable state		
Antiphospholipid antibodies	Associated with recurrent thrombosis	Anticoagulation with warfarin
	Embolic and thrombotic strokes occur	
Oral contraceptive agents	Relative risk increased 4 times over controls	Stop oral contraceptives
	Thought to be caused by hypercoagulability	
Sickle cell disease	Microvascular occlusion caused by sickled cells	No good treatments exist
	Seen in 5% to 17% of patients with sickle cell disease	
Polycythemia	Vascular occlusion caused by increased viscosity and hypercoagulability	Treat underlying cause (if known)
Inherited thrombotic tendencies	Include many familial clotting abnormalities	Treat abnormality (if possible)
		Anticoagulation

*CNS, Central nervous system; TIA, transient ischemic attack.

Continued

Table 1-5

Medical Conditions That Cause Arterial System Disease—cont'd

CONDITION	FEATURES*	TREATMENT
Others		
Venous thrombosis	Seen in meningitis, hypercoagulable states, and after trauma	Anticoagulation
	Increased intracranial pressure, headache, seizures	May need surgical decompression
	Focal neurological signs, especially in legs more than arms	
	Diagnosed with angiography	
Arterial dissection	More common in children and young adults	Surgical treatment as needed
	May present with TIA	Anticoagulation after acute state
	Often preceded by trauma, mild to severe	

based on the clinical history and examination can a further diagnostic evaluation be performed. Modern technology has improved the tools available for the accurate diagnosis of stroke and includes an armamentarium of imaging studies to identify the exact nature of the lesions that may cause neurological deficits. Each imaging study available has benefits and limitations that are useful to know for assessing a patient who has had a stroke. The stroke evaluation also should include an evaluation for the cause of the stroke.

Cerebrovascular Imaging

The main tool used in stroke diagnostic evaluations is cerebral imaging, which historically included pneumoencephalography and other studies no longer performed. CT is probably the most common and the best known of the studies. MRI is now more common and has some advantages over CT, but availability and cost are still prohibitive in some areas. Positron emission tomography scans and single-photon emission CT scans are just being introduced and may have a role in stroke diagnosis.

Computerized Axial Tomography

CT is a readily available and useful technique that has become the standard for the evaluation of a patient experiencing an acute onset of stroke. The most important functions of CT scanning in an acute patient are ruling out other conditions (e.g., tumor or abscess) and helping identify whether evidence exists of hemorrhage into the infarction. In the acute phase of stroke, most CT scans are actually negative with no clear evidence of abnormalities. A negative immediate CT scan with an acute neurological deficit determined by physical examination actually can verify the impression of stroke because it rules out tumors, hemorrhages, and other brain lesions. The few changes seen in an acute stroke by CT are subtle and can include loss of distinction

between gray and white matter and sulcal effacement. Acute bleeding, however, is visible on CT scanning and can be present in as many as 39% to 43% of patients.[29] By definition, hemorrhagic infarction occurs within 24 hours of infarction, and hemorrhagic transformation occurs after 24 hours of infarction. The cause of the hemorrhagic change is thought to result from reperfusion into areas of damaged capillary endothelium and is common in large infarcts with extensive injury. Hemorrhagic transformation occurs equally in all distributions of infarcts[113] and is not associated necessarily with hypertension or with older age.[27] Hemorrhagic transformation can be detected in the acute phase by CT; in this case, one should not use anticoagulants because they may increase in the severity of the cerebral hemorrhage.

In the subacute phase, the findings from CT clearly show the development of cerebral edema within three days, which then fades over the next two to three weeks; then a decrease in the signal intensity occurs over the infarction. This decrease corresponds with the change from the positive mass effect (swelling) of the acute phase to the negative mass effect (shrinkage) of the chronic phase. The infarct actually may be difficult to see again in two to three weeks but is clearly visible with the addition of contrast material. Long-term parenchymal enhancement develops, which is consistent with the scar formation that becomes the permanent CT finding. The loss of tissue volume (negative mass effect) and the permanent scar tissue are the characteristic features of a chronic infarct (Figs. 1-4 to 1-8).

Magnetic Resonance Imaging

MRI is now as commonly used in acute patients as CT, because cost and availability have improved. The MRI also has the advantage of allowing earlier detection of

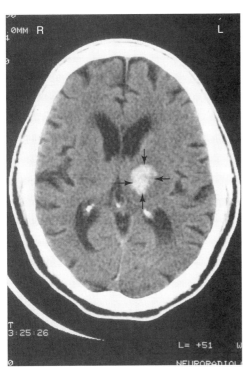

Figure 1-4   Magnetic resonance image of brain without gadolinium demonstrates an acute large left basal ganglia infarct. An acute infarct on the image appears white and is indicated by arrows.

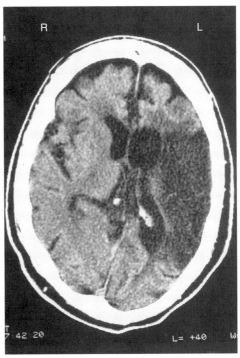

Figure 1-6   Computerized tomography scan of the brain without contrast demonstrates a large, previous, left middle cerebral artery distribution infarction. Loss of mass of brain tissue has occurred with dilated ventricles. Bleeding or acute infarction is not evident.

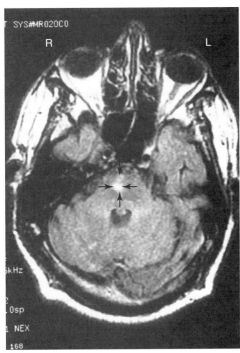

Figure 1-5   Magnetic resonance image of the brainstem and cerebellum without gadolinium demonstrates an acute right pontine infarct. The infarct appears white and is indicated by arrows.

infarcts and, as more acute interventions have become common, allows for better evaluation of the course of acute treatment. Newer techniques such as diffusion-weighted averaging have been used to help in the identification of early infarcts.[58, 141] MRI also can rule out other conditions and can screen for acute bleeding. In addition, MRI can be more sensitive for detecting cerebral infarctions in acute patients. Magnetic resonance images are created by mapping out the relaxation of protons after the imposition of a strong magnetic field. These images are then taken in two ways: T1- and T2-weighted images. In T1 images, fat and tissues with similar proton densities are enhanced (bright). In T2 images, water and tissues rich in water are enhanced. As in CT scans, sulcal effacement can be seen, but hyperintensity is also evident in affected areas on the T1-weighted images. Magnetic resonance images can show meningeal enhancement over the dura, which occurs in 35% of acute stroke cases.[44] MRI also can detect hemorrhage in much the same way as CT does.

The subacute changes of edema and mass effect can be seen with MRI, and use of contrast may be necessary to elucidate an infarct in the two- to three-week window. MRI has an advantage in determining a hemorrhage in a late stage because it can detect the degradation products

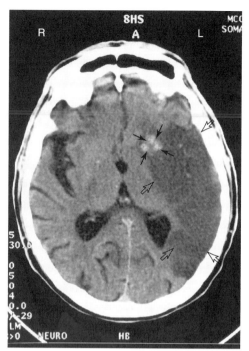

Figure 1-7 Computed tomography scan of the brain without contrast demonstrates a large subacute left middle cerebral artery distribution infarction, indicated by the hollow arrows. No loss of brain tissue mass has occurred compared with Fig. 1–6. Evidence of acute bleeding is in the basal ganglia on the left, which is white on the scan and is indicated with solid arrows.

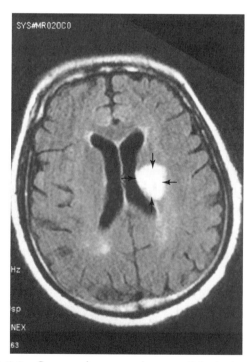

Figure 1-8 Computed tomography scan of the brain without contrast demonstrates a large, acute left thalamic hemorrhage. The acute bleeding in the thalamus on the left is white on the scan and is indicated with arrows.

of hemoglobin (hemosiderin deposits) and show hemorrhage areas well after CT can no longer detect a bleed. The changes on MRI in a chronic infarction are similar to those on a CT scan.

Positron Emission Tomography and Single-Photon Emission Computerized Tomography Scanning

Positron emission tomography and single-photon emission CT scanning are new techniques available only at selected centers. They have no clear role in the acute-stage evaluation of stroke.[2] In the subacute and chronic stages of stroke, these techniques help to distinguish between infarcted and noninfarcted tissue and can help delineate areas of dysfunctional but potentially salvageable brain tissue. These studies can also be used to try to assess brain function in the chronic setting. However, because of cost, limited availability, and an unclear definition of their use, they are essentially only research tools and do not have a role in the routine management of stroke patients.

WORKUP FOR CAUSE OF STROKE

The workup for the diagnosis of stroke is aimed at answering three main questions:
1. Is the stroke thrombotic or embolic?
2. Does an underlying cause require treatment?
3. Do any risk factors require modification?

Transcranial and Carotid Doppler

Transcranial and carotid Doppler studies allow for noninvasive visualization of the cerebral vessels. The advantages are that they provide useful therapeutic information on the state of the cerebral vessels and the blood flow to the brain. Approximately one third of patients who have had ischemic strokes that are cardiac in origin have significant cerebrovascular disease.[25] Patients with symptoms or evidence of posterior circulation disease are tested best with a transcranial Doppler study, including examination of the vertebrobasilar system. The cost is low compared with other tests such as MRA or cerebral angiography, which has significant associated morbidity and mortality. The evidence of carotid disease can help shape the patient's treatment plan and can encourage pursuit of definitive treatments such as carotid endarterectomy.

Magnetic Resonance Angiography

MRA is used to evaluate patients with stroke symptoms to detect any vascular abnormalities that may have caused the stroke or to look for alterations of cerebral blood flow that may have resulted from an embolic or thrombotic event. This is a very common noninvasive technique and is often done at the time of the MRI scan to assess the extent of cerebral injury; MRA is able to image vessels similarly to classical angiography.[160] The newer techniques of MRA have sensitivity for detection of 86% to

90%[111] for detection of severe stenosis, and the earlier issues of relatively low specificity of 64%[13,79] (due to over-detection by the earlier techniques) is now in the range of 89% to 96% for studies done with contrast enhanced MRA.[77] Despite these advantages, the spatial resolution is still less than traditional angiography, which may be an issue in cases where surgical management is planned. However, with constantly improving techniques and increased field strengths and parallel imaging, high resolution MRA may soon equal the resolution seen in CT angiography.[65]

Electrocardiography

Electrocardiography is used to evaluate patients with stroke symptoms to detect dysrhythmias (which may be a source of embolic material) or myocardial infarction or other acute cardiac events that may be related to an acute stroke.

Echocardiography

In patients with a history of cardiac disease and stroke, echocardiography usually is warranted. The types of cardiac disease that usually cause emboli and should be investigated with an echocardiograph include congestive heart failure, valvular heart disease, dysrhythmias, and a recent myocardial infarction. In some individuals, a patent foramen ovale (the fetal opening between the right and left sides of the heart) persists into adulthood and can be the source of a paradoxical embolus from the venous circulation that crosses from the right atrium into the left atrium. A transesophageal echocardiogram can then be useful in combination with a bubble study to assess for a right-to-left shunt. This specialized study also can visualize parts of the heart better in the search for emboli in areas such as the left atrial appendage when the standard transthoracic echocardiogram is inconclusive.

Blood Work

The standard acute evaluation of the stroke patient includes a complete screening set of blood analyses, including hematological studies, serum electrolyte levels (ionizing substances such as sodium and potassium), and renal (e.g., serum creatinine) and hepatic chemical analyses (liver function tests). The typical hematological evaluation has a complete blood count, platelet count, prothrombin time, and partial thromboplastin time. These studies help to rule out other causes of strokelike symptoms, to diagnose complications, and to allow for a baseline analysis before the initiation of therapies such as anticoagulation. The blood chemistry analyses allow metabolic abnormalities to be ruled out, as do the renal and hepatic chemistry analyses. The latter part of the stroke evaluation can involve numerous specialized tests chosen according to the clinical symptoms and development of the differential diagnosis as the evaluation

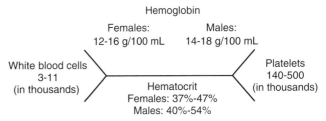

Figure 1-9   Complete blood count.

Table 1-6

Medical Studies Used to Clarify Diagnoses in Stroke Evaluation

SPECIALIZED STUDIES TO EVALUATE STROKE	ASSOCIATED CONDITIONS
Proteins S and C	Hypercoagulable state
Anticardiolipin antibodies (lupus anticoagulant)	Lupus erythematosus, hypercoagulable state
Erythrocyte sedimentation rate	Collagen vascular disease
Rheumatoid factor	Lupus erythematosus, collagen vascular disease
Antinuclear antibody	Lupus erythematosus, collagen vascular disease
Hemoglobin	Polycythemia
Sickle cell preparation	Sickle cell disease
Hemoglobin electrophoresis	Sickle cell disease
Blood and tissue cultures	Infectious emboli

progresses (Fig. 1-9). Table 1-6 provides a sample of some of these studies and their associated conditions.

MEDICAL STROKE MANAGEMENT

Principal Goals

As in the medical management of all patients, the care of stroke management requires good general patient care. All phases include caring for the conditions the patient may have and preventing medical complications and anticipating needs that will arise as the patient progresses through the acute phase into the convalescent, rehabilitative, and long-term maintenance phases after stroke. Care for acute patients is provided best in a specialized stroke unit that commonly deals with the issues and concerns unique to these patients.[2,102] Outcome studies have demonstrated the benefit of these units in the care of stroke patients.[91] Medical rehabilitation units also have been shown to be beneficial in the improvements of outcomes in the subacute and convalescent phases.

Acute Stroke Management

In management of acute stroke patients, basic medical needs have to be addressed and to include essentials such as airway protection, maintenance of adequate circulation, and the treatment of fractures or other injuries and conditions present at the time of admission. The neurological management of the acute stroke problems focus on identifying the cause of the stroke, preventing progression of the lesion, and treating acute neurological complications. Some specific approaches apply to treatment of each of the different types of stroke.

General Principles

The general principles of acute stroke management include attempting to stop progression of the lesion to limit deficits, reducing cerebral edema, decreasing the risk of hydrocephalus, treating seizures, and preventing complications such as DVT or aspiration that may lead to severe illness. (See the previous sections for a discussion of the studies used in acute patients to diagnose stroke.) Once the type of lesion has been defined, specific treatment can be instituted. Although numerous studies have been performed and are underway on the reduction of stroke mortality or disability,[136] no routine medical or surgical treatment has been shown to be effective. Currently, more aggressive methods such as angioplasty and thrombolysis are being studied, and the results of these trials are expected to lead to treatments that actually will improve the outcomes for individuals who have had strokes.

The basic principles in the approach to the treatment of acute stroke include an attempt to achieve improvement in cerebral perfusion by reestablishing blood flow, decreasing neuronal damage at the site of ischemia by modifying the pathophysiological process, and decreasing edema in the area of damaged tissue (which often can lead to secondary damage to nonischemic brain tissue). Many pharmacological and surgical treatments have been targeted toward at least one of these areas. Depending on the stroke mechanism, the agents and techniques of choice are used.

Ischemic Stroke

In patients who have had ischemic strokes, the restoration of blood flow and the control of neuronal damage at the area of ischemia are of the highest priority. In large strokes, edema can play a significant role, and mass shift can even lead to hydrocephalus. The pharmacological therapies are divided broadly into antithrombotic, thrombolytic, neuroprotective, and antiedema therapies. The surgical therapies include endarterectomy, extracranial-intracranial bypass, and balloon angioplasty.

Pharmacological Therapies

Antithrombotic Therapy (Antiplatelet and Anticoagulation). The principal rationale behind the use of antiplatelet and anticoagulation agents is that rapid recanalization and reperfusion of occluded vessels reduces the infarction area. The theoretical benefit also exists of preventing clot propagation and recurring vascular thrombosis. The risks associated with the use of these treatments includes hemorrhagic conversion, hemorrhage, and increased cerebral edema, all of which are associated with worse outcomes.[90] Current research has not established a clear advantage to the use of aspirin or heparin in acute stroke patients, but these agents still are commonly used in the hope that they may decrease injury from acute stroke. Aspirin, an irreversible antiplatelet agent, is administered when symptoms appear. Heparin is administered intravenously in a continuous infusion.[71] Both of these agents are started only after determination by CT or MRI that no hemorrhage is associated with the stroke. Ticlopidine, another antiplatelet agent, has been even less studied, and its role, if any, in acute stroke treatment is unclear. A recent metaanalysis of the trials of heparin and oral anticoagulation therapy in acute stroke treatment showed a marginal benefit from treatments with anticoagulation compared with no treatment at all.[135] Currently, numerous large, multicentric studies in the United States and Europe are examining the best approach to the antithrombotic treatment of stroke that should provide better guidance as their results become known in the next few years.

Thrombolytic Therapy. Thrombolytic therapy is attractive as a therapy for acute stroke, because it opens up occluded cerebral vessels and immediately restores blood flow to ischemic areas. However, a problem in using these agents in stroke treatment is that the treatment must start in six hours from onset of symptoms to be therapeutic. Most patients are symptomatic at a much later stage, and even if they have symptoms early enough, a rapid workup to rule out a cerebral bleed must be performed before initiation of therapy. The successful use of these agents—primarily urokinase, streptokinase, and tissue plasminogen activator—in the treatment of myocardial ischemia has aroused interest in similar use of these agents for acute stroke treatment. The mechanism of action of these agents is to cause fibrin breakdown in the clots that have been formed and thus to lead to lysis of the occlusions in the blood vessels. Reviews of thrombolytic therapy for stroke treatment have shown some reduction in mortality, but no definitive answer is available to date concerning efficacy.[163] Currently, streptokinase is out of favor because of increased mortality and morbidity from intracranial hemorrhage,[123,156] but tissue plasminogen activator, a more specific thrombolytic agent, has been able to achieve favorable results. The National Institute of Neurological Disorders and Stroke trial was the cornerstone trial in approval of treatment of acute ischemic stroke with thrombolytics.[3,6,103,157] The trial was a double-blind, placebo-controlled trial that revealed an improvement in early outcomes in 24 hours of treatment and demonstrated an increase in symptom-free survival from 38% (placebo) to 50% (treatment) at three months. The strict use of a three-hour window from the onset of symptoms and the rigid blood pressure guidelines of the National Institute of Neurological Disorders and Stroke trial are probably contributors to the excellent outcomes; the exact treatment protocols are still being defined. On reexamination at one year, the treated patients continued to show a benefit, and this has encouraged the use of this agent in selected groups.[87] Other thrombolytic agents such as alteplase also have shown benefit and are being used routinely. The results are at the same level of effectiveness as tissue plasminogen activator.[5] Unfortunately, the three-hour window of efficacy limits the number of individuals who can receive benefit, and studies to expand the window of intervention to have hours or more have not shown clear benefits.[30,64] In the patient with stroke beyond three hours, the currently recommended interventions are mostly limited to the use of anticoagulants and antiplatelet agents to prevent further events.[103] Further active investigation continues to search for effective treatments in this large group of individuals with late presentation of stroke.

Other Treatments for Altering Cerebral Perfusion.
A number of different treatments aimed at lowering blood viscosity or cerebral perfusion have been used, including hemodilution with agents such as dextran, albumin, and hetastarch. None of the 12 studies reviewed by Asplund demonstrated any clear benefit.[9] Similarly, studies of prostacyclins and several different types of cerebral vasodilators have also shown no clear evidence of increased survival rates or improvement in outcomes after treatment.[90] Research continues to be active in these areas, but so far none of these alternative treatments for increasing cerebral perfusion has yielded a favorable outcome.

Neuroprotective Agents. Neuroprotective agents are medications that can alter the course of metabolic events after the onset of ischemia and therefore have the potential to reduce stroke damage. No agent has shown clear benefits among this group of treatments. These agents include calcium channel blockers, naloxone, gangliosides, glutamate antagonists, and free-radical scavengers. Each of these agents has had promise in the theoretical or laboratory realm, but none has proved to be clinically efficacious.

The use of naloxone, a narcotic antagonist, is based on the in vitro observation that naloxone has neuroprotective effects. Unfortunately, the clinical trials to date have not demonstrated any benefit.[33] The therapeutic rationale of using calcium channel blockers is that they prevent injury to ischemic neurons by preventing calcium influx, which decreases metabolic activity in the neuron.[90] Initial hope was that the treatment results for SAH, in which nimodipine decreases secondary ischemia, would be similar for stroke. Unfortunately, the results of several studies

have not shown any clear benefits from treatment with these agents,[108] and none of them currently are used routinely for stroke treatment.

In animal experiments, glutamate antagonists decrease the size of infarction area in stroke.[90] However, the few studies done in human beings have been inconclusive and have shown serious neuropsychiatric side effects.[33]

Gangliosides may reduce ischemic damage by counteracting toxic amino acids in ischemic tissue. Despite the many studies that have been performed, no clearly demonstrated benefits have resulted from use of these agents.[33]

The free-radical scavengers include 21-amino steroids (lazaroids), ascorbic acid (vitamin C), and tocopherol (vitamin E). They have not been well-evaluated, and some studies to establish their clinical use are being undertaken.[90] However, vitamin E has been demonstrated clinically to reduce the risk of heart disease, so secondarily its use may decrease the risk of stroke.

Agents for Cerebral Edema. Agents that reduce cerebral edema include corticosteroids, mannitol, glycerol, vinca alkaloids, and piracetam. All the studies done on persons receiving steroids[122] after an acute stroke demonstrated no clear benefits, and steroid use creates a risk of diabetes and DVT.[62] Use of the other agents also has no clear benefit in the treatment of acute stroke and are also not routinely used.

Cooling Therapy. An exciting new development in the treatment of acute stroke has been the initiation of cooling therapy on presentation with the induction of a medical coma to limit the extent of brain injury after stroke. In most patients who present with stroke, there is a natural tendency for the body temperature to be elevated between 4% and 25%, which is associated with increased injury and poorer outcomes.[18,35] Studies have shown that injury could be slowed with supercooling, and the technique has been used in surgery to help limit injury and to prolong safe surgical time in both neurosurgical and cardiothoracic procedures.[28,131,139] The pooled analysis of existing studies does not yet provide convincing evidence that death or long-term disability are significantly changed from the application of mechanical or pharmacological cooling, but the therapy is just starting to be used on a larger scale, and new research findings published in the next several years may show a benefit to routine cooling of acute stroke victims.

Surgical Therapies
Endarterectomy. A carotid endarterectomy is the surgical opening of the carotid arteries to remove plaque. This therapy has been shown to be useful in preventing recurrent strokes or development of stroke in individuals with TIAs, but it has not been used to treat acute stroke. In theory, the opening of the carotids could subject ischemic areas and their blood vessels to excessive pressure from

restored blood flow and lead to hemorrhage.[40] Concerns about using major anesthesia in a patient with a new stroke makes this surgery too risky to treat acute stroke.

Extracranial-Intracranial Bypass. Despite the initial attraction of bringing extracranial blood flow into the intracranial vessels through the use of bypass procedures, the large trial done in the 1980s demonstrated no improvement in patient outcomes, and the procedure has been largely abandoned.[47]

Balloon Angioplasty. Despite its efficacy in opening blocked coronary arteries in patients with heart disease and its successful treatment of acute myocardial infarction, the use of balloon angioplasty in acute stroke has not been studied. Clinical centers are actively investigating its possible uses.

Hemorrhagic Stroke

In patients who have had a hemorrhagic stroke, the size and location of the lesion determines the overall prognosis; supratentorial lesions greater than 5 cm have a poor prognosis, and brainstem lesions of 3 cm are usually fatal.[49] In these cases, the control of edema is important, and the techniques previously described can be used. In patients with SAH, the treatment regimen is usually more aggressive and focuses on several issues, which include the control of intracranial pressure, prevention of rebleeding, maintenance of cerebral perfusion, and control of vasospasm.

Prevention of Rebleeding. Before 1980, six weeks of bed rest were prescribed routinely for the care of patients with acute SAH to prevent rebleeding. In 1981 a study demonstrated that bed rest was inferior to surgical treatment, lowering of blood pressure, and carotid ligation.[158] Antihypertensive medications for the prevention of rebleeding are still controversial, and no consensus exists as to their use. Carotid ligation used to be popular, but more recent reevaluations of the benefits of the technique have not been as conclusive, and because of its surgical risks, direct repair of the aneurysm is a better choice. Antifibrinolytic agents have been studied and have been beneficial for low-risk patients in whom surgery must be delayed, but they seem to increase the risk of ischemic events. The placement of intraluminal coils, balloons, and polymers has shown some benefit in the short-term prevention of rebleeding, but the long-term efficacy is still unclear, and the techniques remain experimental.[102] Because the risk of rebleeding is also very high in post-SAH seizures, even though the incidence of seizure is low, the recommendation is that patients receive antiseizure medications for prophylaxis.

Control of Vasospasm. The treatment of vasospasm is important for the reasons previously outlined. The current treatments include the use of orally administered nimodipine, a calcium channel blocker shown to improve outcomes of patients who have had an SAH with vasospasm. The results of using other calcium channel antagonists are unclear. The use of hypertension/hypervolemia/hemodilution has been recommended by some studies. Creating more volume than normal results in hypertension. The stretch caused by the volume stimulates the smooth muscle pressure receptors that line the vessels. These receptors inhibit muscle action by a protective response, and the blood vessel dilates to accommodate the increased volume. Hypertension/hypervolemia/hemodilution is most effective in preventing vasospasm after surgically clipping the aneurysm. Significant cardiac and hemodynamic risks are associated with this therapy, so intensive care unit (ICU) monitoring is required.[102]

PREVENTION OF STROKE RECURRENCE

Ischemic Stroke

In general, the strategies to prevent recurrence of ischemic stroke can be divided into two areas: risk factor modification (which also applies to primary prevention) and secondary prevention to treat the underlying cause of stroke in individuals with a history of stroke. Following is a discussion of the secondary interventions that can be used to prevent recurrence of stroke.

Hypertension. Although the treatment of hypertension is an important primary preventive measure in the management of stroke, whether blood pressure reduction after stroke is beneficial has not been proved definitively. The transient rise in blood pressure after stroke usually settles without intervention.[164] Because of the uncertainty about whether overaggressive treatment of acute elevated blood pressure is harmful, definitive antihypertensive therapy probably should be delayed for two weeks.[90] At that time, one should follow the usual recommendations regarding adequate control of hypertension because some evidence indicates that it is beneficial. This seems especially appropriate in patients who have had a lacunar stroke because the development of multiple lacunae is related to uncontrolled blood pressure.

Antiplatelet Medications. In patients who have had a TIA or stroke, long-term use of aspirin has been shown to decrease the incidence of death, myocardial infarction, and recurrent events by up to 23%.[7] The doses of aspirin in numerous studies have ranged from 30 mg to 600 mg; all doses resulted in a 14% to 18% reduction in recurrent cerebral events, but gastrointestinal complications increased with the higher doses.[1,48,153] In general, a standard dosage of one regular adult aspirin (325 mg a day) is the usual treatment for recurrent ischemic stroke. Studies are underway that compare the efficacy of warfarin versus aspirin in treating ischemic stroke; the results of these studies are not yet available. Ticlopidine is another antiplatelet medication effective in reducing the incidence of recurrent stroke.[81] Ticlopidine is most efficacious in women, patients who are not helped by aspirin therapy, and patients with vertebrobasilar symptoms, hypertension, diabetes, and no severe carotid disease.[62]

Anticoagulation. The incidence of recurrent stroke and TIA in patients with atrial fibrillation is approximately 7% per year. For patients who have atrial fibrillation with cardiac sources of emboli, warfarin is the clear treatment of choice; this is true for primary and secondary prevention. Although aspirin has some preventive effects, it is not as efficacious. In the presence of structural cardiac disease or atrial fibrillation, aspirin should be used only to treat patients in whom warfarin anticoagulation is contraindicated.[90]

The odds ratio for recurrence is approximately 0.36 in those treated with warfarin versus control and 0.84 for those treated with aspirin versus control.[45] However, problems exist with warfarin anticoagulation in the elderly. Cognitive and compliance difficulties can lead to an increase in complications. Unclear issues in anticoagulation use include when to start anticoagulants after stroke, the safety of anticoagulants in clinical practice, and the optimum anticoagulant blood level. Several studies are currently examining these questions.

Treatment of Dysrhythmias or Underlying Disease. Obviously, primary and secondary prevention should treat the underlying cause of the ischemic stroke. Prevention can include cardioversion to normal sinus rhythm and treatment with antidysrhythmic medications, and treatment of underlying medical conditions if they can be found. Unfortunately, only a small proportion of patients who have had TIAs and strokes can benefit from these specific treatments.

Carotid Endarterectomy. The surgical treatment of carotid artery stenosis has been shown to be beneficial in recent studies of stroke recurrence in patients with severely (greater than 70%) stenosed carotid arteries.[12,46] The data on the intermediate group of patients (stenosis from 30% to 70%) are being collected. For patients with high-grade stenosis, carotid endarterectomy reduces the range of stroke risk from 22% to 26% down to 8% to 12%.

Hemorrhagic Stroke

The mainstay of ICH prevention is controlling systolic and diastolic hypertension. No clear benefit exists for one group of treatment agents versus another as long as adequate hypertension control is maintained. In patients in whom the ICH follows vasculitis or the use of anticoagulants, the treatment for preventing recurrence includes treating the vasculitis or terminating anticoagulant use.[128]

The secondary prevention of recurrent stroke and SAH of AVMs and/or aneurysms includes surgical management of the lesions (the treatment of choice). Clipping or microsurgical dissection of the lesions is performed whenever possible and as soon as the patient is able safely to undergo the procedure.[102,149] In surgically unresectable lesions, alternatives include sclerotherapy, coating, trapping, and proximal arterial occlusion.[102]

PREVENTION OF COMPLICATIONS AND LONG-TERM SEQUELAE

General Principles

To prevent complications and long-term sequelae after a stroke, maximizing function, decreasing morbidity, and preventing rehospitalization from a complication are important. Prevention of these complications begins on the day the patient arrives at the hospital with symptoms of acute stroke. Many complications are associated with bed rest in general, but some are specific to stroke.

Musculoskeletal Complications

Contractures. Contractures are periarticular motion impairments that result from loss of elasticity in the periarticular tissues, which include muscles, tendons, and ligaments. Contractures can occur in any immobilized joint but are particularly prevalent in the paretic limbs after a stroke. In fact, only 10% of stroke patients recover limb strength and mobility rapidly enough to avoid developing contractures.[63] Shoulder pain, contractures, and muscle pain occur in 70% to 80% of patients who have had a hemiplegic stroke.[128] Chapter 10 addresses the management and related issues of the hemiplegic shoulder. Contractures also occur in other areas and begin to be problematic within a few days of onset or several days after the stroke when symptoms of immobility and spasticity may begin to develop. Usually contractures occur in a pattern of flexion, adduction, and internal rotation; muscles that span two joints are more susceptible to contracture formation.[66] To prevent shortening of the connective tissue in muscles and joints, an active range of motion (ROM) program must be initiated. Because certain muscles span two joints, joints must be positioned to allow full physiological stretch of the muscles involved. Once a contracture is present, the mainstay of treatment is gradual, prolonged stretch. The minimal treatment is a sustained stretch greater than 30 minutes.[84] Other treatments include splinting, deep-heating modalities,[23] and possible surgical release for long-standing, tight contractures[66] (see Chapter 13).

Osteoporosis. Bone is a metabolically active tissue normally in a state of equilibrium between active bone resorption and deposition. The ratio of bone formation to bone resorption is influenced by the stressors to which the bone is subjected, a relationship known as Wolff law.[23] The lack of weight-bearing and normal stress on long bones on the hemiplegic side of a stroke patient leads to a predominance of bone resorption. This loss of bone mass can start as early as 30 hours after the beginning of immobility[155] and with bed rest can be as high as 25% to 45% in 30 to 36 weeks.[39] In patients who have had a stroke, osteoporosis is often worse, and the rate of hip fracture is far higher on the side of the hemiplegia.[67]

Osteoporosis prevention is accomplished best with measures that include active weight-bearing exercise and active muscle contraction. Medical therapies for individuals at risk for osteoporosis should be initiated. Therapies include bone-forming agents, calcium and vitamin D supplementation, hormone replacement, and other measures as needed. Box 1-1 shows some of the medical treatments available for osteoporosis.

Heterotopical Ossification. Heterotopical ossification is the deposition of calcium in the form of mature bone in the soft tissues. The condition is not particularly common after stroke but occurs with increased incidence after traumatic brain injury. The incidence ranges from 11% to 76% in various studies.[17] Spasticity is associated with the development of heterotopical ossification as are long-bone fractures and a prolonged coma. Symptoms of heterotopical ossification usually develop one to three months after injury with pain and limited ROM.[24] The diagnosis is based on clinical examination, elevated alkaline phosphatase levels in the serum, and a positive bone scan.

Treatment for heterotopical ossification includes active ROM; no studies indicate that the condition is caused or worsened by active ROM exercises.[17] Pharmacological treatment options include the use of etidronate disodium and nonsteroidal antiinflammatory drugs.[24] Other treatments include radiation therapy and, for refractory cases after the lesion has matured, surgical excision of the heterotopical ossification. Performance of ROM exercises after surgery is particularly important. Low-dose radiation or etidronate disodium can also be used to prevent recurrence.[34]

Box 1-1

Treatments for Osteoporosis

- Bone forming agents (etidronate and others)
- Estrogen replacement
- Calcitonin
- Calcium supplementation
- Vitamin D supplementation
- Fluoride supplementation
- Weight-bearing exercises

Falls. Falls are of particular concern in survivors of stroke. These patients are at increased risk of hip fracture because of developed osteoporosis, and the acuity of their balance, visual perceptions, and spatial perceptions is decreased. The increased risk of falls has been documented in several studies and is greater in patients who have had a right hemispheric stroke.[36,106,118] Fall prevention should emphasize balance and cognitive training, removing environmental hazards, and using adaptive devices. (These measures are reviewed in Chapters 8, 14, 15, 19, 27, and 28.)

Neurological Complications

Seizures. Seizures after strokes have been documented since the nineteenth century. The incidence of late-onset seizures (epilepsy) in the individuals who have had strokes ranges from 6% to 18%,[59,162] whereas the incidence of early seizures is approximately 10%, with reports ranging from 3% to 38%.[14,168] The risk for seizures is highest right after stroke; 57% of seizures occur in the first week, and 88% of all seizures after strokes occur in the first year.[14] Seizures are more common in patients who have had an SAH; 85% of these seizures are early seizures.[148] The timing of seizures that occur after stroke varies according to the mechanism of injury. The timing of seizures after thrombotic and embolic strokes appears about equal. Patients with SAH have more seizures soon after the stroke, whereas patients with ICH are more similar to patients with ischemic stroke and may have more late-onset seizures.[168]

The treatment and management of seizures associated with stroke are usually straightforward, and monotherapy often produces adequate results. If the patient only has acute-onset seizures in the setting of his or her stroke, the patient often does not require long-term antiseizure medication. A single, brief seizure or a nongeneralizing local seizure also can often be managed conservatively. If seizures do require treatment, a single agent usually suffices and is beneficial, because the drug interactions are fewer, and the compliance is better with monotherapy. Carbamazepine and phenytoin are the preferred agents for treating epilepsy after stroke. Management of the medication requires close follow-up to ensure that the desired outcome is achieved: an asymptomatic, seizure-free patient. Excessive medication can lead to a number of symptoms (Box 1-2). Inadequate control of the condition leads to additional seizures. For situations in which seizures become refractory to treatment, one must remember several factors.[168] Intercurrent illness or metabolic disarray that lowers the seizure threshold may make the seizures more frequent and difficult to treat. Patient compliance may be a problem, especially if the stroke created cognitive and behavioral deficits. Progressive lesions or new infarcts are also causes of increasing seizure frequency. Finally, a stroke that occurs in highly epileptogenic areas—such as the hippocampus,

Box 1-2

Signs of Excessive Antiseizure Medication

- Lethargy
- Drowsiness
- Depression
- Nystagmus
- Ataxia
- Irritability
- Distractibility
- Poor cognition
- Poor memory

the parietooccipital cortex surrounding the rolandic fissure, and calcarine cortex—may engender refractory epilepsy and require combination therapy. Table 1-7 lists the common seizure medications and their side effects.

Hydrocephalus. Hydrocephalus can occur acutely, especially in patients with SAH and ICH as discussed previously, or it can develop symptoms insidiously later. Hydrocephalus is usually heralded by the gradual onset of a triad of symptoms, including lethargy with decreased mental function, ataxia, and urinary incontinence. Once hydrocephalus is suspected, one should perform a CT scan promptly because the increasing size of the ventricles is readily visible. Once diagnosed, one should surgically place a ventricular shunt. The procedure is well-tolerated and can lead to resolution of all the symptoms of hydrocephalus if performed promptly. Patients with an occluded shunt have symptoms that mimic the initial symptoms of hydrocephalus.

Spasticity. Spasticity is defined as a motor disorder characterized by a velocity-dependent increase in tonic stretch reflexes with exaggerated tendon jerks. Spasticity results from hyperexcitability of the stretch reflex (which is one component of the upper motor neuron syndrome).[89] In a normal recovery after a flaccid stroke, an initial period occurs with little resistance to passive motion of the muscles and joints. Approximately 48 hours after the stroke, tendon reflexes and muscle resistance to passive motion begin to return.[66] Spasticity is most pronounced in the flexor muscles and occurs throughout the hemiplegic side. The lower extremity later develops a component of extensor spasticity that can assist with function, whereas the upper extremity spasticity is usually in a flexor pattern.[10]

The management of spasticity includes encouraging voluntary movement, ROM exercises, and a functional rehabilitative approach.[66] The research data on the different neurorehabilitative treatment approaches do not define clearly which approach is most effective, so an individualized approach to treating each patient is the best course. Pharmacological treatments for spasticity are numerous, and they need to be tailored to each patient to find the best balance of side effects and efficacy. The most commonly used agents are baclofen, dantrolene sodium, and diazepam. These medications and a representative sample of the other medications used to treat patients who have had a stroke are presented in the table of medications and their side effects on the inside cover of the book. Other treatments for severe spasticity that are more invasive include phenol blocks and neurolysis, botulinum toxin (Botox) injections, and implantable baclofen pumps. Botox injections and baclofen pumps are still experimental approaches, and ongoing studies will elucidate their future roles (see Chapter 10).

Other Complications

Deconditioning. Physiological deconditioning in patients after a stroke results from the acute medical illness and the associated bed rest and immobility that may result. Table 1-8 lists some of the effects of deconditioning. All of these factors can alter the ability of the patient to recover. Therefore, to get the patient out of bed and to increase activity as early and aggressively as possible is important.

Psychological Complications. Stroke is a major life event and is associated with significant alterations in the individual's well-being and independence. Negative emotional reactions are common in patients following a stroke[152] and can have a significant effect on the patient's eventual outcome. After a stroke, patients may go through the four stages of bereavement described by Worden.[172] These include accepting the loss, experiencing the pain of the loss, adjusting to a new environment in which previous abilities are missing, and investing in new activities. Not all patients become depressed, and this lack of depression does not necessarily mean the patient is in denial.[173] Denial is a normal defense mechanism, and as long as it does not interfere with the rehabilitative process, it is not a concern.[152] The indifference reaction, a persistent denial reaction, is more common in patients who have had a right-sided stroke than a left-sided stroke.[53]

Another common consequence of stroke is emotional lability, which is rapidly shifting from one extreme emotion to another. Approximately 20% of patients have emotional lability six months after a stroke, and up to 10% have lability for one year. Emotional lability is more common in patients with pseudobulbar palsy and right hemispheric strokes, particularly if the patient is depressed.[74]

Anxiety is also common after stroke and is more frequent in patients with left hemispheric strokes[94] and cortical lesions.[144] Many sources of anxiety exist, including financial affairs, family issues, and a fear of dying or recurrent stroke. Reassurance and constant positive feedback during rehabilitation can help, and in severe cases, treatment with anxiolytics and psychological support may be needed.

Table 1-7

Medical Management of Seizures: Drug Therapy

MEDICATION	SIDE EFFECTS	PRINCIPAL USES
Phenytoin	Ataxia Incoordination Confusion Rash Gum hyperplasia Hirsutism Osteomalacia	Tonic-clonic (grand mal) Partial
Carbamazepine	Ataxia Dizziness Diplopia Vertigo Bone marrow suppression Hepatotoxicity	Tonic-clonic (grand mal) Partial
Phenobarbital	Sedation Ataxia Confusion Dizziness Depression Decreased libido Rash	Tonic-clonic (grand mal) Partial
Primidone	Same as phenobarbital	Tonic-clonic (grand mal) Partial
Valproic acid	Ataxia Sedation Tremor Bone marrow suppression Hepatotoxicity Weight gain Transient alopecia	Absence (petit mal) Atypical absence Myoclonic Tonic-clonic (grand mal)
Clonazepam	Ataxia Sedation Lethargy Anorexia	Absence (petit mal) Atypical absence Myoclonic
Ethosuximide	Ataxia Lethargy Rash Bone marrow suppression	Absence (petit mal)

Fortunately, outbursts and aggressive behavior are rare after a stroke, but when they occur, they are more common in patients with left-sided infarcts who are more aware of their deficits. The approach to management of these outbursts should not include restraints and threats but should be based on avoiding excessive frustration in the patient by removing emotional triggers and alternating easy and difficult tasks.[152]

Depression is common after stroke, developing in 20% to 50% of stroke survivors, with 30% being the most commonly accepted figure.[152] The depression can be a reaction to the stroke or a neuropsychological sequela of the stroke. The consequences of depression after stroke are numerous: hospital stays are longer,[42] cognitive impairment is greater,[125] and motivation decreases.[140] Depression is more common in patients with left cortical lesions[145] and lesions close to the frontal poles and is shorter in patients with subcortical and brainstem lesions. Depression after stroke often is treated best with antidepressant medications.[152] In patients who are unable to tolerate antidepressants, are unresponsive to therapy, or have active suicidal ideation, electroconvulsive therapy can be a last resort.[110] (See Chapter 2 for more information about the psychological effects of stroke.)

Table 1-8

Deconditioning Effects of Stroke

Musculoskeletal	Atrophy
	↓ Strength of tendons, ligaments, bones, and muscles
	Depression
	Anxiety
	Sleep disturbance
Cardiovascular	↓ Stroke volume
	↑ Heart rate
	↓ VO₂ max
	↑ Respiratory rate
	↓ Lean body mass
	↑ Body fat
	Orthostatic hypotension
Neurological/emotional	Sensory deprivation
	↓ Balance
	↓ Coordination
	Fatigue
Genitourinary	Diuresis
	Difficulty voiding
Endocrine	Impaired glucose tolerance
	Altered regulation of hormones
Body composition and metabolism	Nitrogen loss
	Calcium loss
	Potassium loss
	Phosphorus loss
	Sulfur loss

Urinary Tract Dysfunction. Urinary incontinence is common after stroke, affecting 51% to 60% of patients,[20] and can cause difficulties with rehabilitation, influence eventual discharge location, and place stress on caregivers.[43] One month and six months after stroke, 29% and 14% of patients, respectively, still have urinary incontinence.[11] The usual pathophysiology of incontinence is detrusor hyperreflexia, which is common in patients with cortical lesions. The incontinence assessment includes a thorough history of the urinary symptoms and can include urodynamic studies to help define the problem. Incontinence treatment includes timed voiding and use of pharmacological agents and intermittent catheterization. If these treatments do not work, incontinence may need to be treated by indwelling catheterization. This is performed on patients who cannot independently self-catheterize and do not have caretakers who can provide this care or on patients who have physical barriers such as urethral strictures that prevent regular catheterizations. Unfortunately, indwelling catheters have a high incidence of associated urinary tract infections. Male patients also may use external condom catheters, which can provide socially acceptable continence when the individual is traveling or physically active. Patients with continuous dribbling also benefit from condom catheters. The goal of all of these therapies is to maintain continence and prevent urinary tract infections and other complications such as skin breakdown from skin maceration.

Skin Breakdown and Decubitus Ulcers. Pressure ulcer formation is a serious health problem in debilitated and immobilized patients. After a stroke, patients are at particular risk for pressure ulcers because they have numerous factors contributing to skin breakdown. Abnormal sensation, contracture, malnutrition, immobility, and muscle and soft-tissue atrophy often develop and may be complicated by advanced age. Prevention of pressure ulcers, rather than treatment of developing ulcers, should be the focus of care. Preventive measures include frequent repositioning, keeping skin clean and dry, maintaining an adequate level of nutrition, and, especially in high-risk patients, using pressure-relief mattresses.[132] Once pressure ulcers have formed, in addition to strictly observing the preventive and pressure relieving measures previously noted, treatments include meticulous wound care with a variety of agents and possibly surgical reconstruction.

Dysphagia. Swallowing disorders are common after a stroke. Dysphagia is more common in the elderly, with an incidence of 25% to 45%.[59,61] Aspiration can lead to pneumonia, and a decreased eating ability can lead to dehydration and malnutrition. Chapter 24 covers the details of the pathology of aspiration and the methods of its treatment.

Aspiration. Aspiration causes chemical pneumonitis that can lead to a secondary bacterial infection. Because numerous anaerobic organisms are in the mouth, aspiration pneumonia can develop into an anaerobic abscess.[92] Such abscesses occur less frequently in edentulous individuals because they have less oral flora and can occur in up to a third of cases in hospitalized patients.[97] The treatment of choice is to reduce the risk of aspiration and to administer antibiotics. Examining a radiographic film for evidence of abscess cavities and the sputum for organisms can help one develop a specific medical treatment. Sputum culture growth often requires up to three or four days, so initial treatment is often empirical and should be the administration of a wide-spectrum antibiotic that is effective against hospital-acquired organisms (which are often resistant to certain antibiotics) and anaerobic bacteria.[92] The usual course of antibiotics is seven to 10 days, but cavitary pneumonia may require far longer treatment for eradication of the organism.[93] Determination of which specific antibacterial agents to use depends on the resistance patterns in the institution in which the aspiration takes place; the infectious disease team at that institution should make the decision about which antibiotics to use.

Deep Venous Thrombosis. DVT is a common problem after stroke and has an incidence of 23% to 75% depending on the severity of the stroke. Most of the morbidity and mortality associated with DVT results from venous thromboembolism (VTE). Pulmonary embolism after stroke has an incidence of 10% to 29% and a mortality rate of 10%.[19] The formation of DVT is caused by the triad of risk factors outlined by Virchow postulates: altered blood flow, damage to the blood vessel wall, and altered blood coagulability. Box 1-3 lists the common risk factors for DVT. Of the risk factors for DVT, stasis is one of the most important. After a stroke, DVT is 10 times more common in the paretic leg.[165] DVT usually begins in the calf, and although the emboli from calf thrombi are not dangerous, these thrombi propagate in about 20% of cases, and about 50% of the proximal deep venous thrombi embolize. About 20% of symptomatic pulmonary emboli are fatal.[134] After a stroke, ambulation in itself is not preventive in the subacute setting: pulmonary embolism occurred in 57% of ambulatory patients in the rehabilitation setting.[147] Lower extremity and pelvic DVT are the most common, but proximal upper extremity DVT also can occur, although it is rare. All of the diagnostic and management issues discussed in the section on VTE that follows applies to this condition as well.

The diagnosis of DVT in the clinical setting is unreliable,[19] and many patients with life-threatening embolism and thrombosis have no clinical symptoms of DVT. Other patients with swelling and tenderness may not have DVT at all and may have any of a number of other diagnoses. The differential diagnosis of lower extremity pain and swelling includes trauma, fracture, gout, cellulitis, and superficial phlebitis. The usual clinical signs of DVT include pain and tenderness, swelling, the presence of Homans sign (elicited by dorsiflexion of the ankle while the knee is flexed resulting in pain in the calf), superficial venous distention, a palpable cord, and fever. Some of these signs, such as Homans, are unreliable indicators. Homans sign is present in less than one third of patients with DVT and is present in half of patients without

Box 1-3

Risk Factors for DVT

- Immobilization
- Postoperative state
- Age >40 years
- Cardiac disease
- Limb trauma
- Coagulation disorders
- Obesity
- Advanced neoplasm
- Pregnancy

DVT.[73] Objective testing for DVT has venography as the gold standard, but this procedure is associated with significant risks, including anaphylaxis and causing DVT. More commonly used risk-free procedures are impedance plethysmography, which is a noninvasive test that measures volume changes in the leg with circumferential calf electrodes,[75] and Doppler ultrasound, which is also a noninvasive test that uses a handheld probe to detect blood flow in deep leg veins.[166] Doppler ultrasound and impedance plethysmography have similar sensitivities and specificities for DVT detection, but Doppler ultrasound is not as portable and has a higher cost than impedance plethysmography.[19]

The clinical diagnosis of pulmonary embolism is also unreliable, and only 30% of patients with pulmonary embolism have clinical DVT, even though 70% have venographic evidence of DVT.[19] The symptoms of submassive pulmonary embolism overlap with the symptoms of many other pulmonary conditions, including tachypnea, tachycardia, rales, hemoptysis, pleuritic chest pain, pleural effusion, general malaise, bronchospasm, and fever. In patients with massive pulmonary embolism with greater than 60% of the pulmonary circulation obstructed, patients are critically ill and develop heart failure, circulatory collapse, hypotension, and coma and can die suddenly.[147] The gold standard for testing for pulmonary embolism is the pulmonary angiogram, but its use is associated with significant morbidity and mortality. The preferred noninvasive test is the ventilation/perfusion scan.[105]

The best approach to VTE is to prevent DVT. The National Institutes of Health Consensus Conference on the Prevention of Venous Thrombosis and Pulmonary Embolism recommends using low doses of subcutaneously administered heparin in all stroke patients with no hemorrhagic components.[121] In all other patients, external pneumatic calf compression is recommended. More recently, low-molecular-weight heparin has been introduced and actually may be more effective than standard heparin for DVT prophylaxis.[72] Low doses of warfarin for DVT prophylaxis in stroke patients has not been well-studied, but its use in other conditions has proved its effectiveness in DVT reduction. Dextran, aspirin, and static compression stockings are not effective for preventing DVT.[19] Physical treatments alone, such as ROM exercises, have not been studied. Ambulatory patients must be able to walk at least 50 feet to have a reduction in risk of DVT,[21] but as previously stated, the risk of pulmonary embolism in ambulatory patients is still significant.[147] The length of time prophylaxis should continue is still not definite, but evidence shows that continuing prophylaxis well into the subacute phase is warranted.[19]

The treatment of VTE (DVT and pulmonary embolism) is based on preventing pulmonary embolism, which can be fatal. A patient who is identified with acute VTE is started on intravenous (IV) heparin as long as no contraindications to anticoagulation exist.[70] The effectiveness of the heparin is determined by monitoring the partial thromboplastin time, and the heparin is adjusted to a dose between 1.5 and 2.5 times control. In a patient with only DVT, warfarin can be started on the first day, and the heparin can be discontinued when the warfarin dose is therapeutic as measured by the increase in the prothrombin time or international normalized ratio. Targets are a prothrombin time of 1.25 to 1.5 times control or an international normalized ratio of 2 to 3.[19] In patients with pulmonary embolism, warfarin may be started a few days later, and after management of the acute stage, the patient keeps receiving it longer; patients with DVT receive warfarin for approximately three months, and patients with pulmonary embolism, for six months.[72] All patients who recently have been diagnosed with VTE are placed on bed rest initially and usually are allowed to become mobile two days after the partial thromboplastin time has become therapeutic.[76] The rehabilitation of patients with VTE who are beginning treatment should continue at the bed side, and, in the case of patients with lower extremity DVT, the rehabilitation program should include activity of daily living (ADL) training, upper extremity programs, communication work, and dysphagia treatments.

FUTURE TRENDS IN MEDICAL STROKE MANAGEMENT

Improved Primary Stroke Prevention

Because the treatments for stroke are so limited and the deficits that can result are so devastating, the primary prevention of stroke has to be the essential strategy to decrease morbidity and mortality from stroke. With a good understanding of the risk factors for stroke, risk factor modification can be targeted at groups and individuals who are at risk. Table 1-1 lists the preventable and nonpreventable risk factors for stroke. Fortunately, many of the risk factors are the same as those for myocardial infarction and vascular disease leading to death, so the modification of stroke risk factors also decreases the risk of cardiac-related morbidity and mortality. Due to greater awareness and risk factor modification and largely through the treatment of blood pressure, a decline of greater than 50% in the stroke mortality rate has occurred in the past 20 years.[169] Each of the modifiable risk factors are considered separately.

Hypertension

Diastolic and systolic hypertension are each independently and strongly implicated in causing stroke. Hypertension increases the risk of stroke in all age groups of men and women.[169] In fact, no threshold level of blood pressure exists below which the risk curve plateaus.[98] For every 7.5 mm Hg increase in diastolic pressure is a 46% increase in stroke incidence and a 29% increase in coronary heart disease (CHD). Reducing blood pressure in hypertensive patients has been shown to decrease the risk of stroke significantly, with an average reduction of 5.8 mm Hg leading to a reduction in stroke incidence of 42% but only a 14% reduction in CHD incidence.[32] Because these trials only spanned two to five years, the reduction in stroke incidence is a direct result of decreased blood pressure and not an alteration in atherogenesis (production of plaque in the arteries), which would take longer to develop.[169] Systolic blood pressure is also a factor; the treatment of isolated systolic hypertension (>160 mm Hg) has been shown to reduce the incidence of stroke by 36% and CHD by 27% over 4.5 years.[120] Treating all forms of hypertension in the older age groups is therefore essential because they are at increased risk for stroke, and most strokes occur in this age group. Screening for hypertension and aggressively treating systolic and diastolic hypertension should be the cornerstone of any primary prevention program for stroke.

Cigarette Smoking

The results of the Framingham Study and the Nurses' Health Study demonstrate that the cessation of cigarette smoking should lead to a prompt reduction in stroke mortality.[31,171] Risk of CHD decreases by 50% in one year and reaches the level of a nonsmoker's risk in five years. Smoking increases stroke risk by 40% in men and 60% in women (with no other risk factors being considered), and it seems to follow that smoking cessation leads to a reduction in stroke risk similar to the reduction in CHD incidence.

Cardiac Dysrhythmia and Myocardial Infarction

CHD, atrial fibrillation, and congestive heart failure lead to an increased incidence of stroke.[169] Preventing these conditions by modifying their associated risk factors leads to a reduction in incidence of stroke. In addition, treating patients who have established dysrhythmias and congestive heart failure with anticoagulants such as warfarin decreases the incidence of stroke (as explained previously).

Blood Lipids

The development of carotid artery atherosclerotic disease has been shown to be related to the levels of serum lipids.[133] However, to relate accelerated atherosclerosis clearly to an increase in the incidence of stroke has been difficult because other pathologies related to serum lipids have been observed. Levels of total serum cholesterol less than 160 mg/dL seem to be associated with ICH and SAH, whereas higher levels of serum cholesterol are associated with atherothrombosis. No relationship has been demonstrated between cholesterol and lacunar strokes.[169] This unusual relationship of low serum lipids and higher hemorrhagic infarct has been demonstrated in Japan and also recently in the United States in the group of patients studied in the Multiple Risk Factor Intervention Trial.[78,124] Because of the ambiguity of these data, a clear statement of guidelines for the management of cholesterol to reduce incidence is difficult to make.

Diabetes

The rate of atherosclerosis development in coronary, femoral, and cerebral vessels is increased in diabetics. Stroke is increased 2.5 to 4 times in diabetics compared with nondiabetics.[86] In the Framingham Study, glucose intolerance (a blood sugar greater than 150 mg/mL) is only a significant, independent contributor to stroke in older women and is greater for women than men at any age.[80] Because of the associated risk of stroke, careful management of diabetes in addition to all other risk factors is prudent.

Oral Contraceptives

In female patients over the age of 35 who have other stroke risk factors, oral contraceptive use is associated with increased incidence of stroke.[142] The relative risk for oral contraceptive users is approximately five times greater if they are already in the high-risk group. With the use of lower estrogen formulation oral contraceptives, the risk has decreased substantially in recent years.[143] That the incidence of fatal SAH increased in oral contraceptive-using women with concomitant smoking is noteworthy; in the group over age 35 the incidence is four times higher.[52] Therefore, the recommendation is that women over the age of 35 avoid using oral contraceptives, and younger women who smoke should be advised of the increased risks associated with concurrent oral contraceptive use.

Alcohol

Heavy alcohol consumption is related to an increase in stroke and stroke deaths, whereas light to moderate alcohol consumption is associated with a reduced incidence of CHD.[38,85] Alcohol is clearly related to hemorrhagic stroke events, but the association with thromboembolic events is not definite. Regardless, patients at risk for stroke should avoid heavy alcohol consumption.

Physical Activity

Despite the clear benefits of physical activity in the reduction of CHD morbidity and mortality, no clear association exists between physical activity and the incidence of stroke.[114,115]

Public Education

The primary goal of primary and secondary prevention programs should be to educate individuals about risk factors and then to teach them the way to modify their risks. During routine visits, a physician should be able to identify at-risk patients through a combination of a history and physical. Routine blood pressure screening should be included in all evaluations, and patients who have hypertension should be treated. A stroke risk profile has been assembled from the Framingham Study data and can be used by physicians[170] (e.g., to help a physician decide which borderline hypertensive patients to treat). Education can start in the physician's office and be continued by all the other health professionals with whom the patient comes into contact. If the community at large is educated about the risk factors of stroke, those individuals who are at highest risk can seek out the attention they require. This model has been implemented and supported through research such as the Agency for Health Care Policy and Research Smoking Cessation Clinical Practice Guidelines.[116]

PART TWO: Introduction to Acute Stroke Rehabilitation

Catherine A. Duffy
Heather Edgar Beland

The neuro-ICU may be the starting point of occupational therapy (OT) evaluation and treatment. Many patients are evaluated, by an occupational therapist, within 48 hours of a stroke. The ICU environment is often fast paced with the focus on monitoring the individual patient's medical status. The primary goals of any neuro-ICU are to stabilize the patient medically, progress the patient neurologically, and support the patient and family through this neurological crisis.[137] Medical testing and procedures take precedence over any OT treatment. Scheduling OT services may be difficult, treatments may be interrupted, and flexibility is necessary.

THE IMPORTANCE OF EARLY INTERVENTION

There are many common complications associated with a prolonged ICU stay, which include but are not limited to deconditioning, muscle weakness, contractures, skin impairments, depression, anxiety, and reduced quality of life.[60] Early OT, engaging in ADL and mobilization, can increase a patient's level of consciousness, enhance overall mental well-being, and foster functional independence.[129,146] Occupational therapists provide a variety of treatments in the ICU, including, but not limited to, evaluations, splinting, positioning, cognitive retraining, self-care, and functional mobility training.

TEAM APPROACH

There are many members of the neuro-ICU/acute care team, and the team may vary among settings. They include a primary team of physicians led by an attending neurologist specializing in critical care. Depending on each case, there may be neurosurgeons also involved in patient care. At teaching hospitals, a team of residents may also make medical decisions regarding the patients. Along with the occupational therapist, the ancillary team consists of nursing, including the primary nurse and nurse practitioner, social workers, nutritionist, speech and language pathologist, and physical therapist (Table 1-9). An occupational therapist treating patients in this environment must foster these relationships to safely treat patients.

The relationship between the primary physician, nurse, and the occupational therapist is particular important. Daily communication with the physicians, residents, and primary nurse is necessary prior to initiating an evaluation or treatment session due to the fluctuating physical condition in the ICU phase of hospitalization.[4,137] Physicians, nursing, or the occupational therapist, using their own clinical judgment will determine if intervention should be delayed should a patient's neurological status deteriorate. Once the patient has been medically cleared for OT evaluation, a review of the patient's medical chart should be completed. The therapist can glean information relating to any precautions and complications that may interfere with the OT treatment (Box 1-4).

MONITORING THE ICU/ACUTE STROKE SURVIVOR

Any therapist treating in the ICU should not only be aware of the medical and nursing priorities in the ICU, but also of how to monitor the patient during OT treatment. The therapist needs to be competent in reading ICU monitors and handling ICU related drains and lines, so that appropriate parameters and precautions are adhered to during the treatment session. Common monitors, drains, lines, and clinical implications are listed later.

Table 1-9

Members of the ICU/Acute Team

MEMBER	ROLE
Attending physician	Leads the medical team is medical decision-making. May lead team rounds. Usually interacts with patient at least once a day.
Resident	At a teaching hospital, residents are responsible for the day to day, hour to hour care of patients. May be on the unit at all times to answer clinical questions regarding patients.
Nursing	Multiple responsibilities include but are not limited to: administering medications, ADL assist, education, positioning, and monitoring neurological status.
Nurse practitioner	In some facilities, nursing practitioners take the place of residents, writing orders and providing medical decision-making when needed.
Nutritionist	Usually the nutritionist evaluates the patient on a PRN (as needed) basis. Most patients in the ICU receive a nutrition consult when they are placed on tube feedings. The nutritionist, along with the physicians, will determine which type of tube feeding a patient should receive, along with the speed at which the feedings should be administered.
Social worker	In the ICU, the social workers are also usually a PRN service providing support to family members and beginning the discussion of discharge planning.
Speech and language pathologist	Speech and language pathologists can provide a twofold service in the ICU setting. They may provide therapy services in the form of language and communication evaluation and treatment. They may also provide bed side swallowing evaluations, along with the occupational therapist. See Chapters 20 and 24.
Physical therapist	The physical therapist provides bed side physical therapy services in the form of therapeutic exercise, mobility, and gait training if appropriate. Along with the occupational therapist, he or she also contributes to discharge planning. See Chapter 15.

Box 1-4

Initiating Treatment

1. Check to make sure occupational therapy orders are active. This should be done prior to each and every treatment session
2. Review the patient's medical record. The therapist should evaluate the medical record for potential reasons to hold a patient from therapy. Such reasons may be a change in mental status, development of a deep vein thrombosis or pulmonary embolism, or expansion of the stroke. Every facility has different standards for when therapy is to be held.
3. Review the patient's current status with the medical team. Using clinical reasoning the therapist will determine if the patient is appropriate for an OT session. The therapist should clear any treatment with the patient's nurse to determine if all medical information reviewed from the medical record is most current.
4. Begin evaluation and treatment with a gross assessment of mental status, strength, and vital signs. Great discrepancies from what is reported in the medical record should be reported to the nurse and treatment suspended. Proceed with therapy as indicated.

Basic ICU Monitor

Most ICU patients are connected to a monitor that allows constant display of all vital signs (Fig. 1-10). These include blood pressure, telemetry reading (which include heart rate and rhythm), respiratory rate, and oxygen saturation percentages. For normal versus abnormal vital sign responses to exercises, refer to Table 1-10. Blood pressure can be monitored either noninvasively (automated pressure cuff) or by invasive measures, such as an arterial line reading (also referred to as an A-line). A common insertion site for an A-line is either the radial or femoral artery (Fig. 1-11). With radial artery placement, passive ROM of the wrist should be avoided; with femoral artery placement, no hip ROM is allowed, resulting in bed rest.

Telemetry

Telemetry detects both the heart rate and rhythm and displays this reading on the monitor. Bed side telemetry is similar to an electrocardiogram (ECG). An ECG is read by placing 12 electrical leads to read heart rate and rhythm while the bed side telemetry uses either three or five leads. The primary nurse will set both heart rate and rhythm parameters on the monitor. Should the rate and rhythm become abnormal, an alarm will sound. Physical activity should be monitored accordingly.

Common Lines and Drains

Foley Catheter. A Foley catheter is indwelling and is used to drain urine from the bladder. The therapist should

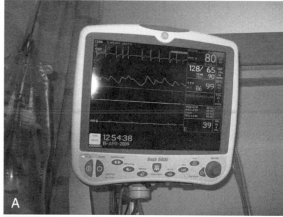

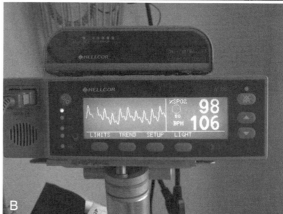

Figure 1-10 **A,** ICU monitoring system, indicating heart rate 80 beats per minute, blood pressure 128/65 (mean arterial pressure 90), oxygen saturation 99, respiratory rate 39. **B,** ICU monitoring system. This system monitors heart rate (106) and oxygen saturation (98%).

avoid clamping the catheter; doing so could result in a backup of urine in the bladder. The bag, which collects the urine, needs to be at a lower level than the patient's bladder for the urine to flow in the correct direction.

External Ventricular Drain. The external ventricular drain (EVD) is a small tube surgically inserted into the ventricles of the brain, which drains cerebral spinal fluid (CSF) (Fig. 1-12). The tube is connected to a device that measures the amount of this fluid. This procedure is used when the intracranial pressure is elevated, and the drain may be clamped for short periods of time by nursing only. Due to specific calibration, function of the drain, and accuracy in measurement the head of the bed must be elevated to a specific level. Unless the drain is clamped, the head of the bed may not be changed, and patients should not be mobilized.

Intracranial Pressure Monitoring Catheter. The intracranial pressure monitoring catheter (ICP) is a catheter passed through a burr hole and placed in the ventricles of the brain.

Table 1-10

Vital Sign Responses

VITAL SIGN	NORMAL RESPONSE TREATMENT	ABNORMAL RESPONSE TO TREATMENT	EXCEPTIONS TO THE RULES
Heart rate			
Normal heart rate 60 to 100 beats per minute. Many patients may have a resting heart rate outside the normal value. Determine the patient's maximum heart rate (220−age)[146] prior to treatment to assess whether or not it is safe to proceed.	Slow and gradual increase in heart rate with activity up to 20 beats higher per minute.	Increase in heart rate greater than 20 beats per minute. A decrease in heart rate or a change in heart rhythm.	At times patients may not be able to tolerate an increase in heart rate that deviates from their baseline. At other times, with young, otherwise healthy, patients, the team may allow the therapist to work patients beyond an increase of 20 beats per minute. Some medications may cause a blunted heart rate response.
Blood pressure			
Normal blood pressure: systolic less than 120 mm Hg, diastolic less than 80 mm Hg. Again many patients may have a resting blood pressure above or below what is considered normal. Check the patient's chart to determine what the patient's blood pressure ratings have been over the past few vital sign cycles. Determine from there if it is safe to proceed.	Slow, gradual, and slight increase in systolic blood pressure with activity. No change or slight decrease in diastolic pressure.	Increase or decrease in systolic blood pressure greater than 20 points and a decrease of diastolic pressure greater than 10 points.[137]	Many times in the ICU, a patient's blood pressure is maintained high (i.e., 200/100) to profuse the brain. It is important to check with the team prior to holding therapy. However, as a general rule, if a patient's systolic blood pressure is greater than 200 and diastolic pressure is greater than 100, check with the team prior to treatment.
Oxygen saturation			
Normal range: 92% to 100% on room air or on supplemental O_2.	Slight drop or increase in O_2 saturation.	Drop in O_2 saturation below 92% (unless that is baseline).	In some cases, the team will allow the therapist to titrate the patient's O_2 needs to the activity by increasing O_2 via nasal cannula. It is important to remember that O_2 is considered a medication, and a written order from the MD is needed to change patient's O_2 consumption.

O_2, oxygen.

It is used with injuries such as hemorrhages, aneurysms, or head trauma that may lead to brain swelling and elevation of the intracranial pressure. This monitor measures any changes in intracranial pressure. The head of the bed is elevated to a set point (usually 30 to 45 degrees), as the intracranial pressure will increase when the head of the bed is lowered. Passive therapy, such as splinting or positioning, may be implemented with physician approval. Generally, ADL treatment and mobilization is held at this time.

Spinal Drain. A spinal drain is a catheter placed in the lumbar spine to drain CSF. It can be used for the treatment of CSF leak or to drain excess CSF fluid. The lumbar drain should be set to drain below the level of the leak. When the drain is open and is draining CSF, the spinal drain is set at a determined level next to the bed. At this time, when the drain is opened, patients are placed flat on their back to allow for drainage. Patients with this drain may get up and out of bed and may engage in ADL

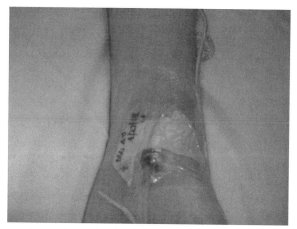

Figure 1-11 Arterial (A) line in the radial artery. (Photo courtesy of Millie Hepburn Smith.)

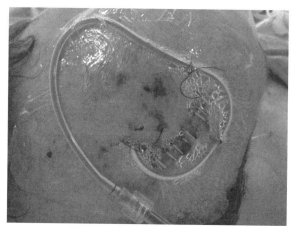

Figure 1-12 Exit site for an external ventricular drain on top of skull. (Photo courtesy of Millie Hepburn Smith.)

treatment only when the drain has been clamped by the nurse. While the drain is open to drain CSF, the patient must remain on bed rest.

Intravenous Line. IV lines are inserted into the peripheral veins and are generally used to administer IV fluids and medications. Because these lines are superficial, care should be taken not to place pressure from the positioning materials or splints directly over the area in order to avoid obstructed or dislodgment.

Feeding Tubes
In the event that a stroke patient is unable to swallow effectively or appears to be a high aspiration risk, alternate methods are used for nutrition intake.

Nasogastric Tube. A nasogastric tube (NGT) is placed through the nostril down the esophagus to the stomach for liquid feeds to pass. It is generally used as a short-term alternative for nutritional intake.

Percutaneous Endoscopic Gastrostomy. A percutaneous endoscopic gastrostomy is a tube inserted surgically with an endoscope through the mouth and into the stomach, exiting out through the stomach wall and dermis (Fig. 1-13).

Precautions for both feeding tubes include elevating the head of bed to 30 degrees or greater while administering the tubes to prevent aspiration. Depending upon the hospital guidelines, the therapist may be allowed to turn off the feeding prior to the therapy session, but it is recommended that the primary care nurse be consulted prior to doing so, for patient safety (see Chapter 24).

Ventilator
At times stroke can result in respiratory failure. When this is the case, patients often require a ventilator to assist them with or to perform the act of breathing for them (Figs. 1-14 and 1-15). When a ventilator is used, the patient also requires an artificial airway. In the first few days after acute stroke, a ventilator can be connected to the patient via an endotracheal tube. A breathing tube is then placed into the patient's mouth and positioned down into the patient's lung systems. If a patient is unable to be weaned from the ventilator, a tracheotomy will be performed. In this procedure, an opening is cut in the patient's trachea and a small endotracheal tube is placed in the opening, which is then attached to the vent via long tubing. Early mobilization of patients on ventilators is encouraged.[112] A recent randomized controlled trial[138] emphasized that early OT/physical therapy (PT) for those ventilated and critically ill is both beneficial and safe, resulting in better functional outcomes, decreased delirium, and more ventilator-free days.

Once the therapist is confident to handle the lines, leads, and monitors in the ICU, the patient's tolerance of the OT intervention should be monitored carefully. Vital signs should be observed during the entire treatment session and should be documented at the beginning, at mid-portion, and at end of treatment. In addition to vital signs, the therapist must also watch for changes in the patient's neurological status during treatment, which may include changes in

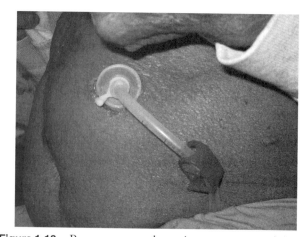

Figure 1-13 Percutaneous endoscopic gastrostomy in abdomen. (Photo courtesy of Millie Hepburn Smith.)

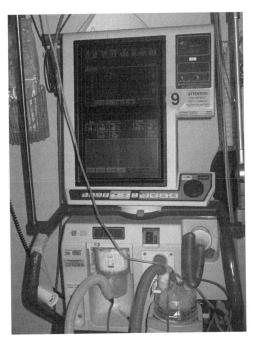

Figure 1-14 This is a commonly used ventilator in the ICU setting. The occupational therapist needs to be aware of the vent setting and alarms while working with the patient.

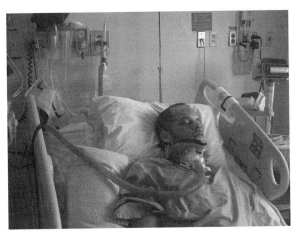

Figure 1-15 The patient is properly positioned on a trach collar and is currently being weaned from the ventilator.

decorticate or decerebrate posturing, tone, pupils, and/or in speech.[137] Patient subjective complaints must be considered. If any changes in the patient's status occur, terminate treatment and inform the medical team immediately.

ASSESSMENTS USED IN ACUTE STROKE REHABILITATION

There are a variety of standardized assessments available[82] to the occupational therapist in the hospital setting. In the acute/ICU setting, it is imperative for the occupational therapist to evaluate motor skills, cognitive function, and ADL. At times it may not be feasible for a patient to

engage in ADL tasks secondary to medical status or sedation. Table 1-11 outlines some of the standardized assessments used during acute rehabilitation.

INTERVENTIONS FOR ACUTE STROKE REHABILITATION

The following sections will describe potential interventions for those in the ICU/acute stage of stroke rehabilitation.

Splinting

The primary goals at this early phase of splinting are to:
1. Correct any biomechanical malalignment and protect joint integrity.
2. Prevent shortening of soft tissues and development of contractures.
3. Maintain skin integrity.

Develop an appropriate wearing schedule to prevent learned nonuse behavior patterns. Splint-wearing at night may be more appropriate than day use, particularly if the patient has begun to initiate movement or attempts to incorporate the hand or upper extremity in functional activities. A wearing schedule should be practical to achieve compliance (Box 1-5; See Chapter 13).

Positioning

Because of the medical complexity of the ICU/acute stroke survivor, many of these patients spend most, if not all, of their time confined to bed. Therefore, positioning has because an integral part of OT treatment plan. The occupational therapist will work to develop a positioning schedule for each individual positioning. The occupational therapist must rely on other members of the interdisciplinary team, including nursing and physical therapists, and the patient's family members, if able, to carry out this portion of the treatment plan (Figs. 1-16 and 1-17).

Different members of the interdisciplinary team have different priorities when it relates to positioning. A primary goal of the team in regards to positioning is to prevent skin breakdown. The occupational therapist is encouraged to teach the team how to position the patient not only to prevent skin breakdown but also to reduce the risk of contractures and encourage joint alignment, and comfort. The occupational therapist should develop a turning schedule for each patient. Patients should alternately be positioned on the affected side, the nonaffected side, and supine. A clock drawn with specific positions can be used as a reminder for the nursing team. See Chapter 10.

When the patient is being positioned, the patient's lines and leads should be carefully observed for they provide vital medications and monitoring of each patient. Careful adjustments need to be made for head of the bed restrictions from feeding tubes or ICP/EVD. When a patient is being positioned with femoral arterial lines, care should be taken to avoid hip flexion, and the wrists of patients with radial A-lines should be maintained in a

Table 1-11

Standardized Assessments Used during Acute Rehabilitation

	ASSESSMENT	DESCRIPTION	SCALES/SCORES	LIMITATIONS
NIH Stroke Scale[22]	Standardized Prognostic Scale Total time to administer: 10 minutes	The NIHSS is a 15-item neurological examination for stroke patients used in many hospitals by physicians, nurses, and therapists. It evaluates levels of consciousness, language, neglect, visual fields, eye movement, motor strength, ataxia, dysarthria, and sensation.[22]	0 = No stroke 1–4 = Minor stroke 5–15 = Moderate stroke 15–20 = Moderate to severe stroke 21–42 = Severe stroke	No evaluation of functional tasks.
MINI FIM[61]	Standardized functional outcome measure. Total time to administer: greater than 30 minutes	Evaluation of functional tasks such as self-care, transfers, mobility, and cognition	Patient receives a score between 0–7 for each functional task. A score of 7 indicates independence while a score of 1 indicates total assist, and a score of 0 indicates the task has not taken place. The Mini FIM includes 7 items from the full 18 item FIM instrument.	Secondary to the medical complexity of ICU patients, many of the ADL or mobility sections may not be able to be completed.
Glasgow Coma Scale[154]	Standardized prognostic scale. Total time to administer: 10 minutes	This scale is used in numerous hospitals by both doctors and therapists. It evaluates best eye opening response, best verbal response, and best motor response.[21]	Each category is given a numeric response with 1 being no response. The responses are added together to create a final score. A score of less than 3 indicates vegetative state, 3–8 severe disability, 9–12 moderate disability, and 13–15 indicates mild injury.[154]	No evaluation of functional tasks.
Orpington Prognostic Scale[88]	Standardized prognostic scale. Total time to administer: 5 to 10 minutes	An evaluation of upper extremity motor function, proprioception, balance, and cognition	The numerical scores of each section are added together for the final score. Lower scores indicate less impairment.	No evaluation of functional tasks. The cognitive evaluation is given verbally and therefore requires language and speech, eliminating patients with aphasia.
Barthel Index[100]	Standardized outcome measure. Total time to administer: greater than 30 minutes	Evaluation of functional tasks such as eating, grooming, bathing, bowel and bladder management, toilet use, dressing, mobility, transfers, and stairs.	Patient receives a score between 0–100, 0 indicating total dependence and 100 total independence with the evaluated activities.	Secondary to the medical complexity of ICU patients, many of the ADL or mobility sections may not be able to be completed (such as eating, toileting, and/or stairs).
JKF Coma Recovery Scale[56,57]	Standardized measure. Total time to administer: 15 minutes.	The scale consists of 23 items within six subscales, evaluating auditory, visual, motor, oral motor, communication, and arousal.	The lowest item on each scale represents reflexive activity, while the highest items represent higher level cognitive behaviors.	No evaluation of functional tasks

Box 1-5

Common Splints Used in Acute Stroke Rehabilitation

Resting hand splint	May be fabricated for the individual but also are available prefabricated.
Cone splint	May prevent long finger flexor tightness when used in conjunction with a wrist extension device and also maintain skin integrity (preventing skin maceration).
Adjustable inflatable hand splint	Contains an air bladder in the palmar surface, which can be adjusted to achieve the level of stretch placed on the long finger flexors. It may be an appropriate choice for the patient who has had more than one stroke and demonstrates increased muscle tone. This type of splint is prefabricated.
Blanket/towel roll	An alternative to a thermoplastic elbow extension or drop arm splint. It is rolled around the patient's arm to help prevent elbow flexion contractures. See Chapter 13 and Fig. 1–16.

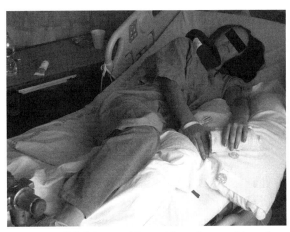

Figure 1-17 Side lying position, with patient positioned on the affected side. Pillow placed under affected upper extremity to maintain proper alignment of the head of the humerus.

neutral position. Foley and rectal tubes should be moved to the same side to which the patient is positioned.

While in the ICU, many patients require a ventilator to provide respiratory assistance. These patients can also be positioned side to side and supine. Care should be taken when moving ventilation tubes. There are many extra articular handles that allow for addition mobility of the patient on a ventilator. If these articular handles do not provide enough length to position a patient in the proper alignment, discuss with the respiratory therapist regarding switching the ventilator from side to side every other day or so.

Functional Activity Suggestions during the Acute Phase

Bed Mobility

Rolling to the Affected Side. Rolling to the affected side promotes early active trunk control and may increase awareness of the weaker side.

Rolling to the Unaffected Side. Rolling to the unaffected side promotes awareness and initial management of the weak upper extremity by teaching the patient to passively guide the arm across the trunk (Fig. 1-18).

Maintaining Side Lying. A rolled pillow placed at the midthoracic spine to the lumbar area may assist the patient in maintaining the side-lying position. A towel roll can be placed under the patient's waist to provide a stretch to the shortened trunk. A primary goal is to assure proper spine alignment, to avoid pressure build up over the bony prominences in the lower extremities (knees and ankles), and to position the scapula in protraction if the patient is positioned on the weakened side.

Bridging. Bridging strengthens the back and hip extensors. From a functional perspective, this movement

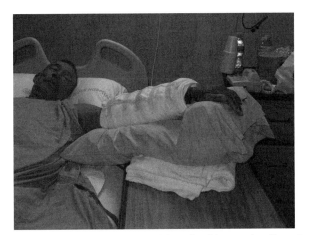

Figure 1-16 Patient's arm positioned with towel roll to increase elbow extension.

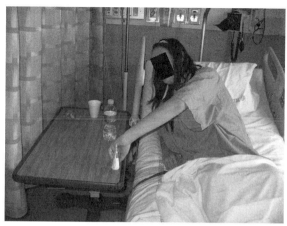

Figure 1-18   Bed level activities. Rolling to the unaffected side and engaging the affected arm in early reaching task and at the same time engaging affected trunk and lower extremity muscles.

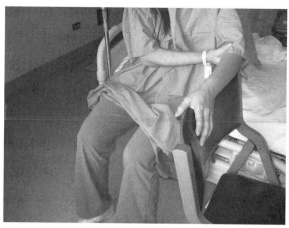

Figure 1-19   While the patient sits on the edge of the bed, a bed side chair is used to facilitate upper extremity weight-bearing activities.

aids in getting on and off the bed pan, can be used during lower body dressing, and also assists moving the lower body toward the side of the bed in anticipation of assuming a sitting position.

Side Lying to Sitting toward the Affected Side. Side lying to sitting toward the affected side promotes early stage weight-bearing on the weak upper extremity. The therapist needs to ensure that the shoulder is properly aligned, and the patient will usually require assistance with initiation of the movement.

Side Lying to Sitting toward the Unaffected Side. Therapists need to be mindful that the involved shoulder remains in a forward position during the motion of side lying to sitting toward the unaffected side.

Weight-Bearing for Function

Upper extremity weight-bearing activities may be done while the patient is side lying as mentioned previously, during bed mobility, or for stabilizing items. It can also be accomplished using the bed side table during meals or grooming tasks. The arm or back rest of a chair can be incorporated in the treatment plan for positioning and setup for weight-bearing (Figs. 1-19 and 1-20). The patient should be taught to push off with both upper extremities when moving from sit to stand. Weight-bearing as a postural support can reverse or prevent tissue shortening of the elbow, wrist, and finger flexors. It can also be used to strengthen the scapula musculature and the triceps. Arm extended weight-bearing can be done in front of the sink during grooming or be done in front of the bed side table while reaching for items nearby (Fig. 1-21).

For the lower extremity, bed level activities include: bridging, sitting at the edge of the bed with both feet on the floor, and early transfer training once patients are medically stable.

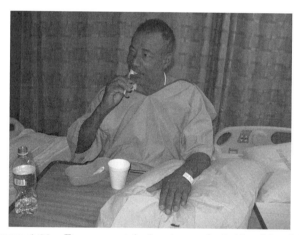

Figure 1-20   Forearm weight-bearing on bed side table while patient dangles off edge of bed.

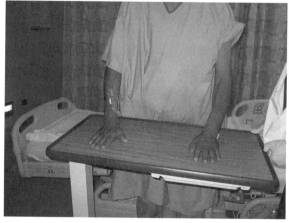

Figure 1-21   Supported standing with bed side table to facilitate upper extremity involvement in activity. Early upright ADL training can be initiated, and weight shifting through the lower extremities is encouraged.

Graded Sitting and Standing Activities

Supported Sitting in Bed. For the supported sitting in bed position, the head of the bed should gradually be raised in approximately 30- to 40-degree increments to avoid an orthostatic hypotensive response. As the patient tolerates the change in degrees of elevation, the therapist should continue to monitor vital signs. If there appears to be no change in the patient's blood pressure, the therapist should continue to elevate the head of the bed to approximately 80 degrees. Sitting at a slightly reclined position is less taxing on the patient's energy and requires less recruitment of the neck, trunk, and back musculature to maintain an upright position. At this point, the patient should be engaged in functional activities, such as feeding, light grooming, upper body bathing and dressing, and leisure activities.

Supported Sitting in a Chair. If the patient is well-supported and can endure sitting in a chair at the bed side, "sitting tolerance" or "out of bed tolerance" can be increased. Pillows may be useful at this early stage to support the lumbar spine and weaker upper extremity. When a therapist is placing a pillow under the upper extremity, he or she should make sure the shoulder alignment is in neutral. Adequate postural support may reduce pain and fatigue. Focus of treatment can include but is not limited to the patient performing self-care tasks, visual scanning activities, and weight-bearing through the upper and lower extremity.

Unsupported Sitting. Unsupported sitting may be done in the bed in a "tailor" (crossed legged) position, depending on the amount of ROM the patient has in the lower extremities. The head of the bed can be elevated, but should not touch the back of the patient. It is used as a safety catch should the patient lose his or her balance in a posterior direction. Pillows may be propped against the bed rails to protect the patient if he or she leans or falls laterally to the weaker side. While seated in this position, the patient can practice righting himself or herself or maintaining a midline position, and the patient should then be engaged in functional activities as tolerated.

Unsupported Sitting at the Edge of the Bed with Feet Dangling. In this position, the patient can be challenged with increased demands on alignment, trunk control, and forward and lateral weight shifts. Scooting to the edge of the bed can be introduced in anticipation of progressing to sit to stand. Postural control may be noticeably improved once the patient's feet contact the floor. The therapist should ensure equal weight-bearing on both lower extremities. See Chapter 7.

Sit to Stand: Pretransfer Phase. To prepare for the sit-to-stand pretransfer phase, therapists should ensure that all lines and IVs have enough length to eliminate pulling or tension. Increasing the surface height the patient rises from will require less work. This transition may require the assistance of more than one person to gain the patient's confidence and safety. The therapist should assure appropriate alignment of both lower extremities with feet placed firmly on the floor and then have the patient begin with several partial sit-to-stand trials. Assess how the weaker lower extremity reacts to weight-bearing, provide appropriate blocking or support to prevent collapse, and check vital signs while the patient is upright.

Supported Standing in Front of a Raised Bed. To initiate supported standing in front of a raised bed, the therapist should position the patient in a chair that faces the side of the bed. With appropriate assistance, the therapist should stand the patient and sit in a chair on the patient's weakened side to support the hip and knee extensors. In this standing position, the patient may practice early weight shifting through the lower extremities and bear weight on the upper extremities in either forearm or arm extended positions (see Fig. 1-21).

EDEMA MANAGEMENT

Evaluate the potential cause if edema is present. Discuss with nursing whether the swelling may be associated with the presence of a blood clot or an IV infiltrate. Check to see if the patient's limb is cool or warm to the touch, observe the skin color, and assess the firmness of the swelling (soft, fluidlike, or pitting).

In the ICU, the preferred method for treating edema is positional elevation, as compression garments or ace wraps may not be appropriate due to various IVs and line access needed by nursing. The extended limb should be positioned above the heart. Active or active assistive ROM should be encouraged and followed by manual massage (Fig. 1-22). See Chapter 12.

SHOULDER MANAGEMENT

Many patients may experience upper extremity edema, pain, humeral head subluxation, and/or impingement after a stroke. Many of the upper extremity interventions provided in the ICU/acute stage are prophylactic measures to prevent these problems.

To protect the shoulder against potential pain and subluxation, the team should be educated in proper rolling techniques and bed mobility, so they can avoid pulling on the extremity. The team should be instructed to roll the patient by placing the hands on the trunk rather than pulling on the extremity. Signage can be hung behind the patient's bed indicating the patient may have shoulder subluxation and informing the team to not pull on the patient's arm (Box 1-6).

Due to the medical complexity of the ICU/acute patient, most are not getting out of bed to the chair for prolonged periods or engaging in prolonged upright activities. While supine, out of bed in a chair, or dangling at

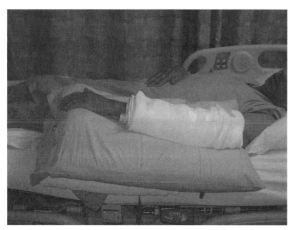

Figure 1-22 Patient's affected upper extremity positioned in towel roll and elevated on pillow to prevent and decrease edema.

Box 1-6

Patient with Right Shoulder Subluxation

Please do not pull on patient's arm. Please contact occupational therapy at 555–8724 with questions or concerns.

---

the bed side, support for a weak shoulder can be provided via proper positioning.

Supine

Provide support to the affected upper extremity with pillows and/or towels. The occupational therapist must use clinical judgment to determine proper positioning for each patient. However, as a general rule, the affected scapula should be protracted, the arm in a forward position, with the wrist neutral and fingers extended.[26]

Edge of Bed

The affected upper extremity is supported on the bed side table or on numerous pillows.

Out of Bed in a Chair

The affected upper extremity is supported on the bed side table, on numerous pillows, or on the arm support of the chair.

Most ICU/acute patients do not require supplemental shoulder supports such as sling, clavicle strap, and/or taping. These supports may be used once patients are performing ADL upright and are spending more time out of bed. See Chapter 10.

In addition to positioning, the occupational therapist will provide the ICU patient with passive and active ROM and will engage the affected upper extremity in functional tasks. The therapist should mind lines and leads while providing these services. When an A-line is present in the radial artery, wrist flexion/extension should be avoided.

INCREASING SPATIAL AWARENESS BY ARRANGING THE ENVIRONMENT

Although the ICU environment may be more restrictive than a rehabilitation setting, there are subtle yet important interventions that can be implemented to increase spatial awareness. Strategically place items of common use, such as the television remote control, on the involved side while providing cues to assist the patient in locating them. Strategically place food items on the meal tray during feeding to encourage scanning and locating desired items to eat. Verbal cues should be diminished as the patient's awareness increases. Reverse the position of the bed, if able, so that the patient's involved space is stimulated (e.g., facing the hallway instead of facing a blank wall). Position the bed side table and phone on the neglected or weaker side of the patient. Use brightly colored bands tied to the bed side rails on the involved side as cues to attend to this side. Hang pictures of family and friends on the involved side while providing cues for the patient to locate them.

EARLY COGNITIVE MANAGEMENT

Patients may spend numerous days to weeks in the ICU. A well-known phenomenon called ICU psychosis can develop within days of being admitted to the ICU.[55,99] ICU psychosis has been defined as a fluctuating state of consciousness characterized by fatigue, distraction, confusion, disorientation, restlessness, clouding of consciousness, incoherence, fear, anxiety, excitement, hallucinations, and delusions.[41] Many factors related to the ICU environment can contribute to the development of ICU psychosis. Some include psychosocial stress, sleep deprivation, sensory overload or underload, and immobilization.[41] Many patients are unable to differentiate between day and night secondary to lighting in most ICU.[41]

The occupational therapist can assist the primary nursing team in a variety of ways to help lessen the effects of ICU psychosis. Some measures that nursing may implement are providing tactile and verbal stimulation, involvement of the patient in his or her care, and supplying effective rest periods.[99] The occupational therapist can minimize environmental monotony and mobilize and engage the patient in familiar self-care tasks. When providing a patient with OT services, communication with patient via gentle touch and voices can help calm patients. Incorporating music and massage into OT treatments can also help reduce anxiety, fear, and depression.[99] See Box 1-7 for treatment ideas.

SKIN PROTECTION AND PREVENTION OF BREAKDOWN

Skin breakdown and development of pressure ulcers are common complications associated with an ICU/acute admission. After stroke, patients are at risk for developing

Box 1-7

Treatment Ideas to Manage ICU Psychosis

- Mobilize and engage in self-care.
- Engage patient in time appropriate tasks (if it is 8 AM complete oral care with window shades open and lights on).
- Use a calm gentle voice and touch when engaging patients.
- Decrease or increase sensory stimulation during OT treatment session depending on patient's needs.
- Educate patient's family in orientating patient not only to date and place but also to time of day.
- Keep clocks and calendars in view.

pressure ulcers due to prolonged bed rest and immobility. Other risk factors include poor circulation, poor nutrition, edema, low level of arousal, confusion, and incontinence.[8] Pressure management and skin protection should become a part of each treatment session. See Table 1-12 for a review of the stages of pressure ulcers.

Prevention of skin breakdown is a team responsibility. The occupational therapist has a unique set of skills to assist the team in protecting the patient's skin. The occupational therapist is often the first team member to mobilize patient and can observe the entire body for signs of skin breakdown. Areas of concern for the ICU patient include sacrum, occiput, heels, greater trochanter, and elbows. Therapist can suggest elbow and heel pads to protect these areas from pressure and friction. Heels can also be floated via positioning or multipodis boots (Fig. 1-23). The therapist can develop positioning devices to assist the nurse with elevating pressure on the occiput (Fig. 1-24) and the sacrum. The occupational therapist can also recommend specialized mattresses to best serve the patient's needs.

COMMUNICATION

For the patient unable to communicate verbally, whether due to mechanical ventilation or aphasia, alternative methods of communication will be necessary. Options may include use of a communication board. Single word choice or pictures that represent feelings or needs can be placed strategically on a small poster board. Examples may include Nurse, Doctor, Pain, Thirst, etc., to which the patient can then point. Alphabet boards are generally not used, as they require energy and time for the patient to "spell" words. For the aphasic patient, words might be eliminated altogether. Other alternatives may include signals for Yes/No questions, such as head nodding or thumbs up or down, and an eye blink system. Working in conjunction with the speech-language pathologist, the occupational therapist may assist with facilitating a communication system that is consistently used by other staff and family members (Box 1-8; see Chapter 20).

DYSPHAGIA SCREENING

Acute swallowing difficulties or dysphagia are often associated with stroke.[159] The risk of aspiration is high and often leads to pneumonia. Other medical complications associated with dysphagia include malnutrition and dehydration.

During the initial admission to the hospital, patients may be placed on "NPO" (nothing by mouth) precautions. Under these circumstances an NGT is usually inserted through the nose and down the esophagus to the stomach. If the patient is conscious, the occupational therapist may initiate a swallowing or dysphagia screening at the bed side.

Before beginning the assessment, the therapist should be aware of the patient's level of alertness, fatigue, and ability to follow commands, as these factors may significantly influence the ability to participate safely. An oral motor examination should precede administration of foods and liquids. The assessment should begin with the patient seated with the head of the bed elevated. If an oral suction device is available at the bed side, it should be turned on (Box 1-9; Fig. 1-25).

Based on the results of the bed side assessment, instrumental testing may be necessary to further evaluate the phases of swallowing that cannot be seen at a bed side oral motor examination. If the patient appears to have adequate oral and swallowing function and a physician's order has been obtained, a feeding trial may be initiated using graded food textures and liquids of various thickness (Box 1-10; see Chapter 24).

SELF-CARE TRAINING

Training in ADL is an integral part of OT treatment. It is important to engage the patient in self-care tasks as soon as they are medically stable.

Energy expenditure is often an issue for the low level patient, so grading the self-care task is as important as the choice of activity. The acute patient may also be limited by IVs, lines, and artificial ventilation. If the patient is having difficulty managing secretions, begin by teaching them how to use an oral suctioning device. Using an adapted call light to request assistance from nursing is also an appropriate goal.

For those with limited motor return, the upper extremity should at least be used as a stabilizer. ADL compensatory strategies can be initiated. If the patient demonstrates active movement, the upper extremity should be incorporated into the self-care task (see Chapter 28).

Table 1-12

Pressure Ulcer Stages

STAGE	DESCRIPTION	ADDITIONAL INFORMATION
Stage I	Intact skin with nonblanchable redness of a localized area usually over a bony prominence. Darkly pigmented skin may not have visible blanching; its color may differ from the surrounding area.	The area may be painful, firm, soft, warmer, or cooler as compared to adjacent tissue. Stage I may be difficult to detect in individuals with dark skin tones. May indicate "at risk" persons (a heralding sign of risk).
Stage II	Partial thickness loss of dermis presenting as a shallow open ulcer with a red pink wound bed, without slough. May also present as an intact or open/ruptured serum-filled blister.	Presents as a shiny or dry shallow ulcer without slough or bruising. This stage should not be used to describe skin tears, tape burns, perineal dermatitis, maceration, or excoriation. Bruising indicates suspected deep tissue injury.
Stage III	Full thickness tissue loss. Subcutaneous fat may be visible, but bone, tendon, or muscle are not exposed. Slough may be present but does not obscure the depth of tissue loss. May include undermining and tunneling.	The depth of a stage III pressure ulcer varies by anatomical location. The bridge of the nose, ear, occiput, and malleolus do not have subcutaneous tissue, and stage III ulcers can be shallow. In contrast, areas of significant adiposity can develop extremely deep stage III pressure ulcers. Bone/tendon is not visible or directly palpable.
Stage IV	Full thickness tissue loss with exposed bone, tendon, or muscle. Slough or eschar may be present on some parts of the wound bed. Often include undermining and tunneling.	The depth of a stage IV pressure ulcer varies by anatomical location. The bridge of the nose, ear, occiput, and malleolus do not have subcutaneous tissue, and these ulcers can be shallow. Stage IV ulcers can extend into muscle and/or supporting structures (e.g., fascia, tendon, or joint capsule), making osteomyelitis possible. Exposed bone/tendon is visible or directly palpable.
Unstageable	Full thickness tissue loss in which the base of the ulcer is covered by slough (yellow, tan, gray, green, or brown) and/or eschar (tan, brown, or black) in the wound bed.	Until enough slough and/or eschar is removed to expose the base of the wound, the true depth, and therefore stage, cannot be determined. Stable (dry, adherent, intact without erythema or fluctuance) eschar on the heels serves as "the body's natural (biological) cover" and should not be removed.

Courtesy of National Pressure Ulcer Advisory Panel

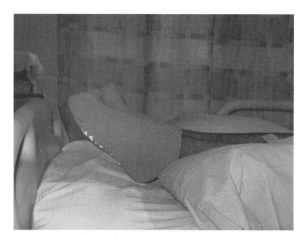

Figure 1-23 This technique is termed "floating the patient heels." It is used while supine in bed to maintain skin integrity and to prevent breakdown.

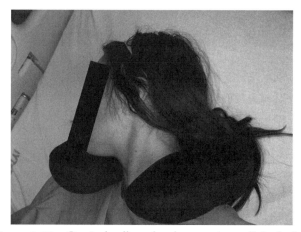

Figure 1-24 Cervical roll used to keep occiput off the bed to decrease pressure that may cause breakdown. The roll allows for head/neck rotation in both directions.

Box 1-8

Communication Keypoints

- Use a normal tone and volume of voice. Avoid shouting at the patient or talking to them in an infantile manner.
- Give the patient enough time to respond to the question.
- Try to stay on the same subject.
- Gesture whenever possible and provide tactile cues as appropriate.
- Speak slowly and directly to the patient's face.
- Simplify questions to Yes/No
- Try to reduce background noise to eliminate distraction. Close the door and turn off the radio or television.
- Only one person should communicate with the patient at one time.
- Be aware of signs of frustration by observing facial expressions.

Box 1-9

Oral Motor Screening

- Observe for the presence of facial asymmetry. Facial drooping or weakness is common in association with the weaker extremities. Foods can pocket in the cheek of the weakened side.
- Observe mouth and lip closure. Can the patient purse his or her lips? Have him or her attempt to blow air into his or her cheeks while keeping his or her lips pursed. Observe if air escapes through one side of the mouth.
- Request the patient to stick out his or her tongue. Does it drift or deviate to one side? Can he or she lick his or her lips and perform lateral movements with the tongue?
- Use a long stick swab to assess the patient's sensation both extra- and intra-orally.
- Use a tongue depressor to assess the patient's gag reflex. Is it present, absent, or delayed?
- Check the soft palate. Use a flashlight to ask the patient to open mouth and say the word "AH." Observe for soft palate elevation.
- Assess the patient's vocal quality. Is it gurgly or wet? Can the patient "clear" his or her voice? Secretions may pool or linger around the vocal cords. Is there hoarseness of the voice? If so, it may be due to inadequate closure of the vocal cords.
- Can the patient demonstrate a volitional cough? Assess the strength of the cough. Is it adequate to clear the airway?
- Is the patient managing his or her own secretions? Does he or she choke or cough on his or her own secretions? Observe whether the swallow is present or delayed.
- A standardized bed side swallowing assessment is recommended (Fig. 1-25).

The initial position may be with the head of the bed elevated. This position provides support of the head and trunk. Vital signs should be monitored throughout the activity. As patients progress, they might be positioned in sitting at the edge of the bed. Demands are greater as patients must maintain their balance while performing the task. Once a patient is able to tolerate sitting at the edge of the bed, the progression should lead to performing tasks seated in a chair. If the patient is able to stand for short periods, then appropriate self-care activities should be performed in standing, such as brushing teeth at the sink or combing hair. Chaining the tasks together will demand more tolerance. Self-care tasks can be graded from simple to complex (Box 1-11).

FAMILY TRAINING

The primary purpose of family training in the ICU/acute setting is to allow for the patient to engage in as many therapeutic activities as possible immediately following the neurological event. Family members should be empowered to assist their loved ones to achieve their therapy goals. Occupational therapists may spend as much time educating the family as they do treating the patients. When training family members, the therapist should demonstrate the tasks and then provide an opportunity for the family member to attempt the tasks. Positive feedback should be provided with corrections given as needed. Families should be provided with written instructions for any tasks they are asked to carry out. During one OT session, no more than three tasks should be given to the family members. This will ensure greater carryover of the tasks provided. The following are suggestions for a family training scheduled in the ICU/acute setting.

Occupational therapists must use their clinical reasoning when providing family training. Many ICU/acute care patients are too medically complex for the family to provide additional therapy services. Such patients may require constant monitoring during physical activity, while other patients may have lines and leads that require a nurse or therapist to handle.

After evaluation patients, family members should be instructed in the following.

- Safely moving noncomplex lines and leads. These may be noninvasive a blood pressure cuff, an O_2 monitor, an IV, and, in certain cases, A-lines.
- Positioning of affected extremities
- Splint wearing schedule, donning and doffing the splint, and performing skin checks
- ROM for elbow, wrist, and hand
- Setting up environment for patient during ADL tasks supine and interacting with patient on affected side (in the case of neglect or sensory loss)

As treatment progresses, the family can be further engaged in the treatment and trained in the following areas:

- Shoulder management: Families must be educated in positioning of the involved upper extremity in bed,

GUSS
(GUGGING SWALLOWING SCREEN)

Name: _____
Date: _____
Time: _____

1. Preliminary Investigation/Indirect Swallowing Test

	YES	NO
Vigilance *(The patient must be alert for at least 15 minutes)*	1 ☐	0 ☐
Cough and/or throat clearing *(voluntary cough)* *(Patient should cough or clear his or her throat twice)*	1 ☐	0 ☐
Saliva Swallow: • Swallowing successful	1 ☐	0 ☐
• Drooling	0 ☐	1 ☐
• Voice change (hoarse, gurgly, coated, weak)	0 ☐	1 ☐
SUM:		(5)
	1–4 = Investigate further[1] 5 = Continue with part 2	

2. Direct Swallowing Test (Material: Aqua bi, flat teaspoon, food thickener, bread)

In the following order:	1→ SEMISOLID*	2→ LIQUID**	3→ SOLID***
DEGLUTITION:			
• Swallowing not possible	0 ☐	0 ☐	0 ☐
• Swallowing delayed (> 2 sec) (Solid textures > 10 sec)	1 ☐	1 ☐	1 ☐
• Swallowing successful	2 ☐	2 ☐	2 ☐
COUGH (involuntary): *(before, during, or after swallowing – until 3 minutes later)*			
• Yes	0 ☐	0 ☐	0 ☐
• No	1 ☐	1 ☐	1 ☐
DROOLING:			
• Yes	0 ☐	0 ☐	0 ☐
• No	1 ☐	1 ☐	1 ☐
VOICE CHANGE: *(listen to the voice before and after swallowing – Patient should speak "O")*			
• Yes	0 ☐	0 ☐	0 ☐
• No	1 ☐	1 ☐	1 ☐
SUM:	(5)	(5)	(5)
	1–4 = Investigate further[1] 5 = Continue liquid	1–4 = Investigate further[1] 5 = Continue solid	1–4 = Investigate further[1] 5 = Normal

SUM: (Indirect Swallowing Test AND Direct Swallowing Test)   _ _ _ _ _ _ (20)

*	First administer ⅓ up to a half teaspoon Aqua bi with food thickener (pudding-like consistency). If there are no symptoms apply 2-5 teaspoons. Assess after the 5th spoonful.
**	3, 5, 10, 20 ml Aqua bi – if there are no symptoms continue with 50 ml Aqua bi (Daniels et al., 2000; Gottlieb et al., 1996) Assess and stop the investigation when one of the criteria is observed.
***	Clinical; dry bread; FEES; dry bread which is dipped in colored liquid
1	Use functional investigations such as Videofluoroscopic Evaluation of Swallowing (VFES), Fiberoptic Endoscopic Evaluation of Swallowing (FEES)

Figure 1-25   The Gugging Swallowing Screen. (From Trapl M, Enderle P, Nowotny M, et al: *Stroke* 38 (11):2948–2952, 2007.)

GUSS
(Gugging Swallowing Screen)
Guss – EVALUATION

	RESULTS	SEVERITY CODE	RECOMMENDATIONS
20	Semisolid/ liquid and solid texture successful	Slight/no dysphagia minimal risk of aspiration	• Normal diet • Regular liquids (First time under supervision of the SLT or a trained stroke nurse!)
15–19	Semisolid and liquid texture successful and solid unsuccessful	Slight dysphagia with a low risk of aspiration	• Dysphagia diet (pureed and soft food) • Liquids very slowly – one sip at a time • Functional swallowing assessments such as Fiberoptic Endoscopic Evaluation of Swallowing (FEES) or Videofluoroscopic Evaluation of Swallowing (VFES) • Refer to Speech and Language Therapist (SLT)
10–14	Semisolid swallow successful and liquids unsuccessful	Moderate dysphagia with a risk of aspiration	Dysphagia diet beginning with • Semisolid textures such as baby food and additional parenteral feeding. • All liquids must be thickened! • Pills must be crushed and mixed with thick liquid. • No liquid medication! • Further functional swallowing assessments (FEES, VFES) • Refer to Speech and Language Therapist (SLT) *Supplementation with nasogastric tube or parenteral*
0–9	Preliminary investigation unsuccessful or semisolid swallow unsuccessful	Severe dysphagia with a high risk of aspiration	• NPO (non per os = nothing by mouth) • Further functional swallowing assessment (FEES, VFES) • Refer to Speech and Language Therapist (SLT) *Supplementation with nasogastric tube or parenteral*

Figure 1-25, cont'd

Box 1-10

Symptoms of Potential Dysphagia

- Facial weakness
- Weak tongue movements
- Poor lip closure
- Drooling
- Coughing on secretions
- Poor or wet voice quality
- Residual food accumulation in mouth

during bed mobility, for transfers, during ADL activities, and while upright. Family members can be instructed to don and doff shoulder supports if needed.

- ADL training: Family members can be trained in setting up the environment using the bed side table, giving simple verbal cues, and providing physical cues to engage the affected upper extremity. If the patient is to go home directly from the acute care setting, family training of both compensatory and remedial techniques for ADL trainings should be initiated.

Box 1-11

Grading ADL during Acute Stroke Rehabilitation

SIMPLE	COMPLEX
Sitting with back supported	Sitting with back unsupported
Finger feeding	Feeding with utensils
Drinking from a cup	Pouring liquids and drinking with a straw
Brushing teeth with set-up	Brushing and cleaning dentures
Washing face with cloth	Washing face and upper body
Donning pullover shirt	Donning a button-down shirt
Donning shorts in bed with bridging	Donning pants while standing to pull up

- Shoulder ROM: Once family members are educated on how to safely handle a subluxed shoulder, they can also be educated to passively range the affected shoulder to 90 degrees of forward flexion. In some cases, occupational therapists can use their clinical judgment and teach the family to perform over head ROM if they can maintain proper alignment of the head of the humerus.
- Positioning: After the family is educated in upper extremity positioning, they should be involved in the patient's positioning schedule. A physically able family member should be trained in proper body mechanics during bed positioning. If a family member is unable to physically complete the positioning himself, he should be educated on the turning schedule and proper positioning. In addition to positioning supine, family should be educated in the proper position of the affected upper extremity while out of bed in a chair. This position should be determined on a case-by-case basis depending on the specific needs of each patient.
- Transfer training: If a patient is to be discharged from the acute care setting to home transfer, training may be appropriate.

GOAL SETTING IN ACUTE CARE

Setting appropriate short-term goals can be challenging in the ICU and acute care environments. Mobility goals should not be omitted as part of the occupational therapist's treatment plan as these mobility skills are a part of not only performing self-care activities but also of enabling the patient to participate in life. Examples of short-term goals are listed in Box 1-12.

DISCHARGE PLANNING

As part of the multidisciplinary team, the occupational therapist should assist and provide input for the patient's discharge plan.[151] The patient's family, support system, and the patient's ultimate destination of home and into the community should be taken into consideration. The goal is for the patient to be safe and as independently functioning as possible. There are several options available for immediate disposition from the ICU and acute care setting (Box 1-13).

Careful consideration should be taken when consulting with the physician and social worker. If the patient appears in need and could benefit from inpatient rehabilitation, the primary care physician may request a physiatry consultation. At this point, the occupational therapist may communicate his or her clinical observations on the patient's progress since admission to the acute care setting.

SUMMARY

In summary acute stroke rehabilitation is multifaceted. Interventions focus on prevention of secondary complications, such as learned nonuse, contracture, and aspiration, and on early attempts at remediation of impairments. Two overarching goals include maximizing participation in appropriate ADL and acting with the team to assure proper discharge planning.

Box 1-12

Acute Goal Setting

Samples of short-term goals for patients with low arousal or in coma	Patient will withdraw from noxious stimuli 1 out of 3 times.
	Patient will open eyes when name is called 1 out of 3 times.
	Patient will turn head away from tactile stimuli.
	Patient will tolerate resting hand splint schedule for 2 hours.
	Patient will tolerate lying on the affected side.
Samples of short-term goals for early stroke rehabilitation	Patient will tolerate sitting in upright in bed at a 60 degree angle for 30 minutes in preparation for engaging in self-care.
	Patient will roll in bed with maximum assistance.
	Patient will tolerate splint wearing schedule for 2-4 hour periods (if appropriate).
	Patient will remove a wash cloth from his or her face independently.
	Patient will wash face with minimal assistance.
	Patient will manage oral secretions with an oral suctioning device with minimal assistance.
	Patient will use call light for nursing attention independently.
	Patient will tolerate dangling at the bed side for 15 minutes with close supervision in preparation for self-care training.
	Patient will feed self 25% to 50% of a meal independently.
	Patient will brush teeth with set-up assistance.
	Patient will don hospital gown with moderate assistance.
	Patient will tolerate sitting in a chair for 60 minutes.

Box 1-13

Discharge Planning

Inpatient rehabilitation	In this setting the patient must be able to tolerate a minimum 3 hours of therapy 6 days per week. The therapy is more aggressive, and length of stay is usually shorter than other settings. The patient's length of stay is dependent upon the rate of progress and attaining established goals.
Subacute rehabilitation	This setting usually occurs in a skilled nursing facility. The patient may receive 90 minutes of therapy 5 times per week. The length of stay may be longer dependent upon tolerance and progress in therapy. Medical insurance coverage may also dictate how long the patient can remain in a subacute center.
Home care services	In some instances, a patient may recover enough function to return home with services. In this case, a referral for visiting nurse and therapy services may be recommended.
Outpatient therapy	If the patient has sufficient recovery to return home and can enter and exit the home with ease, outpatient therapy may be an appropriate option for discharge planning.

CASE STUDY 1

Ischemic Stroke: Management of Acute Case and Complications with Workup

G.H. is a 76-year-old woman who has a history of hypertension and diabetes mellitus and had a myocardial infarction two years ago. She arrives at her local emergency room four hours after an acute onset of weakness in her left arm and leg. She fell at home after trying to get up, and it was only after her neighbors heard her calls for help that the emergency services rescue team came to her aid. On admission to the emergency room, she has an elevated blood pressure of 200/100 and is alert and oriented. Her initial physical examination reveals left-sided weakness and sensory loss that is greater in her arm than her leg. The emergency room team has the impression that she has an acute stroke in evolution, so an emergency CT scan is ordered. The initial blood work and electrocardiogram are unremarkable. While she is in the CT scanner, the on-call resident is paged and asked to come see her because the radiology technician notes that she has become unable to move while in the machine. She now has a dense left hemiplegia. Because of fear of stroke progression, she is admitted to the ICU.

Review of the CT scan shows some mild effacement of the sulci on the right side of the brain and no other clear abnormalities. The neurological consultant advises that G.H.'s treatment that night be conservative and supportive and recommends that G.H. be given an enteric-coated aspirin each day. By the next morning, she has had no further progression of her symptoms but has flaccid left hemiplegia and hemineglect. She remains medically stable during the next several days but is unable to achieve adequate oral intake and has to have an NGT placed for enteral feeding. A physiatric consultation is obtained, and physical and occupational therapy is started at the bed side in the ICU.

Another CT scan is performed on the third hospital day, which reveals a clear, acute infarct in the right temporoparietal area with associated edema and no mass effect or hemorrhage, so the neurologist recommends an extended workup. Carotid Doppler images are normal, and the electrocardiogram indicates stability, but the echocardiogram reveals that G.H. has a decreased ejection fraction of 25% with a visible apical thrombus in the area of her previous myocardial infarction. The neurologist and cardiologist concur on anticoagulation with heparin followed by conversion to warfarin. Anticoagulant therapy is initiated, and the aspirin is no longer administered.

On the sixth hospital day, G.H. is started successfully on warfarin, her hemiparesis has improved, and she is able to move her leg against gravity and with gravity eliminated. However, she is still unable to swallow safely and still has an NGT. G.H. is accepted for inpatient rehabilitation and is transferred to the rehabilitation service on the eighth hospital day.

G.H.'s rehabilitation course is notable because of swelling and pain in her left leg, which is found by duplex Doppler scanning to result from a DVT. Because she developed the thrombosis while receiving adequate anticoagulation medication, she has an umbrella filter placed in her inferior vena cava to prevent development of a pulmonary embolus. G.H. becomes severely depressed and after consultation with the psychiatry service begins receiving antidepressant medication, which has good results. G.H. progresses in therapy, but her left shoulder becomes painful because of a shoulder-hand syndrome, which responds well to aggressive therapeutic intervention. She also develops a progressive increase in skeletal muscle activity, particularly in her left hand, which can only be kept under control with aggressive ROM exercises. At the

Continued

Ischemic Stroke: Management of Acute Case and Complications with Workup—cont'd

time of her discharge, she is able to move short distances with a hemiwalker and needs assistance with dressing her lower extremities and setting up for her basic ADL.

G.H.'s one-year follow-up is notable for the continuing intractable painful spasticity in her left arm, so treatment with Botox is instituted and results in adequate pain relief. She remains stable until five years after her stroke when she suffers a fall with a subsequent hip fracture. Evaluation of bone density shows accelerated osteoporosis in the left hip. She needs left hip hemiarthroplasty but is unable to regain her previous level of function, despite aggressive therapy, and finally has to be admitted to a nursing home when discharged from the hospital.

Hemorrhagic Stroke: Management of Acute Case with Workup

C.C. is a 25-year-old man who works as a sales manager in a local retail store. While dismissing a store clerk whom he caught stealing from the store safe, he suddenly complains of a severe headache, sinks to the chair in his office, and slumps over to the right. Within a few minutes, he is unconscious, and the staff calls the ambulance. C.C. is admitted to the emergency room within 20 minutes, accompanied by the fired clerk who is proclaiming loudly that she has done nothing to him. In the emergency room, C.C. is in a deep coma, breathing deeply, and has dilated pupils and absent reflexes. He is intubated immediately for airway protection and is taken for an emergency CT scan. The study is not completed because C.C. has a seizure while in the CT scanner, but the partially completed study shows a great deal of blood in the ventricles. C.C. is diagnosed with a presumed SAH, and treatment is started. Hyperventilation and treatment with mannitol begin. An intracranial pressure monitor is inserted, and C.C. is given phenytoin and nimodipine. C.C. is managed closely in the ICU and after three days comes out of the coma. He remains intubated and has an MRI/MRA performed that shows a probable berry aneurysm on the anterior communicating artery.

A cerebral angiogram is performed, and a 2-cm aneurysm is clearly visible. C.C. has a good response to the treatment and is extubated on the sixth hospital day. His neurological examination reveals mild disorientation, dysarthria, and tetraparesis more pronounced on the right than the left.

The neurological and neurosurgical team, patient, and family have a discussion and decide that surgical clipping of the aneurysm is the best approach to treating the lesion. C.C. is scheduled for operative intervention the next day. However, in the middle of the night, he suddenly loses consciousness and stops breathing. He has a cardiac arrest but is resuscitated successfully. An emergency CT scan reveals a large recurrent hemorrhage that extends into the cerebral cortex and a herniated brainstem. Aggressive treatments are instituted, but despite all measures the herniation progresses, and C.C. lapses into an irreversible coma. One week later C.C. is declared brain dead, and according to his family's wishes, his organs are donated for transplantation.

REVIEW QUESTIONS

1. Which stroke risk factors are considered modifiable?
2. Which procedures are used to diagnose a stroke?
3. Which clinical signs indicate a patient is receiving excessive seizure medication?
4. What are the risk factors and recommended treatments for DVTs?
5. Other than neurological, what are the common complications that follow a stroke?

REFERENCES

1. The Dutch TIA Trial Study Group: A comparison of two doses of aspirin (30 mg versus 283 mg a day) in patients after a transient ischemic attack or minor ischemic stroke. *N Engl J Med* 325(18):1261–1266, 1991.
2. Adams HP Jr, Brott TG, Crowell RM, et al: Guidelines for the management of patients with acute ischemic stroke: a statement for healthcare professionals from a special writing group of the Stroke Council, American Heart Association. *Circulation* 90(3):1588–1601, 1994.
3. Adams HP Jr, Brott TG, Furlan AJ, et al: Guidelines for thrombolytic therapy for acute stroke: a supplement to the guidelines for the management of patients with acute ischemic stroke—a statement for healthcare professionals from a Special Writing Group of the Stroke Council, American Heart Association. *Circulation* 94(5):1167–1174, 1996.
4. Affleck AT, Liberman S, Polon J, et al: Providing occupational therapy in the intensive care unit. *Am J Occup Ther* 40(5):323–332, 1986.
5. Albers GW, Bates VE, Clark WM, et al: Intravenous tissue-type plasminogen activator for treatment of acute stroke: the standard treatment with alteplase to reverse stroke (STARS) study. *JAMA* 283(9):1145–1150, 2000.
6. Alberts MJ: Diagnosis and treatment of ischemic stroke. *Am J Med* 106(2):211–221, 1999.
7. Antiplatelet Trialists' Collaboration: Collaborative overview of randomized trials of antiplatelet therapy. I. Prevention of death, myocardial infarction, and stroke by prolonged antiplatelet therapy in various categories of patients. *BMJ* 308(6921):81–106, 1994.
8. Antle D, Leafgreen P: Reducing the incidence of pressure ulcer development in the ICU. *AJN* 101(5):24EE–24GG, 2001.
9. Asplund K: Hemodilution in acute stroke. *Cerebrovasc Dis* 1(suppl):129, 1991.

10. Bach-y-Rita P: Process of recovery from stroke. In Brandstser ME, Basmajian JV, editors: *Stroke rehabilitation*, Baltimore, 1987, Williams & Wilkins.

11. Barer DH: Continence after stroke: useful predictor or goal of therapy? *Age Ageing* 18(3):183–191, 1989.

12. Beneficial effect of carotid endarterectomy in symptomatic patients with high grade stenosis, North American Symptomatic Carotid Endarterectomy Trial Collaborators. *N Engl J Med* 325(7):445–453, 1991.

13. Berry E, Kelly S, Westwood ME, et al: The cost-effectiveness of magnetic resonance angiography for carotid artery stenosis and peripheral vascular disease: a systematic review. *Health Technol Assess* 6(7):1–155, 2002.

14. Black SE, Norris JW, Hachinski VC: Post stroke seizures. *Stroke* 14: 134, 1983.

15. Bonita R: Epidemiology of stroke. *Lancet* 339(8789):342–344, 1992.

16. Bonita R, Beaglehole R, North JD: Event, incidence and case fatality rates of cerebrovascular disease in Auckland, New Zealand. *Am J Epidemiol* 120(2):236–243, 1984.

17. Bontke CF, Boake C: Principles of brain injury rehabilitation. In Braddom RL, editors: *Physical medicine and rehabilitation*, Philadelphia, 1996, Saunders.

18. Boysen G, Christensen H: Stroke severity determines body temperature in acute stroke. *Stroke* 32(2):413–7, 2001.

19. Brandstater ME, Roth EJ, Siebens HC: Venous thromboembolism in stroke: literature review and implication for clinical practice. *Arch Phys Med Rehabil* 73(suppl 5):S379–S391, 1992.

20. Brockhurst JC, Andrews K, Richards B, et al: Incidence and correlates of incontinence in stroke patients. *J Am Geriatr Soc* 33(8):540–542, 1985.

21. Bromfield EB, Reding MJ: Relative risk of deep venous thrombosis or pulmonary embolism post-stroke based on ambulatory status. *J Neurol Rehab* 2(2):51, 1988.

22. Brott T, Adams HP Jr, Olinger CP, et al: Measurements of acute cerebral infarction: a clinical examination scale. *Stroke* 20(7):864–870, 1989.

23. Bushbacher RM: Deconditioning, conditioning, and the benefits of exercise. In Braddom RL, editor: *Physical medicine and rehabilitation*, Philadelphia, 1996, Saunders.

24. Bushbacher R: Heterotopic ossification: a review. *Crit Rev Phys Med Rehabil* 4:199, 1992.

25. Caplan LR: Diagnosis and treatment of ischemic stroke. *JAMA* 266(17):2413–2418, 1991.

26. Carr EK, Kenney FD: Positioning of the Stoke Patient: a review of the literature. *J Nurs Stud* 29(4):355–369, 1992.

27. Cerebral Embolism Study Group: Immediate anticoagulation of embolic stroke, Brain Hemorrhage and Cerebral Embolism Task Force: cardiogenic brain embolism—the second report of the Cerebral Embolism Task Force. *Arch Neurol* 46(7):727, 1989.

28. Chyatte D, Elefteriades J, Kim B: Profound hypothermia and circulatory arrest for aneurysm surgery. Case report. *J Neurosurg* 70(3):489–491, 1989.

29. Cinnamon J, Viroslav AB, Dorey JH: CT and MRI diagnosis of cerebrovascular disease: going beyond the pixels. *Semin Ultrasound CT MRI* 16(3):212–236, 1995.

30. Clark WM, Wissman S, Albers GW, et al: Recombinant tissue-type plasminogen activator (alteplase) for ischemic stroke 3 to 5 hours after symptom onset. The ATLANTIS study: a randomized controlled trial. Alteplase thrombolysis for acute noninterventional therapy in ischemic stroke. *JAMA* 282(21):2019–2026, 1999.

31. Colditz GA, Bonita R, Stampfer MJ, et al: Cigarette smoking and risk for stroke in middle-aged women. *N Engl J Med* 318(15):937–941, 1988.

32. Collins R, Peto R, MacMahon S, et al: Blood pressure, stroke, and coronary heart disease. II. Short-term reductions in blood pressure: overview of randomised drug trials in an epidemiological context. *Lancet* 335(8693):827–838, 1990.

33. Counsel C, Sandercock P: The management of patients with acute ischemic stroke. *Curr Med Lit Geriatr* 7:99, 1994.

34. Coventry MB, Scanlon PW: The use of radiation to discourage ectopic bone: a nine-year study in surgery about the hip. *J Bone Joint Surg Am* 63(2):201–208, 1981.

35. Den Hertog HM, van der Worp HB, Tseng MC, et al: Cooling therapy for acute stroke. *Cochrane Database Syst Rev* 21(1): CD001247, 2009.

36. DeVincenzo DK, Watkins S: Accidental falls in a rehabilitation setting. *Rehabil Nurs* 12(5):248–252, 1987.

37. Dichter MA: The epilepsies and convulsive disorders. In Isselbacher KJ, Braunwald E, Wilson JD, et al, editors: *Harrison's principles of internal medicine*, New York, 1994, McGraw-Hill.

38. Donahue RP, Abbott RD, Reed DM, et al: Alcohol and hemorrhagic stroke: the Honolulu Heart Program. *JAMA* 255(17):2311–2314, 1986.

39. Donaldson CL, Hulley SB, Vogel JM, et al: Effect of prolonged bed rest on bone mineral. *Metabolism* 19(12):1071–1084, 1970.

40. Dyken ML: Overview of trends in management and prognosis in stroke. *Ann Epidemiol* 3(5)535, 1993.

41. Dyson M: Intensive Care Unit psychosis, the therapeutic nurse-patient relationship and the influence of the intensive care setting: analyses of interrelating factors. *J Clin Nurs* 8:284–290, 1999.

42. Ebrahim S: *Clinical epidemiology of stroke*, Oxford, 1995, Oxford University Press.

43. Ebrahim S, Nouri F: Caring for stroke patients at home. *Int Rehabil Med* 8(4):171–173, 1987.

44. Elster AD, Moody DM: Early cerebral infarction: gadopentetate dimeglumine enhancement. *Radiology* 177(3):627–632, 1990.

45. European Atrial Fibrillation Trial Study Group: Secondary prevention in nonrheumatic atrial fibrillation after transient ischemic attack or minor stroke. *Lancet* 342(8882):1255–1262, 1993.

46. European Carotid Surgery Trial Collaborative Group: Medical research council carotid surgery trial: interim results for patients with severe (70% to 90%) or with mild (0% to 30%) carotid stenosis. *Lancet* 334(8655):175, 1989.

47. Failure of extracranial-intracranial arterial bypass to reduce the risk of ischemic stroke: results of an international randomized trial, the EC/IC Bypass Study Group. *N Engl J Med* 313(19):1191–2000, 1985.

48. Farrell B, Godwin J, Richards S, et al: The United Kingdom transient ischaemic attack (UK-TIA) aspirin trial: final results. *J Neurol Neurosurg Psychiatry* 54(12):1044, 1991.

49. Fisher CM: Clinical syndromes in cerebral thrombosis, hypertensive hemorrhage, and ruptured saccular aneurysm. *Clin Neurosurg* 22:117–147, 1975.

50. Fisher CM: Pathological observations in hypertensive cerebral hemorrhage. *J Neuropathol Exp Neurol* 30(3):536–550, 1971.

51. Fisher CM: Atherosclerosis of the carotid and vertebral arteries: extracranial and intracranial. *J Neuropathol Exp Neurol* 24(3):455, 1965.

52. Further analyses of mortality in oral contraceptive users, Royal College of General Practicioners' Oral Contraceptive Study. *Lancet* 1(8219):541–546, 1981.

53. Gainotti G: Emotional behavior and hemispheric side of the lesion. *Cortex* 8(1):41–55, 1972.

54. Garraway WM, Whisnant JP, Drury I: The changing pattern of survival following stroke. *Stroke* 14(5):699, 1983.

55. Geary SM: Intensive care unit psychosis revisited: Understanding and managing delirium in the critical care setting. *Crit Care Nurs Q* 17(1):51–63, 1994.

56. Giancio JT, Kalmar K, Whyte J: The JFK Coma Recovery Scale-Revised: measurement characteristic and diagnostic utility. *Arch Phys Med Rehabil* 85(12):2020–2029, 2004.

57. Giancino J, Kalmar K: Coma Recovery Scale-Revised, *The Center for Outcome Measurement in Brain Injury* (website). www.tbims.org/combi/crs. Accessed 7/12/09.

58. Gonzalez RG, Schaefer PW, Buonanno FS, et al: Diffusion weighted MR imaging: diagnostic accuracy in patients imaged within 6 hours of stroke symptom onset. *Radiology* 210(1):155–162, 1999.

59. Gordon C, Hewer RL, Wade DT: Dysphagia in acute stroke. *Br J Med* 295(6595):411–414, 1987.

60. Gosselink R, Bott J, Johnson M, et al: Physiotherapy for adult patients with critical illness: recommendations of the European Respiratory Society and the European Society of Intensive Care Medicine Task Force on Physiotherapy for Critically Ill Patients. *Intensive Care Med* 34(7): 1188–1199, 2008.

61. Groher ME, Bukatman R: The prevalence of swallowing disorders in two teaching hospitals. *Dysphagia* 1(1):3, 1986.

62. Grotta JC, Norris JW, Kamm B: Prevention of stroke with ticlopidine: who benefits most? TASS Baseline and Angiographic Data Subgroup. *Neurology* 42(1):111–115, 1992.

63. Hachinski V, Norris JW: *The acute stroke*, Philadelphia, 1985, FA Davis.

64. Hacke W, Kaste M, Fieschi C, et al: Randomized double-blind placebo-controlled trial of thrombolytic therapy with intravenous alteplase in acute ischemic stroke (ECASS II), Second European-Australian Acute Stroke Study Investigators. *Lancet* 352(9136):1245–1251, 1998.

65. Hadizadeh DR, Gieseke J, Lohmaier SH, et al: Peripheral MR angiography with blood pool contrast agent: prospective intra individual comparative study of high-spatial-resolution steady-state MR angiography versus standard-resolution first-pass MR angiography and DSA. *Radiology* 249(2):701–711, 2008.

66. Harburn KL, Potter PJ: Spasticity and contractures. *Phys Med Rehabil State Art Rev* 7(8):113, 1993.

67. Hassenfeld M: Increased incidence of hip fracture on the hemiplegic side of post stroke patients. Unpublished work presented at Columbia Presbyterian Medical Center, May 1993, New York.

68. Hauser WA, Ramirez-Lassepas M, Rosenstein R: Risk for seizures and epilepsy following cerebrovascular insults. *Epilepsia* 25(5):666, 1984.

69. Heros RC, Zervas NT, Varsos V: Cerebral vasospasm after subarachnoid hemorrhage: an update. *Ann Neurol* 14(6):599–608, 1983.

70. Hirsh J: Heparin. *N Engl J Med* 324(22):1565–1574, 1991.

71. Hirsh J: From unfractionated heparins to low molecular weight heparins. *Acta Chir Scand Suppl* 556:42–50, 1990.

72. Hirsh J, Genton E, Hull R: *Venous thromboembolism*, New York, 1981, Grune & Stratton.

73. Hirsh J, Hull R: Natural history and clinical features of venous thrombosis. In Coleman RW, Hirsh J, Marder V, et al, editors: *Haemostasis and thrombosis: basic principles and clinical practice*, Philadelphia, 1982, Lippincott.

74. House A, Dennis M, Molyneux A, et al: Emotionalism after stroke. *BMJ* 298(6679):991–994, 1989.

75. Hull R, Hirsh J: Diagnosis of venous thromboembolism. In Coleman RW, Hirsh J, Marder V, et al, editors: *Haemostasis and thrombosis: basic principles and clinical practice*, Philadelphia, 1982, Lippincott.

76. Hull RD, Raskob GE, Rosenbloom D, et al: Heparin for 5 days as compared with 10 days in the initial treatment of proximal venous thrombosis. *N Engl J Med* 322(18):1260–1264, 1990.

77. Huston J 3rd, Fain SB, Riederer SJ, et al: Carotid arteries: maximizing arterial to venous contrast in fluoroscopically triggered contrast-enhanced MR angiography with elliptic centric view ordering. *Radiology* 211(1): 265–273, 1999.

78. Iso H, Jacobs DR Jr, Wentworth D, et al: Serum cholesterol levels and six year mortality from stroke in 350,977 men screened for the multiple risk factor intervention trial. *N Engl J Med* 320(14):904–910, 1989.

79. Kallmes DF, Omary RA, Dix JE, et al: Specificity of MR angiography as a confirmatory test of carotid artery stenosis. *Am J Neuroradiol* 17(8):1501 1506, 1996.

80. Kannel WB, McGee DL: Diabetes and cardiovascular disease: the Framingham Study. *JAMA* 241(19):2035–2038, 1979.

81. Kanter MC, Sherman DG: Strategies for preventing stroke. *Curr Opin Neurol Neurosurg* 6(1):60–65, 1993.

82. Kasner SE: Clinical interpretation and use of stroke scales. *Lancet Neurol* 5(7):603–612 2006.

83. Kistler JP, Ropper AH, Martin JB: Cerebrovascular disease. In Isselbacher KJ, Braunwald E, Wilson, JD, et al, editors: *Harrison's principles of internal medicine*, New York, 1994, McGraw-Hill.

84. Kottke FJ, Pauley DL, Ptak RA: The rationale for prolonged stretching for correction of shortening of connective tissue. *Arch Phys Med Rehabil* 47(6):345–352, 1966.

85. Kozararevic D, McGee D, Vojvodic N, et al: Frequency of alcohol consumption and morbidity and mortality: the Yugoslavia Cardiovascular Disease Study. *Lancet* 1(8169):613–616, 1980.

86. Kuller LH, Dorman JS, Wolf PA: Cerebrovascular disease and diabetes. In *Diabetes in America: diabetes data compiled for 1984*, National Diabetes Data Group, NIH Pub No 85–1468, Bethesda, MD, August 1985, Department of Health and Human Services.

87. Kwiatkowski TG, Libman RB, Frankel M, et al: Effects of tissue plasminogen activator for acute ischemic stroke at one year, National Institute of Neurological Disorders and Stroke Recombinant Tissue Plasminogen Activator Stroke Study Group. *N Engl J Med* 340(23):1781–1787, 1999.

88. Lai S, Duncan PW, Keighley J: Prediction of functional outcome after stroke comparison of the Orpington Prognostic Scale and the NIH Stroke Scale. *Stroke* 29(9):1838–1842, 1998.

89. Lance JW: Pathophysiology of spasticity and clinical experience with baclofen. In Feldman RG, Young RR, Koella P, editors: *Spasticity-disordered motor control*, Chicago, 1980, Year Book.

90. Langhorne P, Stott DJ: Acute cerebral infarction: optimal management in older patients. *Drugs Aging* 6(6):445–455, 1995.

91. Langhorne P, Williams BO, Gilchrist W, et al: Do stroke units save lives? *Lancet* 342(8868):395–398, 1993.

92. Levison ME: Pneumonia, including necrotizing pulmonary infections (lung abscesses). In Isselbacher KJ, Braunwald E, Wilson JD, et al, editors: *Harrison's principles of internal medicine*, New York, 1994, McGraw-Hill.

93. Levison ME, Bush L: Pharmacodynamics of antimicrobial agents: bactericidal and postantibiotic effects. *Infect Dis Clin North Am* 3(3):415–421, 1989.

94. Lezak MD: *Neuropsychological assessment*, ed 2, New York, 1983, Oxford University Press.

95. Locksley HB: Natural history of subarachnoid hemorrhage, intracranial aneurysms, and arteriovenous malformations: based on 6368 cases in a cooperative study. In Sahs AL, Perret G, Locksley HB, et al, editors: *Intracranial aneurysms and subarachnoid hemorrhage: a cooperative study*, Philadelphia, 1969, Lippincott.

96. Longstreth WT Jr, Nelson LM, Koepsell TD, et al: Clinical course of spontaneous subarachnoid hemorrhage: a population based study in King County, Washington. *Neurology* 43(4):712–718, 1993.

97. Lorber B, Swenson RM: Bacteriology of aspiration pneumonia: a prospective study of community and hospital acquired cases. *Ann Intern Med* 81(3):329–331, 1974.

98. MacMahon S, Peto R, Cutler J, et al: Blood pressure, stroke, and coronary heart disease. I. Prolonged differences in blood pressure: prospective observational studies corrected for regression dilution bias. *Lancet* 335(8692):765–774, 1990.

99. Maddocks W: The role of the nurse in preventing intensive care psychosis. *Nurs Prax N Z* 10(3):12–15, 1995.

100. Mahoney FI, Barthel DW: Functional evaluation: the Barthel index. *Maryland State Med J* 14:61–65, 1965.

101. Marmot MG, Poulter NR: Primary prevention of stroke. *Lancet* 339(8789):344–347, 1992.

102. Mayerberg MR, Batjer HH, Dacey R, et al: Guidelines for the management of aneurysmal subarachnoid hemorrhage: a statement

for healthcare professionals from a special writing group of the Stroke Council, American Heart Association. *Stroke* 25(11):2315–2328, 1994.

103. McCullough LD, Beauchamp NB, Wityk R: Recent advances in the diagnosis and treatment of stroke. *Surv Ophthalmol* 45(4):317–330, 2001.

104. McGill HC Jr: The pathogenesis of atherosclerosis. *Clin Chem* 34(8B):B33–B39, 1988.

105. McNeil BJ, Bettman MA: The diagnosis of pulmonary embolism. In Coleman RW, Hirsh J, Marder V, et al, editors: *Haemostasis and thrombosis: basic principles and clinical practice*, Philadelphia, 1982, Lippincott.

106. Mion LC, Gregor S, Buettner M, et al: Falls in the rehabilitation setting: incidence and characteristics. *Rehabil Nurs* 14(1):17–22, 1989.

107. Mohr JP: Lacunes. *Stroke* 13(1):3–11, 1982.

108. Mohr JP, Orgogozo JM, Harrison MJG, et al: Meta-analysis of nimodipine trials in acute ischemic stroke. *Cerebrovasc Dis* 4:197, 1994.

109. Murray CJ, Lopez AD. Mortality by cause for eight regions of the world: Global Burden of Disease study. *Lancet* 349(9061):1269–1276, 1997.

110. Murray GB, Shea V, Conn DK: Electroconvulsive therapy for post-stroke depression. *J Clin Psychiatry* 47(5):258, 1986.

111. Nederkoorn PJ, Van Der Graaf Y, Hunink MG, et al: Duplex ultrasound and magnetic resonance angiography compared with digital subtraction angiography in carotid artery stenosis: a systematic review. *Stroke* 34(5):1324–1331, 2003.

112. Needham D: Mobilizing patients in the intensive care unit improving neuromuscular weakness and physical function. *JAMA* 300(14):1685–1689, 2008.

113. Okada Y, Yamaguchi T, Minematsu K, et al: Hemorrhagic transformation in cerebral embolism. *Stroke* 20(5):598–603, 1989.

114. Paffenbarger RS Jr, Laughlin ME, Gima AS, et al: Work activity of longshoremen as related to death from coronary heart disease and stroke. *N Engl J Med* 282(20):1109–1114, 1970.

115. Paffenbarger RS, Wing AL, Hyde RT: Physical activity as an index of heart attack risk in college alumni. *Am J Epidemiol* 108(3):161–175, 1978.

116. Perry RF: Clinical practice guidelines for smoking cessation. *JAMA* 276(6):448, 1996.

117. Pessin MS, Duncan GW, Mohr JP, et al: Clinical and angiographic features of carotid transient ischemic attacks. *N Engl J Med* 296(7):358–362, 1977.

118. Poplingher AR, Pillar T: Hip fracture in stroke patients: epidemiology and rehabilitation. *Acta Orthop Scand* 56(3):226–227, 1985.

119. *PORT Study (funded by the Agency for Health Care Policy and Research)*, Durham, NC, 1994, Duke University Medical Center.

120. Prevention of stroke by antihypertensive drug treatment in older persons with isolated systolic hypertension: final results of the Systolic Hypertension in the Elderly Program (SHEP), SHEP Cooperative Research Group. *JAMA* 265(24):3255–3264, 1991.

121. Prevention of venous thrombosis and pulmonary embolism, NIH Consensus Development. *JAMA* 256(6):744–749, 1986.

122. Quizilbash N, Murphy M: Meta-analysis of trials of corticosteroids in acute stroke. *Age Ageing* 22(suppl):2, 1993.

123. Randomised controlled trial of streptokinase, aspirin, and combination of both in treatment of acute stroke, Multicenter Acute Stroke Trial: Italy (MAST-I) Group. *Lancet* 346(8989):1509–1514, 1995.

124. Reed DM: The paradox of high risk of stroke in populations with low risk of coronary heart disease. *Am J Epidemiol* 131(4):579–588, 1990.

125. Robinson RG, Bolla-Wilson K, Kaplan E, et al: Depression influenced intellectual impairment in stroke patients. *Br J Psychiatry* 148:541, 1986.

126. Ropper AH, Davis KR: Lobar cerebral hemorrhages: acute clinical syndromes in 26 patients. *Ann Neurol* 8(2):141–147, 1980.

127. Rosamond W, Flegal K, Friday G, et al: Heart disease and stroke statistics—2007 update: a report from the American Heart Association Statistics Committee and Stroke Statistics Subcommittee. *Circulation* 115(5):e69–e171, 2007.

128. Roth EJ, Harvey RL: Rehabilitation of stroke syndromes. In Braddom RL, editor: *Physical medicine and rehabilitation*, Philadelphia, 1996, Saunders.

129. Rowland TJ, Cooke DM, Gustafsson LA, Role of occupational therapy after stroke. *Ann Indian Acad Neurol* [serial online] 11(5):99–107, 2008.

130. Rutan GH, Kuller LH, Neaton JD, et al: Mortality associated with diastolic hypertension and isolated systolic hypertension among men screened for the Multiple Risk Factor Intervention Trial. *Circulation* 77(3):504–514, 1988.

131. Saccani S, Beghi C, Fragnito C, et al: Carotid endarterectomy under hypothermic extracorporeal circulation: a method of brain protection for special patients. *J Cardiovasc Surg (Torino)* 33(3):311–314, 1992.

132. Salcido R, Hart D, Smith AM: The prevention and management of pressure ulcers. In Braddom RL, editor: *Physical medicine and rehabilitation*, Philadelphia, 1996, Saunders.

133. Salonen R, Seppanen K, Rauramaa R, et al: Prevalence of carotid atherosclerosis and serum cholesterol levels in eastern Finland. *Atherosclerosis* 8(6):788–792, 1988.

134. Salzman EW, Hirsh J: Prevention of venous thromboembolism. In Coleman RW, Hirsh J, Marder V, et al, editors: *Haemostasis and thrombosis: basic principles and clinical practice*, Philadelphia, 1982, Lippincott.

135. Sandercock PA, van den Belt AG, Lindley RI, et al: Antithrombotic therapy in acute ischemic stroke: an overview of the randomized trials. *J Neurol Neurosurg Psychiatry* 56(1):17–25, 1993.

136. Sandercock PAG, Willems H: Medical treatment of acute ischemic stroke. *Lancet* 339(8792):537–539, 1992.

137. Schwartz Cowley R, Swanson B, Chapman P, et al: The role of rehabilitation in the intensive care unit. *J Head Trauma Rehabil* 9(1): 32–42, 1994

138. Schweickert, WD, Pohlman MC, Pohlman AS, et al: Early physical and occupational therapy in mechanically ventilated, critically ill patients: a randomised controlled trial. *Lancet* 373(9678):1874–1882, 2009.

139. Shankaran S, Laptook AR, Ehrenkranz RA, et al: Whole-body hypothermia for neonates with hypoxic-ischemic encephalopathy. *New Engl J Med* 353(15):1574–1584, 2005.

140. Sinyor D, Amato P, Kaloupek DG, et al: Post-stroke depression: relationships to functional impairment, coping strategies and rehabilitation outcome. *Stroke* 17(6):1102–1107, 1986.

141. Sorenson AG, Buonanno FS, Gonzalez RG, et al: Hyperacute stroke: evaluation with combined multisection diffusion-weighted and hemodynamically weighted echo-planar MR imaging. *Radiology* 199(2):391–401, 1996.

142. Stadel BV: Oral contraceptives and cardiovascular disease. *N Engl J Med* 305(12):672–677, 1981.

143. Stampfer MJ, Willett WC, Colditz GA, et al: A prospective study of the past use of oral contraceptive agents and the risk of cardiovascular diseases. *N Engl J Med* 319(20):1313–1317, 1988.

144. Starkstein SE, Cohen BS, Fedoroff P, et al: Relationship between anxiety disorders and depressive disorders in patients with cerebrovascular injury. *Arch Gen Psychiatry* 47(3):246–251, 1990.

145. Starkstein S, Robinson R, Price TR: Comparison of cortical and subcortical lesions in the production of post stroke mood disorders. *Brain* 110(Pt 4):1045, 1987.

146. Stiller K, Phillips A: Safety aspects of mobilising acutely ill inpatients. *Physiother Theory Pract* 19(4): 239–257, 2003.

147. Subbarao J, Smith J: Pulmonary embolism during stroke rehabilitation. *Ill Med J* 165(5):328–332, 1984.

148. Sundaram MB, Chow F: Seizures associated with spontaneous subarachnoid hemorrhage. *Can J Neurol Sci* 13(3):229–231, 1986.

149. Sundt TM Jr, Kobayashi S, Fode NC, et al: Results and complications of surgical management of 809 intracranial aneurysms in 722 cases: related and unrelated to grade of patient, type of aneurysm, and timing of surgery. *J Neurosurg* 56(6):753–765, 1982.

150. Sundt TM Jr, Whisnant JP: Subarachnoid hemorrhage from intracranial aneurysms. *N Engl J Med* 299(3):116–122, 1978.

151. Sutton S: An acute medical admission unit: is there a place for an occupational therapist. *Br J Occup Ther* 61(1):3–7, 1998.

152. Swartzman L, Teasell RW: Psychological consequences of stroke. *Phys Med Rehabil State Art Rev* 7(1):179, 1993.

153. Swedish Aspirin Low-Dose Trial (SALT) of 75 mg aspirin as secondary prophylaxis after cerebrovascular ischemic events, the SALT Collaborative Group. *Lancet* 338(8779):1345–1349, 1991.

154. Teasdale G, Jennett B. Assessment of coma and impaired consciousness. A practical scale. *Lancet* 2(7872):81–84, 1974.

155. Thompson DD, Rodan GA: Indomethacin inhibition of tenotomy induced bone resorption in rats. *J Bone Miner Res* 3(4):409, 1988.

156. Thrombolytic therapy with streptokinase in acute ischemic stroke: the Multicenter Acute Stroke Trial—Europe Study Group. *New Engl J Med* 335(3):145–150, 1996.

157. Tissue plasminogen activator for acute ischemic stroke, the National Institute of Neurological Disorders and Stroke rt-PA Stroke Study Group. *New Engl J Med* 333(24):1581–1587, 1995.

158. Torner JC, Nibbelink DW, Burmeister LF: Statistical comparisons of end results of a randomized treatment study. In Sahs AL, Nibbelink DW, Torner JC, editors: *Aneurysmal subarachnoid hemorrhage: report of the cooperative study*, Baltimore, 1981, Urban & Schwarzenberg.

159. Trapl M, Enderle P Nowotny M, et al: Dysphagia bedside screening for acute stroke patients: the Gugging Swallowing Screen. *Stroke* 38(11):2948, 2007.

160. U-King-Im JM, Young V, Gillard JH: Carotid-artery imaging in the diagnosis and management of patients at risk of stroke. *Lancet Neurol* 8(6):569–580, 2009.

161. Uniform Data System for Medical Rehabilitation: *The Guide for the Uniform Data Set for Medical Rehabilitation (Including the FIM™ Instrument)*, Version 5.1. Buffalo, NY, 1997, Research Foundation, State University of New York at Buffalo.

162. Viitanen M, Eriksson S, Asplund K: Risk of recurrent stroke, myocardial infarction and epilepsy during long-term follow-up after stroke. *Eur Neurol* 28(4):227–231, 1988.

163. Wardlaw JM, Warlow CP: Thrombolysis in acute ischemic stroke: does it work? *Stroke* 23(12):1826–1839, 1992.

164. Warlow C: Disorders of the cerebral circulation. In Walton J, editor: *Brain's disease of the nervous system*, ed 10, Oxford, England, 1993, Oxford University Press.

165. Warlow C, Ogston D, Douglas AS: Deep venous thrombosis of the legs after strokes. I. Incidence and predisposing factors; II. Natural history. *BMJ* 1(6019):1178–1181, 1976.

166. Wheeler HB, Anderson FA Jr: Diagnostic approaches for deep vein thrombosis. *Chest* 89(suppl 5):407S–412S, 1986.

167. Whisnant JP, Matsumotoa N, Elveback LR: The effect of anticoagulant therapy on the prognosis of patients with transient cerebral ischemic attacks in a community: Rochester, Minnesota, 1955–1969. *Mayo Clinic Proc* 48(12):844–848, 1973.

168. Wiebe-Velasquez S, Blume WT: Seizures. *Phys Med Rehabil State Art Rev* 7(1):73, 1993.

169. Wolf PA, Belanger AJ, D'Agostino RB: Management of risk factors. *Neurol Clin* 10:177, 1992.

170. Wolf PA, D'Agostino RB, Belanger AJ, et al: Probability of stroke: a risk profile from the Framingham Study. *Stroke* 22(3):312–318, 1991.

171. Wolf PA, D'Agostino RB, Kannel WB, et al: Cigarette smoking as a risk factor for stroke: the Framingham Study. *JAMA* 259(7):1025–1029, 1988.

172. Worden JW: *Grief counseling and grief therapy*, New York, 1982, Springer.

173. Wortman CB, Silver RC: The myths of coping with loss. *J Consult Clin Psychol* 57(3):349–357, 1989.

janet falk-kessler

chapter 2

Psychological Aspects
of Stroke Rehabilitation

key terms

anxiety
caregivers
coping

cultural factors
defense mechanisms
depression

personality traits
self-efficacy

chapter objectives

After completing this chapter, the reader will be able to accomplish the following:

1. Understand the psychological manifestations of stroke in both children and adults.
2. Understand how a variety of psychological impairments affect the recovery process.
3. Understand how personality traits impact rehabilitation.
4. Understand the effect of stroke on family members and those in the caregiver role.
5. Understand the importance of participation in recovery.

Understanding the relationship between psychological factors and stroke is a complex undertaking. Anxiety, depression, aggression, and emotional lability are commonly seen in persons who have sustained a stroke, as each takes its toll on adjustment and each affects functional outcome. Psychiatric conditions restrict recovery and restrain quality of life, making assessment and treatment of paramount importance. When considering the psychological consequences of stroke, observing physiological changes, and emotional reactions to this life-altering event, one's personality constructs and cultural background play a role in recovery and outcome. The purpose of this chapter is to review the relationship between stroke and its psychological consequences in adults; the impact on the family's and on the caregiver's well-being; and how to understand the implications for occupational therapy.

In addition, pediatric stroke and the psychological consequences that may result are reviewed.

It is well-documented that nearly 800,000 persons each year suffer a stroke, and of those it is the first attack for almost 600,000.[60] These statistics are especially significant when considering that there is a decrease in stroke incidence, particularly in high income countries, due to attention to cardiovascular risk factors.[32] In the United States, stroke continues to be a leading cause of death, yet more than four million stroke individuals who have had a stroke survive.[60] Stroke is a leading cause of disability and has a major impact on participation as it compromises activities of daily living (ADL) and social roles.[22] Stroke survivors, even in this climate of health care change, continue to receive and to benefit from services offered by occupational therapists.[80]

Stroke is a leading cause of disability and death in individuals over 65-years-old, but 25% of those with stroke are younger,[14] as stroke can occur at any age. In addition to stroke afflicting adults, it has been estimated that stroke affects children at a rate of at least two to three per 100,000.[46] These statistics are further compounded by the significant psychological impact of stroke on the survivors and their families.

It is well established that adults who have sustained a stroke are at high risk for psychological consequences. As many as 30% to 50% of stroke survivors have been estimated to have had some significant psychological disorder following stroke,[96] even in the absence of a disabling condition.[91] In fact, the risk for developing a psychological disorder persists long after the stroke event.[127] Given the profound impact psychological disorders have on recovery, understanding the relationship, the range, and the effect these disorders have on individuals with stroke is paramount, for psychological factors may be antecedents, consequences, and/or reactions to the traumatic neurological experience.

Clearly, a complex relationship exists between psychological factors and medical conditions, and "Psychological Factors Affecting Medical Condition" is even recognized as a diagnostic category.[1] Undesirable psychological features may have an adverse effect on recovery and outcome or may place an individual at risk for an unwanted outcome. Specific psychological symptoms, such as anxiety or depression; specific personality traits or coping styles, such as aggressive personality traits[29,128]; maladaptive health behaviors, such as tobacco or alcohol abuse; and stress-related physiological responses,[116] have been linked to stroke.[69]

Stress of illness and disability affects not only the person but also one's family. An unexpected serious and disabling illness results in the need for all family members to cope and find new ways of relating to one another. Previously established roles, authority relationships, family-based activities, and occupations may change,[71] resulting in a structural shift that puts the entire family at risk for significant distress. Due to the disability, the potential for increased alienation of the individual and of the family adds to the psychological distress already being experienced.[48] When a stroke happens to a child, the implications can be devastating for the family[92] and can result in increased mental health disorders in a parent.[39]

PSYCHOLOGICAL FACTORS AS PREDICTORS OF STROKE

The examination of psychological factors as predictors of stroke has received attention. This area of inquiry is difficult to investigate because the psychological variables typically identified are linked to lifestyle behaviors considered risk factors for coronary heart disease, such as tobacco and alcohol use, and decreased physical activity, and to physiological risk factors (e.g., hypertension).[69,128] Even so, evidence indicates that personality traits may be associated with increased risk for stroke. Longitudinal population based studies have been conducted linking emotion to stroke onset. One study showed that participants with a pattern of outward expression of anger were twice as likely to sustain a stroke compared with even-tempered individuals; individuals with a pattern of inward expression and those who were able to control their anger were not at any higher risk for stroke.[29] Another study also linked anger to stroke, but only in the younger participants, suggesting that the influence of anger on stroke decreases as one ages.[128] Individuals with psychological distress are at greater risk for fatal stroke,[69] as are those who reported high, frequent levels of stress. No relationship exists between reported stress levels and nonfatal stroke. The speculation is that individuals with better coping skills may be able to handle stressful situations and may have fewer associated lifestyle risk factors, thereby reducing their risk.[116]

PRESTROKE PSYCHOLOGICAL FACTORS AS PREDICTORS OF RECOVERY AND REHABILITATION

A series of studies have been done that examine prestroke personality and psychological variables on poststroke recovery and rehabilitation. In one study, a history of either an affective disorder or an anxiety disorder was demonstrated to put a person at increased risk for developing major depression. The severity of the depression symptoms also depended on a personal or family history of affective or anxiety disorders.[74] Personality traits, such as introversion and depression, may increase the mortality risk following a stroke,[75] as may a history of depression.[100] An impaired social relationship with a significant other before a stroke also puts individuals at significant risk for depression during the acute phase following a stroke and during the long term after the stroke.[99]

Personality factors are associated with the ability to resume independence. As a character trait, individual's self-esteem has been linked with recovery and independence,[13] and as such is critical to consider in the rehabilitation process.[119] Personality factors along with occupational status, educational level, workplace accommodation, and occupational choice play a significant role in the ability to return to work.[71] One's ability to handle life events, classified into coping strategies, also affects one's ability to resume daily living function. Individuals with a preference for active coping styles or with an extrovert personality trait show greater improvements in activities of daily living function than those individuals with passive or avoidant coping styles. These individuals are speculated to be more highly motivated and have a more realistic appraisal of their potential, which results in improved activities of daily living function.[27]

EMOTIONAL REACTION TO STROKE

For any individual hospitalized after a traumatic event, a barrage of emotion is likely to develop. When faced with an acute illness with chronic consequences, compounded by being acutely aware of the physical changes occurring and by being surrounded by a foreign and controlling environment adds to ones emotional reaction.[38] During an acute phase of the illness, one is concerned with survival, is often confused with what is happening, and may be the recipient of poor communication from hospital staff. This results in feelings of being overwhelmed; in experiences of loss of control over personal care, which affects one's sense of dignity; and often in experiences of the hospital environment being dissatisfying, inadequate, and insensitive.[17] During the rehabilitation phase, an individual's anxiety may increase if one is not progressing as quickly as one hoped. Depression and social isolation may set in, as family members need to resume normalcy and may not visit as often as they initially did.[17] Fear and anxiety, a sense of powerlessness, and even psychological regression can result from stressors that include a threat to one's integrity, dependence on strangers, separation from home and family, fear of loss of approval, fear of loss of control, fear of loss of control of body parts, and guilt. The initial loss of control (not knowing what is happening), integrity (wearing a hospital gown or using a bedpan), and freedom (given a schedule to follow, transported by others, told what to eat and when to eat) are values underscored by society and, when challenged, further add to stigma, shame, and a sense of isolation.[92] This experience of hospitalization contributes to a diminished sense of self. When patients face discharge from the hospital and/or rehabilitation program, they may feel abandoned by the medical system. Reality of their abilities with their ADL and instrumental ADL, the role changes that occur, and their participation in their activities may all be very challenging. They experience loss, especially around driving (as is symbolizes independence, self-esteem, social support, participation), previously enjoyed hobbies and activities, loss of role, and loss of future plans. They may also feel unattractive and self-conscious as change in their relationship with their partner occurs.[17] See Chapters 23, 25, and 29.

As one's condition begins to stabilize, emotional reactions continue. Research has shown that depression and other psychological conditions may result from physiological damage caused by stroke and from an emotional consequence of the often resultant physically disabling condition and subsequent social disruption. One's reaction to illness and disability, to loss of function, to change in body image, and to role change and possible social alienation can give rise to reactions of grief, anger, guilt, and fear,[31] all of which contribute to a sense of social stigma[46] and produce a myriad of feelings that contribute to depression and anxiety. Indeed, stroke has been suggested to be "an overwhelming psychological event that triggers a depressive episode in predisposed individuals."[125]

If an individual seeks treatment early enough in the development of a nonhemorrhagic stroke, medication is available that may halt the progression of the stroke and even reverse the damage to the brain. However, the medication available is not without potentially fatal consequences. Whether the individual or the individual's family makes the decision for treatment with the medication, if the outcome is poor, the family may be left with feelings of anger and guilt in addition to feelings of grief. If the individual delayed seeking treatment and did not avail himself or herself of potential medication, family members may attribute blame to the patient for the condition with which they now must cope.[110]

Certainly physical recovery plays a major role in one's emotional reaction and in psychological adaptation. The actual experience of stroke, as it is happening, brings forth fear of the unknown and distress that this experience actually is occurring. Although the initial recovery phase may be marked by some improvement in one's physical status, a plateau period during which progress is slowed often follows and may lead to frustration and sadness. One's emotional recovery is marked by a mix of emotions, including uncertainty, hope, loss of control, anger, and frustration. Social recovery similarly is challenged, as one needs to adjust to changing roles, isolation, and the perceived dissonance between past and current/future life.[10]

Lack of control over one's body, fear and shock of the rapidity of the physical changes, and feelings of loss around three particular areas—activities, abilities, and independence—contribute to the emotional challenge of accepting that one's life is changed in significant ways.[42] One may argue that for individuals to make the transition toward recovery, they must assess the psychological meaning of loss as it relates to self-concept. How might the loss of ability as it affects activity engagement affect one's personal meaning of quality of life?[11] To eventually accept a changed self, one's self-concept goes through a process of transformation.

Framed in terms of stages, issues of recovery reflect the interplay among physical recovery, emotional recovery, and psychological adaptation. Although progress takes different forms for each individual, survivors tend to deal with common themes, and each has its impact on adaptation. It has been suggested that the transition from a healthy being to a stroke survivor occurs in stages. Keeping in mind that stroke survivors are often discharged home relatively quickly, there is great impact on family members and consequently everyone's role transition.[119]

To have a successful transition, there are stages in which the survivor and the family go through. One model suggests stages that include denial, which protect one from initial overwhelming emotion; grieving (as distinguished from depression), in which one mourns the loss of function; role transition, to include "care-receiver"; the development of optimal independence, which includes compensatory techniques and adjustment to a new body; rebuilding a social support system; and reintegration into the community via instrumental ADL.[11] It has also been suggested that there are three domains in recovery: physical, psychological, and social. Important to these domains is self-worth, which is related to participation and to quality of life. While stroke has great impact on cognition and physical function, it is also critical to address self-image and sense of being (psychological domain), and changes in relationships (social domain). As family members also change roles due to stroke, it is important to promote a positive self-concept and positive social support; both will have an impact on function.[119] The goal with each of these models is toward acceptance of any remaining disability and the return to a satisfying quality of life. See Chapter 3. Emotional reaction following stroke has significant implications for recovery. Feelings of helplessness or hopelessness affect survival rate,[63] apathy affects functional ability,[47] and depression and anxiety affect function and recovery.[2,14-16,45,50]

One's cultural background also may play a role in how one copes with illness, disability, and rehabilitation. As stated earlier, cultural values and attitudes may devalue any form of dependency. Consequently, a disability may add to feelings of alienation. From a cultural perspective, psychological conditions also may be viewed as a weakness of character. This further stigmatizes the individual and leads to the avoidance of acknowledging feelings and of being treated.[70]

Health professionals, without intending to do so, may become enablers of the loss of personal identity and dignity and contribute to a diminished self-esteem. When an individual is referred to in terms of a disabling condition (e.g., "a right hemi"), one's dignity and sense of personal worth are challenged. This adds to what may be emerging as a damaged sense of self within the context of social stigma. Many individuals go to great lengths to conceal their disabilities from others to avoid being identified as having had a stroke.[90] Although much has been written regarding the negative emotional reaction to stroke, the suggestion also has been made that for individuals whose lives ordinarily are characterized by crises, dealing with the consequences of stroke is not considered an extraordinary event but just another life change.[89] Although this challenges the general assumption that anyone who has experienced a stroke also will experience grief, loss, and distress,[96] considering the context of one's life in which stroke occurs is important.[66]

PERSONALITY CHANGE FOLLOWING STROKE

While it has been noted that a change in personality may follow a stroke, and this may be related to lesion location,[8] the change is characterized as any of the following types: aggressive, disinhibition, paranoid, labile, and apathetic.[33] Although some of the symptoms may appear to be consistent with the signs and symptoms of specific psychiatric conditions, they often emerge as negative emotions or behaviors that do not meet the criteria for particular diagnoses. These can range from euphoria to uncontrollable tears, from worry to agitation, from disinterest to hostility, or from paranoia and guarded behavior to excessive dependency. Despite the behavioral expression of these emotions, they tend not to reflect an underlying mood and may add to the embarrassment experienced by the patient.[8] These behavioral changes are particularly difficult for the caregiver to manage, and they do not respond to medication.[33]

Apathy is a common change that occurs, with some studies suggesting between 20% to 40% of stroke survivors display some apathetic behavior.[33] Although apathy can be a symptom of depression, it can also be a separate construct, occurs more frequently than depression, and affects rehabilitation and recovery.[43] By its very nature, the impact of apathy on energy and motivation clearly effects engagement in the recovery and rehabilitative process.

DEPRESSION

Among the most significant considerations in understanding the characteristics and consequences of stroke is the relationship of depression to onset, recovery, and rehabilitation of persons with stroke. Because of the neurophysiological changes and because of the reaction to the consequences of stroke, depression has major implications for the course of recovery. Despite the causes of depression, assessment and treatment of depression affects psychological, functional, and medical health.

The relationship between cerebrovascular disease and depression has long been studied. Depression is both a risk factor for stroke[33,55] and a major consequence of stroke.[126] For nearly three quarters of a century, the assumption held that depression following a stroke was related only to the functional and social consequences of the disability and not to the neurological damage of the stroke itself. Three decades ago, however, a study compared depression in individuals with stroke to individuals with orthopedic conditions, with both groups matched for functional ability. The significant increase of depression in the group with stroke led the researchers to believe that depression was related to something more than a reaction to functional inability.[35] More recent studies show that depression in stroke can occur at any time; during the acute phase, or two to three years later; and may not reflect functional independence.[127] It is also often accompanied by anxiety.[4] With the acknowledgment that depression is a major complication for individuals with stroke, attention is paid to both the prevention and treatment of poststroke depression.[41,126]

During the past three decades, links have been made between lesion location and depression onset. Past studies have noted that an association exists between lesion location, particularly left anterior lesions, with onset of depression during the acute phase; and an increased severity of depression the closer the lesion is to the left frontal pole,[62,96] and right parietal lesions with depression during the subacute period.[99] Studies suggest that there is not only a neuroanatomical basis of depression following stroke;[79] but also a pathophysiological basis for depression, which may result from a chemical change following brain infarction.[99,101] This avenue of inquiry continues, with attention recently being paid to lesions associated with vascular depression.[100] Lesion location is not without controversy, however. Studies have demonstrated that depression occurs in individuals without regard to location of lesion;[79] often occurs within the acute phase (first three months);[4] and despite its etiology (biological or psychosocial),[115] is a significant consequence of stroke and requires treatment.[116] It is important to view poststroke depression as multifactorial when planning treatment.[115]

Whether poststroke depression is characterized by depressive features or meets criteria for major depression,[33] there are implications for recovery and rehabilitation. Associated with poorer outcomes, as reflected by overall functional impairment, diminished quality of life, and mortality,[76] depression is specifically linked with increased impairment in ADL and is linked with more severe neurological deficits.[50] Any form of depression has an effect on functional status in individuals with stroke and that depressive symptoms; even in the absence of any depression diagnosis, it affects functional status.[45] The duration of depression varies from months to years.[6,14,62] Depression accompanied by cognitive impairment has a longer duration.[42] Any poststroke depression that does not remit leads to a poorer, long-term functional outcome.[15,16,88] In addition, changes in social support add to depression.[17]

Poststroke depression is characterized by unrelenting feelings of sadness, anhedonia, helplessness, worthlessness, and/or hopelessness; loss of pleasure or interest in all activities; change in appetite, weight, or sleep pattern; psychomotor retardation or agitation; loss of energy; loss of concentration; or suicidal ideation.[14,33] Indeed, suicidal ideation, although prevalent in individuals with a variety of acute medical conditions,[53] is also prevalent in medical conditions that become chronic. For individuals with stroke, the prevalence of suicidal ideation increases over time.[52]

Depression also may be characterized by isolative behavior and irritable, angry, or hostile expression. These symptoms can occur to a lesser extent and have a less debilitating effect. When the symptoms are less frequent and less severe, one may have a dysthymia disorder or minor depression.[1] A history of depression has been noted to be a risk factor for stroke,[30] a risk that may exceed the general risk by two to three times.[55] It also is a risk factor for not surviving a stroke.[30] Even an attitude of helplessness affects one's survival rate.[58]

Other psychological diagnoses sometimes are confused with depression, can occur concomitantly, and have a prevalence rate of between 19% and 22%. These diagnoses include apathy (low motivation and/or energy) and various anxiety disorders.[99]

Any form of depression can occur at any time following stroke, and the symptoms used to diagnose depression may depend on whether the depression onset is early or late.[87,114] Regardless of onset or symptom clusters, poststroke depression, whether related to the clinical diagnosis of depression or with the number of clinically significant symptoms associated with depression,[33,41,55,127] has been found to negatively affect the physical recovery from stroke[16] and independence in ADL.[15,16]

ANXIETY DISORDERS

It is well-documented that a significant comorbidity exists between poststroke depression and anxiety.[14] Anxiety disorders, most commonly generalized anxiety disorder, can emerge during any phase of recovery, from the acute phase to the rehabilitation phase. Like depression, the cause may vary. Although compelling evidence suggests anxiety is often a reaction to loss of anticipated or actual functional ability,[14] other evidence links early onset with a previous history of psychiatric conditions.[33] It also may accompany poststroke depression.[33]

Some instances of anxiety may have an anatomical basis and may be associated with left hemisphere lesions.[4] Emotional lability, characterized by extreme expression of emotion such as crying or laughing, but without the underlying feelings of sadness or depression, occurs independent of depression and may be associated with lesions in the anterior regions of the cerebral hemispheres.[99] Excessive worrying, restlessness, irritability and/or tension, and catastrophic reactions (sudden onset of anxiety, hostility, or crying) may be linked with lesion location, specifically the left posterior internal capsule, left cortex, and left anterior subcortex, respectively.[99] Regardless of its cause, anxiety tends to remain stable over time, while depression may decrease.[76] Anxiety, if coupled with depression, impairs functional ability; and by itself, affects quality of life and social functioning.[2,33]

Recent attention has been paid to recognizing post traumatic stress disorder (PTSD) in stroke survivors.

When conceptualizing stroke as an emotionally traumatic event, it is easy to see why it may give rise to symptoms consistent with PTSD. It has been estimated that PTSD occurs in as many as 30% of stroke survivors, the greatest risks related to number of previous strokes one has had, a premorbid negative affect,[72] and cognitive appraisals that also tend to be negative.[34,72] The onset of PTSD tends to occur shortly after the stroke event, as the risk diminishes with time. Anxiety and depression is not predictive of PTSD, although there is an association between number and severity of PTSD symptoms.[72]

Catastrophic reactions in which individuals experience sudden and extreme feelings of anxiety are related to anxiety disorders. Although these reactions typically occur after the acute poststroke phase, the responses may be in reaction to frustration and depression and have implications for rehabilitation.[14] Catastrophic reactions are distinguished from emotional lability in that an underlying emotion is associated with it. The affect expressed with emotional lability, that is, sudden outbursts of laughter or crying, is not associated with one's mood.[75]

OTHER PSYCHOLOGICAL/EMOTIONAL CONDITIONS

Psychotic conditions are rare consequences of stroke, but they can occur. Symptoms can include delusions and hallucinations,[94] paranoia, and mania.[59] Poststroke mania, for example, may occur in up to 2% of stroke survivors and might be related to a previous history.[33] There is some evidence that associates these symptoms with preexisting neuroanatomical risk factors, older age,[94] and lesion location.[99] Most psychotic conditions that emerge after stroke are believed to emerge in individuals with a history of psychotic conditions or in individuals predisposed to developing these conditions.[8]

Poststroke dementia, also known as multiinfarct dementia or vascular dementia, has been diagnosed in many individuals, although the consistency of diagnostic criteria has not been applied.[95] Depending upon the criteria used, anywhere from 6% to 32% of stroke survivors may have signs of dementia.[104] This is especially important, as the risk for dementia even 10 years poststroke is higher than in the nonstroke population.[104] Poststroke dementia occurs more frequently in those over 60-years-old.[104] It has been argued that memory loss need not be a criteria for dementia, particularly when one's executive functioning is impaired and one's mental speed is diminished. It has also been argued that dementia may have a slow onset, starting with cognitive disorders of the nondementia type.[95]

Cognitive deficits, even those not associated with dementia, are common consequences of stroke.[119] Although cognitive deficits may be related directly to lesion, the effect between depression and cognition is interactive, and distinguishing one from the other is sometimes difficult. Some evidence suggests that depression leads to cognitive impairment[81] that might be classified as a pseudodementia[9] and that these conditions can benefit from adequate treatment of depression.[31]

Cognitive ability is linked with one's ability to live independently, as it is directly related to one's ability to learn skills, have insight into one's condition, and to participate in the overall rehabilitation process.[119] Not surprisingly, cognitive ability is a significant predictor of functional outcome and the ability to live independently.[64,119] See Chapters 17, 18, and 19.

Being able to control one's emotions is an important characteristic, and emotional responses to situations or events are expected. Yet, for many stroke survivors, pathological laughter or crying occurs. It has been estimated that between 11% to 40% have this involuntary expression of emotion, an expression unrelated to a situation or event.[33]

Discreet expression of emotion is exhibited by many stroke survivors. While some have been associated with personality change, it has also been argued that emotions may be early indicators of psychological disorders. These emotions include sadness, passivity, aggressiveness, indifference, disinhibition, denial, and adaptation. While a previous psychiatric history is linked with these emotions, family history is not linked, nor is degree of impairment. Linking emotional behaviors to lesion location is inconclusive.[3]

It has been noted that people with stroke have a lowered self-esteem. Self-esteem, which reflects one's sense of worth, may assist or inhibit one's emotional adjustment to illness and disability.[121] While it may coexist with depression, it should also be viewed as a separate entity. Addressing issues of self-esteem has implications for recovery and function. Table 2-1 identifies the prevalence of some of these disorders.

BIOLOGICAL INTERVENTION

A number of factors are associated with the cause of psychological conditions following stroke. Social and psychological stressors play a major role in the development of these conditions, as do anatomical lesions. Despite the debate regarding the primary cause of psychological conditions, leading some to conclude that no evidence supports a single theory on the origin of psychological conditions in persons with stroke;[125] no debate exists regarding the importance of taking a bio-psycho-social approach in understanding and treating stroke, as psychological conditions take their toll on recovery and functional ability.

Medication is not sufficient to counter the effect of stroke on daily function,[16] but it is a critical weapon in the treatment of psychological conditions. Without regard to the cause of the conditions, a number of studies have been conducted to determine the use of psychopharmacological

Table 2-1

Psychiatric Conditions Associated with Stroke

CONDITION	APPROXIMATE PREVALENCE RATE IN ADULTS	APPROXIMATE PREVALENCE RATE IN CHILDREN	FEATURES
Poststroke depression	35%[14] Suicidal ideation: 7% during acute phase 11% within 2 years after stroke[56]	21%[67]	Features consistent with major (20% to 23%[4,102] in adults) or minor (21%[102] in adults) depression
Apathy	22% (half with no depression comorbidity[109]	—	Low motivation and/or energy Affects rehab and recovery, and happens more frequently than depression[43]
Personality change	20% to 40%[33]	17%[67]	Aggressive, disinhibited, paranoid, labile, and apathetic types of changes
Anxiety disorders	Generalized anxiety disorder: 21% to 28% during acute phase,[2] 22% 3 months after stroke[2] 13% with no depression comorbidity[2] PTSD: 30%[72] State of worry: 14%[12] Emotional lability: 18%[73] Catastrophic reaction: 19%[109]	31%[67]	Excessive anxiety and worry Reexperiencing symptoms Expressed anxiety but not fulfilling generalized anxiety disorder criteria Awareness of uncontrollable emotion (pathological laughing or crying) inconsistent with mood Sudden onset of anxiety, hostility, or crying
Attentional deficit hyperactivity disorder		46%[67, 68]	This includes inattention and apathy
Dementia	6% to 32%[104]	—	Cognitive deficits, including executive function, mental speed, and memory loss
Poststroke mania	2%[33]	—	Mood and thought disturbance

PTSD, post traumatic stress disorder.

agents in treating psychological conditions. Antidepressants have been used in individuals with depression or with pathological affect; benzodiazepines have been used for generalized anxiety disorder, with limited success because of side effects; and poststroke psychosis appears to respond to neuroleptic medication.[14,33]

A Cochrane review has examined the effect of medication on preventing and treating poststroke depression.[41] While many of the studies reviewed through metaanalysis have limitations that preclude definite recommendations, it appears that medication will not prevent poststroke depression,[41] but may be useful treating poststroke depression.[41] The opposite may be true for psychosocial interventions; it may be useful in preventing depression,[41] but not in treating depression.[41] Using medication, however, should be done with caution, as side effects can have significant consequences.[41]

COPING WITH ILLNESS, RECOVERY, AND REHABILITATION

The relationship between psychosocial factors and sustaining a stroke is compounded by the role emotion, personality, and culture have in how one copes with traumatic illness. Defense mechanisms, which serve to protect the individual from the overwhelming emotions that may arise, may add to one's difficulty in coping with illness and disability.[78] Defense mechanisms typically used include denial, which negates the reality of what is happening and has happened; avoidance, in which the individual is aware of what is happening and has happened but avoids the implications; regression, in which one exhibits increased emotion and/or increased dependent behavior not characteristic of one's developmental level; compensation, in which one becomes adept in an area to counter an inability of another area; rationalization, which provides reasons or excuses for not being able to accomplish tasks or goals; and diversion of feelings, in which unacceptable feelings are altered into socially appropriate behaviors.[31] How defenses are used also can give rise to how one is viewed by the treating therapist. The therapist may misinterpret behavior guided by maladaptive defense mechanisms and label the individual as a difficult patient.[78]

As the chronicity of the disability becomes apparent, the individual and one's social network must deal with the long-term effects of the stroke. Most immediate is the perceived change in oneself. Because role, lifestyle, and where one is in one's life cycle affect one's emotional reaction, trauma brings forth changes in what one can do and in how one sees oneself. Although time may enable one to develop the adaptive defenses necessary to deal with the anxiety surrounding illness, disability, and the unknown, one's psychological adaptation may be undermined if the symptoms are not alleviated. The resultant reaction to stress is often a universal loss of self-esteem followed by depression. Maladaptive uses of defenses may then ensue.[111]

Psychological adjustment to illness and disability also depends on personality constructs; consequently, individuals who have had strokes need to be understood from the perspective of their character traits, their cultural background, and the psychological consequences that are reactionary and physiologically based. Some evidence exists that personality characteristics play a role in the development of stroke, in the recovery from stroke, and in how one participates in treatment.

Almost a half a century ago, it was suggested that personality constructs characterize how one copes with illness and engages in treatment, and that health care professionals should understand and adapt their interactive styles based on the patient's character.[49] One approach to understanding personality is by using the classification system typical of those with personality disorders, such as the dependent and overdemanding personality, the controlling personality, or the dramatic personality. How individuals use those characteristics to cope with the stress and anxiety associated with illness can assist the therapist implement treatment.[78] For example, patients with compulsive personalities who ask for details and facts will benefit when the therapist provides adequate information to calm any anxiety, and when the therapist encourages the patient to take charge of certain aspects of treatment.[38] A second approach to understanding personality is based on coping styles used in stressful situations. This approach allows one to shape the rehabilitation process so that it reflects the patients' coping style.[19,96] A third approach is to identify whether an individual has certain emotional characteristics, characteristics which are thought to reflect positive

rehabilitation outcomes: ability for reality testing, ability to self-reflect, and ability to acknowledge and grieve for loss.[9] Individuals who have sustained a significant physical illness or injury are struggling with emotional crises and revert to using characteristics from past situations.[38] Understanding personality and its role in coping is critical for rehabilitation, for different styles promote functional adjustment and improved quality of life.[27]

Culture is a major determinant of one's beliefs and attitudes, plays a major role in how one perceives illness and disability, and may influence how one interacts with health care providers. The meaning one ascribes to illness and how one behaves toward illness may be a function of personal and cultural health traditions. Assuming the sick role, which demands that one adjust to the role of patient and then relinquish that role to resume independence, may be determined culturally. For some, one's cultural background may promote motivation toward rehabilitation and recovery; for others, it might obstruct progress. Culture dictates how one interacts in any social organization (a clinic or hospital is a social organization); how and when one communicates; how one deals with personal space, particularly as others intrude on it; and how one considers future goals.[108] Cultural habits may influence how one expresses oneself and, if one is reserved, may be misperceived as one being unmotivated, guarded, or disrespectful.[70] Like personality traits, one's cultural habits may be expressed as a means to deal with stressful situations.

It may seem logical for an individual who has suffered a stroke to be open with health care providers with one's feelings, goals, and concerns. In patient-centered practice, health care professionals expect to rely on patients to inform and instruct them as they evaluate and plan treatment for optimal occupational performance. However, some cultures prefer the health care provider to assume somewhat of an authoritarian role,[57] others may express respect through the avoidance of eye contact yet expect the health care provider to be solicitous in recognition of social worthiness,[37] and others may appear mistrustful and uncommunicative.[70]

Having a disability that challenges one's independence is particularly difficult for those individuals for whom independence, control, and individuality are important values.[70] Indeed, these attributes eventually may motivate one in the rehabilitative process but initially make it more difficult to deal with a trauma that robs one of these values. In addition, culture often prescribes the roles one assumes in a social or family structure. For these individuals, coping with role change becomes even more challenging.

The psychological conditions so prevalent following stroke are particularly difficult for individuals to deal with if their cultural heritage is intolerant of psychological conditions. Although some cultural groups rely on verbal expression and take pride in expressing their feelings, others are embarrassed to discuss personal issues with outsiders,[70] feel guilty if they share feelings with strangers, view any mental condition as one that would bring shame on a family, and expect only willpower and character to overcome psychological problems.[57] Psychological issues for some are viewed from a spiritual context, with the expectation of spiritual interventions.[37] For others, psychological issues are expressed in physical terms; headaches or backaches, for example, may be how one communicates depression.[56] For many individuals, the ability to accept treatment for a mental health condition happens only when all other interventions have failed.[57]

Cultural attitudes add to the emotional reaction one might have to the physical consequences of stroke and make one more resistant to understanding the psychological implications. One also must remember that not everyone from a particular cultural heritage shares the stereotypical cultural beliefs. The imperative, therefore, is that all health care providers understand what the meaning of illness and recovery is for individuals, from their particular personal and cultural perspectives.

RECOVERY

One of the most important contributors to any recovery process is motivation. Although psychological conditions, particularly depression and apathy, are often characterized by low motivation, personal traits influence one's determination toward recovery.

Four factors affect motivation: locus of control, self-efficacy, self-esteem, and social support.[25] Locus of control deals with where one places the influence of one's future. If, for example, individuals believe they can influence their health by eating right, exercising, and so on, then those individuals are viewed as having an internal locus of control. Individuals with an internal locus of control are thought to be more self-motivated. Self-efficacy relates to one's confidence in what one can do. A strong sense of self-efficacy motivates an individual toward accomplishing a goal. Too strong a sense of self-efficacy, however, may be reflected in misjudging one's capabilities, leading to frustration and anger.

Promoting individual control over lifestyle and by focusing on what one can do and work toward indeed may mediate the negative effects of disability and may promote psychological adaptation.[96,112] This is consistent with the social cognition model of setting personal goals within the context of appropriate outcome expectations, a model used successfully in rehabilitation.[97] Developing or maintaining a positive emotional outlook may mediate depression and lead to better functional outcomes.[84] Also important in the transition to recovery is an emphasis on health promotion. Because stroke survivors sometimes return to an unhealthy lifestyle,[97] fostering the psychological skills that can promote self-efficacy becomes even more important.

As previously noted, individuals with depression have difficulty with self-efficacy, and individuals with poststroke depression have more negative cognitions than do individuals without depression who have had a stroke. Although individuals with stroke tend to focus on what they can no longer do, they may not recognize those qualities and abilities they do have.[96] Given the effectiveness of cognitive behavioral approaches in treating depression, cognitive behavioral approaches have been suggested to be efficacious with poststroke depression.[81]

Self-esteem deals with one's perception of one's own worth. An adequate sense of self leads to pride of accomplishment and active participation in the recovery process. Coping strategies focused on personal worth and control help diminish the stress related to illness. These strategies include taking positive action to regain control of one's life.[10] Use of adaptive coping strategies that have worked in the past[30,78,96] also promotes adaptation.

Social support has a major influence on motivation. By not feeling isolated or abandoned, one is more likely to consider the future and work toward goals. The importance of social support to the recovery process cannot be understated. Individuals are able to cope better with their changed self and show adequate self-esteem when their social environment is perceived as adequate. Social support is considered essential in the initial recovery stage following stroke.[102] Psychological adaptation and improvement in function, even if affected by depression, is fostered when family is involved in rehabilitation efforts.[42]

One of the measures of quality of life is social participation.[22,63] If health is influenced by satisfaction with what one does, then engaging in and feeling competent in activity participation, both social and ADL, is often a positive sign.[24] Yet despite the return of or compensation for physical or cognitive functioning, most patients who have sustained a stroke report a decreased involvement in social activities.[42,82] Although there is some evidence that engaging in activities lessens as one ages and evaluating reduced participation in an older individual who has survived stroke from the context of normal aging is useful,[22] participation should always be a goal. Not being content with how one uses one's time may reflect difficulty reengaging in meaningful occupations and may contribute to either boredom or depression.[24] Diminished participation may also result from changed body image, the stigma of evident disability, and dependence on others for transportation as isolation and frustration results.[42] Although physical changes may set in motion the factors that can decrease social involvement, the resultant inability to resume previously held roles, inability to work, and diminished social interaction may have the greatest impact on quality of life.[10,82] Attention to social involvement after rehabilitation becomes especially important in the maintenance of function and in leading a meaningful and fulfilling life . Participation may reflect one's ability to do for oneself.[5] See Chapter 3.

Equally important, families are expected to cope with the immediate health needs and subsequent rehabilitation needs of the family member who has had the stroke, and sometimes they feel unsupported. This is especially true if there is poor communication between health care professionals and family members, or when family member's knowledge about the stroke survivor is ignored or devalued.[86] Entire families undergo role and status change, and for family members to experience depression and anxiety is not unusual.[122] Depression in the primary support person is higher than in the general population.[36] Families as a whole also perceive a decreased quality of life because their social and leisure activities are affected when a family member has had a stroke.[82] In addition, they are now meeting health care needs and not affection needs, which further affects their well-being. The shift in one's relationship can promote tension; a spouse no longer shares occupations, but instead assists with ADL.[24] When the needs of the family are addressed, an individual is better able to handle community reintegration. Family members need honest information, must have accessible health professionals, and must receive support for themselves.[118] Although social support for family members influences how satisfied they are with quality of life, the ability to problem-solve shapes depressive behavior.[41]

Children of stroke survivors can be especially vulnerable. Often, children participate in caregiving activities. For some children, this has positive consequences, as they may feel needed and responsible in a mature way;[117] however, between 30% and 50% of children of survivors exhibit behavior problems.[124] Specifically influencing how well a child of a stroke survivor does is the health status of the healthy parent, rather than the severity of the stroke and the health of the stroke survivor.[123,124] Caregiver strain and/or depression is linked with emotional health in the child.[123] Children, regardless of the severity of the parent's stroke, benefit from support from health care professionals.[123] Exhibited behavioral problems and depression can improve over time.[117,124]

Caregiver's Emotional Well-Being

It is becoming more and more apparent that the emotional health of caregivers, who are usually family members, is being compromised. Often referred to as caregiver burden or strain, the health status of caregiver impacts patient outcome, both functionally and emotionally. Although most caregivers are women and family members,[40] men assume this role as well. The caregiver is at great risk for stress, depression, and anxiety.[122] This may result from feelings of confinement and being overwhelmed with responsibilities,[47] having decreased energy, lack of sleep, dealing with ADL,[28] the sudden change in how one's family functions, changes in personal plans, the overall experience of loss,[47,122] and even unrealistic expectation caregivers have in what to expect.[24]

The caregiver/spouse, particularly if female, is at higher risk for depression due to diminished social interaction with friends and family.[54] Caregiver strain does not seem to change over time.[47]

Taking on the role of caregiver, whether forced or by choice, has emotional consequences for the caregiver, and functional consequences for the stroke survivor. Emotional health of the carer will impact the patient's functional outcome,[40,122] just as the patient's functional status may impact the carer's emotional well-being.[28,47,88] The carer's emotional health also impacts other family members, and emotional or behavioral consequences may be exhibited by children.[123]

Many studies have been done to ascertain the relationship of caregiver strain with factors such as hours spent in the caregiver role and physical and cognitive functional status of the patient. Studies on the relationship of burden to personal strain/stress and role strain have mixed results. Some studies support the notion that decline in the caregiver's health correlates with hours of caregiving,[28] the survivor's decreased ADL function, negative health status,[28,47,77] decreased cognitive ability, and compromised communication skills.[93] There is also evidence that caregivers of relatively functional stroke survivors, i.e., good physical and cognitive function, also have a high incidence of depression.[113] If there is a preexisting depression, it worsens as caregiver responsibilities increase.[28] This supports the notion that all caregivers, regardless of the health and functional status of the survivor, are at risk for emotional distress.

When the caregiver is a family member, one maintains three roles: caregiver, that client in the health care system, and family member.[122] These roles add to the psychological burden the carer experiences.[40] The role shifts required are shifts that affect the entire family, and as family function affects the stroke survivor's outcomes, intervention must include a focus on the family needs.[122]

The American Occupational Therapy Association has underscored the importance of addressing caregiver needs.[85] Much of the research on caregiver intervention is compatible with occupational therapists' domain of practice and should be considered when treating the stroke survivor. This research is not specific to Western countries, as caregiver strain is not bound by culture.[77,93,113] Two areas for intervention have been delineated: social support and participation, and coping strategies.

Social support is critical for caregivers.[28,118] Whether providing resources to assist the caregiver in carrying out responsibilities, resources to provide respite, or resources to simply give emotional support,[28,40,47] maintaining one's quality of life helps reduce or even prevent depression in the carer.[36] Social support plays an important role in reducing caregiver strain,[40,41] and assessing one's social network is the first step toward intervention.

Social participation is equally important. Women may be particularly vulnerable to the effects of decreased social participation, as assuming the role of caregiver may represent a dramatic shift from one's social routine.[54] Reports of participation of carers of patients from many diagnoses have noted that social participation and involvement with meaningful occupations contribute to the caregiver's well-being.[28,44] Community reintegration and social participation of survivors also helps caregivers.[47]

Various models of interventions for caregivers have been proposed and are all aimed at reducing and decreasing burden. Each pays attention to social support and participation. While studies support almost any intervention as positive in improving the psychological health of the carer and reducing the negativity associated with caring, the studies themselves are not methodologically rigorous. This has implications for the findings, but intervention should be provided, as there are positive effects.[26]

Coping strategies also contribute to the emotional health of the carer and begin when the stroke occurs. Just as the stroke survivor's personality and culture contribute to one's reaction to illness, they also have implications for how the individual handles stress and anxiety. Maladaptive coping styles, such as denial and self-blame, used by the caregiver lead to depression, but so might positive coping strategies, particularly early in the recovery process.[93] For example, positive coping styles can include planning, active coping, acceptance, and positive reframing. If planning is based on unrealistic expectations during the acute phase when progress is unpredictable, depression can develop.[93] Nonetheless, coping strategies have been effective in helping the caregiver adjust.

Emotion-focused strategies may be effective when dealing with problems. Positive coping styles[122,40] versus pessimism and negative styles may reduce stress, and addressing social problems may be more effective than social support.[40] Helping the carer set realistic goals when solving problems is also effective.[40,83,122]

Children with Stroke

Too often pediatric stroke is overlooked, and as a result, has not been extensively studied.[51] Two to three children in 100,000 are diagnosed each year,[46] although that estimate may be low,[65] as studies have suggested a rate as high as of 13 in 100,000 children, and one in 5000 live births.[2] Typically associated with clinical conditions, such as congenital heart disease, sickle cell anemia, and infection,[2,61,98] nearly three quarters of pediatric cases have no known preexisting condition.[61] Compounding the ability to diagnose children are "silent brain lesions" that may occur in as many as 20% of children with sickle cell anemia,[98] which affect cognition and behavior, and conditions that "mimic" stroke, such as hemiplegic cerebral palsy, and complicated migraine or seizure.[2]

Pediatric stroke is distinguished from adult stroke in other ways as well. Lifestyle, such as smoking, and risk factors, such as high blood pressure, are not associated with childhood stroke;[2] some studies report functional recovery to be better in children than adults due to the plasticity of the brain,[46] while other studies suggest almost all children who survive stroke have residual impairments[42] as the immature brain is more vulnerable to damage;[51] and survivors of childhood arterial ischemic stroke have poor outcomes.[7] Finally, lesion location does not seem to influence cognitive or psychological outcome.[2] While the most prevalent psychiatric disorder in adults is poststroke depression, which occurs in over 30% of the cases,[14] attentional deficit hyperactivity disorder is the most prevalent in children, occurring in 46% of the cases.[68] Children have impairments that affect a variety of functional domains and that limit activity involvement,[39] and when stroke is compounded by any number of psychiatric conditions, their functional ability is significantly impaired.[67]

The psychological implications of pediatric stroke may best be understood when considering that estimates of between 50% to 80% of all surviving children have attention, behavior, and quality of life deficits.[36,21] Being able to return to and complete school[50,51] is a goal for many survivors and appears to be an indicator of function. Nonetheless, psychological manifestations are apparent in many children and affect functional outcome.

It has been suggested that the child's emotional health is related to the parent's well-being, and that social emotional function and activity limitation are linked to a parent's increased emotional distress.[39] In addition, a family history of psychological conditions is an important risk factor for a child's psychiatric disorder.[67] A high rate of attentional deficit hyperactivity disorders (46%), anxiety disorders (31%), and mood disorders including depression (21%) occur in children.[67] Parents also report a personality change[67,86] and an increase of emotional difficulty and behavioral change.[21,86] Children who have a psychological disorder following stroke are more impaired functionally than those with stroke who do not have a psychological disorder.[67] These children are more impaired in IQ testing, academic functioning, and social functioning.[67]

Despite the barriers, children with stroke tend to have a good quality of life,[21] and many if not most return to school.[46] However, social functioning remains a concern, because of the residual intellectual and language challenges.[46] These children especially benefit when treatment is oriented toward "sameness," i.e., to ensure that the child perceives oneself not a different from one's peers, but similar in both function and in appearance.[7] Acceptance by one's social peer group is an important rehabilitation goal.

OCCUPATIONAL THERAPY PRACTICE

Throughout this chapter, reference has been made to the effect of psychological conditions and psychiatric disorders on recovery and rehabilitation. Personality traits[80] and levels of stress,[69,94] have been linked with mortality rates from stroke, as have severe forms of depression.[30] Personality traits related to self-esteem and coping style have been linked with ability to resume independence.[13,27] Participation in meaningful activities may be the best indicator of recovery.[5,19,22,28,46]

Depression and anxiety have perhaps the greatest impact on recovery and rehabilitation. Depression has been linked in general with recovery from stroke, with deficits in physical function,[50] and with deficits in impairment in daily living.[15,16,88] Even depressive symptoms without a clear diagnosis are linked to poorer functional status.[45] The presence of anxiety also reduces functional ability and diminishes social networks.[3]

Assessment and treatment of psychological conditions and psychiatric disorders is critical when working with individuals who have had a stroke and with their families. As reviewed elsewhere, studies have repeatedly demonstrated that medication is effective in the prevention[84] and treatment of these conditions[16] but should be coupled with psychological and social interventions.

In 2008, the American Occupational Therapy Association published its *Occupational Therapy Practice Framework*, 2nd edition.[103] Critical to the framework, which delineates the focus of practice and links evaluation and intervention with occupation, is the interdependency of performance in areas of occupation, skills, and patterns with context/environment, activity demands, and client factors. Key to the practice of occupational therapy is the understanding of how illness or disability affects occupation and how engagement in occupation depends on the interaction of physical, psychological, emotional, and social conditions.

When using the framework as a guide, one is compelled to evaluate all the patterns and skills necessary to engage in activity and occupation.[103] Ability to engage in everyday activities leads to participation in patient-selected contexts and results in satisfactory quality of life. Because quality of life is measured through physical, psychological, and social indicators,[63,120] the areas identified within this chapter require attention: personality traits; cultural attitudes and beliefs; psychological and cognitive consequences of stroke; emotional reactions to illness, disability, and recovery; and social context and support. This information has a direct bearing on the occupational profile developed, and it affects physical, psychological, and social functioning and the potential for independence.

The patient-centered focus of practice[103] is consistent with what should be the focus of evaluation and intervention. Patients measure success not by the therapist's standards but by their personal goals.[42] Indeed, the benchmarks that professionals use to determine functional ability is typically related to physical performance, whereas patients use quality of life measures.[10]

The Therapeutic Relationship

There is some evidence that psychosocial intervention may indeed prevent poststroke depression.[41] Given this, it is paramount to consider every interaction between the patient and therapist as a context for assessment and intervention.[96] The relationship that develops presents an ongoing opportunity to consider personal and social needs, to clarify and refine goals, and to address the ambient emotional conditions affecting progress. The relationship between therapist and patient may even predict positive functional outcome.[9] The therapeutic relationship begins the moment the patient and therapist interact. This may precede face-to-face contact, as each may have preconceived notions of what to expect. These notions may impede the therapeutic process if they lead to inaccurate or unrealistic assumptions, or they may facilitate the process if they promote the awareness of conditions and contexts that must be considered.

Fundamental to the relationship is respect, trust, concern for dignity, honesty, and the ability to be empathetic.[106] As the therapist and patient work to develop a collaboration that can result in optimal occupational performance, each needs to engage in the therapeutic process to provide meaning and value for the patient. Above all, this engagement is based on respecting the patient's individuality, making it possible for the patient to identify valued goals, and maintaining sensitivity for the fears, concerns, frustrations, and disappointments that emerge. A significant communicative tool in this relationship is empathy: the ability to convey an understanding of another's condition. Not to be confused with sympathy, pity, or identification, each of which can interfere with the therapeutic relationship,[20] empathy advances the helpful nature of the relationship. Conveying empathy, along with informing patients of the processes and rationale behind treatment, anticipating possible difficulties or obstacles, and soliciting social support from family or friends, improves cooperation and compliance in treatment.[107]

Evaluation

Evaluating the psychological conditions in an individual with stroke should be part of every therapist's assessment procedures. In addition to using specific measurement tools that target psychological and cognitive functions, the therapist should seek to answer a series of questions via interview of the patient and family and through observation. This process may be a challenge, particularly if speech, language, or visual spatial impairments are evident.

Psychological conditions may present at any time and with varying degrees of intensity. A change when participating in treatment (e.g., sudden disinterest in activities or goals, decreased energy, difficulty concentrating, increased worrying or agitation, or change in interpersonal interactions) may be indicators of the onset of depression or anxiety.

The mental status examination provides the initial and the ongoing evaluation of mental states. In addition to the examination providing a beginning assessment of a patient's cognitive state (orientation, memory, and attention), it provides the therapist with an assessment of mood and affect, speech and perceptual disturbances, thought processes, concentration ability, abstract thinking, judgment and insight, and reliability.[105] Although one's mental state can change from day to day, it is an important indicator of psychological functioning and provides the therapist with an understanding of the patient factors and performance skills that must be considered when planning treatment.

Character style plays a role in how one approaches illness and recovery, and as a result, understanding a patient's style should affect how the therapist interacts with the patient. If, for example, one is excessively dependent, the patient may be fearful of being left alone, abandoned, or unprotected and would benefit from the therapist's ability to set limits while conveying the intent to help. For those who require details and facts, the therapist should provide adequate information to calm any anxiety, while encouraging the patient to take charge of certain aspects of treatment.[38] Giving the patient a structured way of keeping track of progress outside of the treatment session would engage the patient in a productive way.

The following questions reflect the different personality styles that one may exhibit:[38]

- Does he/she need/demand special attention or appear particularly dependent?
- Does he/she seek out as many facts as possible about the illness or recovery?
- Is he/she particularly personable, and does the patient use charm to form relationships with the therapist?
- Does he/she dwell on difficulties and suffering and not react positively to good news?
- Does he/she overreact to criticism or feedback?
- Does he/she act in a superior manner or seem entitled to special status?
- Is he/she aloof, uninvolved, or appear excessively calm?

In addition to identifying personality styles, being able to identify who can and cannot cope may depend on a series of exhibited characteristics.[38] Table 2-2 lists the traits that reflect positive and negative coping characteristics.

To assess the meaning of illness, from a personal perspective and from a cultural perspective, is important. The meaning of health and illness may be related to having the physical and emotional capacity to do what one wants to do, when one wants to do it, and brings forth behaviors that support one's attitudes and values.[108] Personality and mental conditions may influence this assessment; depression, for example, may lessen one's energy, interest, and commitment to engage in treatment or plan for the future. In addition, how one values and manages time and space, illness and loss, role and family, and work and leisure; how one interacts with others; and most importantly, how one defines self-worth may be determined culturally.[70,108] Part of this process, however, is the recognition that the therapist is using one's own culture and personality through which to consider the patient, to define illness and health, and to develop a therapeutic relationship. Just as understanding the patient's personal and cultural view of illness and health is important to maintain a truly objective patient-centered approach, the therapist has an obligation for self-reflection on these same areas to avoid imposing one's own values and attitudes on evaluation and treatment.

Table 2-2

Characteristics of Coping[38]

POSITIVE CHARACTERISTICS	NEGATIVE CHARACTERISTICS
Focused on immediate problems	Intolerant of others
Flexible optimism	Excessive use of defenses such as denial or rationalization
Resourceful in selecting strategies	Impulsive judgments
Conscious of emotions that can impair judgment	Rigid or inflexible
	Tendency toward preconceived notions
	Passive

Intervention

Much has been presented on the likelihood of psychological conditions emerging at any point of the recovery and rehabilitation process. Indeed, such conditions can emerge after one is discharged home. While emotional needs should be addressed during rehabilitation, it is vital to assess one's emotional status near discharge,[17] as fears reemerge. Emotional distress of any sort, depression, and difficulty accepting one's condition all lead to diminished participation.[23] This is of concern since numerous studies have noted that meaningful engagement in activities and participation in one's community affects the stroke survivor's quality of life[5,10,24,63,82,119] and diminishes caregiver strain.[28,44,47]

The ability to cope with trauma and life-altering events is important in one's recovery. Coping strategies have been found to influence rehabilitation with many chronic conditions and may be affected by personality.[18] Coping may be focused on the meaning of an event or situation, the problems that need to be solved, or the emotions elicited. Using social support, behavioral strategies, and cognitive strategies enable one to deal with stressors.[17] This is consistent with other studies in which clusters of coping behavior have been categorized as active, passive, emotional, and avoidant,[27] or reflect defense mechanisms.[18] Effective coping bolsters a sense of self-worth, which adds to diminishing the stress of illness.[89] Facilitating coping styles that reflect positive emotion is also important in recovery.[83,84] Problem-solving coping strategies result in less distress, as does social support, information seeking, and engagement in activities. It is also useful to help the survivor use positive reinterpretation,[17] which, like the other coping strategies, reflect positive emotion.

Recognizing and addressing the symptoms of emotional and psychological issues should be part of all treatment approaches, and in all phases of care. Attention to self-esteem by building competencies, setting realistic goals, and planning for the future, is an important consideration. Specifically focusing on role transition[21] is also critical, as role satisfaction contributes to one's sense of self. Surprisingly, occupational therapists, despite knowing that practice includes addressing community participation, are not attending to this area when providing treatment.[19] Enabling one to engage in meaningful activities adds to quality of life. Working with family members, especially the caregiver, is important as they are at risk for psychological distress.

SUMMARY

From the initial onset of a stroke through the process of recovery, one follows an unpredictable path. The individual is faced with a plethora of choices and challenges that are as unexpected as they are difficult. One is asked to relearn the activities one has always taken for granted, to assume new roles that may be unfamiliar or that challenge one's self-worth, and to rewrite the future. Although patients aspire to return to their prestroke existence, their struggles are compounded by the emotional reactions to the loss of activities, abilities, and independence,[42] by the potential of social stigma,[88] and for some, by the real presence of psychiatric conditions.[14]

The psychological effects of stroke, whether directly related to the neurological insult or related to the emotional reaction to a disabling condition, must be assessed and treated to ensure optimal functional performance. Because stroke survivors are concerned not only with what they can do, but also with how others perceive and accept them,[96] addressing the psychological, social, and physical concerns with equal value results in a satisfactory quality of life.

REFERENCES

1. Amlie-Lefond C, Sébire G, Fullerton HJ: Recent developments in childhood arterial ischaemic stroke. *Lancet* 7(5):425–435, 2008.
2. Åström M: Generalized anxiety disorder in stroke patients: a 3-year longitudinal study. *Stroke* 27(2):270–275, 1996.
3. Aybek S, Carota A, Ghika-Schmid F, et al: Emotional behavior in acute stroke: the Lausanne emotion in stroke study. *Cogn Behav Neurol* 18(1):37–44, 2005.
4. Barker-Collo SL: Depression and anxiety 3 months post stroke: Prevalence and correlates. *Arch Clin Neuropsychol* 22(4):519–531, 2007.
5. Beckley MN: Community participation following cerebrovascular accident: impact of the buffering model of social support. *Am J Occup Ther* 60(2):129–135, 2006.
6. Berg A, Paolmski H, Lehtihalmes M, et al: Poststroke depression: an 18-month follow-up. *Stroke* 34(1):138–143, 2003.
7. Bernard TJ, Goldenberg NA, Armstrong-Wells J, et al: Treatment of childhood arterial ischemic stroke. *Ann Neurol* 63(6):679–696, 2008.
8. Birkett DP: *The psychiatry of stroke*, Washington, D.C., 1996, American Psychiatric Press.
9. Burbidge A: Recent advances in predicting the response to clinical rehabilitation. *Clin Med* 3(2):172–175, 2003.
10. Burton CR: Living with stroke: a phenomenological study. *J Adv Nurs* 32(2):301–309, 2000.
11. Buscherhof J: From abled to disabled: a life transition. *Top Stroke Rehabil* 5(2):19–29, 1998.
12. Castillo C, Starkstein S, Fedoroff J, et al: Generalized anxiety disorder after stroke. *J Nerv Ment Dis* 181(2):100–106, 1993.
13. Chang A, Mackenzie A, Yip M, et al: The psychosocial impact of stroke. *J Clin Nurs* 8(4):477478, 1999.
14. Chemerinski E, Robinson RG: The neuropsychiatry of stroke. *Psychosomatics* 41(1):5–14, 2000.
15. Chemerinski E, Robinson RG, Kosier JT: Improved recovery in activities of daily living associated with remission of poststroke depression. *Stroke* 32(1):113–117, 2001.
16. Chemerinski E, Robinson RG, Arndt S, et al: The effect of remission of poststroke depression on activities of daily living in a double-blind randomized treatment study. *J Nerv Ment Dis* 189(7):421–425, 2001.
17. Ch'ng A, French D, McLean N: Coping with the challenges of recovery from stroke long term perspectives of stroke support group members. *J Health Psychol* 13(8):1136–1146, 2008.

18. Cipher DJ, Kurian AK, Fulda KG, et al: Using the Millon Behavioral Medicine Diagnostic to delineate treatment outcomes in rehabilitation. *Clin Psychol Med Settings* 14(2) 102–112, 2007.

19. Cott C, Wiles R, Devitt R: Continuity, transition and participation: Preparing clients for life in the community post-stroke. *Disabil Rehabil* 29(20):1566–1574, 2007.

20. Davis CM: *Patient practitioner interaction: an experiential manual for developing the art of health care*, ed 3, Thorofare, NJ, 1998, Slack.

21. De Schryver E, Kappelle LJ, Jennekens-Schinkel A: Prognosis of ischemic stroke in childhood: a long-term follow-up study. *Dev Med Child Neurol* 42(5):313–318, 2000.

22. Desrosiers J, Bourbonnais D, Noreau L, et al: Participation after stroke compared to normal aging. *J Rehabil Med* 37(6):353–357, 2005.

23. Desrosiers J, Demers L, Robichaud L, et al: Short-term changes in and predictors of participation of older adults after stroke following acute care or rehabilitation. *Neurorehabil Neural Repair* 22(3): 228–297, 2008.

24. Doble SE, Shearer C, Lall-Phillips J, et al: Relation between post-stroke satisfaction with time use, perceived social support and depressive symptoms. *Disabil Rehabil* 31(6):476–483, 2009.

25. Drench ME, Noonan AC, Sharby N, et al: *Psychosocial aspects of health care*, Upper Saddle River, NJ, 2003, Prentice Hall.

26. Eldred C, Sykes C: Psychosocial interventions for carers of survivors of stroke: A systematic review of interventions based on psychological principles and theoretical frameworks. *Br J Health Psychol* 13(Pt 3):563–581, 2008.

27. Elmståhl S, Sommer M, Hagberg B: A 3-year follow-up of stroke patients: relationships between activities of daily living and personality characteristics. *Arch Gerontol Geriatr* 22:233–244, 1996.

28. Evercare & National Alliance for Caregiving Study of Caregivers in Decline: *A Close-up Look at the Health Risks of Caring for a Loved One Findings from a National Survey*, Bethesda, 2006, National Alliance for Caregiving.

29. Everson SA, Kaplan GA, Goldberg DE, et al: Anger expression and incident stroke: prospective evidence from the Kuopio ischemic heart disease study. *Stroke* 30(3):523–528, 1999.

30. Everson SA, Roberts RE, Goldberg DE, et al: Depressive symptoms and increased risk for stroke mortality over a 29 year period. *Arch Intern Med* 158(10):1133–1138, 1998.

31. Falvo DR: *Medical and psychosocial aspects for chronic illness and disability*, ed 2, Gaithersburg, MD, 1999, Aspen.

32. Feigin VL, Lawes CM, Bennett DA, et al: Worldwide stroke incidence and early case fatality reported in 56 population-based studies: a systematic review, *Lancet Neurol* 8(4):355–369, 2009.

33. Ferro JM, Caeiro L, Santos C: Poststroke emotional and behavior impairment: a narrative review. *Cerebrovasc Dis* 27(Suppl 1):197–203, 2009

34. Field EL, Norman P, Barton J: Cross-sectional and prospective associations between cognitive appraisals and posttraumatic stress disorder symptoms following stroke. *Behav Res Ther* 46(1):62–70, 2008

35. Folstein M, Maiberger R, McHugh P: Mood disorder as a specific complication of stroke. *J Neurol Neurosurg Psychiatry* 40(10):1018–1020, 1977.

36. Franzén-Dahlin Å, Larson J, Murray V, et al: A randomized controlled trial evaluating the effect of a support and education programme for spouses of people affected by stroke. *Clin Rehabil* 22(8):722–730, 2008.

37. Garcia-Preto N: Peurto Rican families. In McGoldrick M, Giordano J, Pearce J, editors: *Ethnicity and family therapy*, ed 2, New York, 1996, Guilford Press.

38. Gazzola L, Muskin P: The impact of stress and the objectives of psychosocial interventions. In Schein L, Bernard H, Spitz H, et al, editors: *Psychosocial treatment for medical conditions*, New York, 2003, Brunner-Routledge.

39. Gordon AL, Ganesan V, Towell A, et al: Functional outcome following stroke in children. *J Child Neurol* 17(6):429–434, 2002.

40. Grant JS, Elliott TR, Weaver M, et al: Social support, social problem-solving abilities, and adjustment of family caregivers of stroke survivors. *Arch Phys Med Rehabil* 87(3):343–350, 2006.

41. Hackett ML, Anderson CS, House A, et al: Interventions for preventing depression after stroke (review. *Cochrane Database Syst Rev* (3):CD003689.

42. Hafsteinsdottir T, Grypdonck M: Being a stroke patient: a review of the literature. *J Adv Nurs* 26(3):580–588, 1997.

43. Hama S, Yamashita H, Shigenobu1 M, et al: Depression or apathy and functional recovery after stroke. *Int J Geriatr Psychiatry* 22(10):1046–1051, 2007.

44. Hasselkus BR, Murray BJ: Everyday occupation, well-being, and identity: the experience of caregivers in families with dementia. *Am J Occup Ther* 61(1):9–20, 2007

45. Herrmann N, Black S, Lawrence J, et al: The Sunnybrook Stroke Study: a prospective study of depressive symptoms and functional outcome. *Stroke* 29(3):618–624, 1998.

46. Hurvitz EA, Beale L, Ried S, et al: Functional outcome of paediatric stroke survivors. *Ped Rehabil* 3(2):43–51, 1999

47. Ilse IB, Feys H, de Wit H, et al: Stroke caregivers' strain: prevalence and determinants in the first six months after stroke. *Disabil Rehabil* 30(7):523530, 2008.

48. Imber-Black E: Creating meaningful rituals for new life cycle transitions. In Carter B, McGoldrick M, editors: *Expanded family life cycle*, ed 3, Boston, 1999, Allyn & Bacon.

49. Kahana R, Bibring G: Personality types in medical management. In Zinberg N: *Psychiatry and medical practice in a general hospital*, New York, 1964, International University Press.

50. Kauhanen M-L, Korpelainen JP, Brusin E, et al: Poststroke depression correlates with cognitive impairment and neurological deficits. *Stroke* 30(9):1875–1880, 1999.

51. Kim CT, Han J, Kim H: Pediatric stroke recovery: a descriptive analysis. *Arch Phys Med Rehabil* 90(4):657–662, 2009.

52. Kishi Y, Robinson RG, Kosier JT: Suicidal ideation among patients during the rehabilitation period after life-threatening physical illness. *J Nerv Ment Dis* 189(9):623–628, 2001.

53. Kishi Y, Robinson RG, Kosier JT: Suicidal ideation among patients with acute life-threatening physical illness: patients with stroke, traumatic brain injury, myocardial infarction, and spinal cord injury. *Psychosomatics* 42(5):382–390, 2001.

54. Larson J, Franzén-Dahlin Å, Billing E, et al: The impact of gender regarding psychological well-being and general life situation among spouses of stroke patients during the first year after the patients' stroke event: A longitudinal study. *Int J Nurs Stud* 45:257–265, 2008.

55. Larson SL, Owens PL, Ford D, et al: Depressive disorder, dysthymia, and risk of stroke thirteen-year follow-up from the Baltimore epidemiologic catchment area study. *Stroke* 32(9):1979–1983, 2001.

56. Lee E: Asian American families: an overview. In McGoldrick M, Giordano J, Pearce J, editors: *Ethnicity and family therapy*, ed 2, New York, 1996, Guilford Press.

57. Lee E: Chinese families. In McGoldrick M, Giordano J, Pearce J, editors: *Ethnicity and family therapy*, ed 2, New York, 1996, Guildford Press.

58. Lewis SC, Dennis MS, O'Rourke SJ, et al: Negative attitudes among short-term stroke survivors predict worse long-term survival. *Stroke* 32(7):1640–1645, 2001.

59. Liu CY, Wang SJ, Fuh JL, et al: Bipolar disorder following a stroke involving the left hemisphere. *Aust N Z J Psychiatry* 30(5):688–691, 1996.

60. Lloyd-Jones D, Adams R, Carnethon M, et al: Heart disease and stroke statistics—2009 update: A report from the American Heart Association Statistics Committee and Stroke Statistics Subcommittee. *Circulation* 119(3):182, 2009.

61. Lo W, Stephens J, Fernandez S: Pediatric stroke in the United States and the impact of risk factors. *J Child Neurol* 24(2):194–203, 2009.

62. Lyketsos C, Treisman G, Lipsey JR, et al: Does stroke cause depression? *J Neuropsychiatry* 10(1):103–107, 1998.

63. Mackenzie AE, Chang AM: Predictors of quality of life following stroke. *Disabil Rehabil* 24(5):259–265, 2002.

64. MacNeill SE, Lichtenberg PA, LaBuda J: Factors affecting return to living alone after medical rehabilitation: a cross-validation study. *Rehabil Psychol* 45(4):356–364, 2000.

65. Massicotte MP, Yager JY: Stroke in children. First steps on the road to intervention. *Circulation* 119(10):1361–1362, 2009.

66. Mattingly CE, Lawlor MC: Disability experience from a family perspective. In Crepeau EB, Cohn ES, Schell BAB, editors: *Willard & Spackman's occupational therapy*, ed 10, Philadelphia, 2003, Lippincott Williams & Wilkins.

67. Max JE, Mathews K, Lansing AE, et al: Psychiatric disorders after childhood stroke. *J Am Acad Child Adolesc Psychiatry* 41(5):555–562, 2002.

68. Max JE, Mathews K, Manes F, et al: Attention deficit hyperactivity disorder and neurocognitive correlates after childhood stroke. *J Int Neuropsychol Soc* 9(6):815–829, 2003.

69. May M, McCarron P, Stansfeld S, et al: Does psychological distress predict the risk of ischemic stroke and transient ischemic attack? The Caerphilly Study. *Stroke* 33(1):7–12, 2002.

70. McGoldrick M: Overview: ethnicity and family therapy. In McGoldrick M, Giordano J, Pearce J, editors: *Ethnicity and family therapy*, ed 2, New York, 1996, Guilford Press.

71. McMahon R, Crown DS: Return to work factors following stroke. *Top Stroke Rehabil* 5(2):54–60, 1998.

72. Merriman C, Norman P, Barton J: Psychological correlates of PTSD symptoms following stroke. *Psychol Health Med* 12(5):592–602, 2007

73. Morris PL, Robinson RG, Raphael B: Emotional lability after stroke. *Aust N Z J Psychiatry* 27(4):601–605, 1993.

74. Morris PL, Robinson RG, Raphael B, et al: The relationship between risk factors for affective disorder and poststroke depression in hospitalised stroke patients. *Aust N Z J Psychiatry* 26(2):208–217, 1992.

75. Morris PL, Robinson RG, Samuels J: Depression, introversion and mortality following stroke. *Aust N Z J Psychiatry* 27(3):443–449, 1993.

76. Morrison V, Pollard B, Johnston M, et al: Anxiety and depression 3 years following stroke: Demographic, clinical, and psychological predictors. *J Psychosom Res* 59(4): 209–213, 2005.

77. Muraki I, Yamagishi K, It Y, et al: Caregiver burden for impaired elderly Japanese with prevalent stroke and dementia under long-term care insurance system. *Cerebrovasc Dis* 25(3):234–240, 2008.

78. Muskin P, Haase E: Personality disorders. In Noble J, editor: *Textbook of primary care medicine*, ed 3, St Louis, 2001, Mosby.

79. Nelson LD, Cicchetti D, Satz P, et al: Emotional sequelae of stroke: a longitudinal perspective. *J Clin Exp Neuropsychol* 16(5):796–806, 1993.

80. Ngo L, Latham NK, Jette AM, et al: Use of physical and occupational therapy by Medicare beneficiaries within five conditions: 1994–2001. *Am J Phys Med Rehabil* 88(4):308–321, 2009.

81. Nicholl CR, Lincoln NB, Muncaster K, et al: Cognitions and post-stroke depression. *Br J Clin Psychol* 41(3):221–231, 2002.

82. O'Connell B, Hanna B, Penney W, et al: Recovery after stroke: a qualitative perspective. *J Qual Clin Pract* 21:120–125, 2001.

83. Ostir GV, Berges I, Ottenbacher M, et al: Association between positive emotion and recovery of functional status following a stroke. *Psychosom Med* 70(4):404–409, 2008.

84. Ostir GV, Berges I, Ottenbacher M, et al: Positive emotion following a stroke. *J Rehabil Med* 40(6)477–481, 2008.

85. O'Sullivan A: AOTA's statement on family caregivers. *Am J Occup Ther* 61(6):710, 2007.

86. Paediatric Stroke Working Group: *Stroke in childhood. Clinical guidelines for diagnosis, management and rehabilitation.* Clinical effectiveness and evaluation unit, Royal College of Physicians, 2004 London (website). www.differentstrokes.co.uk. Assessed June 3, 2009.

87. Paradiso S, Ohkubo T, Robinson RG: Vegetative and psychological symptoms associated with depressed mood over the first two years after stroke. *Int J Psychiatry Med* 27(2):137–157, 1997.

88. Pohjasvaara T, Vataja R, Leppsvuori A, et al: Depression is an independent predictor of poor long-term functional outcome post-stroke. *Eur J Neurol* 8:315–319, 2001.

89. Pound P, Gompertz P, Ebrahim S: Illness in the context of older age: the case of stroke. *Sociol Health Illn* 20(4):489–506, 1998.

90. Pound P, Gompertz P, Ebrahim S: Social and practical strategies described by people living at home with stroke. *Health Soc Care Community* 7(2):120, 1999.

91. Prince M, Patel V, Saxena S, et al: No health without mental health, *Lancet* 370(9590):859–877, 2007.

92. Purtilo R, Haddad A: Challenges to patients. In Purtilo R, Haddad A, editors: *Health professional and patient interaction*, ed 6, Philadelphia, 2002, Saunders.

93. Qiu Y, Li S: Stroke: coping strategies and depression among Chinese caregivers of survivors during hospitalization. *J Clin Nurs* 17(12):1563–1573, 2008.

94. Rabins PV, Starkstein SE, Robinson RG: Risk factors for developing atypical (schizophreniform) psychosis following stroke. *J Neuropsychiatry Clin Neurosci* 3(1):6–9, 1991.

95. Rasquin SMC, Lodder J, Verhey FRJ: The effect of different diagnostic criteria on the prevalence and incidence of post-stroke dementia. *Neuroepidemiology* 24(4):189–195, 2005.

96. Remer-Osborn J: Psychologicalal, behavioral and environmental influences on post-stroke recovery. *Top Stroke Rehabil* 5(2):45–53, 1998.

97. Rimmer JH, Hedman G: A health promotion program for stroke survivors. *Top Stroke Rehabil* 5(2):30–44, 1998.

98. Roach ES, Golomb MR, Adams R, et al: Management of stroke in infants and children: a scientific statement from a special writing group of the American Heart Association Stroke Council and the Council on Cardiovascular Disease in the Young. *Stroke* 39(9): 2644–2691, 2008.

99. Robinson RG: An 82-year-old woman with mood changes following a stroke. *JAMA* 283(12):1607–1614, 2000.

100. Robinson RG: Vascular depression and poststroke depression: where do we go from here? *Am J Geriatr Psychiatry* 13(2):85–87, 2005.

101. Robinson RG, Chemerinski E, Jorge R: Pathophysiology of secondary depressions in the elderly. *J Geriatr Psychiatry Neurol* 12(3):128–136, 1999.

102. Robinson R, Murata Y, Shimoda K: Dimensions of social impairment and their effect on depression and recovery following stroke. *Int Psychogeriatr* 11(4):375–384, 1999.

103. Roley SS: Occupational therapy practice framework revision update. *Am J Occup Ther* 62(6):625–683, 2008.

104. Sachdev PS, Brodaty H, Valenzuela MJ, et al: Clinical determinants of dementia and mild cognitive impairment following ischaemic stroke: the Sydney Stroke Study. *Dement Geriatr Cogn Disord* 21(5–6):275–283, 2006.

105. Sadock VJ, Sadock BA, editors: *Kaplan and Sadock's synopsis of psychiatry*, ed 9, Philadelphia, 2003, Lippincott, Williams, and Wilkins.

106. Schwartzberg S: *Interactive reasoning in the practice of occupational therapy*, Upper Saddle River, NJ, 2002, Prentice Hall.

107. Sheridan CL, Radmacher SA: Significance of psychological factors to health and disease. In Schein L, Bernard H, Spitz H, et al, editors: *Psychosocial treatment for medical conditions: principles and techniques*, New York, 2003, Brunner-Routledge.

108. Spector RE: *Cultural diversity in health and illness*, ed 4, Stamford, Conn, 1996, Appleton & Lange.

109. Starkstein SE, Fedoroff JP, Price TR, et al: Catastrophic reaction after cerebrovascular lesions: frequency, correlates, and validation of a scale. *J Neuropsychiatry Clin Neurosci* 5(2): 189–194, 1993.

110. Stevens L, Schulman J: Neurological illness. In Schein L, Bernard H, Spitz H, et al, editors: *Psychosocial treatment for medical conditions: principles and techniques*, New York, 2003, Brunner-Routledge.

111. Strain JJ, Grossman S: Psychologicalal reactions to medical illness and hospitalization. In Strain JJ, Grossman S, editors: *Psychological care of the medically ill*, New York, 1975, Appleton-Century-Croft.

112. Stuifbergen AK, Gordon D, Clark AP: Health promotion: a complementary strategy for stroke rehabilitation. *Top Stroke Rehabil* 5(2):11–18, 1998.

113. Suh M, Kim K, Kim I, et al: Caregiver's burden, depression and support as predictors of post-stroke depression: a cross-sectional survey. *Int J Nurs Stud* 42(6):611–618, 2005.

114. Tateno A, Kimura M, Robinson RG: Phenomenological characteristics of poststroke depression: early-versus late-onset. *Am J Geriatr Psychiatry* 10(5):575–582, 2002.

115. Tharwani HM, Yerramsetty P, Mannelli P, et al: Recent advances in poststroke depression. *Curr Psychiatry Rep* 9(3):225–231, 2007.

116. Truelsen T, Nielsen N, Boysen G, et al: Self-reported stress and risk of stroke: the Copenhagen City Heart Study. *Stroke* 34(4):856–862, 2003.

117. van de Port IGL, Visser-Meily A, Post M, et al: Long-term outcome in children of patients after stroke. *J Rehabil Med*, 39(9):703–707, 2007.

118. van der Smagt-Duijnstee ME, Hamers JPH, Abu-Saad HH, et al: Relatives of hospitalized stroke patients: their needs for information, counseling and accessibility. *J Adv Nurs* 33(3):307–315, 2001.

119. Vanhook P: The domains of stroke recovery: a synopsis of the literature. *J Neurosci Nurs* 41(1):6–17, 2009.

120. van Straten A, de Haan RJ, Limburg M, et al: Clinical meaning of the stroke-adapted sickness impact profile-30 and the sickness impact profile-136. *Stroke* 31(11):2610–2615, 2000.

121. Vickery CD, Sepehri A, Evans CC: Self-esteem in an acute stroke rehabilitation sample: a control group comparison. *Clin Rehabil* 22(2):179, 2008.

122. Visser-Meily A, Post M, Gorter JW, et al: Rehabilitation of stroke patients needs a family-centred approach. *Disabil Rehabil* 28(24):1557–1561, 2006.

123. Visser-Meily A, Post M, Meijer AM, et al: Children's adjustment to a parent's stroke: determinants of health status and psychological problems, and the role of support from the rehabilitation team. *J Rehabil Med* 37(4):236–241, 2005.

124. Visser-Meily A, Post M, Meijer AM, et al: When a parent has a stroke: clinical course and prediction of mood, behavior problems, and health status of their young children. *Stroke* 36(11):2436–2440, 2005.

125. Whyte EM, Mulsant BH: Post stroke depression: epidemiology, pathophysiology, and biological treatment. *Biol Psychiatry* 52:253–264, 2002.

126. Whyte EM, Mulsant BH, Rovner BW, et al: Preventing depression after stroke. *Int Rev Psychiatry* 18(5):471–481, 2006.

127. Whyte EM, Mulsant BH, Vanderbilt J, et al: Depression after stroke: a prospective epidemiological study. *JAGS* 52(5):774–778, 2004.

128. Williams J, Nieto J, Sanford C, et al: The association between trait anger and incident stroke risk: the Atherosclerosis Risk in Communities (ARIC) Study. *Stroke* 33(1):13–19, 2002.

timothy j. wolf
carolyn m. baum

chapter 3

Improving Participation and Quality of Life through Occupation

key terms

client-centered care   participation   quality of life
occupation

chapter objectives

After completing this chapter, the reader will be able to accomplish the following:

1. Describe key concepts of participation, occupation, and quality of life in stroke.
2. Understand key measures occupational therapists can use to address participation, occupation, and quality of life in practice.
3. Address participation in the continuum of care from the acute episode to community reintegration.
4. Describe barriers that threaten participation and quality of life.
5. Identify the key role that therapists have in fostering participation through occupation.

CONCEPTS CENTRAL TO ENABLING PARTICIPATION

In the *Occupational Therapy Practice Framework*, second edition, the definition of "participation" is adopted from the World Health Organization definition in the International Classification of Functioning, Disability, and Health (ICF) and is said to be the "*involvement in a life situation.*"[2,59] The term *participation* encompasses the concepts of personal independence and social and community integration.[59]

Participation must be considered across the life span. A child plays with friends, engages in sports, goes to school, and is a member of a family; an adult participates in family, work, leisure, and community activities; an older adult may want to continue to work, to travel, to do volunteer work, and to spend time with family. These activities reflect the individual's desire to participate fully in society, performing the occupations that are meaningful and important to them

Participation is supported or limited by the physiological, psychological, cognitive, sensory, and motor capacities of the individual. Likewise, participation is supported or limited by environmental factors. Obvious environmental factors include the physical and social factors associated with accessibility and access to social support; others include governmental and organizational policies, especially as they affect employment.

Participation is easily taken for granted. Being able to do what one wants to do, go where one wants to go, and have freedom in the choice of activities at the time at which one wants do them is central to personal independence. Participation can be compromised after a stroke. Others obviously see that an individual's participation will be difficult if mobility problems impair balance or if the individual uses a wheelchair and faces stairs, narrow doorways, and steep inclines. What may not be so obvious are impairments not so visible, such as spatial neglect, depression, and loss of executive control.

In recent years, the concept of participation has become much more visible, for it is a central concept in the new *Occupational Therapy Practice Framework*, second edition (Framework-II) and ICF. Within the Framework-II, supporting health and participation through in engagement in occupation is defined as the overarching goal of occupational therapy intervention.[2] The ICF defines health as the interaction of body function with engagement in activity and participation as influenced by environmental factors and personal choice (Fig. 3-1).[59] The link between health and participation, as defined by these two frameworks, will eventually lead professionals from all of the health fields to eventually organize their services to support participation. One must understand some key concepts to practice with participation as a central concept and outcome. These terms include *occupation*, *client-centered care*, and *quality of life*.

OCCUPATION

To participate fully in a life that has meaning, independence, and choice, the individual engages in "occupations." *Occupation* has been defined as the "ordinary and familiar

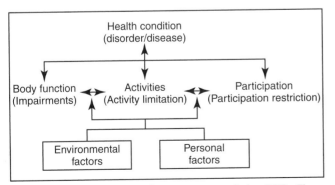

Figure 3-1 Interaction of components of the ICF. (From International Classification of Functioning, Disability, and Health, 2001: World Health Organization, pg. 18, Figure 1.)

things that persons do every day."[16] Occupations have purpose, and perhaps most importantly, they have meaning for the person engaged in them. When individuals engage in occupations, they are engaged in activities that are directed by goals or are purposeful, are performed in situations or contexts that influence them, can be identified by the doer and others, and are meaningful.[15]

Occupations usually are classified into general categories; the most common classifications fall into the domains of work (or productivity), play or leisure, and self-maintenance (also referred to as self-care and instrumental tasks). These categories account for the cycle of activities that constitutes the typical day, regardless of the culture being studied.[39]

Work

Work contributes significantly to life satisfaction, well-being, self-worth, and social identity following stroke.[4,30,46,52] Work is difficult to classify, for what is work to one may be play or leisure to another. Primeau points out that some may derive relaxation and enjoyment in performing household chores, whereas others detest the experience.[44] She asks readers to consider professional athletes who are paid well to exhibit their skills in tennis, golf, baseball, hockey, and other sports. These same occupations are pursued by amateurs as freely chosen recreational and leisure pastimes. The Canadian Association of Occupational Therapists has used the term *productivity* as a more useful alternative to *work*. Productivity is defined as "those activities and tasks which are done to enable the person to provide support to the self, family, and society through the production of goods and services."[12]

Play/Leisure

Play is a term used interchangeably with *leisure* to describe the nonwork activities of adults in addition to play as the chosen activities of children. Takata asks one to consider that play is not defined by specific behaviors or activities but rather by attitudes and behavioral styles.[47] Because of these characteristics, playfulness (or moments of play) can be experienced during (or enfolded within) work. Play and leisure must be considered central to the activities of individuals following stroke.

Leisure is thought to be a class of activities carried out in discretionary time.[22] Freedom of choice in participation without a particular goal other than enjoyment seems to be the defining characteristics of leisure activity.[25] No one can imagine lives devoid of play or leisure, and neither should a person who has had a stroke. That person's engagement in play and leisure should be enabled with tools, skills, and environments (see Chapter 29).

Self-Care

Those activities necessary for maintenance of the self within the environment constitute another major classification of occupation. Often included in this category are activities related to personal care (eating, grooming, and hygiene), getting around (mobility), and communicating. For a person to be self-reliant in any community, a level of competence is required that enables the accomplishment of tasks beyond those of basic self-care (which are referred to as physical self-maintenance). For this reason, M. Powell Lawton identified the use of the telephone, food preparation, housekeeping, laundry, shopping, money management, driving or use of transportation, and medication management as important daily activities and proposed the term *instrumental activities of daily living* (ADL) to describe them[35] (see Chapters 14, 21, 22, 23, and 28).

Often when persons are hospitalized, the focus is on achieving independence in self-care. Christiansen suggested that self-care tasks must be viewed as necessary from a societal point of view.[14] Although eating and hygiene tasks are essential for survival and health, dressing and grooming are important to social interaction and participation. Some expect persons to care for themselves. Sometimes therapists go too far in expecting an individual to perform self-care; some individuals prefer to spend their time in other occupations and accept the help of others to do basic self-care. Therapists are familiar with the use of personal attendants with persons following spinal cord injuries; persons who have had a stroke benefit from a personal attendant, so that they have choice in how they spend their time in occupations more important and meaningful to them.

A discussion of occupation cannot be complete without a discussion of self-efficacy and self-determination. Bandura used the term *self-efficacy* to describe the extent to which successes or failures influence expectations of future success or failure.[3] The experience of success in doing things (occupations) contributes to a positive sense of oneself as effective or competent. In contrast, a negative view of self and one's ability to influence events can lead to perceptions of helplessness. Gage and Polatajko observed that perceived self-efficacy has been shown to influence perseverance and well-being and that it can be modified through successful experiences.[21]

According to self-determination theory, intrinsic sources of motivation lead persons to encounter new challenges.[45] An important (and logical) part of this theory is the claim that settings in which persons experience success helps them feel good about themselves. This enables persons to face their daily challenges more readily and in the process to develop an understanding of who they are and their place in the world.

Following stroke, many individuals are not able to engage in their occupations as they have in the past. Therapy must create the environment for learning that fosters a person's view of self so that successful experiences can be experienced and sustained. Opportunities

for success must be fostered as well, so that these persons are motivated to face their daily challenges.

Occupation is a concept that must be understood in terms of planning and describing the activities of an individual; it provides an important process that can and should be used in the rehabilitation program to improve a person's recovery. Box 3-1 highlights key statements that identify the importance of occupation; these can be translated directly into outcomes that practitioners can address today as they plan client-centered care.

CLIENT-CENTERED CARE

Clients who have had strokes need support to return to their lives as they lived them before the stroke. They require services that help them build endurance, increase movement and strength, increase awareness, obtain assistive devices such as wheelchairs and self-care tools, acquire accessible housing, and gain access to barrier-free workplaces and communities. These needs challenge rehabilitation professionals to extend their interventions beyond the clients' immediate impairments to focus on their long-term health needs by helping them develop healthy behaviors to improve their health and well-being and to minimize long-term health care costs associated with dysfunction.[7]

Rehabilitation traditionally has occurred in institutions and is a time-limited process aimed at helping a person with a stroke reach an optimum level of self-care function. This approach labels the recipient of service as a patient, has led the patient to understand that the therapist would

---

Box 3-1

The Importance of Occupation

- Occupation is the vehicle to acquire, maintain, or redevelop skills necessary to fulfill occupational roles and to provide satisfaction.[20]
- The lack of occupation leads to a breakdown in habits and physiological deterioration, which lead to loss of ability and competency to support daily life.[28]
- Individuals with cognitive loss who remain engaged in occupations retain higher levels of functional status and demonstrate fewer disturbing behaviors.[6]
- Engagement in individually motivating and ongoing occupations supplies sustenance for survival, safety, and enhanced health.[54]
- Meaningful occupations provide individuals with exercise to maintain homeostasis and to keep body parts and neuronal physiology and mental capacities functioning at peak efficiency and enable maintenance and development of satisfying and stimulating social relationships.[54]

fix the problem, and has led the therapist to expect patients and their families to comply with his or her recommendations.[38] This approach does not reflect client-centered care. Within the Framework-II, client-centered care must begin with the occupational therapist gathering information to understand what is currently important and meaningful to the client before beginning to address any impairments.[2] To move from the traditional approach to a client-centered approach, practitioners must shift from focusing on impairments to understanding why problems occur, what the client views as a problem, and what might be done about them.

A client-centered approach requires a different orientation, one that engages the assistance and support of a therapist to facilitate the client's problem-solving and goal achievement.[38] In a client-centered program, the practitioner and the client bring important information to the partnership. For clients to understand why the practitioner is involved in their care and what they can expect to achieve through therapy is as important as for the therapist to understand the issues and needs of the clients. For clients to understand the scope of the therapist's knowledge is also important. The client's knowledge of his or her condition and experience with the problem must become clear for the relationship to progress. If a person has a cognitive limitation, the person selected to be the guardian or caretaker must participate in treatment planning[7] to ensure protection of the client's rights.

Early in the interaction, practitioners should obtain information from clients about their perception of the problem, needs, and goals. The implementation of a client-centered approach requires the use of a top-down approach[37,49] in which clients identify what they perceive to be the important issues causing them difficulty in carrying out their daily activities in work, self-maintenance, leisure, and rest.[7]

A client-centered approach requires practitioners to view clients in the contexts of their lives and help them not only to acquire the skills to handle the immediate issues influencing their health but to also learn strategies and link with community resources that promote, protect, and improve their health over the long term. This approach extends from the agency or institution into the community, requiring the practitioner to take an active role in advocating for healthy communities by removing attitudinal, economical, and physical barriers.[7]

QUALITY OF LIFE

How do we think about the quality of our lives? In a recent discussion the authors had with students, not one student mentioned quality of life issues related to his or her health. Students' descriptions included being satisfied with their lives and doing what they want to do when and how they want to do it. In other words, they were expressing terms that relate to life satisfaction, well-being, and participation.

Rehabilitation professionals must think about their clients in terms of what will be the outcome of services as they affect the daily lives of the clients they serve, not merely the outcome achieved in a short-term goal. The client's perceived quality of life is increasingly being used as a determinant of outcome in health care.[2] Quality is not achieved with improved strength, range, coordination, and balance but by having meaningful relationships, having a job, being a good parent, and engaging in leisure interests, all which depend on having cognitive capacity, strength, endurance, and mobility and may require new skills and new ways of doing things.

The concept of life satisfaction is subjective; what is satisfying to one is not necessarily satisfying to another. The concept reminds one of the importance of implementing a client-centered plan to help the person do what he or she wants and needs to do. The concepts central to life satisfaction are happiness, having plans for the future, and engaging in meaningful interests and experiences.[42] All of these concepts are threatened when an individual's life changes abruptly with a stroke.

Well-being is one of the concepts that contributes to the individual's perception of quality of life. In addition to happiness, well-being includes the person's perception of confidence and self-esteem. Wilcock encourages practitioners to consider relationships (including social friends, family, partnerships, neighbors, and strangers) and the availability of surroundings (including home, school, place of worship, peace, and weather and terrain) as central to the individual's perception of well-being.[54] The World Health Organization Quality of Life Group defines *quality of life* as one's perceptions of one's position in life in the context of the culture and value systems in which one lives and in relation to one's goals, expectations, standards, and concerns.[61]

Being able to go where one wants to go and do what one wants to do is central to personal freedom. Participation should be the ultimate goal of medical and rehabilitative care and social services, for it describes the extent to which a person is engaged in life situations in a societal context.[59] Interventions must help clients participate in daily life, enabling them to develop the skills or build the adaptive strategies to do what is necessary for them to carry out their occupational roles. Practitioners carrying out their roles and doing what clients want and need them to do makes it possible for them to play a role in the clients' life satisfaction and sense of well-being. Such an approach contributes to the health and well-being of clients, and collectively to society, for it enables quality in the lives of those served.

With the revisions to the ICF, activity and participation have become issues central to care and must be included in treatment planning.[59] Effective rehabilitation treatment begins with a sound assessment. In addition to determining the physical, cognitive, and psychological problems resulting from stroke, one must determine the client's prior activities to establish the individual's identity, so the person's interests are clear to all members of the team, for these interests serve to motivate the person during the rehabilitation.

ASSESSMENT OF PARTICIPATION

A variety of measures are available to determine a client's prior level of activity.[33] Traditionally, therapists have relied on activity checklists and open-ended interviews to obtain information regarding participation before stroke. Unfortunately, these interviews are limited by the client's memory. Measures have been developed to provide therapists with a systematical and consistent method for evaluating participation. One such measure is the *Activity Card Sort*, second edition, developed by Baum and Edwards (Fig. 3-2).[5] The Activity Card Sort uses a sorting methodology to assess participation in 89 instrumental, social, and high- and low-demand physical leisure activities. Clients sort the cards into different piles to identify activities that were done before stroke, those activities

they are doing less often, and those they have given up since their stroke. The Activity Card Sort uses cards with pictures of tasks that people do in their daily lives.

These activities are documented in categories of instrumental, leisure, and social activities. Different versions of the card sort are available for the different contexts in which rehabilitation is occurring. The institutional version (for use in hospitals and nursing homes) sorts 89 cards into categories of activities done before illness and not done afterward. The recovering version identifies activities not done before the illness or injury, those given up because of illness, those one is beginning to do again, and those activities the client is doing now. All versions allow one to determine a current activity level. The card sort takes approximately 30 minutes to administer and results in a score of percent of activities retained. The Activity Card Sort has been found to be a reliable and valid measure and is available in several culture-specific formats.[27]

The *Canadian Occupational Performance Measure*, or COPM, is an interview used to assess a client's perception of recovery and goals.[32,34] The COPM is based on a client-centered practice framework. The COPM crosses all diagnoses and is not specific to any age group. The three primary areas identified are self-care, productivity, and leisure. The interview allows identification of problem areas. Satisfaction and importance of the problem areas are

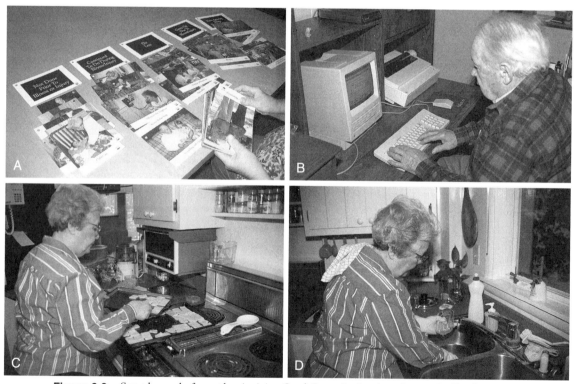

Figure 3-2   Sample cards from the Activity Card Sort. **A,** Sorting the cards. **B,** Computer card. **C,** Cooking card. **D,** Dishwashing card.

rated on a scale from 1 to 10. The COPM takes approximately 45 minutes to administer, but time can vary greatly with the interview. For this reason, the test may be difficult with individuals with cognitive deficits. Despite the length and cognitive difficulty, the assessment validity is good, and the COPM is a client-centered tool that facilitates development of treatment plans and therapeutic goals.[13]

The *Community Integration Questionnaire* was originally designed for individuals with traumatic brain injury and is particularly useful with younger stroke clients.[55] The Community Integration Questionnaire measures handicap as a function of community integration.[36] The questionnaire has 15 items including questions such as "Who does the shopping in your household?" and "How many times a month do you leave the house to go shopping?" Four scores are calculated: home integration, community integration, productivity, and a total score. Each item has a possibility of three responses, with responses weighted numerically. A higher score indicates greater independence.

ASSESSMENT OF QUALITY OF LIFE

The stroke outcome literature historically has reported survival from stroke. Medical advances may prolong life, but knowing how individuals feel regarding their lives after stroke is important.[39] A normal neurological examination may not equate to good quality of life for the client. Therefore, well-designed quality of life measures are essential.

The *Reintegration to Normal Living*[57,58] was developed to document reentry into everyday life following a sudden illness or event. The instrument is a functional status measure that quantitatively assesses the degree of reintegration to normal living achieved by clients after illness or trauma and is useful for individuals with physical or cognitive disabilities. The Reintegration to Normal Living assesses global function and the individual's satisfaction with basic self-care, in-home mobility, leisure activities, travel, and productive pursuits. The client is provided with 11 statements. Some examples include "I am able to participate in recreational activities," "I assume a role in my family that meets my needs and those of the other family members," and "I am comfortable with how my self-care needs are met." The test can be completed using a pencil and paper format or an interview format. Reliability and validity have been established for persons with stroke.

The *Medical Outcomes Study 36-item Short-Form Health Survey*, or SF-36, is the most commonly used life satisfaction scale.[53] The SF-36 has been used extensively with many diagnoses, including stroke, and is quick and easy to administer. The SF-36 is a self-report measure of eight subcategories: physical functioning, physical role limitations, bodily pain, general health perceptions, energy/vitality, social functioning, emotional role limitations, and mental health.

Another quality of life scale is the *Stroke Impact Scale* (SIS). The SIS is a stroke-specific measure that incorporates function and quality of life into one measure.[31] The SIS III is a self-report measure including 59 items that form eight subgroups: strength, hand function, basic and instrumental ADL, mobility, communication, emotion, memory and thinking, and participation. Duncan and colleagues have found the SIS to be valid, reliable, and sensitive to change in stroke populations.[19] Furthermore, the SIS is reliable when responses are provided by proxy.[18]

The *Stroke Adapted Sickness Impact Profile* (SA-SIP) is a shortened form of the more commonly known Sickness Impact Profile.[9,51] The SA-SIP has 30 true/false statements regarding a person's function and stroke-related symptoms. The statements are separated into seven categories: body care and movement, social interaction, mobility, emotional behavior, household management, alertness behavior, and ambulation. The SA-SIP has good reliability and validity

The World Health Organization Quality of Life Scale (WHOQOL-BREF)[40] was derived from the original WHOQOL-100. It includes 26 items as compared to the original with 100 items. It produces scores for four domains related to quality of life: physical health, psychological health, social relationships, and environment. It also includes one facet on overall quality of life and general health. It has been translated into multiple languages (Table 3-1).

BARRIERS TO PARTICIPATION AND QUALITY OF LIFE

Once the practitioners identify problems with participation and quality of life, they must address barriers to resumption of activities, which can be divided into several subgroups, including disability in basic and complex instrumental ADL, decreased cognition, impaired motor function and balance, limited mobility, urinary incontinence, poor speech and language function, depression, decreased resource use, environmental inaccessibility, and diminishing social and community support. Each is discussed to highlight how rehabilitation can address the issues that may limit an individual's participation after stroke.

Persons who have had a stroke have impairments that limit their ability to participate in activities outside the home. To go to the grocery store or to church, the individual must be dressed. Dinner with friends requires the motor ability to feed oneself, the cognitive capacity to carry on a conversation, and the judgment to select the appropriate diet. Difficulty with instrumental or more complex ADL affects the person's ability to return to work, to drive, to manage finances, or to take the bus. See Chapters 21 and 23.

Table 3-1

Summary of Tests and Availability

NAME OF TEST	REFERENCE	TIME TO ADMINISTER	SOURCE
Participation measures			
Activity Card Sort	5	30 minutes	American Occupational Therapy Association, AOTA Press
Canadian Occupational Performance Measure	13	approx 45 minutes	Law M, Baptiste S, Carswell A, et al: *Canadian occupational performance measure manual*, ed 3, Ottawa, 1998, CAOT Publications ACE.
Community Integration Questionnaire	55	10 minutes	Willer B, Rosenthal B, Kreutzer JS, et al: Assessment of community integration following rehabilitation for traumatic brain injury, *J Head Trauma Rehabil* 8(2):75–87, 1993.
Quality of life measures			
Stroke Adapted Sickness Impact Profile	51	15 minutes	van Straten A, de Haan RJ, Limburg M, et al: A stroke-adapted 30–item version of the Sickness Impact Profile to assess quality of life (SAS-SIP30), *Stroke* 28(11):2155–2161, 1997.
Stroke Impact Scale Version 3	19	30 minutes	User agreement and forms available at the following website: www2.kumc.edu/coa/SIS/Stroke-Impact-Scale.htm.
Reintegration to Normal Living	57	10 minutes	Wood-Dauphinee SL, Opzoomer MA, Williams JI, et al: Assessment of global function: the Reintegration to Normal Living Index, *Arch Phys Med Rehabil* 69(8):583–590, 1988.
Medical Outcomes Study Short-Form Health Survey (SF-36)	53	15 minutes	RAND Corporation, Santa Monica, California.
World Health Organization Quality of Life Scale (WHOQOL-BREF)	40	10 minutes	World Health Organization, 1993

Even in the absence of motor impairment, a cognitive deficit can greatly impair the ability of an individual to return to tasks done before the stroke.[23] Cognitive deficits incorporate areas of attention, orientation, perception, praxis, visuomotor organization, memory, executive function, problem solving, planning, reasoning, and judgment.[29] Tatemichi and colleagues showed that cognitive dysfunction was a significant predictor for dependent living after discharge and found that quality of life is related to sequential aspects of behavior.[48] Reading the newspaper, watching a movie, finding items on a grocery list, or knowing what to do if lost in the mall can be a challenge for some individuals following stroke.[26] Clients often report feeling overwhelmed with things that came automatically before the stroke. See Chapters 17, 18, and 19.

Impaired balance is cited in the literature as a key variable to independence in the community because of an increased risk of falls. For someone with impaired balance, a trip to the kitchen for a drink of water is a daunting task. Taking out the trash or resuming bowling may provoke enough fear to stop these activities. Addressing balance impairments in the hospital setting may not transfer to ability in the community, so testing of the individual's abilities outside of a sheltered rehabilitation clinic is essential. Decreased motor function and coordination contributes to poor participation in prior activities by limiting the ability to write, cut food, or resume playing tennis. See Chapters 8 and 9.

For individuals with limited mobility, home and community access is problematic. Difficulty with stairs or the inability to ambulate long distances limits the scope of activities for survivors of stroke. A home visit before discharge is recommended to resolve any immediate issues with inaccessibility, as individuals commonly receive equipment that does not fit in their homes. Obstacles including stairs, furniture, power cords, lighting, and noise affect the ability to participate in activities inside and outside of the home. For working clients, job site evaluations are necessary for vocational success. For a full-time mother, this may include a comprehensive evaluation of the home and learning what tasks she performs to fulfill her roles. See Chapters 14 and 27.

Speech and language deficits occur in as many as 40% of individuals with strokes.[1] Poor speech and language functions deter clients from situations in which conversation is unavoidable. Persisting consequences adversely affect quality of life, ranging from loss of employment to feelings of isolation and depression. Therefore, addressing language barriers and educating clients and families in compensatory strategies alleviates some distress associated with speech and language deficits. Occupational therapists should address participation issues in addition to the interventions provided by speech language pathologists. See Chapter 20.

Depression is another common barrier to participation after stroke. The cause may be directly biological, depending on the location of the lesion in the brain or may be a reaction to a sudden catastrophic event in the client's life. Depression may affect participation and long-term outcomes adversely,[1] and it has been associated with longer hospital length of stay, poor performance in ADL, and decreased socialization. Emotional issues such as fear and depression can lead to decreased reintegration into previous roles and occupations and to decreased quality of life. Following a life-altering event such as a stroke, a person may fear additional illness, injury, or another stroke. For this reason, clients may be hesitant to leave their homes and resume prior roles. In a study by Clarke and colleagues, community-dwelling stroke survivors reported a lower sense of well-being than their healthy community-residing counterparts.[17] Clients and their families should be educated regarding risk factors of stroke rehabilitation strategies and medical management following a stroke. Additional education may decrease anxiety regarding a future stroke. Referral to a psychologist may be indicated for some individuals. See Chapter 2.

Urinary incontinence is a barrier to participation frequently overlooked by rehabilitation teams, although it is generally agreed to have a considerable effect on a person's quality of life and well-being. Between 9% and 40% of the individuals with stroke develop incontinence.[10,43] Incontinence has been identified as a predictor for nursing home placement and is associated with poor recovery from stroke.[10] Studies in the general population have shown that incontinence is associated with depression[50] and higher levels of anxiety.[8] Urinary incontinence often leads to a reduction in social activities and re-

lationships, changes in physical activities, and elaborate planning and forethought before activities that previously could be done spontaneously.[24,41]

Although physical and cognitive impairments constrain the subjective well-being of stroke survivors living in the community, social resources can moderate the adverse effects of residual disabilities. Survivors who have adequate social support are less affected by functional dependence.[17] Social supports have been found to be associated with a higher quality of life in stroke survivors.[29] *Social participation* is defined as socially oriented sharing of resources and is an essential component of quality of life.[11] Therefore, poor resource use may be predictive of decreased quality of life following stroke. Individuals without family or close friends have difficulty reintegrating into prior roles after stroke. Many family members and friends must return to their prior roles several weeks after their loved one's stroke. This produces a gradual decrease in support over time. This decrease often occurs when home health staff have discharged the client, and additional resources such as transportation are required for outpatient therapy, grocery shopping, and medical appointments. This is a critical time for case management to secure the support of community organizations, transportation agencies, and outpatient therapy services. Too often, home health care is discontinued without further referral to a nearby outpatient facility. Although clients are no longer homebound following home care services, they are often in need of further rehabilitation to address the cognitive and emotional issues to help them return to activities, tasks, and roles in the family, work, and the community.

The overarching barrier to addressing these limitations in participation following stroke is the fact that rehabilitation services are overly focused on addressing the motor and self-care impairments. Therefore, the needs of the younger, less neurologically impaired stroke survivors are typically overlooked. This was confirmed in a recent study conducted by the Cognitive Rehabilitation Research Group (CRRG) at Washington University School of Medicine who assessed all individuals with stroke being served by Barnes-Jewish Hospital Stroke Service over a 10-year period. The CRRG found that in their stroke population (N=7740): (1) 45% of the patients are under the age of 65-years-old and nearly 27% are under the age of 55-years-old; (2) of all the patients who had strokes, 49% had a mild stroke, 32.8% had moderate strokes, 17.9% had a severe stroke, and 6% did not live, as defined by the National Institute of Health Stroke Scale (NIHSS); and (3) of the individuals who had a mild to moderate stroke, 71% were discharged directly home, were discharged with home services only, or were discharged with outpatient services only, because they did not typically display motor or self-care deficits.[56] These same individuals have been found to report problems in their ability to reintegrate into their prestroke activities, community roles, and work following their stroke.[56] Since it is known that all of the limitations discussed previously can result from a stroke, it is absolutely essential in a client-centered stroke rehabilitation model to identify these limitations across the continuum of care in order to best support clients.

HOW TO FOSTER PARTICIPATION THROUGHOUT THE CONTINUUM OF CARE

No one method of treatment fosters participation in all avenues of rehabilitative care. The stroke team requires commitment and creativity to address the issue. The specific modality applied is not what enhances participation (and hopefully quality of life). Enhancement comes through the activities selected and the contexts in which they are performed. Only with a client-centered plan and the incorporation of meaningful activities in rehabilitation can the team foster participation to bring meaning to the individual in the rehabilitation program.

ACUTE CARE

In the acute care setting, acting as a triage team member is essential. This requires a thorough assessment battery. Identifying all the impairments that can improve performance in this setting allows for better discharge planning. Detailed evaluation improves the therapists' abilities to identify impairments from severe to subtle. Too often, assessments in the acute care setting are brief, increasing the potential for error in discharge placement, because at times it is difficult to assess the presence or absence of the more subtle complex impairments (i.e., cognitive dysfunction) in the acute care setting. If it is not possible to do a complete assessment, then it is imperative for the team member to recommend a follow-up assessment before discharge. Sending the individual home with a "clean bill of health" when in fact these subtle impairments may be present can have a devastating effect on the mental and physical health of the individual. The assessment in this phase of treatment must include not only basic measures of motor impairment, cognition, and language, but also those of higher level functions, including balance, visual perception, and executive function. These elements are key to successful reentry into the community, participation in roles and activities done before the stroke, and maintenance of quality of life. Often the most problematic deficits are those not physically obvious. Clients and families are less likely to understand the impact of poor memory, impaired judgment, decreased language function, and limited

balance. Translating these deficits to real-life tasks increases the tangibility for clients and their families and facilitates the transition through other avenues of care. Each level of rehabilitation encompasses increasingly complex tasks in varying contexts.

In some instances, clients do not move through acute care quickly. If treatment time is available, performance of basic tasks is critical. The most basic of self-care is required to go to church, to school, or to work. The acute setting is ideal for beginning of basic ADL including bathing, transfers, eating, and toileting, as they are identified as meaningful for the client. Some clients may choose to have an attendant help them with basic ADL. In such cases, goals can evolve around other client-centered tasks. Goals should include items important to the client, such as talking on the phone or visiting with family. Emotional attachment to such activities is great, and a loss or decrease in independence can produce an emotional response that increases disability (see Chapter 1).

INPATIENT REHABILITATION

According to the Agency for Healthcare Quality and Research, rehabilitation seeks to help the person with disabilities achieve the highest possible degree of performance. Rehabilitation is comparable to school in which the client is provided an opportunity for instruction, support, protected practice, education, reassurance, direct assistance, and feedback. This is the "planned withdrawal" of support in which services are provided as needed and are removed when no longer needed. The modalities of inpatient rehabilitation treatment are no different from acute care therapy or outpatient therapy; however, the tasks progress to be more difficult. Once the client has mastered a task in a therapeutic context, the conditions are altered to more real-life situations. Inherent in this progression is that the client is the leader. The therapist must recognize the need for preparing clients to go home beyond using basic ADL performance as a discharge criterion, because this prepares clients to do well inside their homes but does not prepare clients to shop, go to work, or to baby-sit a grandchild. The key to remember in the goal-setting process is the full range of tasks and roles to which the client is returning. Furthermore, a prior level of function must be established and well-documented. An occupational history makes it possible to integrate prior activities into the care plan. If the stroke is impairing prior function, the impairment is treatable and reimbursable. If the prior level of function is documented only in terms of basic self-care, clients will not have access to rehabilitation to return them to community life. By identifying what the person did before admission, one identifies goals to achieve after the prior level of function is achieved. The therapist has more time to achieve those goals once an independent level of self-care is achieved. Response to treatment is better if the client is put in the context of something important to them. For example, a client wants to work on writing. The practitioner provides handwriting exercises every day to complete as homework. However, the client never completes the homework. The client often is labeled unmotivated or uncooperative. The key question to ask is the type of writing the client enjoys. Does the client keep a journal? Does the client enjoy crossword puzzles? These require different writing skills.

When a client enters inpatient rehabilitation, an ongoing evaluation of capacities and client goals is imperative. Through identification of higher-level tasks, clients can be challenged outside the walls of the rehabilitation hospital. For example, a client walks down the hallway of the hospital. What is the response of the other therapists, nurses, and housekeepers in the hallway? What if, one week after discharge, an individual is negotiating a shopping mall? Will the persons in the mall have the same response as the hospital staff? A colleague of the author once referred to this concept as "rehab without walls;" providing rehabilitation in the community rather than restricting it to the hospital setting is the best preparation for life after discharge.

HOME HEALTH

The advantage to home health therapy is that the intervention takes place in the setting where the skills will be applied as they are being learned. One of the obvious goals of home health is to identify the physical barriers to the client's success in the home environment. However, identification of the cognitive and perceptual barriers that limit performance in the home setting is critical. In addition, clients may perform better in a familiar environment. As in inpatient rehabilitation, therapeutic activities should evolve around client-centered goals and may include yard work, laundry, or cooking. The therapist has a dual role in home health therapy. In addition to helping remediate impairments from the stroke, the therapist modifies the environment to achieve maximum participation in goals. The environmental approach also involves educating those in the home to the person's capabilities and how they can enable the person to be active to continue the recovery and help the person gain self-management skills. Preparing the client in the home environment is the first step in preparing the client for community reentry. The downfall of home health therapy is the lack of peer support from other stroke clients and minimal client-team interaction. Referral of the client to outpatient therapy or a community support group once the client is no longer restricted to the home setting is recommended.

OUTPATIENT THERAPY

A good outpatient program involves a multidisciplinary team working with the client to achieve maximum independence in all aspects of life the client indicates as important. Outpatient therapy forces the client to maintain a schedule of therapies, get ready in time for the appointment, arrange transportation to and from the appointment, and follow through with home programs jointly designed with the therapists. To get to therapy, the client must have the physical endurance to participate in the preparation, the travel, and the therapy itself. The cognitive process involves initiation, planning, attention, organization, and sequencing. Before the client reaches the door of the clinic, therapy has already begun.

A complete assessment includes an inventory of activities, responsibilities, and roles the client likes to do and needs to do every day. Clients can identify the activities most important to them. Often outpatient therapy is difficult because of the broad spectrum of possibilities for clients in this setting. Generating a list of the client's top five goals is recommended. From that point, additional goals can be formulated. In this setting, vocational issues can be addressed. Meeting with the client's employer is important to address barriers in the workplace. Meeting with and educating the caregiver assists with the identification of barriers the client may not see in the home. Addressing social support issues with family and friends is also important. An important strategy is to find activities that are enjoyable to the client and the caregiver, so they can be involved in activities that they enjoy doing together.

COMMUNITY REINTEGRATION

As depicted in Fig. 3-3, an often overlooked but important component to the continuum of care is taking rehabilitation services out into the community. With the age of stroke decreasing, the population of individuals having strokes is increasing engaged in community roles and in particular employment. Inherent in these roles is the need to address more complex activities such as driving, home management, self-management of symptoms, and physical activity. In order to provide client-centered care, this stage in the continuum must be addressed.

CASE STUDY

Improving Participation through Occupation

Rosemary awoke one Saturday morning with slurred speech and difficulty walking. She decided to return to bed for additional rest. After sleeping for several more hours, she awoke with left-sided weakness and facial droop, worsening speech, and an inability to walk. She lived alone, was not married, and had no children. She

Continued

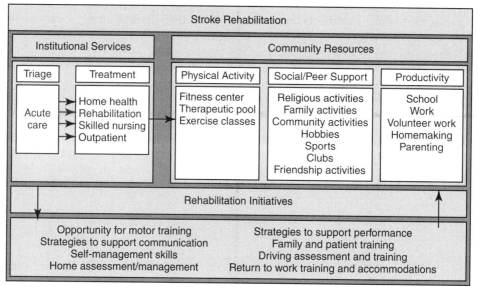

Figure 3-3   Continuum of care in stroke rehabilitation.

Improving Participation through Occupation—cont'd

promptly called 911. When paramedics reached her, the dysarthria was severe and she had complete left hemiplegia. She was oriented to her name and where she was but not to the date. In the emergency room, Rosemary was determined to have sustained a large right middle cerebral artery stroke. She was admitted immediately to the hospital and was referred to the stroke team for evaluation and treatment.

Rosemary's deficits included the following. She was unable to move her left arm or leg. She could roll in bed to her left side using the bed rail, but required maximum assistance to roll to the right. She was dependent with her transfers and basic ADL. She had a left visual inattention and decreased sensation on the left side of her body. She was sleepy and was unable to work with a therapist for more than 30 minutes at a time.

Over her first few days in the hospital, Rosemary began to improve. She was able to tolerate more time in therapy. She could support herself while sitting on the edge of the bed and began to play an active role in her ADL. Rosemary was able to move from her bed to a chair with 75% assistance from the nursing and therapy staff. She was tolerating sitting up in bed and a chair for extended periods throughout the day. The team met to determine the course of Rosemary's rehabilitation. At the team meeting, Rosemary's living alone in a two-story home located in the city was revealed. Multiple steps were required to enter. She had two bathrooms in the house; however, the bathroom with a

shower was located on the second floor. She had no family locally. Her home was located within walking distance of the doctor and a large grocery store.

Rosemary was a violinist in a local quartet and taught violin on the side. She had few friends other than those in the group with whom she worked. In addition, she was driving (and using public transportation), cooking, shopping, and managing her finances independently before her stroke. Because of these responsibilities and her lack of support at discharge, the team decided Rosemary would benefit from inpatient rehabilitation.

On admission to inpatient rehabilitation, Rosemary was evaluated by nursing, physical therapy, occupational therapy, and speech therapy staff members. She required moderate to maximum assistance with basic ADL and transfers. She required 100% assistance to walk using a walker and an ankle/foot orthotic. She was able to move from her bed to a chair and back with 75% assistance. Her memory was good; however, she indicated that her attention was not, and she appeared easily distracted in the clinic. She was oriented to person, place, date, and situation. Her speech remained slurred, but her swallow was normal. Rosemary's endurance improved greatly. She continued to show subtle signs of a left visual inattention, and her left arm continued to be weak throughout. Manual muscle tests indicated strength at the shoulder and elbow was $\frac{3}{5}$. Strength in the wrist and hand was $\frac{2}{5}$. Sensation was normal to pin prick and temperature. She was diagnosed with depression and was treated medically. The only interests stated in her chart included playing and teaching violin and playing bridge.

Following initial evaluation, the team met to discuss her goals and plans for discharge. Although she was improving daily, her ability to live alone was questionable because of her poor balance, limited attention, and decreased strength. Rosemary and the team set goals for her to be independent with basic ADL and transfers from her bed, the bathtub, and the car. The team chose to address her ability to grocery shop and prepare a simple meal in the microwave. The case manager discussed these goals with Rosemary, and she agreed with the team's priorities.

At her second week of inpatient rehabilitation, Rosemary was able to dress herself independently using an adaptive strategy. She was walking with some assistance using an ankle/foot orthotic and a walker. She was able to prepare a bowl of cereal, a sandwich, and a microwave dinner. She was taken on trips to the gift shop and grocery store to evaluate her ability to follow a list, obtain objects on the list, and exchange money correctly. These trips were overstimulating to Rosemary, and her depression worsened. She missed her music and felt that her only love in life was the violin. She lived close to the hospital but did not have close friends or family to get her violin. Rosemary desperately wanted to do a home visit and wanted to get her violin; however, the team thought it would increase her depression because her motor impairment would make it impossible for her to play. Despite the discouragement of the team, one of the therapists brought in a violin for Rosemary to play. The therapist went to a quiet treatment room with Rosemary.

Although Rosemary was hesitant, she removed the violin from the case and asked the therapist to leave the room. She did not want anyone else to hear her attempts to play the violin for the first time. As the therapist closed the door, she could see the fear on Rosemary's face. The therapist returned to the room after 10 minutes. What she heard was amazing. When she opened the door, Rosemary was playing the violin. Her face beamed with pride as the team came in to hear her play. What they all felt was impossible was the key motivator for Rosemary. She began to practice several times a day.

At week 3 of her impatient rehabilitation, the team decided that Rosemary's progress had reached a plateau and that it was time to schedule discharge. Rosemary did not want to burden her small group of friends. She made the decision to transfer to a residential facility until her status improved. At discharge, she was independent with ADL using some adaptive strategies and independent with transfers using adaptive equipment. Some assistance was required with walking using a quad cane and an ankle/foot orthotic, her speech remained slurred, and her facial droop persisted. Muscle strength throughout her arm was 4/5, with poor coordination distally. She was able to balance a simulated checkbook, prepare simple meals independently (she was most comfortable with the microwave), and play her violin, but she could not drive. Rosemary had difficulty with higher-level tasks involving complex sequencing and organization, and performing multiple tasks at once was difficult for her.

Rosemary transferred to a residential facility for two months before returning home. At that time, she was referred to outpatient therapy. Rosemary remained unable to drive but was proficient at using public transportation. She was independent with most basic and instrumental ADL. A friend would pick her up weekly to take her to the grocery store. Her motor status was unchanged from her inpatient rehabilitation discharge. She continued to show 4/5 muscle strength proximally and improved coordination in her hand and fingers. Her speech was normal, and speech therapy was not required. Her higher-level executive functions were nearly normal. Her balance continued to be problematic, but she was walking with a straight cane and an ankle/foot orthotic. A comprehensive evaluation of her activities and quality of life revealed the following. Her Activity Card Sort showed that she had retained only 35% of the activities she had done before the stroke, with the greatest loss in the areas of social activity and high-demand leisure activity. Rosemary's priorities indicated by the Activity Card Sort included the following (in order of importance): playing a musical instrument (her violin), driving, shopping, visiting with friends, and traveling. The Stroke Adapted Sickness Impact Profile (SA-SIP) revealed a score of 15 out of 30. Her score was in the midrange, indicating a decreased quality of life. Some of the problematic areas included "body care and movement," "mobility," and "ambulation." Rosemary received a score of 28 on the Reintegration to Normal Living Index. The scoring range of the index is from 11 to 55. A lower score indicates lower satisfaction. Rosemary's score was in the midrange, indicating some difficulty. Low scores included items regarding travel, spending days occupied with work that is important, getting around the community, and being comfortable in the company of others. The Community Integration Questionnaire indicated some severe difficulties in areas of home, social, and productivity. Rosemary's home integration score was a 3.6 out of 10 points, her social integration score was a 3 out of 12 points, her productivity score was a 1 out of 6 points, and her total score was 7.75 out of 28 points, indicating a poor level of independence. The team met with Rosemary to set her goals for outpatient therapy. Scores from her assessments were discussed. Rosemary identified that her primary barriers to satisfaction were her decreased ability to

Continued

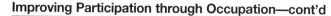

CASE STUDY

Improving Participation through Occupation—cont'd

play her violin and her inability to drive. Because she was unable to drive, she had difficulty shopping, meeting friends, and traveling. Although she had friends to drive her to events or was able to use public transportation close to home, Rosemary felt a decrease in autonomy. This decrease in autonomy and an inability to continue her work added to her depression. Goals were set according to priorities outlined by Rosemary in her Activity Card Sort. The team set goals with Rosemary to improve her motor performance to improve her violin playing and walking independently while carrying a violin case. A driving evaluation was completed and indicated that she was able to return to driving. A trip to the grocery store and the mall allowed the therapists to determine her best method of negotiating the mall and for carrying bags to the car after shopping. Rosemary returned to therapy the second week with her violin. After an additional week of therapy, Rosemary had met her goals for playing the violin, driving, shopping, and visiting with friends. On discharge from outpatient therapy, Rosemary was able to teach violin again and hoped to return soon to concert performances. Her scores on the SA-SIP had increased to 3 out of 30. Her Community Integration Questionnaire scores returned to normal, and her activity level as measured by the Activity Card Sort returned to 85% of what it was before her stroke.

REVIEW QUESTIONS

1. Describe the concepts encompassed in the word *participation* and the factors that affect participation.
2. What are the categories of occupation?
3. How may self-efficacy affect a client's recovery?
4. Define quality of life. What is the relationship between quality of life and activity and participation?
5. Describe some common assessments of participation and quality of life.
6. What are some common barriers limiting participation and quality of life?
7. How can therapists address participation through the continuum of care from acute care to the community?
8. What may have been done differently with Rosemary's care to facilitate her recovery? What did the therapists do well with Rosemary?

ACKNOWLEDGMENTS

The authors acknowledge with appreciation the contributions to earlier versions of this chapter by Michelle Hahn.

REFERENCES

1. Agency for Health Care Policy and Research: *Post-stroke rehabilitation*, Rockville, MD, 1995, US Department of Health and Human Services, Public Health Service, Agency for Health Care Policy and Research.
2. American Occupational Therapy Association (AOTA): Occupational therapy practice framework: Domain and process (2nd ed.). *Am J Occup Ther* 62(6): 625–683, 2008.
3. Bandura A: *Social learning theory*, Englewood Cliffs, NJ, 1977, Prentice Hall.
4. Banks P, Pearson C: *Improving services for younger stroke survivors and their families* (website). www.chss.org.uk/pdf/research/Young_stroke_study_2003.pdf. Accessed October 30, 2007.
5. Baum CM, Edwards DF: *Activity card sort*, ed 2, Bethesda, MD, 2008, AOTA Press.
6. Baum CM, Edwards DF, Morrow-Howell N: Identification and measurement of productive behaviors in senile dementia of the Alzheimer type. *Gerontologist* 33(3):403–408, 1993.
7. Baum CM, Law M: Occupational therapy practice: focusing on occupational performance. *Am J Occup Ther* 51(4):277–288, 1997.
8. Berglund AL, Eisemann M, Lalos O: Personality characteristics of stress incontinent women: a pilot study. *J Psychosom Obstet Gynaecol* 15(3):165–170, 1994.
9. Bergner M, Bobbitt RA, Carter WB, et al: The Sickness Impact Profile: development and final revision of a health status measure. *Med Care* 19(8):787–805, 1981.
10. Brittain KR, Peet SM, Castleden, CM: Stroke and incontinence. *Stroke* 29(2):524–528, 1998.
11. Bukov A, Maas I, Lampert T: Social participation in very old age: cross sectional and longitudinal findings from BASE. *J Gerontol B Psychol Sci Soc Sci* 57(6):510–517, 2002.
12. Canadian Association of Occupational Therapists: *Guidelines for the client-centered practice of occupational therapy*, Toronto, 1995, The Association.
13. Chan C, Lee T: Validity of the Canadian occupational performance measure. *Occup Ther Int* 4:229–247, 1997.
14. Christiansen, CH: A social-psychological approach to understanding self-care. In Christiansen CH, editor: *Ways of living: self-care strategies for special needs*, Bethesda, MD, 1994, American Occupational Therapy Association.
15. Christiansen CH, Baum C: *Occupational therapy: overcoming human performance deficits*, Thorofare, NJ, 1997, Slack.
16. Christiansen CH, Clark F, Kielhofner G, et al: Position paper: occupation. *Am J Occup Ther* 49(10):1015–1018, 1995.
17. Clarke P, Marshall V, Black SE, et al: Well-being after stroke in Canadian seniors: findings from the Canadian study of health and aging. *Stroke* 33(4):1016–1028, 2002.
18. Duncan PW, Lai SM, Tyler D, et al: Evaluation of proxy responses to the Stroke Impact Scale. *Stroke* 33(11):2593, 2002.
19. Duncan PW, Wallace D, Lai SM, et al: The Stroke Impact Scale version 2.0: evaluation of reliability, validity, and sensitivity to change. *Stroke* 30(10):2131–2140, 1999.
20. Fidler GW, Fidler JW: Doing and becoming: purposeful action and self-actualization. *Am J Occup Ther* 32(5): 305–310, 1978.
21. Gage M, Polatajko H: Enhancing occupational performance through an understanding of perceived self-efficacy. *Am J Occup Ther* 48(5):452–461, 1994.
22. Gunter BG, Stanley J: Theoretical issues in leisure study. In Gunter BG, Stanley J, St Clair R, editors: *Transitions to leisure: conceptual and human issues*, Landham, MD, 1985, University Press of America.
23. Hochstenbach J, Anderson P, van Limbeek J, et al: Is there a relation between neuropsychologic variables and quality of life after stroke? *Arch Phys Med Rehabil* 82(10):1360–1366, 2001.
24. Hunskaar S, Vinsnes A: The quality of life in women with urinary incontinence as measured by the Sickness Impact Profile. *J Am Geriatr Soc* 39(4):378–382, 1991.

25. Iso-Ahola SE: Basic dimensions of definitions of leisure. *J Leisure Res* 1:28–39, 1979.
26. Katz N: *Cognitive rehabilitation: models for intervention in occupational therapy*, Boston Mass. 1992, Butterworth-Heinemann.
27. Katz N, Karpin H, Lak A, et al: Participation and occupational performance: reliability and validity of the Activity Card Sort. *Occup Ther J Res* 23(1):10–17, 2003.
28. Kielhofner G: *Conceptual foundations of occupational therapy*, Philadelphia, 2004, FA Davis.
29. King RB: Quality of life after stroke. *Stroke* 27(9):1467–1472, 1996.
30. Koch L, Egbert N, Coeling H, Ayers D: Returning to work after the onset of illness: experiences of right hemisphere stroke survivors. *Rehabil Couns* 48(4):209–218, 2005.
31. Lai S, Studenski S, Duncan P, et al: Persisting consequences of stroke measured by the stroke impact scale. *Stroke* 33(7):1840–1850, 2002.
32. Law M, Baptiste S, Mills J: Client–centred practice: what does it mean and does it make a difference? *Can J Occup Ther* 62(5): 250–257, 1995.
33. Law M, Baum CM, Dunn W: *Measuring occupational performance: supporting best practice in occupational therapy*, Thorofare, NJ, 2001, Slack.
34. Law M, Cooper BA, Strong S, et al: The person-environment-occupation model: a transactive approach to occupational performance. *Can J Occup Ther* 63(1):9–23, 1996.
35. Lawton MP: The functional assessment of elderly people. *J Am Geriatr Soc* 19(6):465–481, 1971.
36. Levine MN: Quality of life in stage II breast cancer: an instrument for clinical trials. *J Clin Oncol* 6(12):1798–1810, 1988.
37. Mathiowetz V, Bass-Haugen J: Motor behavior research: implications for therapeutic approaches to central nervous system dysfunction. *Am J Occup Ther* 48:733–745, 1994.
38. McColl MA, Gerein N, Valentine F: Meeting the challenges of disability: models for enabling function and well-being. In Christiansen CH, Baum CM, editors: *Occupational therapy: enabling function and well being*, ed 2, Thorofare, NJ, 1997, Slack.
39. Moore A: The band community: synchronizing human activity cycles for group cooperation. In Zemke R, Clark F, editors: *Occupational science: the evolving discipline*, Philadelphia, 1996, FA Davis.
40. Murphy B, Herrman H, Hawthorne G, et al: *Australian WHOQoL instruments: User's manual and interpretation guide*, Melbourne, 2000, Australian WHOQoL Field Study Centre.
41. Naughton J, Wyman JF: Quality of life in geriatric patients with lower urinary tract dysfunction. *Am J Med Sci* 314(4):219–227, 1997.
42. Neugarten BL, Havinghurst RJ, Tobin SS: Measure of life satisfaction. *J Gerontol* 16(2):134–143, 1961.
43. Patel M, Coshall C, Lawrence E, et al: Recovery from poststroke urinary incontinence: associated factors and impact on outcome. *J Am Geriatr Soc* 49(9):1229–1233, 2001.
44. Primeau L: Work versus non-work: the case of household work. In Zemke R, Clark F, editors: *Occupational science: the evolving discipline*, Philadelphia, 1996, FA Davis.
45. Ryan RM, Deci EL: Self-determination theory and the facilitation of intrinsic motivation, social development, and well-being. *Am Psychol* 55(1):68–78, 2000.
46. Stuart H: Stigma and work. *Healthcare Papers* 5(2):100–111, 2005.
47. Takata N: The play milieu: a preliminary appraisal. *Am J Occup Ther* 25:281–284, 1971.
48. Tatemichi T, Desmond D, Stern Y, et al: Cognitive impairment after stroke: frequency, patterns, and relationship to functional abilities. *J Neurol Neurosurg Psychiatry* 57:202–207, 1994.
49. Trombly CA: Occupation: purposefulness and meaningfulness as therapeutic mechanisms. The 1995 Eleanor Clarke Slagle Lecture. *Am J Occup Ther* 49:960–972, 1995.
50. Valvanne J, Juva K, Erkinjuntti T, et al: Major depression in the elderly: a population study in Helsinki. *Int Psychogeriatr* 8(3): 437–443, 1996.
51. van Straten A, de Haan RJ, Limburg M, et al: A stroke-adapted 30–item version of the Sickness Impact Profile to assess quality of life (SAS-SIP30). *Stroke* 28:2155–2161, 1997.
52. Vestling M, Tufvesson B, Iwarsson S: Indicators for return to work after stroke and the importance of work for subjective well-being and life satisfaction. *J Rehabil Med* 35(3):127–131, 2003.
53. Ware JE, Sherbourne CD: The MOS 36–item Short-Form Health Survey (SF-36). I. Conceptual framework and item selection. *Med Care* 30(6):473–483, 1992.
54. Wilcock, A: A theory of the human need for occupation. *Occup Sci Aust* 1(1):17–24, 1993.
55. Willer B, Linn R, Allen K: Community integration and barriers to integration for individuals with brain injury. In Finlayson M, Garner S, editors: *Brain injury rehabilitation: clinical considerations*, Baltimore, 1993, Williams & Wilkins.
56. Wolf T, Baum CM, Connor L: Changing face of stroke: Implications for occupational therapy practice. *Am J Occup Ther* 63(5):621–625, 2009.
57. Wood-Dauphinee SL, Opzoomer MA, Williams JI, et al: Assessment of global function: The Reintegration to Normal Living Index. *Arch Phys Med Rehabil* 69(8):583–590, 1988.
58. Wood-Dauphinee SL, Williams J: Reintegration to normal living as a proxy to quality of life. *J Chronic Dis* 40(6):491–502, 1987.
59. World Health Organization: *The International Classification of Function, Disability and Health*, Geneva, 2001, World Health Organization.
60. Deleted.
61. World Health Organization Quality of Life Group: Development of the 3 WHO quality of life assessment. *Psychol Med* 28(3):551–558, 1998.

virgil mathiowetz

chapter 4

Task-Oriented Approach to Stroke Rehabilitation

key terms

model of motor behavior
motor control
motor development

motor learning
task-oriented evaluation
framework

task-oriented treatment
strategies

chapter objectives

After completing this chapter, the reader will be able to accomplish the following:

1. Describe the motor behavior (i.e., motor control, motor learning, and motor development) theories and model that support the occupational therapy task-oriented approach to persons after stroke.
2. Describe the evaluation framework for the occupational therapy task-oriented approach and identify specific assessments that are consistent with the approach.
3. Describe general treatment principles for the occupational therapy task-oriented approach and their application to persons after stroke.
4. Given a case study of a person after stroke, describe occupational therapy task-oriented approach evaluation and treatment strategies that you would use.

This chapter provides a theoretical foundation for the occupational therapy (OT) task-oriented approach or a function-based approach for persons after stroke. Mathiowetz and Bass-Haugen[56] proposed this approach in 1994 based on the motor behavior/motor control, motor development, and motor learning-theories and research of that time. Motor behavior, OT theories, and research have evolved since then, so the OT task-oriented approach has evolved as well.[5,54] This chapter represents the most recent thinking regarding this approach.

The theoretical assumptions of the neurophysiological approaches, which include Rood sensorimotor approach,[71] Knott and Voss proprioceptive neuromuscular facilitation,[48] Brunnstrom movement therapy,[12] and Bobath neurodevelopmental treatment[8,9] were based on the empirical experience and research of their time. However, as the motor behavior theories changed in the 1980s and 1990s, the assumptions of the neurophysiological approaches were challenged,[34,77] and alternative approaches were proposed.[14,15,40,54-56] Recently the theoretical assumptions of the neurodevelopmental treatment approach were updated with current motor behavior theories.[42] However, many of the neurodevelopmental treatment techniques have changed little, despite the changed theoretical assumptions. This may reflect the fact that neurodevelopmental treatment was developed empirically first, and then theoretical assumptions of the time were used to explain why it might work. In contrast, the OT task-oriented approach evaluation and interventions strategies emerged primarily from its theoretical assumptions (see Chapter 6).

THEORETICAL ASSUMPTIONS AND MODEL UNDERLYING THE OCCUPATIONAL THERAPY TASK-ORIENTED APPROACH

Systems Model of Motor Control

In the past 25 to 30 years, new models of motor control have evolved from the ecological approach to perception and action[29,83] and from the study of complex, dynamical systems in mathematics and the sciences.[33] The new models emphasize the interaction between persons and their environments and suggest that motor behavior emerges from persons' multiple systems interacting with unique tasks and environmental contexts.[62] "Thus, the systems model of motor control is more interactive or heterarchical and emphasizes the role of the environment more than the earlier reflex-hierarchical model."[54]

In the systems model, the nervous system is viewed differently from earlier reflex-hierarchical models. Instead of being the primary system controlling movement, the nervous system now is considered only one system among many systems that affect motor behavior. "The nervous system itself is organized *heterarchically* such that higher centers interact with the lower centers but do not control them. Closed-loop and open-loop systems work cooperatively and both feedback and feedforward control are used to achieve task goals."[54] The central nervous system interacts with multiple personal and environmental systems as a person attempts to pursue a functional goal.

Ecological Approach to Perception and Action

The ecological approach "emphasizes the study of interaction between the person and the environment during everyday, functional tasks and the close linkage between perception and action (i.e., purposeful movement)."[54] Gibson described the role of functional goals and the environment in the relationship between perception and action. He stated that direct perception involves the active search for affordances[30] or the functional use of objects for a person with unique personal characteristics.[87] Therefore, Gibson's concept of affordances recognizes the close linkage between perception and action in terms of what the information available in the environment means to a specific person.[30]

Bernstein[7] also recognized the importance of the environment and personal factors other than the central nervous system in motor behavior. He explained the role that a particular muscle has in a movement is influenced by the context or circumstances and described three potential sources of variability in muscle function. Variability is due to anatomical factors. For example, from kinesiology one knows that in a standing position, the shoulder flexor muscles contract concentrically to bring the humerus to the 90-degree position. However, in the prone position with one's arm at one's side, shoulder extensor muscles contract eccentrically until reaching the 90-degree position. Thus, which muscles are activated depends on the initial position of the body. Another example relates to extending the shoulder from the 90-degree position when standing. If one wants to extend it quickly or against resistance, the shoulder extensor muscles contract. In contrast, if one extends the shoulder slowly against no resistance, the shoulder flexor muscles contract eccentrically, and the shoulder extensor muscles do not need to contract at all. In both cases, the role of the muscle is determined by the context in which it is used. A second source of variability is due to mechanical factors. Many nonmuscular forces, such as gravity and inertia, determine the degree to which a muscle needs to contract. For example, a muscle must exert much less force if contracting in a gravity-eliminated plane rather than against gravity. Likewise, the contraction of the elbow extensor muscles would be different if the shoulder were extending or flexing at the same time because of the effects of inertia. Again, the effect of a muscle contraction is related to the context. A third source of variability is due to physiological factors. "When higher centers send down a command for a muscle to contract, middle and lower centers have the opportunity to modify the command. Lower and middle centers receive peripheral sensory feedback. Thus, the impact of the command on the muscle will vary depending on the context and degree of influence of the middle and lower centers. As a result, the relationship between higher center or executive commands and muscle action is not a one-to-one."[54]

Mathiowetz and Wade[57] also demonstrated the influence of context (informational support available in the environment) on movement. They reported that a natural informational support condition (e.g., eating applesauce with a spoon) elicited a smoother and more direct movement pattern than an impoverished informational support condition (e.g., pretending to eat applesauce with a spoon without any of the objects). Many have taken a dynamical systems view as a means to explain the complex person-environment interactions that occur in everyday life.

Dynamical Systems Theory

The study of dynamical systems originated in the disciplines of mathematics, physics, biology, chemistry, psychology, and kinesiology and has been applied to the professions of OT, physical therapy, nursing, adapted physical education, and some areas of medicine.[13,53] Such study has influenced the development of a systems model of motor control as well. Dynamical systems theory proposes that behaviors emerge from the interaction of many systems and subsystems. Because the behavior is not specified but is emergent, it is considered to be self-organizing.[46] Despite the many *degrees of freedom* or ways of performing a task available to persons, they tend to use relatively stable patterns of motor behavior.[81] For example, when one walks or brushes the teeth, one has many choices in how to perform the task, yet one tends to use preferred patterns. These relatively stable patterns of motor behavior, which are unique to each person, provide evidence of *self-organization*.

Behavior can shift between periods of stability and instability throughout life. For example, behaviors can change from being stable to being less stable as a result of a stroke or aging. In fact, "it is during unstable periods, characterized by a high variability of performance, that new types of behaviors may emerge either gradually or abruptly. These transitions in behavior, called *phase shifts*, are changes in preferred patterns of coordinated behavior to another."[54] A gradual phase shift occurs when an infant progresses from walking while holding on to a parent's hands to walking without a helping hand over several months. An abrupt phase shift in prehension pattern occurs when a person changes from picking up a small object such as a peanut to picking up a large object such as a large coffee mug. How can these phase shifts or changes in behavior be explained?

In the dynamical systems view, *control parameters* are variables that shift behavior from one form to another. They do not control the change but act as agents for reorganization of the behavior into a new form.[38] Control parameters are gradable in some way. In the infant example, the degree of parental support influenced the change or phase shift from walking with support to walking without support. As parental support decreases, infants need to rely more on their own ability to maintain balance and need to increase their strength to support and control their own body weight in an upright position. In the other example, increasing the size of the object to be grasped elicited the change in prehension pattern from tip prehension to cylindrical grasp. Consequently, object size also is considered a control parameter.

Explanations of changes in motor behavior in the systems model of motor control are different from earlier reflex-hierarchical models. Thelen[79] stated that an important characteristic of a system perspective is that the shift from one preferred movement pattern to another is marked by discrete, discontinuous transitions. These changes in only one or several personal or environmental systems (i.e., control parameters) can contribute to transitions in motor behavior.[18] In conclusion, no inherent ordering of systems exists in terms of their influence on motor behavior, and systems themselves are subject to change over time.

SYSTEMS VIEW OF MOTOR DEVELOPMENT

A systems view of motor development suggests that changes over time are caused by multiple factors or systems such as maturation of the nervous system, biomechanical constraints and resources, and the impact of the physical and social environment.[38,54] For example, Thelen and Fisher[80] reported that the disappearance of the stepping reflex at 4- to 5-months-old is due to multiple factors internal and external to the child. Internal factors included the strength of the leg muscles, weight of the legs, and arousal level of the child. External factors included the varying effects of gravity in different environments. Thus, maturation of the nervous system alone cannot explain this change in developmental behavior. A systems view also suggests that normal development does not follow a rigid sequence, as the motor milestones would suggest. In fact, children follow variable developmental sequences because of their unique personal characteristics and environmental contexts. If the traditional developmental sequences are no longer sufficient as a guide for working with children, then they are certainly not appropriate as a guide for working with adults after stroke.[85]

In addition, the systems view suggests that behaviors observed after central nervous system damage result from patients' attempts to use their remaining resources to achieve functional goals. For example, the flexor pattern of spasticity often seen after stroke is due to various factors in addition to spasticity, such as weakness, inability to recruit appropriate muscles, biomechanical principles related to lever arms, and/or soft-tissue tightness. Thus, when inefficient/ineffective movement patterns are seen after stroke, therapists need to consider multiple factors as potential contributing variables (see Chapter 10).

CONTEMPORARY VIEW OF MOTOR LEARNING

Schmidt[75] defined motor learning as "a set of processes associated with practice or experience leading to relatively permanent changes in the capabilities of responding." Thus, recent motor learning theories acknowledge that behavior changes observed during practice may be only temporary. As a result, contemporary motor learning research not only evaluates learning after the acquisition phase (i.e., immediate effects) but also after a retention phase (i.e., short-term or long-term effects) or a transfer test (i.e., ability to generalize to new task), and thus new ways of thinking about motor learning have emerged. Motor learning research supports the idea that random practice (i.e., repetitive practice of several tasks in a varied sequence within a practice session) is better than blocked practice (i.e., repetitive practice of the same task within a practice session).[76] Similarly, practicing variations of the same tasks in varied contexts is better than practicing the same task in the same context. In addition, practicing the whole task rather than parts of a task usually is better, especially if the parts are interdependent or relatively fast.[73]

McNevin, Wulf, and Carlson[58] summarized some additional principles. When persons are learning a new task such as golfing, they should focus on the movement effects (external focus on the golf club head) rather than on their own arm movements (internal focus). Self-controlled practice (i.e., a person being trained decides when and how feedback is given and whether assistive devices are used) is better than instructor-controlled practice. Finally, dyad training, in which a person is able to alternate observing and practicing a task, is beneficial to learning a new task.

Research on the role of feedback in learning demonstrates that physical and verbal guidance enhanced immediate performance but interfered with long-term learning.[73] Winstein and Schmidt[88] reported that 50% feedback (i.e., feedback after half of the trials) was better than 100% feedback. Faded or decreasing feedback was better than increasing feedback. Finally, summary feedback after multiple trials is better than immediate feedback after every trial.[74] In all cases, less feedback was better than more feedback.

Most research on motor learning has been performed on persons without disabilities using a brief, contrived task in laboratory environments. Therefore, therapists need to be cautious about applying these principles to persons with disabilities performing functional tasks in everyday, natural environments.

However, several studies have explored whether motor learning principles can be applied to persons after stroke. Hanlon[37] provided some evidence that random practice was better than blocked practice. Merians and colleagues[59] reported that practice in a condition with reduced augmented feedback was beneficial for performance consistency but not for accuracy for persons with and without stroke. Dean and Shepherd[19] reported that task-related training using variable practice and varied contexts improved balance ability during seated reaching activities. Finally, Fasoli and colleagues[22] reported that externally focused (task-related) instructions resulted in faster and more forceful movements than internally focused (movement-related) instructions for persons with

and without stroke. Chapter 5 provides additional discussion of the application of motor learning principles to stroke rehabilitation.

SYSTEMS MODEL OF MOTOR BEHAVIOR

The model in Fig. 4-1 has been updated to include terminology from the Occupational Therapy Practice Framework.[1] The figure depicts the theoretical basis of the OT task-oriented approach. The model illustrates the interaction between the person (client factors, performance skills, and performance patterns) and their environment (context and activity demands). Occupational performance tasks (i.e., activities of daily living [ADL], instrumental activities of daily living [IADL], work, education, play/leisure, rest, and sleep) and role performance (social participation) emerge from the interaction between the systems of the person (cognitive, psychosocial, and sensorimotor) and the systems of the environment (physical, socioeconomical, and cultural). Changes in any one of these systems or subsystems

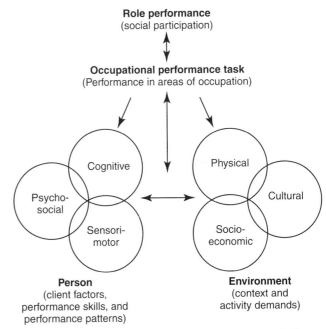

Figure 4-1 The systems model of motor behavior, which supports the occupational therapy task-oriented approach, emphasizes that occupational performance tasks and role performance emerge from an interaction of the person and their environment. In addition, any occupational performance task affects the person and environment. A continuous interaction occurs between role performance and occupational performance tasks. These interactions are ongoing across time. (Adapted from Mathiowetz V, Bass-Haugen J: Assessing abilities and capacities: motor behavior. In Radomski MV, Latham CAT, editors: *Occupational therapy for physical dysfunction,* ed 6, Baltimore, 2008, Lippincott Williams & Wilkins.)

can affect occupational performance tasks and/or role performance. "In some cases, only one primary factor might determine occupational performance. In most cases, occupational performance tasks emerge from the interaction of many systems. The on-going interactions between all components of the model reflect its heterarchical nature."[54]

In addition, any occupational performance task affects the environment in which it occurs and the person acting. For example, if a patient with hemiplegia becomes independent in driving by using assistive technology and adaptive strategies, the patient's ability to drive would free family members from needing to provide transportation for appointments and social events. The patient would be able to resume the role of driver and the task of driving, which were likely meaningful to the patient's life. Thus the occupational performance task of driving affects persons and objects in the environment (i.e., assistive technology added to the car). The task also affects the person and the associated components. The ability to be less dependent on the family may affect the patient's self-esteem positively (i.e., psychosocial subsystem). The process of driving "provides the patient the opportunity to solve problems and to discover optimal strategies for performing tasks. This influences a client's cognitive and sensorimotor subsystems and the ability to perform other functional tasks."[54]

The specific components (subsystems) of the systems, which influence occupational performance tasks, may be framed in OT terminology.[1,2] Components of the cognitive (mental) system include orientation, attention, memory, problem-solving, sequencing, learning, and generalization ability. Components of the psychosocial system include a person's interests, coping skills, self-concept, interpersonal skills, self-expression, time management, emotional regulation, and self-control skills that could affect occupational performance tasks. Strength, endurance, range of motion, sensory functions and pain, perceptual function, and postural control are components associated with the sensorimotor system. The environment includes physical, socioeconomical, and cultural characteristics of the task itself and the broader environment. Components of the physical environment system include objects, tools, devices, furniture, plants, animals, and the natural and built environments, which could limit or enhance task performance. The social supports provided by the family, friends, caregivers, social groups, community, and financial resources are components of the socioeconomical system, which could influence choice in activities. Finally, components of the cultural system include customs, beliefs, activity patterns, behavioral standards, and societal expectations, which also could affect occupational performance tasks.

The inclusion of role performance in this systems model reflects an OT, not a motor behavior perspective.

"Occupational therapists believe the roles that persons want and need to fulfill determine the occupational performance tasks and activities they need to do. Conversely, the tasks and activities persons are able to do determine what roles they are able to fulfill."[54] Box 4-1 summarizes the assumptions of the OT task-oriented approach.

EVALUATION FRAMEWORK USING THE OCCUPATIONAL THERAPY TASK-ORIENTED APPROACH

The therapist conducts the evaluation using a top-down approach as suggested by Latham.[49] Box 4-2 gives a framework for evaluation. Evaluation efforts focus initially on role performance and occupational performance tasks because they are the goals of motor behavior. A thorough understanding of the roles that a patient wants, needs, or is expected to perform and of the tasks needed to fulfill those roles enables therapists to plan meaningful and motivating treatment programs. After a patient has identified the most important role and occupational performance limitations, therapists use task analysis to identify which subsystem of the person or environment is limiting functional performance. This process may indicate the need for evaluation of selected subsystems of the person or environment.[25] The emphasis on role and occupational performance in the OT task-oriented approach is consistent with the idea that OT evaluation should be primarily at the participation and activities level rather than the impairment level, using World Health Organization[90] terminology. The therapist needs to use qualitative and quantitative measures during the evaluation process.[86] "Therefore, therapists use interviews, skilled observations,

---

Box 4-1

Assumptions of the Occupational Therapy Task-Oriented Approach Based on a Systems Model of Motor Behavior

- Personal and environmental systems, including the central nervous system, are heterarchically organized.
- Functional tasks help organize behavior.
- Occupational performance emerges from the interaction of persons and their environment.
- Experimentation with various strategies leads to optimal solutions to motor problems.
- Recovery is variable because patient factors and environmental contexts are unique.
- Behavioral changes reflect attempts to compensate and to achieve task performance.

Data from Mathiowetz V, Bass-Haugen J: Assessing abilities and capacities: motor behavior. In Radomski MV, Latham CAT, editors: *Occupational therapy for physical dysfunction*, ed 6, Baltimore, 2008, Lippincott Williams & Wilkins.

Box 4-2

Evaluation Framework for the Occupational Therapy Task-Oriented Approach Based on a Systems Model of Motor Behavior

Role performance (social participation)	Roles: Worker, student, volunteer, home maintainer, hobbyist/amateur, participant in organizations, friend, family member, caregiver, religious participant, other?
	Identify past roles and whether they can be maintained or need to be changed.
	Determine how future roles will be balanced.
Occupational performance tasks (areas of occupation)	ADL: bathing, feeding, bowel and bladder management, dressing, functional mobility, and personal hygiene and grooming
	IADL: home management, meal preparation and cleanup, care of others and pets, community mobility, shopping, financial management, and safety procedures
	Work and/or education: employment seeking, job performance, volunteer exploration and participation, retirement activities, and formal and informal educational participation.
	Play/leisure: exploration and participation
	Rest and sleep: preparation and participation
Task selection and analysis	What client factors, performance skills and patterns, and/or contexts and activity demands limit or enhance occupational performance?
Person (client factors; performance skills and patterns)	Cognitive: orientation, attention span, memory, problem solving, sequencing, calculations, learning, and generalization
	Psychosocial: interests, coping skills, self-concept, interpersonal skills, self-expression, time management, and emotional regulation and self-control
	Sensorimotor: strength, endurance, range of motion, sensory functions and pain, perceptual function, and postural control
Environment (context and activity demands)	Physical: objects, tools, devices, furniture, plants, animals, and built and natural environment
	Socioeconomic: social supports: family, friends, caregivers, social groups, and community and financial resources
	Cultural: customs, beliefs, activity patterns, behavior standards, and societal expectations

Adapted from Mathiowetz V, Bass-Haugen J: Assessing abilities and capacities: motor behavior. In Radomski MV, Latham CAT, editors: *Occupational therapy for physical dysfunction*, ed 6, Baltimore, 2008, Lippincott Williams & Wilkins.

and standardized assessments to evaluate their clients. Although the client is the primary source of information, other sources including the client's records, caregivers, family members, and the client's environment contribute as well."[54] The evaluation framework is described in more detail subsequently.

The first step in the evaluation process is to assess role performance. "Therapists must determine which roles clients had prior to the onset of disability, and which roles they can and cannot do at this time."[54] A discussion of roles that patients want or must do in the future helps determine which roles are most important to them. In addition, therapists need to explore ways that role changes have affected or will affect patients and their families, especially the primary caregivers. Jongbloed, Stanton, and Fousek[45] recommended that therapists ask questions

such as "How have roles changed since the disability?" "How have family members reacted to these changes?" "Is there role flexibility when needed?" and "How competently do members perform roles?" The therapist may need to adjust these questions to the patient's level of understanding. The patient and significant others must participate in the evaluation of role performance whenever possible.

The therapist may assess role performance using a nonstandardized, semistructured interview. However, a standardized assessment tool such as the Role Checklist[4,63] is suggested. The Role Checklist is a self-report, written inventory designed for adolescent, adult, or geriatric populations. In Part One, patients check the 10 roles (Fig. 4-2) that they have performed in the past, are performing in the present, and plan to perform in the future. In Part Two, patients rate the value of each role to them on a scale from "not at all valuable," "somewhat valuable," to "very valuable." The Role Checklist takes 10 to 15 minutes to complete and has evidence of reliability and validity (see Fig. 4-2).

The therapist may use other assessment tools to gather information on role performance. For example, the Occupational Performance History Interview-II (OPHI-II)[47] is a broad, semistructured assessment of occupational life history including work, leisure, and

ROLE CHECKLIST

NAME _____ AGE _____ DATE _____

SEX: ☐ MALE   ☐ FEMALE   ARE YOU RETIRED?   ☐ YES   ☐ NO

MARITAL STATUS: ☐ SINGLE   ☐ MARRIED   ☐ SEPARATED   ☐ DIVORCED   ☐ WIDOWED

The purpose of this checklist is to identify the major roles in your life. The checklist, which is divided into two parts, presents 10 roles and defines each one.

PART I
Beside each role indicate, by checking the appropriate column, if you performed the role in the past, if you presently perform the role, and if you plan to perform the role in the future. You may check more than one column for each role. For example, if you volunteered in the past, do not volunteer at present, but plan to in the future, you would check the past and future columns.

ROLE	PAST	PRESENT	FUTURE
STUDENT: Attending school on a part-time or full-time basis.			
WORKER: Part-time or full-time paid employment.			
VOLUNTEER: Donating services, **at least once a week,** to a hospital, school, community, political campaign, and so forth.			
CAREGIVER: Responsibility, **at least once a week,** for the care of someone such as a child, spouse, relative, or friend.			
HOME MAINTAINER: Responsibility, **at least once a week,** for the upkeep of the home such as housecleaning or yard work.			
FRIEND: Spending time or doing something, **at least once a week,** with a friend.			
FAMILY MEMBER: Spending time or doing something, **at least once a week,** with a family member such as a child, spouse, or other relative.			
RELIGIOUS PARTICIPANT: Involvement, **at least once a week,** in groups or activities affiliated with one's religion (excluding worship).			
HOBBYIST/AMATEUR: Involvement, **at least once a week,** in a hobby or amateur activity such as sewing, playing a musical instrument, woodworking, sports, the theater, or participation in a club or team.			
PARTICIPANT IN ORGANIZATIONS: Involvement, **at least once a week,** in organizations such as civic organizations, political organizations, and so forth.			
OTHER: _____ A role not listed which you have performed, are presently performing, and/or plan to perform. Write the role on the line above and check the appropriate column(s).			

Figure 4-2   Role Checklist. (Courtesy of Frances Oakley, MS, OTR, FAOTA.)

PART II

The same roles are listed below. Next to <u>each</u> role, check the column that best indicates how valuable or important the role is to you. Answer for <u>each</u> role, even if you have never performed or do not plan to perform the role.

ROLE	NOT AT ALL VALUABLE	SOMEWHAT VALUABLE	VERY VALUABLE
STUDENT: Attending school on a part-time or full time basis.			
WORKER: Part-time or full-time paid employment.			
VOLUNTEER: Donating services, **at least once a week,** to a hospital, school, community, political campaign, and so forth.			
CAREGIVER: Responsibility, **at least once a week,** for the care of someone such as a child, spouse, relative, or friend.			
HOME MAINTAINER: Responsibility, **at least once a week,** for the upkeep of the home such as housecleaning or yard work.			
FRIEND: Spending time or doing something, **at least once a week,** with a friend.			
FAMILY MEMBER: Spending time or doing something, **at least once a week,** with a family member such as a child, spouse, or other relative.			
RELIGIOUS PARTICIPANT: Involvement, **at least once a week,** in groups or activities affiliated with one's religion (excluding worship)			
HOBBYIST/AMATEUR: Involvement, **at least once a week,** in a hobby or amateur activity such as sewing, playing a musical instrument, woodworking, sports, the theater, or participation in a club or team.			
PARTICIPANT IN ORGANIZATIONS: Involvement, **at least once a week,** in organizations such as civic organizations, political organizations, and so forth.			
OTHER: _____ A role not listed which you have performed, are presently performing, and/or plan to perform. Write the role on the line above and check the appropriate column(s).			

Figure 4-2, cont'd

daily life activities. One part of it explores life roles, whereas other parts explore interests, values, organization of daily routines, goals, perceptions of ability, and environmental influences. The complete OPHI-II takes about 50 minutes and has evidence of reliability and validity. The OPHI-II includes information not only on role performance but also on occupational performance tasks, which are the next step of the evaluation process. In conclusion, after patients have identified the roles that they want or need to perform, they more easily can identify the tasks and activities needed to fulfill each role.

The second step in the evaluation process is the assessment of occupational performance tasks: ADL, IADL, work, education, and play/leisure (see Box 4-2). "Because roles, tasks, activities, and their contexts are unique to each person, a client-centered assessment tool such as the *Canadian Occupational Performance Measure* (COPM)[50] is recommended."[54] The COPM uses a semistructured interview to measure a patient's self-perception of occupational performance over time. First, patients identify problem areas in self-care, productivity, and leisure. Second, they rate the importance of each problem area, which assists therapists in setting treatment priorities.

Third, patients rate their own performance and their satisfaction with their performance on the five most important problem areas. Therapists may use these performance and satisfaction ratings again as outcome measures, measuring change across time. If therapists are concerned that a patient cannot rate performance accurately because of a cognitive impairment or age, therapists may use direct observation of selected activities or a caregiver interview to verify the information. The information elicited by the COPM is unique to each patient and the individual's environment, which is an essential part of the OT task-oriented approach (Fig. 4-3).

Another recommended measure of occupational performance specific to ADL and IADL is the Assessment of Motor and Process Skills (AMPS).[24] The assessment is client-centered because the person chooses two or three ADL or IADL tasks to be performed, which ensures that the task or activity is familiar and relevant to the person being evaluated. The purpose of the AMPS is "to determine whether or not a person has the necessary motor and process skills to effortlessly, efficiently, safely and independently perform the ADL tasks needed for community living."[24] The AMPS is appropriate for persons from diverse backgrounds and with diverse needs and interests because it has been standardized internationally and cross-culturally. "A unique feature of the AMPS is that it can adjust, through Rasch analysis, for the difficulty of tasks performed and the severity of the rater who scores the client's performance. In addition, it allows a therapist to compare the performance of clients who performed one set of tasks on initial evaluation with the results of a re-evaluation on a different set of tasks."[54] The primary limitation of the AMPS is that it requires a five-day training workshop to learn how to administer the assessment in a reliable and valid way. Computer software to score the AMPS is provided as part of the workshop. Finally, the AMPS assists in the next step in the evaluation process, because it requires observation of patients performing occupational performance tasks (see Chapter 21).

While evaluating occupational performance tasks, "therapists must observe both the outcome and the process (i.e., the preferred movement patterns, their stability or instability, the flexibility to use other patterns, efficiency of the patterns, and ability to learn new strategies) to understand the motor behaviors used to compensate and to achieve functional goals."[54] Determining the stability of the motor behavior is important to determine the feasibility of achieving behavioral change in treatment. "Behaviors that are very stable will require a great amount of time and effort to change. Behaviors that are unstable are in transition, the optimal time for eliciting behavioral change."[54] Thus, when behaviors are more stable, a compensatory approach may be most appropriate; when behaviors are unstable, a remediation approach may be

more successful. Quantitative and qualitative measures are needed to evaluate the process of task performance.

The third step in the evaluation process involves task selection and analysis. The tasks selected for observation should be ones that patients have identified as important but difficult to do. Task analysis requires therapists to observe their patients performing one or more occupational performance tasks. In most cases, observation of performance happens as part of the second step described previously. Therapists use task/activity analysis to evaluate activity demands, context, patient factors, performance skills, and performance patterns to determine whether a match exists that enables persons to perform occupational tasks within a relevant environment. If the person is unable to perform the task, therapists attempt to determine which person or environment subsystems are interfering with occupational performance. "In dynamical systems theory, these are considered the critical control parameters or the variables that have the potential to shift behavior to a new level of task performance."[54] Each person has unique strengths, limitations, and environmental context after a stroke. Therefore, the critical control parameters that support or limit occupational performance tasks are also unique. An effective intervention strategy for one person after stroke may not be effective for the next person. Another concept of dynamical systems theory is that critical control parameters also change as persons and their environments change over time. Therefore, an intervention that worked well early in a patient's rehabilitation might not work well late in the rehabilitation process or vice versa.

The identification of critical control parameters is the most challenging part of the evaluation process. However, evidence in the research literature indicates that some variables or subsystems of the person and/or environment are potential critical control parameters for persons after stroke. Gresham and colleagues[36] reported that psychosocial and environmental factors were significant determinants of functional deficits in persons for the long term after stroke. In a review, Gresham and colleagues[35] reported that 11% to 68% of persons experience depression after stroke, with 10% to 27% meeting the criteria for major depression. In the cognitive area, Galski and colleagues[28] reported that for persons after stroke, "deficits in cognition, particularly higher-order cognitive abilities (e.g., abstract thinking, judgment, short-term verbal memory, comprehension, orientation) play an important role in determining length of stay and in predicting functional status at the end of hospital stay." In the sensorimotor area, weakness,[65] fatigue,[44] impaired motor function,[6] and visuospatial deficits[82] are associated with poorer functional outcomes. For example, Bernspang and colleagues[6] reported that motor function measured with the Fugl-Meyer Assessment[27] was correlated moderately ($r = 0.64$) with self-care ability.

		IMPORTANCE
STEP 1A: Self-Care		
Personal Care (e.g., dressing, bathing, feeding, hygiene)	STYLING & COMBING HAIR	8
	DRESSING IN A TIMELY MANNER	6
Functional Mobility (e.g., transfers, indoor, outdoor)	GETTING UP SAFELY FROM BATHTUB	8
Community Management (e.g., transportation, shopping, finances)		
STEP 1B: Productivity		
Paid/Unpaid Work (e.g., finding/keeping a job, volunteering)		
Household Management (e.g., cleaning, doing laundry, cooking)	CHANGING SHEETS	9
	PREPARING MEALS FOR FAMILY	10
	FOLDING TOWELS	2
Play/School (e.g., play skills, homework)		
STEP 1C: Leisure		
Quiet Recreation (e.g., hobbies, crafts, reading)	SEWING	8
	NEEDLEPOINT	5
	MAKING X-MAS WREATHS	5
Active Recreation (e.g., sports, outings, travel)	PLAYING WITH GRANDKIDS ON THE FLOOR	9
	BOWLING	4
Socialization (e.g., visiting, phone calls, parties, correspondence)		

Figure 4-3   Identifying problems and rating importance via the *Canadian Occupational Performance Measure*. (Modified from Law M, Baptiste S, Carswell A, et al: *Canadian Occupational Performance Measure*, Toronto, 1994, CAOT Publications ACE.)

Practitioners must use the aforementioned literature on potential control parameters with caution. Most of these were correlation studies, which indicate relationships between these variables and functional performance, but they do not prove a causal link. In addition, most correlations were moderate or low, which suggests that any one variable explains a relatively small percentage of the variance associated with functional performance. However, Reding and Potes[70] provided evidence that as the number of impairments increased, functional outcomes decreased. "Thus, multiple variables contribute to functional performance for most persons with central nervous system dysfunction. The challenge is to identify those variables that are most critical to your clients."[54]

Bobath[9] suggested that spasticity is the primary cause of motor deficits in persons after stroke and that weakness and decreased range of motion are due to spastic antagonists. However, evidence is increasing that indicates that spasticity is not a critical control parameter.[11] For example, Sahrmann and Norton[72] reported electromyography findings that indicated movements were not limited by antagonist stretch reflexes (spasticity) but were limited by delayed initiation and cessation of agonist contraction. Similarly, Fellows, Kaus, and Thilmann[23] found no relationship between movement impairments and passive muscle hypertonia in the antagonist muscles. O'Dwyer, Ada, and Neilson[64] found no relationship between spasticity and either weakness or loss of dexterity. "Thus, research evidence challenges the assumption that spasticity causes the weakness and decreased range of motion often seen in persons with central nervous system dysfunction."[54] Recently, the Neuro-Developmental Treatment Association acknowledged this change in thinking: "There is not a direct relationship between spasticity and constraints on motor impairments or functional performance, as the Bobaths first proposed"[42] (see Chapter 10).

After identifying the critical control parameters that support or constrain occupational performance, the therapist must assess the interactions of these systems. Consider two patients who have complete loss of voluntary control of their dominant hand. The role and occupational performance tasks of the patient as a worker may or may not be affected. If the worker were an automobile mechanic, the interaction of this personal limitation with the activity demands of the work environment would likely make the task of repairing a car engine difficult or impossible to perform. However, if the worker were a self-employed writer, the person could learn to use a one-handed keyboard with the nondominant hand and could continue writing because the interaction of performance skills and activity demands would not interfere with role and task performance. This part of the evaluation requires the therapist to use qualitative and quantitative assessments and clinical reasoning to determine how subsystem of the person and the environment might affect occupational performance.

The fourth step in the evaluation process is to perform specific assessments of client factors, performance skills, and performance patterns, which are thought to be critical control parameters. The critical control variables are the only ones that need to be evaluated. "The evaluation of selected variables according to the OT task-oriented approach contrasts with bottom-up approaches that evaluate all component variables. This selective approach eliminates the need to evaluate variables that have little functional implication and saves therapists' time, which is critical for cost containment."[54]

Occupational therapists use a variety of assessments to evaluate patient factors, performance skills, and performance patterns that support or constrain occupational performance. Some assessments were designed to examine one or more impairments within the context of occupational performance. The Arnadottir OT-ADL Neurobehavioral Evaluation (A-ONE)[3] facilitates evaluation of perceptual and cognitive systems within the context of ADL (see Chapter 18 for details). From a task-oriented perspective, this is a preferred assessment tool because it links impairments more closely to occupational performance. In contrast, most assessments of impairments are conducted independent of occupational performance.

The fifth step of the evaluation process is evaluation of the environment: context and activity demands. The inclusion of physical, social, and cultural environments in American Occupational Therapy Association[2] uniform terminology acknowledges their important impact on occupational performance. A number of OT theories[16,21,51,78] emphasize the importance of assessing environmental context as part of the overall evaluation process. See Radomski[68] and Cooper and colleagues[17] for specific assessments of environmental contexts. See Chapter 27.

TREATMENT PRINCIPLES USING THE OCCUPATIONAL THERAPY TASK-ORIENTED APPROACH

Help Patients Adjust to Role and Task Performance Limitations

Many patients are not able to continue some of the roles and tasks that they performed before their strokes. This is a frustrating and sometimes depressing situation for many persons after stroke. Therapists can help by exploring alternative ways of fulfilling roles and of performing the associated tasks. Therapists also can explore potential new roles and new tasks. For example, in the case study presented at the end of this chapter, an important role for G.W. was continuing to help his son on the farm. The therapist helped the patient identify the tasks with which he had helped in the past and which ones would be impossible or difficult to perform in the future. For G.W., heavy or bilateral tasks (e.g., moving bales of hay and repairing heavy equipment) would fit this category. Brainstorming about alternative tasks that he could do unilaterally or relatively light tasks (e.g., record keeping) that he could still perform would enable him to continue his role as an assistant to his son. Inclusion of the son in this discussion was important, because he had suggestions that G.W. had not considered.

Create an Environment That Uses the Common Challenges of Everyday Life

Therapists need to be creative in creating environments within their clinical settings that provide typical challenges. Some facilities have purchased more real-life environments such as Easy Street, whereas other facilities have remodeled their clinics to simulate environments in which patients typically have to interact. Some have created small apartments to create a more realistic environment, in contrast to a typical hospital room, in which patients can interact before being discharged. Home care settings are ideal situations for following this treatment principle because the patient's own environment and objects can be used for therapy.

A stroke unit provides a more effective environment for improving functional outcomes.[43] The physical environment is set up to enable patients to function more independently. Patients are encouraged to wear their own clothing instead of hospital gowns. Thus, they are confronted with the common clothing of everyday life. In addition, staff members are trained to encourage independent behaviors. In G.W.'s case, nursing staff on the previous unit had assisted him in dressing and bathing. On the rehabilitation unit, nursing staff would encourage him to perform as many self-care tasks as possible. In addition, most rehabilitation units have patients eat together in a dining area instead of in their own rooms. This is a more typical way of eating, plus it facilitates social interaction and support from others struggling with many of the same problems. In addition, dining with others facilitates learning from and problem-solving with each other.

Practice Functional Tasks or Close Simulations to Find Effective and Efficient Strategies for Performance

In all cases, the therapist must use the functional tasks and activities that have been identified as important and meaningful to their patients. This demonstrates to patients that the therapist has listened to them and respects their choices and priorities. As a result, patients more easily understand the relevance of therapy to their lives.

Use of functional, natural tasks rather than rote exercise in treatment is important. A number of studies have demonstrated that the kinematics of movement are different when one performs a real task instead of rote exercise.[57,91] A metaanalytical review[52] provided evidence

that "engagement in purposeful activity produces better quality of movement than concentration on movement per se." Nelson and colleagues[61] demonstrated that after stroke, persons who performed an occupationally embedded exercise had significantly greater supination active range of motion than persons who did rote exercises. These studies support the idea that the use of functional tasks has beneficial therapeutic effects.

Higgins[39] suggested that persons need to practice functional, everyday activities to find the most effective and efficient way of doing the activity. Because persons are unique, their performance patterns and levels of skill vary. Therefore, therapists should not expect that one way of performing a task would be the most effective and efficient way of performing a task for all patients. Thus, therapists should encourage patients to experiment to find the most effective and efficient way of performing functional tasks. In one evidence-based review, the authors concluded, "There is strong evidence that patients benefit from exercise programmes in which functional tasks are directly and intensively trained."[84]

Provide Opportunities for Practice Outside of Therapy Time

Therapists need to recognize that the amount of time they have to work with a patient is short relative to the total time in a day. Therefore, enticing patients to continue therapy on their own time is important. Therapists can provide homework assignments for patients to work on their own. If homework is given, follow-up is important, and therapists should ask their patients how their homework went. What worked for the patients, and what did not work for them? Effective communication with other rehabilitation staff and family members is crucial, so that their attempts to be helpful do not reduce the opportunities for patients to practice outside of therapy time. Most important is for therapists to help patients find new ways to use their involved extremity, even if it is only to stabilize objects. A good homework assignment is to challenge the patient to find a new way to use the involved arm each day.[26] Ultimately, the goal is to get patients to use their involved arm without thinking about it.

Use Contemporary Motor Learning Principles in Training or Retraining Skills

Therapists should consider the following three motor learning principles:

- Use random and variable practice within natural contexts in treatment.
- Provide decreasing amounts of physical guidance and verbal feedback.
- Develop task analysis and problem-solving skills of patients so that they can find their own solutions to occupational performance problems in home and community environments.

Although blocked or repetitive practice of the same task normally is not recommended, such practice may be helpful or necessary when a patient is first learning the requirements of a new task.[74] However, therapists should shift to random and variable practice schedules as soon as possible to enhance motor learning. Random practice involves practicing more than one task within a session (i.e., avoiding repetitive practice of the same task). Variable practice involves experimenting with different tools for completing a task, with different location of the tools relative to the person, or with varied environments for performing a task. In addition, patients should practice tasks in their natural context whenever possible. Therefore, ADL tasks normally done in a patient's room should be practiced there rather than in the OT clinic. Even better would be patients practicing ADL tasks in their own homes.

When therapists are beginning to teach patients new tasks or new ways to perform previously learned tasks, they may need to provide some physical guidance and verbal feedback.[73] However, guidance and feedback should be tapered off quickly so that the person does not become dependent on them. For a therapist not to provide guidance and feedback when a patient is struggling to perform a task is difficult. However, providing physical guidance prevents patients from learning how to use their remaining resources to get the job done, and providing immediate and frequent feedback prevents patients from learning how to use their own feedback mechanisms to monitor and evaluate their own performance. If patients are unaware of a deficit (e.g., neglect to use involved extremity in a task), the use of a videotape of their performance can supplement their usual feedback mechanisms.[69] By the time a patient is approaching discharge, therapists should be providing minimal guidance or feedback. The therapist should remember that the goal of rehabilitation is to train the patient to be independent without the therapist's presence.

In a related issue, patients need to learn how to analyze tasks and to problem-solve on their own. If the therapist always analyzes tasks for patients and solves all their problems, the patients will not learn how to do those things themselves. In the limited therapy time available, preparing patients for all possible tasks, activities, and environments that they will confront after they are discharged is impossible. The therapist's role is to train patients how to do task analysis and problem-solving during the rehabilitation process, so that by the time they are discharged, they are capable of doing those things on their own. From early in rehabilitation, the therapist should involve patients in task analysis and guide them through the process. As occupational problems are addressed, the therapist should keep patients involved in trying to find solutions to problems. Therapists should encourage experimentation to find the optimal solution for that specific person. The therapist should remember that the same solution does not work for all patients (see Chapter 5).

Minimize Ineffective and Inefficient Movement Patterns

As described previously, during observation of a patient performing an occupational performance task, therapists attempt to identify what may be critical personal or environmental factors that are interfering with effective and efficient movement patterns. The following strategies are ways that therapists can intervene to reduce ineffective and inefficient movement.

Remediate a Client Factor (Impairment) if it is the Critical Control Parameter.
When therapists identify person factors in the cognitive, psychosocial, or sensorimotor systems as possible critical control parameters, then they should attempt to remediate those factors, assuming that is possible. For example, Flinn[26] identified decreased strength as one critical control parameter that interfered with occupational performance tasks for a person after stroke. Thus, she attempted to remediate this sensorimotor variable through the use of exercise and increased use of the involved extremity for functional tasks. For this person, the use of exercise was meaningful because she saw a clear connection between her exercise program and her ability to use her involved arm and hand for everyday tasks. The therapist also encouraged her to use her involved extremity whenever possible in therapy and for various homework assignments.

In the case of G.W., decreased strength, impaired sensation, and neglect of the left upper extremity were identified as possible control parameters. Therefore, attempts to remediate these factors were warranted in this case. However, sometimes remediation of a potential control parameter is impossible because of the severity of the disease process or limited time available for therapy. In such cases, a more compensatory approach to treatment is indicated.

Adapt the Environment, Modify the Task, Use Assistive Technology, and/or Reduce the Effects of Gravity.
For many patients, the quickest and most effective approach to improving occupational performance is to adapt the task and/or the environment. For example, Gillen[31] described a patient with severe limitations in self-care activities following multiple sclerosis and ataxia. Tremor, impaired postural control, paraparesis, and decreased endurance limited his occupational performance. The patient's priority was to gain access to the community and community resources. He did not have adequate motor control to operate a manual chair or to control a standard power chair. Therefore, a specialized power chair was prescribed that provided optimal head and trunk stability, allowed independent tilting, included

a joystick with tremor-dampening electronics, and a forearm trough to provide maximal stability to the arm controlling the joystick. A volar wrist splint provided additional stability to the wrist. With training in varied environments, the patient improved from total assistance in mobility to minimal supervision. Thus, the use of assistive technology, task modification, and training in varied environments was the most efficient and effective means of improving the mobility independence of this patient.

For G.W., a standard bath chair enabled independent and safe tub transfers. For shoe tying, G.W. preferred the use of Kno-Bows, an adapted device, for fastening his shoes rather than learning one-handed shoe tying. For cutting meat, an enlarged-handled fork was tried to encourage use of the left hand. However, this was not feasible at the time, so a rocker knife was prescribed. Thus a variety of adapted devices increased the ADL independence of G.W.

For patients unable to raise their arms up against gravity (i.e., grade 2 shoulder flexion and shoulder abduction muscles), the use of technology that minimizes the effects of gravity on their arms may help strengthen those weak muscles and enable increased functional performance. The use of body weight support during treadmill training has resulted in increased lower extremity strength and increased ambulation ability of person's poststroke.[84] Unfortunately, there has been limited application of this concept to the upper extremity. Devices such as mobile arm supports with elevation assist (e.g., Jaeco Multilink Elevation Assist) or deltoid aide counterbalanced slings (e.g., Swedish Help Arm or Mobility Arm) minimize the effects of gravity on a patient's arm and can be graded to provide less assistance as the person increases in strength. When these patients have some hand function, these devices can be used effectively for task-specific training. When these patients have limited hand function, the Armeo or T-WREX (www. hocoma.com) may be effective devices. They enable patients with upper extremity weakness and limited grasp and release to exercise their arm while using virtual reality simulated functional activities such as grocery shopping and cleaning a stove top. These task-specific activities can be adjusted to each patient's ability, and they motivate patients to use the available function in their arms and hands.[41] These devices that minimize the effects of gravity on a patient's arm have the potential to increase upper extremity strength and to improve functional performance. However, more research is needed to evaluate their effectiveness. See Chapters 11 and 28.

For Persons with Poor Control of Movement, Constrain the Degrees of Freedom. Persons learning a new task initially restrict the degrees of freedom at their joints by self-imposing some form of freezing of body segments.[39] As a result, their performance appears stiff and uncoordinated. With practice, the performance becomes smoother and more coordinated as the restrictions on the degrees of freedom decrease. Unfortunately, some persons with central nervous system damage are not able to constrain the degrees of freedom at their joints. For example, Gillen identified poor postural stability and tremor as interfering with the functional performance of a person with multiple sclerosis and ataxia. He speculated "that performance would be improved by increasing postural stability and decreasing the number of joints (decreasing the degrees of freedom) required to participate in chosen tasks."[32] Therefore, he used orthotic devices, assistive technology, and adaptive positioning of the trunk and upper extremity to help his patient constrain the degrees of freedom and to increase stability, which enabled improved ADL performance. Thus, the occupational performance of a patient with tremor was enhanced by strategies to decrease the degrees of freedom at those joints.

For Persons Who Do not Use Returned Function in Their Involved Extremities, Use Constraint-Induced Therapy. A growing body of literature supports the beneficial effects of constraint-induced movement therapy (CIMT) for persons after stroke with active wrist extension and active finger extension.[10,60,89] The original CIMT involves intensive therapy (i.e., about six hours per day for 10 days in a two-week period) while the less involved arm is constrained by a sling or glove. As a result, participants are forced to use their involved extremity to complete functional tasks, and thus CIMT counteracts the learned nonuse seen in many persons after stroke. CIMT is consistent with two assumptions of the OT task-oriented approach: "functional tasks help organize behavior and experimentation with various strategies leads to optimal solutions to motor problems"[54] (see Chapters 6 and 10).

In most clinical settings, CIMT as originally proposed would not fit into the current structure of inpatient rehabilitation programs and current reimbursement practices. However, there is growing evidence that a less intense (i.e., less times per day) and more distributed (i.e., spread out longer than two weeks) form of CIMT is also effective.[20,66,92] Thus, modified CIMT can be used within current rehabilitation programs. However, after stroke many persons do not meet the minimal eligibility requirements during their initial rehabilitation, so most CIMT programs are conducted on an outpatient basis for persons who are six months or more poststroke and who have sufficient return of function to benefit from CIMT. No evidence indicates that CIMT is effective for persons without some active wrist and finger extension. In the case of G.W., with the neglect of his involved extremity, he would not be a good candidate for CIMT now because he does not have sufficient active wrist and finger extension to benefit. At a later time, when that function does return, a trial of CIMT would be indicated. Chapters 6 and 10 contain more detailed discussions of CIMT. For a more detailed discussion of the OT task-oriented approach treatment, see Bass-Haugen, Mathiowetz, and Flinn.[5]

SUMMARY

This chapter describes an OT task-oriented approach for persons after stroke and describes the theoretical basis for and assumptions of the approach, based on contemporary motor control, motor learning, and motor development literature. The chapter also provides a top-down evaluation framework that emphasizes the importance of evaluating role and occupational performance tasks first and then the selective assessment of personal and environmental factors. In addition, the chapter describes the application of treatment principles to various patient problems and, finally, includes a case study describing the application of the OT task-oriented approach to a specific person after stroke.

CASE STUDY

Occupational Therapy Task-Oriented Approach for a Stroke Survivor

G.W. is a 69-year-old retired farmer who suffered a right cerebral vascular accident with resultant left hemiparesis five days ago. He was admitted to the acute care hospital and was then transferred to the rehabilitation unit today.

From the chart, it was learned that he is now medically stable. He is taking angiotensin-converting enzyme inhibitors for high blood pressure and Coumadin for prevention of a second stroke. He has been living in a small town with his wife since moving from their farm three years ago. His son, daughter-in-law, and their three children are farming in the local community.

Initial Evaluation

The Role Checklist was administered to evaluate G.W.'s role performance. Although retired, he continued to help out his son part-time as needed on the farm. He did most of the home maintenance, including the yard and a small garden. He attended church regularly, was a member of the men's club, and volunteered for the annual church dinner. In addition to his son who farms, he has another son and daughter, who are married and live within a two-hour drive. He has eight grandchildren. He and his wife enjoyed traveling with another retired couple from their church.

The COPM was administered to evaluate occupational performance tasks. The following five tasks were rated as most important to him: dressing, bathing, driving, gardening, and helping his son on the farm. His performance and satisfaction for these tasks were rated low. However, he had not had the opportunity to try the latter three tasks since his stroke, and nursing staff assisted him with dressing and bathing. He reported that he was independent in sink hygiene tasks, feeding (except for cutting meat), and toileting (except for pulling up and fastening trousers). He could ambulate 10 feet with a large, quad-based cane with moderate assistance. His wife did all the grocery shopping and cooking. G.W. had helped his wife with the laundry. He was unsure whether he would be able to play cards in the men's club now.

Dressing and bathing were chosen as tasks to be observed on the following day. G.W. was not able to dress himself independently primarily because of inability to use and/or neglect in using his left upper extremity. When cued to use his left arm, he demonstrated some voluntary control of his left shoulder and elbow and limited movement in the wrist and fingers. He complained of numbness in his left hand. During the bathing assessment, he needed assistance getting into and out of a tub. However, he could transfer in and out of the tub using a standard transfer bench. Once in the tub, he could control the water and bathe himself with one hand. He demonstrated good sitting balance during these activities, and he could stand independently when he could hold onto something with his right arm. He complained about the amount of time and energy it took him to perform self-care tasks. He demonstrated no evidence of cognitive or perceptual deficits except for some neglect of his left arm and left visual space. Based on these observations, it appeared that sensorimotor factors (decreased strength, endurance, range of motion, sensation, and neglect) were potential causes of limitations in occupational performance tasks, so these factors were selected for further evaluation. In contrast, cognitive and psychosocial factors appeared to be potential supports for increased independence. In addition, it appeared that modification of the environment (e.g., use of adaptive equipment such as a bath chair, Kno-Bows for shoe fasteners, and rocker knife) could be used to enable occupational performance tasks. However, more information was needed regarding his home and community environment to prepare for his discharge to home.

Tables 4-1 and 4-2 show the results of manual muscle testing, passive range of motion, and hand strength assessments for the left upper extremity only.

Sensory testing indicated a loss of protective sensation and diminished light touch in the left hand (Semmes-Weinstein monofilaments) and impaired proprioception in the left forearm, wrist, and hand. A line bisection test showed moderate visual neglect of the left side.

Home Environment

G.W. and his wife live in a small two-story home. Their bedroom, bathroom, kitchen, living room, and dining room are on the main floor. The upstairs has two bedrooms, a bathroom, and storage space. The washer and dryer are located in the basement. The front and back of the home have five steps with a handrail on one side only. They have a one-car detached garage that is close to the house. They have a 10-year-old car with a stick shift. They have a 10 × 20 foot vegetable and flower garden in their backyard.

Their home is paid for, and they receive modest checks from Social Security and some farm rental income from their son. If they stay healthy, their income is adequate for what they want to do. However, they are worried that if one or both of them were to become disabled and require nursing home care, then their income would not be sufficient to cover expenses.

Community Environment

Their house is lo_____
four blocks from _____
a grocery store, _____
liquor store, and _____
clothing or hardw_____
to a larger town _____
Their son's farm is located five miles from the house. The church has a split-level entrance with 10 steps to church level and 10 steps to the basement where the men's club meets. Fortunately, the church installed a chair glide to assist persons with mobility problems to get into church. However, no chair glide is available for the basement level. At this time, he knows that he cannot get up and down 10 steps, and this is a concern.

After a discussion of the evaluation results, the patient and therapist agreed on the following goals.

Week 1 Treatment Plan

1. Increase active use of the left upper extremity during ADL and leisure tasks (i.e., avoid neglect and learned nonuse of the left arm and hand).

Continued

Table 4-1

Manual Muscle Testing and PROM Assessment

LEFT UPPER EXTREMITY	MMT	PROM	LEFT UPPER EXTREMITY	MMT	PROM
Shoulder flexion	2+	0–155	Pronation	2−	0–75
Shoulder abduction	2+	0–155	Supination	3−	0–80
Shoulder external rotation	2−	0–45	Wrist flexion	2+	0–80
Shoulder internal rotation	2+	0–70	Wrist extension	1+	0–45
Elbow flexion	3−	0–150	Finger and thumb flexion	3+	Full
Elbow extension	2−	0–150	Finger and thumb extension	1+	Full

MMT, Manual muscle test; PROM, passive range of motion (units in degrees).

Table 4-2

Hand Strength Assessment

HAND STRENGTH	RIGHT HAND	INTERPRETATION	LEFT HAND	INTERPRETATION
Grip	102#	WNL	3#	BNL
Key pinch	19#	WNL	2#	BNL
Palmar pinch	17#	WNL	1#	BNL

BNL, below normal limits; WNL, within normal limits.

Occupational Therapy Task-Oriented Approach for a Stroke Survivor—cont'd

2. Increase independence in ADL and leisure tasks.
3. Begin planning for discharge to home and for possible roles for him on his son's farm.

The patient became aware through the evaluation process that he tended to neglect his left arm and hand and was motivated to improve its function. Thus, he was open to experimenting with using his left upper extremity to assist during functional tasks. He was taught one-handed dressing techniques with reminders to use his left arm and hand as much as possible. For example, G.W. was encouraged to raise his left arm as he slid his shirt on and to use his left hand to stabilize his shirt and pants while buttoning. Various options for tying his shoes were explored. He chose to use Kno-Bows because of the ease of using them compared with alternatives. A rocker knife was chosen to enable independent cutting of meat. The therapist communicated with his wife and nursing staff on what he was able to do relative to ADL tasks and what adapted equipment (e.g., bath chair) he needed to be independent. G.W. was independent in bathing himself when the bath chair was available to him. He expressed some concern about slipping and falling when he would get home. Plans were made to order the grab bars, bath chair, and nonskid bath mat.

In addition, various leisure activities including card playing were explored. He was able to pull cards toward himself with his left hand but was unable to pick them up or hold them. A cardholder was prescribed so that he could play cards immediately. Although he only had a mild interest in playing checkers, he found out that he could slide enlarged checkers with his left hand and was willing to work at this activity to improve his left arm and hand function.

During one session, his son and wife came to discuss his roles at home and on his son's farm. Both of them suggested that they could get help for the things that he could not do. Although G.W. agreed that there were some tasks he could no longer do or did not care to do, he still wanted to do some gardening and to help with some things on the farm. He did not want just to sit around and watch television. After brainstorming what roles and tasks might still be possible, the discussion shifted to adapted strategies and equipment that might be needed to make these tasks possible.

At the end of the first week, he was able to perform all ADL task with minimal supervision (i.e., reminders to use his left hand and to search his left visual space). He could now walk 30 feet with his cane and was practicing going up and down steps in physical therapy.

Week 2 Treatment Plan

1. Explore the possibility of driving and continued gardening.
2. Finalize plans for discharge to home, including ordering and installing adapted devices.
3. Finalize home program and follow-ups.

The patient was evaluated on some aspects of driving using a modified car. He was able to transfer in and out of the car with moderate supervision. He was discouraged that he was not able to push in the clutch with his left foot. He preferred driving a stick shift but could see that a car with an automatic transmission would be easier for him. He agreed to discuss getting a different car with his wife and son. Other adaptations that might make driving easier and safer were explored. The issue of neglect of his left visual field was discussed and evaluated using a driving simulator. He did have problems (i.e., simulated crashes) because of neglect. It was decided that additional practice with the simulator and other activities to improve his visual scanning were necessary before he could drive again.

G.W. continued to use various leisure and ADL activities to increase active use of his left arm and hand. Set-up of the activities was structured to require increased visual scanning as he did these activities.

Although G.W. continued to improve in his walking and stair-climbing ability, it was decided that a second handrail should be installed at both entrances to the home and in the basement and upstairs stairways. His son agreed to arrange for someone to do this. In addition, he agreed to install grab bars in the bathroom and in the hallway between the bathroom and bedroom. Sometimes, G.W. needed to use the bathroom at night.

Although he was improving in his performance on the driving simulator, he was told that he was not yet safe to drive. G.W. was referred to a regional driving center, which evaluates and trains persons with disabilities in safe driving. His wife or son would drive him until he could drive again.

A home program was developed with a variety of tasks and activities that required the use of his left arm and hand. He was now approaching the level of function that made him an appropriate candidate for CIMT. Unfortunately, access to this type of program was not feasible for G.W. because of distance and money. The therapist explained the concept of CIMT and developed a modified program that G.W. could do on his own. The modified program was adapted from a small study by Page and colleagues[67] and provided some evidence that an outpatient program of CIMT could be beneficial. Three outpatient follow-ups were scheduled to monitor and upgrade his home program.

REVIEW QUESTIONS

1. What are at least four assumptions of the occupational therapy task-oriented approach?
2. What is the primary focus of an evaluation of persons after stroke using the occupational therapy task-oriented approach?
3. From an occupational therapy task-oriented approach perspective, when is it appropriate to evaluate a performance component?
4. Describe at least four intervention principles of the occupational therapy task-oriented approach and how they could be applied to persons after stroke.
5. Describe at least two ways that contemporary motor learning principles could be applied to persons after stroke.

REFERENCES

1. American Occupational Therapy Association: Occupational therapy practice framework: domain and process, ed 2. *Am J Occup Ther* 62(6):625–683, 2008.
2. American Occupational Therapy Association: Uniform terminology for occupational therapy, ed 3. *Am J Occup Ther* 48(11):1047–1054, 1994.
3. Arnadottoir G: *In The brain and behavior: assessing cortical dysfunction through activities of daily living*, St Louis, 1990, Mosby.
4. Barris R, Oakley F, Kielhofner G: The role checklist. In Hemphill BJ, editor: *Mental health assessment in occupational therapy*, Thorofare, NJ, 1988, Slack.
5. Bass-Haugen J, Mathiowetz V, Flinn N: Optimizing motor behavior using the occupational therapy task-oriented approach. In Radomski MV, Latham CAT, editors: *Occupational therapy for physical dysfunction*, ed 6, Baltimore, 2008, Lippincott Williams & Wilkins.
6. Bernspang B, Asplund K, Eriksson S, et al: Motor and perceptual impairments in acute stroke patients: effects on self-care ability. *Stroke* 18(6):1081–1086, 1987.
7. Bernstein N: *The coordination and regulation of movements*, Elmsford, NY, 1967, Pergamon Press.
8. Bobath B: *Adult hemiplegia: evaluation and treatment*, ed 3, Oxford, 1990, Butterworth-Heinemann.
9. Bobath B: *Adult hemiplegia: evaluation and treatment*, ed 2, London, 1978, William Heinemann Medical Books.
10. Bonaiuti D, Rebasti L, Sioli P: The constraint induced movement therapy: a systematic review of randomized controlled trials on the adult stroke patients. *Eura Medicophys* 43(2):139–146, 2007.
11. Bourbonnais D, Vanden Noven S: Weakness in patients with hemiparesis. *Am J Occup Ther* 43(5):313–319, 1989.
12. Brunnstrom S: *Movement therapy in hemiplegia*, New York, 1970, Harper & Row.
13. Burton AW, Davis WE: Optimizing the involvement and performance of children with physical impairments in movement activities. *Pediatr Exerc Sci* 4:236–248, 1992.
14. Carr JH, Shepherd RB: *Neurological rehabilitation: optimizing motor performance*, Oxford, 1998, Butterworth-Heinemann.
15. Carr JH, Shepherd RB: *A motor relearning programme for stroke*, ed. 2, Rockville, MD, 1987, Aspen.
16. Christiansen C, Baum C: Person-environment occupational performance: a conceptual model for practice. In Christiansen C, Baum C, editors: *Occupational therapy: enabling function and well-being*, Thorofare, NJ, 1997, Slack.
17. Cooper B, Letts L, Rigby P, et al: Measuring environmental factors. In Law M, Baum C, Dunn W, editors: *Measuring occupational performance: supporting best practice in occupational therapy*, Thorofare, NJ, 2001, Slack.
18. Davis WE, Burton, AW: Ecological task analysis: translating movement behavior theory into practice. *Adapted Phys Activity Q* 8(2):154–177, 1991.
19. Dean CM, Shepherd RB: Task-related training improves performance of seated reaching tasks after stroke. *Stroke* 28(4):722–728, 1997.
20. Dettmers C, Teske U, Hamzei F, et al: Distributed form of constraint-induced movement therapy improves functional outcome and quality of life after stroke. *Arch Phys Med Rehabil* 86(2):204–209, 2005.
21. Dunn W: Measurement of function: actions for the future. *Am J Occup Ther* 47(4): 357–359, 1993.
22. Fasoli S, Trombly CA, Tickle-Degnen L, et al: Effect of instructions on functional reach in persons with and without cerebrovascular accident. *Am J Occup Ther* 56(4):380–390, 2002.
23. Fellows SJ, Kaus C, Thilmann A: Voluntary movement at the elbow in spastic hemiparesis. *Ann Neurol* 36(3):397–407, 1994.
24. Fisher A: *Assessment of motor and process skills*, ed 3, Fort Collins, CO, 1999, Three Star Press.
25. Fisher AG, Short-DeGraff M: Improving functional assessment in occupational therapy: recommendations and philosophy for change. *Am J Occup Ther* 47(3):199–201, 1993.
26. Flinn N: A task-oriented approach to the treatment of a client with hemiplegia. *Am J Occup Ther* 49(6):560–569, 1995.
27. Fugl-Meyer AR, Jääskö L, Leyman I, et al: The post-stroke hemiplegic patient: a method for evaluation of physical performance. *Scand J Rehabil Med* 7(1):13–31, 1975.
28. Galski T, Bruno RL, Zorowitz R, et al: Predicting length of stay, functional outcome, and aftercare in the rehabilitation of stroke patients: the dominant role of higher-order cognition. *Stroke* 24(12):1794–1800, 1993.
29. Gibson JJ: *In The ecological approach to visual perception*, Boston, 1979, Houghton Mifflin.
30. Gibson JJ: The theory of affordances. In Shaw R, Bransford J, editors: *Perceiving, acting, and knowing*, Hillsdale, NJ, 1977, Erlbaum.
31. Gillen G: Improving mobility and community access in an adult with ataxia. *Am J Occup Ther* 56(4):462–466, 2002.
32. Gillen G: Improving activities of daily living performance in an adult with ataxia. *Am J Occup Ther* 54(1):89–96, 2000.
33. Gleick J: *Chaos: making a new science*, New York, 1987, Penguin Books.
34. Gordon J: Assumptions underlying physical therapy interventions: theoretical and historical perspectives. In Carr JH, Shepherd RB, Gordon J, et al, editors: *Movement science: foundations for physical therapy in rehabilitation*, Rockville, MD, 1987, Aspen.
35. Gresham GE, Duncan PW, Stason WB, et al: *Post-stroke rehabilitation: clinical practice guidelines*, No 16, AHCPR Pub No 95–0662, Rockville, MD, 1995, US Department of Health and Human Services, Public Health Service, Agency for Health Care Policy and Research.
36. Gresham GE, Phillips T, Wolf P, et al: Epidemiologic profile of long-term stroke disability: the Framingham study. *Arch Phys Med Rehabil* 60(11):487–491, 1979.
37. Hanlon RE: Motor learning following unilateral stroke. *Arch Phys Med Rehabil* 77(8):811–815, 1996.
38. Heriza C: Motor development: traditional and contemporary theories. In Lister MJ, editor: *Contemporary management of motor control problems: proceedings of the II STEP conference*, Alexandria, VA, 1991, Foundation for Physical Therapy.
39. Higgins S: Motor skill acquisition. *Phys Ther* 71(2):123–139, 1991.
40. Horak FB: Assumptions underlying motor control for neurologic rehabilitation. In Lister MJ, editor: *Contemporary management of motor control problems: proceedings of the II STEP conference*, Alexandria, VA, 1991, Foundation for Physical Therapy.
41. Housman SJ, Scott KM, Reinkensmeyer DJ: A randomized controlled trial of gravity-supported, computer-enhanced arm

exercise for individuals with severe hemiparesis. *Neurorehabil Neural Repair* 23(5):505–514, 2009.

42. Howle JM: *Neuro-developmental treatment approach: theoretical foundations and principles of clinical practice*, Laguna Beach, CA, 2002, Neuro-Developmental Treatment Association.

43. Indredavik B, Bakke F, Solberg R, et al: Benefit of a stroke unit: a randomized controlled trial. *Stroke* 22(8):1026–1031, 1991.

44. Ingles JL, Eskes GA, Phillips SJ: Fatigue after stroke. *Arch Phys Med Rehabil* 80(2):173–178, 1999.

45. Jongbloed L, Stanton S, Fousek B: Family adaptation to altered roles following stroke. *Can J Occup Ther* 60(2):70–77, 1993.

46. Kamm K, Thelen E, Jensen JL: A dynamical systems approach to motor development. *Phys Ther* 70(12):763–775, 1990.

47. Kielhofner G: *User's manual for the OPHI-II*, Chicago, 1988, Model of Occupational Performance Clearinghouse.

48. Knott M, Voss DE: *Proprioceptive neuromuscular facilitation*, ed 2, New York, 1968, Harper & Row.

49. Latham CAT: Conceptual foundations for practice. In Radomski MV, Latham CAT, editors: *Occupational therapy for physical dysfunction*, ed 6, Baltimore, 2008, Lippincott Williams & Wilkins.

50. Law M, Baptiste S, Carswell A, et al: *Canadian Occupational Performance Measure*, ed. 3, Ottawa, 1998, CAOT Publications.

51. Law M, Cooper B, Strong S, et al: Theoretical contexts for the practice of occupational therapy. In Christiansen C, Baum C, editors: *Occupational therapy: enabling function and well-being*, ed 2, Thorofare, NJ, 1997, Slack.

52. Lin K-C, Wu C-Y, Tickle-Degnen L, et al: Enhancing occupational performance through occupationally embedded exercise: a meta-analytic review. *Occup Ther J Res* 17(1):25–47, 1997.

53. Lister MJ: *Contemporary management of motor control problems: proceedings of the II STEP conference*, Alexandria, VA, 1991, Foundation for Physical Therapy.

54. Mathiowetz V, Bass-Haugen J: Assessing abilities and capacities: motor behavior. In Radomski MV, Latham CAT, editors: *Occupational therapy for physical dysfunction*, ed 6, Baltimore, 2008, Lippincott Williams & Wilkins.

55. Mathiowetz V, Bass-Haugen J: Evaluation of motor behavior: traditional and contemporary views. In Trombly CA, editor: *Occupational therapy for physical dysfunction*, ed 4, Baltimore, 1995, Williams & Wilkins.

56. Mathiowetz V, Bass-Haugen J: Motor behavior research: implications for therapeutic approaches to CNS dysfunction. *Am J Occup Ther* 48(8):733–745, 1994.

57. Mathiowetz VG, Wade M: Task constraints and functional motor performance of individuals with and without multiple sclerosis. *Ecol Psychol* 7(2):99–123, 1995.

58. McNevin NH, Wulf G, Carlson C: Effects of attentional focus, self-control, and dyad training on motor learning: implications for physical rehabilitation. *Phys Ther* 80(4):373–385, 2000.

59. Merians A, Winstein C, Sullivan K, et al: Effects of feedback for motor skill leaning in older healthy subjects and individuals post-stroke. *Neurol Rep* 19(2): 23–25, 1995.

60. Morris DM, Crago JE, Deluca SC, et al: Constraint-induced movement therapy for motor recovery after stroke. *NeuroRehab* 9(1): 29–43, 1997.

61. Nelson DL, Konosky K, Fleharty K, et al: The effects of occupationally embedded exercise on bilaterally assisted supination in persons with hemiplegia. *Am J Occup Ther* 50(8):639–646, 1996.

62. Newell KM: Constraints on the development of coordination. In Wade MG, Whiting HTA, editors: *Motor development in children: aspects of coordination and control*, Dordrecht, Netherlands, 1986, Martinus Nijhoff.

63. Oakley F, Kielhofner G, Barris R, et al: The Role Checklist: development and empirical assessment of reliability. *Occup Ther J Res* 6(3):157–170, 1986.

64. O'Dwyer NJ, Ada L, Neilson PD: Spasticity and muscle contracture following stroke. *Brain.* 119(pt 5):1737–1749, 1996.

65. Olsen TS: Arm and leg paresis as outcome predictors in stroke rehabilitation. *Stroke* 21(2):247–251, 1990.

66. Page SJ, Levine P, Leonard A, et al: Modified constraint-induced therapy in chronic stroke: Results of a single-blinded randomized controlled trial. *Phys Ther* 88(3):333–340, 2008.

67. Page SJ, Sisto SA, Levine P, et al: Modified constraint induced therapy: a randomized feasibility and efficacy study. *J Rehabil Res Dev* 38(5):583–590, 2001.

68. Radomski MV: Assessing context: personal, social, and cultural. In Radomski MV, Latham CAT, editors: *Occupational therapy for physical dysfunction*, ed 6, Baltimore, 2008, Lippincott Williams & Wilkins.

69. Flinn NA, Radomski MV: Learning. In Radomski MV, Latham CAT, editors: *Occupational therapy for physical dysfunction*, ed 6, Baltimore, 2008, Lippincott Williams & Wilkins.

70. Reding MJ, Potes E: Rehabilitation outcomes following initial unilateral hemispheric stroke: life table analysis approach. *Stroke* 19(11):1354–1358, 1988.

71. Rood MS: Neurophysiological reactions as a basis for physical therapy. *Phys Ther Rev* 34(9):444–449, 1954.

72. Sahrmann SA, Norton BJ: The relationship of voluntary movement to spasticity in the upper motor neuron syndrome. *Ann Neurol* 2(6):460–465, 1977.

73. Schmidt RA: *Motor learning and performance: from principles to practice*, Champaign, IL, 1991, Human Kinetics.

74. Schmidt RA: Motor learning principles for physical therapy. In Lister MJ, editor: *Contemporary management of motor control problems: proceedings of the II STEP conference*, Alexandria, VA, 1991, Foundation for Physical Therapy.

75. Schmidt RA: *Motor control and learning: a behavioral emphasis*, ed 2, Champaign, IL, 1988, Human Kinetics.

76. Shea JB, Morgan R: Contextual interference effects on the acquisition, retention, and transfer of a motor skill. *J Exp Psychol Hum Learn Mem* 5(2):179–187, 1979.

77. Shumway-Cook A, Woolacott M: *Motor control: theory & practical application*, Baltimore, 1995, Williams & Wilkins.

78. Spencer J, Krefting L, Mattingly C: Incorporation of ethnographic methods in occupational therapy assessment. *Am J Occup Ther* 47(4):303–309, 1993.

79. Thelen E: Self-organization in developmental processes: can systems approaches work? In Gunnar MR, Thelen E, editors: *Systems and development*, Hillsdale, NJ, 1989, Erlbaum.

80. Thelen E, Fisher DM: Newborn stepping: an explanation for a "disappearing reflex." *Dev Psychol* 18(5):760–775, 1982.

81. Thelen E, Ulrich BD: Hidden skills. In *Monograph of the Society for Research in Child Development*, 56 (serial no 223), Chicago, 1991, University of Chicago Press.

82. Titus MN, Gall NG, Yerxa EJ, et al: Correlation of perceptual performance and activities of daily living in stroke patients. *Am J Occup Ther* 45(5):410–418, 1991.

83. Turvey MT: Preliminaries to a theory of action with reference to vision. In Shaw R, Bransford J, editors: *Perceiving, acting, and knowing*, Hillsdale, NJ, 1977, Erlbaum.

84. Van Peppen RPS, Kwakkel G, Wood-Dauphinee S, et al: The impact of physical therapy on functional outcomes after stroke: What's the evidence? *Clin Rehabil* 18(8): 833–862, 2004.

85. VanSant A: Should the normal motor developmental sequence be used as a theoretical model to progress adult patients? In Lister MJ, editor: *Contemporary management of motor control problems: proceedings of the II STEP conference*, Alexandria, VA, 1991, Foundation for Physical Therapy.

86. VanSant A: Life-span development in functional tasks. *Phys Ther* 70(12):788–798, 1990.

87. Warren WH: Perceiving affordances: visual guidance of stair climbing. *J Exp Psychol Hum Percept Perform* 10(5):683–703, 1984.

88. Winstein CJ, Schmidt RA: Reduced frequency of knowledge of results enhances motor skill learning. *J Exp Psychol [Learn Mem Cogn]* 16(4):677–691, 1990.

89. Wolf SL, Winstein CJ, Miller JP, et al: Effect of constraint-induced movement therapy on upper extremity function 3 to 9 months after stroke: the EXCITE randomized trial. *JAMA* 296(17):2095–2103, 2006.

90. World Health Organization: *International classification of functioning, disability, and health*, Geneva, 2001, World Health Organization.

91. Wu CY, Trombly CA, Lin KC, et al: A kinematic study of contextual effects on reaching performance in persons with and without stroke: influence of object availability. *Arch Phys Med Rehabil* 81(1):95–101, 2000.

92. Wu C, Chen C, Tsai W, et al: A randomized controlled trial of modified constraint-induced movement therapy for elderly stroke survivors: Changes in motor impairment, daily functioning, and quality of life. *Arch Phys Med Rehabil* 88(3): 273–278, 2007.

joyce s. sabari

chapter 5

Activity-Based Intervention in Stroke Rehabilitation

key terms

function

capacity

performance

neural plasticity

learned nonuse

constraint induced movement
therapy (cimt)

learning

training

practice

kinesiological linkages

generalized motor programs

cognitive strategies

strategies for community
participation

declarative learning

procedural learning

implicit learning

explicit learning

generalization/transfer of learning

intrinsic feedback

extrinsic feedback

knowledge of performance
(kp feedback)

knowledge of results
(kr feedback)

practice conditions

repetitive practice

blocked practice

contextual interference

closed tasks

variable motionless tasks

open tasks

mechanical constraints to
movement

self-monitoring skills

metacognition

task/activity analysis

postural set

postural adjustments

dissociation between body
segments

activity synthesis

practice challenges

compensatory adaptations

chapter objectives

After completing this chapter, the reader will be able to accomplish the following:

1. Apply the principles of the International Classification of Function and the Occupational Therapy Practice Framework to occupational therapy intervention for stroke survivors.
2. Understand implications of neuroscience studies of plasticity and constraint induced movement therapy to activity based interventions in stroke rehabilitation.
3. Design effective practice opportunities for stroke survivors to recover motor, cognitive, and participation skills.
4. Understand the basis of interventions designed to enhance stroke survivors' potential to achieve maximal recovery.
5. Apply principles of activity analysis and synthesis when designing occupational therapy intervention for stroke survivors.

With advances in medical intervention and societal attitudes toward people with disabilities, rehabilitation expectations and outcomes for stroke survivors are continuously improving. In recent years, evidence from the neuroscience and rehabilitation research literature, and shifts in thinking about the definition of health and wellness, have provided increasing support for two major tenets of occupational therapy with stroke survivors: that recovery of function can be enhanced through the therapeutic use of task-based challenges, and that a return to a meaningful lifestyle after a stroke is contingent on complex interactions between multiple factors.

This chapter presents concepts from the International Classification of Function (ICF),[64] the Occupational Therapy Practice Framework,[2] the Occupational Therapy Practice Guidelines for Adults with Stroke,[44] and research literature to provide an evidence-based foundation for the efficacy of activity-based intervention with stroke survivors. In addition, this chapter presents an introduction to salient concepts about practice and learning from the motor learning literature. Finally, this chapter applies the evidence to provide occupational therapists with guidelines for using activity-based intervention in stroke rehabilitation.

BACKGROUND CONCEPTS AND EVIDENCE

International Classification of Function

The ICF reflects a current understanding that health represents far more than the absence of disease (Fig. 5-1). Function, a dynamic interaction between health conditions and contextual factors, is ICF's yardstick for measuring successful rehabilitation outcomes. According to ICF, function is the integrated totality of one's body function, activity, and participation. The term *disability* is used as the antithesis of function and includes impairment, activity limitation, and/or participation restriction. In its discussion of activity and participation, the ICF distinguishes between capacity (the theoretical potential to perform) and performance in a person's actual, current context. This distinction is crucial in occupational therapy with stroke survivors. Demonstrated improvements within a treatment setting are mere changes in capacity. Clearly, the goal must be to promote generalization of regained skills for improvements in actual performance.

ICF integrates medical and social models of disability. While appreciating the medical model's value in promoting change within an individual, ICF also recognizes that social and environmental factors influence performance. Occupational therapists share this dual orientation in stroke rehabilitation. Depending on a person's current potential for skill recovery, occupational therapists adapt tasks and environments to promote optimal practice conditions for internal change or to facilitate task performance within constraints of insurmountable physical or cognitive limitations.

Occupational Therapy Practice Framework

The occupational therapy profession applauds both the vision and semantics of ICF. Accordingly, the Occupational Therapy Practice Framework[44] is structured to synchronize with ICF and thus to highlight that long-standing values within our profession are consistent with contemporary views about health and quality of life.

The Occupational Therapy Practice Framework provides practitioners with a foundation for designing and implementing multidimensional services that enable clients to participate in self-selected life activities within their homes, families, and communities. The Domain of Occupational Therapy[2] requires therapists to include the following components in assessment, planning, treatment, and outcomes:

- Client factors
- Activity demands
- Context
- Performance patterns
- Performance skills
- Actual performance of tasks and roles in real-life situations

Consistent with ICF's dual orientation to medical and social concerns, occupational therapy intervention considers two groups of factors: those within the individual (client factors, performance patterns, and performance skills) and those within the environment (activity demands and context). Some factors contribute to a particular person's capacity to engage in self-selected occupations; others do not. Some factors are amenable to change; others are not. A client may wish to change some factors and may have no incentive to change others. For each

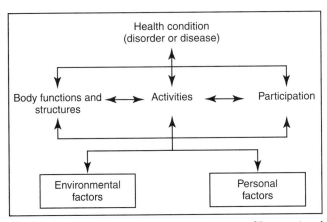

Figure 5-1 Interactions between components of International Classification of Function. (From World Health Organization: International classification of functioning, disability, and health [ICF], Geneva, Switzerland.)

individual, the skilled occupational therapist determines the unique constellation of impact, potential, and desire. Intervention promotes change in those internal and external factors that the therapist and client have collaboratively identified as treatment goals (Fig. 5-2).

Stroke is a complex condition. Depending upon the nature of the cerebrovascular accident (CVA) and immediate medical care, residual neuropathology varies widely among individuals. Consequently, related impairments and potentials for improvement differ significantly. Each person presents with a unique lifetime history of roles, activities, temporal patterns, and culture. Each person and family has unique constraints that govern their willingness to change long-standing routines and environments.

Various chapters in this text explore ways occupational therapists intervene, both to promote change within an individual and to adapt external factors to promote compensation. The ultimate goal of both interventions is participation in valued life activities. A comprehensive occupational therapy program for any stroke survivor will artfully target both internal and external factors. The interaction between internal and external factors is complex indeed. Improvements in motor and cognitive skills alone, unaccompanied by adaptations to family structure or physical accessibility, may fail to lead to an outcome of full, meaningful participation. Correspondingly, an overreliance on compensation, without providing stroke survivors opportunities to improve internal skills, seriously limits clients from reaching their ultimate potentials for engagement in a wide variety of life roles.

Occupational Therapy Practice Guidelines for Adults with Stroke

Practice guidelines are developed by many health professions to promote the use of evidence-based interventions for the goals of improving client care, enhancing consumer satisfaction, and facilitating interdisciplinary

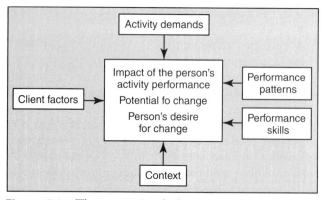

Figure 5-2 The occupational therapist's clinical reasoning process. In determining treatment goals, the therapist considers the three factors in the center square for each of the surrounding domain areas.

communication. The American Occupational Therapy Association (AOTA) has published practice guidelines related to a variety of client populations and areas of occupational therapy intervention. The Occupational Therapy Practice Guidelines for Adults With Stroke[44] presents extensive evidence from research literature in the neurosciences and in clinical rehabilitation that provide significant support for the value of introducing individualized task-based challenges to improve motor, cognitive, and occupational performance in stroke survivors.

NEUROSCIENCE STUDIES OF BRAIN PLASTICITY

It is common knowledge that necrotic tissue in the mammalian central nervous system does not regenerate.[4] This is the greatest challenge in stroke rehabilitation, as compared to rehabilitation for individuals with injuries to the peripheral nervous system or to the musculoskeletal system, where we expect ultimate recovery of damaged tissue. Even so, countless stroke survivors experience significant recovery of motor, language, and cognitive function.

Early, spontaneous recovery is typically attributed to resolution of temporary pathophysiology in regions of the affected hemisphere indirectly damaged by stroke-related sequelae described in Chapter 1. A stroke is a catastrophic physiological event. In addition to cell death in those neurons deprived of oxygen, indirect damage includes changes in cerebral blood flow, cerebral metabolism, edema, and cascading degeneration along neural pathways. The concept of diaschisis, coined by the 19th century Russian neurologist von Monakow has continued to influence neurologists and neuroscientists.[9,40,48] Diaschisis, or transient inhibition, spreads to remote sites in the fiber pathways leading from the site of injury. As diaschisis resolves over time, neural activities return to the temporarily suppressed regions, and the stroke survivor experiences return of function. Diaschisis is a probable explanation for the shift to spontaneous innervation of some flaccid muscles so often seen in the early weeks after a stroke. The phenomenon of "learned nonuse", articulated by Taub and colleagues[39,55] represents a person's inability to functionally use this reemerging motor activation. Occupational therapy intervention can prevent or reverse learned nonuse through interventions described in Chapter 10.

Neuroscience researchers are actively exploring a variety of potential recovery mechanisms after central nervous system damage. The possibility of plasticity, or reorganization of undamaged systems in the brain, has generated a growing body of positive research findings. These studies of humans and other mammals have provided significant evidence that recovery of function after brain lesions is associated with recruitment of brain regions not typically activated for a specified function.[10] These studies consistently find that reorganization of neural mechanisms is a dynamic process that is influenced by the person's active efforts to meet environmental and task demands.[26,30]

Depending on the extent of neuropathology, all stroke survivors have varying potentials for spontaneous recovery and reorganization of neural mechanisms. Using principles presented in this and subsequent chapters, the occupational therapist determines:

- Each client's current potential to relearn motor and cognitive skills
- How to match task-based challenges to each person's current potential
- How to modify each person's environment to provide the appropriate balance between challenge and compensation

CONSTRAINT INDUCED MOVEMENT THERAPY

Constraint Induced Movement Therapy (CIMT), which has yielded the strongest outcomes evidence of any treatment in the history of stroke rehabilitation,[62,63] provides significant support for the therapeutic value of activity-based practice for improving motor function in a select group of stroke survivors. CIMT evolved from the theory of learned nonuse, which postulates that potential motor recovery after unilateral brain lesions is limited by a learned overreliance on the unaffected limbs. Immediately after brain injury, contralateral flaccidity limits functional use of the affected arm and leg. Because motor function remains unaffected on the opposite side, most stroke survivors compensate by relying exclusively on the unaffected limbs to perform tasks. This theory of learned nonuse may explain why upper limb recovery lags behind lower limb recovery. Although each attempt to stand or walk requires bilateral activity in the legs, many upper limb activities may be accomplished by using the unaffected side exclusively.

In CIMT, physical constraint to the unaffected upper limb is provided in an effort to reverse the effects of learned nonuse. The typical research protocol has been for subjects who are at least one year poststroke to wear a mitt on the unaffected arm to remind them not to use this limb during virtually all waking hours for two weeks. On each of the 10 weekdays, subjects spend six hours in a rehabilitation program in which they are challenged with individualized task challenges that elicit repetitive practice in using their paretic arm and hand. In controlled double blind studies at three to nine months[62] and two years after intervention,[63] subjects who participated in CIMT performed significantly better than control participants in the speed and quality of their movement.

More importantly, they reported significant differences in the actual amount of use of the affected upper limb, as compared to control subjects. A note of caution about the use of CIMT in the early stage of stroke recovery emerges from acute animal studies. Studies with lesioned rats[27,42] have found that forced use with these animals during the first seven days after injury leads to degeneration of surrounding, surviving neural tissue.

Proponents of CIMT have never claimed that their approach reverses paralysis. In addition to intact cognitive function, criteria for participation in constraint programs include the minimum requirements that participants exhibit at least 10-degrees of active extension at the wrist, metacarpophalangeal, and interphalangeal joints, and demonstrate ability to maintain standing balance without upper extremity support.[62,63] CIMT is clearly an approach for a select category of stroke patients; but the principles have been successfully applied to several other protocols, which are described in Chapter 10.

In essence, CIMT "forces" the individual to practice using a paretic limb, and thus provides the central nervous system with appropriate challenges for reorganization of motor control. There is another aspect to CIMT never discussed by its proponents, and that may have significance for occupational therapy intervention with stroke survivors. There is a hypothesized link with Seligman's "theory of learned helplessness."[49] First discovered in dogs and later tested in numerous studies of humans,[50] this theory postulates that, after repeated exposure to situations in which actions are ineffective, organisms become passive, even when future actions could be effective. After an initial period of flaccidity following a stroke and subsequent relearning of one-handed task performance, many stroke survivors remain essentially unaware of a return of motor potential. Several factors might explain this phenomenon:

- The person has no reason to try to use the arm and thus remains ignorant about emerging motor potential.
- The person notices isolated abilities to perform specific movements, but doesn't know how to use these movements for integrated functional performance.
- The person experiences mechanical constraints that limit the capacity to use the recovering paretic limb in a functional way.

For those stroke survivors who meet the qualifying criteria, CIMT may be an effective way to improve motor performance. For those whose recovery is more limited, the concept of learned nonuse may still be helpful toward structuring effective therapeutic intervention. Furthermore, the extensive literature about neuroplasticity and CIMT supports the need for therapists to be experts about the role of practice and learning when providing evidence-based intervention to stroke clients.

PRACTICE AND LEARNING

Goals of Training and Learning

Learning and training are two distinct phenomena, each with its own required style of practice. The goal of training is to memorize a prescribed solution to a selected task challenge, whereas the goal of learning is to develop one's own solution, which can be applied in a variety of situations. Based on each client's abilities and role demands, the occupational therapist determines whether the therapeutic goal will be to promote training or learning. In therapeutic training, practice entails repetitive performance of a designated sequence of behaviors. Task performance must occur in the actual setting in which the individual plans to perform the task, because there is no evidence that skills acquired through training can be successfully applied in different environmental contexts.[52,57]

Learning and training are both internal phenomena that cannot be observed directly. Therapists assume that training has occurred if performance of a specific task improves and persists over time. Therapists assume learning has occurred when a person is able to apply a new set of skills within a variety of situations.[46,51] Whenever possible, occupational therapy attempts to promote learning of motor and cognitive skills that will provide the individual with an infinite number of choices for task and role engagement. Practice for learning requires active engagement in tasks that require problem-solving and implementation of effective foundational strategies. Therefore, before providing practice opportunities to stroke survivors, occupational therapists must first prepare the clients with underlying motor, cognitive, and social foundational strategies.

Foundational Strategies for Task Performance

Kinesiological Linkages and Generalized Motor Programs

When the neuromuscular system is functioning optimally, a person can rely on automatic kinematic and kinetic linkages to serve as a foundation for functional movements. Although these linkages are described in a variety of ways,[5,46,51] motor control theorists and kinesiologists agree that they promote optimal mechanical interactions between muscles and body segments.

Often, stroke survivors have lost the automatic kinesiological linkages associated with efficient movement.[13,59] This may be a result of limited mobility of body segments, weakness of specific muscular components, or loss of the motor program that links muscles or joints during a given movement sequence. Several automatic kinematic linkages are commonly observed during optimal movement, but are unavailable to many stroke survivors:

- Pain-free shoulder abduction through the full range of motion relies on scapulohumeral rhythm, a kinematic linkage between the scapula and humerus[41] (Fig. 5-3).
- The deltoid and rotator cuff muscles are kinetically linked to ensure that the deltoid fibers produce the desired rotary force on the humerus. Without this linkage, an attempt to abduct the shoulder will instead result in a nonfunctional upward shrug of the shoulder[41] (Fig. 5-4).
- Glenohumeral external rotation is automatically linked with end-range humeral flexion and abduction.[41]
- Grasp patterns are automatically linked with wrist extension to allow for efficient use of extrinsic finger muscles.[41]
- Lumbopelvic rhythm provides for appropriate interactions between movements at the lumbar spine and adjoining pelvis. When rising to stand from a seated position, for example, forward trunk motion is most efficiently initiated at the hips and is accompanied by simultaneous pelvic anterior tilt.[41] See Chapter 14.

Kinesiological linkages can be conceptualized as generalized motor programs (GMPs).[31,33,46] These "prestructured sets of central commands" govern a particular class of actions. GMPs are designed to be modified in response to continuous changes in environmental and task parameters. Therefore, a unique pattern of activity, with core

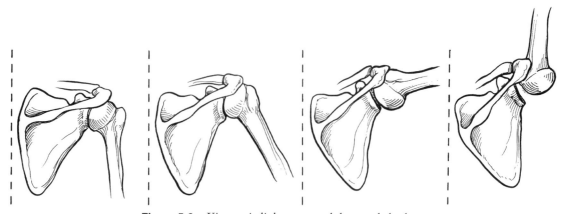

Figure 5-3 Kinematic linkage: scapulohumeral rhythm.

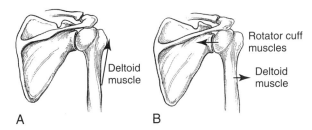

Figure 5-4 Kinetic linkage: relationship between deltoid and rotator cuff muscles. **A,** Deltoid muscle force acting alone. **B,** Deltoid and rotator cuff muscles working together.

foundational characteristics, emerges whenever the GMP is executed. For illustration purposes, a forehand tennis swing may be conceptualized as a GMP. Foundational kinesiological relationships comprise a GMP, but an athlete alters the force characteristics, timing, and spatial details of the forehand swing, depending upon the speed, force, and direction of the tennis ball's trajectory and the player's intentions regarding how to return the ball to the opponent. When designing therapeutic interventions to improve functional motor performance in stroke survivors, therapists determine the GMPs for general categories of movement, such as reach, grasp, balance, standing up, and sitting down. An occupational therapist determines which kinesiological linkages are impaired and intervenes by assisting with reestablishing these general foundations for optimal motor performance. Motion analysis studies of rolling, getting out of bed, standing up from a sitting position, and moving the arms provide useful information that can help an occupational therapist determine which components are essential in a variety of performance contexts.[12,51]

Cognitive Strategies
Just as kinematic linkages serve as foundational strategies for efficient movement, cognitive processing strategies provide individuals with a framework for interpreting and acting on complex information in a variety of situations. These strategies are organized approaches that assist a person in selecting relevant cues from the environment and planning the most appropriate response.[57,58]

Depending on the nature and location of the pathology associated with the CVA, a stroke survivor may demonstrate impairments in selecting and implementing appropriate cognitive strategies for accomplishing complex tasks. If these impairments are severe, they will limit performance of routine self-care tasks. Minimal to moderate impairments become more apparent when the individual attempts to resume more demanding occupations such as home management, work, or school activities. Toglia and Golisz have been particularly influential in designing evaluation and treatment protocols to guide occupational therapists in this aspect of intervention.[19,56,57]

Occupational therapy intervention begins with helping patients develop insight about these deficits through a program that challenges them to estimate task difficulty, predict outcomes, and evaluate personal performance.[20,56] Then the occupational therapist teaches general processing strategies that are practiced in a variety of contexts:

- Occupational therapists structure treatment to help clients develop several types of cognitive strategies.
- Prioritizing information before beginning a task is a strategy that can be applied to activities as varied as grocery shopping (using a list, coupons, and the weekly circular), doing a work-related task, or planning a family outing.
- Clustering related information together may be a useful strategy for a student attempting to master a difficult subject or for a person trying to remember what to purchase in the pharmacy.
- Blocking out irrelevant details is a foundational strategy necessary for reading a map and managing monthly bills.
- A left-to-right scanning strategy can be used to find a certain item in a bathroom cabinet and to check typing for errors. Maintaining a daily notebook of things to do and to remember is a strategy with wide applications in a range of situations.
- Additional strategies and their applications are discussed in Chapters 17, 18, and 19. Each individual tests the strategies introduced by the therapist to determine whether they are effective and in which situations they can be successfully applied.

Strategies for Community Participation
The social and emotional challenges of coping after a stroke are as demanding as the motor and cognitive challenges (see Chapters 2 and 3). Just as therapeutic interventions can improve strategies essential for moving and for processing information, so too can occupational therapists help stroke survivors develop a core of effective strategies that will help them negotiate their interactions with others and return to full participation within their communities. Therapists should introduce practice of these strategies early in the rehabilitation process. This helps stroke survivors understand that they can realistically expect to continue engaging in activities and roles that bring quality to their lives, regardless of the amount of motor recovery.

Types of Learning
Procedural and Declarative Learning
Occupational therapists structure practice opportunities according to the type of learning goal. Declarative learning is needed for tasks in which language skills are used to organize complex sequences of action.[4] Learning a new recipe or a multistep dance routine may require that a person be able to consciously express the processes to be

performed. Mental rehearsal is an effective technique for enhancing declarative learning. During mental rehearsal, the individual practices the sequence by reviewing it silently or by verbalizing the steps in their appropriate order. Most skill development in stroke rehabilitation, however, can be characterized as procedural learning, which is achieved through task practice in a series of varying contexts. For example, a person learns to maneuver a wheelchair through a process of procedural learning. Skill develops through opportunities to experiment with different combinations of arm or arm and leg movements to achieve propulsion in a variety of directions and speeds. Similarly, activities requiring balance or reach and grasp require procedural learning. Chapters 8 and 10 present therapeutic interventions for promoting development of these procedural skills.

Implicit and Explicit Learning Processes

Gentile[16] and others[6] propose that individuals use two distinct but interdependent processes during the acquisition of functional motor skills. An explicit learning process, which is consciously driven, guides the kinematics of the movement. Gentile hypothesizes that people use an explicit process to develop a "ballpark" match between the shape or direction of their movements and the environmental requirements for achieving the goal. External guidance and feedback is likely to have a beneficial impact upon the explicit learning process. Schmidt[46] refers to such intervention as an "instructional set," in which the person is given a general idea or image of the task to be learned.

An implicit learning process guides the kinetics of the movement or the dynamics of force generation. This aspect of movement requires appropriate selection of muscle contraction patterns, which is determined by accurate predictions of how external forces will affect the movement. Implicit learning requires a self-organizing process and may take longer to develop than explicit learning. Furthermore, implicit learning lies beyond conscious awareness and is unlikely to be augmented by external guidance or feedback.[11,38] Historically, neurorehabilitation interventions that attempted to directly influence implicit aspects of motor performance, such as muscle recruitment or force modulation, have failed to achieve functional outcomes. Following evidence from motor learning research, therapists should attempt to influence implicit learning by providing appropriate opportunities for effective practice.

Amount of Practice

Practice is a critical component to learning. Educators, therapists, and neuroscientists universally agree that the amount of practice affects success in skill development.[46,60] Effective protocols in stroke rehabilitation[15,34,35,62,63] all share the common characteristic of maximizing the amount of practice. Occupational therapy provides stroke survivors with structured practice opportunities to maximize emerging skills. This is not nearly as simple as it sounds. When people practice maladaptive strategies, they "learn" patterns of behavior that may be counterproductive to future improvements in functional performance. To provide appropriate practice opportunities, therapists must be able to clearly envision the intended practice outcomes and to skillfully manipulate a variety of factors within each practice session. These factors include instructions, feedback, activity parameters, salient conditions within the practice environment, and practice schedules. Furthermore, therapists must recognize the importance of practice during daily activities outside of therapy sessions and structure feasible independent practice opportunities for patients. Subsequent chapters will emphasize ways occupational therapists structure these factors and their interactions so that stroke survivors can engage in practice that yields desired learning for functional outcomes.

Promoting Generalization of Learning

Three stages of learning are important in the occupational therapy process[46]:

1. The *acquisition phase* occurs during initial instruction and practice of a skill (e.g., the initial treatment sessions in which a person learns to use the left arm for functional reach).
2. The *retention phase* occurs after the initial practice period as individuals are asked to demonstrate how well they perform the newly acquired skill; therapists often refer to this as *carryover* (e.g., a patient's ability to perform previously learned reaching activities).
3. In the *transfer phase* the individual must use the skill in a new context (e.g., the patient's ability to incorporate a reaching strategy when getting dressed or preparing a meal). The stroke survivor can generalize the strategies learned in the therapy setting and use them in real-life situations.

Literature about skill acquisition presents several concepts helpful in guiding therapeutic intervention that promotes generalization of learning. These concepts can be categorized into three major groups: type of feedback, development of underlying strategies, and practice conditions (Fig. 5-5).

Type of Feedback

Feedback, or information about a response, can be intrinsic or extrinsic, concurrent or terminal, and can provide knowledge of performance (KP) or knowledge of results (KR). Intrinsic feedback is a result of an individual's own proprioceptive, tactile, vestibular, visual, and auditory sensory systems. Often after a stroke, somatosensory function is impaired, which limits the effectiveness of intrinsic feedback about motor performance. Extrinsic feedback from a therapist or feedback technology can

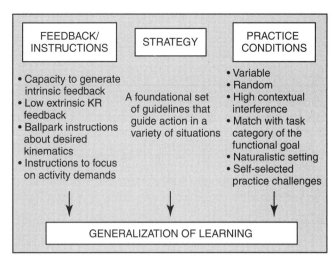

Figure 5-5 Factors that contribute to generalization of learning. KR, Knowledge of results.

provide useful supplementary information to facilitate early awareness and learning. However, extrinsic feedback must be gradually decreased for generalization to occur.[46]

Concurrent feedback is provided during task performance. It includes intrinsic somatosensory feedback and ongoing verbal or manual guidance by a therapist. Terminal, or summary, feedback is given after task completion.[47] There are no published studies that compare the effectiveness of concurrent and terminal feedback, but research has established that excessive external concurrent feedback is clearly distracting to the learner.[47]

Knowledge of Performance. KP feedback is information about the processes used during task performance, such as the way a person moves the pelvis or scapula or whether an appropriate cognitive or social strategy has been implemented. Individuals with intact proprioceptive systems receive concurrent, intrinsic KP feedback as they move. Stroke survivors, however, may no longer have access to this continuous supply of information. Extrinsic KP can be provided before a task is initiated. For example, a therapist can guide a person into assuming a postural set that will facilitate motor performance or in planning a strategy that will enhance performance of a cognitively demanding task. Research literature examining persons without neurological impairments[53,66] and stroke survivors[14] indicates that a focus on internal performance factors may be counterproductive to learning. Instructing the learner to focus on relevant information in the environment (such as the distance or shape of a goal object) seems to be more effective than directing the learner's attention internally toward the key elements of a particular movement pattern or sequence.[14] The skillful therapist must structure selected parameters within the practice tasks to "press" the individual toward using an intended movement pattern.

Knowledge of Results. KR is feedback about the outcome of an action in terms of accomplishing a goal. This information can serve as a basis for correcting errors for more effective performance on future trials. Results of laboratory research with healthy subjects indicates that frequent, accurate, immediate KR tends to promote improved performance during the acquisition phase but poorer performance during the retention and transfer stages of learning.[45,61] Similarly, bandwidth KR, in which feedback is provided only when the performance response is outside a given range of acceptable performance, also leads to better generalization of learning.[61] Schmidt[46] provides the following theoretical explanation of these findings. When limited KR is provided during acquisition, individuals must rely on relevant cues provided by intrinsic mechanisms to improve their performance on future trials, and they tend to develop less dependency on extrinsic feedback. Based on these findings, it is wise for therapists to limit the immediacy and frequency of KR feedback during stroke rehabilitation. Furthermore, therapists are advised to require that patients determine how effectively they performed therapeutic tasks. To generalize their knowledge for use in situations outside the treatment context, stroke survivors need to learn ways to assess their own performance of functional activities.

Strategy Development

Strategies are organized plans or sets of rules that guide action in a variety of situations. New knowledge is more likely to be generalized for use after the acquisition phase if the individual learns a foundational strategy that can be applied to performance of multiple tasks.[52]

Therapeutic approaches that advocate the importance of strategy formulation during task performance[13,57] seek to develop selected motor or cognitive linkages through engagement in a series of tasks that, at a superficial level, may seem unrelated. Each task, however, requires use of the selected strategy. To ensure generalization of the strategy, the selected underlying skill is practiced repeatedly in a variety of contexts during a treatment session. For example, the therapeutic goal may be to develop a selected lumbopelvic linkage as a GMP for forward reach in sitting and standing up from a seated position. The session may begin with the therapist moving the patient's pelvis so that the person understands the kinematic model of action. The therapist may then ask the patient to sit on a therapy ball, which is rocked forward and backward using anterior and posterior pelvic movement. After this, the seemingly unrelated task of reaching for objects from the seated position will emphasize that the patient anteriorly tilt the pelvis by directing attention to "keeping your back straight" and "bringing your nose over your toes." Finally, the patient will practice standing up and sitting down on a variety of surfaces, with an emphasis one the same lumbopelvic interactions previously practiced in different contexts. Research findings from studies with healthy participants provide support for the use of this approach for learning the invariant structure of a GMP.[18,33] In the terminology of motor learning science, these studies found that a constant or blocked practice schedule of the underlying GMP, using varied practice parameters, leads to enhanced transfer benefits.

Carr and Shepherd's program for optimizing motor function after stroke[12,13] uses five major techniques to assist patients with developing motor strategies: (1) verbal instruction, (2) visual demonstration, (3) manual guidance, (4) accurate and timely feedback, and (5) consistency of practice. In addition, patients develop skill in providing themselves with intrinsic feedback about the kinematics of their motor performance. Outcome studies[39] of individuals recovering from stroke provide support for this program's efficacy.[12,13]

Toglia[56,57] and Golisz[19] developed a systematic approach to promote generalization of cognitive strategies, in which the therapist grades treatment by changing certain characteristics of a task but leaving the underlying strategy the same. The following example illustrates a treatment sequence designed to facilitate learning and generalization of a strategy for categorizing information:

The initial task is the first activity performed by the patient, such as sorting a deck of playing cards into a red group (hearts and diamonds) and a black group (spades and clubs). Near transfer is an alternate form of the initial task. Using the previous example, the person might be instructed to sort the playing cards into four groups according to their suits or two groups of odd and even numbers.

Intermediate transfer has a moderate number of changes in task parameters but still has some similarities to the initial task. For example, the same person may be asked to create three categories for sorting a stack of photographs for eventual placement in a photo album.

Far transfer introduces an activity conceptually the same as but physically different from the initial task. Now the person may be asked to organize a collection of magazines into groups based on general interest areas (e.g., news, sports, fashion) for display in a clinic waiting room.

Very far transfer requires spontaneous use of the new strategy in daily functional activities. Before traveling to a neighborhood mall, the person may be asked to categorize items on a shopping list based on the type of store in which they can most likely be purchased.

This "multicontext approach" emphasizes the use of self-assessment and intrinsic KP feedback. Before attempting a new task, patients estimate their performance accuracy and efficiency and determine similarities and differences between the current task and previous activities. After completing a task, patients evaluate their performance and identify techniques that may be helpful

in the future. The therapist's major roles are to structure the activity progression and guide patients in developing insights and strategies. See Chapter 19.

Practice Conditions

Several aspects of practice conditions have been studied under both laboratory and clinical conditions. Occupational therapists can use these findings to structure practice conditions in stroke rehabilitation programs. The key is to structure conditions during the acquisition phase that will produce optimal retention and transfer of the learned skills.

Practice Schedules. During blocked (or repetitive) practice, patients practice one task until they master it. This is followed by practice of a second task until it is also mastered. Random (or variable) practice requires patients to attempt multiple tasks or variations of a task before they have mastered any one of the tasks. In addition, the various trials are performed in a random order. Subjects who participate in variable practice perform better on transfer tests than subjects who participate in repetitive practice.[21] A study of stroke outpatients found that random practice was more effective than blocked practice for long-term retention of improvements in reach and manipulation skills.[22] An explanation is that variable practice facilitates generalization by preventing individuals from developing context-dependent inflexibility when using a newly learned skill.

Contextual Interference. Contextual interference refers to factors in the learning environment that increase the difficulty of initial learning.[7] Research studies consistently find that higher levels of contextual interference promote retention and generalization (transfer) of newly learned skills.[8,29,54] These findings are typically explained with the hypothesis that initial obstacles to skill acquisition prevent individuals from developing context-dependent inflexibility when using the learned skill in new situations.[7] Another explanation is that high contextual interference forces a person to use greater versatility in learning strategies in order to overcome the difficulty of initial practice during the acquisitional learning phase.[28] Limited KR feedback is one example of contextual interference that has already been discussed. Blocked and random practice schedules, described previously, are examples of low and high contextual interference, respectively. Although blocked practice may lead to quicker skill acquisition, random practice results in greater retention and generalization.[46]

Whole versus Part Practice. Therapists may intuitively believe that it will be easier for a client to learn small segments of a task than the task in its entirety. However, breaking a task into its component parts for teaching purposes is useful only if the task can be naturally divided into units that reflect the inherent goals of the task.[37] One reason for this is that continuous skills (or whole-task performance) are easier to remember than discrete responses. For example, once people have learned to ride a bicycle or play tennis, they will retain these motor skills even without practicing them for many years. On the other hand, segmented, laboratory-type motor skills may be acquired easily but are less likely to be retained over time. Therefore, therapists are advised to teach tasks in their entirety rather than in artificial segments. For example, for best retention and generalization, the task of putting on a shirt is best taught all at once rather than in different portions during consecutive therapy sessions. If it is difficult for a stroke survivor to master all the steps simultaneously, the therapist can cue the patient or can provide manual guidance for selected aspects of the task (as is used in backward chaining instruction). The patient will become accustomed to completing the task during each trial. The therapist's assistance can be gradually decreased as practice sessions continue.

Practice in Natural Settings. Transferring skills learned during training to real-life situations is significantly influenced by the degree of similarity between the practice environment and the actual environment.[36] Wu and colleagues[65] provided specific support for the value of using real task performance during therapy sessions to improve motor control in stroke survivors. Their motion analysis studies of persons with and without stroke compared the kinematic parameters of reach patterns when participants reached forward to perform a functional task and when they reached forward with no functional goal. Participants in both the neurologically intact and poststroke groups performed better when real objects were available to shape the reach performance.

Skills for performing tasks such as dressing or bathing are best generalized when the skills have been acquired in a setting that resembles the environment in which the activity will ultimately be performed. Occupational therapy clinics with simulated home and community environments will promote better generalization of performance area skills than clinics in which practice of daily tasks is contrived. However, many stroke survivors can never generalize what they learn in simulated settings; in these cases, home-based occupational therapy is required.

Different Practice Conditions for Different Task Categories. Gentile[16] postulated that motor activities can be classified into four general categories based on environmental pacing conditions and variability between successive trials. Practice conditions for learning will vary depending on the task category.

Closed tasks are activities in which the environment is stable and predictable and methods of performance are consistent over time. Brushing teeth or getting into and out of a bathtub are examples of closed tasks that may be goals for stroke survivors. The best strategy for developing skill in a specific closed task is to develop a narrow and consistent method of performance through repetitive practice of the task.

Variable motionless tasks also involve interacting with a stable and predictable environment, but specific features of the environment are likely to vary between performance trials. Drinking is an example of a variable motionless task because the type of mug, glass, or cup used, and the amount the container is filled will vary in different situations. Dressing is another example because people's wardrobes consist of clothing of varying fabrics, dimensions, and styles. To achieve independence in a variable motionless task, a patient must learn more than one method of performance. The therapist must provide individuals with opportunities to solve the activity's motor problems in a wide variety of contexts.

In consistent motion tasks, an individual must deal with environmental conditions in motion during an activity performance; the motion is consistent and predictable between trials. Stepping on to or off of an escalator or moving through a revolving door are examples of consistent motion tasks. Patients need practice that will enable them to accurately match the timing of their actions to the predictable changes of the moving objects in the environment.

Open tasks require people to make adaptive decisions about unpredictable events because objects within the environment are in random motion during task performance. These activities require appropriately timed movements and spatial anticipation of where the relevant objects will be moving. For example, a passenger who is sitting in a moving train must maintain balance when the supporting surface is moving unpredictably. When crossing a street, a person must anticipate the speed and rhythm of both pedestrians and oncoming traffic. When playing most ball games, people must predict the speed and direction of the ball to position themselves in the right place at the right time. Research has shown that the skills required for successful open-task performance cannot be learned through repetitive practice in a stationary environment.[24,25] Natural practice in an unpredictable environment seems to be the best strategy for developing skill in open-task performance.

Applying Background Concepts to Using Activity-Based Intervention in Occupational Therapy with Stroke Clients

Prerequisites to Engaging in Activity-Based Practice

Depending on the extent of the neuropathology, each stroke survivor has a hypothetical, unknown potential for recovery of function. Although practice is crucial, a variety of factors may impede a person's capacity to benefit from practice opportunities:

- Mechanical constraints to movement
- Inadequate self-monitoring skills
- Inadequate task analysis and problem-solving skills
- Low expectations for goal achievement

A skilled therapist prepares each patient to engage in activity-based practice by directing interventions toward maximizing each factor described in the following sections.

Freedom from Mechanical Constraints to Movement

Stroke survivors encounter several mechanical constraints that limit their ability to move and force them to develop alternative movement strategies. Selected muscle weakness and loss of automatic control over complex postural adjustments are primary impairments, directly related to the stroke pathology. Other mechanical constraints, such as soft-tissue contracture and changes in joint alignment, are secondary to changes in posture and loss of mobility associated with stroke.[12,13,43] As secondary impairments, these losses are preventable and reversible with timely interventions.

Muscles lose their natural distensibility when they cease to be passively lengthened by antagonist muscles or an external force. This loss of passive muscle length may lead to malalignments in posture that contribute to a continuing spiral of increasing and additional abnormalities in soft-tissue flexibility. Without active or passive movement, the person is at risk of developing fixed limitations of joint motion and alignment.[12,13,43] These problems can be prevented by establishing appropriate postural alignment while lying down, sitting, and standing. In addition, shortly after a stroke, individuals are instructed to follow daily routines to maintain optimal muscle length through the practice of a variety of motor tasks. These interventions are discussed in Chapters 7, 10, 14, and 26.

Fluid, efficient movement requires a mechanical capacity for dissociation between body segments. Although body segments may be kinematically linked during certain actions, each segment must also be free to move independently of its adjacent structures. Scapular-humeral rhythm requires full dissociation between the scapula and thorax. Coordinated shoulder movements require that the humerus freely move independently of the scapula. A full repertoire of trunk activity requires mobility between the thoracic and lumbar spine and between the pelvis and lumbar spine. Stroke survivors often experience loss of dissociation between adjacent body segments. This may occur simply because of losses in soft-tissue distensibility, or it may be linked to maladaptive motor strategies people develop in a subconscious effort to solve other problems. For example, individuals with postural adjustment deficits resulting from stroke often feel insecure about their ability to maintain balance, even in routine sitting or standing positions. The strategy of fixating the pelvis on the lumbar spine or the scapula on the thorax may have the short-term benefit of enhancing a person's sense of postural security. A negative consequence is that these habitual postures lead to difficulty dissociating the pelvis and scapula from adjacent proximal structures. This lack of sufficient limb girdle mobility subsequently interferes with the kinematics of upper and lower extremity movement. Current therapeutic approaches advocate the early introduction of techniques to enhance balance and postural control.[13,51] In addition to the inherent advantages of postural security, early recovery of appropriate balance strategies may prevent postural habits that can compromise a stroke survivor's future potential to use reemerging muscle function for functional arm and leg movement. See Chapters 7, 8, and 14.

Other secondary impairments, such as edema and pain, seriously limit a person's potential for movement or functional activity engagement. Therapists are responsible for preventing and minimizing mechanical constraints to movement before introducing practice opportunities for improving motor control. See Chapter 12.

Foundational Strategies

As previously discussed, developing foundational strategies is valuable as an intervention approach designed to maximize generalization of learned skills. GMPs are critical for a variety of motor actions. In addition, foundational strategies for classes of cognitive and social skills enable stroke survivors to meet current and unanticipated, future activity demands. Explicit learning, combined with structured demands to enhance self-monitoring of salient features in a desired strategy, establishes an underlying framework for a foundational strategy. Implicit learning, through participation in selected, graded task challenges, promotes development of higher order skills associated with the strategy. Practice opportunities for implementing a strategy under varying parameters promotes flexibility in modifying the strategy to accommodate to ever changing environmental demands.

Self-Monitoring Skills

Stroke survivors face the challenge of resuming their lives in a body quite different from the one they inhabited before; sensory information may be difficult to interpret, muscles may no longer work in effortless synchrony, and postural preparation for movement may no longer be automatic.

Before stroke survivors can begin to learn effective strategies for movement and task performance, they need to become acutely aware of the way their bodies work, which movements are possible at different body segments, when their postures are optimally aligned, and when they are efficiently "set" to perform particular activities. These understandings are critical for redeveloping appropriate kinesiological linkages that will serve as motor foundations for task performance.

Metacognition[1] is the knowledge and regulation of personal cognitive processes and capacities. It includes an awareness of personal strengths and limitations and the ability to evaluate task difficulty, plan ahead, choose appropriate strategies, and shift strategies in response to environmental cues. The multicontext approach to cognitive perceptual impairment emphasizes developing insight about personal deficits (and strengths) as a first step toward developing strategies for functional performance after brain injury. See Chapter 19.

Understanding the concept of metacognition is important for understanding movement as well. Before individuals can generalize the way to use scapulohumeral rhythm in tasks requiring functional reach, they must first understand the amount of mobility their unaffected scapula has. Then they must acknowledge when their affected scapula is not moving freely so that they can develop internal feedback mechanisms that will enable them to correct their scapula movements when those movements are insufficient for accomplishing a given task. The ultimate goal is to use this personal knowledge of movement to change the foundational strategy used for reaching tasks in a variety of contexts. "The individual's degree of effectiveness in the learning process (and thus in problem solving in general) will be limited by his or her ability for critical self-analysis and environmental analysis in light of the problems encountered and by his or her ability to generate and control the solutions to these problems."[25]

Finally, stroke survivors must know how to monitor their own recovery of motor function. As illustrated in the theory of learned nonuse, many individuals fail to use the hemiparetic arms, even when muscle activity is available. Therapists can teach patients how to actively check for changes in ability to recruit specific muscles. Therapy sessions must be viewed as opportunities for stroke survivors to share their new discoveries with their therapists. In turn, the occupational therapist structures activities for the patient to practice emerging skills, both during the therapy session and as "homework" challenges.

Task Analysis and Problem-Solving Skills

Occupational therapists have always recognized that they need to be skillful at analyzing tasks. Task analysis enables an occupational therapist to establish treatment goals, synthesize treatment activities, and develop compensatory strategies.[2] Rehabilitation professionals realize more often that clients must also learn to analyze activities. Without this skill, the clients would be perpetually dependent on their therapists for successful task achievement. A stroke survivor must learn to determine which motor, cognitive-perceptual, and psychological challenges a task presents. Only then can effective strategies be chosen to "solve the problems"[44] inherent in the infinite variety of tasks encountered while actively engaging in meaningful life roles.

While reading subsequent chapters in this text, it should be remembered that occupational therapists strive to develop patients' insight and problem-solving skills, regardless of whether the intervention relates to balance, gross motor function, limb movement, visual skills, neurobehavioral performance, or daily living tasks.

Expectation for Goal Achievement

Stroke is a catastrophic event, often leading to depression and despair. Suddenly, a person finds himself in an unfamiliar body. His arms and legs no longer respond to willed commands. Small movements pose a threat to balance. Simple tasks are impossible to perform.

Studies of recovery after brain damage consistently show that a drive to perform functional tasks serves as the challenge that may be crucial for cortical remodeling. Most stroke survivors want desperately to move, but in the first few weeks after the CVA, their flaccid muscles prohibit them from acting on this desire. By the time diaschisis begins to subside, many of them have learned not to expect anything of their paretic limbs. They settle for letting others help them perform daily tasks, or they settle for accomplishing activities without the contributions of their paretic arm or leg.

Occupational therapists play a critical role in empowering stroke survivors to be active agents in their recovery and to return to valued activity engagement. Without making false promises, the therapists can challenge their patients to be vigilant for incremental returns in function. Without implying that full motor recovery is essential to a meaningful life style, they can encourage their patients to look for ways to use small improvements in functional ways. Without blaming future limitations in recovery on the stroke survivor, therapists can teach the patients ways to prevent secondary impairments, and to thus maximize their own potentials for recovery, whatever that potential might be.

It is a serious error to present occupational therapy as "therapy for your arm." Statistically, far fewer stroke survivors experience significant motor recovery in arm use, as compared to lower limb function.[23,32] When occupational therapy's focus is on the broader goals of returning to independent, safe performance of valued activities, patients can take pride in their reemerging abilities in a variety of physical, cognitive, and social domains. Those fortunate enough to detect emerging innervation to muscles of the arm and hand should be challenged to translate this motor recovery into functional performance. Those who do not enjoy such motor return must be presented with other goals toward which they will direct their serious efforts.

STRUCTURING ACTIVITY DEMANDS TO PROVIDE EFFECTIVE PRACTICE OPPORTUNITIES

Activity-based intervention is a foundation of occupational therapy in stroke rehabilitation. During the evaluation process, an occupational therapist determines:

- Which activities are important to the stroke survivor as determined by the individual's roles, interests, and anticipated environment
- Which activities the stroke survivor can or cannot perform
- Which internal and external factors impede the survivor's ability to complete the identified activities

During treatment, occupational therapists use activities in two major ways.

1. Some activities may be designed to provide structured challenges to improve internal skills. For example, an occupational therapist may engage a stroke survivor in a modified card game. Depending on the skill-related goals for this individual, the occupational therapist may structure the activity so that it requires forward reach with a hemiparetic arm. Alternatively, the card game may require the person to place the cards along a wide horizontal surface while standing. This modification in activity parameters provides opportunities for learning balance strategies while shifting the center of gravity in a lateral direction.

2. Other activities are designed to provide practice of actual task performance in real-life situations. Examples include direct practice in performing a morning self-care routine or getting into and out of an automobile. Practice of individualized roles in real-life situations is critical, but typically unfeasible during therapy sessions. Therefore, therapists need to structure homework assignments for stroke survivors to practice at home and to discuss at the next therapy session.

Task Analysis

An occupational therapist assesses tasks of daily living in the environmental context in which the individual plans to perform each task. The therapist determines which skills are necessary for task performance and compares this analysis to the functional strengths and limitations exhibited by an individual stroke survivor. This task analysis enables the occupational therapist to plan an individualized treatment program that will improve relevant performance skills and enable the person to use compensatory strategies to overcome those limitations that show weak potential for significant improvement.

Analyzing an Activity's Requirements for Postural Set

The occupational therapist determines the optimal "postural set" for performing a selected motor task. To perform the simple act of standing up, individuals must posturally set themselves in several ways. Both feet must be positioned on the floor in an appropriate base of support; perpendicular angles are established at the ankle, knee, and hip joints; and the pelvis is tilted anteriorly to free the lumbar spine for forward movement.[13,51]

When standing, people automatically change the configuration of their bases of support in anticipation of the direction toward which they expect to shift their body weight. If they plan to shift forward, as is done when reaching ahead, they will establish an anterior-posterior base of support. If they plan to shift to the left or right, as is done when stepping laterally to position their bodies in front of a bathtub, they will establish a medial-lateral base of support. Persons with hemiplegia often assume postural support bases inappropriate for the upcoming activity. The occupational therapist facilitates future task performance by determining and then instructing the individual in choosing appropriate postural sets for specific activities. For example, assuming the most efficient postural set for standing in front of a toilet can determine whether a man will be able to safely urinate independently.

Just as appropriate postural sets are important precursors to efficient motor performance, preplanning is also instrumental in determining the success of cognitively or visually challenging tasks. Activity analysis includes a determination of preliminary cognitive strategies that will facilitate task performance. For example, a person with right hemisphere dysfunction may experience difficulty in spatially orienting a blouse or slacks for independent dressing. The individual may be unaware that, prior to the stroke, he used a quick and automatic process to visualize and orient the garments in relation to the body segments. The occupational therapist's skill in activity analysis enables this person to develop a "set up" strategy, such as lining up each garment before attempting to complete the additional steps of dressing.

Analyzing Activity Requirements for Weight Shift and Balance

Postural adjustments that serve as balance mechanisms during weight shift are often impaired after stroke.[13,43,51] Understanding a task's inherent balance challenges is critical for developing treatment goals and compensatory strategies. Success in shifting weight during activity performance can be facilitated greatly through appropriate postural sets. The importance of this class of prerequisite skills is important when bathing. If patients use a tub bench, they will need to posturally set themselves for a posterior weight shift from stand to sit onto the bench. Once sitting, they will need to rotate their pelvis and bring both legs into the tub. The next step will be to shift their weight laterally, while sitting, to position themselves on the tub bench. A forward weight shift will often be required to adjust the water, and significant challenges to a lateral weight shift when sitting may be presented when patients must wash their genitals. If patients step into the bathtub and stand under a shower, they must posturally set themselves for a lateral weight shift for entrance and exit to and from the tub or shower. Reaching up and down from the standing position will be a critical performance component for safe, independent completion of this activity. These performance component skills may be practiced often in other contexts, such as in activities that require similar balance adjustments while sitting and standing. However, they must ultimately be practiced in the context in which the actual bathing activity will take place.

Analyzing Activity Requirements for Dissociation between Body Segments

Difficulty with dissociation between body segments is commonly associated with stroke.[13,43,51] The occupational therapist assesses the type and magnitude of such dissociations in each analyzed performance area task. For example, to put on shoes and socks, patients must be able to dissociate their pelvis from the lumbar spine to anteriorly and posteriorly tilt the pelvis to cross one leg over the other. They will also need to dissociate their lumbar from their thoracic spine to achieve the trunk rotation required to reach their left hand to their right foot. If they use their paretic arm to assist with the task, disassociation between the scapula and thorax will be required, as will disassociation between the humerus and scapula. Determination of these requirements through activity analysis guides treatment and helps the stroke survivor understand the therapist's rationale for choice of treatment methods.

Other Aspects of Task Analysis

Various tasks require different levels of motor planning and motor sequencing. For patients with impairments in these areas, the therapist will determine the nature of each of their challenges within specific performance area activities. Finally, when stroke survivors demonstrate impairments in visuospatial or cognitive skills, the occupational therapist will carefully analyze each task's unique challenges and assist individuals in developing strategies to meet these specific performance component requirements.

Activity analysis also enables the occupational therapist to determine strategies for task performance that will promote efficient movement patterns and be least likely to contribute to the development of secondary impairments. Strategies for relaxing excessive skeletal muscle activity and preventing abnormal postures are described in Chapters 10 and 13. The occupational therapist instructs the stroke survivor to incorporate these strategies into the routine performance of daily activities. In addition, activity analysis assists the therapist in determining which compensatory strategies or adaptive equipment will be most effective

for each individual stroke survivor. See Chapters 15, 27, and 28.

Using Activity to Assess a Client's Skills

Activity analysis enables occupational therapists to evaluate skill levels through observation of patients as they participate in selected tasks. The Árnadóttir OT-ADL Neurobehavioral Evaluation (A-ONE)[3] provides a systematic framework for assessing cognitive and perceptual function through structured observations of activities of daily living performance. This tool is discussed further in Chapter 18.

Carr and Shepherd's program for optimizing motor function after stroke[12,13] describes a therapeutic strategy for evaluating motor skills in the context of task performance. The therapist analyzes a patient's performance of a specific task and compares it with the optimal kinesiology associated with that task. A major focus of this analysis is to identify those factors that serve as obstacles (or blocks) to moving in efficient kinesiological patterns. When some patients with hemiparesis try to reach forward to grasp for a cup, they tend to use the entire shoulder girdle as one tightly bound unit instead of disassociating the scapula from the thorax or the humerus from the scapula.

Intervention strategies are directly determined from task analysis. In the previous example, the therapist would provide passive mobilization to reduce mechanical constraints and to enhance the patient's internal awareness of available scapular motion. The patient would then practice reaching forward in a variety of contexts while the therapist provides manual guidance and structures placement of goal objects to maximize appropriate kinematic linkages. Strong backgrounds in kinesiology and movement analysis are helpful to the therapist when implementing a motor relearning approach.

Helping Patients Develop Their Own Skills in Activity Analysis

An ultimate goal in stroke rehabilitation is for individuals to learn the strategy of analyzing activities in reference to their own functional strengths and impairments. During the occupational therapy process, therapists share their strategies for activity analysis and challenge patients to develop their own skills in this area. Midway through the treatment process, therapists present new tasks and require the stroke survivors to analyze each task's inherent performance requirements. In addition, occupational therapists encourage individuals to develop their own alternative strategies for task performance. The therapist's major role at this stage is to provide feedback about the safety and efficacy of the person's ideas. Before treatment is terminated, stroke survivors should develop skill in activity analysis so that they have the confidence and capability to attempt an infinite variety of new tasks and roles.

Activity Selection and Synthesis

Occupational therapists select activities and modify task demands:

- To structure specific practice components within an activity, with the goal of improving internal skills
- To adapt tasks so they will be easier or safer to perform, according to each individual's demonstrated internal capacities, limitations, and interests

The following game of dominoes is an example of modifying activity parameters to elicit specific demands for motor practice. With full knowledge by the patient that the primary purpose of engaging in this game is to practice skills of forward reach and lateral pinch, the therapist modifies the height and distance of the table surface to provide sufficient, but not excessive, challenges to the GMP for forward reach. The therapist purposely places the dominoes on their sides, rather than flat, to encourage external rotation at the glenohumeral joint and supination at the forearm. The therapist also considers the interaction between the person's balance adjustments and ability to control increasing numbers of degrees of freedom in movements of the hemiparetic arm. Based on prior and ongoing assessment, the therapist determines whether the person will perform the task while sitting or standing, and the amount of shift in center of gravity that will be required by positioning of the dominoes on the table.

When an occupational therapist modifies an activity to facilitate current performance, the focus is on external adaptations to compensate for unchanging internal limitations. Such modifications are discussed in Chapters 27 and 28. It is important for therapists to understand that both types of activity modification may be appropriate for a single individual. It is equally important that the stroke survivor clearly understands the purpose of each therapeutic activity.

Activity synthesis is unique for each individual. Although the occupational therapist applies carefully considered, general foundational concepts when planning treatment for stroke survivors, no textbook can provide specific activity formats that will be appropriate for groups of individuals, even if they all have the same diagnosis. Each stroke survivor has an individual constellation of abilities, limitations, interests, roles, and personal goals. Occupational therapists synthesize activities by modifying parameters of specific tasks in specific contexts to provide practice challenges or compensatory adaptations. This requires flexibility, creativity, and sensitivity to individual needs.

REVIEW QUESTIONS

1. How do the ICF and the Occupational Therapy Practice Framework each integrate medical and social models of disability? What interventions do occupational therapists provide to promote internal change within stroke survivors? What interventions do occupational therapists provide to change factors in a stroke survivor's external environment?

2. How do "patterns of use" influence central nervous system reorganization after injury? What are implications to occupational therapy intervention with stroke survivors?

3. Which stroke survivors are candidates for CIMT? How can the theory of learned nonuse influence occupational therapy intervention for other stroke survivors?

4. From your knowledge of kinesiology, give specific examples of kinematic or kinetic linkages during normal movement.

5. Give two examples of strategies for community participation that will be valuable for stroke survivors to develop.

6. What aspects of motor skills are learned through implicit learning processes? What occupational therapy interventions are most effective in facilitating implicit learning?

7. What is contextual interference and how does it affect retention and transfer of learning? Describe three ways an occupational therapist can modify feedback or practice schedules to promote contextual interference.

8. What are the necessary substrates for stroke survivors to meet their maximal potential for recovery? How can therapeutic intervention influence these substrates?

9. Describe the difference between modifying activities to promote practice for skill recovery and modifying activities to help stroke survivors compensate for current limitations.

REFERENCES

1. Akama K, Yamauchi H: Task performance and metacognitive experiences in problem solving, *Psychol Rep* 94(2):715–722, 2004.
2. American Occupational Therapy Association: Occupational therapy practice framework: Domain and process (2nd ed.), *Am J Occ Ther* 62: 625–683, 2008.
3. Árnadóttir G: *The brain and behavior: assessing cortical dysfunction through activities of daily living*, St Louis, 1990, Mosby.
4. Bear MF, Connors BW, Paradiso MA: *Neuroscience: exploring the brain*, ed 3, Baltimore, 2007, Lippincott Williams and Wilkins.
5. Bernstein N: *The coordination and regulation of movements*, Elmsford, NY, 1967, Pergamon.
6. Boyd LA, Winstein CJ: Implicit motor-sequence learning in humans following unilateral stroke: The impact of practice and explicit knowledge, *Neurosci Lett* 298(1):65–69, 2001.
7. Brady F: A theoretical and empirical review of the contextual interference effect and the learning of motor skills, *Quest* 50:266–293, 1998.
8. Brady F: Contextual interference: A meta-analytic study, *Percept Mot Skills* 99:116–126, 2004.
9. Brodtmann A, Puce A, Darby D, Donnan G: fMRI demonstrates diaschisis in the extrastriate visual cortex, *Stroke* 38(8):2360–2363, 2007.

10. Butefisch CM: Plasticity in the human cerebral cortex: Lessons from the normal brain and from stroke, *Neuroscientist* 10(2):163–173, 2004.

11. Candler C, Meeuwsen H: Implicit learning in children with and without developmental coordination disorder, *Am J Occup Ther* 56(4):429–435, 2002.

12. Carr J, Shepherd R: *Neurological rehabilitation: Optimizing motor performance*, Oxford, 1998, Butterworth-Heinemann.

13. Carr JH, Shepherd RB: *Stroke rehabilitation: Guidelines for exercise and training to optimize motor skill*, Boston, 2003, Butterworth-Heinemann.

14. Fasoli SE, Trombly CA, Tickle-Degnen LT, Verfaellie MH: Effect of instructions on functional reach in persons with and without cerebrovascular accident, *Am J Occup Ther* 56(4):380, 2002.

15. French B, Thomas LH, Leathley, MJ, et al: Repetitive task training for improving functional ability after stroke, *Cochrane Database Syst Rev* 17(4):CD006073, 2007.

16. Gentile AM: A working model of skill acquisition with application to teaching, *Quest* 17(1):3–23, 1972.

17. Gentile AM: Implicit and explicit processes during acquisition of functional skill, *Scand J Occup Ther* 5(1):7–16, 1998.

18. Giuffrida CG, Shea JB, Fairbrother JT: Differential transfer benefits of increased practice for constant, blocked, and serial practice schedules, *J Mot Behav* 34(4):353–365, 2002.

19. Golisz KM: Dynamic assessment and multicontext treatment of unilateral neglect, *Top Stroke Rehabil* 5(1):11–28, 1998.

20. Goverover Y, Johnston MV, Toglia J, Deluca J: Treatment to improve self-awareness in persons with acquired brain injury, *Brain Inj* 21(9):913–923, 2007.

21. Hall KG, Magill RA: Variability of practice and contextual interference in motor skill learning, *J Mot Behav* 27(4):299–309, 1995.

22. Hanlon R: Motor learning following unilateral stroke, *Arch Phys Med Rehabil* 77(8):811, 1996.

23. Hendricks HT, van Limbeek J Geurts AC, Zwartz MJ: Motor recovery after stroke: A systematic review of the literature, *Arch Phys Med Rehabil* 83(11):1629, 2002.

24. Higgins JR, Spaeth RK: Relationship between consistency of movement and environmental condition, *Quest* 17(1):61, 1972.

25. Higgins S: Motor skill acquisition, *Phys Ther* 71(2):123, 1991.

26. Hoffman AN, Malena RR, Westergom BP, et al: Environmental enrichment-mediated functional improvement after experimental traumatic brain injury is contingent on task-specific neurobehavioral experience, *Neurosci Lett* 431(3):226–230, 2008.

27. Humm JL, Kozlowski DA, James DC, et al: Use-dependent exacerbation of brain damage occurs during an early post-lesion vulnerable period, *Brain Res* 783(2):286–292, 1998.

28. Jarus T, Goverover Y: Effects of contextual interference and age on acquisition, retention, and transfer of motor skill, *Percept Mot Skills* 88(2):437–447, 1999.

29. Jarus T: Motor learning and occupational therapy: the organization of practice, *Am J Occup Ther* 48(9):810, 1994.

30. Jones TA, Allred RP, Adkins DL, et al: Remodeling the brain with behavioral experience after stroke, *Stroke* 40(3):S136–S138, 2009.

31. Kelso JAS: Relative timing in brain and behavior: Some observations about the generalized motor program and self-organized coordination dynamics, *Human Movement Science* 16(4):453–460, 1997.

32. Kwakkel G, Kollen B: Predicting improvement in the upper paretic limb after stroke: A longitudinal prospective study, *Restor Neurol Neurosci* 25(5-6): 453–460, 2007.

33. Lai Q, Shea CH, Wulf G, Wright DL: Optimizing generalized motor program and parameter learning, *Res Q Exerc Sport* 71(1):10–24, 2000.

34. Lin KC, Wu CY, Tickle-Degnen L, Coster W: Enhancing occupational performance through occupationally embedded exercise: A meta-analytic review, *Occup Ther J Res* 17(1):25–47, 1997.

35. Ma HI, Trombly C: A synthesis of the effects of occupational therapy for persons with stroke, part II: Remediation, *Am J Occ Ther* 56(3):260–274, 2002.

36. Ma HI, Trombly CA, Robinson-Podolski C: The effect of context on skill acquisition and transfer, *Am J Occup Ther* 53(2):138–144, 1999.

37. Ma HI, Trombly CA, The comparison of motor performance between part and whole tasks in elderly persons, *Am J Occup Ther* 55(1):62–67, 2001.

38. Magill RA: Knowledge is more than we can talk about: Implicit learning in motor skill acquisition, *Res Q Exerc Sport* 69(2):104–110, 1998.

39. Mark VW, Taub E: Constraint-induced movement therapy for chronic stroke hemiparesis and other disabilities, *Restor Neurol Neurosci* 22(3-5): 317–336, 2004.

40. Mountz JM: Nuclear medicine in the rehabilitative treatment evaluation in stroke recovery. Role of diaschisis resolution and cerebral reorganization, *Eura Medicophys* 43(2):221–239, 2007.

41. Neumann DA: *Kinesiology of the musculoskeletal system: Foundations for physical rehabilitation*, St Louis, 2002, Mosby.

42. Riesdal A, Zeng J, Johansson BB: Early training may exacerbate brain damage after focal brain ischemia in the rat, *J Cereb Blood Flow Metab* 19(9):997–1003, 1999.

43. Ryerson S, Levit K: *Functional movement reeducation: A contemporary model for stroke rehabilitation*, NewYork, 1997, Churchill Livingstone.

44. Sabari JS: Occupational therapy practice guidelines for adults with stroke, Bethesda, MD, 2008, AOTA Press.

45. Salmani AW, Schmidt RA, Walter CB: Knowledge of results and motor learning: a review and critical reappraisal, *Psychol Bull* 95(3):355, 1984.

46. Schmidt RA, Lee TD: *Motor control and learning: a behavioral emphasis*, ed 4, Champaign, IL, 2005, Human Kinetics.

47. Schmidt RA, Wulf G: Continuous concurrent feedback degrades skill learning: implications for training and simulation, *Hum Factors* 39(4): 509–525, 1997.

48. Seitz RJ, Azari NP, Knorr U, et al: The role of diaschisis in stroke recovery, *Stroke* 30(9):1844–1850, 1999.

49. Seligman ME, Weiss J, Weinraub M, Schulman A: Coping behavior: learned helplessness, physiological change and learned inactivity, *Behav Res Ther* 18(5):459–512, 1980.

50. Seligman ME: Learned helplessness, *Annu Rev Med* 23:407–412, 1972.

51. Shumway-Cook A, Woollacott M: *Motor control: theory and practical applications*, ed 2, Philadelphia, 2001, Lippincott Williams & Wilkins.

52. Singer RN, Cauraugh JHL: The generalizability effect of learning strategies for categories of psychomotor skills, *Quest* 37(1):103, 1985.

53. Singer RN, Lidor R, Cauraugh JH: To be aware or not aware? What to think about while learning and performing a motor skill, *Sport Psychol* 7(1):19, 1993.

54. Ste-Marie DM, Clear SE, Findlay LC, Latimer AE: High levels of contextual interference enhance handwriting skills acquisition, *J Mot Behav* 36(1): 115–126, 2004.

55. Taub E: Movement in nonhuman primates deprived of somatosensory feedback. Exerc Sport 4:335–74, 1976.

56. Toglia JP: *A dynamic interactional model to cognitive rehabilitation*. In Katz N: *Cognition and occupation across the life span*, Bethesda, MD, 2005, AOTA Press.

57. Toglia JT: Generalization of treatment: a multicontext approach to cognitive perceptual impairment in adults with brain injury, *Am J Occup Ther* 45(6):505, 1991.

58. Toglia J, Kirk U: Understanding awareness deficits following brain injury. *Neurorehabilitation* 15(1):57–70, 2000.

59. Trombly CA: Foreword. In Smits JG, Smits-Boone EC: *Hand recovery after stroke*, Boston, 2000, Butterworth Heinemann.

60. Trombly CA: Observations of improvement of reaching in five subjects with left hemiparesis, J Neurol Neurosurg Psychiatry 56(1):40, 1993.

61. Winstein CJ: Knowledge of results and motor learning—implications for physical therapy, *Phys Ther* 71(2):140, 1991.

62. Wolf SL, Winstein CJ, Miller JP, et al: Effect of constraint-induced movement therapy on upper extremity function 3 to 9 months after stroke: The EXCITE randomized clinical trial, *JAMA* 296(17):2095–2104, 2006.

63. Wolf SL, Winstein CJ, Miller JP, et al: Retention of upper limb function in stroke survivors who have received constraint-induced movement therapy: The EXCITE randomized trial, *Lancet Neurol* 7(1):33–40, 2008.

64. World Health Organization: *International classification of function,* Geneva, 2001, The Organization.

65. Wu CY, Trombly CA, Lin LC, Tickle-Degnen L: A kinematic study of contextual effects on reaching performance in persons with and without stroke: Influences of object availability. *Arch Phys Med Rehabil* 81(1):95–101, 2000.

66. Wulf G, Hoss M, Prinz W: Instructions for motor learning: Differential effects of internal versus external focus of attention, *J Mot Behav* 30(2):169, 1998.

ashwini k. rao

chapter 6

Approaches to Motor Control Dysfunction: An Evidence-Based Review

key terms

body weight support and tread-mill training

constraint induced movement therapy

evidence-based practice

neurotherapeutic approach

robot-aided motor training

task-oriented approach

chapter objectives

After completing this chapter, the reader will be able to accomplish the following:

1. Understand principles of evidence-based practice and criteria of evaluating research.
2. Understand the rationale behind the various techniques described in this chapter.
3. Evaluate the evidence testing the effectiveness of the approaches in stroke rehabilitation.

The therapeutic professions are in the midst of a paradigm shift with regard to stroke rehabilitation. This chapter examines the evidence for a traditional approach in stroke rehabilitation (Bobath approach or neurodevelopmental treatment [NDT]). The overwhelming lack of evidence for this approach has led to the articulation of a new clinical paradigm based on a functional task-oriented approach. Evidence for specific therapeutic applications within this task-oriented paradigm is evaluated to help determine the best (most effective) practices for rehabilitation of sensorimotor dysfunction following stroke.

UNDERSTANDING EVIDENCE-BASED PRACTICE

Evidence-based practice has become integrated in occupational therapy (OT) and physical therapy (PT) education and practice in the past few years. Its importance stems from the need to choose the best (most effective and current) available intervention techniques, which is a fundamental ethical responsibility of clinical practice. Sackett coined the term *evidence-based medicine* and defined it as "the conscientious, explicit, and judicious use of current best evidence in making decisions about the care of individual patients. The practice of evidence-based medicine means integrating individual clinical expertise with the best available external clinical evidence from systematic research."[72]

Evidence-based rehabilitation is the application of the principles of evidence-based medicine to problems in the field of rehabilitation. According to Law,[44] evidence-based rehabilitation practice is based on a self-directed learning model in which practitioners must take responsibility for continuously evaluating their techniques in an effort to improve them.

Mohide[56] identified three basic components of evidence-based practice:

1. Best research evidence: A first step in evidence-based practice is to identify rigorous, clinically relevant research studies that apply to the clinical problem at hand. For this chapter, this would imply an examination of the best available evidence in the rehabilitation of sensorimotor dysfunction following stroke.
2. Clinical expertise: The second step is using one's clinical expertise and experience to identify patients' strengths and weaknesses and the risks and benefits of potential interventions. Once the clinician has identified the best research evidence, the next step is to determine if the techniques described in studies apply to the individual patient, given his or her strengths and weaknesses. A focus on the inclusion and exclusion criteria that the studies used is important to determine if the individual patient in question would benefit from the techniques.
3. Patient values: The final step is to incorporate a patient's values into clinical decision-making.

This chapter examines the best research evidence for stroke rehabilitation. To do so requires first defining criteria by which clinical outcome studies were evaluated.

CRITERIA FOR EVALUATING RESEARCH ARTICLES

For each specific intervention technique, the authors searched databases (such as Medline, Pubmed, CINAHL, PEDro) for randomized controlled trials (or high quality nonrandomized studies with low bias) published in the past decade, i.e. between 1999 and 2009. The analysis was restricted to studies published in English.

Once studies describing clinical trials on the effectiveness of specific techniques were chosen, two criteria were used to rank each study. The first ranking criteria were developed by the Centre for Evidence Based Medicine, Oxford, UK.[11] The criteria are based on guidelines proposed by Sackett.[72] In this framework, research articles are ranked as follows: (1a) systematic review of randomized clinical trials; (1b) individual randomized clinical trial with narrow confidence interval; (2a) systematic review of cohort studies; (2b) individual cohort study or low quality randomized clinical trial; (3a) systematic review of case-control studies; (3b) individual case-control study; (4) case series, poor quality cohort and case-control studies; (5) expert opinion.

The second criterion was the Physiotherapy Evidence Database (PEDro) score.[12] In this 10-point scale, one point is scored if each of the following criteria are satisfied: (1) random allocation of subjects; (2) allocation concealment; (3) baseline similarity across groups; (4) subject blinding; (5) therapist blinding; (6) tester blinding; (7) measures of a key outcome obtained from at least 85% of subjects; (8) intention to treat analysis; (9) between-group statistical comparisons reported; (10) point estimate and measures of variability for at least one key outcome measure.

For this evidence-based review, the selected studies had a score of at least 4/10 on the PEDro score, which is used as an indicator of good quality studies. The PEDro scale was used because its validity and reliability are established.[51]

Before reviewing the evidence, a brief description of research designs is provided to help the reader understand the terms used in the evidence tables. For more detailed descriptions of research designs, the reader is referred to Helewa and Walker[26] and Law.[44]

Randomized controlled trials or randomized clinical trials (RCT) are the most rigorous way of determining whether a cause-and-effect relationship exists between treatment and outcomes. Some of the important features of randomized trials are:

- Random assignment of subjects to experimental and control groups. Randomization ensures that groups are similar at the beginning of intervention.
- Subject, therapist, and tester blinding: Patients and experimenters should remain unaware of which treatment was given until the study is completed in order to prevent bias.
- All intervention groups are treated identically except for the experimental treatment.

A cohort study involves studying groups of individuals who share some common characteristics, such as positive history of stroke. In this case, subjects are not allocated to different groups at random, making them less rigorous than RCT.

The before-and-after design is a study of one group of patients without a control group. When a control group is included, the design is called *case control design*. Because the control group in this case consists of healthy subjects, the two groups are different at the outset of the study.

Descriptive designs are not rigorous but are useful in describing a disorder in detail.

PARADIGM SHIFTS IN STROKE REHABILITATION

The therapeutic professions of OT and PT have witnessed two paradigm shifts related to the treatment of neurological dysfunction. According to Gordon,[22] paradigm shifts within therapeutic practice can occur for two reasons: (1) because the theoretical model underlying a therapeutic approach does not fit with current knowledge, and (2) because existing approaches do not appear adequate to solve clinical problems. The past 60 years have witnessed two distinct paradigm shifts in the treatment of stroke.

The first shift occurred in the years immediately following World War II; at that time the dominant therapeutic paradigm was muscle reeducation, which was used extensively to treat peripheral nerve disorders such as poliomyelitis. Although useful for polio, muscle reeducation was not adequate to treat individuals with disorders of the upper motor neuron, such as paresis following stroke. As a result, a few therapists began studying how the nervous system controls movements and began to apply these principles into clinical practice. This approach heralded the development of techniques such as proprioceptive neuromuscular facilitation, Bobath approach or neurodevelopmental treatment (NDT), Brunnstrom movement therapy and sensory integration, to name a few of the prominent approaches.

The Neurotherapeutic Approaches: The First Paradigm Shift

Principles of Neurotherapeutic Approaches. Although each neurotherapeutic approach is different from each other, all approaches share some common elements.[22,23] This section and the subsequent review of the evidence focuses on the Bobath approach/NDT because this approach historically has been the most widely used in stroke rehabilitation. However, the assumptions underlying the Bobath approach also hold true for the other approaches mentioned previously. Some of the common elements of the neurotherapeutic approaches are as follows:

1. The central nervous system is organized hierarchically, with higher centers such as the cerebral cortex exerting a controlling influence over the lower centers (such as the spinal cord). When a deficit occurs in the motor system, more primitive forms of movement (such as reflexive postures and movements), controlled by the lower centers (spinal cord and brainstem), are released from their normal inhibition from the higher centers.[7] Thus, treatment within this framework was aimed at reestablishing control by the higher centers.
2. Normal movement can be facilitated by providing specific patterns of sensory input, particularly through the proprioceptive and tactile sensory systems. Under this assumption, sensory stimulation was proposed to produce long-term effects of reestablishing normal sensorimotor neural connections.
3. Recovery from brain damage follows a predictable sequence that mimics normal development. Treatment used developmental postures in an effort to facilitate recovery. This principle has since been eliminated in current concepts of Bobath therapy.[69]
4. Reflexes were used to facilitate or inhibit motor activity. Experience of normal movement patterns must be provided so that the patient does not learn abnormal patterns of posture and movement after stroke. Reflex inhibitory movement patterns, which were opposite to the pattern of spasticity observed in patients, were used to prevent learning of abnormal movements.
5. Sequelae of stroke can be understood through a neurophysiological explanation. This assumption means that sensorimotor impairments seen after stroke result primarily from the damaged motor system.

The original principles that defined Bobath approach have been adapted and tailored to suit the current knowledge of the functioning of the central nervous system.[53] Core theoretical assumptions of the Bobath approach includes an appreciation of task and context specificity of motor learning (a concept associated with a task-oriented approach), neuroplasticity, systems approach that highlights the interaction of the person, task, and environment in producing functional behavior.[34,69] This amalgam of old and new conceptual principles have produced a high variability and confusion in practice patterns among therapists using the Bobath approach.[53]

Outcome Studies on Neurotherapeutic Techniques. This section evaluates the evidence for the effectiveness of the Bobath approach in stroke rehabilitation. Table 6-1 presents the details of seven RCT and two high quality nonrandomized trials that compared the effectiveness of the Bobath approach with usual care, task-oriented therapy, or orthopedic approach. The studies in the evidence table are listed chronologically.

Timing of Therapy. Of the nine studies related to NDT, two included patients in the acute stage,[41,42] three included patients in the subacute stage,[67,86,91] two studies included patients in the acute and subacute stages,[24,25] one study included patients in the subacute or chronic stage,[97] and one study included patients from acute, subacute, and chronic stages.[81]

Outcomes Measures. Three of the nine studies on the Bobath approach measured outcomes at the impairment level only.[67,81,86] Given the importance of testing outcomes at multiple levels of the International Classification of Function (ICF) model, it is important that a majority of studies (six) included outcomes at the impairments and activity levels.[24,25,41,42,91,97] Outcome measures at the impairment level ranged from quantitative analysis of gait, Arm Research Action Test, Nine or Ten Hole Peg Test, Stroke Impairment Assessment Scale, Berg Balance Scale, Modified Ashworth Scale, six-minute walk test, and Stroke Rehabilitation Assessment of Movement. The most common outcome measures at the activity limitation level were the Barthel index, Extended ADL Scale, Motor Assessment Scale, and Rivermead Motor Assessment.

Text continued on p.124

Table 6-1

Evidence Table for the Neurodevelopmental Treatment/Bobath Approach

AUTHOR/ YEAR	AIMS AND RATIONALE	DESIGN, SUBJECTS, OXFORD RATING, AND PEDRO SCORE	INTERVENTION	COMPARISON INTERVENTION	ASSESSMENT	OUTCOMES	RESULTS	COMMENTS
Langhammer et al, 2000	Compare outcome of Bobath therapy with motor learning program	Double blind RCT; 61 patients acute stage 1b; 6/10	Bobath therapy (N=28); 5 days a week for duration of hospital stay	MRP (N=33)	3 days post-admission, 3 weeks, and 3 months poststroke	1. MAS 2. SMES 3. BI 4. NHP 5. Length of stay, assistive device	Both groups improved at 3 months on MAS, SMES, and Barthel Index. MRP had better improvement on MAS and had shorter hospital stay.	Well-designed study; MRP better than Bobath approach
Langhammer et al, 2003	Evaluate effectiveness of Bobath and MRP 1 and 4 years after stroke	Double blind RCT; 61 patients acute stage 2b; 4/10	Bobath therapy (N=28); No intervention following initial therapy during acute stage	Motor Learning Program (N=33); No intervention following initial therapy during acute stage	1 and 4 year follow-up of patients from Langhammer et al, 2000	1. MAS, SMES 2. SMES 3. BI 4. Nottingham Health Profile 5. Length of stay, assistive device, mortality 6. BBS	No difference in mortality rate; motor function decreased from year 1 to year 4 on MAS and SMES for both groups; independence in ADL decreased; QOL better at 1 and 4 years than at 3 months	Initial benefit of MRP not maintained in the long term, partly because therapy was discontinued.
Tang et al, 2005	Compare Bobath approach (NDT) with POWM therapy	RCT; 47 patients acute, subacute, or chronic stage; 2b; 6/10	Bobath therapy (N=22); 50 min. sessions 5× week; mat activity, sitting, standing, walking, stair climbing; focus on movement normalization	POWM therapy (N=25); using cognitive skills to focus attention and train memory	Pretreatment and post-treatment	1. Mini Mental State Exam; 2. STREAM	Both groups improved on STREAM; POWM better than Bobath on overall score, mobility, and lower extremity scores of STREAM	Well designed study; NDT not as good as active willed movement therapy, a form of task-oriented approach

Study	Purpose	Design/Subjects	Intervention	Comparison	Timing	Outcome Measures	Results	Comments
Wang et al, 2005	Compare Bobath therapy with orthopedic approach	Single blind RCT; 44 patients at subacute or chronic stage; subjects categorized by function into spasticity group (Brunnstrom stage 2 to 3), or relative recover stage (Brunnstrom stage 4 to 5); 2b; 5/10	Bobath treatment (N=21) included normalization of tone, postural reeducation, manual facilitation, key points of control; 40 min, 5 × week for 4 weeks	Orthopedic approach (N=23) included passive, active, assistive exercise; practice of functional activities (rolling, sitting, transfers, walking) 40 min, 5 × week for 4 weeks	Pretreatment and post-treatment;	1. SIAS 2. MAS 3. BBS 4. SIS	Lower functioning group improved with either the Bobath or orthopedic approach; Bobath group had better scores on SIAS tone and SIS; higher functioning group improved with either treatment, Bobath group had better scores on MAS	No follow-up assessment; did not address ceiling effect for MAS, BBS, and SIS scores. Bobath group marginally better than orthopedic treatment, which is not a treatment of choice in stroke.
Van Vliet et al, 2005	Compare Bobath with Movement Science approach	Double blind RCT; 120 patients at subacute stage; 1b; 6/10	Bobath (N=60) Median 23 min/day; no details on treatment, manual strategy used. Treatment continued as long as patients required	Movement Science (N=60), median 23 min/day; no details on treatment, cognitive strategy used; treatment continued as long as patients required	Pretreatment, 1, 3, and 6 months after randomization.	1. RMA 2. MAS, Secondary: 3. Ten-hole peg test 4. 6 min walk, 4. Modified Ashworth Scale 5. Nottingham Sensory Assessment 6. BI 7. EADL	At baseline Bobath group had better lower extremity scores on the RMA, MS group had better upper limb RMA scores. Bobath group spent more time with therapist, MS group spent more time with PT Assistant. No differences seen in any outcomes across the two groups.	Baseline differences between groups; time spent with therapist not equivalent across groups. Bobath therapy no different than movement science approach. Duration of therapy less than standard practice

Continued

Table 6-1

Evidence Table for the Neurodevelopmental Treatment/Bobath Approach—cont'd

AUTHOR/ YEAR	AIMS AND RATIONALE	DESIGN, SUBJECTS, OXFORD RATING, AND PEDRO SCORE	INTERVENTION	COMPARISON INTERVENTION	ASSESSMENT	OUTCOMES	RESULTS	COMMENTS
Platz et al, 2005	Evaluate effect of augmented exercise therapy; compare Bobath with Arm BASIS training (repetitive training to restore ROM)	Single blind RCT, multicenter; 60 subacute patients; 1b; 8/10	Bobath group (N=20) focused on control of muscle tone, recruitment of arm during functional tasks (45 min/day, 4 weeks)	Arm BASIS group (N=20) received repetitive training of arm movement with to improve ROM (45 min/day, 4 weeks); Usual treatment (N=20) had ADL, arm activities, stance and gait, speech, and cognition (30 min/day, 4 weeks)	Pretreatment and post-treatment	1. Arm motor section of Fugl Myer test 2. ARAT 3. Ashworth Scale for elbow flexors	Arm BASIS group performed better than Bobath group on Fugl Myer motor score, ARAT, and Ashworth scale; Bobath group was similar to usual treatment	Well-designed study; Bobath therapy not as effective as repetitive training of arm movement; Bobath approach similar to usual care
Hafsteinsdottir et al, 2005	Investigate effects of Bobath therapy/NDT on functional status and quality of life in acute and subacute stroke	Nonrandomized parallel design, multicenter; 324 patients with acute and subacute stroke (<1 year); 2b; 5/10	Bobath group (N=223) received intervention from nurses and PTs trained in the Bobath approach; no details of treatment provided	Control group (N=101) received conventional PT and OT treatment; no details of treatment provided	Pretreatment, 12 month follow-up	1. BI (<12 or death defined as poor outcome) 2. SIP 3. Visual Analog Scale	Bobath group received higher number of sessions. At 12 months, higher percentage of subjects in Bobath group had poor outcome; no differences were seen in quality of life between groups.	Despite limitation of nonrandomization, this is the most definitive study on the lack of effect of the Bobath approach

Study	Purpose	Design	Intervention (Bobath) group	Control group	Measurement	Outcome measures	Results	Comments
Hafsteinsdottir et al. 2005	Investigate effects of Bobath therapy on depression, shoulder pain and quality of life in acute and subacute stroke	Nonrandomized parallel design, multicenter; 324 patients with acute and subacute stroke (<1 year); 2b; 5/10	Bobath group (N=223) received intervention from nurses and PTs trained in the Bobath approach; no details of treatment provided	Control group (N=101) received conventional PT and OT treatment; no details of treatment provided	Pretreatment and post-treatment, 6 and 12 month follow-up	1. SF-36 2. CES-D 3. Visual Analog Scale for pain	No differences between groups in shoulder pain and quality of life. Fewer patients in Bobath group depressed at 1 year follow-up	Nonrandomized study; large study clearly shows no benefit of Bobath approach on shoulder pain and quality of life
Thaut et al, 2007	Compare effectiveness of RAS with Bobath approach/NDT for gait training	Single blind RCT; 78 patients at subacute stage; 1b; 7/10	Bobath group practiced gait without rhythmic cues (N=35); 30 min/day, 5 days/week, for 3 weeks	RAS group (N-43) practiced gait with metronome and music; 30 min/day, 5 days/week, for 3 weeks	Pretreatment and post-treatment	1. Quantitative Gait Analysis (velocity, cadence, stride length, swing symmetry)	RAS group had greater improvement on all four gait measures and patient satisfaction	Well-designed RCT; Bobath approach not as effective as RAS for gait training

ADL, Activities of daily living; ARAT, Action Research Arm Test; BBS, Berg Balance Scale; BI, Barthel Index; CESD, Center for Epidemiological Studies Depression Scale; EADL, Extended Activities of Daily Living Scale; MAS, Motor Assessment Scale; MRP, Motor Learning Program; NDT, neurodevelopmental treatment; NHP, Nottingham Health Profile; OT, occupational therapy; POWM, problem oriented willed movement; PT, physical therapy, QOL, quality of Life; RAS, rhythmic auditory stimulation; RCT, Randomized Controlled trial; RMA, Rivermead motor assessment; ROM, range of motion; SIAS, Stroke Impairment Assessment Scale; SIP, Sickness Impact Profile; SIS, Stroke Impact Scale; SMES, Sodring Motor Evaluation Scale; STREAM, Stroke Rehabilitation Assessment of Movement

Study Designs. The designs included in this review were seven RCT and two high-quality nonrandomized parallel design studies with a large number of subjects. All the studies were classified as either 1b or 2b on the Oxford levels of evidence scale.

Results of the Review. Of the nine trials examining the effect of Bobath approach, one compared Bobath to an orthopedic approach to stroke rehabilitation,[97] two studies compared Bobath with usual care including conventional PT and OT[24,25] and the other five compared Bobath approach with the task-oriented approach[41,42,67,86,91] or a variant of a task-oriented approach called the problem oriented willed movement therapy.[81]

The Bobath approach was marginally better than an orthopedic approach,[97] which is not the therapy of choice in stroke rehabilitation. When compared with conventional PT and OT, Bobath approach was no better for impairment or activity limitation outcomes.[24,25] When compared with a task-oriented approach, which represents a novel approach to stroke rehabilitation, Bobath approach was clearly less effective in four of the six studies.[41,67,81,86] There were two exceptions to this pattern: one study[42] found no differences in outcomes evaluated at one and four years after the initial therapy was administered, perhaps because patients did not receive therapy in the interim period. The other study[91] had methodological limitations that may explain the lack of differences. For instance, at baseline testing, there were differences across the two groups, the amount of time patients spent with the therapist was not the same, and finally the duration of therapy was much less compared with all other studies. Despite these two studies, the evidence overwhelmingly points to the lack of effectiveness of the Bobath approach when compared with a task-oriented approach.

Implications for Practice. Three recent systematic reviews have reported no evidence for the superiority of the Bobath approach.[34,48,62] The present review extends the results of the previous systematic reviews to demonstrate that the use of the Bobath approach needs to be reconsidered in stroke rehabilitation.

In the past few years, an attempt has been made among proponents of neurofacilitation approaches to integrate established techniques of NDT with the language of newly emerging knowledge in motor control and motor learning. This is readily seen in a recent text describing the theoretic basis of NDT.[30,34] Although this is typical during paradigm shifts, the amalgamation of old techniques with new theoretical knowledge is not useful either theoretically (since established Bobath techniques are not consistent within the new paradigm of motor control and learning) or for clinical practice (since numerous studies have demonstrated that there is indeed little evidence). The challenge for therapists is to design and evaluate techniques within the newly emerging paradigm of task-oriented training.

Functional Task-Oriented Training: The Second Paradigm Shift

The second paradigm shift in the treatment of neurological disorders began in the 1990s. Therapists began to regard neurotherapeutic approaches with less optimism. The dissatisfaction with the neurotherapeutic approaches is due, in part, to the fact that retraining normal movement patterns do not carry over into the performance of functional daily living skills, which is the ultimate goal of rehabilitation. In addition, there is a greater demand on therapists to use interventions that have demonstrated effectiveness. Evidence that demonstrates a lack of effectiveness of neurotherapeutic approaches, particularly the Bobath approach, has led to the development of novel training regimens based on what has been termed the *task-oriented approach*.[75]

Principles of the Functional Task-Oriented Approach. The task-oriented approach is based on a systems model of motor control and theories of motor learning. The approach attempts to understand the problems faced by the nervous system to control movements. This field of motor neuroscience represents a multidisciplinary approach to understanding motor control and learning from the perspectives of neurophysiology, biomechanics, and behavioral sciences. Within this framework, motor control is understood as an attempt by the nervous system to adapt movements to constraints imposed by the mechanics of the motor apparatus (including length, mass of limbs, and intersegmental dynamics of moving segments), constraints imposed by the environment (open or closed environment), and constraints imposed by the behavioral context. Studies on motor control often analyze movements at the biomechanical and behavior levels. See Chapters 4 and 5 for a detailed description.

Chapter 4 provides the reader with a more comprehensive description of the task-oriented approach. What follows is a brief description of some of the incipient principles of treatment, based on suggestions by Carr and Shepherd[10] and Gentile.[21] Within this framework, the responsibility of the therapist as a teacher of motor skills is to select contextually appropriate functional tasks, vary task parameters to ensure greater transfer of learning, structure practice schedules to encourage active participation of the patients, structure the environment so that all regulatory conditions of a given task are present, and provide feedback. To apply a task-oriented approach to treatment successfully, therapists need to become familiar with analyzing tasks and the processes underlying skill acquisition. The following two sections evaluate the literature on task-oriented approach to stroke rehabilitation.

Outcome Studies Using a Task-Oriented Approach. For the purpose of this review, the author chose eleven RCT that explicitly tested a task-oriented intervention for rehabilitation of upper limb function (Table 6-2). Length of the training programs across the studies varied from two to six weeks, the number of sessions ranging from 10 to 20.

Timing of Intervention. Of the eleven trials, one study tested patients in the acute stage,[58] five tested patients in the subacute stage,[5,16,17,60,100] one study trained patients in the acute and subacute stages,[38] and four tested patients in the chronic stage.[29,54,87,88]

Outcome Measures. Four of the eleven studies only measured outcomes at the impairment level,[16,54,60,88] whereas six studies measured outcomes at the impairment and activity limitation levels.[5,17,38,58,87,100] Only one study measured outcomes at all three levels of the ICF model.[29] Variables at the impairment level commonly tested were gait velocity, endurance, ground reaction forces, kinematic variables in reaching, Action Research Arm Test, and positron emission tomography (PET) scan. Variables related to activity limitation were measured using the 36-item Short-Form Health Survey, Barthel index, and the Functional Ambulation Classification. The only outcome at the participation level was the OARS-IADL and SF-36.

Study Designs Used. All eleven studies included in the review were RCT, of which three were rated as 1b and the other eight rated as 2b, according to the Oxford criteria. The PEDro score ranged from 4 to 8, indicating that all were high quality studies.

Results of the Review. Task-oriented training demonstrated positive outcome when compared with immobilization,[38] resistance training,[87,88] Bobath approach,[58,100] and usual PT and OT.[16,60] Task-oriented therapy was effective in the acute (one study) and subacute stages of stroke (five out of six studies). In the chronic stage, two studies documented effectiveness primarily for lower functioning subjects.[54,87] One study did not find arm training better than lower limb training,[29] and one study found modest gains.[88]

Table 6-2 shows substantial evidence to suggest that task-oriented training leads to improvement of outcomes at the impairment and activity limitation levels. However, since some studies showing a positive effect of task-oriented therapy tested outcomes at the impairment level only, it will be useful for future randomized trials to include outcome measures at multiple levels of the ICF model.

Clinical Implications. The present review of task-oriented training studies confirms the results of two recent reviews,[31,70] there is very good evidence for the effectiveness of this approach in comparison with traditional therapy, Bobath approach, or immobilization. These studies demonstrate that improvement in motor skills and function depends on contextually appropriate task-specific practice of functional skills. Given that this approach is relatively new, additional RCT with larger number of subjects are needed. It will also be important to have control groups that receive dose equivalent standard care.

A number of studies were not included under the general category of task-oriented approach because these studies tested a specific type of task-oriented therapy called constraint-induced movement therapy (CIMT), described in detail in the subsequent section.

Constraint-Induced Movement Therapy

Rationale and Principles. *Constraint-induced movement therapy* is a term used for a family of intervention techniques that aim to decrease the effects of learned nonuse of a paretic limb. This family of techniques involves two basic features: (1) discouraging the use of the unaffected or less affected limb through verbal prompt but more often by applying some form of restraint to the unaffected limb with a sling, splint, or a mitten, and (2) intensive training of the paretic arm through active participation in functional activities.[8,89,90]

Some authors have proposed that the inability to move the paretic limb may arise, at least in part, from a phenomenon termed *learned nonuse*. The proposal is based on experiments in which deafferentation was performed in one limb in primates through dorsal rhizotomy.[82] Following surgery, monkeys did not use their affected limbs because of the lack of sensory feedback, and they preferentially used their unaffected limbs. When the monkeys were forced to use their affected limbs, greater recovery of movement was seen. This indicates that the inability to use the affected limb may be a behavioral learned response to paresis. See Chapters 4, 5, and 10.

Outcome Studies. In the past decade, a large number of studies have been conducted on the effects of CIMT. As seen in Table 6-3, eighteen RCT and one dose-equivalent placebo-controlled trial were identified. All nineteen studies scored either 1b or 2b on the Oxford levels of evidence scale, and the PEDro score ranged from 4 to 8 out of a score of 10. This indicates that all studies were high quality trials. CIMT studies are unique because all studies were careful in subject selection: all subjects included required a minimum of 10-degrees of active extension at the metacarpophalangeal joint and 20-degrees of active extension at the wrist. In addition, a number of studies excluded patients with excessive spasticity and sensory deficits. The narrow specification of inclusion and exclusion criteria may have led to the selection of a highly homogeneous

Text continued on p.142

Table 6-2

Evidence Table for Task-Oriented Training

AUTHORS AND YEAR	AIMS AND RATIONALE	DESIGN, SUBJECTS, OXFORD RATING, PEDRO SCORE	INTERVENTION	COMPARISON INTERVENTION	ASSESSMENT	OUTCOME MEASURES	RESULTS	COMMENTS
Kwakkel et al, 1999	Evaluated different intensities of functional training of the lower and upper limbs in acute and subacute stroke	Single blind RCT; 101 subjects with acute stroke (<14 days of stroke); 1b; 7/10	Arm training group (N=33) practiced functional skills such as reaching, grasping, punching a ball; leg training group (N=31) practiced sitting, standing and weight bearing exercises in sitting and standing; 30 min/day; 5 days/week for 20 weeks	Control group (N=37) had their upper and lower limbs immobilized by a pressure splint	Stroke onset, weekly for 10 weeks, then once in 2 weeks from week 11-20; 26 week follow-up	1. BI 2. FAC 3. ARAT	All groups were similar at baseline; compared with control group, arm training group had better scores on dexterity; leg training group had better scores on ADL, walking and dexterity for all assessments until 20 weeks; At 26 weeks, arm and leg training groups had better score on dexterity.	Well-designed study; functional training of upper and lower limb skills produced task specific improvement.
Nelles et al, 2001	Investigate the effects of intensive arm training on neuronal plasticity in subacute stroke	RCT; 10 subjects with subacute stroke (<30 days) and 5 healthy control subjects; 2b; 4/10	Experimental group (N=5) received task-oriented training including practice of reaching for objects in different directions, to different distances; 45 minutes/day, 5 days a week for 3 weeks	Control group (N=5) received nonspecific rehabilitation program including ROM, stretching, soft-tissue mobilization; 45 minutes/day, 5 days a week for 3 weeks	Pretreatment and post-treatment	1. PET regional cerebral blood flow 2. FM 3. NIHSS	Experimental group showed a trend for greater improvement on FM and NIHSS compared with control group; Experimental group had greater activation of bilateral inferior parietal and premotor areas and contralateral sensorimotor cortex.	Small sample; task-oriented training promotes neuronal plasticity; however, task-oriented group improvement was not significantly different on clinical outcomes compared with control group

Study	Purpose	Design/Subjects	Intervention	Timing	Outcome Measures	Results	Comments
Mudie et al, 2002	Compare effects of task-related reach training, Bobath training, and feedback training on sitting weight distribution	RCT blocked randomization using 2:1 ratio; 40 subjects with acute stroke; 2b; 4/10	Task related group (N=10) practiced reaching to functional objects beyond arm length in sitting; Feedback training group (N=10) trained on reaching to targets and were provided error feedback using the BPM; both groups received OT and PT; daily treatment for two weeks	Bobath group (N=10) received tone normalization, trunk and pelvic ROM, and balance in sitting; Bobath group received standard OT and PT; control group (N=10) received only standard OT and PT treatment; daily treatment for two weeks	Pretreatment and post-treatment, 2 and 12 week follow-up	1. Balance in sitting using the BPM 2. Balance in standing using the BPM 3. BI	Weight distribution was better for BPM, Bobath, and control groups at the end of treatment; all four groups improved at 2 week follow-up; BPM and task-related group maintained improvement at 12 weeks; BPM, task related training and control group performed better on BI	Small sample; task-related training or balance training with feedback better for sitting symmetry in the long term
Thielman et al, 2004	Compare effectiveness of task-related training and PRE in chronic stroke	RCT; 12 subjects with chronic stroke (5 to 18 months); 2b; 4/10	Task-related group (N=6) practiced reaching to functional objects with the trunk restrained in sitting; 35 minutes/day, 3 days/week for 4 weeks	PRE group (N=6) practiced whole arm pulls using a theraband in sitting; movement amplitude was similar to task-related group; 35 minutes/day, 3 days/week for 4 weeks	Pretreatment and post-treatment	1. Kinematic measures (movement time, peak velocity, movement units, curvilinearity ratio) 2. MAS 3. RMA	Low level subjects in the task-related group improved on the RMA; no training effect was seen for MAS; Low level subjects in task-related group improved hand curvilinearity after training	Small sample; lower functioning subjects benefited most from task-related training

Continued

Table 6-2

Evidence Table for Task-Oriented Training—cont'd

AUTHORS AND YEAR	AIMS AND RATIONALE	DESIGN, SUBJECTS, OXFORD RATING, PEDRO SCORE	INTERVENTION	COMPARISON INTERVENTION	ASSESSMENT	OUTCOME MEASURES	RESULTS	COMMENTS
Winstein et al, 2004	Evaluate effects of task-related training and strength training (ST) in acute and subacute stroke	Nonblinded RCT; 60 subjects with acute or subacute stroke (2 to 35 days); 1b; 6/10	Task-related training group (N=20) received SC plus repetitive practice of functional tasks; ST group (N=20) received SC plus resistive movements using theraband; Both groups received therapy 1 hour/day, 5 days/week for 4 weeks	SC group (N=20) included facilitation, neuromuscular electric stimulation, stretching, using an NDT approach and ADL training.	Pretreatment and posttreatment, 6 and 9 month follow-up	1. FM 2. FTHUE 3. FIM	Task-related training and ST groups had better FM and Isometric torque at posttreatment primarily in less severe patients; Isometric torque improvement was maintained at 9 months	Well-designed study; task-related training was better than ST in the long-term
Blennerhasset et al, 2004	Investigate whether additional practice of upper or lower limb task improves function in subacute stroke	Single blind RCT; 30 subjects with subacute stroke (11 to 49 days); 2b; 8/10	Upper limb group (N=15) received usual PT for 1 hour/day, 5 days/week, and additional circuit training involving practice of functional tasks; 1 hour/day, 5 days/week for 4 weeks	Mobility group (N=15) received usual PT for 1 hour/day, 5 days/week, and additional training on bikes and treadmill, and practice of sit-to-stand, obstacle course walking, standing balance; 1 hour/day, 5 days/week for 4 weeks	Pretreatment and posttreatment, 6 month follow-up	1. Six-minute walk test 2. TUG 3. Step Test 4. MAS 5. JTHFT	Upper limb group performed better on the MAS and JTHFT; lower limb group had better mobility scores on the TUG	Well-designed study shows the task specificity of training; small sample

Study	Design/Subjects/Level	Experimental group	Control group	Measurement	Outcome measures	Results	Conclusions
Desrosiers et al, 2005	Evaluate effect of arm training program (unilateral and bilateral) in subacute stroke	Single blind; 47 subjects with subacute stroke (10 to 47 days); 2b; 6/10	Experimental group (N=20) received usual OT and PT, plus practiced symmetrical bilateral and unilateral functional tasks; 45 minutes/day, 4 days/week for 5 weeks	Control group (N=21) received usual OT and PT, plus functional activities to enhance strength, active assistive and passive movements; 45 minutes/day, 4 days/week for 5 weeks	Pretreatment and post-treatment	1. FM 2. Grip strength 3. Manual dexterity (Box and Block Test) 4. PPT 5. Finger to Nose Test 6. TEMPA 7. FIM	Both groups improved as a result of therapy; no differences were seen between groups	Task training did not enhance motor function above usual and customary care in subacute stroke
Higgins et al, 2006	Evaluate efficacy of a task-oriented program on arm function in chronic stroke	Single blind RCT; 91 subjects with chronic stroke (< 1 year); 1b; 8/10	Arm training group (N=47) practiced functional upper limb tasks; 1.5 hours/day, 3 days/week for 6 weeks	Mobility training (N=44) practiced functional mobility and balance tasks; 1.5 hours/day, 3 days/week for 6 weeks	Pretreatment and post-treatment	1. Box and Block Test 2. NHPT 3. TEMPA 4. Grip Strength 5. STREAM 6. BI 7. Older Americans Resources and Services Scale (OARS-IADL) 8. SF-36 9. Geriatric Depression Scale	No differences were seen between groups on motor performance or function at posttreatment	Well-designed study; upper limb task-oriented intervention no better than lower limb intervention

Continued

Table 6-2

Evidence Table for Task-Oriented Training—cont'd

AUTHORS AND YEAR	AIMS AND RATIONALE	DESIGN, SUBJECTS, OXFORD RATING, PEDRO SCORE	INTERVENTION	COMPARISON INTERVENTION	ASSESSMENT	OUTCOME MEASURES	RESULTS	COMMENTS
Michaelson et al, 2006	Compare effects of task-related training with TR compared with training without TR in chronic stroke	Double blind RCT; 30 subjects with chronic stroke (6 to 48 months); 2b; 7/10	TR group (N=15) practiced functional unimanual and bimanual reaching tasks; trunk movement restrained with belts; 1 hour/day, 3 days/week for 5 weeks	Control group (N=15) practiced functional unimanual and bimanual reaching tasks; 1 hour/day, 3 days/week for 5 weeks	Pretreatment and post-treatment, 1-month follow-up	1. FM 2. TEMPA 3. Isometric force 4. Manual dexterity (Box and Block Test) 5. Kinematic analysis (trunk displacement and elbow extension range)	TR group did better on FM and increased elbow extension range at posttest and follow-up; both groups improved on TEMPA and Box and Block test	Task-related training using TR improves motor function in low functioning subjects; small sample
Dean et al, 2007	Compare effects of task-related reaching training with sham training on sitting ability and quality in subacute stroke	Single blind RCT; 12 subjects with subacute stroke (<3 months); 2b; 7/10	Task-related reaching group (N=6) received regular PT and additional sitting training protocol (coordination of trunk and arm in reaching; loading of affected foot, prevention of maladaptive strategies); 0.5 hours/day, 5 days/week over 2 weeks	Control group (N=5) received regular PT and sham treatment (completing cognitive manipulation tasks in sitting); 0.5 hours/day, 5 days/week over 2 weeks	Pretreatment and post-treatment, 6 month follow-up	1. Sitting ability (maximum reach distance for forward and across reaches in sitting); 2. Sitting quality (reach movement time, average peak vertical force through affected foot)	Maximum reach distance was higher for task-related reaching after treatment and at follow-up; movement time and peak vertical force were better for task-related reaching at posttreatment; task-related reaching group had better carry over (peak vertical force in standing)	Small sample; well-designed study showing that task-related training is better for sitting ability and quality

| Thielman et al, 2008 | Compare effect of task-related training with RE on reaching in chronic stroke | RCT; 11 subjects with chronic stroke (>6 months); 2b; 5/10 | Task-related training group (N=5) practiced reaching movements to objects placed at different distances and directions; TR in sitting; 45 minutes/day, 3 days/week for 4 weeks | Control group (N=6) practiced arm movements against resistance of theraband in sitting with TR; 45 minutes/day, 3 days/week for 4 weeks; | Pretreatment and post-treatment | 1. Kinematic analysis of arm movement (amplitude, time to peak velocity, movement time, wrist displacement and curvilinearity ratio)
2. WMFT
3. F
4. Active ROM | Task-related training group had straighter hand path and lower deceleration time after training; both groups improved on the FM and active ROM; no improvement on WMFT | Small sample; task-related training leads to modest gains in arm function |

ADL, Activities of daily living; ARAT, Action Research Arm Test; BI, Barthel Index; BPM, balance performance monitor; FAC, Functional Ambulation Category; FIM, Functional Independence Measure; FM, Fugl-Myer Assessment; FTHUE, Functional Test of the Hemiparetic Upper Extremity; JTHFT, Jebsen Taylor Hand Function Test; MAL, Motor Activity Log; MAS, Modified Ashworth Scale; NDT, neurodevelopmental therapy; NHPT, None Hole Peg Test; NIHSS, National Institute of Health Stroke Scale; OT, occupation therapy; PET, positron emission tomography; PPT, Purdue Pegboard Test; PRE, progressive resistive training; PT, physical therapy; RMA, Rivermead Motor Assessment; RCT, randomized controlled trial; RE, resistive exercise; ROM, range of motion; SC, standard care; ST, strength training; STREAM, Stroke Rehabilitation Assessment of Movement; TEMPA, Upper Extremity Performance test; TR, trunk restraint; TUG, Timed UP and Go; WMFT, Wolf Motor Function Test.

Table 6-3

Evidence Table for Constraint-Induced Movement Therapy

AUTHORS AND YEAR	AIMS AND RATIONALE	DESIGN, SUBJECTS, OXFORD RATING, PEDRO SCORE	INTERVENTION	COMPARISON INTERVENTION	ASSESSMENT	OUTCOME MEASURES	RESULTS	COMMENTS
Dromerick et al, 2000	Examine if CIMT is more effective than conventional therapy in acute stroke	Single blind RCT; 20 subjects with acute stroke (<14 days); 2b; 5/10	OT treatment focused on ADL, functional upper limb training with affected arm; unaffected hand in padded mitten for 6 hours a day; 2 hours/day, 5 days/week for 2 weeks	Standard OT treatment including compensatory treatment for ADL, upper limb strength, ROM, and positioning; 2 hours/day, 5 days/week for 2 weeks	Pretreatment and posttreatment	1. ARAT 2. BI 3. FIM	ARAT scores were higher for CIMT group at discharge; no differences were seen for BI score; CIMT group had higher scores on the FIM UL dressing	Low dosage CIMT (2 hours) shows improvement only in impairment level measures in acute stroke; small sample
Page et al, 2002	Test efficacy of modified CIMT in subacute stroke	Single blind, multiple baseline RCT; 14 subjects with subacute stroke (1 to 6 months poststroke); 2b; 4/10	Modified CIMT group (N=7) treated in 30 min OT sessions for functional training of upper limb using shaping; 30 min PT sessions to improve balance and mobility; less affected limb restrained in hemisling for 5 hours of frequent arm use each day; 1 hour/day, 3 days/week for 10 weeks	Traditional therapy group (N=4) received OT and PT based on Proprioceptive Neuromuscular Facilitation; and compensatory training; Control group (N=6) received no therapy; 1 hour/day, 3 days/week for 10 weeks	Two pretreatment, posttreatment	1. FM 2. ARAT 3. MAL	Modified CIMT group improved more than traditional therapy and no therapy group on FM, ARAT, and MAL	Modified CIMT, based on distributed practice over 10 weeks, better than traditional therapy based on PNF or no therapy in subacute stage; small sample size

Study	Design/Subjects	CIMT	Control	Timing	Outcome Measures	Results	Conclusions
Wittenberg et al, 2003	Determine if CIMT is more effective than less intensive control intervention in changing motor function and brain physiology in chronic stroke	Single blind RCT; 16 subjects with chronic stroke (>12 months since stroke); 2b; 6/10	CIMT included task-oriented training of upper limb; restraint of unaffected limb using hand splint and sling; 6 hours/day during weekdays and 6 hours/day on weekend over 10 consecutive days	Control group received passive therapy and task performance using unaffected hand; 3 hours/day during weekdays and no therapy on weekend over 10 consecutive days	Pretreatment and post-treatment and 6 month follow-up	1. WMFT 2. MAL 3. AMPS 4. PET 5. TMS	No differences were seen on WMFT and AMPS. CIMT had better performance on MAL. No differences were seen across groups on physiological measures	CIMT produced increased use of the affected arm but this did not result in decreased impairment or improved function despite greater intensity of CIMT; small sample
Suputtitada et al, 2004	Evaluate the effectiveness of CIMT on hand dexterity in chronic stroke	Single blind RCT; 69 patients with chronic stroke (1 to 10 years since stroke); 1b; 6/10	CIMT group (N = 33) treated in groups of 3 to 4; practice of functional tasks with affected hand; unaffected hand in glove; 6 hours/day, 5 days/week for 2 weeks	Control group (N = 36) treated in groups of 3 to 4; therapy based on Bobath approach including practice of bimanual tasks; 6 hours/day, 5 days/week for 2 weeks	Pretreatment and post-treatment	1. ARAT 2. Hand grip strength 3. Pinch strength	Both groups improved on the primary outcome (ARAT), with CIMT group showing more improvement; CIMT group had greater improvement on hand and pinch strength	CIMT produces greater improvement in hand function, grip and pinch strength compared with Bobath approach of comparable intensity and duration

Continued

Table 6-3

Evidence Table for Constraint-Induced Movement Therapy—cont'd

AUTHORS AND YEAR	AIMS AND RATIONALE	DESIGN; SUBJECTS, OXFORD RATING, PEDRO SCORE	INTERVENTION	COMPARISON INTERVENTION	ASSESSMENT	OUTCOME MEASURES	RESULTS	COMMENTS
Page et al, 2004	Determine efficacy of modified CIMT as compared with traditional therapy or no therapy in chronic stroke	Single blind, multiple baseline RCT; 17 subjects with chronic stroke (> 1 year); 2b; 6/10	Modified CIMT group (N=7) treated in 30 min OT sessions for functional training of upper limb using shaping and approximation; 30 min PT sessions to improve balance and mobility and upper limb stretching; less affected limb restrained in hemisling for 5 hours of frequent arm use each day; 1 hour/day, 3 days/week for 10 weeks	Traditional therapy group (N=4) received OT and PT based on PNF; and compensatory training; control group (N=6) received no therapy; 1 hour/day, 3 days/week for 10 weeks	Two pretreatment and posttreatment	1. FM 2. ARAT 3. MAL	Modified CIMT group improved more than traditional therapy group on FM, ARAT, and MAL. Control group performed worse at posttreatment	Modified CIMT, distributed over 10 weeks, is better than traditional therapy based on PNF or no therapy; small sample size
Page et al, 2005	Compare effectiveness of modified CIMT to traditional rehabilitation in acute stroke	Single blind, multiple baseline RCT; 10 subjects with acute stroke (<14 days); 2b; 5/10	Modified CIMT (N=5) included practice of functional tasks with affected upper limb; unaffected hand was restrained in a padded mitt for 5 hours/day of frequent time use; 0.5 hours/day, 3 times/week for 10 weeks	Traditional rehabilitation (N=5) included stretching, weight bearing, manual dexterity exercises and ADL training with unaffected limb; 0.5 hours/day, 3 times/week for 10 weeks	Two pretreatment and posttreatment	1. FM 2. ARAT 3. MAL	Modified CIMT group performed better than traditional rehabilitation group on FM, ARAT, and MAL	Small sample; No statistical analysis;

Author, Year	Purpose	Design, Sample, Level	CIMT Group	Control Group	Measures	Results	Comments
Wolf et al, 2006	Compare effects of CIMT versus customary care in subacute and chronic stroke patients in multisite trial	Single blind RCT; 222 stroke patients (>12 months) 1b; 6/10	CIMT group received shaping, practice of functional tasks and additional practice at home (N=106); unaffected limb in instrumented mitt worn for 90% of waking hours; 6 hours/day, 5 days/week for 2 weeks	Usual and customary care ranged from no treatment to orthotics, OT and PT either at home, day program	Pre treatment and post treatment, 4, 8, and 12 month follow-up 1. WMFT 2. MAL 3. SIS	CIMT group showed greater improvement than controls on WMFT (log performance time, functional ability) at post-treatment; CIMT group showed more improvement than controls on MAL at 12 months; no differences WMFT functional ability at 12 months	Control group received less therapy, no standardization of control group treatment; large sample size; multicenter trial; greater effect of CIMT may be due to massed practice
Taub et al, 2006	Compare effectiveness of CIMT with dose equivalent placebo control group in chronic stroke	Placebo controlled trial; 41 patients chronic stroke (>1 year) assigned to groups in blocks; 2b; 4/10	CIMT group (N=21) practiced functional tasks with paretic limb, received shaping and performance feedback; unaffected limb in resting hand splint for 90% of waking hours; 6 hours/day; 5 days/week for 2 weeks	Control group (N=20) received general fitness program including strength, balance, stamina training, and relaxation exercises; 6 hours/day; 5 days/week for 2 weeks	Pretreatment and post-treatment, week 1, 2, 3, 4, 3 months, and 2 year follow-up 1. MAL 2. AAUT 3. WMFT	The CIMT group had more females, increased arm strength and better mood at baseline; CIMT group had better scores after treatment on MAL, AAUT and WMFT performance; no difference in functional ability; improvement maintained up to 2 years	Groups not randomized and not similar at baseline; CIMT is more effective than dose-equivalent control treatment in chronic stroke

Continued

Table 6-3

Evidence Table for Constraint-Induced Movement Therapy—cont'd

AUTHORS AND YEAR	AIMS AND RATIONALE	DESIGN, SUBJECTS, OXFORD RATING, PEDRO SCORE	INTERVENTION	COMPARISON INTERVENTION	ASSESSMENT	OUTCOME MEASURES	RESULTS	COMMENTS
Boake et al, 2007	Evaluate the effectiveness of CIMT on motor function of the upper limb in subacute stroke	RCT; 23 patients with subacute stroke (<14 days of stroke); 2b; 6/10	CIMT group practiced reaching, grasping, lifting, and placing objects with affected hand (N=10); shaping and approximation; unaffected limb in mitt for 90% of waking hours; 3 hours/day; 6 days/week for 2 weeks	Control group practiced daily living tasks with either hand to improve strength, muscle tone and ROM (N=13); 3 hours/day; 6 days/week for 2 weeks	Pre-treatment and post treatment 3- to 4-month follow-up	1. FM of motor recovery 2. Grooved Pegboard Test 3. MAL 4. Transcranial Magnetic Stimulation	Both groups improved on primary outcome (FM); no differences between groups at posttreatment or follow-up; CIMT group reported better outcome in quality of movement during ADL performance; no differences in motor threshold at posttreatment or follow-up	Same dosage did not highlight benefit of CIMT; small sample size
Wu et al, 2007a	Evaluate effect of mCIMT on motor control of upper limb and functional change in chronic stroke	Single blind RCT; 30 subjects with chronic stroke (12 to 36 months); 1b; 7/10	Modified CIMT (N=15) received OT treatment including practice of functional tasks using shaping, and normalization of tone; unaffected hand restrained in a mitt for 5 hours/day at time of frequent use; 2 hours/day, 5 days/week for 3 weeks	Traditional rehabilitation group (N=15) received OT using Bobath approach including balance, stretching, weight-bearing of affected limb; fine motor tasks and ADL skills using unaffected arm; 2 hours/day, 5 days/week for 3 weeks	Pretreatment and post-treatment	1. Kinematic analysis of arm movement 2. MAL 3. FIM	Modified CIMT group had lower movement time and displacement and higher percentage of movement time at peak velocity; modified CIMT had better arm use and quality of movement in MAL and better FIM scores	Well designed study; modified CIMT better than Bobath approach for improving arm kinematics and functional gains in chronic stroke; no follow-up assessment

| Wu et al. 2007 b | Examine benefits of mCIMT on motor and daily function, quality of life in elderly patients with subacute and chronic stroke | RCT single blind; 26 elderly subjects (>65 years) with subacute or chronic stroke (0.5–31 months); 2b; 6/10 | mCIMT (N=13) received OT treatment including practice of functional tasks using shaping, and normalization of tone; unaffected hand restrained in a mitt for 5 hours/day at time of frequent use; mCIMT 2 hours/day, 5 days/week for 3 weeks | Traditional rehabilitation group (N=13) received OT using Bobath approach including balance, stretching, weight bearing of affected limb; fine motor tasks and ADL skills using unaffected arm; 2 hours/day, 5 days/week for 3 weeks | Pretreatment, post-treatment | 1. FM
2. FIM
3. MAL
4. Stroke Impact Scale (SIS) | mCIMT group performed better on FM, FIM, MAL and SIS compared with traditional rehabilitation | Small sample; no follow up; Modified CIMT better than Bobath approach for improving hand function and quality of life in elderly subjects with stroke |
| Wu et al, 2007c | Evaluate effect of modified CIMT on motor control of upper limb and functional change in subacute and chronic stroke | RCT single blind; 47 subjects with chronic stroke (3 weeks to 37 months); 2b; 6/10 | Modified CIMT (N=24) received OT treatment including practice of functional tasks using shaping and normalization of tone; unaffected hand restrained in a mitt for 5 hours/day at time of frequent use; Modified CIMT 2 hours/day, 5 days/week for 3 weeks | Traditional rehabilitation group (N=23) received OT using Bobath approach including balance, stretching, weight-bearing of affected limb; fine motor tasks and ADL skills using unaffected arm; 2 hours/day, 5 days/week for 3 weeks | Pretreatment and post-treatment | 1. Kinematic analysis of arm movement
2. FM
3. MAL | Modified CIMT group had lower movement time, displacement, and movement units; modified CIMT had better arm use and quality of movement in MAL and better FM scores | Well-designed study; modified CIMT better than Bobath approach for improving arm kinematics and functional gains in subacute and chronic stroke; no follow-up assessment |

Continued

Table 6-3

Evidence Table for Constraint-Induced Movement Therapy—cont'd

AUTHORS AND YEAR	AIMS AND RATIONALE	DESIGN, SUBJECTS, OXFORD RATING, PEDRO SCORE	INTERVENTION	COMPARISON INTERVENTION	ASSESSMENT	OUTCOME MEASURES	RESULTS	COMMENTS
Lin et al, 2007	Evaluate effect of modified CIMT on motor control of upper limb and functional change in chronic stroke	Single blind RCT; 32 subjects with chronic stroke (13 to 26 months); 2b; 6/10	Modified CIMT (N=15) received OT treatment including practice of functional tasks using shaping and normalization of tone; unaffected hand restrained in a mitt for 5 hours/day at time of frequent use; Modified CIMT 2 hours/day, 5 days/week for 3 weeks	Traditional rehabilitation group (N=17) received OT using Bobath approach including balance, stretching, weigh-bearing of affected limb, fine motor tasks and ADL skills using unaffected arm; 2 hours/day, 5 days/week for 3 weeks	Pretreatment and post-treatment	1. Kinematic analysis of arm movement 2. MAL 3. FIM	Modifieds CIMT group had lower reaction time and higher percentage of movement time at peak velocity; modified CIMT group had better arm use and quality of movement in MAL and better FIM scores	Modified CIMT better than Bobath approach for improving arm kinematics and functional gains in chronic stroke; no follow-up assessment; small sample
Myint et al, (2008)	Compare the effects of CIMT with control treatment in outpatient subacute stroke	Single blind RCT; 43 patients at subacute stage (2 to 16 weeks post-stroke); 2b; 7/10	CIMT upper limb training with OT including shaping, task-oriented training (N=23); unaffected limb placed in shoulder sling 4 hours/day, 5 days/week for 2 weeks	OT and PT using an Bobath approach including bimanual tasks, strengthening, ROM, positioning and mobility training (N=20); 4 hours/day 5 days/week for 2 months	Pretreatment and post-treatment and 12 week follow-up	1. Functional test for hemiparetic upper extremity 2. Action Research Arm Test (ARAT) 3. Motor Activity Log (MAL) 4. Nine-hole Peg Test 5. Barthel Index	While both groups improved at posttest and follow-up, CIMT group performed better on all impairment level outcome measures at 12 week follow-up. No differences seen on BI at 12 week follow-up	Well-designed study; CIMT better than Bobath approach in subacute stroke; small sample size; no benefit of CIMT on functional skills

Study	Design	Intervention	Comparison	Timing	Measures	Results	Conclusion
Dahl et al, (2008)	Examine feasibility and effect of CIMT compared with traditional rehabilitation in the short-term and long-term in an inpatient setting	Double blind RCT; 30 patients at subacute and chronic stage (>2 weeks post stroke); 1b, 8/10	CIMT in groups including practice of ADL and leisure skills, (N=18); unaffected limb in mitt; 6 hours/day, 5 days/week for 2 weeks	Standard PT and OT including upper and lower extremity training for 55 minutes and robot exposure for 5 minutes at each session; 30 minutes/day, 5 days/week for 2 weeks	Pretreatment and post-treatment and 6 month follow-up	1. WMFT 2. MAL 3. FIM 4. SIS	CIMT group showed greater improvement than control group at posttest on WMFT and MAL, but differences washed out at 6 month follow-up. Both groups improved comparably on SIS.	Small sample size, CIMT group received more treatment than control group. Since no differences seen at 6 months, CIMT not better than conventional treatment in the long-term
Sawaki et al, 2008	Determine if CIMT is more effective than less intensive control intervention in changing motor function and brain physiology in subacute stroke	Single blind RCT; 30 subjects with subacute stroke (3 to 9 months since stroke); 2b; 5/10	CIMT (N=15) included unimanual skill acquisition and functional training (object manipulation); restraint of unaffected limb using hand splint and sling; no information on dosage; therapy given for 10 consecutive weekdays	Control group (N=15) received usual and customary care ranging from no treatment to application of orthotics or OT and PT; no information on dosage; therapy given for 10 consecutive weekdays	Pretreatment and post-treatment and 4-month follow-up	1. WMFT 2. TMS	Both groups improved on WMFT CIMT group had better grip strength at posttreatment and follow-up; no differences seen across groups on other WMFT items or TMS measures	CIMT resulted in modest improvement only in grip strength did not lead to improvement in function or cortical reorganization
Brogårdh et al, 2009	Examine the effect of using a mitt during CIMT in subacute stroke	RCT 24 patients (1 to 3 months poststroke); 2b; 6/10	CIMT mitt group wore mitt for 90% of waking hours; training included practice of fine motor skills, strength training, stretching; 3 hours/day; 5 days/week for 2 weeks	CIMT no Mitt group had training including practice of fine motor skills, strength training, stretching; 3 hours/day; 5 days/week for 2 weeks	Pretreatment and post-treatment, 3 month follow-up	1. Modified Motor Assessment scale 2. Sollerman Hand function test 3. 2-point discrimination test 4. MAL	Both groups improved their hand and arm function but no differences were seen between groups posttreatment or at follow-up	There is no effect of wearing a mitt during CIMT in subacute stroke

Continued

Table 6-3

Evidence Table for Constraint-Induced Movement Therapy—cont'd

AUTHORS AND YEAR	AIMS AND RATIONALE	DESIGN, SUBJECTS, OXFORD RATING, PEDRO SCORE	INTERVENTION	COMPARISON INTERVENTION	ASSESSMENT	OUTCOME MEASURES	RESULTS	COMMENTS
Lin et al, 2009	Compare modified CIT intervention with a dose-matched control intervention in chronic stroke	Single blind RCT; 32 subjects with subacute and chronic stroke (6 to 40 months post-stroke); 1b; 7/10	Modified CIMT group (N=16) received OT with functional training of upper limb using shaping, normalization of tone; unaffected hand in mitt for 5 hours/day; modified CIMT 2 hours/day, 5 days/week for 3 weeks	Control group (N=16) received OT focused on Bobath approach and functional task training and weight-bearing; unaffected hand in mitt for 5 hours/day; control group 2 hours/day, 5 days/week for 3 weeks	Pretreatment and post-treatment	1. FM 2. FIM 3. MAL 4. NEADL 5. SIS	Modified CIMT group performed better on FM, FIM (self-care and locomotion) and SIS (ADL, mobility, and hand function), on the mobility domain of the NEADL	Modified CIMT better than Bobath approach in improving motor function and quality of life in subacute and chronic stroke

| Dromerick et al, 2009 | Compare CIMT with traditional OT and examine if effect of CIMT is dose dependent in very early stroke | Single blind RCT; 52 subjects with stroke (<28 days of admission to inpatient rehabilitation); 1b; 7/10 | Dose matched CIMT group (N=19) received 2 hours of shaping (5 days/week for 2 weeks) and wore a mitt for 6 hours/day; higher intensity CIMT group (N=16) received 3 hours (5 days/week for 2 weeks) of shaping and wore a mitt 90% of waking hours; both groups practiced functional tasks. | Traditional OT group (N=17) including compensatory techniques for ADL, ROM, strengthening; upper limb bilateral activities; 2 hours/day, 5 days/week for 2 weeks | Pretreatment and post-treatment, 3 month follow-up | 1. ARAT 2. NIHSS 3. FIM 4. SIS | All three groups improved on the ARAT; no differences were seen between control and dose matched CIMT group; high intensity CIMT had lower gains on ARAT; no differences seen across groups on FIM score; SIS score was highest for the dose matched CIMT group at 90 days | Excellent study; CIMT was no more effective than control OT of same intensity; high intensity CIMT led to less improvement in upper limb function. |

AAUT, Actual Amount of Arm Use Test; ADL, activities of daily living; AMPS, Assessment of Motor and Process Skills; ARAT, Action Research Arm Test; BI, Barthel Index; CIMT, Constraint Induced Movement Therapy; FIM, Functional Independence Measure; FM, Fugl-Myer Assessment; MAL, Motor Activity Log; MAS, Modified Ashworth Scale; NDT, neurodevelopmental therapy; NEADL, Nottingham Extended Activities of Daily Living Scale; NIHSS, National Institute of Health Stroke Scale; OT, occupational therapy; PET, positron emission tomography; PNF, Proprioceptive Neuromuscular Facilitation; PT, physical therapy; RCT, randomized controlled trial; RMA, Rivermead Motor Assessment; ROM, range of motion; SIS, Stroke Impact Scale; TMS, Transcranial Magnetic Stimulation; WMFT, Wolf Motor Function Test; UL, upper limb group of patients most likely to recover from stroke based on spontaneous recovery.[32,36]

There was tremendous variability in the form of CIMT and the dosage of intervention. Seven of the nineteen trials tested the standard version of CIMT, which included six hours of practice in each session. The other three trials of standard CIMT included either two hours,[18] three hours,[9] or four hours of training in each session.[59] However, all the ten trials of standard CIMT provided massed practice over 10 sessions across two weeks. Nine trials tested a modified version of CIMT, in which practice was distributed over sessions ranging from 12 to 30. Modified CIMT trials have been designed to replicate therapeutic dosage similar to standard practice. However, as Table 6-3 demonstrates, there is tremendous variability in dosage, ranging from 30 minutes to six hours of practice per session.

Since one of the major principles of CIMT is constraint of the unaffected hand, all studies included some form of constraint using a mitt, sling, hemisling, or splint. There was a large variability across studies in terms of the hours of restraint (from five hours to 90% of waking hours).

Timing of Intervention. Four CIMT trials were conducted in the acute stage,[6,18,19,66] four trials were conducted in the subacute stage,[9,59,63,73] and six trials were conducted in the chronic stage.[46,65,80,85,101,104] Five trials included subjects both in the subacute and the chronic stage.[14,46a,103,105,106]

Outcome Measures. Most of the studies reviewed measured outcomes at the impairment and activity limitation level. Typical instruments used to measure impairment level measures were the Action Research Arm Test (which measures upper limb dexterity), the Fugl-Meyer Assessment (which measures the ability of the arm to move against the typical synergistic pattern), the Wolf Motor Function Test (which quantifies motor function after stroke), PET scan, and Transcranial Magnetic Stimulation. Activity limitation was measured by measures such as the Rehabilitation Activities Profile (based on the ICF and, which assesses disability and handicap), Motor Activity Log (which measures actual amount of use and quality of movement), Barthel index, and the Functional Independence Measure (which measures activity limitation). Participation restriction was measured by administration of the Stroke Impact Scale in a few studies.

Results of the Review. The results are equivocal at present. CIMT is clearly better than the Bobath approach either in the subacute or chronic stages. When compared with usual care or conventional functional OT and PT, CIMT is more beneficial in studies where the CIMT group received a higher dosage of therapeutic intervention. When compared with dose equivalent functional training, CIMT does not seem more effective. The one exception was the study by Taub and colleagues[85] who found CIMT to be more effective than general fitness. However, the results of this study have to interpreted with caution as there were differences between groups at baseline, and subjects were not randomized. In the acute stage, CIMT is no more effective than dose equivalent functional OT treatment. Higher dose CIMT was less beneficial as compared with low dose CIMT.[19] In the subacute stage, when CIMT is compared with dose equivalent functional training, both interventions result in similar improvement (see Table 6-3).

Clinical Implications. CIMT appears to be a beneficial approach, but future studies need to compare CIMT with dose equivalent functional task-oriented training, which is shown to be effective. Such a study may address the criticism that the improvements demonstrated are due to a nonspecific effect of increased intensity of treatment rather than to a specific effect of constrained-induced training. Most of the studies reported in Table 6-3 used a standard CIMT training protocol in which training was massed over a period of two weeks and was compared with a control group that received less intense conventional training or ineffective traditional approaches, such as the Bobath approach. Studies using a modified CIMT protocol, while demonstrating some benefits, had the limitation of small sample size or comparison with traditional therapy known to be less effective (Bobath approach).

According to Taub and Uswatte,[84] the improvements seen with CIMT could be a result of massing of practice. Given that similar positive results have been obtained by increasing the intensity of traditional therapy, van der Lee[90] argues that using traditional therapeutic procedures that often may be less frustrating to patients than CIMT may be just as effective.

Robot-Aided Motor Training for Upper Limb Function
Rationale and Principles. A recent addition to the arsenal of techniques for stroke rehabilitation is the use of robotic manipulators for providing training of arm movements. Robot manipulators have been used successfully in experimental paradigms that attempted to elucidate the mechanisms underlying normal motor control and learning[74] and also to clarify mechanisms underlying disorders of upper limb movements in patients with movement disorders.[76]

The rationale for using a robotic device in rehabilitation is to decrease the labor-intensive nature of therapy and to provide a device that could be used for quantitative evaluation and treatment.[40] Proponents of this approach contend that current therapeutic evaluations are usually subjective and that therapists spend much time on one-on-one interaction with patients. The idea is to have devices available at rehabilitation centers for use when the patient is not in therapy sessions. Given that patients spend a large percentage of time outside therapist interaction, an attempt at facilitating practice during this time should be beneficial. Robot-assisted training attempts to provide intensive practice of repetitive and stereotyped movements. See Chapter 11 for a full discussion of this topic.

Outcome Studies. A review of studies testing the effectiveness of robot assisted training revealed ten RCT, as listed in Table 6-4. Typical training with this approach involves the patient making horizontal plane movements while grasping the handle of the robot manipulator. Target locations and patient movement are displayed on a computer screen in front of the patient. Typically, patients are trained to produce movements of the shoulder and elbow joints while the wrist and hand joints and the trunk are immobilized with restraints. The robot is typically programmed to either passively move the paretic limb or produce an assistive force during movements. The number of sessions (12 to 60) and the total training time (eight hours to 300 hours) varied tremendously across studies.

Timing of Intervention. Two studies tested patients in the acute stage,[52,68] four studied patients in the subacute stage,[20,28,50,93] and four studies tested patients at the chronic stage.[15,33,49,95]

Outcome Measures. Most of the studies reviewed measured outcome variables at the impairment and activity limitation levels. The exceptions were studies that tested outcomes only at the impairment level.[15,28] Typical instruments used to measure impairments included the Fugl-Meyer Assessment, Action Research Arm Test, Trunk Control Test, and kinematic analysis of arm movement. Instruments used to measure activity limitation were the Functional Independence Measure, Chedoke-McMaster Stroke Scale, and the Barthel index.

Results of the Review. The results of effectiveness of robot assisted training are fairly clear; when compared with robot exposure,[20,92] traditional therapy using the Bobath approach[49,50,52] or neuromuscular facilitation,[15,28] robot training is more effective in improving function. This result can be explained by the fact that subjects in the robot groups received more training of upper limb movements compared with the control groups. However, when robot assisted training is compared with dose equivalent functional training, robot assisted training offers no additional benefits.[33,68,95]

Clinical Implications. The results highlight that robot assisted training offers no advantage to functional training with a therapist. Its effectiveness is limited to studies where robot assisted training was compared with traditional approaches that have been shown to be ineffective (such as the Bobath approach). Given the expense and extensive training of personnel to use the robot device, and its limited effectiveness, it may be beneficial to

think of testing robotic devices as an adjunct to therapy rather than as a primary method of therapy delivery. Before additional RCT are implemented, the rationale and experimental procedures need to be clarified. For instance, at present, robot training provides practice of pointing movements (movements of the shoulder and elbow) on the horizontal plane. In an effort to isolate movements to these two joints, the trunk and distal extremities are often stabilized by constraints producing rather unnatural conditions for practice of arm movements. Functional reaching movements involve coordinated movement of the trunk-arm complex and of the wrist-hand complex. Whether practice of isolated components of the shoulder-elbow complex would transfer to real-world situations is unclear, given the task-specific nature of transfer of training. The responsibility of therapists is to select appropriate, challenging functional tasks, vary task parameters, progress to more difficult tasks, and test for transfer. Given the complexity of therapeutic training, robot manipulators can perhaps serve best by providing quantitative evaluation of impairments rather than as a therapeutic tool.

Body Weight Support and Treadmill Training to Improve Gait

Rationale and Principles. Approximately half the individuals who suffer a stroke do not recover their ability to walk independently.[32] Given that independent walking is a necessary prerequisite to successful community reintegration, not surprisingly gait training has occupied an important role in therapeutic practice following stroke. Gait training following stroke involves practice of individual segments of walking, practice of walking over ground with assistance of therapists and/or assistive devices, or more recently, practice of walking on a treadmill with partial body weight support.

Experiments on animals have shown that the basic neural circuitry for producing the rhythmic alternating movements of the lower limb is at the spinal cord level. Locomotor training with weight support of the hindlimbs has been shown to improve gait to near normal levels in cats whose spinal cords have been transected at thoracic levels, thereby isolating lower cord segments from the rest of the central nervous system.[2] In fact, patients with spinal cord injury have been shown to improve after treadmill training with body weight support.[99] Apart from the limited early evidence of the benefit of treadmill training in patients with spinal cord injury, the rationale for this approach is that it removes some of the biomechanical and equilibrium constraints of weight-bearing and facilitates walking by activation of spinal locomotor circuits. See Chapter 15.

Outcome Studies. A review of studies testing the effectiveness of body weight support training revealed six RCT listed in Table 6-5. Typical training with this approach involves beginning gait training on a treadmill by

Text continued on p.152

Table 6-4

Evidence Table for Robot-Assisted Therapy

AUTHORS AND YEAR	AIMS AND RATIONALE	DESIGN, SUBJECTS, OXFORD RATING, PEDRO SCORE	INTERVENTION	COMPARISON INTERVENTION	ASSESSMENT	OUTCOME MEASURES	RESULTS	COMMENTS
Volpe et al, 2000	Test whether additional robotic training of the paretic limb enhances motor outcome in subacute stroke	RCT; 56 patients in subacute stage 2b; 7/10	Robot training involved pointing to a series of targets using motion at shoulder, elbow, or both joints; 1 hours, 5 days a week for 5 weeks	Robot exposure; 1 hour/week on robot	Beginning and end of training (5 weeks)	1. FM 2. MSS 3. Motor Power Score 4. FIM	Experimental group had better motor outcome related to shoulder and elbow movements and better FIM scores than control group	Robot training group had more training. Results show limited improvement in function. No follow-up
Lum et al, 2002	Compare robotic training with conventional PT (NDT) in chronic stroke	RCT; 27 subjects, chronic hemiparesis (>6 months), 2b, 6/10	Standard rehabilitation and robot-aided therapy that included pointing movements involving shoulder and elbow joints, 1 hour session/day for 24 days	Standard rehabilitation (Bobath approach) for 55 minutes and robot exposure for 5 minutes at each session; 1 hour session/day for 24 days	Beginning of training, one month, end of training (2 months) and 6 month follow-up	1. FM 2. BI 3. FIM (self-care and transfer sections) 4. Strength measured through force transducer 5. Reaching kinematics	Robot-assisted group had larger improvements on proximal FM at 1 and 2 months and higher FIM scores at 6 months	Small sample size, robot training better than Bobath approach at improving proximal movements
Fasoli et al, 2004	Examine effects of robotic training in subacute stroke	RCT retrospective, 56 patients with sub-acute stroke (>3 weeks); 2b; 6/10	Robot training group (N = 30) received passive or active assistive practice of planar arm movements involving the shoulder and elbow joints with the MIT-Manus; 1 hour/day, 5 days/week for 5 weeks	Robot exposure group (N=26) received training for 1 hour/ week; subjects practiced planar arm movements without assistance	Beginning of training, during training and at discharge	1. FM 2. MSS 3. MRC test of motor power 4. FIM	Robotic group performed better on the FM, Motor Status Score, and MRC test of motor power; both groups improved scores on FIM; no differences were seen across groups	Control group did not receive dose equivalent practice; robotic therapy better than robotic exposure on impairment level measures

Author	Purpose	Design/Subjects	Intervention		Timing	Outcome Measures	Results	Comments
Daly et al, 2005	Compare effects of task-oriented plus robotic therapy in chronic stroke patients	RCT; 12 chronic stroke patients (>12 months) 2b; 5/10	In-motion robot training (1.5 hours/day) focused on shoulder and elbow movement accuracy and smoothness. Subjects also practiced functional upper limb tasks (3.5 hours/day). Training for 5 hours/day, 5 days/week for 12 weeks.	Functional neuromuscular stimulation (1.5 hours/day) involving wrist and finger activation. Subjects also practiced functional upper limb tasks (3.5 hours/day). Training for 5 hours/day, 5 days/week for 12 weeks.	Beginning of training, end of training (12 weeks) and 6 month follow-up	Baseline, end of treatment and 6 month follow up 1. AMAT functional ability 2. AMAT shoulder-elbow 3. AMAT wrist-hand 4. FM coordination scale 5. Target accuracy 6. Movement smoothness	The robot group showed improvement on the AMAT, the AMAT shoulder-elbow, FM, and movement accuracy and smoothness; the stimulation group improved on AMAT wrist-hand	Small sample size; addition of robot training to functional training is beneficial for improving performance at the impairment level.
Hesse et al, 2005	Compare computerized AT with ES in subacute stroke patients	RCT; 44 subacute stroke patients (4< 8 weeks); 1b; 7/10	Standard rehabilitation based on Bobath approach (45 minutes of PT, 30 minutes of OT), plus practice with arm trainer for pronation-supination and wrist flexion and extension movements; 20 min/day, 5 days/week for 6 weeks	Standard rehabilitation based on Bobath approach (45 minutes of PT, 30 minutes of OT), plus electrical stimulation of wrist extension movements; 20 min/day, 5 days/week for 6 weeks	Beginning of training, end of training (6 weeks) and 3-month follow-up	1. FM upper extremity 2. MRC Scale 3. MAS	AT group had higher BI score at baseline; no FM, MRC scores improved more for AT group	Well-designed study; no functional outcomes measured; additional robot training improved motor performance

Continued

Table 6-4

Evidence Table for Robot-Assisted Therapy—cont'd

AUTHORS AND YEAR	AIMS AND RATIONALE	DESIGN, SUBJECTS, OXFORD RATING, PEDRO SCORE	INTERVENTION	COMPARISON INTERVENTION	ASSESSMENT	OUTCOME MEASURES	RESULTS	COMMENTS
Lum et al, 2006	Compare unilateral and bilateral robotic training with conventional PT in subacute stroke	RCT; 30 subacute patients (1 to 5 months poststroke); 2b; 4/10	Three groups of robot training; unilateral, bilateral or combined group had 50 minutes of robot training; 1 hour/day for 4 weeks	Conventional therapy (Bobath approach); 1 hour/day for 4 weeks	Beginning of training, end of training (4 weeks) and 6 month follow-up	1. FM upper extremity 2. MSS 3. FIM 4. Motor Power exam	Baseline differences in MAS and MSS scores; combined robot group better scores on FM and MSS score at 4 weeks but not at 6 months; no improvement on FIM	Small sample size per group; baseline differences; no functional improvement
Kahn et al, 2006	Examine effects of active-assistive robot training in chronic stroke	RCT; 19 patients with chronic stroke (>1 year); 2b; 4/10	Active-assistive robot training including reaching to different directions; 24 sessions (45 min) over 8 weeks	Training of free reaching (unassisted) movements; 24 sessions (45 min) over 8 weeks	3 tests before training; 3 tests after training; 6 month follow-up	1. Pointing movement outcomes including stiffness, range, speed, smoothness and straightness 2. Chedoke McMaster score 3. Rancho Los Amigos Functional Test time to completion	No baseline differences between groups; both groups improved ROM speed; smoothness better for control group	Small sample size; no benefit of robot training over practice of reaching movements. No functional outcomes tested

Study	Purpose	Design	Intervention		Assessment	Measures	Results	Conclusions
Masiero et al, 2007	Examine effects of additional early robotic therapy on impairments and functional recovery	RCT; 35 patients with acute stroke (≤1 week); 1b; 6/10	Standard PT and OT (Bobath treatment); additional training with NeRebot, active assisted shoulder and elbow movements; 4 hours/week for 5 weeks	Standard PT and OT (Bobath treatment); additional robot exposure; (NeRebot) 1 hour/week for 5 weeks	Beginning of training, end of training (5 weeks); 3 and 8 month follow-up	1. MRC score 2. FM 3. FIM 4. Trunk control test 5. MAS	Robot training well tolerated; robot group performed better on FM, FIM, proximal MRC scores at the end of training; on follow up benefits sustained on FM, MRC deltoid and FIM	Robot group had higher baseline FIM score; control group had less exposure than experimental group; robot therapy may complement early rehabilitation
Rabadi et al, 2008	Determine the effect of activity based therapy using either an ergometer, robotic device or occupational therapy in acute stroke	RCT; 30 subjects with acute stroke (<4 weeks); 2b; 6/10	Robot group (N=10) used the MIT-Manus to practice passive and active assistive planar movements involving the shoulder and elbow joints; 1024 movements in 40 min session, 5 days/week for 12 days Ergometer group (N=10) used a bidirectional pedal for aerobic exercise of the upper limb; 2200 movements in 40 min session, 5 days/week for 12 days. Both groups received, in addition, standard rehabilitation for 3 hours/day.	Control group (N=10) received OT including ROM and active movements during functional activity; 640 movements in 40 min session, 5 days/week for 12 days, in addition to standard rehabilitation for 3 hours/day.	Beginning and end of training	1. FM 2. MSS 3. FIM total 4. FIM motor 5. FIM cognitive	All three groups improved on FM, MSS, and FIM scores. No differences were seen across groups. OT group had better scores on the FIM and FM compared with ergometer and robotic groups	Robotic therapy not better than functional OT training in acute stroke

Continued

Table 6-4

Evidence Table for Robot-Assisted Therapy—cont'd

AUTHORS AND YEAR	AIMS AND RATIONALE	DESIGN, SUBJECTS, OXFORD RATING, PEDRO SCORE	INTERVENTION	COMPARISON INTERVENTION	ASSESSMENT	OUTCOME MEASURES	RESULTS	COMMENTS
Volpe et al, 2008	Compare intensive PT with robotic training in chronic stroke	RCT; 21 patients with chronic stroke (>6 months); 2b; 6/10	Robot group (N=11) used the MIT-Manus to practice passive and active assistive planar movements involving the shoulder and elbow joints; 1 hour/day, 3 days/week for 6 weeks	Therapy group (N=10) practiced active assistive and goal directed functional arm movements; treatment based on motor learning approach; 1 hour/day, 3 days/week for 6 weeks	Pretreatment and post-treatment, 3 month follow-up	1. FM Shoulder elbow 2. FM wrist hand 3. MAS 4. SIS 5. ARAT	Both groups improved over duration of treatment and maintained improvement at 3 months; no differences between groups	Robot training no better than task-oriented training in chronic stroke

AMAT, Arm Motor Ability Test; ARAT, Action Research Arm Test; AT, arm trainer; BI, Barthel index; ES, electrical stimulation; FIM, Functional Independence Measure; FM, Fugl-Myer Assessment; MAS, Modified Ashworth Scale; MIT, Massachusetts Institute of Technology; MRC, Medical Research Council score; MSS, Motor Status Score; NDT, neurodevelopmental treatment; OT, occupational therapy; PT, physical therapy; RCT, randomized controlled trial; RMA, Rivermead Motor Assessment; ROM, range of motion; SIS, Stroke Impact Scale;

Table 6-5

Evidence Table for Treadmill Training with Body Weight Support

AUTHORS AND YEAR	AIMS AND RATIONALE	DESIGN, SUBJECTS, OXFORD RATING, AND PEDRO SCORE	INTERVENTION	COMPARISON INTERVENTION	ASSESSMENT	OUTCOME MEASURES	RESULTS	COMMENTS
Nilsson et al, 2001	Compare walking training over ground (based on a motor relearning approach) with treadmill training in subacute stroke stage	Double blind RCT; 73 patients at subacute stage (<8 weeks); 1b; 7/10	Treadmill training with BWS (N= 36); 30 minutes/day 5 days/week for 2 months	Walking training (N= 37); 30 minutes/day 5 days/week for 2 months	Pretreatment and post-treatment, 10 month follow-up	1. FIM 2. FM 3. FAC 4. Walking velocity (10 meters) 5. BBS	Both groups improved performance on the FIM, walking velocity, FAC, and balance. No differences were seen across groups.	Good study RCT 10-month follow-up; no benefit of BWS training
da Cunha et al, 2002	Compare BWS treadmill training and typical therapy with only typical therapy	RCT; 13 patients in subacute stage (<6 weeks) 20 minutes/day 5 days/week for 3 weeks 2b; 4/10	Supported treadmill training group (N=6) received regular PT which included stair climbing and walking on uneven surfaces and supported treadmill training; 3 hours/day of total therapy; 20 min/day treadmill training	Control group (N=7) received regular PT, OT, which included gait training and stair climbing; 3 hours/day of total therapy	Pretreatment and post-treatment	1. FAC 2. Gait speed 3. Walking distance 4. Energy expenditure	Differences were seen in walking energy cost and walking distance. No differences were seen for other outcome measures.	Small sample size; no follow-up; BWS not more effective than regular therapy

Continued

Table 6-5

Evidence Table for Treadmill Training with Body Weight Support—cont'd

AUTHORS AND YEAR	AIMS AND RATIONALE	DESIGN, SUBJECTS, OXFORD RATING, AND PEDRO SCORE	INTERVENTION	COMPARISON INTERVENTION	ASSESSMENT	OUTCOME MEASURES	RESULTS	COMMENTS
Werner et al, 2002	Compare BWS treadmill training with electromechanical gait trainer in subacute stroke patients	RCT crossover trial; 30 patients in subacute stage (4 to 12 weeks); 2b; 7/10	BWS treadmill training (N=15); 15 to 20 min/day × 7 days/week × 6 weeks.	Electromechanical gait trainer (N=15); 15 to 20 min/day × 7 days/week × 6 weeks.	Pretreatment, 1, 2, 3, 4, 5 weeks of treatment, posttreatment, 6 month follow-up	Measured at baseline, 6 wks and 6 months. 1. FAC 2. Gait Velocity 3. RMA 4. MAS	Both groups improved in 6 weeks; subjects in electromechanical trainer group had better FAC scores at 6 weeks; and required use of 1 therapist assistance; treadmill group required 2 therapist assistance; no differences between groups at 6 months.	Good study. electromechanical trainer as good as BWS treadmill training and requires fewer therapists.
Barbeau and Visintin, 2003	Compare treadmill training plus BWS with treadmill training without BWS in subacute stroke	Single blind RCT; 100 chronic subacute patients (1 to 5 months); 2b; 4/10	BWS (with 2 therapists) treadmill training with 40% of body weight support; 20 min × 4 days/week × 6 weeks	Treadmill training without BWS; 20 min × 4 days/week × 6 weeks	Pretreatment and posttreatment, 3 month follow-up	Baseline, end of training (6 weeks) and 3 month follow-up 1. BBS 2. STREAM 3. Overground walking speed; 4. Endurance (walk distance)	Both groups improved over 6 weeks; greater improvement seen in BWS group for severely impaired patients on all outcomes.	Moderate quality study shows that BWS may be appropriate for severely impaired patients in chronic stage

Author	Purpose	Study design; quality	Intervention	Timing	Outcome measures	Results	Comments
Sullivan et al, 2007	Compare BWS with lower extremity strength training in chronic stroke	Single blind RCT; 80 chronic stroke patients (4 months to 5 years); 1b; 7/10	BWS with 30% to 40% weight; Group 1: BWS + UE 2: BWS + UE 3: BWS + Lower extremity progressive resistive exercise; 1 hour session, 4 × week, 6 weeks	Limb loaded cycling + UE; 1 hour session, 4 × week, 6 weeks	Pretreatment and post-treatment, 6 month follow-up	Baseline, after 12 and 24 treatment sessions; 6 month follow-up; 1. Overground self selected walking speed 2. Fast walking speed 3. 6-minute walk distance 4. FM 5. SIS; 6. SF-36; 7. Lower extremity peak torque	BWS treadmill groups improved on self-selected and fast walking speed; whereas limb loaded cycle group improved only on 6 min walk distance and flexor torque after 24 sessions and at 6 month follow-up	High quality study; shows that task-specific BWS training beneficial for chronic stroke patients compared with resistive cycling.
Yen et al, 2008	Examine effects of additional BWS training on motor performance and cortical excitability	RCT nonblinded; 14 chronic stroke patients (>6 months); 2b; 7/10	50 min PT session (stretching, strengthening, balance, overground walking) 2 to 5 sessions/week for 4 weeks + BWS (30 min session 3 days/week for 4 weeks) with 1 to 2 therapists	50 min PT session (stretching, strengthening, balance, overground walking) 2 to 5 sessions/week for 4 weeks	Pretreatment and post-treatment	Baseline and post-treatment; 1. BBS 2. Gait analysis (GAITRite); 3. Cortical area and motor threshold using TMS	PT + BWS group improved their BBS score, gait speed and step length and decreased motor threshold; control group improved in gait speed and cadence.	Study shows that additional training using BWS improves balance, gait and cortical excitability. Did not test additional PT in control group, so improvements may be a result of nonspecific additional training

BBS, Berg Balance Scale; BWS, body weight support; FAC, Functional Ambulation Classification; FIM, Functional Independence Measure; FM, Fugl-Meyer Assessment; MAS, Modified Ashworth Scale; OT, occupational therapy; PT, physical therapy; RCT, randomized controlled trial; RMA, Rivermead Mobility Assessment; SIS, Stroke Impact Scale; STREAM, Stroke rehabilitation assessment of movement; TMS, Transcranial Magnetic Stimulation; UE, upper extremity ergometry.

supporting the body in a harness. The initial support given was generally 40% of the body weight, which is gradually decreased as the patient improves. The length of training ranged from 12 to 42 sessions conducted across four to eight weeks. In two of the studies, body weight support treadmill training was coupled with gait training.

Timing of Intervention. Treadmill training was initiated in the subacute stage in four studies[3,13,61,98] and in the chronic stage in two studies.[79,107]

Outcome Measures. Most of the studies reviewed measured outcome variables at the impairment and activity limitation levels. Only one study measured outcomes at all three levels of the ICF.[79] Typical instruments used to assess impairment level measures were the Stroke Rehabilitation Assessment of Movement (which evaluates voluntary movement of the limbs and mobility), Berg Balance Scale (which evaluates balance during sitting and standing activities), walking speed, distance and endurance, the Fugl-Meyer Assessment (which evaluates locomotor function and control, sensory quality, and balance), and kinematic analysis of walking. Instruments used to measure activity limitation were the Functional Independence Measure, Functional Ambulation Classification (which quantifies amount of assistance needed in walking), and the Rivermead Motor Assessment. Instruments used to measure participation limitation were Stroke Impact Scale and SF-36.

Results of the Review. When compared with functional training of ambulation or training with an electromechanical trainer, body weight supported treadmill training was no more effective, all interventions producing similar, but positive, outcomes. When compared with control groups that did not have training of walking, body weight support was more effective in outcomes related to walking and balance. When body weight support was added to the PT intervention, it was more effective.[107] However, this benefit may be the result of additional training since the control group did not receive dose equivalent therapy. The clearest evidence for the benefit of body weight support treadmill training was seen for severely impaired patients.[3]

Clinical Implications. The review suggests that training of walking and balance may be task-specific, and body weight support treadmill training may not be more effective compared with functional training without body weight support. When examined in the context of the high cost associated with body weight support apparatus, and the number of therapists required to administer therapy, functional training may be more cost-effective and equally beneficial. The only indication for body weight support training may be in the case of severely impaired patients who may benefit from relearning the walking movement patterns without being encumbered with controlling their body weight and forward progression.

SUMMARY

A challenging yet exciting period for stroke rehabilitation is occurring as occupational and physical therapists are being asked to provide training based on sound scientific principles and with demonstrated effectiveness. The lack of support for traditional neurotherapeutic approaches, such as Bobath approach, recent advances in understanding of motor control and dyscontrol, and emerging technologies have facilitated a second paradigm shift toward a functional task-oriented approach. At present, the literature suggests that task-oriented training of the upper limb and functional walking training is the most effective method in stroke rehabilitation. The challenge for the next decade is to develop more creative, functional, task-oriented intervention techniques that will maximize the independent functioning of patients within their natural contextual settings[10] and to test these techniques in a systematical manner at different stages of the recovery process, in different practice settings, and at different intensities. Most likely, no one technique will offer a panacea for stroke rehabilitation given the varied nature of impairments and activity limitations.

ACKNOWLEDGMENTS

The author dedicates this chapter to the memory of his uncle Dr. Sangameshwar who lost his battle to stroke during the writing of this chapter. The author acknowledges Glen Gillen and Clare Bassile for helpful discussions.

REVIEW QUESTIONS

1. What is evidence-based practice?
2. What are the principles of evidence-based practice?
3. What are the criteria for reviewing articles on treatment outcomes?
4. Describe the most common research designs used in outcome studies.
5. What are some of the basic principles of neurotherapeutic approaches?
6. Is there evidence to support the application of neurotherapeutic approaches?
7. What are some of the basic principles of the functional task-oriented approach?
8. Describe the evidence to support the task-oriented approach, CIMT, treadmill training and body weight support, and robot-assisted training.

REFERENCES

1. Aisen ML, Krebs HI, Hogan N, et al: The effect of robot-assisted therapy and rehabilitative training on motor recovery following stroke. *Arch Neurol* 54(4):443–446, 1997.

2. Barbeau H, Rossignol S: Recovery of locomotion after chronic spinalization in the adult cat. *Brain Res* 412(1):84–95, 1987.

3. Barbeau H, Visintin M: Optimal outcomes obtained with body-weight support combined with treadmill training in stroke subjects. *Arch Phys Med Rehabil* 84(10):1458–1465, 2003.

4. Blanton S, Wolf SL: An application of upper-extremity constraint-induced movement therapy in a patient with subacute stroke. *Phys Ther* 79(9):847–853, 1999.

5. Blennerhassett J, Dite W: Additional task-related practice improves mobility and upper limb function early after stroke: a randomised controlled trial. *Aust J Physiother* 50(4):219–224, 2004.

6. Boake C, Noser EA, Ro T, et al: Constraint-induced movement therapy during early stroke rehabilitation. *Neurorehabil Neural Repair* 21(1):14–24, 2007.

7. Bobath B: *Adult hemiplegia: evaluation and treatment*, ed 3, Oxford, 1990, Butterworth-Heinemann.

8. Bonaiuti D, Rebasti L, Sioli P: The constraint induced movement therapy: a systematic review of randomised controlled trials on the adult stroke patients. *Eura Medicophys* 43(2:139–146, 2007.

9. Brogårdh C, Vestling M, Sjölund BH: Shortened constraint-induced movement therapy in subacute stroke— no effect of using a restraint: a randomized controlled study with independent observers. *J Rehabil Med* 41(4):231–236, 2009.

10. JH Carr, RB Shepherd: *Stroke rehabilitation: guidelines for exercise and training to optimize motor skill*, Oxford, 2003, Butterworth-Heinemann.

11. Centre for Evidence Based Medicine. Levels of evidence(website). www.cebm.net/index.aspx?o=1025. AccessedNovember 2009.

12. Centre of Evidence-Based Physiotherapy. Physiotherapy evidence database (website). www.pedro.org.au/english/downloads/pedro-scale/. AccessedNovember 2009.

13. da Cunha IT Jr , Lim PA, Qureshy H, et al: Gait outcomes after acute stroke rehabilitation with supported treadmill ambulation training: a randomized controlled pilot study. *Arch Phys Med Rehabil* 83(9):1258–1265, 2002.

14. Dahl AE, Askim T, Stock R, et al: Short- and long-term outcome of constraint-induced movement therapy after stroke: a randomized controlled feasibility trial. *Clin Rehabil* 22(5):436–447, 2008.

15. Daly JJ, Hogan N, Perepezko EM, et al: Response to upper-limb robotics and functional neuromuscular stimulation following stroke. *J Rehabil Res Dev* 42(6):723–736, 2005.

16. Dean CM, Channon EF, Hall JM: Sitting training early after stroke improves sitting ability and quality and carries over to standing up but not to walking: a randomised trial. *Aust J Physiother* 53(2):97–102, 2007.

17. Desrosiers J, D Bourbonnais D, Corriveau H, et al: Effectiveness of unilateral and symmetrical bilateral task training for arm during the subacute phase after stroke: a randomized controlled trial. *Clin Rehabil* 19(6):581–593, 2005.

18. Dromerick AW, Edwards DF, Hahn M: Does the application of constraint-induced movement therapy during acute rehabilitation reduce arm impairment after ischemic stroke? *Stroke* 31(12):2984–2988, 2000.

19. Dromerick AW, Lang CE, Birkenmeier RL, et al: Very Early Constraint-Induced Movement during Stroke Rehabilitation (VECTORS): A single-center RCT. *Neurology* 73(3):195–201, 2009.

20. Fasoli SE, Krebs HI, Ferraro M, et al: Does shorter rehabilitation limit potential recovery poststroke? *Neurorehabil Neural Repair* 18(2):88–94, 2004.

21. Gentile AM: Skill acquisition: action, movement and neuromotor processes. In Carr J, Shepherd RB, editors: *Movement science: foundations for physical therapy in rehabilitation*, Gaithersburg, MD, 2000, Aspen.

22. Gordon J: Assumptions underlying physical therapy intervention: theoretical and historical perspectives. In Carr J, Shepherd RB, editors: *Movement science: foundations for physical therapy in rehabilitation*, Gaithersburg, MD, 2000, Aspen.

23. Hafsteinsdottir TB: Neurodevelopmental treatment: application to nursing and its effects on the hemiplegic stroke patient. *J Neurosci Nurs* 28(1):36–47, 1996.

24. Hafsteinsdottir TB, Algra A, Kappelle JL, Grypdonck MHF: Neurodevelopmental treatment after stroke: a comparative study. *J Neurol Neurosurg Psychiatry* 76(6):788–792, 2005.

25. Hafsteinsdottir TB, Kappelle JL, Grypdonck MHF, Algra A: Effects of Bobath-bed therapy on depression, shoulder pain and health-related quality of life in patients after stroke. *J Rehabil Med* 39(8):627–632, 2007.

26. Helewa A, Walker JM: *Critical evaluation of research in physical rehabilitation*, Philadelphia, 2000, Saunders.

27. Hesse SA, Bertelt C, Schaffrin A, et al: Restoration of gait in non-ambulatory hemiparetic patients by treadmill training with partial body-weight support. *Arch Phys Med Rehabil* 75(10):1087–1093, 1994.

28. Hesse S, Werner C, Pohl M, et al: Computerized arm training improves the motor control of the severely affected arm after stroke: a single-blinded randomized trial in two centers. *Stroke* 36(9):1960–1966, 2005.

29. Higgins J, Salbach NM, Wood-Dauphinee S, et al: The effect of a task-oriented intervention on arm function in people with stroke: a randomized controlled trial. *Clin Rehabil* 20(4):296–310, 2006.

30. Howle JM: *Neuro-developmental treatment approach: theoretical foundations and principles of clinical practice*, Laguna Beach, CA, 2002, Neuro-Developmental Treatment Association.

31. Hubbard IJ, Parsons MW, Neilson C, Carey LM: Task-specific training: evidence for and translation to clinical practice. *Occup Ther Int* 16(3–4):175–189, 2009.

32. Jørgensen HS, Nakayama H, Raaschou HO, et al: Outcome and time course of recovery in stroke. Part I: Outcome. The Copenhagen Stroke Study. *Arch Phys Med Rehabil* 76(5):399–405, 1995.

33. Kahn LE, Zygman ML, Rymer WZ, Reinkensmeyer DJ: Robot-assisted reaching exercise promotes arm movement recovery in chronic hemiparetic stroke: a randomized controlled pilot study. *J Neuroeng Rehabil* 3:12, 2006.

34. Kollen BJ, Lennon S, Lyons B, et al: The effectiveness of the Bobath concept in stroke rehabilitation. *Stroke* 40(4): 89–97, 2009.

35. Krebs HI, Hogan N, Aisen ML, et al: Robot-aided neurorehabilitation. *IEEE Trans Rehabil Eng* 6(1):75–87, 1998.

36. Kreisel SH, Hennerici MG, Bäzner H: Pathophysiology of stroke rehabilitation: the natural course of clinical recovery, use-dependent plasticity and rehabilitative outcome. *Cerebrovasc Dis* 23(4):243–255, 2007.

37. Kunkel A, Kopp B, Muller G, et al: Constraint-induced movement therapy for motor recovery in chronic stroke patients. *Arch Phys Med Rehabil* 80(6):624–628, 1999.

38. Kwakkel G, RC Wagenaar RC, Twisk JW, et al: Intensity of leg and arm training after primary middle-cerebral-artery stroke: a randomised trial. *Lancet* 354 (9174):191–196, 1999.

39. Kwakkel G, Kollen BJ, Wagenaar RC: Long term effects of intensity of upper and lower limb training after stroke: a randomised trial. *J Neurol Neurosurg Psychiatry* 72(4):473–479, 2002.

40. Kwakkel G, Kollen BJ, Krebs HI: Effects of robot-assisted therapy on upper limb recovery after stroke: A systematic review. *Neurorehabil Neural Repair* 22(2):111–121, 2008.

41. Langhammer B, Stanghelle JK: Bobath or motor relearning programme? A comparison of two different approaches of physiotherapy in stroke rehabilitation: a randomized controlled study. *Clin Rehabil* 14(4):361–369, 2000.

42. Langhammer B, Stanghelle JK: Bobath or motor relearning programme? A follow-up one and four years post stroke. *Clin Rehabil* 17(7): 731–734, 2003.

43. Laufer Y, Dickstein R, Chefez Y, et al: The effect of treadmill training on the ambulation of stroke survivors in the early stages of rehabilitation: a randomized study. *J Rehabil Res Dev* 38(1):69–78, 2001.

44. Law M: In *Evidence-based rehabilitation: a guide to practice*, ed 2, Thorofare, NJ, 2008, Slack.

45. Liepert J, Bauder H, Wolfgang HR, et al: Treatment-induced cortical reorganization after stroke in humans. *Stroke* 31(6):1210–1216, 2000.

46. Lin KC, Wu CY, Wei TH. et al: Effects of modified constraint-induced movement therapy on reach-to-grasp movements and functional performance after chronic stroke: a randomized controlled study, *Clin Rehabil* 21(12): 1075–1086 2007.

46a. Lin K, Wu C, Liu J, et al: Constraint-induced therapy versus dose-matched control intervention to improve motor ability, basic/extended daily functions, and quality of life in stroke. *Neurorehab Neural Repair* 23(2):160-165, 2009.

47. Lord JP, Hall K: Neuromuscular reeducation versus traditional programs for stroke rehabilitation. *Arch Phys Med Rehabil* 67(2):88–91, 1986.

48. Luke C, Dodd KJ, Brock K: Outcomes of the Bobath concept on upper limb recovery following stroke. *Clin Rehabil* 18(8):888–898, 2004.

49. Lum PS, Burgar CG, Shor PC, et al: Robot-assisted movement training compared with conventional therapy techniques for the rehabilitation of upper-limb motor function after stroke. *Arch Phys Med Rehabil* 83(7): 952–959, 2002.

50. Lum PS, Burgar CG, Van der Loos M, et al: MIME robotic device for upper-limb neurorehabilitation in subacute stroke subjects: A follow-up study. *J Rehabil Res Dev* 43(5):631–642, 2006.

51. Maher CG, Sherington C, Herbert RD, et al: Reliability of the PEDro scale for rating quality of randomized controlled trials. *Phys Ther* 83(8):713–721, 2003.

52. Masiero S, Celia A, Rosati G, Armani M: Robotic-assisted rehabilitation of the upper limb after acute stroke. *Arch Phys Med Rehabil* 88(2):142–149, 2007.

53. Mayston M. Editorial: Bobath concept: Bobath@50: mid-life crisis—what of the future? *Physiother Res Int* 13(3):131–136, 2008.

54. Michaelsen SM, Dannenbaum R, Levin MF: Task-specific training with trunk restraint on arm recovery in stroke: randomized control trial. *Stroke* 37(1):186–192, 2006.

55. Miltner WH, Bauder H, Sommer M, et al: Effects of constraint-induced movement therapy on patients with chronic motor deficits after stroke: a replication. *Stroke* 30(3):586–592, 1999.

56. Mohide EA: What is EBP: how do we facilitate its use? In Wong R, editor: *Evidence-based healthcare practice: general principles and focused applications to geriatric physical therapy*, Arlington, VA, 2002, Marymount University.

57. Monger C, Carr JH, Fowler V: Evaluation of a home-based exercise and training programme to improve sit-to-stand in patients with chronic stroke. *Clin Rehabil* 16(4):361–367, 2002.

58. Mudie MH, Winzeler-Mercay U, Radwan S, Lee L: Training symmetry of weight distribution after stroke: a randomized controlled pilot study comparing task-related reach, Bobath and feedback training approaches. *Clin Rehabil* 16(6):582–592, 2002.

59. Myint JM, Yuen GF, Yu TK, et al: A study of constraint-induced movement therapy in subacute stroke patients in Hong Kong. *Clin Rehabil* 22(2):112–124, 2008.

60. Nelles G, Jentzen W, Jueptner M, et al: Arm training induced brain plasticity in stroke studied with serial positron emission tomography. *Neuroimage* 13(6 pt 1):1146–1154, 2001.

61. Nilsson L, Carlsson J, Danielsson A, et al: Walking training of patients with hemiparesis at an early stage after stroke: a comparison of walking training on a treadmill with body weight support and walking training on the ground. *Clin Rehabil* 15(5):515–527, 2001.

62. Paci M: Physiotherapy based on the Bobath concept for adults with post-stroke hemiplegia: a review of effectiveness studies. *J Rehabil Med* 35(1):2–7, 2003.

63. Page SJ, Sisto SA, Johnston MV, et al: Modified constraint-induced therapy after subacute stroke: a preliminary study. *Neurorehabil Neural Repair* 16(3):290–295, 2002.

64. Page SJ, Sisto SA, Levine P, et al: Modified constraint induced therapy: a randomized feasibility and efficacy study. *J Rehabil Res Dev* 38(5):583–590, 2001.

65. Page SJ, Sisto S, Levine P, McGrath RE: Efficacy of modified constraint-induced movement therapy in chronic stroke: a single-blinded randomized controlled trial. *Arch Phys Med Rehabil* 85(1):14–18, 2004.

66. Page SJ, Levine P, Leonard AC Modified constraint-induced therapy in acute stroke: a randomized controlled pilot study. *Neurorehabil Neural Repair* 19(1):27–32, 2005.

67. Platz T, Eickhof C, van Kaick S, et al: Impairment-oriented training or Bobath therapy for severe arm paresis after stroke: a single-blind, multicentre randomized controlled trial. *Clin Rehabil* 19(7):714–724, 2005.

68. Rabadi M, Galgano M, Lynch D, et al: A pilot study of activity-based therapy in the arm motor recovery post stroke: a randomized controlled trial. *Clin Rehabil* 22(12): 1071–1082, 2008.

69. Raine S: The current theoretical assumptions of the Bobath approach as determined by the members of the BBTA. *Physiother Theory Pract* 23(3):137–152, 2007.

70. Rensink M, Schuurmans M, Lindeman E, Hafsteinsdóttir T: Task-oriented training in rehabilitation after stroke: systematic review. *J Adv Nurs* 65(4):737–754, 2009.

71. Reinkensmeyer DJ, Kahn E, Averbuch M, et al: Understanding and treating arm movement impairment after chronic brain injury: progress with the ARM guide. *J Rehabil Res Dev* 37(6): 653–662, 2000.

72. Sackett DL: *Clinical epidemiology: a basic science for clinical medicine*, ed 2, Boston, 1991, Little, Brown.

73. Sawaki L, Butler AJ, Leng X, et al: Constraint-induced movement therapy results in increased motor map area in subjects 3 to 9 months after stroke. *Neurorehabil Neural Repair* 22(5):505–513, 2008.

74. Shadmehr R, Donchin O, Hwang EJ, et al: Learning to compensate for dynamics of reaching movements. In Vaadia E, editor: *Motor cortex and voluntary movements*, Boca Raton, FL, 2005, CRC Press.

75. Sumway-Cook A, Woollacott MH: *Motor control: Translating research into clinical practice*, ed 3, Philadelphia, 2007, Lippincott Williams & Wilkins.

76. Smith MA, Brandt J, Shadmehr R: Motor disorder in Huntington's disease begins as a dysfunction in error feedback control. *Nature* 403(6769): 544–549, 2000.

77. Smith GV, Silver KHC, Goldberg AP, et al: "Task-oriented" exercise improves hamstring strength and spastic reflexes in chronic stroke patients. *Stroke* 30(10):2112–2118, 1999.

78. Sullivan KJ, Knowlton BJ, Dobkin BH: Step training with body weight support: effect of treadmill speed and practice paradigms on poststroke locomotor recovery. *Arch Phys Med Rehabil* 83(5):683–691, 2002.

79. Sullivan KJ, Brown DA, Klassen T, et al: Effects of task-specific locomotor and strength training in adults who were ambulatory after stroke: results of the STEPS randomized clinical trial. *Phys Ther* 87(12):1580–1602, 2007.

80. Suputtitada A, Suwanwela NC, Tumvitee S: Effectiveness of constraint-induced movement therapy in chronic stroke patients. *J Med Assoc Thai* 87(12):1482–1490, 2004.

81. Tang QP, Yang QD, Wu YH, et al: Effects of problem-oriented willed-movement therapy on motor abilities for people with poststroke cognitive deficits. *Phys Ther* 85(10):1020–1033, 2005.

82. Taub E: Movement in non-human primates deprived of somatosensory feedback. *Exerc Sport Sci Rev* 4:335–374, 1977.

83. Taub E, Miller NE, Novack TA, et al: Technique to improve chronic motor deficit after stroke. *Arch Phys Med Rehabil* 74(4):347–354, 1993.

84. Taub E, Uswatte G: Constraint-induced movement therapy and massed practice. *Stroke* 31(4):983–986, 2000.

85. Taub E, Uswatte G, King DK, et al: A placebo-controlled trial of constraint-induced movement therapy for upper extremity after stroke. *Stroke* 37(4):1045–1049, 2006.

86. Thaut MH, Leins AK, Rice RR, et al: Rhythmic auditory stimulation improves gait more than NDT/Bobath training in near-ambulatory patients early poststroke: A single-blind, randomized trial. *Neurorehabil Neural Repair* 21(5):455–459, 2007.

87. Thielman GT, Dean CM, Gentile AM: Rehabilitation of reaching after stroke: task-related training versus progressive resistive exercise. *Arch Phys Med Rehabil* 85(10): 1613–1618, 2004.

88. Thielman G, Kaminski T, Gentile AM: Rehabilitation of reaching after stroke: Comparing 2 training protocols utilizing trunk restraint. *Neurorehabil Neural Repair* 22(6):697–705, 2008.

89. Tuke A: Constraint-induced movement therapy: a narrative review. *Physiotherapy* 94(2): 105–111, 2008.

90. van der Lee JH: Constraint-induced therapy for stroke: more of the same or something completely different? *Curr Opin Neurol* 14(6):741–744, 2001.

91. van Vliet PM, NB Lincoln NB, Foxall A: Comparison of Bobath based and movement science based treatment for stroke: a randomized controlled trial. *J Neurol Neurosurg Psychiatry* 76(4):503–508, 2005.

92. Visintin M, Barbeau H, Korner-Bitensky N, et al: A new approach to retrain gait in stroke patients through body weight support and treadmill stimulation. *Stroke* 29(6):1122–1128, 1998.

93. Volpe BT, Krebs HI, Hogan N, et al: A novel approach to stroke rehabilitation: robot-aided sensorimotor stimulation. *Neurology* 54(10):1938–1944, 2000.

94. Volpe BT, Krebs HI, N Hogan N, et al: Robot training enhanced motor outcome in patients with stroke maintained over 3 years. *Neurology* 53(8):1874–1876, 1999.

95. Volpe BT, Lynch D, Rykman-Berland A: Intensive sensorimotor arm training mediated by therapist or robot improves hemiparesis in patients with chronic stroke. *Neurorehabil Neural Repair* 22(3):305–310, 2008.

96. Wagenaar RC, Meijer OG, van Wieringen PC, et al: The functional recovery of stroke: a comparison between neuro-developmental treatment and the Brunnstrom method. *Scand J Rehabil Med* 22(1):1–8, 1990.

97. Wang RY, Chen HI, Yang YR: Efficacy of Bobath versus orthopedic approach on impairment and function at different motor recovery stages after stroke: a randomized controlled study. *Clin Rehabil* 19(2):155–164, 2005.

98. Werner C, Von Frankenberg S, Treig T, et al: Treadmill training with partial body weight support and an electromechanical gait trainer for restoration of gait in subacute stroke patients: a randomized crossover study. *Stroke* 33(12):2895–901, 2002.

99. Wernig A, Muller S: Improvement of walking in spinal cord injured persons after treadmill training. In Wernig A, editor: *Plasticity of motoneuronal connections*, Berlin, 1991, Elsevier.

100. Winstein CJ, Rose DK, Tan SM, et al: A randomized controlled comparison of upper-extremity rehabilitation strategies in acute stroke: A pilot study of immediate and long-term outcomes. *Arch Phys Med Rehabil* 85(4):620–628, 2004.

101. Wittenberg GF, R Chen R, Ishii K, et al: Constraint-induced therapy in stroke: magnetic-stimulation motor maps and cerebral activation. *Neurorehabil Neural Repair* 1(1):48–57, 2003.

102. Wolf SL, Lecraw DE, Barton LA, et al: Forced use of hemiplegic upper extremities to reverse the effect of learned nonuse among chronic stroke and head-injured patients. *Exp Neurol* 104(2):125–132, 1989.

103. Wolf SL, Winstein CJ, Miller JP, et al: Effect of constraint-induced movement therapy on upper extremity function 3 to 9 months after stroke: the EXCITE randomized clinical trial. *JAMA* 296(17):2095–2104, 2006.

104. Wu CY, Lin KC, Chen HC, et al: Effects of modified constraint-induced movement therapy on movement kinematics and daily function in patients with stroke: a kinematic study of motor control mechanisms. *Neurorehabil Neural Repair.* 21(5):460–466, 2007.

105. Wu CY, Chen CL, Tsai WC, et al: A randomized controlled trial of modified constraint-induced movement therapy for elderly stroke survivors: changes in motor impairment, daily functioning, and quality of life. *Arch Phys Med Rehabil* 88(3):273–8, 2007.

106. Wu CY, Chen CL, Tang SF, et al: Kinematic and clinical analyses of upper-extremity movements after constraint-induced movement therapy in patients with stroke: a randomized controlled trial. *Arch Phys Med Rehabil* 88(8): 964–970, 2007.

107. Yen CL, Wang RY, Liao KK, et al: Gait training induced change in corticomotor excitability in patients with chronic stroke. *Neurorehabil Neural Repair* 22(1):22–30, 2008.

glen gillen

chapter 7

Trunk Control: Supporting Functional Independence

key terms

activities of daily living	static balance	trunk
limits of stability	postural control	anticipatory postural control
hemiplegia	dynamical balance	stability

chapter objectives

After completing this chapter, the reader will be able to accomplish the following:

1. Understand the functional anatomy of the trunk.
2. Understand the control requirements for various movement patterns and activities.
3. By activity analysis, understand key components of trunk control required for independence in various activities of daily living.
4. Comprehensively evaluate trunk control and its effect on function.
5. Implement interventions to improve and compensate for loss of trunk control.

Loss of trunk control commonly occurs in patients who have had a stroke and persists into the chronic stage of recovery.[52] The recovery of trunk control is varied, but during the first month after stroke, significant improvements may be observed. In contrast to common beliefs, the time course of recovery of the trunk is similar to the recovery of arm, leg, and functional ability.[51]

Impairments in trunk control include weakness (both contralesional and, to a lesser extent, ipsilesional), loss of stability, stiffness, and loss of proprioception, and may lead to the following:

- Dysfunction in upper and lower limb control
- Increased risk of falls
- Potential for spinal deformity and contracture

- Impaired ability to interact with the environment
- Visual dysfunction resulting from head/neck malalignment
- Symptoms of dysphagia because of proximal malalignment
- Decreased independence in activities of daily living (ADL) and other meaningful tasks
- Decreased sitting and standing tolerance, balance, and function

For a comprehensive review of this topic, see Chapters 4 and 5 for incorporating task-oriented, learning and environmental strategies into treatment plans focused on improving trunk control, Chapter 8 for a complete overview of the multiple variables that affect balance skills, Chapter 10 for a review on the interdependence of trunk control and upper extremity function, and Chapter 14 for an overview of mobility impairments.

Regaining trunk control has been a major focus of stroke rehabilitation for many years. Until more recently, the majority of the literature focusing on trunk control/postural control was based on expert clinicians' observations of and treatment philosophies about trunk dysfunction after stroke. The traditional approaches to treatment[7,8,17,22,40] have emphasized improved trunk control as a key element of focus in the stroke population, and this focus continues as therapists integrate current models of motor control and learning (see Chapters 4 and 6).

AN OVERVIEW OF COMMON TRUNK IMPAIRMENTS THAT MAY INTERFERE WITH DAILY FUNCTION

While motor control studies after stroke focus primarily on upper extremity function and/or gait (see Chapters 10 and 15), there is a body of descriptive evidence that aims to give clinicians insight into the various specific trunk impairments observed after stroke.

Dickstein and colleagues[20] examined anticipatory postural adjustment in trunk muscles during the performance of upper and lower limb flexion tasks in patients with hemiparesis secondary to stroke. The researchers recorded electromyographic activity of the lumbar erector spinae and of the latissimus dorsi muscles bilaterally during flexion of either arm and from the two rectus abdominis and obliquus externus muscles during flexion of either hip. The authors documented impairments in the activity of trunk muscles in the hemiparetic subjects. This was manifested in the reduced activity level of the lateral trunk muscles, in delayed onset, and in reduced synchronization between activation of pertinent muscular pairs. Further, they documented that these impairments were associated with motor and functional deficits.

Bohannon, Cassidy, and Walsh[11] have studied trunk muscle strength impairments after stroke (specifically forward and lateral trunk flexion strength). Their study included 20 patients with stroke and resultant hemiparesis and 20 control subjects. Trunk strength was measured with a handheld dynamometer; subjects were seated upright during the study. Results indicated that trunk strength, whether lateral or forward, was significantly decreased in the patients relative to controls. The greatest difference in strength was in forward flexion strength. The patients demonstrated trunk weakness on the paretic side relative to the nonparetic side. The conclusion was that trunk muscle strength was impaired multidirectionally in the stroke population.

Bohannon[10] studied 11 stroke patients and evaluated lateral trunk flexion strength and the effect of trunk muscle strength on sitting balance and ambulation. His results indicated that the mean lateral flexion force on the paretic side was 32.1%, which was significantly less than the mean lateral flexion force on the nonparetic side. His study further demonstrated a statistically significant correlation between sitting balance and strength of the lateral trunk flexors.

Bohannon[9] also studied the recovery of trunk muscle strength after stroke in 28 subjects. Subjects' strength was tested in a variety of directions, including forward flexion, movement toward the paretic side, and movement toward the nonparetic side. Statistical analysis demonstrated that trunk muscle strength increased significantly over time. The greatest recovery was in the direction of forward flexion. This study again verified a strong correlation between trunk muscle strength and sitting balance at the initial and final assessments.

Esparza and colleagues[23] examined hemispheric specialization and the coordination of arm and trunk movements during pointing in subjects with strokes. They concluded that arm and trunk timing was disrupted compared with healthy controls, temporal coordination of trunk and arm recruitment is mediated bilaterally by each hemisphere, and that the differences they found in the range of trunk displacement between subjects with right and left lesions suggest that left hemisphere plays a greater role than the right in controlling complex arm-trunk movements.

Ryerson and colleagues[43] documented trunk position sense impairments in those with poststroke hemiparesis. Specifically, individuals exhibited greater trunk repositioning error than age-matched controls. Based on this finding, the authors recommended trunk position sense retraining emphasizing sagittal and transverse movements as a potential poststroke intervention strategy to improve trunk balance and control.

In addition to the mentioned studies, several studies have focused on documenting electromyographic activity in normal subjects during a variety of tasks including trunk displacements.[1,5,19,25,50,58] See Basmajian's and DeLuca's[5] classic text for a comprehensive review of electromyographic studies performed during functional tasks.

FUNCTIONAL TRUNK ANATOMY

Skeletal System

This section reviews the bony components of trunk anatomy, including articulations and range of motion (ROM).

Vertebral Column. The vertebral column is made up of 26 vertebrae, which are classified as follows:

- Cervical: 7
- Thoracic: 12
- Lumbar: 5
- Sacral: 5 (fused into one bone, the sacrum)
- Coccygeal: 4 (fused into one or two bones, the coccyx)

As a whole, the vertebral column from sacrum to skull is equivalent to a joint with three degrees of freedom[33] in the directions of flexion and extension, right and left lateral flexion, and axial rotation. Kapandji[33] has documented the ROM throughout the vertebral column (Table 7-1).

An understanding of spinal alignment is necessary for effective evaluation and treatment planning. Normal alignment of the vertebral column implies that the appropriate spinal curvatures are present. In the sagittal plane, the vertebral column shows four curvatures[33] (Table 7-2 and Fig. 7-1).

Pelvis

According to Kapandji,[33] "The bony pelvis constitutes the base of the trunk. It supports the abdomen and links the vertebral column to the lower limbs. It is a closed osteo-articular ring made up of three bony parts and three joints." The three bony parts include the two iliac bones and the sacrum. The three joints of the pelvis include two sacroiliac joints and the symphysis pubis. It is critical to remember that because of the firmness of the sacroiliac and lumbosacral junctions, every pelvic movement is

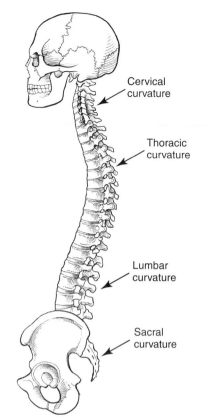

Figure 7-1   Lateral view of spine with spinal curvatures.

accompanied by a realignment of the spine predominantly in the lumbar region.[47]

Pelvic tilt can occur anteriorly or posteriorly. In an anterior tilt, the anterior superior iliac spines of the ilia migrate anteriorly to the foremost part of the symphysis pubis. This pelvic motion accentuates the lumbar curve and results in increased hip flexion. In contrast, posterior pelvic tilt results in a "flattening" of the lumbar curve and an increase in hip extension. Lateral pelvis tilting results in a height discrepancy of the iliac crests and is accompanied by lateral spine flexion and a lateral rib cage displacement.

Rib Cage

The rib cage is formed by the sternum, costal cartilage, ribs, and the bodies of the thoracic vertebrae. The rib cage protects the organs in the thoracic cavity, assists in respiration, and provides support for the upper extremities. During inspiration the ribs are elevated, and during expiration the ribs are depressed.

Although each rib has its own ROM (occurring primarily at the costovertebral joint), rib cage shifts occur with movement of the vertebral column. During column extension, the rib cage migrates anteriorly, and the ribs are elevated. During spinal flexion, the rib cage moves posteriorly, and the ribs are depressed. Lateral flexion results in a right or left shift of the rib cage in the frontal

Table 7-1

Range of Motion of the Vertebral Column

MOVEMENT	RANGE OF MOTION
Flexion	Cervical: 40 degrees
	Thoracolumbar: 105 degrees
	Total: 145 degrees
Extension	Cervical: 75 degrees
	Thoracolumbar: 60 degrees
	Total: 135 degrees
Lateral flexion	Cervical: 35 to 45 degrees
	Thoracic: 20 degrees
	Lumbar: 20 degrees
	Total: 75 to 85 degrees
Rotation	Cervical: 45 to 50 degrees
	Thoracic: 35 degrees
	Lumbar: 5 degrees
	Total: 85 to 90 degrees

Table 7-2

Spinal Curvatures

CURVATURE	POSTERIOR MOVEMENT	
	CONVEX	CONCAVE
Sacral (fixed)	X	
Lumbar		X
Thoracic	X	
Cervical		X

plane. Finally, rotation of the vertebral column results in one side of the rib cage moving posteriorly and movement of the opposite side anteriorly in the transverse plane.

Muscular System

Muscles of the Abdominal Wall

The general functions of the abdominal muscles are as follows:

- Abdominal viscera support
- Respiration assistance
- Trunk control in the directions of flexion, lateral flexion, and rotation

Although these muscles are situated primarily on the anterior aspect of the trunk, they also are situated laterally and slightly posteriorly, forming a girdle around the abdomen. The abdominal muscles consist of three groups: the rectus abdominis, the obliques (internal and external), and the transversus abdominis (Fig. 7-2).

Rectus Abdominis. The rectus abdominis consists of right and left sides that are separated by a fibrous band called the *linea alba*, which runs from the xiphoid process to the pubis.

The proximal attachment is the xiphoid process of the sternum and adjacent costal cartilage, whereas the distal attachments are the pubic bones near the pubic symphysis.[47]

The muscle is palpated easily in the following two cases:

1. When the subject is supine and is asked to lift the head and shoulders off the support surface in a straight plane (sit-up)
2. During backward sway in sitting or standing position

When this muscle is activated and not opposed by the extensors, the pelvis and sternum are approximated, the pelvis is pulled into a posterior tilt, and the lumbar curves flatten. Because of its multisegmental arrangement, the rectus abdominis can contract in part or as a whole, making a variety of postures possible. De Troyer's work[19] demonstrated that "abdominal muscle recruitment which naturally occurs in response to posture in most individuals does not uniformly involve the whole of the muscles."

The rectus abdominis (and the other muscles of the trunk) require a stable origin to function efficiently.[17] This stable origin can be the pelvis or thorax, depending on the posture and which part of the trunk is moving. Davies[17] further explains, "The pelvis is stabilized in lying, sitting, and standing by the activity of the muscles around the hips, and in sitting and lying the stabilization is helped by the weight of the legs themselves. Stabilization of the thoracic origin for activities in which the abdominals contract to move or prevent movements of the pelvis requires selective extension of the thoracic spine." Davies further points out that the abdominal muscles cannot function effectively when their origin and insertion are approximated (e.g., in patients with an exaggerated thoracic kyphosis). Winzeler-Mercay and Mudie[57] noted weakness based on electromyographic recordings in the rectus abdominis after stroke during dynamic trunk movements such as donning shoes. The weakness was noted particularly on the involved side. Similarly, Tanaka, Hachisuka, and Ogata[49] found that peak torque of the flexors was significantly less than in healthy controls.

The rectus abdominis can be self-palpated by assuming a recumbent posture in a chair (slumping in the chair) and then pulling up and forward to an aligned position. One should notice that the burst of activity diminishes when leaning forward (shoulders move in front of hips).

Obliques. The obliques consist of three interwoven muscles: internal obliques, external obliques, and transversus abdominis.

External Obliques. The external oblique forms the superficial layer of the abdominal wall. Its fibers run an oblique course superoinferiorly and lateromedially.[33] The muscle is lateral to the rectus abdominis and covers the anterior and lateral regions of the abdomen. The attachments are as follows:[47]

- **Proximal attachment:** Anterolateral portions of ribs where the muscle interdigitates with serratus anterior and slips from latissimus dorsi
- **Distal attachment:** Upper fibers run down and forward and attach to an aponeurosis that connects them to the linea alba; lower fibers attach to the crest of the ilium

If the external oblique contracts unilaterally, the trunk rotates to the opposite side. Therefore, if one rotates to

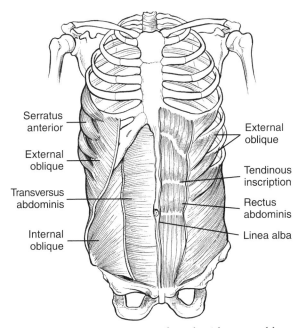

Figure 7-2 Anterior anatomy of trunk with resected layers.

Serratus anterior

External oblique

Transversus abdominis

Internal oblique

External oblique

Tendinous inscription

Rectus abdominis

Linea alba

the left, the right external oblique is active and vice versa. Bilateral contraction assists in trunk flexion and a resultant posterior pelvic tilt. This muscle is also active during straining and coughing.[47] The muscle is palpated easily while rotating the trunk to the opposite side.

Internal Obliques. The internal obliques also are located laterally and are covered by the external obliques. In essence, the internal obliques constitute the second layer of muscles on the abdominal wall. This muscle covers the same area as the external oblique, but its fibers cross those of the external oblique. Attachments are as follows:[47]

- **Proximal attachment:** Inguinal ligament, crest of ilium, and thoracolumbar fascia
- **Distal attachments:** Pubic bone, an aponeurosis connecting to linea alba, and last three or four ribs

This muscle groups is activated during trunk rotation, but contraction occurs toward the same side (i.e., rotation to the left occurs following contraction of the left internal oblique). Clearly the external and internal obliques are synergists in the action of trunk rotation. The right external and left internal oblique work together to rotate the trunk to the left and vice versa. "The efficient action of the muscles of one side of the abdominal wall is therefore very much dependent upon the fixation or anchorage provided by the activity of the muscles on the other side, particularly for activities involving rotation of the trunk."[16]

Tanaka, Hachisuka, and Ogata[49] examined trunk rotation performance in poststroke hemiplegic subjects and found significantly lower muscle performance in the subjects compared with the health controls. No differences were found when comparing right and left rotation in terms of angular velocities, the side of hemiplegia, or gender, but muscle performance in both directions was decreased compared with controls.

The internal obliques are difficult to palpate. However, the therapist may feel tension under the fingertips when palpating the lateral abdominal wall on the side toward which the trunk is rotating. This tension is due in part to activation of the internal obliques.

Transversus Abdominis. The transversus abdominis is the deepest layer of the abdominal wall. Its fibers run transversely, and the muscle has been called the corset muscle because it encloses the abdominal cavity like a corset. Attachments are as follows:[47]

- **Proximal attachments:** Lower ribs, thoracolumbar fascia, crest of the ilium, and inguinal ligament
- **Distal attachments:** Via an aponeurosis fuses with other abdominal muscles into linea alba

The main action of the transversus abdominis is forced compression; the muscle acts like a girdle to flatten the abdominal wall and compress the abdominal viscera.

Weakness of this muscle permits bulging of the anterior abdominal wall, thereby indirectly leading to an increase in lordosis.[38] The therapist may palpate this muscle between the lower ribs and the crest of the ilium during forced expiration.

Posterior Trunk Muscles

The posterior trunk muscles include the quadratus lumborum, the erector spinae group, and latissimus dorsi (Fig. 7-3). The actions of this group of muscles include trunk extension, lateral flexion, rotation of the trunk, and assistance with balancing the vertebral column.

Quadratus Lumborum. The quadratus lumborum is lateral and posterior (i.e., on the posterior abdominal wall); it lies between the psoas major and the erector spinae group. The attachments are as follows:[47]

- **Proximal attachment:** Crest of ilium
- **Distal attachments:** Twelfth rib and transverse processes of first to third lumbar vertebrae

The main action of this muscle is to assist in "hip hiking." Therefore, the muscle is active during lateral trunk flexion. The easiest way to palpate the quadratus lumborum is to have the subject prone, to palpate superior and lateral to the iliac crest, and to ask the subject to hike the hip.

Erector Spinae Group. The erector spinae group of muscles is a large mass that fills the spaces between the transverse and spinous processes of the vertebrae and extends laterally covering a large portion of the posterior thorax. Multiple muscles make up this group, and they are named according to attachments, shape, and action. Muscles such as the transversospinales, the interspinales,

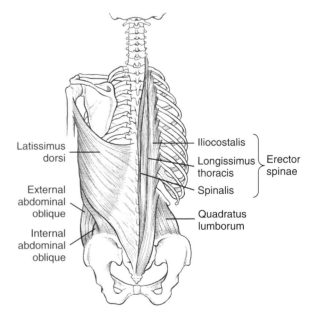

Figure 7-3   Posterior anatomy of trunk.

the longissimus, and the iliocostalis are included in this group.

Collectively, these muscles connect the back of the skull to the posterior iliac crest and sacrum. Unopposed contraction of the back extensors approximates the head and the sacrum. The pelvis is pulled into an anterior tilt (accentuating the lumbar curve), and the ribs are forced to flare. These muscles also contract during lateral flexion (to balance the abdominals), and they may assist in trunk rotation during unilateral contraction (e.g., assist the trunk with rotating to the ipsilateral side). The therapist easily can palpate this muscle group with patients in the prone position if the head and shoulders are lifted from the support surface;[47] palpation also is possible during forward sway in sitting or standing. The therapist easily can palpate the lower back extensors during low back extension (accentuating the lumbar curve) while the patient is sitting.

Winzeler-Mercay and Mudie[57] found increased activity in the erector spinae on both sides during work activities (such as reaching and donning shoes) and at rest. This increased activity was particularly evident on the involved side. They hypothesized that this abnormal response might reflect a disruption of cortical influences on motor unit activity. Similarly, Tanaka, Hachisuka, and Ogata[48] found that peak torque of the extensors was significantly less than in healthy controls.

Latissimus Dorsi. The latissimus dorsi is superficial and covers the posterior/lateral trunk. Its attachments include the following:[47]
- **Proximal attachments:** Spinous processes of T6 down, dorsolumbar fascia, posterior crest of ilium, lower ribs, interdigitations with external oblique; fibers converge toward axilla, passing over the inferior angle of the scapula.
- **Distal attachments:** Tendon attaches to crest of lesser tubercle of humerus, proximal to the teres major.

Acting unilaterally, the latissimus dorsi adducts, extends, and internally rotates the humerus and laterally flexes the trunk (approximates the shoulder and the pelvis). Bilateral contraction helps hyperextend the spine and anteriorly tilt the pelvis.

MOTOR CONTROL CONSIDERATIONS

Trunk Muscle Contractions

To achieve full trunk control and to use this control during functional tasks, patients must regain the ability to contract their trunk muscles under three different circumstances outlined by Davies.[17] The task of lower extremity bathing from a seated position illustrates these points:
1. Contracting to move opposite the pull of gravity: When the trunk is moving in a direction that is opposite to gravitational pull, the muscles on the uppermost side of the trunk are contracting concentrically.

For example, after washing feet, the trunk is straightened from a bent-over position by concentric contraction of the back extensors (the uppermost muscles). Therefore, the muscles are shortening actively. The one exception to the rule that the uppermost muscles are active during this type of contraction is bridging. In this case, movement does occur in a direction opposite the pull of gravity (back and buttocks moving away from the support surface), but the underside muscles (the extensors) are contracting concentrically and are responsible for the success of this task. Concentric contractions are used functionally to reposition the trunk during or after task completion.

2. Preventing movement that would occur because of gravitational pull: This type of muscle contraction (usually isometric) prevents falling toward the pull of gravity, stabilizes the trunk for successful completion of tasks, and forms the basis of many balance reactions. During lower extremity washing, the back extensors contract to stabilize (isometrically hold) the trunk as one washes the lower leg, allowing proximal stabilization for distal function. As a note, when one leans all of the way forward (extreme flexion), the back extensors become inactive, and the vertebral ligaments become responsible for holding the trunk in this posture.[5]

3. Controlling the speed of trunk movements in the direction of gravitational pull: In this type of contraction, the muscles are contracting eccentrically (in controlled and active elongation). The muscles responsible for this contraction are on the side of the trunk that is opposite the pull of gravity. When one leans forward to wash the feet during lower body washing, the back extensors contract eccentrically to control the speed and range of the forward trunk movement. This muscle contraction has a braking effect as the large mass of the trunk moves into the pull of gravity.

The previous examples show that functional independence requires control of all three trunk muscle contractions and combinations. Successful treatment plans must include activities that elicit a variety of trunk muscle contractions. Self-care training inherently challenges a variety of trunk postures and muscle contractions.

Musculoskeletal Components

Control of the trunk depends on several musculoskeletal variables including ROM, biomechanical alignment, strength, and muscle length. These variables are interdependent and can create a vicious circle in stroke patients.

Postural Malalignment

Stroke patients commonly assume postural malalignments that first must be identified via observations and palpations. After identification, the causative factors must be determined before determining the most appropriate intervention (Table 7-3).

Prolonged postural malalignment results in muscle shortening on one side of the trunk and muscle overstretching on the opposite side. For example, a posterior pelvic tilt with lumbar flexion results in shortening of the anterior musculature and elongation (overstretching) of the posterior muscles. Lateral flexion on the right side results in muscle shortening on the right side and muscle elongation on the left side of the trunk.

Postural malalignment may occur because of unilateral weakness (specifically around the pelvis), unbalanced skeletal muscle activity, perceptual dysfunction and an inability to perceive midline, and soft-tissue shortening.

Prolonged postural malalignment can result in soft-tissue shortening, loss of ROM, and an inability to generate enough force to contract the muscle group in question. The total force of muscle (active tension) is high at the rest length of the muscle (i.e., when the trunk is aligned properly) and less when the muscle is tested at shorter lengths. Therefore, the force-generating mechanism within the muscle works optimally at the rest length of the muscle[38] (i.e., a symmetrical and aligned trunk).

Managing Stiffness and the Degrees of Freedom Problem

Mohr[40] states, "Normal control in any body part demands the ability to dissociate (separate) different parts of the body." She gives the examples of dissociating the head from the body, one side of the body from the other, and the upper trunk from the lower trunk. Instead, patients often appear stiff, have nonfluid movements, and move their body segments as a unit

Examples of dissociation during functional tasks include upper trunk rotation with lower trunk stability while reaching for toilet paper, counterrotation of the trunk during ambulatory activities, and upper trunk rotation with concurrent lower trunk lateral flexion to increase the range of reach beyond the arm span when reaching for a phone positioned on the left side of a desk with the right hand.

Difficulty with dissociation/postural stiffness may result from soft-tissue tightness, bony contracture, or efforts by the patient to decrease the degrees of freedom in the trunk[45] during functional activities. It is critical to determine why the person is not able to dissociate. A typical clinical problem is determining if trunk stiffness and lack of dissociation is due to soft-tissue tightness (which may require soft tissue stretching and mobilization) or if the person is freezing the degrees of freedom in an effort to maintain stability (which requires core stabilization activities). One method to differentiate the cause is to provide various levels of postural support, for example, sitting in a high back chair versus sitting unsupported on a therapy table, or side lying versus sitting unsupported. If the underlying cause of the stiffness is related to freezing the degrees of freedom, substantial differences will be noted for both passive and active

Table 7-3

Common Postural Alignments and Potential Causes

Posterior pelvic tilt/lumbar spine flexion (loss of the lumbar curve)	■ Weakness in back lower back extensors ■ Abdominal weakness (as this position requires little abdominal control) ■ Generalized weakness in the trunk ■ Shortened or overactive hamstrings mechanically pulls the pelvis into a posterior tilt.
Pelvic obliquity characterized by unequal weight-bearing through the ischial tuberosities	■ Shortened or overactive muscle activity on one side of the trunk ■ Weakness on one side of the trunk ■ Visual-perceptual deficits (i.e., unilateral neglect or impaired processing of body and spatial relationships)
Increased kyphosis	■ Weakness in back lower back extensors ■ Abdominal weakness (as this position places the persons weight anteriorly, i.e., a position that requires little abdominal control) ■ Exacerbation of premorbid kyphosis
Sitting off midline and/or lateral spine flexion	■ Shortened or overactive muscle activity on one side of the trunk ■ Weakness on one side of the trunk ■ Visual-perceptual deficits (i.e., unilateral neglect or impaired processing of body and spatial relationships)
Rib cage rotation	■ Asymmetrical strength in the trunk rotators (i.e., oblique musculature) ■ Overactive unilateral trunk rotators
Head/neck malalignment (rotation away from and lateral flexion toward the involved side)	■ Unilateral neglect ■ Shortened or overactive neck musculature such as the sternocleidomastoid

movements under the various conditions of postural support. In the situations in which the patient has the most support (side lying and supported seating), he or she will be able to "free" the degrees of freedom and move with increased ease and fluidity, and will be able to separate body parts. If the same person is placed in a condition of decreased postural support, the system will respond by "freezing" the degrees of freedom, and stiffness will emerge.

Motor Adaptation

Concerning motor adaptation, Smith, Weiss, and Lehmkuhl[47] state, "Normal postural control requires the ability to adapt responses to changing tasks and environmental demands. This flexibility requires the availability of multiple movement strategies and the ability to select the appropriate strategy for the task and environment. The inability to adapt movements to changing task demands is a characteristic of many patients with neurological disorders. Patients become fixed in stereotypical patterns of movement, showing a loss of movement flexibility and adaptability."

Motor adaptation can occur in response to an external perturbation or in anticipation of potentially destabilizing forces. Unexpected external perturbations include bumping into someone in a crowded lobby, being in a vehicle that unexpectedly turns or decelerates, and being on a moving platform, such as an escalator, that stops unexpectedly.

Activities that lead to trunk movements in anticipation of destabilizing forces (i.e., internal perturbations) include reaching for a heavy book on a shelf, reaching beyond the arm span, and preparing to push or pull a chair into place. Shumway-Cook and Woollacott[46] point out that anticipatory postural control depends heavily on previous experience and learning. Research focusing on anticipatory postural responses during reach activities is presented in Chapter 10.

GENERAL CONSIDERATIONS FOR EVALUATION AND TREATMENT OF THE TRUNK

Therapists should consider the following points during evaluation of the trunk and treatment planning:

1. Proper evaluation and treatment of the trunk result from use of keen observational skills. Patients should be undressed (shirtless or in sports bra or bathing suit top), so that movements are more easily observed during functional tasks. Clothing folds, wrinkles, and crooked seams can lead to incorrect observations.
2. The therapist must realize that the slightest change in posture can change trunk muscle activity and alignment completely.[16] For example, a subtle anterior shift of the shoulders results in extensor activation, whereas a subtle posterior shift of the shoulders results in trunk flexor activation.
3. The therapist should evaluate the trunk in a variety of postures that coincide with ADL. Trunk adjustments are task specific; therefore, a trunk evaluation of a patient who is supine should include activities such as rolling, assuming/maintaining side lying, bridging, and transitions to sitting (see Chapter 14). Evaluations of seated patients should include activities such as upper and lower extremity dressing, scooting, and bathing; evaluations of standing patients should include reaching for items in medicine cabinets, on bookshelves, and in kitchen cabinets (see Chapter 8).

EVALUATION PROCESS

Subjective Interview

Therapists should question patients about their perceived stability limits. Stability limits have been defined as the "boundaries of an area of space in which the body can maintain its position without changing the base of support."[47] Patients' perceived stability limits may or may not be consistent with their actual limits. If patients' perceived limits of stability are greater than their actual limits, they are at risk for falls. If their perceived limits of stability are less than their actual limits, they may be reluctant to attempt tasks with progressively greater demands on their postural system (e.g., lower extremity dressing without assistive devices and picking up objects from the floor without a reacher).

Perceived stability limits may have a direct correlation with observed neurobehavioral deficits. Body scheme disorders commonly occur in the stroke population. These deficits include body neglect, somatoagnosia, and impaired right/left discrimination.[2] Ayres[3] has defined body scheme as a postural model on which movements are based. Knowledge of body parts and their relationships are necessary for deciding what and where to move and in what way to perform.[2] Spatial relation deficits including spatial neglect, depth perception, and spatial relation disorders also may have an effect on patients' perceived stability limits (gaining and regaining midline orientation and position in space) (see Chapter 18).

Other components of the subjective interview include determining patients' insights into their trunk malalignments and their ability to perceive and assume midline positions.[43] The therapist's goal in this interview is to gain insight into the patients' ability to make accurate observations about their postural dysfunction. This is difficult for many patients because trunk control does not occur at a conscious level in the majority of daily tasks.

Standardized Assessments

The use of valid and reliable tools is always recommended. The following section reviews available measurement instruments related to trunk control. The first three instruments specifically evaluate trunk control after stroke and are therefore highly recommend for this area of practice/research, while the others are comprehensive measures that include items related to the trunk. See Table 7-4 for a review of the psychometric properties of these three measures.

Table 7-4

Psychometric Properties of the Trunk Control Test and Two Trunk Impairment Scales

PSYCHOMETRIC CHARACTERISTICS	TRUNK CONTROL TEST	TRUNK IMPAIRMENT SCALE (VERHEYDEN)	TRUNK IMPAIRMENT SCALE (FUJIWARA)
Number of items	4	17	7
Score of each item	0, 12, or 25	0 to 1, 0 to 2, or 0 to 3	0 to 3
Total score range	0 to 100	0 to 23	0 to 21
Test-retest reliability	Not available	Kappa and weighted kappa values, percentage of agreement, ICC (kappa between 0.46 and 1, % of agreement between 82% and 100%, ICC between 0.87 and 0.96)	Not available
Interrater reliability	Spearman rho correlation coefficient ($r = 0.76$)	Kappa and weighted kappa values, percentage of agreement, ICC (kappa between 0.7 and 1, % of agreement between 82% and 100%, ICC between 0.85 and 0.99)	Weighted kappa values (between 0.66 and 1)
Measurement error	Not available	Inter- and test-retest examiner measurement error (inter: -1.84 to 1.84, test-retest: -2.90 to 3.68)	Not available
Responsiveness	Not available	Not available	Standardized response mean value (0.94)
Internal consistency	Cronbach α (0.83 and 0.86)	Cronbach α (between 0.65 and 0.89)	Rasch analysis (all but three items showed mean square fit statistic within 1.3)
Content validity	Not available	Literature review, observing stroke patients, clinical experience and discussion with specialists in stroke rehabilitation	Principal component analysis (three factors identified)
Construct validity	Correlation with gross motor function subscale of the Rivermead Motor Assessment (between 0.70 and 0.79)	Correlation with Barthel Index ($r = 0.86$)	Not available
Concurrent validity	Not available	Correlation with Trunk Control Test ($r = 0.83$)	Correlation with Trunk Control Test ($r = 0.91$)
Predictive validity	Significant predictor on admission of (motor part of the) FIM at discharge ($R^2 = 0.54$ when predicting FIM, $R^2 = 0.71$ when predicting motor FIM)	Significant predictor on admission of Barthel Index score at six months poststroke (unpublished data)	Significant predictor on admission of motor part of the FIM at discharge (added $R^2 = 0.09$)
Discriminant ability	Not available	Significant differences between stroke patients and healthy individuals ($P < 0.0001$)	Not available

FIM, Functional Independence Measure; ICC, intraclass correlation.
From Verheyden G, Nieuwboer A, Van de Winckel A, De Weerdt W: Clinical tools to measure trunk performance after stroke: a systematic review of the literature. *Clin Rehabil* 21(5):387-394, 2007.

Trunk Control Test

The Trunk Control Test[14] examines four functional movements: roll from supine to the weak side, roll from supine to the strong side, sitting up from supine, and sitting on the edge of the bed for 30 seconds (feet off the ground). Each of the four tasks are scored as follows: 0, unable to perform with assistance; 12, able to perform but in an abnormal manner; and 25, able to complete movement normally. The range of scores is 0 to 100.

The Trunk Control Test has been shown to be sensitive to change in assessing recovery of stroke patients, to correlate with the Functional Independence Measure, and to predict motor Functional Independence Measure items at discharge better than motor Functional Independence Measure Scores.[12,14] In addition, Duarte and colleagues[21] found that the Trunk Control Test significantly correlated with length of stay, discharge motor Functional Independence Measure scores, gait velocity, walking distance, and the Berg Balance Scale. They also found that the Trunk Control Test predicted 52% of the variance in length of stay and 54% of the discharge Functional Independence Measure (Table 7-5).

Trunk Impairment Scale (A)

This scale evaluates motor impairment of the trunk after stroke. The tool scores static (3 items), dynamical sitting balance (10 items), and trunk coordination (4 items). It also aims to score the quality of trunk movement and to be a guide for treatment. The scores range from a minimum of 0 to a maximum of 23[53] (Table 7-6).

Trunk Impairment Scale (B)

This tool consists of seven items. Abdominal muscle strength and verticality items were derived from the Stroke Impairment Assessment Set, and the other five items consist of the perception of trunk verticality, trunk rotation muscle strength on the affected and the unaffected sides,

and righting reflexes both on the affected and the unaffected sides. The seven items are scored on four-point scale with 0 indicated poor performance and 3 indicated best performance[28] (Box 7-1 and Table 7-7).

Postural Assessment Scale for Stroke Patients

The Postural Assessment Scale for Stroke Patients includes items related to trunk control. Overall, the scale contains 12 four-point items graded from 0 to 3. Higher scores indicate better performance. Items include sitting without support, standing with and without support, standing on the nonparetic leg, standing on the paretic leg, supine to affected side, supine to nonaffected side, supine to sit, sit to supine, sit to stand, stand to sit, and standing and picking up a pencil from the floor. The Postural Assessment Scale for Stroke Patients has been found to be highly valid and reliable during the first three months after stroke.[6]

Five items have been suggested[31] to measure trunk control: sitting without support, supine to affected side, supine to nonaffected side, supine to sitting on the edge of the bed, and sitting to supine. Recent work on this instrument has demonstrated that while the tool can predict performance in ADL at one year poststroke, a ceiling effect was noted at various points in recovery indicating a limited discriminative ability between individuals and a limited responsiveness over the first six months after stroke.[56]

Chedoke-McMaster Stroke Assessment

The Chedoke-McMaster Stroke Assessment is used to assess physical impairment and disability in clients with stroke. It has two components including the Impairment Inventory (which determines the presence and severity of physical impairments in the six dimensions of shoulder pain, postural control, arm, hand, foot, and leg quantified in a seven-point staging system) and the Activity Inventory (which measures the client's functional ability). The Activity Inventory has two components: the Gross Motor Function Index (with items including moving in bed and transferring to a chair) and the Walking Index (with items including walking on rough ground and climbing stairs). The maximum score that a client can obtain is 100 as there are 14 items with a seven-point scale and a two-point score awarded for age-appropriate walking distance.[30]

Motor Assessment Scale

The Motor Assessment Scale[12] is a comprehensive assessment of motor behavior and includes items related to trunk control. Overall, the scale consists of eight items: supine to side-lying (onto intact side), supine to sit, balanced sitting, sit to stand, walking, upper arm function, hand movements, and advanced hand activities. Each item is scored on seven-point scale from 0 to 6. Higher scores indicate better performance.

Table 7-5

Trunk Control Test

TESTS (ON BED)	SCORING 0—UNABLE TO 12—ABLE TO DO WITH NONMUSCULAR HELP 25—NORMAL
1. Rolling to weak side	
2. Rolling to strong side	
3. Balance in sitting position	
4. Sitting up from lying down	

From Collin C, Wade D: Assessing motor impairment after stroke: a pilot reliability study. *J Neurol Neurosurg Psychiatry* 53(7):576-579, 1990.

Table 7-6

Trunk Impairment Scale (A)

The starting position for each item is the same. The patient is sitting on the edge of a bed or treatment table without back and arm support. The thighs make full contact with the bed or table, the feet are hip width apart and placed flat on the floor. The knee angle is 90°. The arms rest on the legs. If hypertonia is present the position of the hemiplegic arm is taken as the starting position. The head and trunk are in a midline position.

If the patient scores 0 on the first item, the total score for the TIS is 0. Each item of the test can be performed three times. The highest score counts. No practice session is allowed. The patient can be corrected between attempts. The tests are verbally explained to the patient and can be demonstrated if needed.

ITEM

Static sitting balance

1. Starting position	Patient falls or cannot maintain starting position for 10 seconds without arm support	□0
	Patient can maintain starting position for 10 seconds	□2
	If score = 0, then Trunk Impairment Scale (TIS) total score = 0	
2. Starting position	Patient falls or cannot maintain starting position for 10 seconds without arm support	□0
Therapist crosses the unaffected leg over the hemiplegic leg	Patient can maintain starting position for 10 seconds	□2
3. Starting position	Patient falls	□0
Patient crosses the unaffected leg over the hemiplegic leg	Patient cannot cross legs without arm support on bed or table	□1
	Patient crosses the legs but displaces the trunk more than 10 cm backward or assists crossing with the hand	□2
	Patient crosses the legs without trunk displacement or assistance	□3
	Total static sitting balance	/7

Dynamical sitting balance

1. Starting position	Patient falls, needs support from an upper extremity, or the elbow does not touch the bed or table	□0
Patient is instructed to touch the bed or table with the hemiplegic elbow (by shortening the hemiplegic side and lengthening the unaffected side) and return to the starting position	Patient moves actively without help, elbow touches bed or table	□1
	If score = 0, then items 2 and 3 score = 0	
2. Repeat item 1	Patient demonstrates no or opposite shortening/lengthening	□0
	Patient demonstrates appropriate shortening/lengthening	□1
	If score = 0, then item 3 scores = 0	
3. Repeat item 1	Patient compensates. Possible compensations are: (1) use of upper extremity, (2) contralateral hip abduction, (3) hip flexion (if elbow touches bed or table further than proximal half of femur), (4) knee flexion, (5) sliding of feet	□0
	Patient moves without compensation	□1
4. Starting position	Patient falls, needs support from an upper extremity, or the elbow does not touch the bed or table	□0
Patient is instructed to touch the bed or table with the unaffected elbow (by shortening the unaffected side and lengthening the hemiplegic side) and return to the starting position	Patient moves actively without help, elbow touches bed or table	□1
	If score = 0, then items 5 and 6 score = 0	
5. Repeat item 4	Patient demonstrates no or opposite shortening/lengthening	□0
	Patient demonstrates appropriate shortening/lengthening	□1
	If score = 0, then item 6 scores = 0	
6. Repeat item 4	Patient compensates. Possible compensations are: (1) use of upper extremity, (2) contralateral hip abduction, (3) hip flexion (if elbow touches bed or table further than proximal half of femur), (4) knee flexion, (5) sliding of feet	□0
	Patient moves without compensation	□1
7. Starting position	Patient demonstrates no or opposite shortening/lengthening	□0
Patient is instructed to lift pelvis from bed or table at the hemiplegic side (by shortening the hemiplegic side and lengthening the unaffected side) and return to the starting position	Patient demonstrates appropriate shortening/lengthening	□1
	If score = 0, the item 8 scores = 0	

Table 7-6

Trunk Impairment Scale (A)—cont'd

ITEM

8. Repeat item 7	Patient compensates. Possible compensations are: (1) use of upper extremity, (2) pushing off with the ipsilateral foot (heel loses contact with the floor)	☐0
	Patient moves without compensation	☐1
9. Starting position	Patient demonstrates no or opposite shortening/lengthening	☐0
Patient is instructed to lift pelvis from bed or table at the unaffected side (by shortening the unaffected side and lengthening the hemiplegic side) and return to the starting position	Patient demonstrates appropriate shortening/lengthening	☐1
	If score = 0, then item 10 scores = 0	
10. Repeat item 9	Patient compensates. Possible compensations are: (1) use of upper extremity, (2) pushing off with the ipsilateral foot (heel loses contact with the floor)	☐0
	Patient moves without compensation	☐1
	Total dynamical sitting balance	/10

Coordination

1. Starting position	Hemiplegic side is not moved three times	☐0
Patient is instructed to rotate upper trunk 6 times (every shoulder should be moved forward 3 times), first side that moves must be hemiplegic side, head should be fixated in starting position	Rotation is asymmetrical	☐1
	Rotation is symmetrical	☐2
	If score = 0, then item 2 scores = 0	
2. Repeat item 1 within 6 seconds	Rotation is asymmetrical	☐0
	Rotation is symmetrical	☐1
3. Starting position	Hemiplegic side is not moved three times	☐0
Patient is instructed to rotate lower trunk 6 times (every knee should be moved forward 3 times), first side that moves must be hemiplegic side, upper trunk should be fixated in starting position	Rotation is asymmetrical	☐1
	Rotation is symmetrical	☐2
	If score = 0, then item 4 scores = 0	
4. Repeat item 3 within 6 seconds	Rotation is asymmetrical	☐0
	Rotation is symmetrical	☐1
	Total coordination	/6
	Total trunk impairment scale	/23

From Verheyden G, Nieuwboer A, Mertin J, et al: The Trunk Impairment Scale: a new tool to measure motor impairment of the trunk after stroke, *Clin Rehabil* 18(3):326-334, 2004.

Fugl-Meyer Assessment

The Fugl-Meyer Assessment[27] evaluates five areas: joint motion and pain, balance, sensation, upper extremity motor function, and lower extremity motor function. The balance subscale includes seven functions related to postural control: sit without support, protective reactions on affected and nonaffected sides, stand with support, stand without support, stand on nonaffected leg, and stand on affected leg.

Mao and colleagues[39] compared the psychometric properties of the balance subscale of the Fugl-Meyer Assessment, the Berg Balance Scale (see Chapter 8), and the Postural Assessment Scale for Stroke Patients. They concluded

that all three tests showed acceptable levels of reliability, validity, and responsiveness with the Postural Assessment Scale for Stroke Patients showing slightly better psychometric characteristics. The reader is referred to Chapter 8 for a review of other standardized assessments of postural control. In addition, the reader should review Chapter 21 concerning use of the Assessment of Motor and Process Skills. The assessment includes motor skill items such as stabilizes, aligns, and positions. The Assessment of Motor and Process Skills is unique and highly recommended, for the therapist can gather information related to motor skills during ADL performance.

Box 7-1

Trunk Impairment Scale (B)
Trunk Impairment Scale Items and Criteria for Scoring

PERCEPTION OF TRUNK VERTICALITY

While the patient is sitting on the edge of a bed or on a chair without a backrest, with the feet off the ground, the examiner holds both sides of the patient's shoulders and makes the patient's trunk deviate to the right and left. The examiner asks the patient to indicate when he or she feels the trunk is in a vertical position. The examiner then records the degree of trunk angle deviation from the vertical line drawn from the midpoint of the Jacoby line.

    0 = The angle is ≥30 degrees.
    1 = The angle is <30 degrees and ≥20 degrees.
    2 = The angle is <20 degrees and ≥10 degrees.
    3 = The angle is <10 degrees.

TRUNK ROTATION MUSCLE STRENGTH ON THE AFFECTED SIDE

The patient is asked to roll the body from the supine position to the unaffected side. The arms should be crossed in front of the chest and legs kept extended. The patient is asked to roll his or her body without pushing the floor with his or her limbs or pulling on the bed clothes. Isometric contractions for stabilization and other muscles than external oblique (e.g., pectoralis major) activation during rolling are allowed.

    0 = No contraction is noted in external oblique muscles on the affected side.
    1 = External oblique muscle contraction is visible on the affected side, but the patient cannot roll his or her body.
    2 = The patient can lift the affected side scapula but cannot fully rotate the body.
    3 = The patient can fully rotate the body.

TRUNK ROTATION MUSCLE STRENGTH ON THE UNAFFECTED SIDE

The patient is asked to roll the body from the supine position to the affected side. Scoring is the same as for the trunk rotation muscle strength on the unaffected side.

RIGHT REFLEX ON THE AFFECTED SIDE

The patient sits on the edge of a bed or a chair without a backrest. The examiner pushes the patient's shoulder laterally (about 30 degrees) to the unaffected side and scores according to the degree of the reflex elicited on the affected side of the patient's trunk.

    0 = No reflex is elicited.
    1 = The reflex is poorly elicited, and the patient cannot bring his or her body back to the erect position as before.
    2 = The reflex is not strong, but the patient can bring his or her body back to the erect position almost as before.
    3 = The reflex is strong enough, and the patient can immediately bring his or her body back to the erect position as before.

RIGHTING REFLEX ON THE UNAFFECTED SIDE

The examiner pushes the patient's shoulder laterally (about 30 degrees) to the affected side. Scoring is the same as for the righting reflex on the affected side.

STROKE IMPAIRMENT ASSESSMENT SET VERTICALITY

    0 = The patient cannot maintain a sitting position.
    1 = A sitting position can only be maintained while tilting to one side, and the patient is unable to correct the posture to an erect position.
    2 = The patient can sit vertically when reminded to do so.
    3 = The patient can sit vertically in a normal manner.

STROKE IMPAIRMENT ASSESSMENT SET ABDOMINAL MUSCLE STRENGTH

Stroke Impairment Assessment Set abdominal muscle strength is evaluated with the patient resting in a 45-degree semireclining position in either a wheelchair or a high-back chair. The patient is asked to raise the shoulders off the back of the chair and assume a sitting position.

    0 = Unable to sit up
    1 = The patient can sit up provided there is no resistance to the movement.
    2 = The patient can come to a sitting position despite pressure on the sternum by the examiner.
    3 = The patient has good strength in the abdominal muscles and is able to sit up against considerable resistance.

From Fujiwara T, Liu M, Tsuji T, et al: Development of a new measure to assess trunk impairment after stroke (trunk impairment scale): its psychometric properties. *Am J Phys Med Rehabil* 83(9):681-688, 2004.

Table 7-7

Comparison of the Trunk Impairment Scale (B) and the Trunk Control Test

CONTENT	TRUNK IMPAIRMENT SCALE	TRUNK CONTROL TEST
Practicality		
No. of items	7	4
Score of each item	0 to 3	0, 12, 25
Score range	0 to 21	0 to 100
Reliability		
Interrater reliability	Yes, weighted kappa	Yes, Spearman rank correlation
Internal consistency	Yes, Rasch analysis (mean square fit index)	Yes, Cronbach α
Validity		
Content validity	Yes, principal component analysis	No
Construct validity	Yes, Rasch analysis (logits)	Yes, correlation of individual items
Concurrent validity	Yes, with TCT	Yes, with RMA GF
Predictive validity	Yes, discharge Functional Independence Measure motor score	Yes, discharge FIM motor score

FIM, Functional Independence Measure.
RMA GF, Rivermead Motor Assessment gross function scores.
From Fujiwara T, Liu M, Tsuji T, et al: Development of a new measure to assess trunk impairment after stroke (trunk impairment scale): its psychometric properties. *Am J Phys Med Rehabil* 83(9):681-688, 2004.

Observations of Trunk Alignment/Malalignment

For the purposes of this chapter, observations concern the seated posture. The patient's trunk should be exposed as much as possible, and the patient should be asked to "sit up nice and straight and gently rest your hands in your lap." (Table 7-8 outlines the ideal alignment of the trunk and extremities and common asymmetries observed after stroke during static sitting.)

Following the evaluation of postural malalignments during static sitting, the therapist should begin to hypothesize the cause of these malalignments. Causes may include increased skeletal muscle activity on one side of the trunk, inability to recruit muscle activity or weakness, soft-tissue shortening, fixed deformity, body scheme disorder, and inability to perceive midline.

The therapist must remember that observed postures may be caused by more than one impairment (see Table 7-3). For example, stroke patients tend to sit in a posterior pelvic tilt position with resultant hip extension and thoracic spine flexion. This posture may result from one of or a combination of the following:

- Weakness or lack of activity in the trunk extensors, especially in the lower back
- Fixed contracture of the hamstrings and/or thoracic spine
- Abdominal weakness: The mentioned posture changes the center of gravity and decreases the potential to fall backward. The abdominal muscles are primarily responsible for preventing backward sway, therefore assuming a flexed posture reduces the chance of having to activate the abdominals to prevent falls.

Another example of a commonly observed malalignment is trunk shortening on the side affected by the stroke. The patient may assume this posture for several reasons:

- Inactive shoulder elevators on the side affected by the stroke that let the shoulder depress[16]
- Increased muscle activity of the scapula depressors that pull the shoulder down on the affected side
- Perceptual dysfunction resulting in an inability to find midline, bearing the most weight on the stronger side and resulting in a shortening of the affected side
- Increased muscle activity or shortening of the affected lateral flexors resulting in a shortening response
- Fear of shifting weight to the affected side, with the majority of weight on stronger side, resulting in shortening of the affected side

Following the observation of the patient in a static posture, the occupational therapist must observe trunk responses during functional activities. The two most effective methods of making these observations are observing patients during self-care and mobility in a variety of positions and controlled reach pattern activities (Table 7-9). During functional reach patterns, trunk responses are required to provide proximal stability for distal function, enhance the ability to interact with the environment by increasing reaching distance (i.e., extend the arm span with an appropriate trunk response), and prevent falls.

An individual's reaching ability is limited to within the arm span by static trunk postures. When an object is placed beyond arm's length (e.g., on a floor, across a dining table, or under a sink), a trunk response is required to pick up the object successfully.

Table 7-8

Typical Alignment and Common Malalignments after Stroke

	NORMAL ALIGNMENT	COMMON MALALIGNMENT
Pelvis	Equal weight-bearing through both ischial tuberosities	Asymmetrical weight-bearing
		Posterior pelvic tilt
	Neutral to slight anterior tilt	Unilateral retraction
	Neutral rotation	
Vertebral column	Straight from posterior view	Scoliosis
	Appropriate curves from lateral view	Loss of lumbar curve; increased thoracic kyphosis
		Shortening on one side; elongation on opposite side
Rib cage	Neutral in terms of lateral tilt	Lateral tilt
	Neutral rotation	Flaring on one side
	Alignment over pelvis and under shoulders	Unilateral retraction
Shoulders	Symmetrical height	Asymmetrical height
	Alignment over pelvis	Unilateral retraction
Head/neck	Neutral	Protraction
		Flexion to weak side
		Rotation away from weak side
Upper extremities	Resting in lap; if weight-bearing, effortless and symmetrical	Use of stronger extremity as postural support to maintain alignment
		Too little or too much activity in more involved extremity
Lower extremities	Hips at 90 degrees	Hips toward extension because of posterior pelvic tilt
	Knee aligned with hips	Hip adduction resulting in knee contact
	Feet in full contact with floor, accepting weight; feet under knees	"Windswept" hips
		Feet not equally bearing weight, or "pushing"; foot placed in front of knee

In general, picking up an object from the floor or from in front of an individual requires an anterior trunk shift. Picking up objects placed beyond the arm span to the right or left of the individual requires a lateral weight shift from the trunk primarily onto one of the ischial tuberosities. Retrieving objects placed behind the trunk requires a posterior weight shift. Rotational trunk responses result from reaching across the midline or for objects posterior to the shoulders or hips.

The therapist's goals while observing the patient perform functional reach patterns are the following:

- Ensure that trunk and upper extremity patterns are coordinated to result in successful task completion.
- Note any fall potential.
- Note asymmetries during reaching.
- Objectively evaluate the perceived and actual stability limits of the patient.
- Note in which directions the patient is or is not able to reach beyond the arm span.
- Note factors such as trunk stiffness and decreased ROM.

Evaluation of Specific Trunk Movement Patterns

In addition to performing each movement pattern, the reader should refer to the appropriate figures while reading this section. The following evaluation procedures are based on the work of Mohr,[40] Boehme,[8] Davies,[16] and Basmajian and DeLuca.[5]

Trunk Flexor Control

The trunk flexors are evaluated by the five different methods that follow:

1. Patients assume a seated, upright position. The therapist asks them to move their shoulders behind their hips slowly and with control (Fig. 7-4, *A*); this movement pattern occurs in the sagittal plane, is initiated from the upper trunk,[40] and elicits an eccentric contraction of the trunk flexors.[25,50] Holding the end range of this posture results in an isometric contraction of the trunk flexors. Observations should include resistance to movement, fall potential, and symmetry of the posterior weight shift. Unilateral weakness causes the weak side to become posterior to the stronger side (i.e., it results in rotation of the trunk).

2. From the end position of the first movement pattern, the therapists asks patients to move their shoulders forward so that they are sitting in proper alignment within the sagittal plane (see Fig. 7-4, *B*); this movement pattern is achieved by a concentric contraction of the trunk flexors.[25] The therapist should note symmetry during the movement pattern. Unilateral weakness causes the stronger side to lead the pattern.

Table 7-9

Effects of Object Positioning on Trunk Movements and Weight Shifts during Reaching Activities*

POSITION OF OBJECT	TRUNK RESPONSE/WEIGHT SHIFT
Straight ahead at forehead level, past arm's length 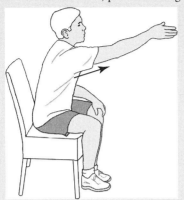	Trunk extension, anterior pelvic tilt Anterior weight shift
On floor, between feet 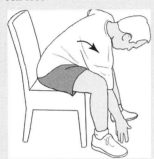	Trunk flexion Anterior weight shift
To side at shoulder level, past arm's length 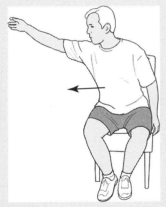	Left trunk shortening, right trunk elongation, left hip hiking Weight shift to right
On floor, below right hip 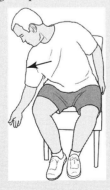	Right trunk shortening, left trunk elongation Weight shift to right

*These examples are for a patient with left hemiplegia. The left-hand column indicates where to position objects during a reaching task (using the right upper extremity). The right-hand column indicates the resultant trunk position and weight shift.

Continued

Table 7-9

Effects of Object Positioning on Trunk Movements and Weight Shifts during Reaching Activities—cont'd

POSITION OF OBJECT	TRUNK RESPONSE/WEIGHT SHIFT
Behind right shoulder, at arm's length 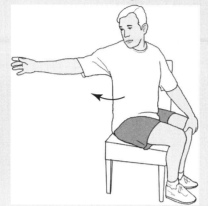	Trunk extension and rotation (right side posteriorly) Weight shift to right
At shoulder level, to left of left shoulder 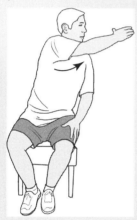	Trunk extension and rotation (left side posteriorly) Weight shift to left
On floor, to left of left foot 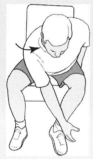	Trunk flexion and rotation (left side posteriorly) Weight shift to left
Above head, directly behind 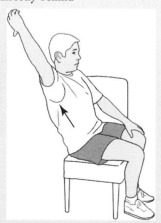	Trunk extension, shoulders move behind hips Posterior weight shift

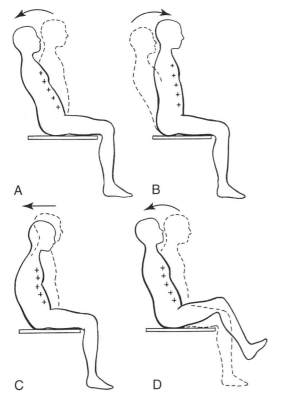

Figure 7-4 Trunk flexor control. Dotted lines indicate trunk starting position, solid lines indicate trunk final position, arrows indicate movement direction, and plus signs indicate muscle groups primarily responsible for control of pattern. (Skeletal muscle activity occurs on both sides of the trunk; that is, reciprocal innervation.)

3. In an aligned, seated position, patients assume a controlled lumbar flexion posture (posterior tilt with flattening of the lumbar curve and spinal flexion) (see Fig. 7-4, *C*). Mohr[40] states that this movement pattern is initiated by the lower trunk and pelvis. If this pattern is performed actively, the final posture is assumed by concentric flexor contraction. Patients also may achieve this posture by a relaxation response of the low back extensors, so the therapist should palpate the flexors to ensure the pattern is due to active movement. At the end range of this pattern—posterior tilt and spinal flexion (a recumbent posture)—little to no muscle activity exists, and patients maintain this posture by support of their vertebral ligaments.[5]

4. The therapist also should evaluate control of the trunk flexors when the patient is supine (during rolling and bed mobility activities). While the patient is in a supine position, the therapist asks the patient to sit up in a straight plane. This movement pattern, which is controlled primarily by the rectus abdominis, allows the therapist to evaluate antigravity control of the trunk flexors. The therapist also can ask the patient to roll by lifting one shoulder up and across the trunk in a position of trunk flexion and rotation. This movement pattern also gives the therapist insight into the antigravity control of the flexors (primarily the obliques).[38]

5. Although the first four movement patterns to test flexor control were initiated by the patient, testing the response of the flexors to being moved by the therapist also is useful. The therapist lifts the lower legs of the patient into a position of increased hip flexion. For the patient to refrain from falling backward, the trunk flexors must be activated isometrically (see Fig. 7-4, *D*).

As a rule of thumb the trunk flexors are activated in the seated position when the shoulders move posterior to the hips (backward sway), when the trunk is moving away from the support surface (supine starting point), and during rotational activities.

Trunk Extensor Control

The following four movement patterns are used to evaluate trunk extensor control during seated activities and bridging.

1. To start this movement pattern, the patient assumes a flexed spine posture with a posterior pelvis tilt (the resting posture for many stroke survivors). The patient initiates the movement with the lower trunk and pelvis[40] and assumes an extended spine posture with a neutral to slight anterior tilt, which accentuates the lumbar curve (Fig. 7-5, *A*). The patient completes the movement pattern by a concentric contraction of the trunk extensors, which is the trunk pattern required for forward reach.

2. Patients assume an aligned, seated starting position and are asked to keep their spine straight as they lean forward, keeping the shoulders in front of the hips in the sagittal plane (see Fig. 7-5, *B*). They assume this posture by an eccentric contraction of the trunk extensors,[5,25,50] and if they hold the posture between the middle to end range, the back extensors isometrically contract. The patient has unilateral weakness if the trunk moves forward asymmetrically. Unilateral weakness causes the weaker side to lead the movement pattern (e.g., to fall into gravity). If the movement continues in a forward direction (e.g., patient reaches down to the floor), the back extensors become inactive at the end range, and the tension of the vertebral ligaments maintains the position.[5]

3. While patients are in the end posture of the second movement pattern, the therapists asks them to move their shoulders back to assume a seated, aligned position (see Fig. 7-5, *C*). To assume this posture, the trunk extensors contract concentrically, although the hip extensors initiate the movement;[5,50] this movement occurs in the sagittal plane.

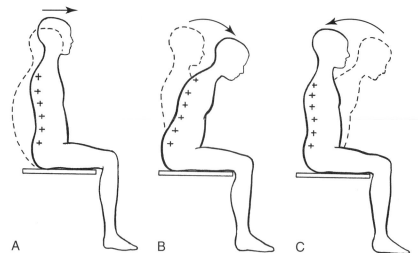

Figure 7-5   Trunk extensor control. Dotted lines indicate trunk starting position, solid lines indicate trunk final position, arrows indicate movement direction, and plus signs indicate muscle groups primarily responsible for control of pattern. (Skeletal muscle activity occurs on both sides of the trunk; that is, reciprocal innervation.)

4. The therapist also should test the back extensors by observing the patient in a bridge posture. While the patient is in a supine position with the hips and knees flexed, the therapist asks the patient to assume a bridge position, which is accomplished by a concentric contraction of the back and hip extensors[16] and is maintained by an isometric contraction of the same muscles. The release of the posture is controlled by eccentric contraction of the back and hip extensors.

As a rule of thumb, in the seated posture the back extensors are active during anterior weight shifts (in which the shoulders move in front of the hips), during correction of posture to a position of alignment from an anterior weight shift, and during bridging activities.

Control of the Lateral Flexors

Lateral flexion occurs in the coronal plane; therefore, a balance of control between the flexors and extensors is required to maintain movement. Electromyographic studies have demonstrated that dorsal and ventral muscles coactivate during lateral flexion.[50] Electromyographic activity of the right and left erector spinae has been documented during lateral trunk flexion.[5,25]

Mohr[40] states, "Two different movement strategies occur when you reach down to the side: (1) the initiation may occur in the upper trunk and the ipsilateral spine shortens, or (2) the movement can be initiated with your lower trunk and pelvis, resulting in ipsilateral elongation." Three movement patterns are used to evaluate control of lateral trunk flexion:

1. The first movement pattern is initiated from an aligned, seated position. The pelvis remains stable, and the upper trunk initiates lateral flexion toward the floor with the shoulder approximating the hip (Fig. 7-6A). The end posture (one of ipsilateral trunk shortening) occurs by an eccentric contraction of the side of the elongating trunk.[40,50] In Fig. 7-6, *A*, the right side of the trunk is shortening, but the predominant control is on the left side, which is elongating eccentrically. Holding this posture between the middle and end ranges allows evaluation of isometric lateral flexion control. Therapists should evaluate both sides of the trunk using this movement pattern.

2. While patients are in the end position of the first movement pattern, the therapist asks them to realign themselves by sitting up straight (see Fig. 7-6, *B*). The trunk is realigned by a concentric contraction of the lateral flexors[38] (the left lateral flexors in Fig. 7-6, *B*).

3. The last movement pattern evaluates lateral flexion, which initiates the movement from the lower trunk and pelvis.[40] This movement pattern allows reach beyond the arm span in the frontal plane. During this movement, the majority of weight is shifted to one ischial tuberosity; the shoulder and hip approximate in this pattern. In the resulting posture the trunk is elongated on the weight-bearing side, and trunk shortening occurs on the nonweight-bearing side (see Fig. 7-6, *C*). The predominant control comes from concentric contraction of the lateral flexors on the shortening side. Fig. 7-6, *C*, illustrates the contraction on the right side of the trunk. The therapist must evaluate both sides of the trunk.

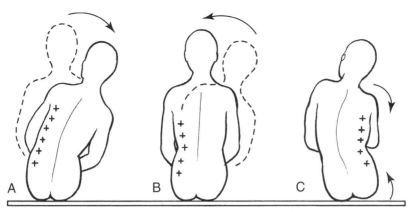

Figure 7-6 Lateral flexor control. Dotted lines indicate trunk starting position, solid lines indicate trunk final position, arrows indicate movement direction, and plus symbols indicate muscle groups primarily responsible for control of pattern. (Skeletal muscle activity occurs on both sides of the trunk; that is, reciprocal innervation.)

Rotation Control

Concerning rotation control, Kapandji[33] states, "Rotation of the vertebral column is achieved by the paravertebral muscles and the lateral muscles of the abdomen. Unilateral contraction of the paravertebral muscles causes only weak rotation... During rotation of the trunk, the main muscles involved are the oblique muscles. Their mechanical efficiency is enhanced by their spiral course around the waist and by their attachments to the thoracic cage away from the vertebral column, so that both the lumbar and lower thoracic vertebral columns are mobilised." During rotation of the trunk to the left, the right external and left internal obliques are activated (Fig. 7-7). The fibers of both of these muscles run in the same direction and are synergistic. Basmajian's[4] review of the literature on electromyography demonstrates that bilateral activity in the extensors at the thoracic level is evident during rotation.

Mohr[40] states, "Stroke patients will very rarely rotate because normal rotation requires extensors and flexors to be active simultaneously on opposite sides of the trunk." Rotational trunk control depends on muscle fixation on one side of the trunk, resulting in efficient muscle action on the opposite side.

Trunk rotation can occur in two positions: flexion with rotation and extension with rotation.[7] Mohr[40] points out that rotation can be initiated by the upper trunk or the lower trunk/pelvis. Rotation control is evaluated by five movement patterns:[8,40]

1. In the first movement pattern, the patient sits upright, and the pelvis remains stable on the support surface. The patient reaches across midline so that the shoulder moves toward the opposite hip (e.g., reaching with the right arm across the body toward the floor). The result is a position of flexion and rotation. The primary control is by concentric contraction of the

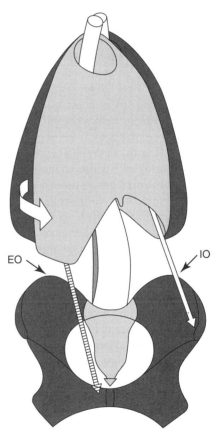

Figure 7-7 Rotation control. *IO,* Internal oblique; *EO,* external oblique. (From Kapandji IA: *The physiology of the joints,* vol 3, *The trunk and vertebral column,* New York, 1974, Churchill Livingstone.)

obliques and contraction of the back extensors (especially at the thoracic level). The therapist must evaluate both sides of the trunk.

2. In the second movement pattern, the upper trunk remains stable, and the lower trunk and pelvis

initiate a forward movement on one side (e.g., scooting forward). The result is a position of extension with rotation.

3. In the third movement pattern the patient reaches behind at the shoulder level (upper trunk initiation), and the resulting posture is rotation and extension.

4. The fourth movement pattern involves initiating a backward shift with the lower trunk and pelvis (scooting backward) while shifting to one side and rotating the opposite side posteriorly; this posture is flexion with rotation.

5. The final movement pattern is similar to a pattern reviewed in the section on trunk flexion control. The patient is supine and initiates a segmental roll by lifting the shoulders up from the support surface and toward the opposite side of the body. This pattern is controlled by a concentric contraction of the abdominal muscles (the obliques).

Trunk Control during Activities of Daily Living

There is a clear relationship between the loss of trunk control and the loss of functional independence. Conclusions from empirical research include:

- Franchignoni, Tesio, and Ricupero[26] stated that trunk control appears to be an obvious prerequisite for the control of more complex limb activities that, in turn, constitute a prerequisite for complex behavioral skills.
- Hsieh and colleagues[31] affirmed that strong evidence exists for the predictive value of trunk control on comprehensive ADL, and they recommended early assessment and management of trunk control after stroke.
- Karatkas and colleagues[34] concluded that trunk flexion and extension muscle weakness in unihemispheric stroke patients can interfere with balance, stability, and functional disability.
- Verheyden and colleagues[52] asserted that measures of trunk performance are significantly related with values of balance, gait, and functional ability.

The previous section focused on select movement patterns of the trunk. Evaluating the trunk in this manner is useful for identifying specific problem areas and focusing treatment plans. However, the impact that impaired trunk control has on functional tasks is more relevant to all rehabilitation professionals. Most, if not all, of the reviewed movement patterns (and combinations of them) are used during ADL performance. Therefore, the evaluation of trunk control can take place during skilled observations of ADL.

For clarification, an infinite number of variations are observed in movement patterns during task performance. Therefore, the focus of evaluation and treatment should be on observing, evaluating, and treating the patient in a variety of different environments and with tasks that include multiple variables. The situational context and task demands determine which components of trunk control are necessary for successful task performance. Box 7-2 has an example of task variables that affect trunk control patterns.

The list of trunk control variations during ADL performance in the following section are not considered exhaustive, but are guidelines for observing trunk patterns and inherent variations during various tasks. The reader should mimic performing each task to ensure understanding of the posture descriptions (Table 7-10).

Upper Extremity Dressing

Pullover Shirt. Putting on a pullover shirt requires the following movements:

- *Trunk flexion:* Required for the patient to manipulate the shirt in the lap and reach down toward the lap to insert an arm into the sleeve
- *Trunk extension:* Observed as the patient realigns the trunk, continues to pull up the sleeve, and inserts the head into the shirt
- *Trunk rotation with extension:* May be necessary for reaching posteriorly and adjusting the orientation of the shirt and/or tucking the shirt into the pants

Button-Down Shirt. Putting on a button-down shirt requires the following movements:

- *Trunk flexion:* Used to orient the shirt correctly on the lap for preparation of donning and to guide the arm into the sleeve when the trunk is inclined forward
- *Trunk extension:* Required to realign the trunk from the previous position
- *Trunk rotation with extension:* Used to reach with the more functional arm behind the head and to the opposite shoulder to grasp the collar of the shirt and pull it to the opposite side (Fig. 7-8); also used to

---

Box 7-2

Variables of Eating That Affect Required Trunk Control Patterns

- Size of table
- Type of seating surface (e.g., presence of armrests or backrest, cushions, chair height, distance person is from table)
- Placement of items such as condiments, utensils, and serving bowls (e.g., near or far, right or left)
- Type of food (e.g., hot soup, cold fruit)
- Solitary or group dining (e.g., may get assistance with passing needed items)
- Errors (e.g., dropping fork, spilling beverage)

Table 7-10

Trunk Control to Support Participation

ACTIVITY	POSSIBLE NECESSARY MOVEMENTS
Bridging	Bridging requires trunk extension, which is necessary at the trunk and hips to assume a functional bridge position. (The height of the bridge depends on the task. For example, bridging to use a bedpan requires more extension than bridging to don/doff pants.) See Chapter 14.
Scooting	Scooting requires the following movement: ■ **Trunk flexion and extension:** Must be balanced for successful scooting. (The efficiency of the scooting pattern is compromised if the patient maintains a flexed trunk with a posterior pelvic tilt or a hyperextended trunk.) ■ **Lateral flexion:** Lower trunk initiation is used to clear the buttocks from the support surface, which is required to advance the hip forward. ■ **Trunk rotation with extension:** Lower trunk initiation allows the patient to achieve the goal of scooting forward
Toileting	Using the toilet requires the following movements: ■ **Lateral flexion:** Lower trunk initiation may be used depending on the sequence of clothing management for toileting and the type of transfer being used (for example, if patients are performing a sit-pivot transfer, clothing usually is managed from the seated position. Therefore, lateral flexion is necessary so that pants and underwear can clear the hips/buttocks); may also be used for wiping after toileting. ■ **Trunk rotation with extension:** Used to reach across the body for toilet paper ■ **Trunk flexion:** May be used for self-catheterization, application of a condom-style catheter, management of feminine hygiene products, and wiping after toileting
Bathing (seated on a tub seat or bench).	Bathing requires the following movements: ■ **Trunk flexion and extension:** Required to reach toward the lower extremities and then realign ■ **Trunk rotation:** Trunk rotation with flexion is used to reach down toward the opposite lower extremity for lower leg and foot washing; trunk rotation with extension may be used when reaching posteriorly to wash back and neck. (In general, trunk rotation is used when reaching across the midline of the trunk. The amount of flexion and extension depends on the area of the body being washed [e.g., flexion for lower body washing; extension for upper body washing].) ■ **Lateral flexion:** Lower trunk initiation is required to wash the perineum and rectal areas; upper trunk initiation may be used to wash the sides of the lower legs or to pick up a bar of soap from the bottom of the tub. (Bathing activities place extra demands on trunk control because of the slippery nature of the support surface.)
Grooming	**Oral care** Hygiene of the mouth requires the following movements: ■ **Trunk flexion:** Isometric control commonly used to position the head over the sink to preventing spillage of toothpaste and saliva onto clothing; increased trunk flexion for expectorating (toothpaste and mouthwash) after completion of tooth brushing ■ **Trunk extension:** Used to realign body from previous position; also used to reach for supplies in a medicine cabinet over a sink and during gargling ■ **Trunk rotation with flexion:** May be used to reach toward and adjust the faucet opposite the arm being used **Hair care** Hair care requires the following movements: ■ **Trunk flexion or extension:** May be used isometrically during hair washing; trunk flexion is used if patients prefer to lean forward and allow the lather to be rinsed off in front of them; trunk extension (and head/neck extension) is used if patients prefer to lean back and allow the lather to be rinsed off behind them; both may be used during hair combing to accentuate the position of the head and optimally position the brush or comb to make contact with the scalp. ■ **Lateral flexion:** May be used during hair washing or combing (initiated by upper trunk) as the head is tilted to the right or left side; also may be used for optimal head placement.

Table 7-10

Trunk Control to Support Participation—cont'd

ACTIVITY	POSSIBLE NECESSARY MOVEMENTS	
Dressing	Upper extremity	*Pullover shirt* Putting on a pullover shirt requires the following movements: ■ **Trunk flexion:** Required for the patient to manipulate the shirt in the lap and reach down toward the lap to insert an arm into the sleeve ■ **Trunk extension:** Observed as the patient realigns the trunk, continues to pull up the sleeve, and inserts the head into the shirt ■ **Trunk rotation with extension:** May be necessary for reaching posteriorly and adjusting the orientation of the shirt and/or tucking the shirt into the pants *Button-down shirt* Putting on a button-down shirt requires the following movements: ■ **Trunk flexion:** Used to orient the shirt correctly on the lap for preparation of donning and to guide the arm into the sleeve when the trunk is inclined forward ■ **Trunk extension:** Required to realign the trunk from the previous position ■ **Trunk rotation with extension:** Used to reach with the more functional arm behind the head and to the opposite shoulder to grasp the collar of the shirt and pull it to the opposite side (see Fig. 7-8); also used to move the second arm through the sleeve and tuck the shirt into the pants ■ **Trunk flexion:** Used as the patient attempts to button the shirt; more often used as relaxation position (a slumped posture) rather than an active flexion pattern
	Lower extremity (seated)	Putting on pants, underwear, shoes, and socks requires the following movements: ■ **Trunk flexion:** Required to reach down toward the feet (see Fig. 7-9) ■ **Trunk rotation with flexion:** Required to reach the more functional arm toward the opposite foot ■ **Trunk extension:** Required to realign the trunk from the previous positions ■ **Lateral flexion:** Required when using a crossed-leg method to don/doff pants, underwear, or footwear (the crossed-leg position shifts the patients' center of gravity posteriorly, placing increased demand on the abdominal muscles [i.e., controlling the trunk in flexion while preventing a posterior fall]) (see Fig. 7-10); also required to pull pants and underwear up or down over the buttocks and hips successfully
Eating		Eating requires the following movements: ■ **Trunk flexion and extension:** Used in varying degrees with a hand-to-mouth pattern in which an anterior weight shift of the trunk toward the table occurs (see Fig. 7-11) to position the mouth over the plate as food enters. (The degree to which this weight shift occurs depends on the type of food being eaten. Food that is hot or liquid requires increased flexion toward the plate or bowl. The increased flexion reduces the distance the food must be transported, thereby reducing spillage opportunities.) ■ **Trunk rotation:** May be used in flexion and extension to reach for condiments that are across the midline of the trunk ■ **Lateral flexion:** Lower trunk initiation may be used in reaching for condiments that are positioned to the side of the place setting and beyond arm's length and also may be used with trunk rotation postures (see Fig. 7-12); upper trunk initiation may be used when reaching for an object that drops on the floor to the side of the patient.

move the second arm through the sleeve and tuck the shirt into the pants
■ *Trunk flexion:* Used as the patient attempts to button the shirt; more often used as relaxation position (a slumped posture) rather than an active flexion pattern

Lower Extremity Dressing (Seated). Putting on pants, underwear, shoes, and socks requires the following

movements:
■ *Trunk flexion:* Required to reach down toward the feet (Fig. 7-9)
■ *Trunk rotation with flexion:* Required to reach the more functional arm toward the opposite foot
■ *Trunk extension:* Required to realign the trunk from the previous positions
■ *Lateral flexion:* Required when using a crossed-leg method to don/doff pants, underwear, or footwear

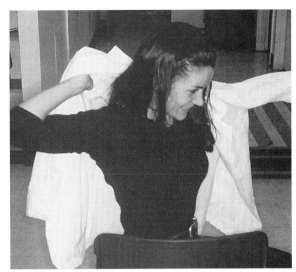

Figure 7-8 Trunk control during upper extremity dressing.

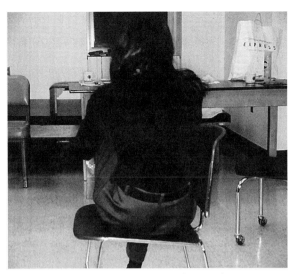

Figure 7-10 Trunk adjustments during lower extremity dressing.

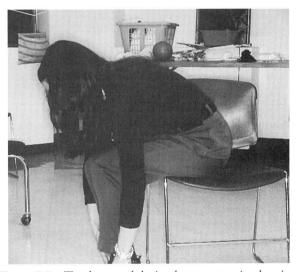

Figure 7-9 Trunk control during lower extremity dressing.

(the crossed-leg position shifts the patients' center of gravity posteriorly, placing increased demand on the abdominal muscles [i.e., controlling the trunk in flexion while preventing a posterior fall]) (Fig. 7-10); also required to pull pants and underwear up or down over the buttocks and hips successfully

Grooming

Oral Care. Hygiene of the mouth requires the following movements:

- *Trunk flexion:* Isometric control commonly used to position the head over the sink to preventing spillage of toothpaste and saliva onto clothing; increased trunk flexion for expectorating (toothpaste and mouthwash) after completion of tooth brushing

- *Trunk extension:* Used to realign body from previous position; also used to reach for supplies in a medicine cabinet over a sink and during gargling
- *Trunk rotation with flexion:* May be used to reach toward and adjust the faucet opposite the arm being used

Hair Care. Hair care requires the following movements:

- *Trunk flexion or extension:* May be used isometrically during hair washing; trunk flexion is used if patients prefer to lean forward and allow the lather to be rinsed off in front of them; trunk extension (and head/neck extension) is used if patients prefer to lean back and allow the lather to be rinsed off behind them; both may be used during hair combing to accentuate the position of the head and optimally position the brush or comb to make contact with the scalp
- *Lateral flexion:* May be used during hair washing or combing (initiated by upper trunk) as the head is tilted to the right or left side; also may be used for optimal head placement

Eating

Eating requires the following movements:

- *Trunk flexion and extension:* Used in varying degrees with a hand-to-mouth pattern in which an anterior weight shift of the trunk toward the table occurs (Fig. 7-11) to position the mouth over the plate as food enters. (The degree to which this weight shift occurs depends on the type of food being eaten. Food that is hot or liquid requires increased flexion toward the plate or bowl. The increased flexion reduces the distance the food must be transported, thereby reducing spillage opportunities.)

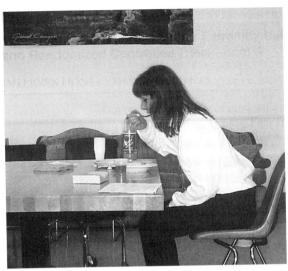

Figure 7-11 Trunk control while eating.

- *Trunk rotation:* May be used in flexion and extension to reach for condiments that are across the midline of the trunk
- *Lateral flexion:* Lower trunk initiation may be used in reaching for condiments that are positioned to the side of the place setting and beyond arm's length and also may be used with trunk rotation postures (Fig. 7-12); upper trunk initiation may be used when reaching for an object that drops on the floor to the side of the patient.

Bathing (Seated on a Tub Seat or Bench). Bathing requires the following movements:
- *Trunk flexion and extension:* Required to reach toward the lower extremities and then realign

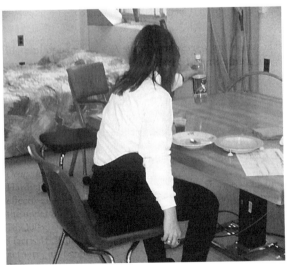

Figure 7-12 Trunk adjustments while reaching for utensils or condiments.

- *Trunk rotation:* Trunk rotation with flexion is used to reach down toward the opposite lower extremity for lower leg and foot washing; trunk rotation with extension may be used when reaching posteriorly to wash back and neck. (In general, trunk rotation is used when reaching across the midline of the trunk. The amount of flexion and extension depends on the area of the body being washed [e.g., flexion for lower body washing; extension for upper body washing].)
- *Lateral flexion:* Lower trunk initiation is required to wash the perineum and rectal areas; upper trunk initiation may be used to wash the sides of the lower legs or to pick up a bar of soap from the bottom of the tub. (Bathing activities place extra demands on trunk control because of the slippery nature of the support surface.)

Toileting. Using the toilet requires the following movements:
- *Lateral flexion:* Lower trunk initiation may be used depending on the sequence of clothing management for toileting and the type of transfer being used (for example, if patients are performing a sit-pivot transfer, clothing usually is managed from the seated position. Therefore, lateral flexion is necessary so that pants and underwear can clear the hips/buttocks.); may also be used for wiping after toileting.
- *Trunk rotation with extension:* Used to reach across the body for toilet paper
- *Trunk flexion:* May be used for self-catheterization, application of a condom-style catheter, management of feminine hygiene products, and wiping after toileting

Bridging. Bridging requires trunk extension, which is necessary at the trunk and hips to assume a functional bridge position. (The height of the bridge depends on the task. For example, bridging to use a bedpan requires more extension than bridging to don/doff pants.) See Chapter 14.

Scooting. Scooting requires the following movement:
- *Trunk flexion and extension:* Must be balanced for successful scooting (The efficiency of the scooting pattern is compromised if the patient maintains a flexed trunk with a posterior pelvic tilt or a hyperextended trunk.)
- *Lateral flexion:* Lower trunk initiation is used to clear the buttocks from the support surface, which is required to advance the hip forward.
- *Trunk rotation with extension:* Lower trunk initiation allows the patient to achieve the goal of scooting forward.

TREATMENT TECHNIQUES TO ENHANCE TRUNK CONTROL DURING TASK PERFORMANCE

Assuming an Appropriate Starting Posture

Before initiation of tasks and retraining of trunk control, the trunk must be in a proper biomechanical alignment. Therapists should observe patients anteriorly, posteriorly, and laterally to detect deviations from normal alignment (see Table 7-8).

Physically or verbally cueing patients to assume an appropriate starting posture should place them in a position of readiness for function-optimal symmetry in the trunk that is usually in midline, depending on the task (Box 7-3).

This neutral starting posture is similar to the position the trunk and lower extremities assume when a person begins a typing task.

An aligned and upright trunk posture has been shown to recruit muscle activity in the trunk. Floyd and Silver's electromyographic studies[25] demonstrated that a "slumped" position while sitting (simultaneous trunk flexion and extension of the hip joint) resulted in trunk extensor relaxation. In contrast, sitting upright in a chair without a backrest resulted in increased activity of the erector spinae muscle group. This muscle activity persisted as long as the trunk remained in extension, despite adjustments of the head and shoulders. A "slumped" posture, which consists of trunk flexion, posterior pelvic tilt, and resulting hip extension, is observed commonly during evaluation of posture in the stroke population; the position requires minimal skeletal muscle activity.

Andersson and Ortengren's review of the literature[1] demonstrated that the position of the feet had an effect on the myoelectric activity of the trunk extensors. Knee flexion (causing the feet to come toward the chair) increased muscle activity in the trunk, whereas knee extension resulted in a decrease in muscle activity. Stroke patients commonly assume a seated posture in which their feet (especially the more affected lower extremity) are positioned on the floor in front of their knees (e.g., in knee extension). The position of the feet tends to have an effect on pelvic tilt and resultant trunk postures. When the feet are positioned under the knees and toward the chair, an anterior pelvic tilt and trunk extension are enhanced. The opposite is also true: when the feet are positioned in front of the knees and the knees are extended, a posterior pelvic tilt and resulting trunk flexion are enhanced.

More recently, there is further empirical evidence that a neutral spine/starring position should be encouraged from both a neuromuscular and functional perspective. Cholewicki and colleagues[13] demonstrated that antagonistic trunk flexor-extensor muscle coactivation was present around the neutral spine posture in healthy individuals, and this coactivation increased with added mass to the torso. Gillen and colleagues[29] examined the effects of various seated trunk postures on upper extremity function. Fifty-nine adults were tested using the Jebsen Taylor Hand Function Test while in three different trunk postures. Significant mean differences between the neutral versus the flexed and laterally flexed trunk postures were noted during selected tasks. Specifically, dominant hand performance during the tasks of feeding and lifting heavy cans was significantly slower while the trunk was flexed and laterally flexed than when performed in the neutral trunk position. Performance of the nondominant hand during the tasks of picking up small objects, page turning, and the total score was slower while the trunk was flexed compared with performance in the neutral trunk position. These findings support the assumption that neutral trunk posture improves upper extremity performance during daily activities, although the effect is not consistent across tasks.

Patients should be encouraged to feel the difference between an aligned and a malaligned posture. The patient should be able to assume an appropriate posture automatically. Demonstration of the effect that a slumped posture has on reaching activities performed with the side less affected by the stroke may be helpful. Patients may realize that the distance and quality of their reach is enhanced when they are sitting in a proper alignment.

Although the use of mirrors for visual feedback may be appropriate for some patients, mirrors should be used with caution for patients with neurobehavioral deficits. Another technique for assisting patients with gaining symmetry is to have the therapist positioned in front of the patient and to assume the patient's postures to provide feedback for the patient. Therapists should slowly correct their posture, instructing the patient to mimic the movement. The therapist may state, "Keep your shoulders in line with mine" or "Keep your forehead at the same level as mine."

Mohr[40] emphasizes use of activities that encourage rotation and lateral flexion to gain midline control: "the active movements of the trunk into rotation and lateral flexion are caused by the same muscles that flex and extend the trunk. The different movements occur as a

---

Box 7-3

Seated Position of Readiness for Function

- Pelvis is in neutral to anterior tilt
- Equal weight-bearing on both ischial tuberosities
- Trunk erect and midline with appropriate spinal curves
- Shoulders symmetrical and over the hips
- Head/neck neutral
- Hips slightly above the level of the knees
- Knees in line with the hips
- Feet equally weight-bearing and underneath the knees

result of different interactions of these muscles with each other . . . In order for patients to achieve midline postural control, the therapist must work with the patient in the higher levels of lateral and rotational planes of movement."

Maintaining or Increasing Trunk Range of Motion through Mobilization and Movement

Concerning ROM in the trunk, Mohr[40] states, "If there is not full range in all trunk movements (flexion extension, lateral flexion, and rotation), it will be more difficult to gain full control of the trunk. Any lack of ROM in the trunk will lead to decreased function."

Although limited ROM in the extremities is commonly evaluated and treated, the ROM in the spine often is overlooked. After acute strokes, patients lose the ability to shift their weight and make postural adjustments. Evaluating patients who have trunks influenced completely by gravity and who demonstrate only static trunk postures is common. In these cases, prolonged immobilization of the trunk because of loss of control can result in loss of soft-tissue elasticity, joint play, and ultimately function. These problems, compounded by inappropriate trunk positioning and support in upright postures, lead to a cycle of immobility, soft-tissue changes, loss of range, and impaired functional abilities.

Specific trunk mobilization techniques are beyond the scope of this chapter but are discussed in the literature.[8,16,22,40] Just as therapists train patients to perform self-ROM activities for their extremities, therapists must promote patient awareness of trunk mobility and educate them about specific movement patterns that maintain and/or increase their trunk ROM. Following are examples of movement patterns that patients can perform to meet this goal:

1. While supine, patients flex their hips and knees as if preparing to bridge. Patients are instructed to keep their shoulders flat on the bed and simultaneously allow their knees to fall slowly from one side and then the other. This movement pattern encourages dissociation from the upper and lower trunk (rotation).
2. While supine, patients keep their hips and knees straight while cradling their more affected upper extremity. The goal is to lift and rotate the upper trunk as if initiating a roll with the upper trunk (rotation).
3. While sitting, patients cradle their more affected upper extremity against their chest. The therapist encourages patients to move the upper trunk in a twisting motion without letting the pelvis move (rotation).
4. While sitting, patients practice moving from an upright posture to a posture of lateral flexion on one side so that they are bearing weight on their forearm to the side of their trunk. The pelvis should

remain stable on the support surface for optimal stretch (lateral flexion).
5. While sitting, patients hold their more affected wrist and reach to the floor between their feet. The therapist also encourages them to allow their head to drop and dangle (flexion).
6. While supine, patients assume a bridge posture and hold the position as able (extension).
7. While sitting, patients practice lifting their hip from the support surface. This movement can be enhanced by having the patient reach up and to the side with the opposite upper extremity. Reaching beyond the arm span in this posture requires lateral flexion for the reach pattern to be successful (lateral flexion).

Using Various Postures

Therapists may use various postures as an adjunct treatment during patients' performance of functional tasks. Therapists should select postures based on specific patient needs. The chosen posture should accentuate and challenge the movement and control patterns interfering with independent performance of life activities. If the patient is not engaging in a specific activity (self-care tasks, games, and adapted sports), the use of these postures in isolation is not encouraged. Examples of varying postures include the following:

- **Seated with legs crossed:** Use of this posture is appropriate for patients whose inability to control lateral flexion and flexion patterns and to shift their weight is preventing functional independence. Working with patients in this posture encourages weight transference to one ischial tuberosity and has the added effect of challenging abdominal control. This occurs because the crossed leg is in a position of hip flexion. When the hips are flexed, the traction on the hamstrings tends to tilt the pelvis posteriorly,[33] resulting in a posterior shift in the center of gravity. Abdominal control therefore is required to prevent a posterior loss of balance. Participation in tasks such as lower extremity dressing, lower body washing, and activities such as modified volleyball place extra demands on patients who are in this position.
- **Sitting in front of a table while bearing weight on both forearms:** Ryerson and Levit[44] recommend this posture during the acute stage of hemiplegia when little postural control is evident. In this posture, patients use their upper extremities as a point of proximal stability. The therapist should stress that the arm should be active and the trunk should not be allowed to "hang" on an inactive arm. Patients are encouraged to practice anterior, posterior, and lateral shifting in this posture to reestablish postural control; coordinate trunk, scapula, and humerus patterns; and to establish weight-bearing of the upper

extremities. Because both arms are engaged in a weight-bearing activity, patient participation in functional tasks is difficult. Immediately following use of this posture, the therapist must engage the patient in a follow-up activity such as reaching to ensure the postures can be incorporated into ADL.

- **Prone on elbows:** Although effective for gaining trunk extension, this position should be used with caution. The position may compromise respiratory status, cause shoulder pain if upper extremity alignment is not considered, and be generally uncomfortable for older stroke patients. The position may be effective for some patients and may be a required posture for some transitional movements such as floor-to-chair transfers.
- **Kneeling:** This posture is appropriate for patients having trouble in gaining trunk/hip extension. Patients also may find this posture uncomfortable, but it may be necessary for transitional patterns.
- **Variations on the degree of hip flexion while seated:** Changing the position of the lower extremities can challenge the performance of specific trunk patterns. Being in a position with the knees below the hips, such as sitting on a high stool, decreases the amount of hip flexion and has a tendency to place the trunk in increased extension.

Conversely, positioning the patient with the knees above the hips (increasing the amount of hip flexion) results in a position of trunk flexion and a posterior weight shift, which places greater demands on the trunk flexors.

Treating the "Pusher Syndrome" or Contraversive Pushing

The "pusher syndrome" is a phrase coined by Davies,[19] who derived the name from what she felt was the most striking aspect of this syndrome: the patient pushes heavily toward the hemiplegic side in all positions and resists any attempt at passive correction (i.e., a correction that would bring the weight toward or over the midline of the body to the unaffected side). This phenomenon has been documented in patients with both right and left hemispheric lesions. Further analysis has revealed that the brain structure typically damaged in patients with pusher syndrome is the left or right posterolateral thalamus.[36]

Danells and colleagues[15] defined pushing as "resistant to accepting weight on and actively 'push' away from the nonparetic side." The authors identified pushers (n=65) from stroke patients with moderate to severe hemiparesis and examined longitudinal changes in symptoms, level of impairment, and functional independence. Assessments were performed within 10 days postonset, at six weeks, and at three months. The authors found:

- At one week after stroke, 63% of patients demonstrated features of pushing.

- In 62% of pushers, symptoms resolved by six weeks, whereas in 21%, pushing symptoms persisted at three months.
- Motor recovery and functional abilities at three months were significantly lower among the pushers compared with the nonpushers.
- Pushers also had a significantly longer hospital length of stay (89 days versus 57 days).
- Motor and functional recovery improved significantly over the three-month study period for both pushers and nonpushers.
- Although the pushers had greater lengths of stay in both acute care and rehabilitation facilities, they were discharged home with similar frequency to the nonpushers.

Perennou and colleagues[42] investigated whether the pusher syndrome affects only the trunk for which gravitational feedback is given by somesthetic information, or the head as well (gravitational information given by the vestibular system). The results of their pilot study indicated that that the pusher syndrome does not result from disrupted processing of vestibular information but from a higher-order disruption in the processing of somesthetic information originating in the left hemibody, which could be an extinction phenomenon. The authors felt that this disruption leads pushers actively to adjust their body posture to a subjective vertical bias to the side opposite the lesion.

Pedersen and colleagues[41] also examined the pusher syndrome. The study examined the incidence of the syndrome, the relation of this syndrome to neurobehavioral deficits, and the effect of the syndrome on the rehabilitation process in 327 patients. The study revealed a 10% incidence and found no significant differences in hemineglect or anosognosia in patients with and without ipsilateral pushing. The study discovered that patients who demonstrated ipsilateral pushing required 3.6 weeks longer to reach the same outcome as patients who did not demonstrate ipsilateral pushing. Of note in this study are the Barthel index scores at admission and discharge. On admission, patients who demonstrated ipsilateral pushing scored an average of 13.7 on the Barthel index compared with 46.8 for patients without evidence of pushing. On discharge, the average score for pushers was 43.9 compared with 66.8 for patients without pushing. The discharge scores (in terms of ADL function) of the patients who were pushers were still below the admission scores for patients who did not push.

Davies[17] summarizes the typical signs of the pusher syndrome as the following:

- Head turned away from affected side and laterally flexed toward stronger side
- Decreased ability to perceive stimuli from affected side
- Lack of facial expression

- Poor breath control with monotone, hypophonic voice
- An elongated affected side
- Evidence of pushing with stronger leg while supine
- Holding onto side of bed or mat as if falling
- Shortening of stronger side of trunk with elongation of hemiplegic side while sitting
- Marked resistance to attempts to transfer weight to stronger side
- Pushing with stronger arm and leg to more affected side
- Difficulty transferring, especially to stronger side
- All weight shifted to affected side while standing; leaning against therapist's supporting arm or flexing forward at hips
- Hemiplegic leg adduction (scissors) when walking; difficulty taking a step with affected leg because of an inability to shift weight to stronger side

Pushing can be quantified via the Scale for Contraversive Pushing (SCP).[35] It is scored 0 to 6 with higher the scores indicating a greater severity of pushing. There are three domains (posture, extension, and resistance) that are assessed for both sitting and standing positions (i.e., six scored items) (Box 7-4). Using a cut score of greater than 0 in each section appears to increase the agreement of clinical and SCP observations and has been suggested.[4]

Unfortunately at this point, specific interventions are based on anecdotal evidence only, but they may still be helpful to clinicians. Davies[17] recommends the following specific treatments for the pusher syndrome:

- Restore head movements: maintain full passive ROM, stretch, and encourage active ROM by scanning activities.
- Activate the side flexors (see activities described in previous sections).
- Use functional activities to regain midline while standing.

Karnath and Broetz[37] recommend the following intervention sequence:

- Realize the disturbed perception of erect body position.
- Visually explore the surroundings and the body's relation to the surroundings. Ensure that the patient sees whether he or she is oriented upright. The therapist should use visual aids that give feedback about body orientation (i.e., the therapist's arm) and work in a room containing many vertical structures, such as door frames, windows, pillars, and so on.
- Learn the movements necessary to reach a vertical body position.
- Maintain the vertical body position while performing other activities.

Box 7-4

The Scale for Contraversive Pushing

	Sitting	Standing
(A) Posture (symmetry of spontaneous posture)		
Score 1 = severe contraversive tilt with falling to the contralesional side	☐	☐
Score 0.75 = severe contraversive tilt without falling	☐	☐
Score 0.25 = mild contraversive tilt without falling	☐	☐
Score 0 = no tilt/upright body orientation	☐	☐
Total (max = 2):		
(B) Extension (use of the arm/leg to extend the area of physical contact to the ground)		
Score 1 = performed already in rest	☐	☐
Score 0.5 = performed not until position is changed	☐	☐
Score 0 = no extension	☐	☐
Total (max = 2):		
(C) Resistance (resistance to passive correction of posture to an upright position)		
Score 1 = resistance is shown	☐	☐
Score 0 = resistance is not shown	☐	☐
Total (max = 2):		

Max, maximum.

Translated from Karnath HO, Ferber S, Dichgans J: The origin of contraversive pushing. *Neurology* 55(9):1298-1304, 2000.

Note: For section B: For sitting, ask the patient to glide the buttocks on the mattress toward the nonparetic side, to transfer from bed to wheelchair toward the nonparetic side, or both. For standing, ask the patient to start walking. If pushing already occurs when the patient is rising from the sitting position, section B is given the value of 1 for standing.

For section C: Touch the patient at the sternum and the back. Give the following instructions: "I will move your body sideward. Please permit this movement."

A hands-on approach does not seem to be effective with patients who have the pusher syndrome; therapists' attempts to assist patients with gaining midline by handling is met by further patient resistance. Manipulating the environment and providing external cues (verbal) seem to be more effective. Examples include the following:

- Have patients reach with their stronger upper extremity for objects beyond their arm span to encourage a weight shift to the stronger side.
- Provide verbal cues to realign the trunk, such as, "Bring your head toward mine" and "Bring your left shoulder toward the wall."
- Provide a target toward which patients can move their trunk and maintain the position as long as possible. For example, place a bolster on patients' stronger side, and cue them to lean against the bolster and hold the position.
- Remove surfaces from which to push. For example, raise the hospital bed or therapy table, so that the person's foot is not on the floor and place a movable surface (e.g., small ball) under the less affected foot to prevent pushing.

Further empirical intervention studies are needed in this area of practice.

Engaging in Reaching Tasks

Therapists can use placement of objects in reaching activities as a way to place a variety of demands on the trunk. The key to eliciting a trunk response is to place the object slightly beyond the arm's reach. Fisher[24] observes that when subjects without brain injuries reach, they anteriorly tilt the pelvis, slightly extend the upper back, and move the trunk in the direction of the arm. Patients with brain injuries do not incorporate trunk movements into arm movements and reach only to arm's length as they maintain a slumped posture.

Therapists have the ability to control the desired response by the way they set up the activity. Setting up the activity includes placing items required during ADL in specific places, choosing the appropriate environment (e.g., kitchen with upper and lower shelves, bookcase, desk space, meal table), deciding how far beyond the arm span the activity should be placed, and deciding on the characteristics of the objects the patient is reaching for (number of objects, weight of the objects, and whether objects require one or two hands). Table 7-11 includes examples of activity placement and resulting trunk response.

Dean and Shepard[18] investigated, via a randomized placebo-controlled trial of task-related training after stroke, the effect of a training program designed to improve the ability to balance in sitting after stroke. The training program was designed to improve sitting balance and involved emphasis on appropriate loading of the affected leg while at the same time practicing reaching tasks using the unaffected hand to grasp objects located beyond arm's length. The reaching tasks were performed under varied conditions. Changing the location of the object that the subject was reaching for varied the distance and direction of reach. Seat height, movement speed, object weight, and extent of thigh support were also varied. Increasing the number of repetitions and complexity of the tasks advanced the training. The authors found that after training, subjects were able to reach faster and farther, increase load through the affected foot, and increase activation of affected leg muscles compared with the control group (highlighting the critical contribution of the lower extremities in promoting sitting balance). The experimental group also improved in sit to stand. The control group did not improve in reaching or sit to stand, and finally, neither group improved in walking. See Tables 7-9 and 7-11 for suggestions to grade reaching tasks.

Using Movable Surfaces

Several authors have advocated the use of movable surfaces to challenge trunk control.[8,16,32] Movable surfaces used in treatment include items such as therapy balls, bolsters, and rocker boards. Movable surfaces can be used in treatment in a variety of ways, including the following:

- To grade the difficulty of the task
- To challenge the patient to maintain control of the surface without outside assistance (challenge isometric patterns)
- To allow the patient to respond to the therapist's perturbation of the movable surface

Table 7-11

Examples of Grading Activities during Reaching Tasks

	EASIER	MORE DIFFICULT
Sitting surface	Firm and stable surface	Cushioned or unstable surface
	Full thigh support	Partial thigh support
Object	Within arm's reach	Beyond arm's reach
	Light (e.g., a pencil)	Heavy (e.g., bag of flour)
Use of arms	Reach with one arm	Reach with both arms
External support	Maximum via therapist, bolsters, and so on	None
Prediction	Predictable (e.g., lift stationary object)	Unpredictable (e.g., catch a ball)

- To allow the patient to initiate moving the surface
- To enhance stretching and mobilization of the trunk by using a particular surface such as a large ball
- To add variety to treatment sessions
- To focus on isolated trunk control

Use of movable surfaces may be appropriate for patients who are experiencing difficulty controlling their trunk in environments with external perturbations (e.g., trains, automobiles, and buses). Although movable surfaces are used commonly in the clinic, research concerning the effectiveness of this type of treatment compared with other types is lacking. One may argue that when patients master trunk control on a movable surface (a difficult situation), their control will improve on less demanding surfaces (surfaces that do not move). Unfortunately, this argument is not supported by current research that advocates task-specific training.

Handling

Handling is a common technique used in the clinic. This intervention commonly is associated with neurodevelopmental therapy[7] and may allow the patient to feel the desired movement pattern, gain range, assist weak movement patterns, and provide external support to prevent falls. To be effective, the patient must be aware of the goal associated with handling, and the therapist should use handling within the context of a functional task. In addition, the handling from the therapist should be graded to allow the patient to perform as much of the movement pattern as possible. A variety of texts that review specific techniques of handling are available.[7,8,16,17,22,32] Although handling is commonly used, research does not support use of this technique (see Chapter 6).

Using Activities of Daily Living and Mobility Tasks

Clearly the most effective tools that occupational therapists can use to help patients regain trunk control are self-care, instrumental ADL, and mobility tasks.

The therapist first must perform a thorough evaluation as described in previous sections. Following the evaluation, therapists and patients should identify the most problematic movement patterns that occur during the patients' daily activities. At this point, therapists use their activity analysis skills to choose appropriate tasks that incorporate the desired patterns and postures as described previously. For example, if the identified problematic patterns are lateral flexion and lateral weight shifts, therapists may choose the following activities for the patient to practice:

- Lower extremity dressing
- Weight shifting for pressure relief
- Scooting
- Assuming a sitting position from side-lying position
- Reaching for objects that are positioned above and to the side of the patient opposite the side where lateral flexion is desired

- Reaching for objects on the floor that are on the side of the patient

The majority of ADL and mobility tasks encompass a variety of postures and movements. For the mentioned strategies to be effective, therapists should initially focus patients' attention on the desired components of trunk movements. As the patient progresses, the obvious goal is for the trunk responses to be relearned and become automatic.

Therapeutic Exercise

A recent pilot randomized controlled trial[55] (N = 33) documented that conventional occupational and physical therapy combined with additional trunk exercises aimed at improving sitting balance and selective trunk movements has a positive effective on the selective performance of lateral flexion after stroke. Specifically, the experimental group received 10 hours of additional trunk exercises that included:

- **Supine exercises with legs bent and meet on the therapy table:** anterior/posterior pelvic movements, bridging, and trunk rotation, initiated from the upper and lower trunk
- **In sitting:** flexion and extension of the trunk without moving the trunk forward or backward, flexion/extension of the lumbar spine, flexion/extension of the hips with the trunk extended, lateral flexion of the trunk initiated from the shoulder and pelvic girdle, upper and lower trunk rotation, and scooting forward and backwards.

Adapting the Environment

Some patients may have little improvement in trunk control. Environmental adaptations are necessary for these patients to enhance independent performance. Examples include

- Use of outside supports can help maintain trunk stability while the extremities are engaged in functional tasks. Supports such as lateral supports, anterior chest straps, arm chairs, pillows and cushions for propping, and lap trays are examples of equipment used to compensate for compromised trunk control (see Chapter 26).
- Rearrangement of the environment can decrease demands on the trunk. Placing required equipment within the patient's reach (arm reach) not only increases independence but also may prevent falls. Storing dishes on the counter instead of in a cabinet, placing utensils in front of the patient, and keeping grooming items on top of the sink instead of in a medicine cabinet are examples of this strategy.
- Provision of adaptive equipment is a common strategy to increase independent performance and minimize safety risks. ADL equipment issued to compensate for poor trunk control may include the

following: long-handled shoe horns, elastic laces, adapted bath brushes, soap on a rope, reachers, tub seats, and commodes. See Chapter 28 for more information on adaptive devices.

- Home modifications such as grab bars and bed rails also may be indicated. See Chapter 27 for a full review of home adaptations and equipment recommendations.

CASE STUDY

Regaining Trunk Control after a Stroke

S.G. is a 64-year-old female who came to the rehabilitation unit after a right middle cerebral artery cerebrovascular accident. The following data were collected from the initial evaluation (specific to the trunk):

- Sensation was intact.
- Static postural malalignments included posterior pelvic tilt, retracted left rib cage, and increased weight-bearing on left ischial tuberosity.
- Dynamical posture was difficult to assess because the patient was afraid to move. The patient could not reach beyond her arm span when reaching with her right arm. She had a tendency to fall backward and to the left during lower extremity dressing and when reaching for objects behind her.
- S.G.'s personal occupational therapy goals were to be able independently to don her shoes, be able to reach for objects she had dropped without falling, and decrease the amount of spillage that occurred during meals.

The initial treatment plan included adapting her wheelchair with lateral supports (which were removed when she was supervised by friends, family, and staff) and a lumbar roll to maintain optimal alignment while functioning in the wheelchair, trunk mobilizations (specifically in the directions of extension and lateral flexion to both sides), activities to recruit abdominal activity (rolling, games that encouraged trunk rotation, reaching for objects positioned overhead and behind her), and activities that presented unexpected challenges to her trunk control (e.g., balloon volleyball and catch). During the initial stages of treatment, the therapist sat behind S.G. in a straddle position, which increased feelings of security and allowed the therapist to provide outside assistance with difficult patterns and to prevent falls. S.G. was observed while eating, and the therapist noted that she did not shift her weight anteriorly when bringing food to her mouth. Instead she kept her trunk supported against the back of the chair. Because of the increased distance the food had to travel to reach her mouth, spillage was considerable, especially of liquids on a spoon (e.g., soup and cereal milk). S.G. was trained to shift her weight forward as she brought food to her mouth. Although spillage still occurred, it happened less frequently, with the food falling to the plate or table and not in her lap.

As S.G. progressed, the therapist was able to sit next to or in front of her during activities. She engaged in graded reaching activities in which the distance S.G. was required to reach was increased progressively. Activities included reaching to lower shelves in the refrigerator and reaching for objects positioned at specific levels (e.g., knee level, midshin level, and floor level).

On discharge from inpatient rehabilitation, S.G. was able to perform all basic ADL with distant supervision and without assistive devices, reach to the floor when she propped her upper trunk with her more affected forearm against her knees, and eat independently by using a rocker knife to cut her food, with spillage occurring only 10% of the time.

REVIEW QUESTIONS

1. What is considered an aligned posture in preparation for engagement in functional tasks? What are the common deviations from this posture after stroke?
2. Name three ADL tasks that require control in the rotation plane.
3. What are advantages and disadvantages of using movable surfaces in trunk control treatment?
4. What are appropriate treatment activities for patients who lack trunk extensor control?
5. Explain the reason an appropriate starting alignment is considered a prerequisite for initiating functional activities.
6. Which trunk patterns are required for donning a button-down shirt?

REFERENCES

1. Andersson BJ, Ortengren R: Myoelectric back activity during sitting. *Scand J Rehabil Med* Suppl 3:73–90, 1974.
2. Árnadóttir G: *The brain and behavior: assessing cortical dysfunction through activities of daily living*, St. Louis, 1990, Mosby.
3. Ayres AJ: *Developmental dyspraxia and adult onset apraxia*, Torrance, CA, 1985, Sensory Integration International.
4. Baccini M, Paci M, Rinaldi LA. The Scale for Contraversive Pushing: a reliability and validity study. *Neurorehabil Neural Repair* 20(4): 468–472, 2006.
5. Basmajian JV, DeLuca CJ: *Muscles alive: their functions revealed by electromyography*, ed 5, Baltimore, 1985, Williams & Wilkins.
6. Benaim C, Perennou DA, Villy J, et al: Validation of a standardized assessment of postural control in stroke patients. *Stroke* 30(9): 1862–1868, 1999.
7. Bobath B: *Adult hemiplegia: evaluation and treatment*, ed 3, London, 1990, Butterworth-Heinemann.
8. Boehme R: *Improving upper body control: an approach to the treatment of tonal dysfunction*, Tucson, AZ, 1988, Therapy Skill Builders.
9. Bohannon RW: Recovery and correlates of trunk muscle strength after stroke. *Int J Rehabil Res* 18(2):162–167, 1995.

10. Bohannon RW: Lateral trunk flexion strength: impairment, measurement reliability and implications following unilateral brain lesion. *Int J Rehabil Res* 15(3):249–251, 1992.

11. Bohannon RW, Cassidy D, Walsh S: Trunk muscle strength is impaired multidirectionally after stroke. *Clin Rehabil* 9(1):47, 1995.

12. Carr JH, Shepherd RB, Nordholm L, et al: Investigation of a new motor assessment scale for stroke patients. *Phys Ther* 65(2):175–180, 1985.

13. Cholewicki J, Panjabi M, Khachatryan A. Stabilizing function of trunk flexor and extensor muscles around a neutral spine posture. *Spine* 22(19):2207–2212, 1997.

14. Collin C, Wade D: Assessing motor impairment after stroke: a pilot reliability study. *J Neurol Neurosurg Psychiatry* 53(7):576–579, 1990.

15. Danells CJ, Black SE, Gladstone DJ, et al: Poststroke "pushing": natural history and relationship to motor and functional recovery. *Stroke* 35(12):2873–8, 2004.

16. Davies PM: *Right in the middle: selective trunk activity in the treatment of adult hemiplegia*, New York, 1990, Springer-Verlag.

17. Davies PM: *Steps to follow: a guide to the treatment of adult hemiplegia*, New York, 1985, Springer-Verlag.

18. Dean CW, Shepard RB: Task-related training improves performance of seated reaching tasks after stroke: a randomized controlled trial. *Stroke* 28(4):722–728, 1997.

19. De Troyer A: Mechanical role of the abdominal muscles in relation to posture. *Respir Physiol* 53(3):341–353, 1983.

20. Dickstein R, Sheffi S, Markovici E, et al: Anticipatory postural adjustment in selected trunk muscles in post stroke hemiparetic patients. *Arch Phys Med Rehabil* 85(2):261–7, 2004.

21. Duarte E, Marco E, Muniesa JM, et al: Trunk control test as a functional predictor in stroke patients. *J Rehabil Med* 34(6):267–272, 2002.

22. Eggers O: *Occupational therapy in the treatment of adult hemiplegia*, New York, 1983, Springer-Verlag.

23. Esparza DY, Archambault PS, Winstein CJ, et al: Hemispheric specialization in the co-ordination of arm and trunk movements during pointing in patients with unilateral brain damage. *Exp Brain Res* 148(4):488–497, 2003.

24. Fisher B: Effect of trunk control and alignment on limb function. *J Head Trauma Rehabil* 2(2):72, 1987.

25. Floyd WF, Silver PHS: The function of the erector spinae muscles in certain movements and postures in man. *J Physiol* 129(1):184, 1955.

26. Franchignoni FP, Tesio L, Ricupero C, et al: Trunk control as an early predictor of stroke rehabilitation outcome. *Stroke* 28(7):1382–1385, 1997.

27. Fugl-Meyer AR: Post-stroke hemiplegia: assessment of physical properties. *Scand J Rehabil Med* 7(suppl):85–93, 1980.

28. Fujiwara T, Liu M, Tsuji T, et al: Development of a new measure to assess trunk impairment after stroke (trunk impairment scale): its psychometric properties. *Am J Phys Med Rehabil* 83(9):681–8, 2004.

29. Gillen G, Boiangiu C, Neuman M, et al: Trunk posture affects upper extremity function of adults. *Percept Mot Skills* 104(2):371–380, 2007.

30. Gowland C, Stratford P, Ward M, et al: Measuring physical impairment and disability with the Chedoke-McMaster Stroke Assessment. *Stroke* 24 (1):58–63, 1993.

31. Hsieh CL, Sheu CF, Hsueh IP, et al: Trunk control as an early predictor of comprehensive activities of daily living function in stroke patients. *Stroke* 33(11):2626–2630, 2002.

32. Hypes B: *Facilitating development and sensorimotor function: treatment with the ball*, Hugo, MN, 1991, PDP Press.

33. Kapandji IA: *The physiology of the joints, vol 3, The trunk and vertebral column*, New York, 1974, Churchill Livingstone.

34. Karatas M, Cetin N, Bayramoglu M, et al: Trunk muscle strength in relation to balance and functional disability in unihemispheric stroke patients. *Am J Phys Med Rehabil* 83(2):81–87, 2004.

35. Karnath HO, Ferber S, Dichgans J. The origin of contraversive pushing. *Neurology* 55(9):1298–1304, 2000.

36. Karnath H-O, Ferber S, Dichgans J: The neural representation of postural control in humans. *Proc Natl Acad Sci USA* 97(25):13931–13936, 2000.

37. Karnath HO, Broetz D: Understanding and treating "pusher syndrome." *Phys Ther* 83(12):1119–1125, 2003.

38. Kendall FP, McCreary EK, Provance P: *Muscles testing and function*, ed 4, Baltimore, 1993, Lippincott Williams & Wilkins.

39. Mao HF, Hsueh IP, Tang PF, et al: Analysis and comparison of the psychometric properties of three balance measures for stroke patients. *Stroke* 33(4):1022–1027, 2002.

40. Mohr JD: Management of the trunk in adult hemiplegia: the Bobath concept. *Top Neurol* 1(1):1–12, 1990.

41. Pedersen PM, Wandel A, Jorgensen HS, et al: Ipsilateral pushing in stroke: incidence, relation to neuropsychological symptoms, and impact on rehabilitation: the Copenhagen stroke study. *Arch Phys Med Rehabil* 77(1):25–28, 1996.

42. Perennou DA, Amblard B, Laassel el M, et al: Understanding the pusher behavior of some stroke patients with spatial deficits: a pilot study. *Arch Phys Med Rehabil* 83(4):570–575, 2002.

43. Ryerson S, Byl NN, Brown DA, et al: Altered trunk position sense and its relation to balance functions in people post-stroke. *J Neurol Phys Ther* 32(1):14–20, 2008

44. Ryerson S, Levit K: The shoulder in hemiplegia. In Donatelli RA, editor: *Physical therapy of the shoulder*, ed 2, New York, 1991, Churchill Livingstone.

45. Sabari JS: Motor learning concepts applied to activity-based intervention with adults with hemiplegia. *Am J Occup Ther* 45(6):523–530, 1991.

46. Shumway-Cook A, Woollacott M: *Motor control: theory and practical applications*, Baltimore, 1995, Williams & Wilkins.

47. Smith LK, Weiss EL, Lehmkuhl, LD: *Brunnstrom's clinical kinesiology*, ed 5, Philadelphia, 1996, FA Davis.

48. Tanaka S, Hachisuka K, Ogata H: Muscle strength of trunk flexion-extension in post-stroke hemiplegic patients. *Am J Phys Med Rehabil* 77(4):288–290, 1998.

49. Tanaka S, Hachisuka K, Ogata H: Trunk rotary muscle performance in post-stroke hemiplegic patients. *Am J Phys Med Rehabil* 76(5):366–369, 1997.

50. Thorstensson A, Oddsson L, Carlson H: Motor control of voluntary trunk movements in standing. *Acta Physiol Scand* 125(2):309, 1985.

51. Verheyden G, Nieuwboer A, De Wit L, et al: Time course of trunk, arm, leg, and functional recovery after ischemic stroke, *Neurorehabil Neural Repair* 22(2):173–9, 2008.

52. Verheyden G, Vereeck L, Truijen S, et al: Trunk performance after stroke and the relationship with balance, gait and functional ability, *Clinical Rehabilitation* 20(5):451–8, 2006.

53. Verheyden G, Nieuwboer A, Mertin J, et al: The Trunk Impairment Scale: a new tool to measure motor impairment of the trunk after stroke. *Clin Rehabil* 18(3):326–34, 2004.

54. Verheyden G, Nieuwboer A, Van de Winckel A, et al: Clinical tools to measure trunk performance after stroke: a systematic review of the literature. *Clinical Rehabilitation* 21(5):387–94, 2007.

55. Verheyden G, Vereeck L, Truijen S, et al: Additional exercises improve trunk performance after stroke: a pilot randomized controlled trial. *Neurorehabil Neural Repair* 23(30):281–286, 2009.

56. Wang CH, Hsueh IP, Sheu CF, et al: Discriminative, predictive, and evaluative properties of a trunk control measure in patients with stroke. *Phys Ther* 85(9):887–94, 2005.

57. Winzeler-Mercay U, Mudie H: The nature of the effects of stroke on trunk flexor and extensor muscles during work and rest. *Disabil Rehabil* 24(17):875–886, 2002.

58. Woodhull-McNeal AP: Activity in torso muscles during relaxed standing. *Eur J Appl Physiol* 55(4):418–424, 1986.

susan m. donato
karen halliday pulaski

chapter 8

Overview of Balance Impairments: Functional Implications

key terms

balance

base of support

center of mass

gaze stabilization

limits of stability

posture

chapter objectives

After completing this chapter, the reader will be able to accomplish the following:

1. Identify the systems involved in balance, and understand the assessment and evaluation of component balance skills and balance during functional activity.
2. Provide examples of treatment plans and ideas based on specific balance dysfunctions to allow the therapist to implement focused intervention.
3. Participate in the development of goals and documentation systems with emphasis on the setting for service delivery and the effect of the current health care environment.

THEORY

Balance is the ability to control the center of mass over the base of support within the limits of stability; balance results in the maintenance of stability and equilibrium. A person's ability to maintain balance in any position depends on a complex integration of multiple systems. Many theories have been proposed to explain the ability to maintain balance. In the now outdated reflex or hierarchical model, balance was considered the interaction of reflexes and reactions, which are organized hierarchically, that result in the support of the body against gravity.[22,32] In this model, balance deficits result from eliminating higher central nervous system control, resulting in the release of spinal and supraspinal reflexes. This model has declined in popularity in recent years because common opinion embraces the idea that the nervous system more likely is comprised of complex interactions of multiple systems rather than organized as a distinct hierarchy. See Chapter 4.

The systems or distributed control model introduced by Bernstein describes balance as a complex interaction of musculoskeletal and neural systems.[50] The ability to maintain balance is specific to and modified around the constraints of the environment and task. Within this system a disruption of balance (or instability) results from a malfunction in or disruption of any one or more of the elements of the postural control system. Likewise, balance is maintained through the interaction of sensory organization and postural control systems. The information is combined and integrated in the central nervous system.

SENSORY ORGANIZATION

According to the systems model, information from three sensory systems is used for maintaining balance. Information from the visual, vestibular, and somatosensory systems is critically important.

The visual system (see Chapter 16) provides information regarding vertical orientation and visual flow. Visual or optical flow information, which describes movement of an image on the retina, is important input that aids detection of personal and environmental movement. Information provided by the visual system can be ambiguous and must be compared with other sensory information to determine accuracy. For example, a person sitting in a stationary car next to another stationary car at a red light then may receive optical flow information that indicates the other car is moving backward. This information alone is not adequate for determining which vehicle is moving; it only reveals relative movement. The information must be compared with the other sensory information to determine which car has moved.

Somatosensory information is comprised of cutaneous and pressure receptors on the soles of the feet and of muscle and joint receptors. This information helps determine characteristics of and the relationship of the individual to the support surface. During most tasks, somatosensory information may be the most heavily relied on input in the adult population. Like visual input, somatosensory input can be ambiguous. For example, dorsiflexion at the ankle indicates that the body is displaced anteriorly over the base of support. However, when standing on an incline, this ankle position may coincide with midline posture. The individual must consider other senses to determine which position is accurate.

Information from the vestibular system helps determine head position and head motion in space relative to gravity. This information generally plays a minor role in balance control, unless somatosensory and visual inputs are inaccurate or unavailable. The vestibular system is the only sensory reference that is not ambiguous because it depends on gravity, which is consistent in the environment. The vestibular system (see Chapter 9) is composed of the otolith and semicircular canals. The semicircular canals sense angular acceleration, which is a change in velocity along a curved path (e.g., shaking or nodding the

head). The canals are capable of detecting movement in all planes because all three are oriented in different planes (Fig. 8-1). Input from the semicircular canals influences postural responses and drives compensatory eye movements.

The otolith is composed of the utricle and saccule. Together they are responsible for determining changes in head position in the linear plane or translational movement of the head. Specifically, the utricle responds to head tilt and translations along the horizontal plane. In addition, the utricle appears to play an important role in producing small, torsional eye movements, which keep the eyes level when the head is tilted laterally. This helps with maintaining postural control and vertical orientation in space. The saccule appears to be instrumental in detecting vertical translations of the head.

In addition to these three systems, individuals' internal representations or perceptions influence the interactions of information. Each individual possesses an internal perception related to the task, themselves, and the environment, which in turn influences sensory interactions and responses.

To use sensory information appropriately, each individual develops what is referred to as a *sensory strategy*. A sensory strategy is formulated when the central nervous system integrates, evaluates, and selects information received from the visual, somatosensory, and vestibular systems. The information is evaluated according to internal and external constraints, including availability of sensory information and the accuracy of environmental information. Information evaluation also may depend on the occurring movement strategy occurring. The development of a sensory strategy results in a sensory-motor interaction. The central nervous system determines the most efficient use of sensory input, which then allows for generation of appropriate motor output to complete the

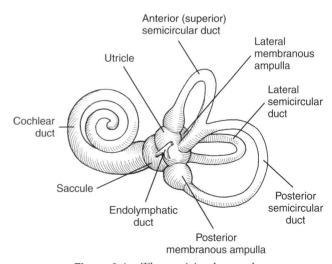

Figure 8-1   The semicircular canals.

necessary task or reach a desired goal. This rapid process is not detectable when no deficits exist.

POSTURAL CONTROL

An individual's ability to maintain equilibrium depends not only on accurate evaluation and use of sensory information but also on the implementation of effective movement strategies. Movement strategies are stereotyped or synergistic patterns used to maintain the center of mass over the base of support; they are characterized as automatic, not reflexive or voluntary. Movement strategies occur too quickly to be under voluntary control but are too slow to be considered reflexive. Synergistic movement patterns are useful in that they reduce the degrees of freedom, thus decreasing the response time. Postural actions are reduced or absent when an individual uses an external support such as a cane or countertop to help maintain postural control. Automatic postural responses include ankle, hip, and stepping strategies.[47]

An ankle strategy is used to maintain the center of mass over the base of support when movement is centered on the ankles. Knee, hip, and trunk stability is necessary for this strategy to be effective. Ankle strategies are used to control small, slow swaying motions. They are effective when the surface area is firm and long in relation to foot length. Muscular activation while using the ankle strategy occurs in a distal to proximal sequence. Timing of muscular contractions is important to generate sufficient torque about the ankles and to maintain adequate stability at the hips, knees, and trunk. Ankle strategies frequently are used during "quiet" standing. For example, this strategy is effective in controlling the small, slow swaying motions that occur when a person stands in line (e.g., at a bank or grocery store).

Hip movement that maintains or restores equilibrium is a hip strategy. This strategy is most effective in maintaining stability when the support surface is short in relation to foot length or is compliant. Hip movement is used to control large or rapid swaying motions or when an ankle strategy is ineffective (i.e., unable to occur rapidly enough or generate adequate torque). Muscle activation while using hip strategies occurs in a proximal to distal sequence. This strategy is used more frequently than ankle strategies when the center of mass approaches the outer limits of the base of support and is more effective because of the ability to generate greater speed and range. An example of a situation in which persons would use a hip strategy would be a circumstance that requires them to stand on a narrow beam.

When ankle and hip strategies are or are perceived to be ineffective, the base of support is expanded in the direction of center of mass movement, resulting in the use of what is called a *stepping strategy*. In this case the person

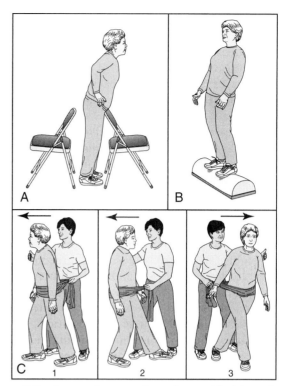

Figure 8-2 Automatic postural reactions: ankle, hip, and stepping strategies. (From Cameron MH, Monroe LG: *physical rehabilitation: evidence-based examination, evaluation, and intervention*, St. Louis, 2007, Saunders.)

takes a step to widen the base of support. This is the strategy used effectively when taking each step while walking. The person shifts weight outside the existing base of support and takes a step to bring the base of support back under the center of mass (Fig. 8-2).

Each of the preceding movement strategies is a reactive response to center of mass movement. Anticipatory control is postural muscular activity that precedes and decreases center of mass movement. Previous experience weighs heavily in the determination of the appropriate sequence and degree of muscle activity required to maintain stability when anticipating a perturbation. Because anticipatory activities precede destabilization, misperceiving the needed amount of muscle activity may result in too much or too little correction. For example, when persons pull a door open, they initiate a posterior weight shift to counteract the weight of the door. If the weight of the door is lighter than anticipated, too much correction might occur and may result in a posterior perturbation of balance.

CENTRAL NERVOUS SYSTEM STRUCTURES

Maintaining equilibrium involves the precise integration of sensory information and the generation of appropriate and effective motor responses. Specific central nervous system structures are responsible for performing these complex tasks. The cerebellum is the primary integrating and modulating force in balance control. The cerebellum receives information from structures such as the cortex, basal ganglia, spinocerebellar tract, vestibular nuclei, and vestibular pathways. Input is modulated, interpreted, and sent out to the cortex; basal ganglia; thalamus; fourth, fifth, and sixth cranial nerves; vestibular nuclei and pathways; and indirectly to the spinal cord, providing the regulatory input needed to control movement. Damage to any one of these structures can result in difficulties with balance and postural control. Through this complex network of central nervous system interactions the cerebellum facilitates smooth coordination of movement. The cerebellum influences the timing and synergy of muscle groups during synergistic movements and muscle tone or stiffness. Symmetrical, appropriate, balanced skeletal muscle activity is necessary for maintaining postural alignment and is required for smooth, coordinated movements and stability. An example of a disorder involving the cerebellum is ataxia (poor coordination of agonist and antagonist muscles that results in jerky, poorly controlled movements). An individual with cerebellar dysfunction might have an unsteady gait or visual disturbances. See Chapter 15.

The basal ganglia are also involved in integrating information used for postural control and in a series of complex pathways, much of the exact nature of which is uncertain.

The basal ganglia receive information from the cortex and cerebellum and then output information to the motor cortex via the thalamus. The basal ganglia work closely with the cerebellum and are believed to influence the sequencing of automatic postural reactions including the ankle, hip, and stepping strategies previously discussed. The continuous postural adjustments that play a role in smooth, coordinated movement are also controlled by the basal ganglia. Examples of disorders involving the basal ganglia include but are not limited to rigidity, bradykinesia (slowness of movement), akinesia, resting or intention tremors, chorea, and athetosis.

The brainstem also is involved in balance control because it houses the vestibular nuclei, which receive input from the cerebellum and the vestibular system. Information is output to the vestibulospinal tract, oculomotor complex, cerebellum, and parietal lobe. The brainstem is instrumental in the integration of the vestibular input and influences compensatory eye movements (Table 8-1).

COMPREHENSIVE EVALUATION

A comprehensive evaluation is crucial in helping the therapist understand specific balance problems patients may be experiencing. A comprehensive evaluation always should include a subjective client interview, an assessment of balance skills within the context of meaningful functional tasks, and an assessment of balance component

Table 8-1

Central Nervous System Structures Involved in Balance Control

STRUCTURE	INPUT	OUTPUT	FUNCTION	INDICATION OF DYSFUNCTION
Cerebellum	Cortex Basal ganglia Spinocerebellar tract Vestibular nuclei Vestibular pathways	Cortex Basal ganglia Thalamus Cranial nerves: IV, V, VI Vestibular nuclei Vestibular pathways	Integrates and modulates information. Regulates input to control movement. Influences muscle tone/stiffness. Inputs timing and synergy of muscle groups during synergistic movements.	Ataxia Unsteady gait Visual disturbance
Basal ganglia	Cortex Cerebellum	Motor cortex Thalamus	Sequences automatic postural reactions.	Rigidity Bradykinesia Akinesia Tremors (resting/intention) Chorea Athetosis
Brainstem	Cerebellum Vestibular system	Vestibulospinal tract Oculomotor complex Cerebellum Parietal lobe	Integrates vestibular input. Initiates compensatory eye movements.	Dysfunctional compensatory eye movements Vestibular dysfunction

skills. Evaluations may vary depending on the acuteness of the neurological insult, severity of the stroke, and setting in which care is provided (e.g., acute care, inpatient rehabilitation, skilled nursing facility/subacute unit, outpatient rehabilitation, or home health care).

Subjective Interview

When conducting a subjective interview, the clinician must keep in mind that patients who have had an acute stroke may not be able to provide accurate information during the interview process due to cognitive and/or language impairments. Clinicians may need to use other sources of information, including family members, significant others, and information from the medical chart to supplement, clarify, or verify information a patient provides. Patients may improve in their ability to provide information as cognitive and language deficits improve. Patients often also demonstrate a greater awareness of their situation and surroundings as they improve and become more fully integrated into the home and community environments.

Subjective patient interviews allow patients to describe in their own words and from their own perception just how the stroke has affected their level of functioning. The interview should allow the therapist to obtain the following information about the patient:

1. Premorbid health history

   The patient's premorbid health history can have a significant impact on prognosis and thus appropriate goals. Having a thorough understanding of any premorbid conditions that could affect a patient's balance functioning is important for the therapist. Examples include diabetic neuropathies, vision disturbances, vertigo, prior stroke or head injuries, prior lower extremity range of motion or strength problems, or other orthopedic issues such as lower back dysfunction.

2. Prior lifestyle

   As more details are added to this portion of the interview, the therapist will be better equipped to create an individualized treatment plan to meet the individual patient needs. The interview should include information such as the following:

   - What time does the patient generally wake each morning?
   - Did the patient bathe at sponge level, shower level, or bathtub level? A sponge bath may indicate a prior history of balance issues that resulted in a fear of falling in the shower.
   - Did the patient need to take rest breaks or spread his or her basic activities of daily living out of a period of time? Again, this may indicate a premorbid issue with endurance related to balance.
   - What household chores did the patient engage in? Outlining a schedule of a typical day at home may be helpful to the therapist in designing goals and a

customized treatment plan. The therapist's attendance to the specifics of performing tasks and to the order in which tasks occur is important for treatment planning and goal setting purposes.

3. Prior functional status

   The therapist must have a thorough understanding of the patient's functional level before the stroke. This portion of the interview should include information such as the following:

   - Whether the patient ambulated independently and what device if any was necessary for ambulation
   - Whether the patient required any assistance with performing daily tasks and, if so, what specific help did was required
   - Whether the patient was able to function independently in the community (including specifics about activities) and whether any change in activity was experienced in the past six months. Attention should be focused on life roles the patient was engaged in (e.g., spouse, caregiver, parent, grandparent, etc.).

4. Patient's perspective of current functioning

   This area may be difficult for patients who have just had a stroke, but understanding what patients consider as problems resulting from balance deficits and what goal areas are relevant for the patient is important for the therapist to grasp. Early in the rehabilitation process, patients may cite self-care and mobility as problem areas. Later, when patients are receiving home health or outpatient services, they may no longer experience difficulty in these basic areas but may cite problems with household or community activities. This portion of the interview is important for determining patients' awareness level about the way their balance deficit limits their participation in normal activities and for determining appropriate and meaningful goals.

Clinically, occupational therapists use a different approach to evaluation than other allied health professionals. After a complete review of the medical chart and a subjective interview, occupational therapists would next assess functional activities that are meaningful and relative to a specific patient based on the patient's perception, the life roles a patient engages in and the specific functional goals important to the patient. Following assessment of functional activity, the occupational therapist would then complete a full assessment of component skills necessary to complete these activities. This process is more fully discussed later in this chapter. However, for the purposes of this chapter, the reader will first be introduced to the various component areas that should be assessed and that are specifically related to balance. A therapist must have a comprehensive understanding of the component skills that contribute to typical balance in order to effectively engage in skilled clinical observation during assessment of functional activity.

Component Assessment

Component assessment focuses on numerous isolated skills and processes that contribute to balance. Thorough range of motion testing of active and passive range of motion, particularly of the trunk and lower extremities, must be completed and helps determine whether a patient has any biomechanical constraints that might have an effect on postural control. The therapist must evaluate the patient's strength and appropriate patterns of skeletal muscle activity, particularly of the lower extremities and trunk, to determine neuromotor influences on postural control. The therapist also must examine the sensory systems that play a role in maintaining equilibrium. One such system is the visual system (see Chapter 16) and includes visual acuity and oculomotor function assessments. Oculomotor function includes eye movements such as voluntary movements, smooth pursuits, saccadic eye movements, and gaze stabilization. Assessment of sensation, particularly of the lower extremities, is also critical and should include light touch, deep pressure, proprioception, and kinesthesia assessments. Assessment should focus on both the ability for the patient to interpret the sensory stimulation and the ability for the brain to organize and use the sensory information available. The vestibular system is a third system that should be fully assessed. The function of the vestibular system is to provide information about head position and head motion in space relative to gravity. The vestibular system is difficult to evaluate in isolation but is discussed more fully within the context of sensory organization. The reader is also referred to Chapter 9 for a more in-depth review of vestibular assessment and rehabilitation.

As an occupational therapist, the clinician must examine more complex tasks that integrate the specific balance components. The therapist should evaluate patients' postural alignment while they are seated and standing. Skilled observation while a patient is engaged in functional activity is critical in performing these and subsequent assessments. Symmetrical alignment and appropriate positioning of body parts over the base of support are the goals. The therapist should note any asymmetry in alignment or bias over the base of support. In general, the posture for static standing or the "starting or ready position" should be symmetrical; the head should be in midline, centered over the shoulders; the shoulders should be centered and aligned over the pelvis; under "normal" conditions, the feet should be approximately hip distance apart; and the pelvis should be centered over the base of support created by the feet (Figs. 8-3 and 8-4). Postural alignment and symmetry is directly related to what specific activity a patient is engaged in as well. This means as a patient begins to move and engage in functional activity, the alignment and symmetry will change to allow the patient to complete the activity. For example, the postural alignment and symmetry needed to unload a dishwasher and put dishes away in an overhead

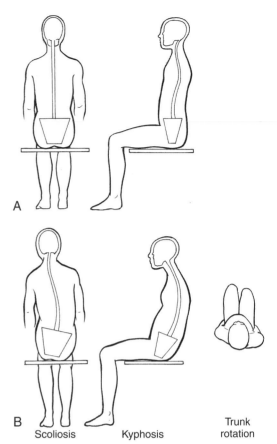

Figure 8-3 **A,** Correct alignment during sitting. **B,** Common asymmetries assumed after stroke.

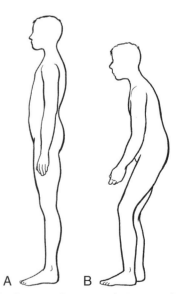

Figure 8-4 **A,** Correct alignment during standing. **B,** Flexed posture. (Note hip/knee flexion, kyphosis, forward head posture, and change in center of gravity.)

cabinet is different than if the patient is vacuuming the living room rug. Skilled observation requires the therapist to have a solid understanding of both activity analysis and postural alignment and symmetry relative to that activity.

Each individual also possesses an area about which the center of mass may be moved over any given base of support without disrupting equilibrium. This is referred to as the *limits of stability*. Assessment of patients' ability to move within their limits of stability and noting the symmetry and extent of those limits is necessary. Because of the biomechanical constraints of the foot and ankle, the limits are greatest in the anterior/posterior direction and smaller in the lateral direction. The greatest degree of movement usually occurs anteriorly. The area created by the limits of stability is in the form of an ellipse (Fig. 8-5). Therapists need to assess both actual and perceived limits of stability. Actual limits of stability are the true ellipse that a patient can achieve relative to foot length and available motor control. Perceived limits of stability are the

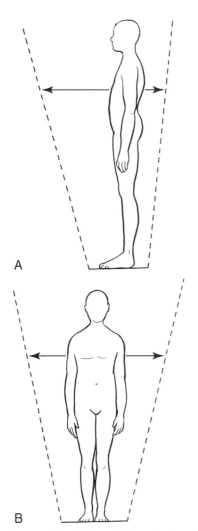

Figure 8-5 Limits of stability. **A,** Lateral view. **B,** Anterior view.

ellipse a patient perceives he or she can move; patients may underestimate or overestimate this area. If patients underestimate the limit, usually due to fear of falling, it results in an inability to weight shift normally to complete the activity. If the patient overestimates this area, usually due to sensory or perceptual deficits, it results in a fall.

The limits of stability may be measured in a number of ways. An experienced evaluator with a strong understanding of typical limits of stability might ask patients to shift their weight as far as they can in all directions and then observe and note the patients' ability to move over their base of support. The therapist also may ask patients to perform a task that requires the center of mass to move over the base of support while observing their performance. Several computerized pressure plate systems on the market are able to compute an individual's "normal" limits of stability based on height by force plate analysis. The therapist then can compare normal and actual figures. These pieces of equipment are costly and are not available in all clinics. It is crucial that therapists determine if the patient is actually shifting the center of mass over the base of support or substituting abnormal movement patterns, such as bending at the hips or shifting at the shoulders, in an attempt to accomplish the task.

Postural Control System

Information regarding biomechanical and neuromuscular parameters available to the patient has been established through the comprehensive component evaluation. Integration and the effectiveness of these capabilities in the central nervous system are tested by assessing automatic postural responses; patients must be exposed to conditions that normally would elicit particular responses.

Ankle strategies are most effective when used with a firm support surface that is long in relation to foot length. They are used to control small, slow swaying motions. For an initial assessment, the patient should be standing on a firm surface with the feet approximately hip distance apart. The therapist should note oscillations about the ankles. If the patient is able to perform this task effectively, increasing the demands of the task by narrowing the base of support may be necessary. The therapist may ask patients to place their feet together to decrease the size of the base of support, narrow the limits of stability, and increase the need to control center of mass oscillations. The therapist should note increased use of ankle strategies, and if swaying increases in speed or magnitude, the patient may initiate a hip strategy.[47] Individuals should be able to maintain their balance in this position with an ankle strategy and perhaps with minimal use of a hip strategy. Not using ankle strategies or using stepping strategies in this position indicates a disturbance in the ability to generate automatic postural responses.

Several methods exist for assessing hip strategies. Hip strategies are most effective when used with a support surface that is short in relation to foot length, the support surface is compliant, or ankle strategies are (or are perceived to be) ineffective. Simulation of each of these conditions should result in the use of a hip strategy. For higher level patients, the therapist may ask the patient to stand on a 4-inch balance beam so that only the middle of the foot receives support. Ankle strategies are ineffective under these circumstances because adequate torque cannot be produced around the ankle when the support surface is this short. The therapist should note use of primarily anterior/posterior hip strategies. Attempts to use ankle strategies only or any use of stepping strategies indicates a dysfunction in the ability to generate an appropriate hip strategy. Compliant support surfaces also result in use of hip strategies in "normal" subjects. The therapist can simulate this condition by having the patient stand on a 4-inch-thick piece of medium-density foam. Adequate torque around the ankles is not possible under this condition, and the patient uses hip strategies in all planes/directions. As stated previously, excessive attempts to use ankle strategies or exclusive use of stepping strategies indicates dysfunction.

The therapist may assess lateral hip strategies by having the patient assume a tandem stance (a heel-toe position in which one foot is directly in front of the other). This position significantly narrows the lateral limits of the base of support; because ankle strategies have a limited lateral range of effectiveness, the patient uses hip strategies. This position on a firm support surface would not be challenging enough to elicit hip strategy use in some patients. These patients could perform the same task on a 4-inch balance beam to further narrow the base of support.

When one assesses use of hip strategies in any of these conditions, observation of strategy sequence is important. The therapist also should note the effectiveness of the target strategy. Use of ineffective strategies (i.e., loss of balance) indicates that a particular strategy has failed.

The therapist may elicit use of the stepping strategy[47] by further challenging the postural control system (e.g., by combining all of the previous test conditions). For example, the therapist may ask patients to stand with feet together or in tandem on a compliant surface. A delay in or lack of a stepping strategy that results in a loss of balance indicates dysfunction. (See Fig. 8-2.)

Sensory Organization

In addition to automatic postural response assessments, assessments of sensory organizational abilities are also important. In other words, therapists must assess patients' abilities to organize and evaluate the orientationally correct sense used to generate appropriate responses. Six test conditions are considered acceptable for thoroughly assessing sensory organization. Computerized tests of sensory organization are available commercially and often are combined with force plates that can measure motor responses to test conditions (to a degree). The sensory organization portion of the apparatus usually consists of a safety harness, movable foot plate, and a movable visual screen that surrounds the subject. Test conditions also have been simulated in the clinic by using 4-inch medium-density foam as a compliant surface, and a visual "dome" that encompasses the patient's visual field and is worn on the head.[48]

The first condition for testing sensory organization allows subjects to receive accurate input from all sensory systems. Patients stand on a firm support surface with their eyes open, and the therapist records responses.

During the second condition, the therapist asks patients to close their eyes, which deprives them of visual input. Therefore, only somatosensory and vestibular inputs are available to help patients maintain equilibrium. Under this test condition, patients may have a postural response if conflicting information is received from the available sources or the individual is accustomed to relying heavily on visual input.

In the third test condition, patients wear the visual screen or dome and thus receive conflicting visual information. The screen or dome is "sway referenced," which means that it moves along with the individual's naturally occurring sway and provides the visual system with the illusion that no sway is occurring: optical flow input indicates that the environment and the individual are stationary. In this test condition, the support surface is firm and fixed, so somatosensory and vestibular information is accurate; although visual information is available, it is inaccurate. The patient must check and evaluate incoming sensory information and use only the accurate information. Too heavy a reliance on visual input might result in increased sway caused by delayed identification of the need to adjust to spontaneous sway.

The fourth condition uses a sway-referenced support surface; the support surface is sway referenced to naturally occurring sway. The therapist also may use the 4-inch foam to provide inaccurate somatosensory information. Under these circumstances, visual and vestibular information are accurate, and somatosensory information is available but inaccurate. Once again, an inappropriate postural response indicates an inability to use accurate information or identify and censor inaccurate somatosensory information.

The fifth and sixth test conditions are the most complex and require patients to use vestibular information. During the fifth test condition, patients must close their eyes, which deprive them of visual information. The support surface is sway referenced or foam is used, thus the only accurate information that helps maintain postural control is vestibular. Difficulty maintaining balance may result from a disturbance in the vestibular system or ability to integrate the information.

The sixth test condition uses sway-referenced visual and somatosensory information; vestibular information is the only accurate input. Disruption of the postural control may result because of the inability to evaluate the information (a more difficult process because two systems are providing inaccurate information) or a disruption of the central or peripheral vestibular system[48] (Fig. 8-6).

This hierarchy of test conditions (Table 8-2) allows therapists to assess the ability of the central nervous system to integrate information appropriately. The hierarchy is also a method for determining whether a person is relying too heavily on a particular source of information. These tests also can provide preliminary information about vestibular system function and may indicate a need for further testing.

Balance Assessments

In addition to those mentioned, numerous other functional balance assessments have been developed.[21,24,34,47] A large body of evidenced based research is available for many of these assessments. Discussed next is a brief overview of the more commonly used standardized or formal assessments used with either the stroke population or the neuro population in general. It is at times difficult to balance the restricted amount of time clinicians have with their patients with the need to use more standardized and formal assessments tools to assist with such things as predicting length of stay, establishing appropriate treatment plans and long term goals, justification of skilled intervention, recommendations for adaptive equipment, risk of

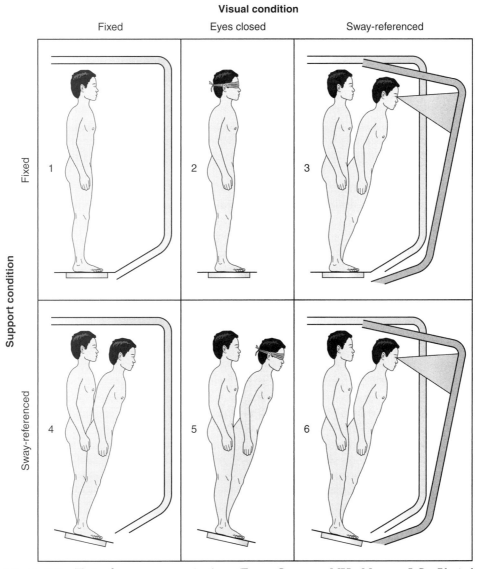

Figure 8-6 Test of sensory organization. (From Cameron MH, Monroe LG: *Physical rehabilitation: evidence-based examination, evaluation, and intervention*, St. Louis, 2007, Saunders.)

Table 8-2

Test of Sensory Organization

TEST CONDITION	ACCURATE SENSORY INFORMATION	INACCURATE OR ABSENT SENSORY INFORMATION
1	Visual, vestibular, somatosensory	
2	Somatosensory, vestibular	Absent vision
3	Somatosensory, vestibular	Inaccurate vision
4	Visual, vestibular	Inaccurate somatosensory
5	Vestibular	Absent vision, inaccurate somatosensory
6	Vestibular	Inaccurate vision, inaccurate somatosensory

falls, and discharge planning. Each venue of care and each provider of service must weigh and decide for themselves what tools are most useful and most efficient for their specific patient population. There is no one single assessment tool that clinicians can use to fully assess balance, and therefore clinicians should consider using a variety of tools.

The Berg Balance Scale[4] is by far the most commonly used balance assessment. This assessment tool can assist with predicting fall risk, determining lengths of stays, and determining adaptive equipment and discharge planning recommendation.[1,7,23,30,35,51,56,61] The test does not help the therapist in determining why patients might lose their balance and therefore is limited in its ability to assist with treatment planning. The test examines a number of factors, such as unsupported sitting and standing, transfers, reaching forward, picking objects up from the floor, turning 360 degrees, and standing on one foot, and each is graded on a 5-point scale. The assessment outlines the specific scoring criteria. This test examines many aspects of balance and has been shown to have high interrater reliability and validity in older adults.[5,7,14,35,51] This test has been developed primarily for and used with the older population and stroke patients.[3,14,51] The Berg can be time consuming, however. A new, shorter version of the Berg, referred to as the Berg Balance Scale 3P (7 item) Test, has been developed. Tasks in the shortened version include reaching forward with outstretched arm, standing with eyes closed, standing with one foot in front, turning to look behind, retrieving object from floor, standing on one foot, and sitting to standing. Available research suggests that this shortened version demonstrates similar psychometric properties as the original Berg Assessment.[14,60]

The Timed Up and GO (i.e., TUG) test is another common, highly used evaluation. The TUG has three subtests. The TUG Alone requires the patient to stand up from a chair with armrests, walk a short distance, turn around, return to the chair, and sit again.[34] The TUG Cognitive requires the same activity while the patient counts backward from 20. The Tug Manual again requires the same basic activity while the patient carries a full glass of water. These three subtests have established cut-offs to assist the therapist in predicting likelihood of falls under different conditions and therefore can be useful in recommnendations.[1,46] Performance is rated on a somewhat nonspecific 5-point scale. This test is used with the older adult population and, because of its varying rating criteria, the criteria should be evidence-based and consistent in use within a facility if used as an assessment tool.[42]

The Clinical Test of Sensory Organization and Balance,[49] which was described previously, uses six test conditions to assess an individual's ability to access, use, and organize sensory information. Within this formalized procedure, the therapist times the tests, measures the amount of sway, and records complete loss of balance falls. This test is also appropriate for use in children, patients with hemiplegia,[19] and patients with vestibular disorders.[15]

This formalized assessment provides specific information to the therapist about why patients may lose their balance and is therefore is very useful in developing individualized treatment plans. This test can be time consuming, however (see Fig. 8-6).

The functional reach test[21] requires the patient to stand next to a wall with a yardstick placed parallel to the floor. The patient is asked to reach as far forward as possible, and the reach length is measured. This test is quick and easy to perform and does not require expensive equipment. Test/retest and interrater reliability are high.[21,51,62] The test has been used with a variety of populations spanning children through the elderly.[20,21,62] The disadvantage of this examination is that it only measures one functional task and only assesses skills in the anterior direction.[63]

The Postural Assessment Scale for Stroke Patients (PASS)[9,30,35] tests the ability for patients to maintain a given posture as well as to maintain equilibrium while changing positions. Specifically, this test is a 12-item test that looks at various postures and transitions of postures including lying, sitting, and standing, and uses a 0-3 rating scale. Research indicates that this test has high construct validity, high correlation with functional measures such as the Functional Independence Measure, high interrater reliability, and test-retest qualities. This test is most predictive in the first 30 days poststroke and takes approximately 10 minutes to administer. A short form of the PASS has been developed and tested, and it contains only five items and uses the 0-3 scale for scoring; initial research indicates that the short form may also demonstrate high interrater reliability and validity.[13,60]

The Activities Specific Balance Confidence Scale (ABCS)[9,41,44,45] is a patient perception test that attempts to capture the patient's view of his or her disability related to functional activities and perceived fall risk. It is a 16-item test that asks patients to score their perception of their risk of falling when engaging in a particular task. This test is best used in an outpatient or home health setting. Research suggests that perception of fall risk may be positively related to functional mobility and greater community reintegration.[41,45] The Falls Efficiency Scale (FES) is also a confidence assessment scale used in much the same manner.[40]

The Brunnel Balance Assessment Scale (BBAS) is a scale that measures balance at three levels: sitting, standing, and stepping. The entire assessment scale can be administered at the same time, or it may be administered in sections. The advantage of this assessment is that it can be used repetitively as the patient progresses in mobility; because of this, the assessment easily lends itself to one that can be used across an entire continuum of care and across a wide range of patients with varying levels of mobility. Research suggests that this assessment tool demonstrates high reliability and validity and is a potentially useful predictive validity.[55,57]

The Motor Assessment Scale (MAS) is a relatively lengthy assessment (15 to 60 minutes depending on the patient's participation) that focuses on supine to sidelying, supine to sitting edge of bed, sitting balance, sit to stand, walking, and effect of upper arm function, hand movements, and advanced hand movements on balance. It uses a 1- to 6-point scale. This assessment is reliable, valid, and sensitive to change over time.[23,25,56] Disadvantages include the amount of time needed to administer the test, especially with more mobile patients and a more in-depth training needed for consistent therapist use. Advantages are similar to the Brunnel Balance Assessment Scale.

The assessment and treatment of balance disorders for recovering stroke patients are complex. Therapists need to understand the balance system and have a comprehensive way to assess balance function and dysfunction. They then determine realistic short- and long-term goals that are appropriate for each patient based on diagnostic and evaluation information. The therapist should devise a comprehensive treatment plan to improve specific balance deficits and ultimately assist the patient with transitioning to a more independent lifestyle.

Assessment of Balance in Relation to Function

Occupational therapists should complete the initial assessment of function in relation to balance in the same way they assess all functional activities. A thorough understanding of typical movement and excellent observation skills are essential when assessing balance through functional activity. As with any skill therapists acquire, these abilities develop and improve as the therapists gain experience. Patients should attempt the activity, and therapists should determine whether patients can do the task, the quality of the performance, and whether patients are unsuccessful and why. Therapists may not have determined the specific balance deficits yet, but they can look for a pattern of dysfunction. Observations during functional activities should focus on when patients lose and do not lose their balance. Therapists should then determine what might be causing the loss of balance.

Specifically, therapists should observe what happens during functional activities when patients have to move their center of mass over their base of support, move their head, stand on uneven surfaces, function in lower lighting, move from one type of surface to another, or function on a narrower base of support. Therapists also should observe patients' postural alignment, whether a bias in posture exists and in which direction that bias occurs, patients' limits of stability, the width between their feet during functional tasks, and what patients do after losing their balance (e.g., use ankle, hip, or step strategy or no strategy at all). The initial contact with patients engaged in functional tasks should involve only observations (and guarding for safety). Therapists must allow patients to "fail" or lose their balance in a safe way, so that they can determine what patients do during functional tasks.

The specific functional tasks to be used during evaluation depends on what the patient's goals are at the time of intervention and the setting in which treatment is being received. Stroke survivors may receive rehabilitation services in a number of settings. Inpatient settings would include acute care, acute inpatient rehabilitations settings, a skilled nursing facility or a subacute unit within a hospital or skilled nursing facility. Follow-up services may be received by home health therapists or in an outpatient rehabilitation setting. Often, patients will initially receive home health services and then transition to an outpatient center based on individual need and patient progress. Determination of where a patient receives services depends on many factors, including medical necessity, ability to tolerate at least three hours of therapy a day, discharge plan and availability for a 24-hour caregiver, availability of transportation, and health insurance policies.

As lengths of stays in all inpatient settings have dramatically shortened, as have the number of approved visits for outpatient and home health services, it is imperative for therapists to be aware of what the focus should be, based on the venue of care in which they work, the patients' goals, and the discharge plan and situation. Acute and inpatient therapists usually focus on bathing and dressing; basic transfers including bed, toilet, and shower (if applicable); and basic home management tasks if the patient will be required to complete these tasks at discharge. Given that the average length of stay in acute care is three to five days and the average length of stay in an inpatient rehab setting is 14 days, patients rarely return home independent in these basic areas. This means that many outpatient or home health therapists may still need to focus on basic self-care and mobility tasks. As the patient progresses, outpatient and home health therapists may also have the opportunity to address home management tasks such as meal preparation, cleaning, and doing laundry, and community tasks such as grocery shopping, banking, going to church, using public transportation, and participating in leisure activities. See Chapters 3 and 21. Patients receiving services in a skilled nursing facility may be eligible to receive up to a 100 days of therapy services; given this, the focus of treatment for therapists and patients in this setting would begin with basic self-care and mobility and, as the patient progresses, graduate to addressing home management tasks and community reentry activities as appropriate.

After therapists have had an opportunity to observe patients during functional activities, they should begin to develop hypotheses about the reasons patients are losing their balance during various activities. The component evaluation and the diagnostic information can assist therapists in determining whether their hypotheses are substantiated. For example, patients may lose their balance when attempting to put on their pants while standing. Therapists may hypothesize that the loss of balance results from a poor ability to shift weight accurately, poor postural alignment when attempting to shift weight, and a lack of lateral hip strategy used when standing on one leg. These hypotheses can be supported by testing patients' limits of stability, evaluation of their postural alignment, and assessment of whether they are using an available hip strategy. These steps allow therapists to develop individualized treatment plans and set realistic short- and long-term goals for each patient.

Therapists must keep in mind that they do not treat balance deficits separately from other deficits a stroke survivor may have. The treatment of balance dysfunction obviously is affected by any existing cognitive, visual perceptual, motor, or sensory deficits, such as memory deficits or a left neglect. For example, patients with cognitive deficits undoubtedly benefit more from a treatment program that incorporates familiar, repetitive functional tasks rather than an exercise program with activities that are meaningless to them. Therapists should incorporate multiple goals into each treatment session.

Because of current, ongoing changes in health care reimbursement, therapists' collaboration with patients to focus treatment around goals that enable discharge home, often with family supports, is crucial. This approach allows patients to transition as quickly as possible to less restrictive environments. Failure to focus on goals may result in patients being discharged to more restrictive environments that allow less independent lifestyles (e.g., to a nursing home instead of home or an assisted living arrangement). Therapists should also focus on treating specific balance deficits to develop an individualized treatment plan that will assist patients with becoming independent as soon as possible. The balance between remediation versus compensation will be influenced by many factors, including patient prognosis for recovery, the discharge environment (physical environment and the availability of a caregiver), and the period in which a therapist is given to work with a patient.

ESTABLISHING GOALS AND TREATMENT PLANS

Setting goals for patients with balance disorders can be difficult. Therapists must have a thorough understanding of patients' specific neuropathological condition. Although a complete neuroanatomy review is beyond the scope of this chapter, appropriate resources are listed in the references. Several factors contribute to whether patients receive a positive or poor prognosis and may include size and location of the lesion and any secondary factors that have developed, such as extensions of the original stroke, brain edema, and anoxia. The clinical presentation of the patient following a stroke will also affect the ability for patients to make realistic progress; for example, a patient with a pure motor stroke would likely have a better prognosis for recovery than a patient who also has sensory and cognitive impairments. Typically, the more skill areas influenced, the poorer the prognosis. Age and prior lifestyle of the patient may also affect prognosis. The previous medical history must also be considered for determining eventual functional outcomes. Factors to consider include any prior stroke, a history of alcohol use, any head trauma, diabetic neuropathies, age-related changes (such as the loss of inner ear hairs), orthopedic issues and balance problems (such as vertigo). Prior problems may interfere with a patient's ability to compensate for the new neurological insult.

Ideally, a treatment team consists of an otolaryngologist or neurologist, a physical therapist, an occupational therapist, the patient, and the patient's family (if applicable). The occupational therapist is not responsible for prognosticating, but to set realistic goals and an appropriate treatment plan, the therapist must have input from the otolaryngologist or neurologist concerning prognosis. If therapists are not fortunate enough to work directly with an otolaryngologist, they should contact the neurologist treating the patient for the stroke. Occupational therapists also must work closely with physical therapists to ensure that the treatment plans of both disciplines support and reinforce each other rather than work against or duplicate each other.

After receiving the prognosis, the therapist must decide whether to design a treatment plan that focuses on remediation, compensation, or both. The plan may be affected greatly by the setting in which the therapist provides treatment, the amount of time a therapist has to work with a patient, and, if it is inpatient setting, the discharge plan. If the prognosis indicates considerable improvement within two weeks, a therapist providing inpatient services may decide to emphasize remediation initially and then compensation just before discharge to ensure that the patient is functional in basic tasks. A therapist providing outpatient treatment for the same patient may focus solely on remediation because the patient already has established a safe way to function in the environment and is now focusing on improving balance deficits. If a patient has a poor prognosis for recovery of balance function, the inpatient therapist may emphasize compensation early in treatment to ensure functional success at discharge, especially if the support at home is an elderly spouse. A patient's cognitive status also significantly affects when compensatory devices are introduced into treatment. A patient with memory loss requires more repetition and time to learn to use a walker while performing kitchen tasks than a patient without memory loss. Introducing devices and training the patient and his or her family or significant other in their use early in treatment is more likely to facilitate learning specific techniques.

Despite the decision therapists make regarding compensation versus remediation, therapists need to understand the implications of prescribing use of compensatory devices for patients with balance deficits. When a walker or cane is introduced into treatment before a patient is even given a chance to function without it, the therapist cannot accurately assess the patient's ability to remediate the balance deficits. A walker or cane instantly increases the base of support and thus decreases the demand on the patient's balance system to improve. It also greatly changes the way in which a patient moves during functional activities and alters normal movement. The patient no longer has to shift weight in a normal way. Instead, weight is shifted through the upper extremities during ambulation. Postural muscle activity has been shown to be altered even with light upper extremity support. See Chapter 15.

Therapists must make informed decisions about using equipment during treatment. They must take into consideration all of the factors discussed previously when choosing a treatment plan. Tub seats and reachers may be appropriate for patients with orthopedic limitations or who have a poor prognosis for recovery of balance function; however, introducing too many devices too early in treatment may in fact hinder recovery of balance function. For example, if patients are given tub benches or shower seats and are never given the opportunity to attempt to stand for brief periods in the shower, they may not be able to reach their full level of independence. This is not to suggest that devices should not be considered or recommended—numerous patients are able to function only because of their adaptive equipment and devices—it is only to suggest that when planning treatment, therapists should be aware of the implications of using each device. Therapists may consider training patients to use devices outside of therapy that provide greater independence but limit their use during actual therapy sessions. Patients then can maintain their independence while still working toward improving their balance. Therapists may help patients function more safely and become more active, even if they continue to use a device. Decisions regarding equipment, as with all treatment decisions, should be carefully thought-out relative to each individual patient. See Chapter 28.

Using functional activities and emphasizing functional outcomes always have been basic principles of occupational therapy, and they are now beginning to be embraced by many other disciplines. Hsieh and colleagues[27] stated that using added-purpose occupation is motivating during performance. They added that numerous studies suggest that using meaningful tasks in treatment improves movement and performance.[6,26,28,29,31,36-38,43,52,53,64,65] Traditional treatment of balance disorders has been focused on exercise with the hope and assumption that patients would carry over what they learned in exercise into daily function. Although occupational therapists always have centered treatment on functional activities, during the past few decades therapists may have treated daily activities as secondary in their attempt to integrate older neurophysiological treatment approaches. Currently available information supports the use of functional tasks as primary intervention tools (Boxes 8-1 and 8-2). The tasks specifically should address the balance component disturbances that have been identified during evaluation, so that occupational therapists can provide individualized and functional treatment.

TREATING ASYMMETRICAL WEIGHT DISTRIBUTION

Patients who have had a stroke often have an impaired ability to control their center of mass over their base of support, both in sitting and standing. These patients often

Box 8-1

Sample Treatment Activities and Goals While in Standing Postures

- Static standing (no engagement in activity) graded by timed tolerance for the posture
- Static standing while holding a glass of water
- Standing while fastening shirt closures
- Retrieving an object (graded by size and weight of object) from a shelf at chest level
- Retrieving an object from a shelf at knee level (graded by weight and size of object)
- Pulling up pants from ankles while standing
- Setting table, including covering table with table cloth
- Opening refrigerator and retrieving object from top shelf
- Opening refrigerator and retrieving object from bottom shelf
- Removing shoes while standing
- Donning pajama pants while standing
- Picking up phone book from floor
- Placing full pet food bowl on floor
- Retrieving pot or pan from lower cabinet

These treatment activities do not necessarily represent a progression of difficulty.

Box 8-2

Sample Treatment Activities and Goals for Ambulatory Patients

- Carrying empty shopping bag 30 feet (graded by distance and surface)
- Carrying bag of groceries 30 feet (graded by weight, distance, and surface)
- Carrying a half-full glass of water 30 feet
- Carrying a full glass of water 30 feet
- Carrying a full cup on a saucer 30 feet
- Walking upstairs without upper extremity support
- Walking upstairs carrying laundry basket

These treatment activities do not necessarily represent a progression of difficulty.

assume an asymmetrical posture during activities that require static and dynamical balance skills. Asymmetrical posture and poor upright stability have been correlated with an increased risk for falls.[63] In addition, an unstable upright posture also has been correlated with diminished functional assessment on the Barthel index.[33] Wu and colleagues[63] indicated that one functional goal in rehabilitating persons with hemiplegia should be "to improve symmetrical characteristics of postural control." The most common form of treatment for asymmetrical weight-bearing and poor postural control is using passive and active weight shifting. This treatment traditionally has been provided in the form of exercise or introduction of outside perturbations to encourage postural reactions. The underlying assumption is that practicing the repetition of postural adjustments will result in long-term improvements in balance during functional sitting balance, ambulation, and functional activities.[18] Numerous authors have advocated the use of passive and active weight shifting as a viable treatment approach.[8,10,11,59] If patients are not able actively to shift their weight, they initially may need guidance from the therapist and assistance with moving in effective patterns. Ultimately, patients also must be able to actively shift their weight. Active weight shifting requires postural adjustments that are intrinsic to the activity being performed.[18] Patients must be able to initiate and execute a skilled weight shift that is an appropriate response to the perturbation actually experienced to maintain balance. Patients who experience difficulty with perceiving weight shifts and limits of stability may overestimate or underestimate the amount of weight shift required to adjust to the perturbation. Other patients may know a weight shift is needed, but may not be able to execute the coordinated motor movements and timing to make it effective.

Treatment for patients should focus on value-added occupations specific to individual patients. The therapist can use information gained during the patient interview to determine in which performance areas a patient is experiencing balance deficits (e.g., weight shifting in sitting to don socks, donning pants while standing or reaching into a lower cabinet during meal preparation) and which activities the patient values. Occupational therapists must perform task analyses to determine which weight shifts are required to complete the tasks patients want to perform. The therapist also should consider information from the component evaluation (e.g., poor ability to shift center of mass laterally and anteriorly when reaching up to a high cabinet in the kitchen) when making the treatment plan.

The Royal College of Physicians in their recommendations for stroke care have included information that skills gained within therapy should be integrated into daily life activities.[58] Incorporating active weight shifting into a specific activity or using weight shifting that is inherent to successful completion of an activity allows patients to learn more normal postural responses to particular activities; therapists should not assume training has transferred from an exercise to an activity. Therapists also must be sure that the type of weight shifting they are asking patients to do is appropriate for particular tasks. Patients then are able to incorporate an anticipatory set based on the specific task, an important component of motor learning. It has been postulated that learning or relearning strategies that reduce simultaneous cognitive demands may be beneficial for stroke rehabilitation.[39] Activities can be graded by the amount of weight shifting required, size of the base of support, and complexity of the task. Weight shifting can occur due to present anticipatory controls (e.g., shifting the center of gravity laterally to prepare to don pants while standing) or outside perturbations (e.g., getting on or off an escalator). Weight shifts also can occur in response to movement initiated by the upper extremities (e.g., putting a table cloth on a table). The therapist can make these activities more difficult by gradually increasing the force required by the upper extremities to perform the task (e.g., picking up an empty suitcase and then a full suitcase). Breaking down activities into a hierarchy of tasks ranging from simple to more complex is advisable, and treatment should involve selection of tasks based on patients' abilities and their typical daily activities. For example, the task of making a bed requires numerous weight shifts but may not necessarily be an appropriate activity for a patient who did not make beds before the stroke.

Patients may be able to use a variety of feedback mechanisms to improve symmetrical postural alignment. Therapists can instruct them to use somatosensory information about pressure they receive through their feet while weight shifting (if sensation is intact). If patients have a lateral bias, the therapist needs to cue them. For example, a therapist can cue a patient with an anterior or posterior bias to locate foot pressure in relation to the balls of the feet. Caution should be used in attempting to use too much conscious cognitive control over these automatic responses; asserting cognitive effort has been shown to slow motor learning. The ultimate goal is to develop an automatic motor response absent of conscious control.

The therapist also may instruct patients to use visual information. Therapists may need to use a mirror for patients with a posterior bias so that the patients can see they are drifting away from the mirror. This method may be most appropriate when performing self-care tasks that normally involve the use of a mirror.

Treatment Planning and Sensory Organization

As stated previously, the central nervous system uses information from the visual, vestibular, and somatosensory systems to maintain balance. Shumway-Cook and Horak[49] stated that the central nervous system uses this feedback to monitor the relationship between the position of the body in space and the forces acting on it. The therapist must incorporate information obtained from all of the component balance assessments, including the test of sensory organization, into the treatment planning process. The therapist usually will be able to establish a correlation among functional observations, the component assessments, and the test for sensory organization. Occupational therapists are in a unique position and require astute critical thinking skills to compile the required information from all assessment procedures and to establish an appropriate treatment plan. Any particular patient following a stroke may present with a conglomerate of functional neuromotor deficits, cognitive impairments, and somatosensory organization difficulties. Careful consideration of the setting of treatment, length of stay, discharge plan, and family support should also be taken into account when planning treatment. Collaboration among other disciplines is critical to a successful treatment as well.

Inclusion of the manipulation of sensory information into treatment of stroke survivors has been shown to increase functional balance.[2] Because of careful analysis of the results of the sensory organization test, the therapist should be able to identify functional tasks that place patients at risk for loss of balance; these activities can become part of the treatment plan (Table 8-3). Patients who lose their balance while transitioning from linoleum to carpet in their house usually perform poorly under testing conditions forcing them to maintain balance on uneven surfaces. Likewise, patients who lose their balance while walking in a mall or busy area with a great deal of peripheral movement usually perform poorly under the testing conditions forcing them to maintain their balance while receiving conflicting visual input. Therapists need to observe patients' performances during component testing and functional tasks. Therapists also must determine possible compensations or strategies patients may use when one or more systems are impaired. Patients with somatosensory dysfunctions usually become visually-dependent, whereas patients with visual disturbances usually become dependent on surfaces. Patients with vestibular dysfunctions may become visually- or surface-dependent. These compensatory strategies can work for patients in isolated environments but prevent true independence and result in a higher risk for falls for patients who are active in the home and/or community. Patients often limit their participation in home activities or simply stop going out into the community to compensate for balance deficits, which results in social isolation or depression. The therapist can obtain this information from the initial patient interview.

After determining which systems are impaired, therapists should identify activities that are both important to the patient and involve those systems. Those impaired systems can be challenged gradually by controlling the conditions in which the activities are performed. Surface-dependent patients may be more likely to lose their balance when transitioning from one surface to another in the home (e.g., from the kitchen linoleum to the living room carpet). Carrying an object from the kitchen into the living room may be a functional task that places patients at risk for loss of balance. Therapists can develop a treatment plan that initially requires patients to practice holding an item while standing on an uneven surface. The next step would be to have patients reach for an item

Table 8-3

Correlation of Component Testing and Functional Activities

SENSORY INFORMATION*	STRATEGIES	TASK
1. Difficulty with 4, 5, and 6 (sway reference support)	Absent hip strategy	Standing on carpet while opening a lower drawer with flexed hips and knees; walking outside on grass or beach and picking up object off ground; getting on or off escalator or moving sidewalk
2. Difficulty with 2, 3, 5, and 6 (visual conflict)	Excessive ankle/step strategies	Walking in mall; scanning items in kitchen cabinets; scanning items in grocery store; hanging clothes on line out of basket; rinsing shampoo out of hair while in shower with eyes closed and head tipped backward
3. Difficulty with 5 and 6 (must rely on vestibular input)	Delayed strategies	Getting up at night to go to bathroom (e.g., walking in low light down carpeted hallway and transitioning to linoleum in bathroom); walking in dark movie theater down incline while searching for seat
4. Difficulty with 4, 5, and 6	None or delayed lateral hip strategies	Standing on one foot to don pants; standing in near tandem to reach up or down into cabinet; walking from one point to another; standing in near tandem to pick something up off of floor (e.g., cat's dish)

*Numbers refer to test conditions (see Table 8-2).

while standing on an uneven surface. Patients would then carry an item as they transitioned from an uneven surface to an even surface and vice versa. These particular patients also would be at risk for loss of balance during other functional tasks that are required for community (beyond the household) ambulation. Sidewalks, gravel, grass, and sand are all uneven surfaces. The somatosensory information received from the feet of surface-dependent patients remains unchecked and may indicate to the central nervous system that the patients are falling. A balance reaction that is inappropriate to the task (e.g., walking on an uneven surface) but appropriate to the information the central nervous system is receiving and processing may result. Therapists first should have patients practice simple functional tasks on uneven surfaces and then increase the challenge by asking them to engage in more complex tasks while transitioning to and from uneven and even surfaces. The tasks should be meaningful to patients and related to their lifestyles.

Visually dependent patients often are at risk for loss of balance when their vision is obscured for any reason (e.g., when they are in the dark or poorly lit areas) or the central nervous system receives "false" visual information (e.g., peripheral images of persons walking past patients telling the central nervous system they are falling forward when they are not).

Patients may be at risk for losing their balance when getting up in the middle of the night to get a drink or go to the bathroom, walking in a movie theater, or taking a nighttime stroll outside if they are too reliant on their vision. Treatment plans can be developed that require patients to perform various activities in low lighting or with obscured vision. Common examples of this include closing the eyes in the shower while rinsing out shampoo, stepping from a brightly lit environment into a darker environment, and carrying a glass of liquid while walking (patients must keep their eyes on the glass rather than on the floor and the environment to make sure they do not spill the contents). Even walking while engaged in conversation can be difficult for visually-dependent patients because persons normally look at one another rather than the environment while talking.

Patients also may lose their balance during functional activities if they have difficulty with head-eye coordination and gaze stabilization. Activities such as walking in a busy mall, scanning the grocery store shelves for items, and placing groceries on various shelves can cause loss of balance. The central nervous system is unable to override the false visual information that results from these tasks, and thus the patients feel like they are losing their balance. Patients then institute postural reactions that are incongruent with the actual events that are occurring. Therapists can develop treatment plans that challenge patients' ability to maintain gaze stability during functional activities requiring coordinated head-eye movements.

Patients with impaired vestibular function are generally visually- and surface-dependent, although they usually rely more heavily on one system. Patients with premorbid health issues may be more reliant on one system for a predetermined reason. For example, patients with diabetic neuropathies may be more visually dependent because they do not have access to somatosensory information through their lower extremities. Most traditional treatment approaches have relied on graded, repetitive head movements in the form of exercise to improve vestibular functions.[12,17] Cohen and colleagues[16] outline a treatment approach that incorporates this basic premise into functional activity. They stress that treatment activities must include head movements and positions that elicit the vestibular dysfunction during assessment. They also stress that activities must be interesting to patients; their use may assist patients with relating to real-life experiences. Suggested activities include retrieving towels in a basket on the floor and hanging them on an overhead clothesline, ambulating in the hallways while scanning and describing objects placed at various heights, playing badminton, and dribbling a basketball back and forth across the room. A thorough and accurate assessment of the specific impaired balance deficit is necessary to design the most efficacious treatment plan. See Chapter 9.

Throughout this process, careful consideration of safety and fall risks must also be considered, especially when treatment occurs in home care or on an outpatient basis. Thorough patient and family education outlining the reasons for particular difficulties and safety modifications to reduce the risk of falls while treatment is ongoing is essential. For example, a person living at home with unreliable somatosensory feedback and on overreliance on visual information may need to have night lights or hallway lights left on to ensure safe walking to the bathroom at night. See Chapter 14.

RETRAINING BALANCE STRATEGIES

As discussed previously, part of the balance assessment is evaluating what patients do to regain their balance. Three strategies were outlined as normal balance strategies: ankle, hip, and step strategies. A component assessment allows therapists to determine whether a strategy is being used, the amount of delay in strategy use (and therefore its effectiveness), and whether the strategy is appropriate. Therapists must be able to complete skilled, accurate task analyses to determine which strategy should be used in

particular activities. Therapists should see a correlation between functional activity observations and the results of component testing. This information can be used to determine which functional activities may place patients at risk for loss of balance. The identified activities then may become part of the treatment plan (see Table 8-3).

Because these strategies are automatic, the therapist should perform careful activity analysis in treatment planning in order for the treatment activities to elicit the appropriate response. Therapists can elicit ankle strategies by asking patients to engage in tasks requiring small weight shifts on solid support surfaces that are larger than their feet. For example, patients could reach up into a cabinet to put away groceries or put away laundry on a shelf in a closet. Therapists can extract hip strategies by asking patients to engage in tasks requiring larger weight shifts on narrow bases of support. These tasks could include playing toss and catch on a balance beam. Therapists also can acquire hip strategies by asking patients to reach into drawers or cabinets without locking their knees in extension; hip flexion is necessary to counteract the resulting anterior weight shift (Fig. 8-7). Therapists can attain step strategies by engaging patients in activities that require them to make weight shifts outside of their base of support, such as hitting a tennis ball against a wall or reaching out of their base of support to pick up work boots off the floor.

OTHER FACTORS AFFECTING TREATMENT PLANNING

Therapists must consider other factors that may impair patients' balance while functioning. A common factor often overlooked, especially early in the rehab process, is endurance. When patients are treated in an inpatient setting, they often are not asked to complete the entire task. For example, when bathing or dressing, the therapist unintentionally may "help" patients who are bathing or dressing by gathering their clothes or getting towels. Inpatient settings also often have large periods between therapy sessions when patients are not engaged in activity. Therefore, a day in an inpatient setting may ask the patient to participate in activity between one to four hours, but this may not accurately reflect patients' daily home life related to the amount or timing of activity a patient engages in.

In an inpatient setting, patients usually have breakfast brought to them and often eat it in bed. They then may have a break before occupational therapists arrive to address self-care tasks. Patients then may have another break before physical therapists arrive to address gait activities. This type of schedule can result in an inaccurate picture of patients' independence and clearly does consider whether patients' endurance levels will affect their balance at home. Therapists need to devise a treatment plan that resembles the patients' typical day at home as closely as possible.

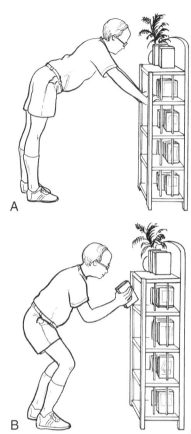

Figure 8-7   A, Knees are hyperextended and locked during functional activity, with weight shifted forward onto the upper extremities. Upper extremities are used as a base of support rather than for function. **B,** Hips and knees are flexed (as during hip strategy use) to allow center of mass to remain over lower extremity base of support. Upper extremities are free to be used for function.

Other factors that can influence a patient's balance during functional activities are cognitive and visual perception impairments. Familiar, functionally based activities can help to reduce the effects of these impairments, but clearly occupational therapists must address these issues during treatment as well.

Medical factors such as fluctuating blood pressures, fluctuating blood sugar levels, infections, metabolic disturbances, and medications also can affect a patient's balance skills. Any significant changes that therapists observe should be reported immediately to the physician. See Chapter 1.

DOCUMENTATION

Accurate and thorough documentation should include a full written evaluation, including a detailed diagnosis at the impairment level, activity participation level, and life role level. It should also include a detailed clinical impression that links diagnosis, specific impairments, comorbidities, current level of function, and anticipated level of function relative to the discharge plan from a particular venue of care. The written evaluation should include a description of the treatment plan based on patient-specific impairments, short- and long-term goals, and patient outcomes, which must be functional and measurable. Because of the current climate of managed health care, documentation should be as streamlined as possible and easily understood by any person who accesses the information, including other team members, case managers, third-party payers, patients, and family members. The documentation format should span the continuum of care where possible and should be adjusted easily to meet the patient's needs and for the setting in which intervention is being provided (e.g., acute care, inpatient rehabilitation, or outpatient clinic). Standardized and formal assessments and treatment interventions should be supported by evidenced-based research as much as possible. Uniformity and consistency of use of evaluation and documentation tools should be a priority if providing care within a continuum.

Documentation tools, if developed appropriately, can help structure thought processes and reinforce clinical reasoning skills in the areas of assessment, treatment planning, and the establishment of goals. The true "skill" of the therapist lies in the ability to assess, synthesize, and develop appropriate overall plans for a specific patient. The more specific the documentation requires the clinician to be, the more directed the treatment plan and goals will be. As length of stays become shorter, it becomes imperative for a documentation tool to function not only as a recording tool, but also as a guide to any therapist using the document, including the novice therapist or the student. Documentation should encompass and reflect information from standardized and formal assessments, functional status, specific impairment deficits, treatment, and goals. Documentation tools should be reliable, valid, sensitive, and specific. They should also reflect real-life situations.

Documentation tools should also easily and quickly convey progress to the reader. Often, the setting determines the frequency of intermittent assessment notes, but each visit or treatment session should be recorded, and evidence of progression should be demonstrated. In the event that a patient fails to progress, documentation should be able to clearly demonstrate why the patient is not progressing, and the intervening timely adjustments in treatment planning, goal setting, and discharge planning that are occurring in response to the lack of progress. Every setting is unique, so therapists should develop documentation formats that meet the needs of the patients served in each particular setting and ensure that documentation focuses on functional outcomes.

SUMMARY

The assessment and treatment of balance disorders for recovering stroke patients are complex. Therapists need to understand the balance system and have a comprehensive way to assess balance function and dysfunction. They then determine realistic short- and long-term goals that are appropriate for each patient based on diagnostic and evaluation information. The therapist should devise a comprehensive treatment plan to improve specific balance deficits and ultimately assist the patient in transitioning to a more independent lifestyle.

CASE STUDY

Improving Function Through Balance Retraining

M.J. is 58-year-old female who was diagnosed with a right middle cerebral artery stroke. She was assessed first by an inpatient rehabilitation occupational therapist who determined that the patient had difficulty controlling her balance during bathing, grooming, and dressing. The patient stated that she wanted to perform all of these activities independently. The therapist noted that M.J. had a postural bias to the right in both sitting and standing, used a wide base of support when standing during functional tasks, and was unable to control her center of gravity when shifting her leg to the left to complete a task. M.J. was able to support weight on her left lower extremity. Sensation was impaired but not absent in her left lower extremity. M.J.'s perceived limits of stability were not congruent with her actual limits of stability. She underestimated her ability to shift weight to the left and thus could not complete tasks that required her to shift weight to the left. When assisted with a left weight shift, M.J. was not able to control the shift because of poor coordination and timing of muscle activation. Because she lost control whenever she shifted weight to the left, M.J. compensated by maintaining an asymmetrical postural alignment. When asked to shift her weight actively to the left, M.J. altered her postural alignment by attempting to shift her shoulders rather than her center of mass.

Inpatient rehabilitation treatment initially centered on assisting M.J. in relearning appropriate motor responses in sitting. Activities that involved reaching and intrinsically incorporated weight shifts to the left were used. Activities of daily living were incorporated with facilitation of midline posture, and weight shifts during this functional task were used. She progressed to standing tasks and incorporating these same principles into standing tasks. The therapist selected parts of self-care tasks that did not require large weight shifts (e.g., combing her hair, washing her face, and selecting clothing from her closet) and focused on maintaining midline. The therapist helped M.J. learn to use visual and somatosensory information when possible to provide information about her position in space. M.J. was discharged home with continued needs in the areas of functional balance skills. Patient and family education focused on appropriate use of adaptive equipment, environmental modifications, and safety in the home.

Following discharge from acute rehabilitation, home care and outpatient therapy services continued. As M.J. improved her ability to achieve and maintain midline during additional static standing tasks, the therapist began to introduce tasks requiring a more significant weight shift from right to left (e.g., putting on her shirt while standing, reaching for objects on the sink, and getting objects out of the closet that were placed to elicit a left weight shift). Emphasis was placed on assisting M.J. with developing an awareness of her actual limits of stability. As M.J.'s control improved, the therapist also focused on narrowing her base of support to the more normal site dictated by particular activities. M.J. improved to the point that she could maintain midline and actively shift weight laterally during self-care activities without assistance from the therapist. Upon discharge from outpatient therapy, M.J. was provided with a comprehensive home program designed to continue to challenge and improve motor control involved in balance skills.

REVIEW QUESTIONS

1. Name the three sensory systems involved in balance control and describe their roles.
2. What purpose do automatic postural responses serve in balance control?
3. What is the role of the cerebellum in balance control?
4. What composes a component assessment of balance skills?
5. Describe three balance assessments.
6. Why should a therapist observe a patient during functional activity? What information should be gathered?
7. In what way does a therapist determine the focus of treatment (e.g., remediation or compensation)?
8. In what way does the treatment of balance deficits by occupational therapy differ from traditional physical therapy treatment?

REFERENCES

1. Andersson AG, Kamwendo K, Siger A, et al: How to identify potential fallers in a stroke unit: a validity indexes of 4 test methods. *J Rehabil Med* 38(3):186–191, 2006.
2. Bayok JF, Boucher JP Leroux, A: Balance training following stroke: effects of task-oriented exercises with and without sensory input. *Int J Rehabil Res* 29(1):51–59, 2006.
3. Berg KO: Balance and its measure in the elderly: a review. *Physiother Can* 41(5):240, 1989.
4. Berg KO, Maki BE, Williams JI, et al: Clinical and laboratory measures of postural balance in the elderly population. *Arch Phys Med Rehabil* 73(11):1073–1080, 1992.
5. Berg KO, Wood-Dauphinee S, Williams J: The balance scale: reliability assessment with elderly residents and patients with an acute stroke. *Scand J Rehabil Med* 27(1):27–36, 1995.
6. Block MW, Smith DA, Nelson DL: Heart rate, activity, duration and affect in added-purpose versus single-purpose jumping activities. *Am J Occup Ther* 43(1):25–30, 1989.
7. Blum L, Korner-Bitensky N: Usefulness of the berg balance scale in stroke rehabilitation: a systematic review. *Phys Ther* 88(5):559–566, 2008.
8. Bobath B: *Adult hemiplegia: evaluation and treatment*, ed 2, London, 1978, William Heinemann.
9. Botner EM, Miller WC, Eng JJ: Measurement properties of the Activities-specific Balance Confidence Scale among individuals with stroke. *Disabil Rehabil* 27(4):156–163, 2005.
10. Brunnstrom S: *Movement therapy in hemiplegia*, New York, 1970, Harper & Row.
11. Carr J, Shepherd R: *Physiotherapy in disorders of the brain*, Rockville, MD, 1980, Aspen.
12. Cawthorne T: The physiological basis for head exercises. *Charter Soc Physiother* 29:106, 1944.
13. Chien C, Lin J, Wang C, et al: Developing a short form of the postural assessment scale for people with stroke. *Neurorehabil Neural Repair* 21(1):81–90, 2007.
14. Chou C, Chien C, Hsueh I, et al: Developing a short form of the berg balance scale for people with stroke. *Phys Ther* 86(2):195–204, 2006.
15. Cohen H, Blatchly CA, Gombash LL: A study of the clinical test of sensory interaction and balance. *Phys Ther* 73(6):346–351, 1993.
16. Cohen H, Miller LV, Kane-Wineland M, et al: Vestibular rehabilitation with graded occupations. *Am J Occup Ther* 49(4):362–367, 1995.
17. Cooksey F: Physical medicine. *Practitioner* 155:300, 1945.
18. Daleiden S: Weight shifting as a treatment for balance deficits: a literature review. *Physiother Can* 42(2):81, 1990.
19. DiFabio RP, Badke MB: Extraneous movement associated with hemiplegic posture sway during dynamic goal-directed weight distribution. *Arch Phys Med Rehabil* 71(6):365–71, 1990.
20. Duncan PW, Studenski S, Chandler J, et al: Functional reach: predictive validity in a sample of elderly male veterans. *J Gerontol* 47(3):93–98, 1992.
21. Duncan PW, Weiner DK, Chandler J, et al: Functional reach: a new clinical measure of balance. *J Gerontol* 45(6):192–197, 1990.
22. Easton T: On the normal use of reflexes. *Am Sci* 60(5):591–599, 1972.
23. English CK, Hillier SL, Stiller K, et al: The sensitivity of three commonly used outcome measure to detect change amongst patients receiving inpatient rehabilitation following stroke. *Clin Rehabil* 20(1): 52–55, 2006.
24. Fregly A, Graybiel A: An ataxia battery not requiring rails. *Aerosp Med* 39(3):277–282, 1968.
25. Gustavsen M, Aamodt G, Mengshoel AM: Measuring balance in subacute stroke rehabilitation. *Adv Physiother* 8(1):15–22, 2006.

26. Heck S: The effect of purposeful activity on pain tolerance. *Am J Occup Ther* 42(9):577–581, 1988.
27. Hsieh C, Nelson DL, Smith DA, et al: A comparison of performance in added-purpose occupations and rote exercise for dynamic standing balance in persons with hemiplegia. *Am J Occup Ther* 50(1):10–16, 1996.
28. Kircher M: Motivation as a factor of perceived exertion in purposeful versus nonpurposeful activity. *Am J Occup Ther* 38(3):165, 1984.
29. Lang E, Nelson D, Bush M: Comparison of performance in materials-based occupation, imagery-based occupation, and rote exercise in nursing home residents. *Am J Occup Ther* 46(7):607, 1992.
30. Liaw L, Hsieh C, Lo S, et al: The relative and absolute reliability of two balance performance measures in chronic stroke patients. *Disabil Rehabil* 30(9): 656–661, 2008.
31. Licht B, Nelson D: Adding meaning to a design copy task through representational stimuli. *Am J Occup Ther* 44(5):408, 1990.
32. Magnus R: Some results of studies in the physiology of posture. *Lancet* 2(5376):531, 1926.
33. Mahoney FI, Barthel DW: Functional evaluation: the Barthel index. *Md State Med J* 14:61, 1965.
34. Mathias S, Nayak USL, Isaacs B: Balance in the elderly patient: the "get up and go test." *Arch Phys Med Rehabil* 67(6):387, 1986.
35. Mao H, Hsueh I, Tang P, et al: Analysis and comparison of psychometric properties of three balance measures for stroke patients. *Stroke* 33(4): 1022–1027, 2002.
36. Miller L, Nelson D: Dual-purpose activity vs. single-purpose activity in terms of duration on task, exertion level, and effect. *Occup Ther Ment Health* 7(1):55, 1987.
37. Morton GG, Barnett DW, Hale LS: A comparison of performance measures of an added-purpose task versus a single-purpose task for upper extremities. *Am J Occup Ther* 46(2):128–133, 1992.
38. Mullins C, Nelson D, Smith D: Exercise through dual-purpose activity in the institutionalized elderly. *Phys Occup Ther Geriatr* 5(3):29, 1987.
39. Orell AJ, Eves F, Masters R. Motor Learning of a dynamic balancing task after stroke: implications for stroke rehabilitation. *Physical Therapy* 86(3):369–380, 2006.
40. Pal J, Hale LA, Skinner MA: Investigating the reliability and validity of two balance measures in adults with stroke. *Int J Ther Rehabil* 12(7):308–315, 2005.
41. Pang MY, Eng JJ, Miller WC: Determinants of satisfaction with community reintegration in older adults with chronic stroke: role of balance efficacy. *Phys Ther* 87(3):282–291, 2007.
42. Poole JL, Whitney SL: *Can balance assessments predict falls in the elderly?* Presentation at the American Occupational Therapy Association Annual Meeting and Conference, Denver, CO, April 9, 1995.
43. Riccia C, Nelson D, Bush M: Adding purpose to the repetitive exercise of elderly women through imagery. *Am J Occup Ther* 44(8):714, 1990.
44. Salbach NM, Mayo NE, Hanley JA, et al: Psychometric evaluation of the original and Canadian French version of the activities-specific balance confidence scale among people with stroke. *Arch Phys Med Rehabil* 87(12):1597–1604, 2006.
45. Salbach NM, Mayo NE, Robichaud-Ekstrand S, et al: Balance self-efficacy and its relevance to physical function and perceived health status after stroke. *Arch Phys Med Rehabil* 87(3):364–370, 2006.
46. Shumway-Cook A, Brower S, Woolacott, M. Predicting the probability for falls in community-dwelling older adults using the timed up and go test. *Physical Therapy* 80(9): 896–903, 2000.
47. Shumway-Cook A, Horak FB: Balance disorders assessment. *NERA*, 1992.
48. Shumway-Cook A, Horak FB: Balance rehabilitation in the neurological patient. *NERA*, 1992.
49. Shumway-Cook A, Horak FB: Assessing the influence of sensory interaction on balance. *Phys Ther* 66(10):1548–1550, 1986.

50. Shumway-Cook A, Olmscheld R: A systems analysis of postural dyscontrol in traumatically brain-injured patients. *J Head Trauma Rehabil* 5(4):51, 1990.

51. Smith PS, Hembree JA, Thompson ME: Berg balance scale and functional reach: determining the best clinical tool for individuals post acute stroke. *Clin Rehabil* 18(7):811–818, 2004.

52. Steinbeck TM: Purposeful activity and performance. *Am J Occup Ther* 40(8):529–534, 1986.

53. Thibodeaux CS, Ludwig FM: Intrinsic motivation in product-oriented and non-product-oriented activities. *Am J Occup Ther* 42(3):169–175, 1988.

54. Tinetti ME: Performance-oriented assessment of mobility problems in elderly patients. *J Am Geriatr Soc* 34(2):119–126, 1986.

55. Tyson, SF, DeSouza, LH: Development of the Brunel Balance Assessment: a new measure of balance disability post stroke. *Clin Rehabil* 18(7):801–810, 2004.

56. Tyson SF, DeSouza LH: Reliability and validity of functional balance tests post stroke. *Clin Rehabil* 18(8): 916–923, 2004.

57. Tyson SF, Hanley M, Chillala J, et al: The relationship between balance, disability, and recovery after stroke: predictive validity of the Brunel Balance Assessment. *Neurorehabil Neural Repair* 21(4): 341–346, 2007.

58. Tyson S, Selley A. A content analysis of physiotherapy for postural control in people with stroke: an observational study. *Disabil Rehabil* 28(13–14): 865–872, 2006.

59. Voss D: Proprioceptive neuromuscular facilitation. *Am J Phys Med* 46:838, 1985.

60. Wang C, Hsueh I, Sheu C, et al: Psychometric properties of 2 simplified 3-level balance scales used for patients with stroke. *Phys Ther* 84(5): 430–438, 2004.

61. Wee JY, Wong H, Palepu A: Validation of the berg balance scale as a predictor of length of stay and discharge destination after stoke rehabilitation. *Arch Phys Med Rehabil* 84(5):731–735, 2003.

62. Weiner DK, Duncan PW, Chandler J, et al: Functional reach: a marker of physical frailty. *J Am Geriatr Soc* 40(3):203–207, 1992.

63. Wu S, Huang HT, Lin CF, et al: Effects of a program on symmetrical posture in patients with hemiplegia: a single-subject design. *Am J Occup Ther* 50(1):17–23, 1996.

64. Yoder RM, Nelson DL, Smith DA: Added-purpose versus rote exercise in female nursing home residents. *Am J Occup Ther* 43(9): 581–586, 1989.

65. Yuen H: *The purposeful use of an object in the development of skill with a prosthesis, master's thesis*, Kalamazoo, MI, 1988, Western Michigan University.

helen s. cohen

chapter 9

Vestibular Rehabilitation and Stroke

key terms

endolymph	vestibular labyrinth	wallenberg syndrome
otoliths	vestibular rehabilitation	
semicircular canals	vestibuloocular reflex	

chapter objectives

After completing this chapter, the reader will be able to accomplish the following:

1. Understand key components of the anatomy and physiology of the vestibular system.
2. Understand stroke syndromes that are associated with vestibular signs and symptoms.
3. Understand general concepts of vestibular rehabilitation.

The vestibular system is one of the special senses; it has receptors on the head and signals the brain via a cranial nerve. The end organs for the vestibular system, the vestibular labyrinths, detect head acceleration, or a change in the rate at which the head is moving. This information is converted to a velocity signal (velocity is speed plus direction), so the signal received by the brain really represents the speed and direction at which the head moves. The labyrinths are located within cavities inside the temporal bones of the skull on either side of the head, so the end organs are inaccessible from the outside world. One cannot see it or otherwise examine it without drilling into the temporal bone to expose it. Because the end organ is not obvious and because the roles of the vestibular system—contributions to postural control, oculomotor control, and spatial orientation, and modulation of some autonomic function—are subtle, the vestibular system was the

last of the special senses to be discovered, and many people still do not understand it.

OVERVIEW OF THE VESTIBULAR SYSTEM

Peripheral Vestibular Labyrinth

A detailed discussion of the anatomy and physiology of the vestibular system is beyond the scope of this chapter. The vestibular system has been reviewed many times in journal articles and textbooks. For excellent reviews, the reader is encouraged to examine other texts. [3,5,7,9,11,24] To put the topic of this chapter in context requires a brief reviews of some main points about the vestibular system.

The vestibular labyrinth has two sets of motion detectors: three semicircular canals (lateral, posterior, and superior) that act as rotatory accelerometers to detect turning motions of the head, and two saclike otoliths (utricle and saccule) that act as linear accelerometers to detect linear acceleration of the head (Fig. 9-1). Since gravity is a fixed linear acceleration, the otoliths also detect static tilt with reference to gravity. This gravitational signal is very important for spatial orientation, because it acts as an earth-fixed reference.

This information, and the complex anatomical structures associated with it, is needed to keep the head erect and see where one are going as one moves through space, plots a course toward a particular location or target, and generates appropriate autonomic responses when one encounters a perturbation; that is, when one is inadvertently thrown off balance for some reason. These motor skills help some lower animals capture and eat their prey and help other animals avoid becoming prey. These skills serve similar purposes in humans as they move through space, while avoiding or encountering obstacles, performing purposeful activities that involve manipulating objects while they move their heads in all planes. People with impaired vestibular systems complain of vertigo and poor spatial navigation skills, blurred vision, impaired postural control, and nausea and other signs of autonomic involvement.

Inertial Mechanism

The mechanism of the vestibular labyrinth is based on the principle of inertia, that is, that an object remains at rest until an asymmetrical force acts on it, and then it continues to move until another asymmetrical force acts on it to stop it. The semicircular canals are narrow (imagine a curved tube approximately the width of a hair on your head), so they provide a large amount of resistance to any fluid that fills it. The canals are then filled with a thick fluid known as *endolymph*. Endolymph has a high specific gravity, so it has high inertia. The inertial properties of endolymph and the high resistance of the canals, combined, mean that the vestibular system is not sensitive to extremely slow head movements. It is somewhat responsive to slow head movements, but it responds most accurately to moderate to rapid head movements in the range of 0.1 to 7.0 Hz. Not surprisingly, this frequency bandwidth is the range of most normal head movements. When an individual rotates his or her head, while shaking his or her head "no," tiny cilia attach to specialized hair cells, located on a miniscule hillock that blocks one end of the canal, and bend backward in response to movement of the endolymph over the gelatinous cup or cupula into which they protrude. This motion of the cilia starts a chain of events within the hair cells in which ions are exchanged; the cell membrane either hyperpolarizes or depolarizes. If the cell membrane depolarizes, then neurotransmitter is released, and the adjacent vestibular nerve fires which signals to the related neurons in the vestibular nuclei, located in the medulla, that the person turned his or her head.

In the otoliths, the hair cells are located in patches either in the base of the utricle or on the side of the saccule. Their cilia protrude into the otoconial membrane, which is a protein matrix containing many

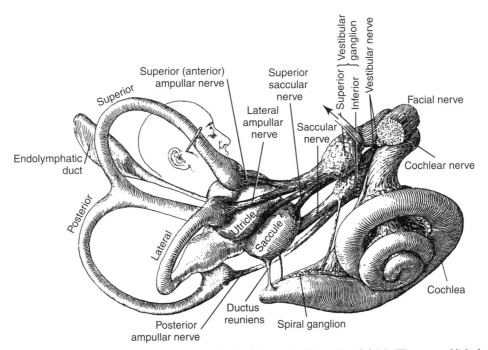

Figure 9-1 Gross anatomy of the vestibular labyrinth. (From Brödel M: *Three unpublished drawings of the anatomy of the human ear,* Philadelphia, 1946, Saunders.)

microscopic crystals of calcium carbonate known as otoconia. The otoconia act as an inertial mass. The otoconial membrane slides back and forth over the cilia in response to linear acceleration. For example, when a person accelerates his or her car going forward, the otoconial membrane virtually slides backward over the underlying cilia, bending them backward and commencing the transduction process described in the preceding paragraph.

Innervation and Blood Supply

All of this hardware in the temporal bone is supplied by nerves and arteries. The vestibular labyrinth is innervated by the vestibular nerve, which is half of cranial nerve VIII. The vestibular nerve has two branches. The superior branch innervates the superior and horizontal semicircular canals and the utricle, and the inferior branch innervates the posterior canal and the saccule.

The arterial supply to the vestibular labyrinth is similar to the innervation. The entire labyrinth receives its blood supply from one artery, the anterior inferior cerebellar artery (AICA), which is a branch off the basilar artery. A major branch from the AICA, the labyrinthine artery, supplies the entire inner ear. Inside the inner ear, it bifurcates to form the common cochlear artery and anterior vestibular artery (AVA). The AVA supplies the area primarily innervated by the superior vestibular nerve, i.e., the superior and horizontal semicircular canals and the utricle. These areas drain into the anterior vestibular vein. The common cochlear artery bifurcates and forms the cochlear artery and the posterior vestibular artery (PVA). The PVA innervates the posterior semicircular canal and the saccule. These areas drain into the posterior vestibular vein. Both veins join with the vein from the round window, elsewhere in the inner ear, and form the vestibulocochlear vein, eventually draining into the cochlear aqueduct and then the inferior petrosal sinus. Other small veins from the semicircular canals join to form the vein of the vestibular aqueduct, eventually draining into the lateral venous sinus (Fig. 9-2).

Interruption to the blood supply to the vestibular labyrinth can cause the usual manifestations of vestibular weakness, including vertigo, disequilibrium, blurred vision, and nausea. The blood supply can be interrupted by ischemia or infarction. When the AVA is involved, the patient does not have hearing loss, since the loss of blood supply is distal to the bifurcation of the labyrinthine artery. When the labyrinthine artery is involved, hearing loss is more likely. During the acute phase of sudden, dramatic, and incapacitating symptoms, which may last hours to days, patients are treated with palliative care. After the acute phase is over, patients who have not compensated spontaneously may be referred for vestibular rehabilitation. These patients are often rehabilitated successfully.

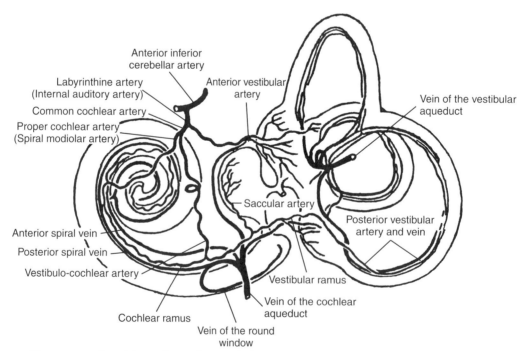

Figure 9-2 Arterial supply to the vestibular labyrinth. (Modified from Nabeya D: Study in comparative anatomy of blood-vascular system of internal ear in mammalian and in homo, *Acta Schol Med Imp Kioto* 6:1, 1923.)

Central Projections

The vestibular nerve projects to the vestibular nuclei in the rostral medulla (Fig. 9-3). The projection has some spatial specificity in that different nerves project to different areas of the vestibular nuclei. From there projections project to the dentate and fastigial nuclei of the cerebellum. Eventually those signals make their way to the flocculus, nodulus, and ventral uvula in the cerebellar vermis, the so-called vestibulocerebellum. Projections out of the cerebellum return to the vestibular nuclei. From there, some signals descend the vestibulospinal tracts to cervical and lumbosacral levels of the spinal cord. Those pathways are involved in postural control and are especially important in the absence of vision. Patients with vestibular weakness caused by peripheral or central lesions often have impaired balance.

After receiving input from oculomotor-related neurons in other nuclei, other tracts ascend the medial longitudinal fasciculus in a complex set of crossed and uncrossed pathways to synapse on the nuclei from cranial nerves III, IV, and IV. Those cranial nerves control the extraocular muscles of the eyes, so those vestibuloocular pathways control the vestibuloocular reflex (VOR). The VOR is an eye movement made in response to head movement, which stabilizes the position of the eye in space. The head is relatively large and sits atop a flexible neck, so as an individual moves his or her body through space, the head moves. To see clearly while the person moves the head, he or she generates the VOR in the direction opposite the head movement. Patients with unilateral vestibular weakness caused by peripheral or central lesions often complain of blurred vision during head movement, due to decreased amplitude of the VOR. Also, some patients with central vestibular lesions have other unusual or abnormal eye movement patterns. Neurologists sometimes use these patterns of eye movements to help localize cerebellar and brainstem lesions.

A few pathways, which are still poorly mapped, ascend via the thalamus to some poorly defined, probably small areas in the cerebral cortex, mostly around some auditory projection areas in the temporal lobe, near the junction of the temporal and parietal lobes and into the insula[8,22] (see Fig. 9-3). The functions of these projections are not clear, but they may mediate the conscious perception of motion or the vestibular contributions to spatial orientation. For example, reports in humans have shown that stimulation to those brain regions in patients undergoing neurosurgery elicits a sense of motion.[26,40] Lesions to the posterolateral thalamus impair upright body orientation[30] and cause perceived tilt of the visual vertical and deviations of the eyes.[44] Lesions to the putative vestibular cortex impair spatial perception by affecting perception of the subjective visual vertical.[43] Research on the ascending projections from the vestibular nuclei has progressed considerably with improvements in brain mapping techniques, so the vestibular thalamic projections and vestibular cortical projections will probably be mapped and studied more thoroughly in the future.

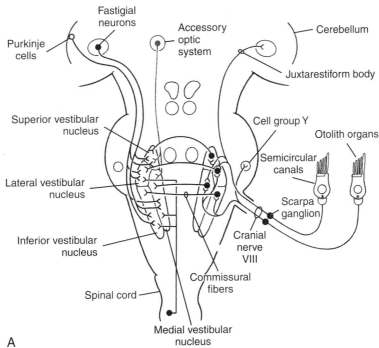

Figure 9-3   Central vestibular projections. Closed cell bodies are excitatory, and open cell bodies are inhibitory. **A,** Afferent projections of the vestibular nerve.

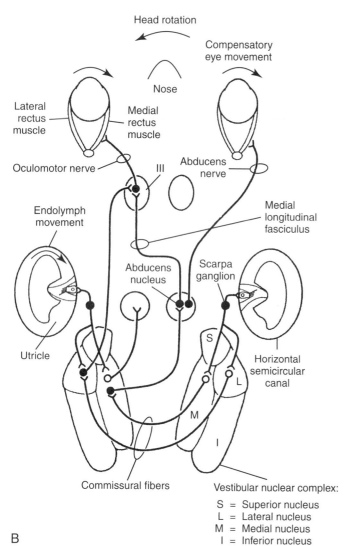

Figure 9-3, cont'd   B, Projections mediating the horizontal vestibulo-ocular reflex.

Continued

A fourth set of projections, also still poorly mapped, are involved in mediating some aspects of autonomic function. Therefore, some patients with vestibular weakness complain of autonomic signs such as nausea, sweating, increased heart rate, or anxiety.[1,2] Recent research has shown differential uses of rotational and linear vestibular inputs in modulating muscle sympathetic nerve activity vs. skin sympathetic nerve activity.[12] For a good review of vestibular autonomic mechanisms and clinical implications, see the paper by Yates and Bronstein.[42]

Central Arterial Supply

The vestibular nuclei receive their blood supply from the anterior and posterior cerebellar arteries (AICA and PICA, respectively). The AICA arises from the basilar artery and supplies the cerebellopontine angle, part of the anterior cerebellum, part of the vermis and the vestibulocerebellum, part of the rostral pons, the middle cerebellar peduncle, and cranial nerve VII (facial nerve) and cranial nerve VIII. The PICA is a branch off the rostral section of the vertebral artery. It supplies the lateral medulla and part of the cerebellum, including part of the vermis, where the nodulus and ventral uvula are located (Fig. 9-4). The vestibular cortical projection is probably supplied by the middle cerebral artery off the branches that supply the temporal lobe. Since the vestibular cortex is still being investigated, the exact blood supply may be a matter for some debate.

STROKE SYNDROMES

In approximately 20% of patients who complain of vertigo, in general, the cause is vascular in nature (stroke, vertebrobasilar migraine headache, or transient ischemic attack).[39] Vestibular lesions in stroke patients, as indicated by complaints of vertigo, are rare, however. In one study of 474 confirmed strokes in which patients were hospitalized, only 2% complained of vertigo.[36] More than half of all brainstem strokes are in the pons,[23] and strokes in that area can cause lesions of the vestibular nuclei. Of the overall population of patients seen in the emergency department and subsequently admitted for stroke, however, the percentage of patients presenting with vertigo is quite small.[32]

Lateral Medullary Syndrome

The most common stroke of the vestibular system, first reported in the late 19th century,[34] is lateral medullary syndrome, also known as Wallenberg syndrome.[3] This syndrome is caused by a stroke of either the PICA or AICA. Therefore, it is a lateral brainstem stroke. Because both arteries that supply the vestibular nuclei also supply other areas, lateral medullary syndrome is manifested by mixed sensory and motor loss, including vertigo, lateropulsion, disequilibrium, ataxia, contralateral loss of pain and temperature sensation in the trunk and limbs, and the following ipsilateral signs: facial numbness, Horner syndrome (drooping of the upper eyelid, constriction of the pupil, and decreased sweating), and dysphagia. Involvement of the PICA also includes hoarseness and skew deviation of the eyes. Involvement of the AICA also includes ipsilateral tinnitus, hearing loss, facial weakness, and reduced peripheral vestibular responses on objective diagnostic tests. These patients have vertigo, difficulty standing and walking, sensory loss on the ipsilateral side of the face and on the contralateral side of the body, difficulty speaking and swallowing, abnormal eye movements, and hearing impairments. In addition to thrombosis and ischemia, dissection of the vertebral artery caused by sports injuries or by chiropractic manipulation of the neck can cause this syndrome.[37]

Lateral medullary syndrome is relatively common. These patients may be referred for rehabilitation, although

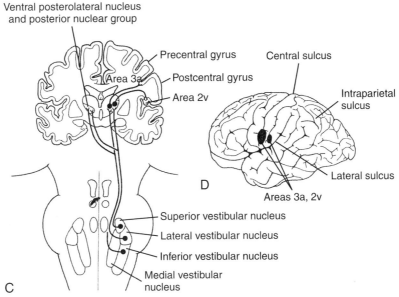

Figure 9-3, cont'd   **C,** Vestibulo-cortical projections. **D,** Likely vestibular projection areas in the cerebral cortex. (From Dickman JD: The vestibular system. In Haines DE, editor: *Fundamental neuroscience,* New York, 1997, Churchill Livingstone.)

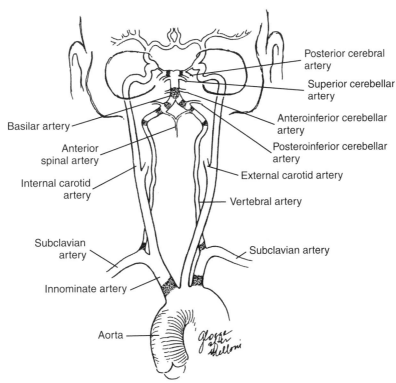

Figure 9-4   Arterial supply to the subcortical central vestibular areas. (From Baloh RW: *Dizziness, hearing loss, and tinnitus: the essentials of neurotology,* Philadelphia, 1983, FA Davis.)

many of them recover spontaneously. No studies have evaluated the effectiveness of rehabilitation in this population, but these patients usually respond well to therapy. Therapy should involve functional skills, balance therapy, and habituation exercises to reduce vertigo, which are the kinds of exercises used to reduce vertigo in patients with peripheral vestibular disorders.[25,31]

Cerebellar Infarcts

Cerebellar lesions without involvement in the brainstem can be caused by occlusion of the PICA, AICA, or vertebral artery. These patients are rarely seen for vestibular rehabilitation. According to noted authorities Baloh and Harker, the acute episodes of vertigo, disequilibrium, and nausea accompanied by typical cerebellar signs, of ataxia, disdiadochokinesia, and gaze nystagmus are often followed by edema of the cerebellum.[4] Cerebellar edema can be fatal because, when the cerebellum becomes compressed, the nearby brainstem structures can be damaged unless the area is surgically decompressed.

Lesions of Vestibular Areas in Cerebral Cortex

Strokes affecting just the insular cortex are rare. One paper reported that, of 4,800 new strokes in a database, four (less than 0.001%) were restricted to the insula. The three patients with anterior insula lesions all had transiently poor balance, and some had transient aphasia and dizziness.[13] These people all recovered spontaneously. More frequently, vertigo and balance problems can be part of the syndrome seen in large middle cerebral artery strokes. In that case, general principles of vestibular rehabilitation should be incorporated in the rehabilitation treatment plan as needed.

VESTIBULAR REHABILITATION

Although isolated central vestibular impairments are unusual, patients with strokes sometimes present with symptoms of vestibular disorder along with their other symptoms. Any patient who complains of vertigo should be evaluated to determine if the problem is central or peripheral. A detailed discussion of vestibular rehabilitation is beyond the scope of this chapter, but many reviews of this topic have been published. The American Occupational Therapy Association has defined the necessary entry-level skills for this subspecialty.[14] A brief overview of this topic follows.

Intervention such as habituation exercises and activities for vertigo,[15,18,19,27] balance therapy, repositioning maneuvers for benign paroxysmal positional vertigo (BPPV),[28] functional skills training (see Chapters 7 and 8), adaptive safety equipment, and home modifications (see Chapters 27 and 28) can be incorporated into the treatment plan for stroke rehabilitation as needed. The goals of vestibular rehabilitation are usually to reduce or eliminate vertigo when present, to reduce oscillopsia (illusory movement of the visual world) when present, to improve safety and to decrease falls (see Chapter 14), and, as in all rehabilitation, to increase independence. Habituation exercises and activities involve repetitive rotations of the head to elicit vertigo in an attempt to desensitize the system to the sensation. Current practice incorporates a visual target, i.e., the patient should be looking at something while moving the head. Therefore, tasks involving repetitive head movements (sorting tasks in which the containers are on different sides) are therapeutic. A recent metaanalysis indicates that habituation treatments are effective, although they have not been tested in stroke patients.[27] This area of practice is dynamic, and new research studies continue to expand our understanding of treatment in this specialty,[16] so the interested therapist should search the literature periodically to learn what is new.

BPPV is a very common peripheral vestibular disorder[35,41] and might occur when small vessels are compromised. This disorder occurs when otoconia, small particles of calcium carbonate located in the otoliths of the vestibular labyrinth, become displaced from the utricle in one of the semicircular canals. Theoretically, disease of the small vessels that supply the vestibular labyrinth could damage the membrane that holds these particles in place and allow them to be released into the semicircular canals. Also, in the emergency department, the physician may not be able to differentiate the acute symptoms of stroke from the acute symptoms of vestibular disorder. Therefore, some patients are admitted to the stroke unit but are later found to have BPPV. For this reason, some therapists in a stroke rehabilitation unit may need to treat patients with BPPV. The "repositioning maneuvers" used to treat BPPV are quite effective and are easily learned,[17,21,28,38] so the astute stroke therapist should learn these techniques. Central positional vertigo has been described in the literature.[6,29] If a stroke patient appears to have BPPV but does not respond to repositioning treatments, the therapist should consult the neurologist to determine if the patient's symptoms might be central in origin.

Graduated balance training exercises and activities are used when patients complain of disequilibrium. These programs usually increase in difficulty from standing still to standing on an unstable surface to moving through space while moving the head about and manipulating objects. Movement in anteroposterior, mediolateral, and off-axis planes should be incorporated.

Patients with vertigo and balance problems are at risk for falling, so therapy should involve some discussion of home modifications, such as bathtub seats, bathroom grab bars, night lights, and tacking down throw rugs (see Chapter 27). These issues can be incorporated into discharge planning for most stroke patients seen as inpatients or during routine discussions during outpatient care.

REVIEW QUESTIONS

1. What is the most common stroke to disrupt the function of the vestibular system? List the symptoms associated with this stroke.
2. What are the signs and symptoms of a cerebellar stroke?
3. What are the two major goals of a vestibular rehabilitation program after a stroke?
4. What are the specific interventions used to improve function during a vestibular rehabilitation program?

REFERENCES

1. Balaban CD: Vestibular autonomic regulation (including motion sickness and the mechanism of vomiting). *Curr Opin Neurol* 12(1): 29–33, 1999.
2. Balaban CD, Thayer JF: Neurological bases for balance-anxiety links. *J Anxiety Disord* 15(1-2):53–79, 2001.
3. Baloh RW, Halmagyi GM, editors: *Disorders of the vestibular system*, New York, 1996, Oxford University Press.
4. Baloh RW, Harker LA: Central vestibular disorders. In Cummings CW, Fredrickson JM, Krause CJ, et al, editors: *Otolaryngology: head & neck surgery*, ed 3, St. Louis, 1998, Mosby.
5. Baloh RW, Honrubia V: *Clinical neurophysiology of the vestibular system*, ed 2, Philadelphia, 1990, FA Davis.
6. Brandt T: Positional and positioning vertigo and nystagmus. *J Neurol Sci* 95(1):3–28, 1990.
7. Brandt T: *Vertigo: its multisensory syndromes*, ed 2, London, 1999, Springer.
8. Brandt T, Dieterich M, Danek A: Vestibular cortex lesions affect the perception of verticality. *Ann Neurol* 35(4):403–412, 1994.
9. Brandt T, Dietrich M, Strupp M: *Vertigo and dizziness: common complaints*, London, 2005, Springer.
10. Brödel M: *Three unpublished drawings of the anatomy of the human ear*, Philadelphia, 1946, Saunders.
11. Bronstein AM, Lempert T: *Dizziness: a practical approach to diagnosis and management*, New York, 2007, Cambridge.
12. Carter JR, Ray CA: Sympathetic responses to vestibular activation in humans. *Am J Physiol Regul Integr Comp Physiol* 294(3): R681–R688, 2008.
13. Cereda C, Ghika J, Maeder P, Bogousslavsky J: Strokes restricted to the insular cortex. *Neurology* 59(12):1950–1955, 1996.
14. Cohen HS, Burkhardt A, Cronin GW, et al: Specialized knowledge and skills in adult vestibular rehabilitation for occupational therapy practice. *Am J Occ Ther* 60(6):669–678, 2006.
15. Cohen H, Kane-Wineland M, Miller LV, Hatfield CL: Occupation and visual/ vestibular interaction in vestibular rehabilitation. *Otolaryngol Head Neck Surg* 112(4):526–532, 1995.
16. Cohen HS: Disability and rehabilitation in the dizzy patient. *Curr Opin Neurol* 19(1):49–54, 2006.
17. Cohen HS, Kimball KT: Effectiveness of treatments for benign paroxysmal positional vertigo of the posterior canal. *Otol Neurotol* 26(5):1034–1040, 2005.
18. Cohen HS, Kimball KT: Increased independence and decreased vertigo after vestibular rehabilitation. *Otolaryngol Head Neck Surg* 128(1):56–66, 2003.
19. Cohen HS, Kimball KT: Changes in gait ataxia and balance after vestibular rehabilitation. *Otolaryngol Head Neck Surg* 130:418–425, 2004.
20. Dickman JD: The vestibular system. In Haines DE, editor: *Fundamental neuroscience*, New York, 1997, Churchill Livingstone.
21. Epley JM: The canalith repositioning procedure: for treatment of benign paroxysmal positional vertigo. *Otolaryngol Head Neck Surg* 107(3):399–404, 1992.
22. Fasold O, von Brevern M, Kuhberg M, et al: Human vestibular cortex as identified with caloric stimulation in functional magnetic resonance imaging. *Neuroimage* 17(3):1384–393, 2002.
23. Fritschi JA, Reulen HJ, Spetzler RF, Zabramski JM: Cavernous malformations of the brain stem. A review of 139 cases. *Acta Neurochirurgica* 130(1-4):35–46, 1994.
24. Furman JM, Cass SP: *Vestibular disorders: a case-study approach*, New York, 2003, Oxford.
25. Furman JM, Whitney SL: Central causes of dizziness. *Phys Ther* 80(2):179–187, 2000.
26. Hawrylyshyn PA, Rubin AM, Tasker RR, et al: Vestibulo-thalamic projections in man—a sixth primary sensory pathway. *J Neurophys* 41(2):394–401, 1978.
27. Hillier SL, Hollohan V: Vestibular rehabilitation for unilateral peripheral vestibular dysfunction. *Cochrane Database Syst Rev* (4):CD005397, 2007.
28. Hilton M, Pinder D: The Epley (canalith repositioning) manoeuvre for benign paroxysmal positional vertigo. *Cochrane Database Syst Rev* (2): CD003162, 2004.
29. Johkura K: Central paroxysmal positional vertigo: isolated dizziness caused by small cerebellar hemorrhage. *Stroke* 38(6):e26–e27, 2007.
30. Karnath HO, Ferber S, Dichgans J: The neural representation of postural control in humans. *Proc Natl Acad Sci USA* 97(25):13931–13936, 2000.
31. Kelly PJ, Stein J, Shafqat S, et al: Functional recovery after rehabilitation for cerebellar stroke. *Stroke* 32(2):530–534, 2001.
32. Kerber KA, Brown DL, Lisabeth LD, et al: Stroke among patients with dizziness, vertigo, and imbalance in the emergency department: a population-based study. *Stroke* 37(1):2484–2487, 2006.
33. Deleted.
34. Lysakowski A, McCrea RA, Tomlinson RD: Anatomy of vestibular end organs and neural pathways. In Cummings CW, Fredrickson JM, Krause CJ, et al, editors: Otolaryngology: head & neck surgery, St. Louis, 1998, Mosby.
35. Neuhauser HK, von Brevern M, Radtke A, et al: Epidemiology of vestibular vertigo: a neurotologic survey of the general population. *Neurology* 65(6):898–904, 2005.
36. Rathore SS, Hinn AR, Cooper LS, et al: Characterization of incident stroke signs and symptoms: findings from the Atherosclerosis Risk in Communities Study. *Stroke* 33(11):2718–2721, 2002.
37. Saeed AB, Shuaib A, Al-Sulaiti G, Emery D: Vertebral dissection: warning symptoms, clinical features and prognosis in 26 patients. *Can J Neurol Sci* 27(4):292–296, 2000.
38. Semont A, Freyss G, Vitte E: Curing the BPPV with a liberatory maneuver. *Adv Otorhinolaryngol* 42:290–293, 1988.
39. Solomon D: Distinguishing and treating causes of central vertigo. *Otolaryngol Clin North Am* 33(3):579–601, 2000.
40. Tasker RR, Organ LW: Stimulation mapping of the upper human auditory pathway. *J Neurosurg* 38(3):320–325, 1973.
41. von Brevern M, Radtke A, Lezius F, et al: Epidemiology of benign paroxysmal positional vertigo. A population based study. *J Neurol Neurosurg Psychiatry* 78(7):710–715, 2007.
42. Yates BJ, Bronstein AM: The effects of vestibular system lesions on autonomic regulation: observations, mechanisms, and clinical implications. *J Vestib Res* 15(3):119–129, 2005.
43. Yelnik AP, Lebreton FO, Bonan IV, et al: Perception of verticality after recent cerebral hemispheric stroke. *Stroke* 33(9):2247–2253, 2002.
44. Zwergal A, Buttner-Ennever J, Brandt T, Strupp M: An ipsilateral vestibulothalamic tract adjacent to the medial lemniscus in humans. *Brain* 131(Pt 11):2928–2935, 2008.

glen gillen

chapter 10

Upper Extremity Function and Management

key terms

biomechanical alignment

complex regional pain syndrome

(modified) constraint-induced movement therapy

contracture

deformity

function

impingement

learned nonuse

manipulation

motor control

orthopedic injuries

pain

positioning

postural control

reaching

shoulder supports

spasticity

subluxation

task-specific training

weakness

weight-bearing

chapter objectives

After completing this chapter, the reader will be able to accomplish the following:

1. Develop evidence-based treatment plans to regain upper extremity function with functional task-related training.
2. Understand the application of adjunct treatments for the upper extremity after stroke, including treatments such as positioning, shoulder supports, electrical stimulation, biofeedback, and stretching programs.
3. Choose functional treatment activities appropriate to the level of available motor control.
4. Understand evaluation and treatment procedures for patients with symptoms of pain syndromes and implement pain prevention protocols into current treatment plans.
5. Identify the common biomechanical malalignments of the upper extremity and trunk after stroke and recognize their effect on function.
6. Prevent secondary complications such as pain, contracture, and learned nonuse.

Impaired upper extremity function is one of the most common and challenging sequelae of a stroke. The Copenhagen stroke study included 515 stroke patients, 71% of whom received occupational and physical therapy and 69% of whom had mild to severe upper extremity dysfunction on admission; all treatment plans included a focus on upper extremity function.[132] Obviously, numerous hours of therapy are spent on this area, as are numerous dollars. This chapter highlights problems associated with upper extremity function after a stroke, research that has been published on upper extremity function/dysfunction after stroke, and suggested evaluation and treatment techniques that focus on acquiring functional use of the extremity and preventing pain syndromes and deformities. Readers should review the concepts in Chapters 4 to 9 and Chapters 11 and 12 for a complete overview of topics related to upper extremity function and motor control.

OVERVIEW OF OCCUPATIONAL THERAPY PERSPECTIVE

"I want to use my arm again" is a goal that occupational therapists hear from stroke survivors during almost every evaluation. For therapists to assist patients with meeting this goal, a thorough understanding of the various problems associated with upper extremity dysfunction after stroke is required. The therapist has the responsibility to stay informed of (and contribute to) the new developments in and information about upper extremity function.

Current models of motor control encompass a variety of neuromotor, biomechanical, behavioral, cognitive, environmental, and learning processes. Mathiowetz and Bass-Haugen[121] have compared and contrasted the various models of motor control therapy in the past and present. Research comparing the effectiveness of various approaches is lacking. However, clearly the current motor behavior research supports a treatment technique well known to occupational therapists: the use of function-based tasks and/or task-specific or task-related training. See Chapters 4, 5, and 6.

The use of functional activities has formed the basis of occupational therapy since its inception.[125] However, the complex problems that interfere with upper extremity function may require an integrated treatment approach that uses functional tasks as the intervention foundation and hands-on approaches/modalities (e.g., mobilization, soft-tissue elongation, and biofeedback) as adjuncts to intervention.

As the body of knowledge concerning motor behavior continues to grow, therapists must analyze research findings their own clinical practices critically. Burgess[38] reminds "A danger in times of transition and rapid change is a distraction from basic principles. When faced with a

choice between conventional and new approaches, the occupational therapist should consider the following questions: Is this treatment effective? How does it work and on what principles is it based? Is it accomplishing what is needed for this patient? Are some of the older treatment methods more solidly based, more effective, or cheaper? Are there other better ways to meet this patient's needs?" This holds true today as new technologies are being developed in an effort to improve upper extremity outcomes after stroke. See Chapter 11.

DEFINITIONS AND CLASSIFICATIONS

A review of the literature on upper extremity function reveals a consistent problem: the lack of a definition for the word *function*. This may be attributed to the fact that a variety of disciplines are contributing information. From an occupational therapy perspective, *function* refers to using the upper extremity to support engagement in meaningful occupations. The International Classification of Function of the World Health Organization is a helpful classification system that includes the following categories:

- Impairment of body systems and body structure: examples include paresis, spasticity, sensory loss, and decreased postural control
- Activity limitations: dysfunction in task performance such as activities of daily living (ADL) and leisure tasks
- Participation restrictions: factor that limits or prevents fulfillment of a role (e.g., parent or worker)[195]

Hughlings Jackson's classification of observed symptoms after a central nervous system lesion is another system helpful for evaluating and treating the upper extremity after stroke. Jackson, a nineteenth-century neurologist, classified symptoms as positive or negative.

Positive symptoms are spontaneous, exaggerated disturbances of normal function and react to specific external stimuli. They include spasticity, increased deep tendon reflexes, and hyperactive flexion reflexes. In contrast, the negative symptoms are deficits of normal behavior or performance. Negative symptoms include loss of dexterity, loss of strength, and restricted ability to move.[107,108]

In the past, the major focus of therapeutic interventions was to decrease the positive symptoms associated with brain lesions. Therapists worked under the assumption that a cause-and-effect relationship existed between the two groups of symptoms. It has become clear that the alleviation of positive symptoms (e.g., spasticity) does not automatically result in an increased ability to move. Therapists therefore must take a broader view when identifying and treating upper extremity problems. A focus on only the positive symptoms (e.g., normalizing tone) does not result directly in increased function. See Chapter 6.

ACTIVITY ANALYSIS OF SELECT UPPER EXTREMITY TASKS

The following examples illustrate the complexity of upper extremity function and should assist in the evaluation process.

Reaching Task/Open Chain Activity

The reaching task described requires the patient to reach for a book on a shelf that is at forehead level. First, initiation of any movement pattern requires a motivational drive to perform; therefore, the activity must have an inherent purpose. The motivation behind and purpose of this activity may be to further knowledge, enhance leisure time, or pass a midterm examination. To complete this activity successfully, the patient must process appropriately the visual/perceptual information collected during the scanning process before initiating the reach pattern. Because the item is above eye level, neck extension with concurrent right and left lateral head and neck rotation and sufficient ocular range of motion (ROM) are required. A person collects a variety of visual information during visual scanning that helps identify particular characteristics of the book (e.g., call number, title, color, and size). This information is interpreted by several visual/perceptual processes (e.g., figure ground, color discrimination, and depth perception). See Chapters 16 and 18.

Before initiation of the reach pattern the lower extremities and trunk undergo several postural adjustments to provide stabilization (anticipatory reactions). The antigravity shoulder muscles prepare to bring the arm to shelf level, and the hand is prepositioned and oriented to prepare for grasping. While the reach pattern is being performed, the scapula protracts and rotates upward by the combination actions of the serratus anterior and upper and lower trapezius muscles. The rotator cuff keeps the humerus in a position biased toward external rotation and seats the head of the humerus in the glenoid fossa. The lower extremities and trunk stay active and stable during the performance of the pattern and may assist with a weight shift toward the shelves depending on the body position.

When the hand makes contact with the book, it is molded to the spine of the book, and the pattern of function is reversed (eccentrically) to return the book to the side of the body. After the person removes the book from the shelf, the grasp and pattern of skeletal muscle recruitment may be adjusted depending on the weight of the book. Although this activity pattern is preplanned based on prior experience, the book may be lighter or heavier than anticipated, so adjustments must be made in response to the feedback. (For example, attempting to pick up a supposedly full suitcase that is actually empty results in an exaggerated lifting motion that may cause a loss of balance.) While the book is being returned to the side, a variety of adjustments may have to be made to allow visualization of the cover of the book or call number (Fig. 10-1).

Weight-Bearing Task/Closed Chain Activity

The weight-bearing task described requires the patient to use one arm as a postural support (i.e., extended-arm weight-bearing to support function) on a kitchen table while the other arm and hand wipe the table. As mentioned previously, motivation and purpose are required. The motivation may be hunger (so the table must be cleaned in preparation for a meal), extrinsic (e.g., visitors), or work-related (e.g., table space needed to balance the checkbook or prepare a lecture). Because the weight-bearing arm is being used as a postural support, a variety of postural adjustments occur in the arm. The weight-bearing arm is active during the task; the active skeletal muscles include (but are not limited to) the scapula muscles biased toward protraction and stabilizing, the elbow extensors, the lower extremities, and the trunk muscles. The amount of skeletal muscle activity in the arm may decrease because of fatigue, resulting in a "locked" elbow, an inactive scapula biased toward an elevated position and retraction, and the trunk inactive and "hanging" on the arm.

The arm wiping the table must stay active (closed chain with superimposed movement) and endure the entire activity if the task is going to be successful. The shoulder complex of this arm glides the hand and sponge along the table surface, so the upper extremity is supported by the environment and is moving simultaneously. The amount of force and pressure exerted on the hand depends on the demands of the task (e.g., wiping crumbs or cleaning off dried syrup). A variety of weight shifts occur during this activity, and they are affected by the size of the table and amount of pressure needed by the wiping hand to accomplish the task.

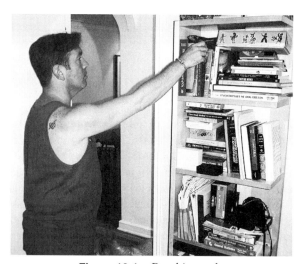

Figure 10-1 Reaching task.

The degree and variety of motor output is specific to the demands of the task.

As with all upper extremity tasks, multiple visual/perceptual processes are required for successful completion of this task. These processes are used to locate the crumbs on the table, clean both sides of the table, and determine when the task is complete (i.e., when the table is clean) (Fig. 10-2).

SELECTED EVALUATION TOOLS

Evaluation tools that are standardized, reliable, and valid can be overlooked no longer. Many therapists continue to use piecemeal evaluations that do not incorporate the use of functional tasks and rely too heavily on evaluation of impairments.

Beyond validity and reliability, when choosing assessments, clinicians must consider time factors, level of motor function, the purpose of the evaluation (clinical, research, or both), and the environment in which the

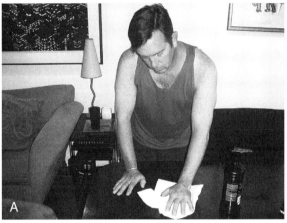
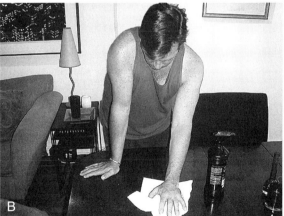

Figure 10-2 **A,** Using the right upper extremity as a postural support while the left upper extremity is supported by the table but moving. Intervention for the involved upper extremities should include engaging the patient in activities that use the upper extremities to support task performance. **B,** An alignment that fosters minimal upper extremity activity. Compare with **A.**

assessment will take place. Many available assessments such as the Fugl-Meyer Assessment only evaluate the impairment level and do not include information regarding how the upper extremity is used during daily occupations. Many use contrived or simulated functional tasks.

Motor Activity Log (Self-Report)

The Motor Activity Log is a self-report questionnaire (report by patient or family) related to actual use of the involved upper extremity outside of structured therapy time. It uses a semistructured interview format. Quality of movement ("How well" scale) and amount of use ("How much" scale) are graded on a 6-point scale. At present, there are 14, 28, and 30 item versions of the tool. Sample items include hold book, use a towel, pick up a glass, write/type, and steady myself, etc.[179-181]

Manual Ability Measure (MAM-36) (Self-Report)

The 36-item Manual Ability Measure (MAM-36) is a new Rasch-developed, self-report disability outcome measure. It contains 36 gender neutral, common performed everyday hand tasks. The patient is asked to report the ease or difficulty of performing such items. It used a 4-point rating scale, with 1 indicating "Unable" (I am unable to do the task all by myself), 2 indicating "Very hard" (It is very hard for me to do the task and I usually ask others to do it for me unless no one is around), 3 indicating "A little hard" (I usually do the task myself, although it takes longer or more effort now than before), and 4 indicating "Easy" (I can do the task without any problem). The MAM-36 can be accessed.[49] A look-up table from raw scores to converted 0-100 Rasch measures is available.[48]

ABILHAND Questionnaire (Self-Report)

The ABILHAND questionnaire asks clients to use a 3-point scale (0 = impossible, 2 = easy) to rate how difficult it would be to complete 23 bimanual tasks (e.g., hammering a nail, wrapping a gift, thread a needle, file nails, cut meat, peel onions, open jar, etc.). Grip strength, motricity, dexterity, and depression are significantly correlated with the ABILHAND measures.[144]

Assessment of Motor and Process Skills

The therapists evaluate motor and process skills[68,69] within the context of basic ADL and instrumental activities of daily living (IADL). The quality of the person's ADL performance is assessed by rating the effort, efficiency, safety, and independence of 16 ADL motor and 20 ADL process skill items, while the person is doing chosen, familiar, and life-relevant ADL tasks. There are more than 100 tasks to choose from, thus promoting a client-centered approach to assessment. Examples of evaluated motor skills include posture, mobility, coordination, strength, reach, manipulation, grip, lifting, effort, and energy expenditure. See Chapter 21.

Arm Motor Ability Test

The Arm Motor Ability Test (AMAT) has been used to determine the effectiveness of constraint-induced movement therapy (CIMT) and includes 13 unilateral and bilateral tasks. Sample items include tying a shoe, opening a jar, wiping up spilled water, using a light switch, using utensils, and drinking. The therapist times task performance and rates movement quality on a 6-point scale. The test is appropriate for evaluating motor skills in high-level clients with active wrist and finger extension. However, most of the AMAT activities are too difficult and frustrating for persons with little motor recovery.[102,146]

Wolf Motor Function Test

The Wolf Motor Function Test has been used to document the outcomes related to CIMT and includes a variety of tasks such basic reaching tasks (e.g., lifting arm from lap to table, extending elbow with and without a weight attached) and more functional activities that involve fine motor control (e.g., picking up a pencil, turning a key in a lock). All tasks but one are unilateral and appropriate for both the dominant and nondominant arm. As many tasks do not require distal control, it is appropriate for people with a more involved upper extremity. The therapist times task performance and qualitatively grades movement.[191]

Chedoke Arm and Hand Activity Inventory

Chedoke Arm and Hand Activity Inventory is a functional measure with 13 items that are assessed using a 7-point quantitative scale, similar to that of the FIM instrument (e.g., 1 = total assist and 7 = independent). It yields a total raw sum of 91 (minimum score = 13) that can be converted to a percentage. Sample items include opening a jar of coffee, dialing 911, zipping a zipper, carrying a bag up the stairs, and drying back with towel.[12,13]

Jebsen Test of Hand Function

The Jebsen Test of Hand Function[97] includes the performance of seven test activities: writing a short sentence, turning over index cards, picking up small objects and placing them in a container, stacking checkers, simulating eating, moving empty large cans, and moving weighted large cans during timed trials. The original paper is based on data collected from 360 normal subjects and patients, including patients with hemiparesis resulting from a stroke. The mean times and standard deviations for normal subjects (with their dominant and nondominant hand) are published in the paper. The test is standardized and reliable and does not have a practice effect. Therapists must be aware that some of the tasks are simulated activities, and some tasks cannot be considered ADL tasks.

Action Research Arm Test

The Action Research Arm Test consists of 19 items in four categories: pinch, grasp, grip, and gross movement. The test is short (approximately 10 minutes). Items are graded on a 4-point scale. Scores for each subtest range from 0 (unable to perform any task) to 6 (able to perform all six tasks). Performance is rated on a 4-point scale ranging from 0 (unable to perform) to 3 (performs normally). The test is most useful for patients with some distal function. The tasks included are contrived.[117]

Motor Assessment Scale

Developed by Carr and Shepherd, the Motor Assessment Scale[44] has been found to be highly reliable, with an average interrater correlation of 0.95 and a 0.98 average test/retest correlation. This evaluation includes sections on upper arm function, hand movements, and advanced hand activities. The upper arm function section includes movement patterns without tasks; the hand sections incorporate the use of objects. Each item is scored on a 7-point scale.

Box and Block Test

The number of wooden blocks ($2.5 \times 2.5 \times 2.5$ cm) that can be transported from compartment of box to another in one minute is counted.[120,145]

Nine-Hole Peg Test

A measure of dexterity, the Nine Hole Peg Test consists of a plastic console with a shallow round dish to contain the pegs on one end of the console and the nine-hole pegboard on the opposite end. Time taken to complete the test is measured as the patient grasps nine pegs and places them in and removes them from the holes on the console.[136]

Functional Test for the Hemiplegic/Paretic Upper Extremity

Although this evaluation[188] is based on Brunnstrom's view that motor recovery takes place in a specific sequence, it does involve functional tasks associated with daily living. This test has been found to be highly correlated with scores on the Fugl-Meyer Assessment and requires approximately 30 minutes to administer. It consists of 17 test items arranged in seven levels according to difficulty. Examples of tasks evaluated include folding a sheet, stabilizing a jar, hooking and zipping a zipper, screwing in a light bulb, and placing a box on a shelf.

Upper Extremity Performance Test for the Elderly/ Test d'Evaluation des Membres Supérieurs de Personnes Agées (TEMPA)

This test consists of four unilateral (pick up and move a jar, pick up a pitcher and pour water into a glass, handle coins, and move small objects) and five bilateral (open a jar and take a spoonful of coffee, unlock a lock and open a pill container, write on an envelope and place a stamp on it, tie a scarf around your neck, and shuffle and deal playing cards) functional tasks. It includes speed of execution and functional ratings. The functional rating is related to level of independence and uses a 4-point scale.[60]

Frenchay Arm Test

This quick test includes five items, such as hair combing with the weak arm and drinking water. Items are graded as successful or unsuccessful.[87]

Motricity Index

This test includes a brief impairment measure of upper extremity function after stroke. Items include pinch strength, elbow flexion, and abduction.[51]

Rivermead Motor Assessment (Arm Section)

This text is part of a comprehensive battery and contains 15 items related to motor recovery of the arm. Sample items include protracting a shoulder girdle while supine, picking up a piece of paper from the table in front and releasing five times, cutting putty on a plate with a knife and fork, and placing string around the head and tying a bow in the back. The scores are dichotomous: success (1) or failure (0).[115]

Fugl-Meyer Assessment (Upper Extremity Motor Function)

Familiarity with this impairment-based test is helpful because the test is used in many research papers to document improvement in function. The assessment is based on the motor recovery model developed by Twitchell and on Brunnstrom's idea that motor recovery occurs in a specific sequence of steps. Improved motor function is considered a deviation from stereotypical synergies defined by Brunnstrom in this test. The test does not involve the use of functional tasks. Sections include ROM, sensation, balance, upper extremity, and lower extremity. Items are graded on a 3-point scale.[72]

USE OF THE INVOLVED UPPER EXTREMITY TO SUPPORT TASK PERFORMANCE: SUGGESTIONS FOR INTERVENTION

The foundation of occupational therapy is built on patients taking an active role in their own recovery by participating in functional activities. In the past, many therapists, while attempting to apply neurophysiological principles to treatment, have limited their use of this modality in favor of more passive techniques that are applied to the patient (e.g., brushing, icing, and neurodevelopmental treatment–based handling techniques performed separately from functional tasks). Occupational therapy now has come full circle, with the most current research

on motor control supporting the use of tasks performed in context-specific situations (see Chapters 4 through 6.) Functional tasks in therapy include occupations that require upper extremity weight-bearing for postural support, reaching, carrying, lifting, grasping, and manipulating of common objects. These types of activities clearly carry over into daily life tasks and are comprehensive enough to treat a variety of problem areas. The importance of using occupation-embedded interventions as opposed to rote exercise has been established.[111,198] Indeed descriptions of the most effective interventions after stroke include task specific, repetitive, intense, active, evidence-based, and function-based. Further task-specific training should be relevant to the patient and context, be randomly ordered from a practice perspective, be repetitive and involve massed practice, focus on whole task practice, and be positively reinforced (Fig. 10-3 and Table 10-1).[89]

Task-Oriented Reaching and Manipulation

The events leading up to a simple voluntary movement such as reaching for a glass of water involve multiple complex processes. Ghez[74] classifies these processes as follows. First, the person needs to identify the glass and its position in space. This first step encompasses a variety of visual and perceptual processes. Second, the person needs to select a plan of action to bring the glass to the mouth. Ghez points out that this step involves specifying which body parts are needed and in which direction they should move. To do this, the person must evaluate the location of the glass in relation to the position of the hand and body. The information collected allows the motor system to determine the appropriate trajectory of the hand. The last step is the execution of the response. Multiple commands are sent to the motor neurons specifying the temporal sequence of muscle activation, the forces to be developed, the changes in joint angles, the orientation of the hand to fit the glass, and the coordination of the shoulder with the distal arm to ensure that the glass will be grasped on contact and immediately. Multiple problems can interfere with these three steps, including the issues discussed in the previous section, visual dysfunction, and praxis deficits.

Two components of upper extremity function have been described by Jeannerod[95,96]: the transportation component, which includes the trajectory of the arm between the starting position and the object, and the manipulation component, which is the formation of grip by combined movements of the thumb and the index finger during arm movement.

In her study of reaching deficits in subjects with left hemiparesis, Trombly[177] used kinematic analysis and electromyography to document impairments in voluntary arm movements. Her analysis demonstrated that the ability to reach smoothly and with coordination was significantly less in the impaired arms than in the unimpaired arms. The continuous movement strategy used during reaching

Text Continued on p.230

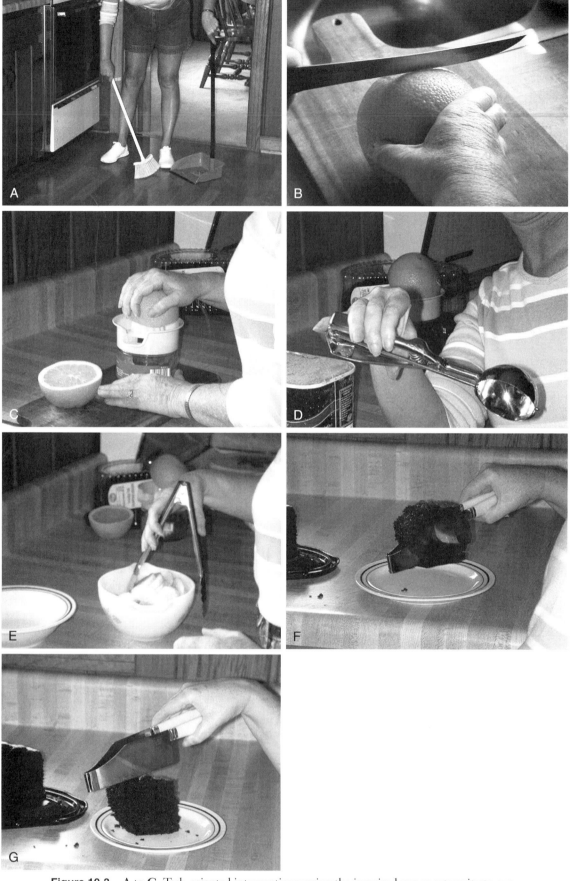

Figure 10-3   **A** to **G,** Task-oriented interventions: using the impaired upper extremity to support participation after stroke. (Courtesy of Yvette Hachtel, JD, MEd, OTR/L)

Table 10-1

Managing the Poststroke Upper Extremity Using Evidence from Systematic Reviews, Meta-analyses, and Randomized Controlled Trials

INTERVENTION	DESIGN/SUBJECTS	CONCLUSIONS
Task-related/ specific practice	A randomized controlled trial comparing standard care (SC), functional task practice (FTP), and strength training (ST).[189]	Compared with SC participants, those in the FTP and ST groups had significantly greater increases in upper extremity function and strength, and decreased upper extremity impairment in the short-term. In the long-term, those in the FTP group benefited the most.
	A prospective, randomized, single blind clinical trial recruited 30 stroke subjects into either an upper limb or a mobility group. All subjects received their usual rehabilitation and an additional session of task-oriented practice using a circuit class format.[17]	Both groups improved significantly between pre- and posttests on all of the mobility measures, while only the upper limb group made a significant improvement on the Jebsen Test of Hand Function and Motor Assessment Scale upper arm items.
	A systematic review of task-oriented training after stroke.[151]	"Studies of task-related training showed benefits for functional outcome compared with traditional therapies. Active use of task-oriented training with stroke survivors will lead to improvements in functional outcomes and overall health-related quality of life." The authors recommended "creating opportunities to practise meaningful functional tasks outside of regular therapy sessions."
	Double-blind randomized control trial. Intervention group (TR group) received progressive object-related reach-to-grasp training with prevention of trunk movements. Control group (C) practiced tasks without trunk restraint.[126]	"TR training led to greater improvements in impairment and function compared with C. Improvements were accompanied by increased active joint range and were greater in initially more severe patients. In these patients, TR decreased trunk movement and increased elbow extension, whereas C had opposite effects (increased compensatory movements). In TR, changes in arm function were correlated with changes in arm and trunk kinematics."
	An investigation of the effects of different intensities of arm and leg rehabilitation training on the functional recovery of activities of daily living (ADL), walking ability, and dexterity of the paretic arm, in a single-blind randomized controlled trial.[105]	Greater intensity of leg rehabilitation improved functional recovery and health-related functional status, and greater intensity of arm rehabilitation resulted in improvements in dexterity.
Constraint induced movement therapy (CIMT)	A systematic review that found 13 randomized controlled trials, 4 of which were excluded because they aimed at comparing different intensity of CIMT.[26]	Findings were positive in all studies, but the minimal clinically important difference, defined as a change of at least 10% of the maximum score of the scale used, was reached only in smaller ones, which may have been influenced by patients' characteristics.

Continued

Table 10-1

Managing the Poststroke Upper Extremity Using Evidence from Systematic Reviews, Meta-analyses, and Randomized Controlled Trials—cont'd

INTERVENTION	DESIGN/SUBJECTS	CONCLUSIONS
	A placebo-controlled trial of CIMT in patients with mild to moderate chronic motor deficit after stroke. The study compared CIMT to a placebo group that received a program of physical fitness, cognitive, and relaxation exercises for the same length of time and with the same amount of therapist interaction as the experimental group.[172]	After CIMT, patients showed large to very large improvements in the functional use of their more affected arm in their daily lives. The changes persisted over the 2 years tested. Placebo subjects showed no significant changes.
	A prospective, single-blind, randomized, multisite clinical trial conducted at 7 U.S. academic institutions.[193]	Among patients who had a stroke within the previous 3 to 9 months, CIMT produced statistically significant and clinically relevant improvements in arm motor function that persisted for at least 1 year.
Modified constraint induced movement therapy (mCIMT)*	Thirty-two patients were randomized to receive mCIMT or traditional rehabilitation for three weeks.[112]	In addition to improving functional use of the affected arm and daily functioning, mCIMT improved motor control strategy during goal-directed reaching.
	This study compared a mCIMT intervention with a dose-matched control intervention that included restraint of the less affected hand and assessed for differences in motor and functional performance and health-related quality of life. N = 32.[113]	Compared with the control group, the mCIMT group exhibited significantly better performance in motor function, level of functional independence, mobility of extended ADL, and health-related quality of life after treatment.
	A single-blinded randomized controlled trial compared mCIMT to a time-matched exercise program for the more affected arm or a no-treatment control regimen.[137]	After intervention, significant differences were observed on the Action Research Arm Test and Motor Activity Log Amount of Use and Quality of Movement scales, all in favor of the mCIMT group.
	Twenty-six patients received either mCIMT or traditional rehabilitation for a period of 3 weeks.[196]	The mCIMT group exhibited significantly greater improvements in motor function, daily function, and health-related quality of life than the traditional rehabilitation group. In addition, those in the mCIMT group perceived significantly greater percent of recovery after treatment than patients in the traditional rehabilitation group.
	Thirty stroke patients were randomly assigned to either an mCIMT or a control group.[201]	Significant differences in favor of mCIMT were found in 6 elements of the Wolf Motor Function Test.
Mental practice	A systematic review of 15 studies of mental practice focused on decreasing impairment and improving function in the poststroke upper extremity.[135]	The results of the majority of the studies suggest mental practice has a positive effect on upper limb recovery at both the impairment and functional levels. However, it is unclear whether the improvements seen are retained over time, or how broad the effects are in terms of improving perceived occupational performance.

*Treatment protocols vary greatly and are discussed in Table 10-3.

Table 10-1

Managing the Poststroke Upper Extremity Using Evidence from Systematic Reviews, Meta-analyses, and Randomized Controlled Trials—cont'd

INTERVENTION	DESIGN/SUBJECTS	CONCLUSIONS
	A randomized placebo controlled trial of mental practice of specific arm movements.[139]	Those receiving mental practice showed significant reductions in affected arm impairment and significant increases in daily arm function. Those in the group receiving mental practice exhibited new ability to perform valued activities.
Combined mCIMT and mental practice	A randomized trial comparing mCIMT versus mCIMT plus mental practice.[138]	All subjects exhibited reductions in affected arm impairment and functional limitation. Those in the mCIMT plus mental practice group exhibited significantly larger changes on both movement measures after intervention.
Electromyographic (EMG) biofeedback	Subjects were randomly assigned to EMG biofeedback or placebo EMG biofeedback groups. Both treatments were applied 5 times a week for a period of 20 days. In addition, the patients in both groups received an exercise program.[7]	"The results showed that there were statistically significant improvements in all variables in both groups, but the improvements in active range of motion and surface EMG potentials were significantly greater in the EMG biofeedback group at the end of the treatment."
	The purpose of this study was to assess electromyographic biofeedback efficacy through meta-analysis. Eight studies met the inclusion criteria (N = 192). Their average effect size was 0.81. The 95% confidence interval for the effect size was 0.5 to 1.12.[161]	"The results indicate that electromyographic biofeedback is an effective tool for neuromuscular reeducation in the hemiplegic stroke patient."
Electrical stimulation	The meta-analysis examined the efficacy of surface electrical stimulation for the prevention or reduction of shoulder subluxation after stroke. Seven (four early and three late) trials met the inclusion criteria.[3]	"Analysis found that, when added to conventional therapy, electrical stimulation prevented on average 6.5 mm of shoulder subluxation (weighted mean difference, 95% CI 4.4 to 8.6) but only reduced it by 1.9 mm (weighted mean difference, 95% CI −2.3 to 6.1) compared with conventional therapy alone. Therefore, evidence supports the use of electrical stimulation early after stroke for the prevention of, but not late after stroke for the reduction of, shoulder subluxation."
	A randomized trial (N= 46). The treatment group received surface neuromuscular stimulation to produce wrist and finger extension exercises. The control group received placebo stimulation over the paretic forearm.[47]	"Data suggest that neuromuscular stimulation enhances the upper extremity motor recovery of acute stroke survivors. However, the sample size in this study was too small to detect any significant effect of neuromuscular stimulation on self-care function."
	This meta-analysis examined the effectiveness of electrical stimulation of subluxation, shoulder pain, range of motion and functional use. The study included 5 papers with 8 data points.[84]	This analysis suggests that electrical stimulation produces positive results including improving subluxation, pain, range of motion, and functional use.

Continued

Table 10-1

Managing the Poststroke Upper Extremity Using Evidence from Systematic Reviews, Meta-analyses, and Randomized Controlled Trials—cont'd

INTERVENTION	DESIGN/SUBJECTS	CONCLUSIONS
	A systematic review of randomized trials related to poststroke shoulder pain. Four trials (a total of 170 subjects) fitted the inclusion criteria.[150]	The review found no significant change in pain incidence or change in pain intensity after electrical stimulation treatment compared with control. There was a significant treatment effect in favor of electrical stimulation for improvement in pain-free range of passive humeral lateral rotation. In these studies, electrical stimulation reduced the severity of glenohumeral subluxation, but there was no significant effect on upper limb motor recovery or upper limb spasticity The authors noted that there does not appear to be any negative effects of electrical stimulation at the shoulder.
EMG-triggered neuromuscular stimulation	This systematic literature search was performed to identify clinical trials evaluating the effect of electrical stimulation. The authors specifically examined the relationship between outcomes and characteristics of the stimulation. 19 clinical trials were included, and the results of 22 patient groups were evaluated.[59]	"A positive effect of electrical stimulation was reported for 13 patient groups. Positive results were more common when electrical stimulation was triggered by voluntary movement rather than when non-triggered electrical stimulation was used." The authors concluded that "triggered electrical stimulation may be more effective than non-triggered electrical stimulation in facilitating upper extremity motor recovery following stroke."
	This meta-analysis assessed the effect of EMG-triggered neuromuscular stimulation on arm and hand functions, specifically the focus was on wrist extension.[25]	The meta-analysis revealed a significant overall mean effect size (delta=0.82, S.D.=0.59). These improved wrist extension motor capabilities findings support EMG-triggered neuromuscular stimulation as an effective poststroke protocol.
	A randomized trial to assess the efficacy of EMG-triggered neuromuscular stimulation (EMG-stim) in enhancing upper extremity motor and functional recovery of acute stroke survivors.[71]	"Subjects treated with EMG-stim exhibited significantly greater gains in Fugl-Meyer (27.0 vs 10.4; $p = .05$), and FIM (6.0 vs 3.4; $p = .02$) scores compared with controls." Data suggest that EMG-stim enhances the arm function of acute stroke survivors."
Bilateral upper extremity training	A systematic review and meta-analysis of 11 studies of bilateral arm training after stroke.[168]	"These findings indicate that bilateral movement training was beneficial for improving motor recovery post-stroke." "These meta-analysis findings indicate that bilateral movements alone or in combination with auxiliary sensory feedback are effective stroke rehabilitation protocols during the sub-acute and chronic phases of recovery."

Table 10-1

Managing the Poststroke Upper Extremity Using Evidence from Systematic Reviews, Meta-analyses, and Randomized Controlled Trials—cont'd

INTERVENTION	DESIGN/SUBJECTS	CONCLUSIONS
	A randomized, single-blind training study comparing bilateral (practice of bilateral symmetrical activities) to unilateral training (performed the same activity with the affected arm only). The activities consisted of reaching-based tasks that were both rhythmic and discrete.[170]	Both groups had significant improvements on the Motor Status Scale and measures of strength. The bilateral group had significantly greater improvement on the Upper Arm Function scale. Both bilateral and unilateral training are efficacious for moderately impaired chronic stroke survivors. Bilateral training may be more advantageous for proximal arm function.
	A randomized controlled trial. Subjects randomized to distributed CIMT, bilateral arm training (BAT), or a control intervention of less specific but active therapy.[114]	BAT may uniquely improve proximal upper limb motor impairment. In contrast, distributed CIMT may produce greater functional gains for the affected upper limb in subjects with mild to moderate chronic hemiparesis.
Mirror therapy	A randomized trial to evaluate the effects of mirror therapy on upper extremity motor recovery, spasticity, and hand-related functioning of inpatients with subacute stroke.[199]	In our group of subacute stroke patients, hand functioning improved more after mirror therapy, in addition to a conventional rehabilitation program, compared with a control treatment immediately after 4 weeks of treatment and at the 6-month follow-up, whereas mirror therapy did not affect spasticity.
	A randomized trial to evaluate the effect of a therapy that includes use of a mirror (MT) to simulate the affected upper extremity with the unaffected upper extremity early after stroke compared to a control (CT).[62]	"In the subgroup of 25 patients with distal plegia at the beginning of the therapy, MT patients regained more distal function than CT patients. Furthermore, across all patients, MT improved recovery of surface sensibility. Neither of these effects depended on the side of the lesioned hemisphere. MT stimulated recovery from hemineglect."
Strengthening interventions for weakness	Systematic review with meta-analysis of randomized trials. 21 trials were identified and 15 had data that could be included in the meta-analysis.[2]	Strengthening interventions increase strength, improve activity, and do not increase spasticity. These findings suggest that strengthening programs should be part of rehabilitation after stroke.
	A review of poststroke strengthening trials.[141]	"While the number of studies is limited, emerging evidence suggests that persons with poststroke weakness can improve strength through resistance exercise in the absence of negative side effects, including exacerbation of hypertonia. Moreover, these improvements in strength appear to transfer to functional improvements. Still, many unresolved issues remain. The potential for strength training to improve the overall outcomes of rehabilitation for persons with poststroke hemiplegia warrants further investigation."
Positioning	A randomized trial to determine the efficacy of positioning the affected shoulder in flexion and external rotation to prevent contracture shortly after stroke.[5]	At least 30 minutes a day of positioning the affected shoulder in external rotation should be started as soon as possible for stroke patients who have little activity in the upper arm.

activities was lost, movement time was longer, peak velocity occurred earlier, and indications of weakness were present.

In a follow-up study, Trombly[176] documented the observed improvements in her subjects' reaching abilities. Her findings indicated that the amplitude of peak velocity improved over time. The level of muscular activity did not improve, but the discontinuity of movements decreased. From her findings, Trombly hypothesized that therapy that allows relearning of sensorimotor relationships is warranted for some patients. She stated that the "level and pattern of muscle activity of these subjects depended on the biomechanical demands of the task rather than any stereotypical neurological linkages between muscles."

From a treatment perspective, research by Trombly and Wu[178] concluded that "Goal-directed reach enabled persons with stroke to display characteristics typical of reach to a target by persons who have not had a stroke better than reaching out in space. These findings support the occupational therapy practice of using objects in a functional context to improve coordinated movement. However, the nature of the objects to be used requires further study."

Van Vliet and colleagues[185] studied subjects in the early months after a stroke. The subjects were able to improve their reaching kinematics during a three- to four-week period; they progressed toward normal performance. Providing the subjects with a meaningful task (e.g., drinking from a cup) helped them perform the reach-to-grasp movement.

Jeannerod[96] stated that "Formation of the finger grip during the action of grasping a visual object involves two main functional requirements, the fulfillment of which will determine the quality of the grasp. First, the grip must be adapted to the size, shape, and use of the object to be grasped. Second, the relative timing of the finger movements must be coordinated with that of the other component of prehension by which the hand is transported to the spatial location of the object." Jeannerod observed that finger posturing anticipates the real grasp and occurs during transportation of the hand. This shaping of the hand is a mechanism independent of the manipulation itself. If treatment programs focused on improved function of the upper extremity are to be designed, then they must include a variety of common objects with different shapes, sizes, and textures to affect this reaching component.

Exner,[66] who defined *in-hand manipulation* as the process of adjusting objects being grasped in the hand, developed a classification system to assist the therapist in activity choice, despite the system not being standardized on stroke survivors (Box 10-1 outlines Exner classification system).

Wu, Trombly, and Lin[198] demonstrated that using material-based occupation (e.g., picking up a pen and

---

Box 10-1

Exner Classification of Manipulation Tasks

TRANSLATION

The object in the hand moves from the finger surface to the palm or vice versa.

SHIFT

Movement occurs at the finger and thumb pads by alternating thumb and radial finger movements (e.g., moving a coin near the distal interphalangeal joints farther out to the pads of the fingers).

SIMPLE ROTATION

The object is turned or rolled between the finger pads and thumb pad by alternating thumb and finger movements (e.g., unscrewing a jar lid).

COMPLEX ROTATION

The object is rotated, which requires isolated, independent movements of the finger or thumb. The object is turned between 180 degrees and 360 degrees (e.g., turning a paper clip so that correct end can be placed on a piece of paper).

---

preparing to write one's name) enhanced quality of movement performance more than imagery-based occupation (e.g., pretending to pick up a pen and preparing to sign one's name) and exercise (e.g., moving the arm forward). Their data suggested that material-based occupation resulted in decreased reaction time, movement time, and movement units. Although this study was performed on normal subjects, they inferred that material-based occupation may be used to elicit efficient and economical preprogrammed movement for performing tasks.

In a study of fine motor coordination training, Neistadt[133] examined the effects of constructing puzzles and performing kitchen activities on fine motor coordination in a group of brain-injured men. Her results demonstrated that the subjects in the functional meal preparation group showed significantly greater improvements in dominant hand dexterity, which is used for picking up small objects, than the subjects in the tabletop puzzle activity group. Her findings suggested that functional activities are more effective (not to mention more meaningful) than tabletop activities for fine motor coordination training in the brain-injured population.

Sietsema and colleagues[163] studied brain-injured patients engaged in rote exercise tasks and occupationally embedded tasks (e.g., reaching out to control a computer game). Their subjects had "mild to moderate spasticity" on evaluation. Their results indicated that the game elicited significantly more ROM during the reach pattern performance than the rote exercise. Their study supported the hypothesis that occupationally embedded interventions promote increased performance. The authors hypothesized that the game provided motivating feedback that enhanced performance.

At this point, research has confirmed that the demands and goals of the task influence motor output.[198] For example, the characteristics of an item being carried across a kitchen influence factors such as how fast a person moves, whether one or two hands are used to grip the object, how close to the body the item is carried, and how stable the arms are held. In daily life, there are many examples of the ways in which movement in daily activities is influenced by the environment (e.g., carrying empty ice trays or full trays, a half-glass of wine or a full cup of coffee, one paper plate or a stack of china plates).

Rosenbaum and Jorgensen[153] have demonstrated that the goal of the task influences motor output. Their subjects were asked to reach for a cylinder and stand it on one end or the other. Depending on the goal of the task (e.g., which side they were to stand the cylinder on), subjects reached with a pronated or supinated grasp pattern. Box 10-2 provides sample activities used to retrain reach patterns. See Chapters 4 and 5.

Weight-Bearing to Support Function

The use of weight-bearing tasks has long been advocated in patients after stroke. Upper extremity weight-bearing has been suggested anecdotally for achieving a variety of therapeutic goals, including inhibiting hypertonus by moving the body proximally against the distal upper extremity[55] and stimulating upper extremity extension during protective responses.[19] Brouwer and Ambury[37] concluded that upper extremity weight-bearing normalizes corticospinal facilitation of motor units in stroke patients. They hypothesized that the mechanism responsible for their results was a sustained increase in motor cortical excitability through augmented afferent input.

McIllroy and Maki[122] and Marsden, Merton, and Morton[118] documented that if the upper extremity is used as a postural support (e.g., during weight-bearing), postural responses to the movements of the opposite arm occur throughout the weight-bearing upper extremity and to other perturbations of posture. Their paper also demonstrated that postural responses from the triceps only occurred when the hand was in contact with a firm object.

Although from a neurophysiological perspective, the effect of weight bearing on upper extremity control (e.g. the "normalization of tone" and "inhibition of spasticity") remains controversial and unproven, the use of weight-bearing patterns is still necessary for treating the upper extremity after a stroke if the goal of treatment is to improve functional performance. Examples include using the more affected upper extremity in a weight-bearing pattern and as a postural support while manipulating clothing during toileting activities or to enhance participation in IADL (e.g., using the more affected extremity as a postural

support during activities requiring standing such as doing the laundry or preparing a meal).

Therapists also can use weight-bearing activities to address impairments that interfere with function. The problem of soft-tissue shortening in the long flexors can be prevented or reversed by bearing weight on extended wrists with extended digits to maintain or increase tissue length. If evaluation reveals that weakness in the extremity is having a limiting effect on function, the therapist can use extended-arm weight-bearing activities to strengthen the

---

Box 10-2

Activities to Retrain Reach Patterns

- With the patient positioned in a supine posture, the therapist supports the weight of the distal extremity with a handhold position. The patient attempts to hold various positions and/or to follow the movements of the therapist's hand. This activity is appropriate for the early motor recovery stage. The degrees of freedom are minimized (with trunk and scapula being supported by the supine posture), and the therapist eliminates the weight of the patient's extremity, maximizing the potential for skeletal muscle recruitment. This activity is easily taught to family members.

- Position the patient in side lying with the patient's arm supported on a table. Practice reaching in multiple directions for various objects or towards various targets while the weight of the limb is supported on the table.

- The patient stands or sits in front of a table with a hand resting on a dust cloth on top of the table. The patient focuses on gliding the hand across the table. The critical pattern consists of humeral flexion, scapula protraction, and elbow extension. The cloth reduces friction, and the weight of the arm is supported on the table (e.g., reach with support).

- The patient is seated, and objects are positioned on the floor in front of patient. The patient reaches for objects on the floor. This downward reach pattern enhances scapula protraction, humeral flexion, and elbow extension by nature of the position of the objects. As the patient gains more control, the objects are raised up to the midshank level, then the knee level, and then the waist level, systematically increasing the motor demands of the task.

- The patient is engaged in the foregoing reach patterns while therapist provides resistance to the functional pattern by tying an elastic band around the palm. The therapist is behind the patient holding the opposite end of the band and is able to grade the level of resistance.

- During the reach activities, the demands of the distal components of movement are systematically increased (e.g., increasing manipulation requirements). Examples include pouring water and opening jars.

triceps and scapula musculature if the weight-bearing activities are performed in appropriate alignment and the weight-bearing pattern remains active during the activity.

To ensure appropriate alignment, the therapists should avoid severe internal rotation, forced elbow extension, and an inactive trunk in patients.[156] During weight-bearing activities, maintenance of palmar hand arches is important for maintaining biomechanical alignment and enhancing active patterns. The points of contact between the weight-bearing surface and the hand include the thenar eminence, hypothenar eminence, metacarpal heads, and palmar surfaces of the phalanges.[100] The arch should be maintained so that therapists can insert a finger between the web space and the first metacarpal head and slide it under the hand until they make contact with the hypothenar eminence.

Although the more affected arm is in a weight-bearing position, the less involved extremity should be engaged in activities that promote weight shifting in all directions (Fig. 10-4). Weight-bearing activities can be performed by the forearm or an extended arm, depending on the demands of the task and the level of available motor control. See Table 10-1 for a review of evidence related to task related training.

GOALS, TASK CHOICES, AND INTERVENTIONS TO PROMOTE FUNCTION

The following goals are examples of treatment activities for different levels and combinations of functional recovery. Using goals and treatments interchangeably ensures a task-specific approach to intervention. These examples should not be interpreted as progression in recovery. Although previous assumptions were that proximal recovery of abilities precedes distal recovery of abilities, this is not always the case. The following activities are graded by increasing the degrees of freedom (e.g., increasing the number of planes of movement that are controlled and integrating hand use), the level of antigravity control, and the objects used in the task. An important note is that the cognitive demands of the task have a substantial effect on the level of upper extremity function. Readers should not consider this list hierarchical. For example, weight-bearing is not a prerequisite to reaching, because the neurological

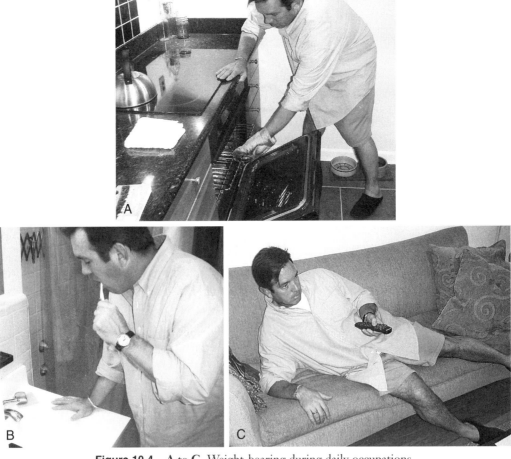

Figure 10-4   **A** to **C,** Weight-bearing during daily occupations.

and biomechanical demands are different. Patients need to be engaged in a variety of tasks that require the use of the upper extremity in a variety ways and engaged in task-specific training.

Focused attention on the more affected upper extremity (no active movement)

- Patient washes upper extremity during upper body bathing activities.
- Patient attends to upper extremity while rolling by passively guiding upper extremity across trunk when preparing to roll.
- Patient prevents arm from dangling while seated in chair.
- Patient positions upper extremity on table during mealtime.

Prevention goals

- Patient stretches arm correctly by reaching to floor and maintaining this position after difficult tasks result in arm posturing.
- Patient's family demonstrates proper guarding techniques for a mobile patient.
- Patient's caretaker demonstrates proper positioning of patient in bed.
- Patient's caretaker demonstrates proper technique to transfer patient from one surface to another (e.g., not by lifting under the axillas).

Forearm weight-bearing as a stabilizer

- Patient stabilizes checkbook with upper extremity while writing checks.
- Patient stabilizes cutting board with upper extremity during meal preparation.
- Patient holds magazine open with upper extremity while doing crossword puzzle.

Using upper extremity for assistance during transitions

- Patient uses upper extremity for assistance with assuming sitting position from side-lying position.
- Patient uses upper extremity to push up into standing position.
- Patient uses upper extremity to reach back before sitting.
- Patient uses upper extremity to lower trunk to mat when assuming supine posture from sitting posture.

Incorporating upper extremity as a postural support when sitting and standing (extended-arm weight-bearing with stabilized hands-on support surface)

- Patient uses upper extremity to assist with lateral shifting while relieving pressure.
- Patient stabilizes upper body with affected upper extremity while wiping and dusting table or ironing with less affected upper extremity.
- Patient uses more affected upper extremity as a stabilizer on a grab bar while manipulating clothing with less affected upper extremity during toileting.
- Patient stabilizes upper body with upper extremity while grooming at sink.

Weight-bearing with superimposed motion (e.g., hand does not leave support surface but slides and pulls objects)

- Patient irons and/or dusts with more affected upper extremity while stabilizing upper body with less affected upper extremity.
- Patient uses affected upper extremity to lock wheelchair brakes with brake extensions.
- Patient uses more affected upper extremity to smooth out laundry.
- Patient uses more affected upper extremity to wax and buff car.
- Patient uses more affected upper extremity to push shopping cart or rolling walker.
- Patient uses affected upper extremity to apply body lotion.
- Patient uses affected upper extremity to wash a mirror or window.

Antigravity shoulder movements without hand function

- Patient initiates roll with more affected upper extremity.
- Patient lifts more affected upper extremity into shirt sleeve.
- Patient lifts more affected upper extremity to countertop.
- Patient pushes drawer closed with back of more affected hand.
- Patient turns off light switch with side of more affected hand.

Initial hand movement (static grasp) with limited shoulder movement (in lap or on work-surface activities)

- Patient adjusts shirt cuff with more affected upper extremity.
- Patient holds book in lap with both hands while reading.
- Patient stabilizes fruits or vegetables with affected hand while cutting with less affected hand.
- Patient holds shopping bag with more affected upper extremity during ambulation.
- Patient holds washcloth with more affected upper extremity and washes mid to lower body.

Reach patterns with hand activity

- Patient picks up sock from floor with more affected upper extremity.
- Patient retrieves item from under sink cabinet with more affected upper extremity.
- Patient opens medicine cabinet with more affected upper extremity.
- Patient retrieves item from top shelf of medicine cabinet with more affected upper extremity.
- Patient drinks out of a cup with more affected upper extremity.

Advanced hand activities

- Patient holds coins in affected palm and slides them to finger tips.
- Patient types 15 words per minute with both upper extremities.

- Patient signs check with more affected upper extremity.
- Patient picks up and reorients paperclip with affected upper extremity.

A benchmarking outcomes system is suggested to track and communicate progress (Box 10-3). Table 10-2 provides further suggestions for choosing tasks for a variety of levels of function.

Constraint-Induced Movement Therapy (Traditional and Modified Protocols)

The term *learned nonuse* was coined by Taub.[171] The learned nonuse phenomenon originally was identified in primate studies and later was applied to chronic stroke patients. With deafferentation of a single forelimb of a monkey, the animal would not use that limb in

Box 10-3

The Australian Therapy Outcome Measures (AusTOMs) for Occupational Therapy: Upper Limb Use

The ability to use one or both upper limbs during activities of daily living include gross and fine manipulative skills and hand and arm use. This may comprise lifting and moving a heavy object while walking; picking up and using a pencil; grasping, using, and releasing objects such as keys, buttons, or taps; throwing and catching an object; and pushing, pulling, twisting, and turning objects.
Scoring: You are able to use half-points.

IMPAIRMENT OF EITHER STRUCTURE OR FUNCTION (AS APPROPRIATE TO AGE)

Impairments are problems in body structure (anatomical) or function (physiological or psychological) as a significant deviation or loss. Impairments may be mental (cognitive/perceptual), sensory, cardiovascular/respiratory, digestive/metabolic/endocrine systems, neurological movement, or musculoskeletal. A variety of impairments may affect ability to use upper limbs (if only one upper limb is affected, then rate the severity of impairments affecting this limb; if both are affected, then rate both). Considering all the impairments an individual may have that affect upper limb use, assess the level of severity of these. Base your assessment on typical presentation of the individual's impairment(s) in an appropriate environment.

0 The most severe presentation of impairment/s., e.g., very dense hemiplegia, severe fixed contractures, unbearable pain, or most severe presentation of cognitive impairment

1 Severe presentation of impairment/s, e.g., dense hemiplegia, severely restricted range of movement, severe pain, or severe cognitive impairment

2 Moderate/severe presentation of impairment/s, e.g., moderate to severe hemiplegia, moderate to severely restricted range of movement, moderate to severe pain, or moderate to severe cognitive impairment

3 Moderate presentation of impairment/s, e.g., moderate hemiplegia, moderately restricted range of movement, moderate pain, or moderate cognitive impairment

4 Mild presentation of impairment/s, e.g., mild hemiplegia, mildly restricted range of movement (e.g., morning stiffness), mild pain, or mild cognitive impairment

5 No impairment/s of structure or function. All structures and functions intact. No pain. Affected arm equal to unaffected arm or norms.

ACTIVITY LIMITATION (AS APPROPRIATE TO AGE)

Activity limitation results from difficulty in the performance of an activity. Activity is the execution of a task by an individual. Assess the individual's ability to use both upper limb/s for tasks and what the client can actually do, e.g., if the client can do all tasks independently with one arm, then score as 5.

0 Does not use upper limb/s. Unable to lift, move, manipulate, use upper limb/s. Full assistance required.

1 Severe limitation in using upper limb/s. Maximum assistance required. Enough function to prevent further injury or to minimize functional restrictions, e.g., shoulder can be slightly abducted to enable clothes to be put on. Client completes some of the movement required for activity.

2 Moderate/severe limitation in using upper limb/s. Needs a person to give some hands on assistance, or requires constant verbal prompting. Can initiate gross motor movements, but difficulty with end of range movements and fine motor control, e.g., consistently spills contents of cup; functional pencil grip but unable to write or form legible letters, can draw. Able to use upper limb for gross function only, such as stabilizing/or able to perform fine grasp but cannot manage gross movements.

3 Moderate limitation in using upper limb/s. Requires verbal cueing, supervision or set-up. Generally, gross movements intact, poor fine motor/dexterity, e.g., reaching for clothesline independently, requiring assistance to manipulate peg on line. Inconsistent completion, e.g., picks up half-full lightweight cup with handles with occasional spills; illegible writing.

4 Mild limitation in using upper limb/s. Able to do but lacking in quality, or extra time required, e.g., clumsy, unreliable grasp/release, reduced carrying capacity, weaker grasp, mildly reduced coordination and dexterity, reduced reach, decreased efficiency and fluency of movement, e.g., holds and raises standard full cup with external support (table, other arm); completes legible writing although may display decreased quality/slow speed/reduced fluency.

5 No limitation in using upper limb/s. Able to lift, move, manipulate, use hand and arm to complete functional tasks bilaterally or unilaterally. May or may not use aids or adaptive equipment such as prosthesis/orthosis, or enlarged/lightweight handle. Completes upper limb activities in reasonable time.

You must also make a rating of the client's participation Restriction and Distress/Wellbeing.

Table 10-2

Suggestions for Categorizing Upper Extremity Tasks

CATEGORY	TASKS
No functional use	Teach shoulder protection Self range of motion Positioning
Postural support/ weight-bearing (forearm or extended arm)	Bed mobility assist Support upright function (work, leisure, activities of daily living) Support during reach with opposite hand Stabilize objects
Supported reach (hand on work surface)	Wiping a table Ironing Polishing Sanding Smoothing out laundry Applying body lotion Washing body parts Vacuuming Locking wheelchair brakes
Reach	Multiple possibilities to engage up- per extremity into activities of daily living, leisure, and mobility; grade tasks by height/distance reached, weight of object, speed, and accuracy

an unrestricted (free) environment. The monkey's initial attempts to use the limb resulted in failures (e.g., dropping food, losing balance, and falling). The monkeys in this study soon found that they could function in their environment with three limbs instead of four. Continued attempts to use the affected limb led to repeated failures at attempted tasks; the effect was suppression of any desire to use that limb. The monkeys *learned* not to use the limb to avoid failure, which masked any future recovery of limb function. Taub and colleagues[171] pointed out that in a free situation, the monkeys did not learn that they could regain use of the forelimb as they recovered function. When the intact forelimb was restrained, the monkeys were forced to use the affected side. This technique converted a useless limb into one capable of function.

Taub[171] hypothesized that the nonuse or limited use of an affected upper extremity in human beings after stroke could in some cases result from a similar phenomenon of learned suppression. To test this hypothesis, Taub[171] studied nine patients with chronic (i.e., greater than one year after stroke) hemiplegia. To be included in this study, patients had to demonstrate

the ability to extend the metacarpophalangeal and interphalangeal joints at least 10 degrees, extend the wrist 20 degrees, and walk without an assistive device. They had to have grossly intact cognitive function, no excess spasticity, be right-arm dominant, and be less than 75-years-old.

Patients were assigned to a control or an experimental group. The experimental group underwent forced-use/CIMT in which the intact limb was placed in a sling and resting-hand splint. The restraint was worn at all times during waking hours except when toileting, when napping, and at times when balance might be compromised. The restraint was worn for 14 days. Each weekday, patients received therapy and were given a variety of tasks—such as eating with utensils, playing ball, playing Chinese checkers and dominoes, writing, and sweeping—to perform with the paretic limb for six hours throughout the day.

The treatment of the control group focused on increasing attention to the paretic limb. This group was told that they had more potential in their extremities than they were using. Therapists performed passive ROM activities, and patients performed ROM activities daily for 15 minutes. The affected limb was not given any training for active movement.

Each group was evaluated before and after intervention with a variety of arm function evaluations and a self-reported Motor Activity Log. The experimental group had significantly faster mean performance speeds from the evaluations, increased quality of movement, and an increased ability to use the extremity in ADL. These improvements were reevaluated two years later; they were at least maintained if not increased. Although the comparison group made subtle gains after intervention, the gains were not retained for the follow-up evaluation. Taub and colleagues[171] concluded that the motor ability of stroke patients who met their inclusion criteria could be increased significantly by the interventions effective for overcoming learned nonuse.

Wolf and colleagues[192] researched forced-use treatment in 25 chronic hemiplegic and stroke patients with minimal to moderate extensor muscle function. The CIMT program lasted for two weeks, with the intact limb being restrained during waking hours. The authors noted significant changes in performance of 19 of the 21 tasks that were evaluated, with most changes persisting for one year after the study. The authors concluded that learned nonuse does occur in select patients with neurological deficits and that this behavior can be reversed through application of a CIMT paradigm.

Van der Lee and colleagues[182] completed an observer-blinded randomized clinical trial with 66 chronic stroke patients who were randomized to two weeks of CIMT or a comparison of equally intensive bimanual training based on two weeks of neurodevelopmental therapy. One week after the last treatment session, the authors found a significant difference in effectiveness in favor of CIMT group compared with the neurodevelopmental therapy group, after correction for baseline differences, on the Action Research Arm Test and the Motor Activity Log amount of use score. One-year follow-up effects were observed only for the Action Research Arm Test. The authors also found that the differences in treatment effect for the Action Research Arm Test and the Motor Activity Log amount of use scores were clinically relevant for patients with sensory disorders and hemineglect, respectively.

The EXCITE trial[193] was a prospective, single-blind, randomized, multisite study and included 222 patients with stroke. Subjects were randomized to either customary care or constraint-induced therapy. Constraint-induced therapy consisted of two components applied over a two-week period; subjects performed intense practice of functional tasks using the affected hand for six hours per day plus subjects reduced use of the unaffected hand by covering it with a mitt for at least 90% of waking hours. The trial found significantly positive results that were maintained in the long term. Outcome measures included:

- The Wolf Motor Function Test, which showed a 52% reduction in time to complete its tasks, significantly better than the 26% reduction found in those in the customary care group.
- The Motor Activity Log, which showed a 76% increase in quantity and a 77% increase in quality of arm use, each significantly better than the 43% and 41% respective increases found in the customary care group.

Dromerick, Edwards, and Hahn[63] questioned whether a CIMT program could be implemented in the acute stroke population (two weeks after stroke) and whether this intervention was more effective than traditional upper extremity interventions (control group) during the acute period. The research team enrolled 23 subjects in a pilot randomized, controlled trial that compared CIMT with traditional therapies. Treatment plans were designed to make sure that patients in both groups received equivalent time and intensity of treatment directly, and an occupational therapist supervised the program. The subjects received routine interdisciplinary stroke rehabilitation, except for the CIMT that occurred during the regularly scheduled occupational therapy sessions. Individualized and circuit-training techniques were used in both groups. All subjects received study treatment for two hours per day, five days per week, for two consecutive weeks. Twenty subjects completed the trial. The CIMT group had significantly higher scores on the Action Research Arm Test and pinch subscale scores. Differences in the mean grip, grasp, and gross movement subscale scores of the Action Research Arm Test did not reach statistical significance. ADL performance was not significantly different between

groups. No subject withdrew because of pain or frustration. The authors concluded that CIMT during acute rehabilitation is feasible. Furthermore, CIMT was associated with less arm impairment at the end of the trial.

Page and colleagues[140] examined the feasibility and efficacy of a modified CIMT protocol administered on an outpatient basis. Their protocol was developed to be more consistent with therapy scheduling and reimbursement patterns, in other words, more user friendly and feasible from the therapist's perspective. They examined six patients who were in a subacute stage of stroke recovery and who exhibited learned nonuse. The patients were assigned to one of three groups; two patients received half-hour physical and occupational therapy sessions three times a week for 10 weeks while they simultaneously had their unaffected arms and hands restrained five days per week during five hours identified as times of frequent use; two patients received regular therapy, and two control patients received no therapy. Outcomes were measured by the Fugl-Meyer Assessment of motor recovery, the Action Research Arm Test, the Wolf Motor Function Test, and the Motor Activity Log. Patients receiving modified CIMT exhibited substantial improvements on the Fugl-Meyer Assessment, Action Research Arm Test, the Wolf Motor Function Test and reported increases in amount and quality of use of the limb based on the Motor Activity Log. Patients receiving traditional or no therapy exhibited no improvements. The author concluded that modified CIMT may be an efficacious method of improving function and use of the affected arms of patients exhibiting learned nonuse. See Table 10-3 for CIMT protocols.

In addition to the apparent functional improvements in the select group of patients who are appropriate for a trial of CIMT, researchers have demonstrated that CIMT produces long-term alteration in brain function. This is the first documented cortical-level change associated with a therapy-induced improvement in the rehabilitation of movement after neurological injury. Liepert and colleagues[110] investigated whether CIMT could produce treatment-induced plastic changes/reorganization of the motor cortex in the human brain. Using focal transcranial magnetic stimulation, the authors mapped cortical motor output area of a hand muscle on both sides in 13 stroke patients in the chronic stage of their illness before and after a 12-day-period of CIMT. The authors found the following:

- Before treatment, the cortical representation area of the affected hand muscle was significantly smaller than the contralateral side.
- After treatment, the muscle output area in the affected hemisphere was significantly enlarged, corresponding to a greatly improved motor performance of the paretic limb.
- Shifts of the center of the output map in the affected hemisphere suggested the recruitment of adjacent brain areas.

Table 10-3

Tested Constraint-Induced Movement Therapy Protocols

TRADITIONAL PROTOCOL	MODIFIED PROTOCOLS
The EXCITE trial defined the intervention as: "Participants in the intervention group were taught to apply an instrumented protective safety mitt and encouraged to wear it on their less-impaired upper extremity for a goal of 90% of their waking hours over a 2-week period, including 2 weekends, for a total of 14 days. On each weekday, participants received shaping (adaptive task practice) and standard task training of the paretic limb for up to 6 hours per day. The former is based on the principles of behavioral training that can also be described in terms of motor learning derived from adaptive or part-task practice. Standard task practice is less structured (i.e., repetition of tasks is not conducted as individual trials of discrete movements); it involves functional activities performed continuously for a period of 15 to 20 minutes (e.g., eating, writing)."[193]	Page and colleagues[137] described the following protocol consisting of 2 components. "The first component consisted of half-hour, one-on-one sessions of more affected arm therapy occurring 3 days per week during a 10-week period. This component included shaping in which operant conditioning was applied in such a way that subjects received positive verbal encouragement to more fully perform selected motor skills with their more affected arm. Shaping was applied with 2 or 3 upper-limb activities (e.g., writing, using a fork) chosen by the subjects with help from their therapist. In the second component of the mCIT intervention, during the same 10-week period, subjects' less affected arms were restrained every weekday for 5 hours identified as a time of frequent arm use, as identified by the subjects with assistance from the therapist. Their arms were restrained using a cotton hemi-sling, while their hands were placed in mesh, polystyrene-filled mitts with Velcro straps around the wrist."
	Lin and colleagues[112] defined their protocol as "restraint of the less affected limb combined with intensive training of the affected limb for 2 hours daily 5 days per week for 3 weeks and restraint of the less affected hand for 5 hours outside of the rehabilitation training."
	Sterr and colleagues[167] defined their protocol as 14 consecutive days; constraint of unaffected hand for a target of 90% of waking hours with 3 hours of shaping training with the affected hand per day. To note they concluded that: "The 3-hour CIMT training schedule significantly improved motor function in chronic hemiparesis, but it was less effective than the 6-hour training schedule."

- In follow-up examinations up to six months after treatment, motor performance remained at a high level.
- At follow-up, the cortical area sizes in the two hemispheres became almost identical, representing a return of the balance of excitability between the two hemispheres toward a normal condition.

Taub and colleagues[171] summarized by stating that if the "neural substrate for a movement is destroyed by CNS injury, no amount of intervention designed to overcome learned nonuse can be successful in helping recover lost function. However, many stroke patients . . . have considerably more motor ability available than they utilize. The suppression of this additional motor capacity is set up by unsuccessful attempts at movement in the acute poststroke phase . . . increased motor activity should then become increasingly possible, but the suppression of movement remains unabated and inhibits use of the limb. However, if individuals are correctly motivated to use this unexpressed ability, they will be able to do so." See Table 10-1 for a review of evidence related to constraint induced movement therapy (Box 10-4). See Chapter 6.

Managing Inefficient and Ineffective Movement Patterns

Being unable to move effectively and therefore unable to interact with the environment is one of the most devastating sequelae of stroke. The loss of the ability to move effectively is a negative stroke symptom.

The movement patterns of stroke survivors have long been discussed in the literature. Controversy continues over the nature of these patterns. These movement patterns have been described as reflex based, a release of abnormal synergies, the result of reversed inhibition or the release of lower patterns of activity from higher inhibitory control, and as learned patterns of movement. Mathiowetz and Bass-Haugen[121] point out that more contemporary models of motor control describe patterns developing after central nervous system damage as results of attempts to use remaining resources to achieve

Box 10-4

Summary of Constraint-Induced Movement Therapy

- Use to counteract learned nonuse. Hypothesized causes of learned nonuse include therapeutic interventions implemented during the acute period of neurological suppression after stroke, an early focus on adaptations to meet functional goals, negative reinforcement experienced by the patients as they unsuccessfully attempt to use the affected limb, and positive reinforcement experienced by using the less involved hand and/or use of successful adaptations.

- Motor inclusion criteria. Control of the wrist and digits is necessary to engage in this type of intervention. Current and past protocols have used the following inclusion criteria: 20 degrees of extension of the wrist and 10 degrees of extension of each finger; or 10 degrees extension of the wrist, 10 degrees abduction of the thumb, and 10 degrees extension of any two other digits; or able to lift a wash rag off a table using any type of prehension and then release it. It is clear that distal function (particularly wrist and digit extension) is a critical factor in being a candidate for the intervention. Therapists should focus on these movements early and intensely. Potential interventions to regain this motor control included electrical stimulation, mental practice, and activities that require distal extension such as reaching for large objects.

- Main therapeutic factor. Massed practice and shaping of the affected limb during repetitive functional activities appears to be the therapeutic change agent. "There is thus nothing talismanic about use of a sling or other constraining device on the less-affected limb."[173]

- Activity choices and therapist's interventions. Select tasks that address the motor deficits of the individual patient, assist the patient to carry out parts of a movement sequence if the patient incapable of completing the movement on is his or her own at first, providing explicit verbal feedback and verbal reward for small improvements in task performance, use modeling and prompting of task performance, use tasks that are of interest and motivating to the patient, ignore regression of function, and use tasks that can be quantified related to improvements.

- Outcome measures. The Motor Activity Log (actual use outside of structured therapy or "real-world use"), Arm Motor Ability Test, Wolf Motor Function Test, and the Action Research Arm Test have been used to document outcomes.

- Cortical reorganization. Constraint-induced movement therapy is the first rehabilitation intervention demonstrated to induce changes in the cortical representation of the affected upper limb.

- The continued rigorous research that has been and continues to be carried out to demonstrate the effectiveness/efficacy of constraint-induced movement therapy should be used as a gold standard for other rehabilitation interventions that are used traditionally (e.g., neurodevelopmental therapy) but have little or no research support.

- Based on available evidence, constraint-induced movement therapy appears to be an effective intervention for stroke survivors who have learned nonuse and who fit the motor inclusion criteria.

---

occupational performance. They give the example of a typical flexor pattern (scapula retraction, internal rotation, elbow/wrist/digit flexion) in the upper extremity; the pattern can stem from factors other than spasticity, such as the inability to recruit appropriate muscles, weakness, soft-tissue tightness, and perceptual deficits.

Carr and Shepherd[42] state that "muscles that are held persistently in a shortened position not only develop contracture but also appear 'easier' for the patients to activate. . . . In the stroke patient such activity appears to become habitual, certain muscle groups, apparently those whose mechanical advantages are greatest (because of their shortened length), contracting persistently to the disadvantage of others." The therapist can observe this phenomenon if a patient is reaching out to a target. Many patients have difficulty with the protraction, elbow extension, and wrist and digit extension patterns of this task. If the therapist observes the patients who have been in a resting posture (e.g., seated in a wheelchair) for a prolonged time, the shortened muscles include the retractors, elbow flexors, and wrist and digit flexors.

Ada and colleagues[1] hypothesize that muscle weakness or paralysis effectively immobilize the upper limb, which results in soft-tissue contracture. The immobility causes length-associated changes in muscles, and persistent positioning results in contracture. These changes in the upper limb result in compensatory movements that generate strong neural connections after frequent repetition, ensuring that the compensatory or adaptive movement patterns become learned rather than more effective and efficient.

A Russian neurologist, Nicoli Bernstein, emphasized a early task-oriented view of motor performance and introduced the concept that purposeful movement is organized to solve motor problems and the concept of degrees of freedom.[158] He hypothesized that the principal problem faced by the central nervous system was the large number of joints and muscles in the human body and the infinite combinations of muscle action. For example, the upper extremity has multiple degrees of freedom if the number of planes through which each joint moves are combined. When contemplating the combinations of degrees of freedom in the trunk, scapula, and shoulder to the hand, it becomes evident that task of controlling them is phenomenal. Bernstein states that "The coordination of a movement is the process of mastering redundant degrees of freedom of the moving organ, that is, its conversion to a controllable system."[158] Bernstein views motor control as a person's ability to coordinate kinematic linkages that limit degrees of freedom. See Chapter 5.

Flinn[70] uses the example of gymnasts learning a new maneuver to apply the concept of degrees of freedom to a task. Gymnasts limit the degrees of freedom in the task by holding some joints rigid while focusing on one specific body part (e.g., foot placement). Although the gymnasts initially may appear stiff, as they become able to control more degrees of freedom, the stiffness disappears and movement relaxes. This example can be applied to learning how to roller-blade, ice-skate, or perform a new swimming stroke. Sabari[158] discusses a patient with hemiplegia who does not dissociate the pelvis from the lumbar spine or scapula from the thorax, which may be an effort to decrease the degrees of freedom.

With this concept in mind, many of the ineffective movement patterns observed in patients can be attributed to attempts to control the degrees of freedom. Therapists need to consider this during treatment planning when choosing activities. The degrees of freedom must be controlled carefully by stabilizing or eliminating use of some of the joints and therefore decreasing the number of joints involved (e.g., supporting the distal extremity on a table or substituting flat-hand stabilization for a hand grasp).[70] Gillen[76,77] has demonstrated a variety of methods to improve task performance in clients with central nervous system dysfunction by manipulating the degrees of freedom via positioning, splinting, movement retraining, and equipment. Further research is required with the stroke population.

Many of the inefficient movement patterns in stroke survivors may result from attempting tasks beyond their level of motor control (Fig. 10-5). Many therapists have watched patients with newly developed motor control proudly show how they can "lift their arm." Of course, the resulting movement is a stereotypical pattern used by stroke survivors. Mathiowetz and Bass-Haugen[121] suggest that the use of these movement patterns is evidence of attempts to use remaining systems to complete tasks. They give the example of a patient with weak shoulder flexors trying to lift an arm. The patient flexes the elbow when trying to raise the arm because this movement strategy shortens the lever arm and makes shoulder flexion easier. This phenomenon can be observed in those with other diagnoses that result in proximal weakness (Fig. 10-6).

Based on these concepts, the roles of the occupational therapist in treating inefficient and ineffective upper extremity patterns are the following:

- To use skills of activity analysis to guide patients' participation in functional upper extremity tasks that correspond to their level of motor control

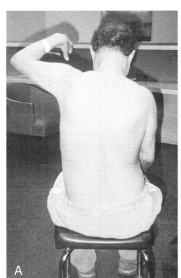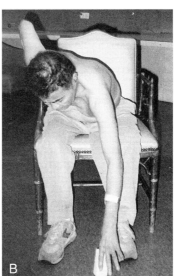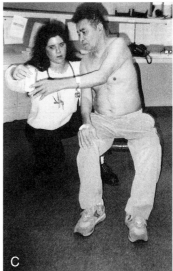

Figure 10-5 **A,** When asked to reach, this patient uses a stereotypical flexor pattern. Note trunk lateral flexion, scapula adduction, humeral abduction, and distal flexion. **B,** When the position of the activity is changed to correspond with the available motor control, and the patient is given a goal (e.g., "Pick up the bottle"), movement pattern is more effective and efficient. **C,** Another position change of same activity results in forward reach with less impact of compensations seen in **A.** The patient reaches with wrist extension, and his hand is prepositioned for successful task completion. The purpose of the activity drives motor output.

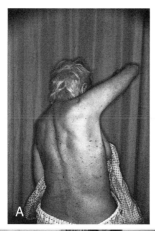

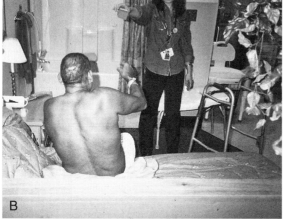

Figure 10-6 Compensatory movements from proximal weakness. **A,** This person's is status post left brain damage resulting in right sided weakness including right scapula instability. Compensatory strategies used to lift her arm include lateral trunk flexion, trunk rotation, scapula adduction and elevation, and elbow flexion. These compensatory movement strategies act to decrease the degrees of freedom, provide proximal stability, and shorten the lever arm of the upper extremity. This person has relatively preserved elbow extension strength, which she cannot use during this movement as it will create a longer lever arm and a loss of control. In the recent past, this movement pattern was attributed to abnormal flexor tone placing the treatment focus on decreasing tone in the antagonistic muscle groups (i.e., elbow flexors). A more current treatment approach includes interventions related to proximal strengthening and practice of graded reach patterns (i.e., a focus on the weak agonists). **B,** This man is using very similar compensatory movements as the woman in **A,** although his diagnosis is a right rotator cuff tear. The inefficient and ineffective movement patterns and the compensatory movements are secondary to proximal weakness.

- Through this process, to enable patients to interact with the environment using their more affected upper extremity
- To use evaluation skills to determine which impairments (e.g., loss of postural control, weakness, pain,

or a combination of components) related to upper extremity function are blocking improvements in occupational performance (e.g., ADL, IADL, work, and leisure)

- To provide function-based activities that focus on improving the identified problem area in an effort to improve task performance
- To provide opportunities to use available motor control throughout the day. Strategies include using devices that unweight the weak upper extremity so that movement can be accessed (Fig. 10-7), providing bedside and home-based activity programs as opposed to only exercise programs, and explicitly teaching stroke survivors how the upper extremity should be used throughout the course of the day to support participation (Fig. 10-8).

In terms of treatment, Mathiowetz and Bass-Haugen[121] suggest that therapists help the patients "find the optimal strategy for achieving functional goals." Goals can be achieved by altering the task requirements, altering the environmental context, and by guiding remediation of the component deficits that interfere with functional performance. The most powerful tools occupational therapists have for intervention are functional activities. Although functional activities have formed the basis of treatment since the profession was developed, only recently has the true impact of functional tasks been evaluated in this area of intervention (Fig. 10-9). See Chapter 4.

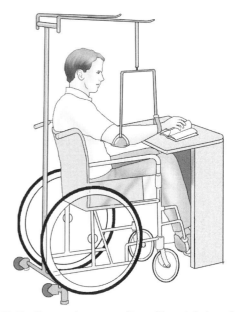

Figure 10-7 Suspension arm sling. Unweighting the upper extremity may promote increased use during the day. The therapist must consider ways in which the patient can move and use the upper extremity outside of therapy. Caution: When evaluating patients using this device, the therapist must make sure that the movement is being generated by the upper extremity as opposed to swinging the arm by moving the trunk.

Daily Planner

8:00 am: Out of bed	Use right arm to push up from side lying to sitting position. Use both arms to push up to stand.
8:15 am: Bathroom	• Use right hand to squeeze out toothpaste (push down through tube while the tube is resting on sink). • Use right arm to stabilize yourself while standing at sink. • Use right arm to stabilize on grab bar during clothing management. • Use wash mitt on right hand to wash legs and chest while sitting on tub bench.
9:15 am: Breakfast	• Use right arm as a stabilizer (ex. stabilize bread when spreading butter with left hand; stabilize fruit while cutting with left hand). • Wipe crumbs off table with right hand after breakfast.
10:00 am: Watching television	• Hold remote in right hand while watching television. • Perform prescribed stretching program during commercials.
11:00 am: Email and computing	Use right arm to control mouse when navigating websites.
11:30 am: Errands/shopping	Hold tote bag using right arm. Loop the tote bag across your forearm and keep your elbow flexed.
12:30 am: Lunch with friends	• Keep right arm positioned on table as opposed to in your lap. • Use right arm to turn menu pages. • Hold napkin in right hand until you are ready to use it.
Etc.	

Figure 10-8 Daily planner to promote upper extremity function throughout the day.

SELECTED ADJUNCT INTERVENTIONS USED WITH A TASK-ORIENTED APPROACH

Mental Practice/Imagery

The use of imagery in treatment has received an increasing amount of support in the literature. Using imagery and mental practice has been shown to do the following:

■ Activate the cortical representation and musculature the correlates with the imagined movements
■ Improve learning and performance
■ Reorganize the motor cortex

Yue and Cole[202] proposed a method for increasing skeletal muscle strength. Healthy subjects were separated into three groups: those receiving imagining training (i.e., training in which the person imagines a muscle is contracting but is not activating the muscle), those receiving contraction training, and a control group. Training resulted in a maximum voluntary contraction force increase of 22% in the imagining group, 30% in the contraction group, and 3.7% in the control group. This study demonstrated that strength increases can be achieved without muscle activation. Early strength increases appear to result from practice efforts on central motor programming. This study adds to the increasing evidence that the neural origin of strength increases before muscle hypertrophy.

In an early study focused on improving upper extremity function after stroke, Page[139] hypothesized that imagery use combined with traditional occupational therapy could enhance motor recovery in patients with upper extremity hemiparesis. He provided eight chronic stroke patients with a four-week course of occupational therapy and imagery (a 20-minute audio tape that consisted of

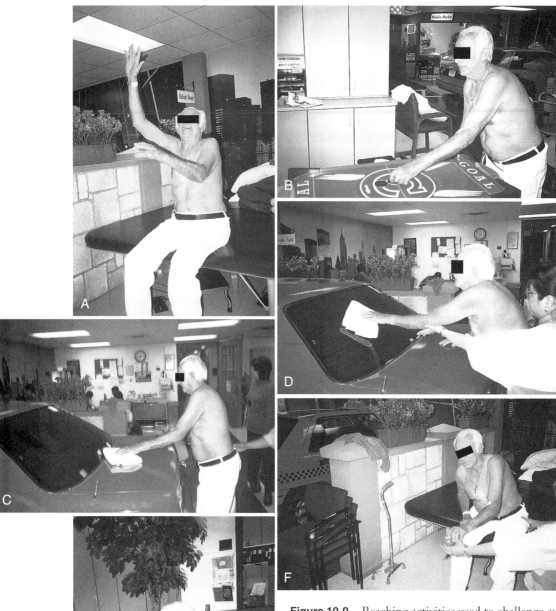

Figure 10-9   Reaching activities used to challenge available motor control appropriately. **A,** When attempting to lift both arms, this man uses an ineffective and inefficient movement pattern. He recruits his available scapula elevators, elbow flexors, trunk extensors, and head/neck extensors. Although it may appear that he lacks elbow extension or that his elbow flexors are "spastic" or "overactive," muscle testing in supine yields a grade of 4 out of 5 for all elbow musculature. His lack of ability to use elbow extension in this movement may indicate an attempt to shorten the lever arm and control the degrees of freedom. **B** and **C,** Using leisure and work tasks that are more appropriate to this man's level of motor control. Both activities are considered supported reach because the hand is in contact with the work surface. Note that the upper extremity patterns are more effective and efficient. **D,** The therapist provides graded physical assist to complete the task as increased biomechanical demands are made using the incline of the car. **E** and **F,** Grading the reaching in space activity using gravity to make the task progressively more difficult.

relaxation followed by cognitive visual images related to the upper extremity being used in weight-bearing tasks and functional tasks that were practiced in occupational therapy). This group was compared with eight controls that received only occupational therapy. He concluded that the patients who received occupational therapy and imagery had significantly more improved function as measured by the upper extremity section of the Fugl-Meyer Assessment. Since then, multiple studies have documented the effectiveness of this adjunctive intervention. See Table 10-1 for a review of evidence related to mental practice (Box 10-5).

Electromyographic Biofeedback

Electromyographic (EMG) biofeedback shows promise and should be studied further for its potential use in treating upper extremity dysfunction after stroke. Biofeedback is provided by electronic instruments that measure and give information about neuromuscular or autonomic activity in the form of auditory or visual feedback signals.

Tries' review[175] of the literature included a variety of rationales for integrating this noninvasive modality, including training voluntary inhibition of spastic muscles and restoring muscle balance, into an upper extremity program. Tries[175] outlined specific techniques for scapula mobility and stability, humeral rotation, integrating

---

Box 10-5

Summary: Using Mental Practice to Improve Upper Extremity Function after Stroke

- During mental practice, an internal representation of the movement is activated and the execution of the movement repeatedly mentally simulated, without physical activity, within a chosen context. It is used for the goal-oriented improvement or stabilization of a given movement.[33] It is cognitive rehearsal of a motor act or task.[94]

- Provides opportunity to promote repetitive task practice

- Most commonly, the mental practice intervention is administered via audiotape. The audiotapes consist of a few minutes of relaxation and focusing followed by several minutes of mental practice of tasks such as turning pages in a book, drinking from a cup, writing, etc. The length of the audiotapes have varied from approximately 10 to 20 minutes.

- Consistent and positive outcomes have been documented, including decreased upper extremity impairment, increased upper extremity function, and increase in everyday use of the limb outside of structured therapy.[135]

- Data from psychophysical, neurophysiological, and brain imaging studies support the existence of a similarity between executed and imagined actions.[94]

---

scapular and humeral rotation with a forward reach pattern, and reinforcement of functional patterns in the elbow, forearm, and hand.

Tries[175] presented a case study outlining the applications of biofeedback for a left-sided hemiplegic patient. Her case study illustrated that despite sensory, cognitive, and perceptual impairments, this patient had significant clinical upper limb functional improvements when combining EMG biofeedback and traditional occupational therapy.

Greenberg and Fowler[80] compared kinesthetic biofeedback (feedback information pertaining to actual movement of a body part rather than the activity of muscle fibers) to conventional occupational therapy. Their results indicated that kinesthetic biofeedback was equally as therapeutic as but no more effective than conventional occupational therapy for increasing elbow extension in hemiplegic subjects.

Crow and colleagues[53] studied two groups (a group receiving biofeedback and a control group) of 20 patients. The patients were studied before and after six weeks of treatment and during a follow-up visit six weeks later. Although the groups did not differ significantly before treatment, the biofeedback group improved significantly on arm-function evaluations. At the six-week follow-up, the beneficial effects were discovered not to have persisted in the experimental group.

Schleenbaker and Mainous[161] concluded from their meta-analysis that biofeedback is an effective tool in neuromuscular reeducation for executing ADL. The use of EMG biofeedback warrants further investigation into its use as an adjunct tool to enhance upper extremity function in select patients with hemiparesis. See Table 10-1 for a review of evidence related to EMG biofeedback.

Electrical Stimulation

Electrical stimulation has been used in poststroke upper extremity rehabilitation for many years. Potential uses have included reduction of shoulder subluxation, reduction of pain, improved motor control, and increasing use of the involved extremity. In general, the effects of electrical stimulation have been the most consistent at improving limb impairments such as ROM and reducing pain. The effects on function and ADL have received less attention and have been inconsistent. See Table 10-1 and Table 10-4 for an evidenced-based review of electrical stimulation.

Electromyographic-Triggered Electrical Stimulation

Electrical stimulation can be triggered by voluntary movement or nontriggered. EMG-triggered stimulation detects underlying muscle activity when it reaches a threshold level prior to providing the stimulation. The stroke survivor must voluntarily activate the correct muscles prior to the stimulation facilitating the motor response. This type of stimulation assures that the intervention is not passive

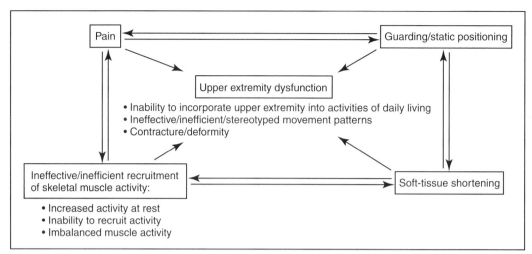

Figure 10-10 Complexity and interdependence of causes of upper extremity dysfunction.

in nature. Triggered electrical stimulation may be more effective than nontriggered electrical stimulation in facilitating upper extremity motor recovery following stroke.[59] This intervention has been shown to be effective at improving wrist extension, a key movement to be considered a candidate for some task oriented approaches such as CIMT. See Table 10-1 for an evidence-based review of EMG-triggered electrical stimulation.

Bilateral Training

Recently, bilateral training (i.e., patients practice identical activities with both upper limbs simultaneously) has been proposed as a strategy to improve upper limb control and function post stroke.[130a] The theory and rationale as to why the intervention may be effective has been described as follows: "Control of bilaterally identical synchronous movement appears to occur centrally through bilaterally distributed neural networks linked via the corpus callosum and involving cortical and subcortical areas. These networks indicate a common facilitatory drive to both motor cortices thought to lead to tight temporal and spatial coupling of limb movement observed during bilaterally identical synchronous voluntary movement. Beneficial effects of bilateral training in stroke are assumed to arise from this coupling effect in which the nonparetic limb provides a template for the paretic limb in terms of movement characteristics, facilitating restoration of movement."[129] Stoykov and Corcos[169] further reviewed neural mechanisms mediating bilateral training including recruitment of the ipsilateral corticospinal track, increased control from the contralesional hemisphere, and a normalization of inhibitory mechanism.

Although some findings have been inconsistent, a recent meta-analysis and randomized controlled trials have demonstrated improvement. Protocols vary but typically use either functional tasks or repetitive arm movements. This technique has been combined with auditory rhythmic cuing and neuromuscular stimulation. Some research has concluded that the technique may be more beneficial for those with proximal limb involvement. See Tables 10-1 and 10-5 for an evidence-based review of bilateral training. See Box 10-6 for a sample protocol.

Mirror Therapy

A relatively new intervention, this intervention appears to be cost-efficient and is able to be done independently. Yavuzer and colleagues[199] describe the intervention as "During the mirror practices, patients were seated close to a table on which a mirror (35×35 cm) was placed vertically. The involved hand was placed behind the mirror and the noninvolved hand in front of the mirror. The practice consisted of nonparetic-side wrist and finger flexion and extension movements while patients looked into the mirror, watching the image of their noninvolved hand, thus seeing the reflection of the hand movement projected over the involved hand. Patients could see only the noninvolved hand in the mirror; otherwise, the noninvolved hand was hidden from sight. During the session patients were asked to try to do the same movements with the paretic hand while they were moving the nonparetic hand" (Fig. 10-11). See Table 10-1 for an evidence-based review of mirror training.

IMPAIRMENTS TO CONSIDER DURING EVALUATION AND INTERVENTION

Evaluation and intervention of the upper extremity are complex tasks that require an understanding of multiple systems. Therapists need to remain open-minded about their interventions and consider the complexity of causes

Table 10-4

Effectiveness of Electrical Stimulation to Decrease Arm Impairment and Improve Function after Stroke

STUDY	SAMPLE	TREATMENT	OUTCOME	d OR EFFECT SIZE	WEIGHT	DW	r INDEX
Chantraine et al. (1999)	N = 115 57 (exp.) 58 (ctrl.)	Both groups rehab using Bobath approach. Exp. Five weeks of FES on muscles surrounding shoulder	At six months Exp. ROM improved Subluxation reduced Pain reduced	.48 .36 .48	29.16 29.52 29.16	14.00 10.63 14.00	.23 .18 .23
Faghri et al. (1994)	N = 26 13 (exp.) 13 (ctrl.)	Experimental group received FES to shoulder muscles	After six weeks of treatment exp. group had significant reduction in subluxation	.82	6.00	4.92	.38
Cauraugh et al. (2000)	N = 11 7 (exp.) 4 (ctrl.)	Both received 30 minutes passive ROM, stretching. Exp. ETNES (1 sec. ramp up 5 sec. biphasic stim. 50 Hz, 1 sec. ramp down, stim.) Range 14-29mA	Post treatment, functional prehension and grasp in hemiplegic hand improved	1.53	2.00	3.06	.61
Wang, Chan, & Tsai (2000)	N = 32 postonset: 16 short duration 16 long duration (each randomly assigned to exp. and ctrl. (8,8)	Exp. Groups both short and long duration, FES 6hr/day for six weeks	Exp. Group, short duration showed improved subluxation, long duration no improvement	1.51 .90	3.11 3.63	4.70 3.27	.60 .41
Linn, Granat, & Lees (1999)	N = 40 Exp. 20 Ctrl. 20	Exp. 4 weeks of electrical stimulation	Less subluxation at end of treatment period	.77	9.31	7.17	.36
				Sum =	111.89	23.12	3.0 (avg. .375)

d. = Σ dw/Σ w 23.12/111.89 = .21

95% Confidence Interval d. +/− 1.96 $\sqrt{1\Sigma w}$ .21 + 1.96* .09 .21 − 1.96* .09 low .04 to high .38

Success rate (Rosenthal, 1991) .50 + avg. r/2 = 69% Treatment Group .50 − avg. r/2 = 31% Control Group

From Hardy J, Salinas S, Blanchard SA, Aitken MJ: Meta-analysis examining the effectiveness of electrical stimulation in improving functional use of the upper limb in stroke patients. *Phys Occup Ther Geriatr* 21(4):61-78, 2003.

Table 10-5

Characteristics of Each Study Used in the Meta-Analysis by Stewart and Colleagues[168]

STUDY	TOTAL N	MEAN AGE: YEARS	LESION LOCATION	MEAN TIME POSTSTROKE (MONTHS)	TRAINING DURATION	LENGTH OF STUDY	TREATMENT PROTOCOL
Mudie and Matyas	8	69.4	Right = 6 Left = 2	4.3	Time ≈ N/A	8 weeks (40 sessions)	Single: bilateral tasks
Mudie and Matyas	4	N/A	N/A	N/A	Time ≈ N/A	6 weeks (30 sessions)	Single: bilateral tasks
Whitall and colleagues	14	63.8	Right = 7 Left = 7	66.9	Time ≈ 50 min	6 weeks (18 sessions)	Coupled: AUD + bilateral movements
Cauraugh and Kim	25	63.7	Right = 12 Left = 13	39.1	Time ≈ 90 min	4 days over 2 weeks	Coupled: ANS + bilateral movements
Cauraugh and Kim	26	66.4	Right = 15 Left = 11	33.6	Time ≈ 90 min	4 days over 2 weeks	Coupled: ANS + bilateral movements
Lewis and Byblow	6	58.7	Right = 5 Left = 1	16.2	33 trials	4 weeks (20 sessions)	Single: bilateral tasks
McCombe-Waller and colleagues	20	N/A	N/A	>12	Time ≈ 50 min	6 weeks (18 sessions)	Coupled: AUD + bilateral movements
Stinear and Byblow	9	62	Right = 3 Left = 6	16.22	Time = 60 min	4 weeks (20 sessions)	Single: bilateral training
Luft and colleagues	21	61.5	Right = 14 Left = 7	50.3 (median)	Time ≈ 50 min	6 weeks (18 sessions)	Coupled: AUD + bilateral movements
Cauraugh and colleagues	26	64.2	Right = 15 Left = 6	50.1	Time ≈ 90 min	4 days over 2 weeks	Coupled: ANS + bilateral movements
Summers and colleagues	12	61.7	Right = 4 Left = 8	62.2	50 trials	6 days	Single: bilateral training

List is in chronological order.

Note. Single = only bilateral training; Coupled = two protocols simultaneously presented; AUD = auditory rhythmic cuing; ANS = active neuromuscular stimulation.

From Stewart KC, Cauraugh JH, Summers JJ: Bilateral movement training and stroke rehabilitation: a systematic review and meta-analysis. *J Neurol Sci* 244(1-2):89-95, 2006.

that interfere with upper extremity use (Fig. 10-10). Many of the various problems associated with upper extremity function overlap and build on each other. The following paragraphs review common impairments in stroke survivors that may or may not interfere with integrating the upper extremity into daily occupations.

Impaired Postural Control

Improving proximal stability to enhance distal mobility has long been a tenet of occupational therapy interventions. Postural adjustments stabilize supporting body parts while other parts (e.g., the upper extremities) are being moved.[73] The following studies describe the effect of postural adjustments on arm function.

In the classic study by Belenkii, Gurfinkle, and Paltsev,[16] unimpaired subjects who were evaluated while standing were asked to raise their arm to a horizontal position after they heard an external signal. Various EMG studies were performed to trace the pattern of muscle activation. The results demonstrated that the postural muscle synergies of

the trunk and lower extremities were activated *before* (by 90 milliseconds) the anterior deltoid, the primary muscle used to perform this motion. The subjects then were evaluated in the supine position while performing the same task. No lower extremity activation was detected in this position (i.e., a different pattern of postural adjustments). The following conclusions can be inferred from this study:

1. Postural adjustments are task-specific.
2. Training of the upper extremity in the supine position does not automatically carry over to activities performed while sitting or standing (if postural control is a limiting factor).
3. Having different disciplines treat one particular half of the body is detrimental to patients' progress because upper extremity function depends on postural support from the lower extremities and trunk.

Bouisset and Zattara[29] replicated the previous study and demonstrated that an upward and forward trunk movement resulting from spine and/or lower limb extension

Box 10-6

Example of Bilateral Training Protocol

TASK PROTOCOL

UNILATERAL TREATMENT ACTIVITIES	BILATERAL TREATMENT ACTIVITIES
1. Pushing and pulling activity (open/close drawer) *Rhythmic task*	1. Pushing/pulling with both arms (open/close 2 identical drawers) *Rhythmic task*
2. Wipe a table with a towel using the affected arm *Discrete task*	2. Wipe a table with both arms using both arms symmetrically *Discrete task*
3. One arm cycling using BTE 181 *Rhythmic task*	3. Bilateral in-phase cycling using BTE *Rhythmic task*
4. Reaching and placing objects. Moving small and medium-sized grocery items from kitchen counter to shelves using only affected arm *Discrete task*	4. Bilateral reaching and placing objects. Moving 2 identical small or medium-sized grocery objects from countertop to shelf with both hands *Discrete task*
5. Shoulder and elbow coupling. Aim to target with affected hand in various areas of work space (using varying levels of arm support, postural sets, and positions in relation to gravity). Includes a total of 4 subtasks *Rhythmic task*	5. Bilateral shoulder and elbow coupling. Aim with both hands to parallel targets (using varying levels of arm support, postural sets, and positions in respect to gravity). Includes a total of 4 subtasks *Rhythmic task*
6. Elbow extension during horizontal reach *Rhythmic task*	6. Bilateral elbow extension during horizontal reach *Rhythmic task*

From Stoykov ME, Lewis GN, Corcos DM: Comparison of bilateral and unilateral training for upper extremity hemiparesis in stroke, *Neurorehabil Repair* 23(9):945-953, 2009.

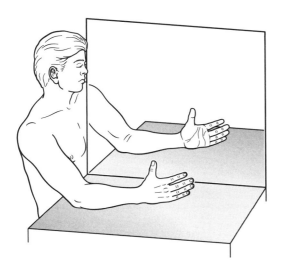

Figure 10-11   Mirror training. Set-up for mirror therapy: The patient's affected arm is hidden behind the mirror. While he is moving his unaffected arm, he is watching its mirror image as if it were the affected one.

precedes upper limb movement. This movement pattern is familiar to therapists who cue their patients to focus on spinal extension and the associated anterior pelvic tilt while treating arm function.

Horak and colleagues[88] compared postural adjustments of subjects with and without hemiplegia during a variety of tasks with different parameters. The hemiplegic subjects demonstrated the same sequence of muscle activation as the subjects without hemiplegia, although activity on the hemiparetic side was delayed. In addition, the hemiparetic individuals were not capable of making rapid movements with the unimpaired arm. This was hypothesized to result from a delay in the anticipatory activity of the contralateral hemiplegic muscles. This study dispels the myth of "good" and "bad" sides after a stroke, especially when postural control is compromised.

In their study of postural adjustments during arm movements, Cordo and Nashner[52] were able to demonstrate that when subjects' postural stability was increased (e.g., by outside shoulder support or placing a finger lightly on a support rail), postural activity was reduced, and voluntary movement enhanced. This concept is crucial to understand when treating upper extremity dysfunction. As support is increased, the postural demands of the task are decreased and vice versa. The therapist can control the patient's level of postural stability by manipulating the following treatment environment factors: positioning—supine to sitting to standing; type of support surface—stationary or unstable surfaces; positioning of objects used in activities—near or far, base of support, and amount of external stability.

Cordo and Nashner[52] also made a critical distinction between associated postural adjustments that *precede* voluntary movements (e.g., reaching) and automatic postural adjustments that *follow* external perturbations (e.g., standing on a bus that stops at a light or being moved by the therapist). Training in one type of adjustment cannot be assumed to carry over into other types of adjustments.

Woollacott, Bonnet, and Yabe[194] demonstrated that their subjects' postural activity varied depending on the task being performed (pushing, pulling) and whether they received information in advance regarding the goal of the task.

Massion[119] points out that voluntary movements are "accompanied by postural adjustments which show three main characteristics: (1) they are 'anticipatory' with respect to movement and minimize the perturbations of posture and equilibrium due to the movement, (2) they are adaptable to the conditions in which the movement is executed, and (3) they are influenced by the instructions given to the subject concerning the task to be performed."

Postural control disorders in stroke patients have been well-documented. Lee[109] emphasized the detrimental impact that postural dysfunction has on free arm movements and therefore ADL. Although a variety of muscles can serve as postural stabilizers, postural control of the trunk is critical for upper extremity function.[19] See Chapter 7.

Occupational therapists must use their activity analysis skills to help patients develop the missing trunk control components. (See Table 7-9 for examples of the effects of object positioning on trunk control and weight shifting during reaching activities.) Functional mobility patterns requiring increased trunk control (e.g., scooting) should be incorporated into treatment plans for upper extremity function. See Chapter 14.

Postural control evaluations should be performed within the context of upper extremity tasks such as reaching or performing ADL and IADL. Evaluating postural control separately does not provide the therapist with sufficient information for intervention. (See Chapters 7 and 8 for more information related to postural control.)

Weakness

Until relatively recently, the impact of weakness (a negative symptom) on stroke patients' functional status has long been ignored. The motor control deficits in patients previously were attributed exclusively to spasticity, which resulted in treatment focused on inhibiting the spasticity. Many therapists considered upper extremity muscle tests for strength difficult to interpret because of common

"synergy patterns." Bourbonnais and colleagues[31] demonstrated that the patterns of activity in the elbow flexor muscles were not consistent with established synergistic patterns. Weakness of the upper extremity musculature plays a major role in upper extremity dysfunction, most likely more than the positive symptoms after stroke. Muscle weakness is reflected by the inability of patients to generate normal levels of muscle force.[30] Stroke survivors who have written about their experiences focus on the difficulty in force production. Brodal[35] reflected on his own stroke: "It was a striking and repeatedly made observation that the force needed to make a severely paretic muscle contract is considerable. . . . Subjectively this is experienced as a kind of mental force, a power of will. In the case of a muscle just capable of being actively moved the mental effort needed was very great."

Bourbonnais and Vanden Noven[30] reviewed the physiological changes in the nervous system that contribute to muscle weakness in patients with hemiparesis. They summarized specific changes at the motor neuron and muscle levels that decrease a patient's ability to produce force. Box 10-7 summarizes these changes.

Bohannon and colleagues[21] found that static strength deficits of the shoulder medial rotator and elbow flexor muscles did not correlate with antagonist muscle spasticity. They concluded that therapists might determine the capacity for force production for an agonist muscle based on its own tone rather than that of its antagonist.

Gowland and colleagues[79] studied agonist and antagonist activity during upper limb movements in stroke patients and concluded that treatment should be aimed at improving motor neuron recruitment rather than reducing antagonist activity. In their study, patients who could not perform select upper extremity tasks had EMG values significantly and consistently lower than those of patients who were successful at the task.

Indeed recent empirical evidence highlights the relationship between weakness and loss of function. Findings include:

- In a study of 93 community dwelling stroke survivors, Harris and Eng[85] concluded that paretic

---

Box 10-7

Physiological Changes Contributing to Weakness

- Motor neuron changes: loss of agonist motor units, changes in recruitment order of motor units, and changes in the firing rates of motor units
- Nerve changes: changes in peripheral nerve conduction
- Muscle changes: changes in the morphological and contractile properties of motor units and in the mechanical properties of muscles

upper limb strength had the strongest relationship with variables of activity and best explained upper limb performance in ADL. Grip strength was also a factor.

- A longitudinal study of 27 stroke survivors found that weakness was the main and only contributor to activity limitations as opposed to spasticity or contracture.[6]
- Chae and colleagues[46] described the relationship between poststroke upper limb muscle weakness and cocontraction, and clinical measures of upper limb motor impairment and physical disability. The authors measured EMG activity of the paretic and nonparetic wrist flexors and extensors of 26 chronic stroke survivors. Upper limb motor impairment and physical disability were assessed with the Fugl-Meyer motor assessment and the arm motor ability test. They concluded that muscle weakness and degree of cocontraction correlate significantly with motor impairment and physical disability in upper limb hemiplegia.
- Mercier and Bourbonnais[123] compared the relative strength of different muscle groups of the paretic upper limb and assess the relationship with motor performance. The maximal active torques of five muscle groups were measured in both upper limbs. Upper limb function was assessed using the Box and Block Test, the Finger-to-Nose Test, the Fugl-Meyer Test, and the TEMPA. They concluded that "the relative forces for shoulder flexion and handgrip are the best predictors of the upper limb function." Additionally, they concluded that the results "do not confirm classical clinical teaching regarding the distribution of weakness following stroke (e.g., proximal to distal gradient; extensors more affected than flexors) but support the hypothesis that strength is related to the function of the paretic upper limb."

From a treatment planning perspective, integrating strengthening interventions is imperative in efforts to regain limb function. Bohannon and Smith[23] analyzed strength deficits in stroke patients and verified that muscle strength improves in stroke patients with hemiplegia who are undergoing rehabilitation. Empirical evidence supports the use of strengthening interventions in this population without deleterious effects:

- Flinn[70] presented a case study of a young female with left-sided hemiplegia. Her treatment program focused on participating in graded functional tasks that systematically increased the motor demands on the more affected upper extremity. Her task-oriented treatment program was augmented by resistive exercises using elastic tubing. Substantial results after six months of therapy included improved level of occupational performance in ADL and IADL, improved manual muscle test scores (which increased from 2/5 to the 4/5 and 5/5 ranges), improved hand function, and improved grip strength scores. Identifying the underlying problems (in this case, weakness and an inability to control excess degrees of freedom) is of utmost importance when planning treatment strategies.
- Bütefisch and colleagues[39] examined the effect of a standardized training on movements of the affected hand in 27 hemiparetic patients using a multiple baseline approach. The training consisted of repetitive hand and finger flexions and extensions against various loads and was carried out twice daily during 15-minute periods. Grip strength, peak force of isometric hand extensions, peak acceleration of isotonic hand extensions, and contraction velocities as indicators of motor performance significantly improved during the training period. Additionally, 24 out of 27 patients improved on the Rivermead Motor Assessment. The authors further challenged traditional therapy (the Bobath concept) aimed at reducing enhanced muscle tone without reinforcing the activity in centrally paretic hand. In the study, patients undergoing this treatment approach alone did not experience a significant improvement in the motor capacity of the hand. The authors emphasized the importance of frequent movement repetition for the motor rehabilitation of the centrally paretic hand and challenge conventional therapeutic strategies that focus on spasticity reduction instead of early initiation of active movements.
- Sterr and Freivogel[166] "assessed whether intensive training increases spasticity and leads to the development of 'pathologic movement patterns,' a concern often raised by Bobath-trained therapists. The authors used a baseline-control repeated-measures test to study 29 patients with chronic upper limb hemiparesis who received daily shaping training. Their results suggest that training has no adverse effects on muscle tone and movement quality."[2]
- A systematic review of multiple studies concluded that "Strengthening interventions increase strength, improve activity, and do not increase spasticity. These findings suggest that strengthening programs should be part of rehabilitation after stroke."
- In their strength training study after stroke, Badics and colleagues[10] concluded that "The extent of strength gain was positively correlated with the intensity and the number of exercising units. Muscle tone, which was abnormally high at baseline, did not further increase in any one case. The results of this study showed that targeted strength training significantly increased muscle power in patients with muscle weakness of central origin without any negative effects on spasticity."

- In their review of weakness and strengthening post stroke, Patten and colleagues[141] identified nine trials of progressive resistive training after stroke. They concluded "All of these studies reported positive adaptations to strength training . . . With one exception, all studies strongly suggest positive effects of strength training on various indices of functional outcome . . ." They further concluded that "while insufficient data exist to draw firm conclusions at this time, functional effects of strengthening appear persistent. Four of the available studies evaluated effects of strength training on spasticity and found no deleterious effects."

The debate about which type of muscle contraction (eccentric, concentric, or isometric) is the most effective in strengthening patients has been long-standing. Muscle groups need to contract in a variety of ways to complete functional tasks successfully. For example, when a person reaches for a can of soup on a high shelf, the shoulder musculature must contract (concentrically) to bring the hand to the level of the shelf, maintain the contraction (isometrically) to locate the correct item, and control the weight of the arm and item in gravity (eccentrically) as the can is placed with control on the countertop.

In a study of dynamical muscle strength training in stroke patients, Engardt and colleagues[65] found that eccentric contractions were more effective than concentric contractions. Twenty patients with hemiparesis resulting from strokes participated in activities that elicited concentric or eccentric contractions. After the treatment, significant improvements resulted in the relative strength of paretic muscles during eccentric and concentric actions in the group that was trained solely with eccentric contractions (i.e., eccentric training increased the strength of both types of contractions); this was not true for the group that only received concentric contraction training. Therefore, the authors determined eccentric contraction training to be more advantageous and efficient (Box 10-8). See Table 10-1 for a review of evidence-based interventions related to strengthening.

Box 10-8

Task Parameters That Can Be Manipulated to Increase Strength

- Gravity: eliminated, assisted, against
- Weight of objects used during tasks
- Amount of external support (e.g., slide hand across table versus reach into space)
- External resistance (e.g., weights, elastic bands, resistance from therapist's hands)

Spasticity

Spasticity, which is a positive symptom according to Jackson classification system, has been a subject of debate by various authors. Although an abundance of research has been done on spasticity, disagreements still exist about its definition, physiological basis, treatment, and evaluation. Glenn and Whyte[75] define spasticity as "a motor disorder with persistent increase in the involuntary reflex activity of a muscle in response to stretch. Four specific phenomena may be variably observed in the constellation of spasticity: hypertonia (frequently velocity dependent and demonstrating the clasp-knife phenomenon), hyperactive (phasic) deep tendon reflexes, clonus, and spread of reflex responses beyond the muscle stimulated." In addition, Babinski sign is characteristic, and hyperactive tonic neck or vestibular reflexes may be present.[116]

Several different phenomena commonly observed in stroke rehabilitation including hyperactive stretch reflexes, increased resistance to passive movement, posturing of the extremities, excessive cocontraction, and stereotypical movement synergies are clumped together in the category of spasticity. Spasticity has become a catchall term for a variety of problems. Rather than being a specific symptom, spasticity is related to a variety of neural and nonneural factors. Therefore, spasticity cannot be treated uniformly by surgical, physical, or pharmacological procedures. *Spastic paresis* is a commonly used term that implies a cause-and-effect relationship (i.e., a cause-and-effect relationship between positive and negative symptoms). This belief has been challenged recently.

Preston and Hecht[147] provide further information regarding the clinical presentation of spasticity to include the following:

- Patients having difficulty initiating rapid alternating movements
- Abnormally timed EMG activation of the agonist and antagonist
- Fluctuation of spasticity as a result of a change in position
- Usual patterns include upper extremity flexion and lower extremity extension

Bobath[18] stated that there is "An intimate relationship between spasticity and movement . . . spasticity must be held responsible for much of the patient's motor deficit." Treatment techniques were based on "helping the patient gain control over the released patterns of spasticity by their inhibition." Patients were treated under the assumption that "Weakness of muscles may not be real, but relative to the opposition by spastic antagonists." A variety of studies have been published that refute these assumptions. See Chapter 6.

Sahrmann and Norton[159] studied normal subjects and subjects with upper motor neuron symptoms. The movement pattern studied was alternating flexion and extension of the elbow. The analysis of their EMG findings showed that the primary cause of impaired movement was not antagonist stretch reflexes but was limited and prolonged agonist contraction recruitment and delayed cessation of agonist contractions after movement had stopped. Rather than focusing treatment on inhibiting spasticity, therapists should train patients to perform alternating movement patterns (e.g., hand-to-mouth patterns) efficiently.

Fellows, Kaus, and Thilmann[67] studied the importance of hyperreflexia and paresis on voluntary arm movements in normal subjects and subjects with spasticity resulting from a unilateral ischemic cerebral lesion. The subjects with spasticity showed a lower maximum movement velocity; the more marked the paresis, the greater the reduction in maximum velocity. No relationship was found between the degree of voluntary movement impairment and level of passive muscle hypertonia in the antagonist. The conclusion was that agonist muscle paresis, rather than antagonist muscle hypertonia, had the most significant effect on impaired voluntary movement.

In their study on overcoming limited elbow movement in the presence of antagonist hyperactivity, Wolf and colleagues[190] concluded that functional elbow improvements could be made without first training the patient specifically to inhibit hyperactivity.

Landau[108] performed pharmacological interventions that effectively abolished the hyperactive stretch reflexes in his patients. This intervention did not result in a corresponding improvement in motor behavior.

Ada, O'Dwyer, and O'Neill[6] examined the relationship between the motor impairments (spasticity and weakness) and their impact on physical activity. They specifically aimed to study the contribution of weakness and spasticity to contracture, and the contribution of all three impairments to limitations in physical activity during the first 12 months after stroke. The authors followed 27 stroke survivors for one year. They found that "the major independent contributors to contracture were spasticity for the first four months after stroke (p = 0.0001-0.10) and weakness thereafter (p = 0.01-0.05). However, the major and only independent contributor to limitations in physical activity throughout the year was weakness (p = 0.0001-0.05)." "For the first time, from a longitudinal study, the findings show that spasticity can cause contracture after stroke, consistent with the prevailing clinical view. However, weakness is the main contributor to activity limitations."

In the traditional evaluation of spasticity, the therapist moves the patient's limb quickly in a direction opposite to the pull of the muscle group being tested, and the examiner feels for a resistance to the movement. The gold standard for rating resistance is the Ashworth Scale[9] or the Modified Ashworth Scale[24] (Box 10-9).

Box 10-9

The Ashworth Scales

ASHWORTH SCALE*

1 Normal tone
2 Slight hypertonus; noticeable catch when limb is moved
3 More significant hypertonus, but affected limb still moves easily
4 Moderate hypertonus; difficulty with passive movement
5 Severe hypertonus; rigid limb

MODIFIED ASHWORTH SCALE†

0 No increase in muscle tone
1 Slight increase in muscle tone, manifested by a catch and release or by minimal resistance at the end of the range of motion when the affected part is moved in flexion or extension
1+ Slight increase in muscle tone, manifested by a catch, followed by minimal resistance throughout the remainder (less than half) of range of motion
2 More significant increase in muscle tone throughout most of the range of motion but affected part is moved easily.
3 Considerable increase in muscle tone; difficult passive movement
4 Affected part in rigid flexion or extension

---

*From Ashworth B: Carisoprodol in multiple sclerosis. *Practitioner* 192:540, 1964.
†From Bohannon RW, Smith MB: Interrater reliability of a modified Ashworth scale of muscle spasticity. *Phys Ther* 67(2):206-207, 1987.

The response of a spastic muscle to stretch has been argued not to be the same during passive and active movement. In addition, spasticity is a multidimensional problem that incorporates neural and nonneural components (e.g., altered soft-tissue compliance). Therefore, some authors have questioned the usefulness of test measures such as the Ashworth Scale and are investigating a more comprehensive evaluation of spasticity.

Although the research on spasticity does not support focusing treatment on suppressing stretch reflexes, it does support treatment focusing on preventing secondary structural muscle changes in patients with spasticity.

Hufschmidt and Mauritz's study[90] suggested that spastic contracture is the result of degenerative changes (e.g., atrophy and fibrosis) and changes of the passive and contractile muscle properties.

In their study on spastic and rigid muscles, Dietz, Quintern, and Berger[61] concluded that the actual muscle fibers undergo changes, which explains the increased muscle tone in spastic patients.

For treating patients with spasticity, Perry[142] emphasized early mobilization and assistance with developing evolving motor control into effective function. These two interventions result in minimal contractures and prevent improper use of patients' available control mechanisms. Hummelsheim and colleagues[91] studied the results of sustained stretch in spastic patients. They found that sustained muscle stretch of approximately 10 minutes led to significant reduction in the spastic hypertonus in the elbow, hand, and finger flexors. They hypothesized that this benefit is due to stretch receptor fatigue or adaptation to the new extended position.

Little and Massagli[116] also emphasized using a stretching program incorporating pain prevention and patient education focusing on the adverse effects of spasticity (contracture), use of slow movements, and importance of daily stretching.

In addition to the mentioned techniques, specific modalities and their physiological bases have been described in the literature and include local cooling, vibration therapy, and electrical stimulation.

Perry[142] summarized the effective rehabilitation of a patient with spasticity by using five categories: contracture minimization, realistic planning, muscle strength preservation and restoration, enhancement of returning control, and substitution for permanent functional loss.

Carr, Shepherd, and Ada[43] summarized their treatment approach based on the assumption that clinical spasticity is a manifestation of length-associated muscle changes and disordered motor control: "The development of spasticity will be less severe if soft-tissue length can be maintained and if motor training emphasizes elimination of unnecessary muscle force and training muscle synergies as part of specific actions."

Again, the point must be emphasized that many of the observed phenomena that occur during treatment should not be attributed automatically to spasticity and require more in-depth evaluations and treatment plans (Box 10-10; Table 10-6).

Preston and Hecht[147] have comprehensively reviewed the literature related to spasticity management, including topics such as oral and intrathecal medications, nerve blocks, orthopedic surgery, and neurosurgical interventions.

Nerve blocks are being used increasingly as an adjunct therapy in the rehabilitation process. Preston and Hecht[147] differentiated between short-term blocks such as procaine and bupivacaine used to diagnose and assist in the evaluation process and long-term blocks such as phenol and botulinum toxin type A (Botox).

Rousseaux, Kozlowski, and Froger[154] assessed the efficacy of Botox treatment on disability, especially in manual activities, and attempted to identify predictive factors of improvement in 20 patients with stroke. They concluded that botulinum toxin A is efficient in improv-

Box 10-10

Treatment of Spasticity

- Prevent pain syndromes.
- Guide *appropriate* use of available motor control.
- Maintain soft-tissue length.
- Avoid using excessive effort during movement.
- Encourage slow and controlled movements.
- Teach specific functional synergies during tasks.
- Avoid use of repetitive compensatory movement patterns.
- Keep spastic muscles on stretch via positioning or orthotics to prevent contracture.
- Teach the patient or caretaker specific stretching techniques targeted at the spastic muscles.
- Use activities to enhance the agonist/antagonist relationship.
- Refer when appropriate for pharmacological or surgical interventions.[147]

ing hand use in patients with relatively preserved distal motricity and in increasing comfort in patients with severe global disorders. Similarly, Bakheit and colleagues[11] completed a randomized controlled trial to assess the efficacy of Botox in decreasing spasticity in stroke survivors. They concluded that treatment with Botox reduced muscle tone in patients with poststroke upper limb spasticity.

While the positive effect at the impairment level (i.e., reduction of spasticity) has been well-documented, the effect on functional limitations is not as clear.[164,183] As spasticity increases, the risk for soft-tissue shortening is heightened, which in fact may lead to a vicious circle of problems such as spasticity, soft-tissue shortening, overrecruitment of shortened muscles, and increased stretch reflexes. Secondary problems that may occur if the spasticity is not managed in a therapy program include the following:

- Deformity of the limbs, specifically the distal upper limb (elbow to digits)
- Impaired upright function caused by soft-tissue contracture (e.g., plantar flexion contractures resulting in a loss of the ankle strategies required to maintain upright stance)
- Tissue maceration of the palm
- Pain syndromes resulting from loss of normal joint kinematics. These syndromes are usually related to soft-tissue contracture blocking full joint excursion. A typical example of this issue is the loss of full passive external rotation of the glenohumeral joint. Attempts at forced abduction in these cases results in a painful impingement syndrome of the tissues in the subacromial space.
- Impaired ability to manage basic ADL tasks, specifically upper extremity dressing and bathing of the

Table 10-6

Suggested Interventions for Problems Commonly Thought to Be Caused by Spasticity*

OBSERVATIONS DURING TREATMENT	SUGGESTED INTERVENTIONS
Posturing of upper extremity—usually consisting of retraction, posterior trunk rotation, internal rotation, elbow flexion, and wrist and digit flexion—during difficult tasks (e.g., gait, transfers, and dressing)	Upper extremity posturing indicates that the task is difficult for the patient. Treatment should include increasing the efficiency of task performance by building in trunk and lower extremity control, incorporating the upper extremity into the task (e.g., by bilateral ironing or using arm as postural support), and teaching the patient to relax the upper extremity after difficult tasks.
Stereotypical flexor patterns when attempting to move arm against gravity	Evaluate components of movement pattern and identify factors that limit efficient movement (e.g., weakness, postural dysfunction, malalignment, and inappropriate task choice). Provide activities that elicit the missing components of movement pattern.
Flexion posture when resting	Implement a contracture prevention program. Provide adequate positioning and teach safe, self range-of-motion exercises.
"Catch" felt during quick-stretch evaluation of upper extremity	Do not assume that this phenomenon is resulting in observed movement dysfunction. Instead, interpret it as a red flag warning that soft-tissue shortening may be present or developing.

*This table represents a variety of functional limitations and problems traditionally considered to be the direct result of spasticity. Although sometimes interconnected, these problems stem from different sources and must be treated accordingly.

affected hand and axilla when flexor posturing is present

■ Loss of reciprocal arm swing during gait activities
■ Risk for falls because of postural malalignment[78]

In summary, although reducing spasticity does not appear to result in automatic improvements related to function, therapists must manage spasticity to prevent soft-tissue contracture, prevent deformity, and maintain a flexible and mobile arm.

Loss of Soft-Tissue Elasticity (Contractures and Deformities)

Contracture in stroke patients results from immobilization and may be attributed to spasticity (particularly during the first four months after stroke) and weakness thereafter,[6] improper positioning, postural malalignment, a lack of variation in limb postures (e.g., prolonged sling use), or a combination of various factors. The formation of contractures indicates a poor prognosis for limb function. Perry[142] discussed the vicious circle of contracture and spasticity: "contractures stiffen tissues, immobility creates contractures. Spasticity preserves the contracture by excluding the intramuscular fibrous tissues from the stretching force."

Botte, Nickel, and Akeson[28] have reviewed the literature correlating spasticity and contracture. As the stroke patient progresses to a state of spasticity, the increased activity of the spastic muscles may result in characteristic posturing of the limb, resulting in increased stiffness of the soft-tissue surrounding the joint and the eventual formation of fixed contracture. The authors further pointed

out that contracture is associated with loss of elasticity and fixed shortening of involved tissues. Contracture may occur in a variety of soft-tissues including the following: skin, subcutaneous tissue, muscle, tendon, ligament, joint capsule, vessels, and nerves.

Halar and Bell[82] categorized contracture as arthrogenic (resulting from cartilage damage, joint incongruency, or capsular fibrosis), soft-tissue related (skin, tendons, ligaments, subcutaneous tissue), and myogenic (shortening of the muscle by intrinsic or extrinsic factors). The therapist must consider the difference between myogenic and joint contracture, especially if the muscle spans two or more joints (e.g., the wrist and hand). The therapist can differentiate contractures by flexing the proximal joint and noting the resulting position of the distal joints. Joint contracture is not affected by changes in proximal joint position. See Chapter 13.

Booth[27] reviewed the physiological and biochemical effects of immobilization on muscle. His findings indicate that muscle strength rapidly declines during limb immobilization because of a decrease in muscle size; muscle fatigability increases rapidly after immobilization. His observations also indicate that muscle atrophy in immobilized limbs begins rapidly, and a decrease in muscle size is greatest in the early phases of immobilization.

Passive Range of Motion. Soft-tissue and joint mobilization are the treatments of choice for preventing contracture. The benefits of mobilization include maintenance of joint lubrication,[28] prevention of secondary orthopedic problems (impingements), maintenance of soft-tissue length, and possible reduction of spasticity by acting on the nonneural components of spasticity.

Contracture is prevented by deliberate and frequent limb movement, with active movement being preferred over passive when possible. Perry[142] pointed out that it is essential to move the patient through complete ROM and not just the middle ranges. Therapists must determine what a full ROM is for each patient and must consider age-related factors. Determining the full ROM on the less affected side may be helpful. A joint that moves or is moved through its full ROM several times daily develops almost no deformities. Although the therapist should maintain the patient's ability to participate in all ranges of trunk and upper extremity activities, the therapist should pay particular attention to the following ranges:

- The mobility of the scapula on the thoracic wall with emphasis on protraction and upward rotation should be maintained because this range is critical in the prevention of soft-tissue impingement in the subacromial space during overhead movements of the arm and in preparation for forward reach patterns. Overhead ranges should not be attempted unless the scapula is freely gliding in upward rotation.

- Maintaining external (lateral) rotation of the glenohumeral joint allows abduction of the arm as the humerus rotates laterally to permit the greater tuberosity of the humerus to clear the acromial process. Bohannon and colleagues,[22] Ikai and colleagues,[93] and Zorowitz and colleagues[203] concluded that loss of external rotation ROM was the factor most significantly correlated to shoulder pain.

- Elbow extension is important because the majority of stroke patients favor elbow flexion as a rest posture.

- The therapists also should maintain wrist extension with concurrent radial deviation. During wrist ROM exercises, therapists must realize that the range of wrist deviation is at a maximum when the wrist is slightly flexed and a minimum when the wrist is fully flexed. Wrist extension is at a maximum during neutral deviation and a minimum during ulnar deviation.[100]

- Composite flexion of the digits leads to collateral ligament elongation. Therapists must maintain this length to prevent deformity and prepare the hand for return of motor function.

- Composite extension of the wrist and digits results in long flexor elongation.

- Digits ranged in intrinsic plus (metacarpophalangeal flexion and interphalangeal extension) and intrinsic minus (metacarpophalangeal extension and interphalangeal flexion).

Halar and Bell[82] recommended active ROM and passive ROM combined with a terminal stretch at least twice per day if contracture is beginning to develop. Therapists must use low-load prolonged stretch if a contracture has developed (see Chapter 13). During the terminal stretch, the therapist should stabilize the proximal body part well. The therapist may distract the joint slightly during the stretch to prevent soft-tissue impingement. The therapist must monitor scapula position during passive ROM activities. If necessary, the therapist should support the scapula in a position of protraction and upward rotation. In addition, the therapist must support the humerus in an external rotation position. The elbow crease should be facing up (not medially toward the trunk) to ensure proper alignment (Fig. 10-12).

Positioning. Positioning is another effective means of maintaining soft-tissue length and can be used to promote low-load, prolonged stretch. Therapists must address positioning needs of patients while they are in bed or wheelchairs/armchairs (see Chapter 26) and anytime they are in a recumbent position. Effective positioning encourages proper joint alignment, variations in joint position, comfort, and the maintenance of stretch in areas at risk for contracture. Common areas of concern during patient positioning include head and neck alignment, trunk alignment, glenohumeral joint alignment, scapula alignment, maintenance of abduction, external rotation, elbow extension, and maintenance of long flexor length.

A thorough literature review comparing authors' strategies on bed positioning has been published.[41] This review found no consensus on some issues and multiple discrepancies on strategies. Many of the positioning protocols are based on the principle of inhibiting primitive reflexes, a topic of considerable debate.

Patients are engaged in therapy only a portion of the day. Studies have shown that patients in rehabilitation

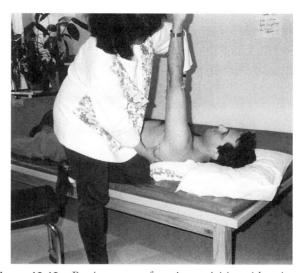

Figure 10-12   Passive range of motion activities with strict attention to the biomechanical alignment of the scapulothoracic and glenohumeral joints. Therapist's right hand assists with mobilization (upward rotation) of the scapula, while left arm keeps humerus externally rotated.

units spend almost half of their days engaged in passive pursuits including sitting unoccupied and lying in bed.[15] Therefore, patients at risk for developing contracture because of limb immobilization are good candidates for participation in a positioning program in addition to therapy.

The positioning suggestions in Box 10-11 are based on Carr and Kenney's review[41] of the positioning literature and highlights the consensus of reviewed authors.

Although the positioning suggestions in Box 10-11 represent the consensus of many authors, major areas of intervention are missing, which result in the controversies surrounding this area of intervention. For example, glenohumeral joint support remains controversial. Although most authors agree that the scapula should be protracted with a pillow, no consensus exists about support of the humerus. If only the scapula is protracted with a pillow, the humerus takes on a position of relative extension. Therefore, only support of both the scapula and humerus achieves the original goal of proper joint alignment (Fig. 10-13).

At this point, no definitive studies support one type of positioning more than another with few exceptions. Ada and colleagues[5] determined that positioning patients in supine with the affected shoulder abducted to 45-degrees and the elbow flexed to 90-degrees and placed in maximum comfortable external rotation, with towels or pillows to support the forearm 30 minutes per day prevented contracture of the internal rotators. Occupational therapists must decide what their intervention goals are and critically analyze their effectiveness. Therapists should not use general, generic strategies for bed positioning; instead, they should evaluate each patient's positioning needs individually.

Patient Management of the Extremity. Strategies to teach patients safe ROM activities they can perform themselves need to be initiated as soon as patients are medically stable. Although the clasped-hand position followed by overhead movements of both extremities has been advocated by some authors, this position may not be the most effective, especially for trauma prevention. This movement pattern does not account for factors such as scapula-humeral rhythm (especially if weakness, malalignment, or tightness around the scapula exists), overzealous patients who do not or cannot respect their pain, or critical shoulder biomechanics. Many patients observed performing this type of ROM activity have their trunk hyperextended, scapula retracted, and humerus internally rotated. This type of alignment does not correspond with an ROM pattern that emphasizes forward flexion of the humerus; it promotes proximal patterns (e.g., retraction) that should be discouraged (Fig. 10-14). Recommended techniques for patients performing ROM activities by themselves safely include the following:

1. "Towel on table": The patient is seated at a table with both arms on top of a towel. The less affected arm guides the towel around the table, with the majority of movement occurring in the trunk and from hip flexion. The patient's goal is to "polish the table" while holding positions at the end of desired ROM. The farther the patient's chair is

---

Box 10-11

Suggested Bed Positioning

POSITIONING OF PATIENT

On unaffected side
- Head/neck: neutral and symmetrical
- Affected upper limb: protracted and forward on pillow-wrist neutral, fingers extended, and thumb abducted
- Trunk: aligned
- Affected lower limb: hip forward, flexed, and supported; knee forward, flexed, and supported

On affected side
- Head/neck: neutral and symmetrical
- Affected upper limb: protracted forward with elbow extended, hand supinated, wrist neutral, fingers extended, and thumb abducted
- Trunk: straight and aligned
- Affected lower limb: knee flexed
- Unaffected lower limb: knee flexed and supported by pillows

In supine
- Head/neck: slight flexion
- Affected upper limb: protracted and slightly abducted with external rotation with wrist neutral and fingers extended
- Trunk: straight and aligned
- Affected lower limb: hip forward on pillow; nothing against soles of the feet

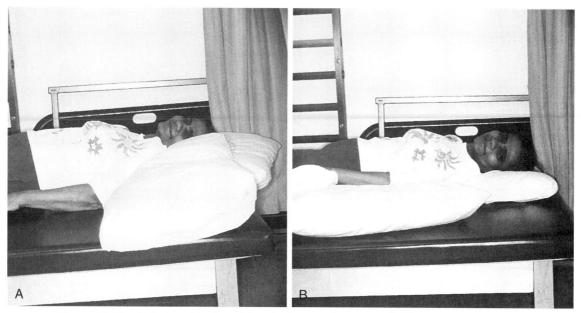

Figure 10-13   A, Bed positioning with only the scapula supported. The humerus takes on a position of relative extension, with the head of the humerus migrating anteriorly. **B,** Proper support of scapula and humerus ensures proper biomechanical alignment of shoulder joint.

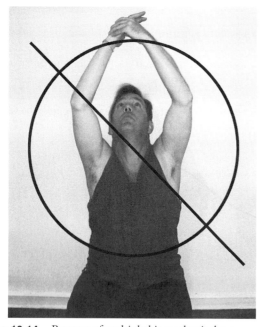

Figure 10-14   Because of multiple biomechanical concerns (e.g., impingement), self-overhead range of motion is discouraged.

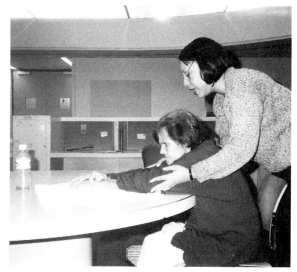

Figure 10-15   "Towel on table." Therapist is training patient to perform safe self range-of-motion activity. As the patient pushes the towel toward bottle, range of motion is gained in humeral flexion, scapular protraction, and elbow extension (which are ranges required for functional reach). Much of the range is gained by hip and trunk flexion.

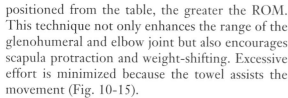

positioned from the table, the greater the ROM. This technique not only enhances the range of the glenohumeral and elbow joint but also encourages scapula protraction and weight-shifting. Excessive effort is minimized because the towel assists the movement (Fig. 10-15).

2. "Rock the baby": The patient's less affected arm cradles the more affected arm, lifts it to 90 degrees,

and places it into positions of horizontal abduction and adduction. Increased horizontal adduction on the more affected side encourages scapula protraction. This technique also encourages trunk rotation (Fig. 10-16).

3. While seated or standing, the patient reaches down to the floor and allows both arms to dangle. This position encourages extension of the elbow, wrist,

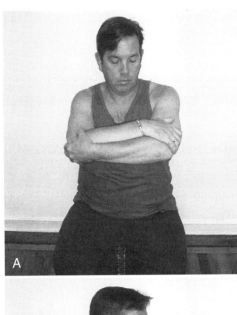

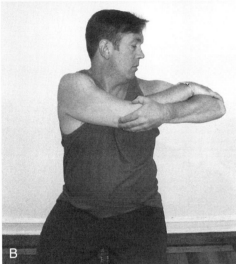

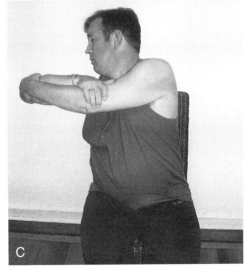

Figure 10-16 "Rock the baby." The patient lifts upper extremity to chest level **(A)** and abducts **(B)** and adducts **(C)** horizontally, allowing trunk rotation.

and digits and forward flexion of the humerus with scapula protraction. The activity is an especially useful technique for patients after they have performed an excessively difficult activity (e.g., gait, transfer, or dressing) that results in stereotypical arm posturing (Fig. 10-17).

4. While seated or standing, the patient places the more affected extremity onto a table or counter so that the forearm is bearing the weight. With the extremity in this position, the patient turns the trunk away from the supported extremity. As the trunk turns farther away and is enhanced by the posterior reach of the less affected arm, the external rotation of the more affected shoulder increases (Fig. 10-18).

5. Davis[57] has advocated rolling over the protracted scapula (from supine to side lying) several times to mobilize the scapula.

6. If the scapula of a patient is mobile and stays mobile, the range of abduction and external rotation may be increased by having the patient lie supine, placing the hands behind the head, and allowing the elbows to fall toward the bed (Fig. 10-19). This is a common resting position for an individual who has unimpaired upper extremity function. This technique should be used judiciously and only for patients who move slowly, respect pain, and have a mobile scapula. Therapists may use the five techniques outlined previously for almost all patients because they inherently follow biomechanical principles.

7. Avoid the use of overhead pulleys.[104]

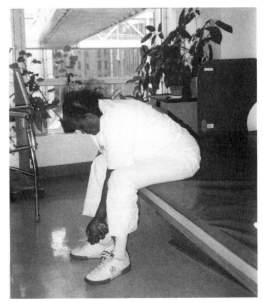

Figure 10-17 Patient performs self range-of-motion activity by reaching to floor. This pattern is especially effective after a difficult task that results in stereotypical posturing.

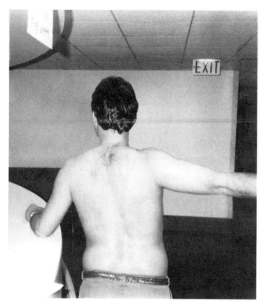

Figure 10-18 External rotation of the left glenohumeral joint is achieved by reaching to side and behind with opposite arm.

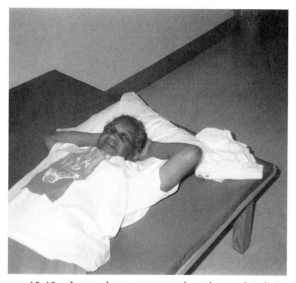

Figure 10-19 Internal rotators stretch to be used judiciously for patients who respect their own pain. This rest posture is effective at maintaining external rotation and abduction of the glenohumeral joint. If range is lacking, the humerus can be supported with a towel until patient gains increased external rotation and horizontal abduction.

The ultimate strategy used to decrease contracture and maintain ROM is encouraging functional use of the trunk and upper extremity. A person who has never had a stroke maintains ROM of an extremity by incorporating it into ADL. Activities that eliminate maladaptive positions during activities, improve balanced muscle activity on both sides of the joints, and focus on activities that encourage ROMs that are commonly decreased in stroke patients (e.g., external rotation, forward flexion, abduction, and protraction) should be incorporated into a comprehensive upper extremity program. (See Chapter 13 for other adjunct treatments to prevent or correct soft-tissue shortening.)

SHOULDER-HAND SYNDROME/COMPLEX REGIONAL PAIN SYNDROME TYPE I

Shoulder-hand syndrome (SHS) is classified as a reflex sympathetic dystrophy disorder or complex regional pain syndrome type I. The painful lesion that precipitates SHS is a proximal trauma such as a shoulder, neck, or rib cage injury or a visceral source such as stroke. The syndrome begins with severe pain and progresses to stiffness in the shoulder and pain throughout the extremity. Other symptoms include moderate to considerable swelling of the wrist and hand, vasomotor changes, and atrophy.[106] If untreated, SHS may result in a frozen shoulder and permanent hand deformity.[34]

Although the cause of SHS remains obscure, most authors associate it with a change in the autonomic nervous system (primarily sympathetic).[50] A study by Braus, Krauss, and Strobel[34] suggested that the SHS in hemiplegic patients is initiated by a peripheral lesion (e.g., a tissue or nerve injury). The authors hypothesized that increased neural activity after a peripheral injury or inflammation leads to a central sensitization responsible for the severe pain associated with SHS. Autopsy data collected by the authors confirmed microbleeding in the area of the suprahumeral joint of the affected side. If the underlying cause is in fact peripheral, then prevention programs theoretically would be effective.

The reported incidence of SHS varies from 27%[34] to 25%[174] to 12.5%[58] to 1.56%.[143] Males seem to be slightly more affected than females.[58,174] The majority of patients with SHS symptoms have partial motor loss, moderate or severe sensory loss, and varying degrees of spasticity.[58] Associated risk factors include subluxation, considerable weakness, moderate spasticity, deficits in confrontational field testing (following hemianopsia or neglect), and altered shoulder biomechanics that may compromise the suprahumeral joint structures.[34]

Daviet and colleagues[56] examined 71 patients with hemiplegia; 34.8% had a complex regional pain syndrome type I. They identified four main clinical factors in the prognosis of complex regional pain syndrome type I as motor deficit, spasticity, sensory deficits, and initial coma. They also concluded that shoulder subluxation, unilateral neglect, and depression did not seem to be determinant predictive factors of complex regional pain syndrome type I severity.

Three stages of SHS have been described (Box 10-12). Davis and colleagues[58] outlined the major diagnostic criteria for SHS based on the following clinical symptoms:

- Shoulder: loss of ROM and pain during abduction, flexion, and external rotation movements
- Elbow: no signs or symptoms
- Wrist: intense pain during extension movements, dorsal edema, and tenderness during deep palpation
- Hand: edema over metacarpals and no tenderness
- Digits: moderate fusiform edema, intense pain during flexion of the metacarpophalangeal and proximal interphalangeal joints, and loss of skin lines

The Tepperman and colleagues[174] study concluded that metacarpophalangeal tenderness during compression was the most valuable clinical sign of reflex sympathetic dystrophy, with a predictive value of 100%. Vasomotor changes and interphalangeal tenderness had the next highest predictive value at 72.7%. Therapists must remember that many of the mentioned signs and symptoms can be found in stroke patients without SHS. If a patient has several characteristic signs and symptoms, one safely can make a diagnosis on clinical grounds alone.[50] Although the diagnosis for SHS is primarily clinical, the most effective way to confirm its presence is to use a differential neural blockade. The physician may use a stellate ganglion block to alleviate the symptoms, which interrupts the abnormal sympathetic reflex; the diagnosis of SHS is confirmed if the block alleviates symptoms.

Box 10-12

Stages of Shoulder-Hand Syndrome/Complex Regional Pain Syndrome Type I

STAGE 1

The patient complains of shoulder and hand pain, tenderness, and vasomotor changes (with symptoms of discoloration and temperature changes). Chances of reversal are high at this stage.

STAGE 2

The patient has early dystrophic limb changes, muscle and skin atrophy, vasospasm, hyperhidrosis (increased sweating), and radiographic signs of osteoporosis. At this stage, shoulder-hand syndrome becomes increasingly difficult to treat.

STAGE 3

Patients rarely have pain and vasomotor changes, but they do have soft-tissue dystrophy, contracture (including a frozen shoulder and clawed hand), and severe osteoporosis. At this stage, shoulder-hand syndrome is irreversible.

Therapists should prevent SHS, so that it will not have to be treated. Davis[57] has developed a prevention protocol that focuses on the following:

- Therapists gaining full understanding of the anatomy and physiology of normal and hemiplegic shoulders
- Proper handling of the upper extremity, including avoiding arm traction during mobility, ADL, and gait activities; supporting the arm as necessary, preventing prolonged arm dangling, and using the trunk and scapula rather than the arm as support during transitional movements
- Staff education focusing on the mentioned handling techniques
- Mobilizing the scapula to ensure gliding when raising or performing ROM activities with the arm
- Family education focusing on proper extremity handling and transfer techniques; training families not to guard at the affected upper extremity during ambulation (because a balance loss would result in an automatic reflex—grabbing the patient's arm)
- Edema control that begins as soon as signs of it are observed (see Chapter 12)
- Training patients to take responsibility for protecting their affected arm

Davis and colleagues[58] hypothesize that therapists can control certain factors contributing to SHS. One factor is the extravasation of intravenous fluids. The team should infuse intravenous fluids into the less affected arm if possible; if not, fluids should be infused proximal to the wrist on the affected side. This strategy prevents infiltration around the needle and a possible edema syndrome. Another contributing factor is poor positioning. Therapists should position patients so that they cannot roll over onto the affected arm, pin it down, and compromise circulation. The other factor is immobilization of a painful shoulder by the patient. Davis[57] wrote, "In this sense, a painful shoulder (but not necessarily SHS) can evolve into SHS through immobility and consequent circulatory problems. Therefore, proper management of the hemiplegic patient in order to prevent trauma to the shoulder is critical."

In a recent prospective, two-part study performed by Braus, Krauss, and Strobel,[34] a prevention protocol was implemented that focused on protecting the affected upper extremity from trauma. All patients, relatives, and members of the therapy and medical teams received detailed instructions when patients initially were hospitalized to avoid peripheral injuries to the affected limb. Wheelchair and bed positioning were modified to ensure no pain resulted from improper positioning. Passive movements of the upper extremity were not made unless the scapula was fully mobilized. Any activity or position that caused pain was changed immediately, and no infusions into the veins of the hemiplegic hands were performed. These strategies alone decreased the incidence of SHS from 27% to 8%.

If symptoms of SHS begin to develop, therapists should make an early diagnosis and begin aggressive treatment. In the study by Braus, Krauss, and Strobel,[34] patients who already had definite SHS symptoms were placed in an experimental group (that received a 14-day treatment with low doses of orally administered corticosteroids and daily therapy) or a placebo group (that received placebo medication and daily therapy). Of the 36 patients in the experimental group, 31 were free of symptoms after 10 days of treatment. Chu, Petrillo, and Davis[50] and Davis[57] also have advocated use of orally administered corticosteroids with therapy.

Kondo and colleagues[103] tested and published a protocol for controlled passive movement by trained therapists and restriction of passive movement by the patients to prevent shoulder hand syndrome (Box 10-13).

Therapy intervention should be symptom specific. Therapists must alleviate edema immediately and maintain joint mobility while preventing pain.[104,187] Davies[55] advocates using activities that result in increased upper extremity ROM but actually result from trunk and hip flexion (e.g., towel exercises, pushing away a therapy ball while seated, and reaching to the floor). Mobilizing the scapula, which can be accomplished by the therapist or having the patient roll onto the protracted scapula from the supine to the side-lying position, also has been described.

Research is beginning to show that peripheral lesions are the cause of SHS in stroke patients, so interventions should incorporate this knowledge. Inappropriate ROM exercises (e.g., overhead ROM activities in patients without scapula mobility or overzealous exercise) and mishandling during ADL (e.g., pulling on the affected arm during transfers, bathing, dressing, and bedtime activities) are factors to consider. In addition to evaluating and treating SHS, occupational therapists play a major role in staff education. All staff and family members who physically move patients need to be aware of appropriate techniques so as to prevent injuries.

Superimposed Orthopedic Injuries

Orthopedic problems associated with stroke have been well-documented. These complications have a negative impact on functional outcomes, prolong rehabilitation, and are one of the main causes of upper extremity pain syndromes after stroke. Indeed a recent magnetic resonance imaging (MRI) study of 89 chronic stroke survivors documented:[162]

- Thirty-five percent of subjects exhibited a tear of at least one rotator cuff, biceps, or deltoid muscle.

Box 10-13

Protocol to Prevent Shoulder Hand Syndrome

The protocol shown below is for prevention of shoulder-hand syndrome in patients in the early stages of recovery after cerebrovascular accident (CVA). Both therapist and patient should follow the instructions and restrictions to passive movement for the first 4 months after CVA. Active movement, however, need not be restricted if the patient can move his or her affected fingers and arm, because active movement effectively diminishes hand edema and stiffness.

PASSIVE RANGE OF MOTION EXERCISES PERFORMED BY THE THERAPIST

1. Shoulder joint
   The shoulder joint should not be moved beyond 90 degrees during abduction and flexion. External and internal rotation should be performed in the adducted position. If the patient complains of pain in a certain position, the exercise must be stopped. During the next session, the therapist should not attempt to move the arm beyond the position that produced pain during the previous session.
2. Elbow joint, forearm (pronation/supination), wrist joint
   There is no restriction to passive movement of these joints by the therapist, but if the patient complains of pain in a certain position, the exercise must be stopped. During the next session, the therapist should not attempt to move the joint beyond this position that produced pain during the previous session.

3. Metacarpophalangeal (MCP) joint and interphalangeal (IP) joint of finger and thumb
   The proximal joint should be supported and held in a neutral position during passive movement of the distal joint. Only 1 joint should be moved at a time. During finger flexion, the wrist must be supported and be held in a neutral position. During finger extension, the wrist must be kept in flexed position.

PASSIVE MOVEMENT BY THE PATIENT

1. Shoulder joint
   The patient should not use the nonaffected arm to move his or her affected shoulder passively. Active movement is encouraged but the range of motion should not go beyond 90 degrees of abduction and flexion. External and internal rotation should be performed in the adducted position.
2. Elbow joint, forearm (pronation/supination), wrist joint
   There are no restrictions for these joints. Active movement is encouraged.
3. MCP joint and IP joint of fingers and thumb
   The patient should not use the nonaffected arm to move his or her affected fingers and thumb passively. Active movement of the affected fingers and thumb is encouraged.

From Kondo I, Hosokawa K, Soma M et al: Protocol to prevent shoulder-hand syndrome after stroke. *Arch Phys Med Rehabil* 82(11): 1619–1623, 2001.

- Fifty-three percent of subjects exhibited tendinopathy of at least one rotator cuff, biceps, or deltoid muscle.
- The prevalence of rotator cuff tears increased with age.
- In approximately 20% of cases, rotator cuff and deltoid muscles exhibited evidence of atrophy. Atrophy was associated with reduced motor strength and reduced severity of shoulder pain.

Rotator Cuff and Biceps Tendon Lesions. The rotator cuff guides and leads the movements of the shoulder joint. The cuff supplies the strength needed to complete the ROM in the shoulder joint and seats the head of the humerus into the glenoid fossa.

Najenson, Yacubovic, and Pikielni[131] studied 32 hemiplegic patients with severe upper limb paralysis; 18 patients served as controls by having their less affected side evaluated. Forty percent of the patients had a rotator cuff tear on the affected side. None of the patients had complaints about the affected shoulder before the stroke. Only 16% of the patients in the control group had ruptured rotator cuffs on the less involved side; all three seemed to be long-standing tears.

Najenson, Yacubovic, and Pikielni[131] also discussed the pathophysiology of a rotator cuff tear in hemiplegic patients. Many older patients are predisposed to rotator cuff ruptures because of degenerative changes associated with aging. Cuff tears commonly result from impingement of the cuff between the greater tuberosity and acromial arch (Fig. 10-20), which occurs when the humerus is forced into abduction without external rotation (e.g., during inappropriate passive ROM activities or activities that are not sensitive to shoulder biomechanics [reciprocal pulleys]). Therapists who have a thorough understanding of joint alignment can prevent impingement during treatment.

Nepomuceno and Miller[134] found seven rotator cuff tears and one a transverse bicipital tendon tear in 24 subjects with painful hemiplegic shoulders. None of the patients had premorbid pathological conditions of the shoulder. With one exception, all patients with soft-tissue lesions had left-sided hemiplegia. (This study did not evaluate the presence of visual field loss or neglect.)

Therapists should note that a relationship between rotator cuff age and wear has been documented. After age 50-years-old, the percentage of lesions significantly increases.

Adhesive Changes. Adhesive changes in the hemiplegic shoulder are considered to result from immobilization, synovitis, or metabolic changes in joint tissue. Hakuno and colleagues[81] studied adhesive changes in hemiplegic shoulders and found that hemiplegia had a significant influence on the prevalence of adhesive changes in the shoulder. Adhesive changes were found in 30% of patients' affected glenohumeral joints as opposed to 2.7% on the less involved side.

Rizk and colleagues[152] examined 30 hemiplegic patients by arthrography of the shoulder and found that 23 patients had capsular constriction typical of frozen shoulder (adhesive capsulitis). Therefore, the authors advocated early passive ROM for the shoulder.

Roy, Sands, and Hill[155] used the following clinical criteria for adhesive capsulitis: shoulder pain, external rotation of less than 20 degrees, and abduction of less than 60 degrees. Ikai and colleagues[93] concluded that adhesive capsulitis is a main cause of shoulder pain and documented adhesive changes in 74% of subjects in their study via shoulder arthrogram. They recommended that "correct positioning and shoulder ROM exercises are advisable in hemiplegic patients with shoulder subluxation."

Brachial Plexus Injury. Kaplan and colleagues[101] identified brachial plexus injury in five of 12 patients in their study. All five had EMG evidence indicating neuropathy of the upper trunk of the brachial plexus on the side affected by the stroke. The deltoid, biceps, and infraspinatus muscles were involved. Moskowitz and Porter[130] also summarized the findings in five stroke survivors with "traction neuropathies" of the upper trunk of the brachial plexus.

Merideth, Taft, and Kaplan[124] reviewed the diagnostic and treatment procedures for stroke survivors with brachial plexus injuries. Physical examination findings included flaccidity and atrophy of the supraspinatus, infraspinatus, deltoid, and biceps muscles in the affected upper extremity with increased muscle tone or distal movement (an atypical pattern of recovery). EMG criteria for diagnosing brachial plexus injuries include the finding of fibrillation

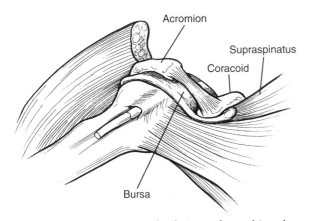

Figure 10-20 Impingement of soft tissues located in subacromial space. Impingement occurs between the head of humerus and acromion/coracoid. Impingement occurs during forced humeral flexion/abduction without concurrent upward rotation of scapula and/or external rotation of humerus.

potentials in the muscles innervated by the upper trunk of the brachial plexus.

Treatment of these patients included positioning and passive and active ROM activities. During active ROM activities, Effects of gravity were monitored to prevent further traction. Using a positioning pillow, the affected upper extremity was positioned as follows: externally rotated 45 degrees, 90 degrees of elbow flexion, and forearm neutral. Patients used slings while ambulating and were educated not to sleep on their affected side, which could result in compression and traction injuries to the upper trunk. (Many authors encourage sleeping on the affected side if this pathological condition is not present.) A major component of the treatment program was the education of the patient, staff, and families regarding proper care and positioning of the upper extremity.

Pain Syndromes

Although pain syndromes have been discussed previously in the context of orthopedic injuries and SHS, their impact on functional recovery is significant, so this section specifically reviews the literature on hemiplegic shoulder pain.

The incidence of shoulder pain in hemiplegic patients has been reported to be as high as 72%.[22,155,184] Roy, Sands, and Hill[155] identified strong associations between hemiplegic shoulder pain and prolonged hospital stays, arm weakness, poor recovery of arm function, ADL, and lower rates of discharge to the home. Those responsible for stroke patients have the onus to be aware of hemiplegic shoulder pain and to diagnose, relieve, and prevent this syndrome. Although shoulder pain is obviously not the only variable leading to prolonged hospital stays, it is a potentially preventable variable over which occupational therapists have much control.

Pain can limit patient's activities, such as rolling in bed, transferring, putting on a shirt or blouse, and bending to reach the feet to put on shoes and socks. The occurrence of shoulder pain also has been linked to depression.[160]

The literature concerning hemiplegic shoulder pain is confusing at times and often contradictory. The following review was obtained from a selection of articles from a variety of disciplines. The focus of the review is clinical correlations associated with hemiplegic shoulder pain.

In their study of 55 patients, Roy, Sands, and Hill[155] found positive correlations between hemiplegic shoulder pain and "glenohumeral malalignment without descent of the humeral head" and between hemiplegic shoulder pain and reflex sympathetic dystrophy (SHS). The study did not confirm a strong association between spasticity (measured by the Ashworth Scale) and hemiplegic shoulder pain.

Joynt[99] found significant correlations between loss of motion and shoulder pain and questioned the relationship between neglect/perceptual dysfunction and pain. His left-sided hemiplegic subjects had a higher incidence of shoulder pain, which led him to question whether the incidence of trauma was increased. He found no correlation between shoulder pain and subluxation, spasticity, strength, or sensation.

Joynt[99] identified the subacromial area as a pain-producing location in a significant number of cases. Of 28 patients who received a subacromial injection of 1% lidocaine, more than half obtained moderate or significant pain relief and improved ROM. The author suggested that physical agent modalities, steroid injections, and careful ROM activities focusing on impingement prevention were significant in reducing pain.

The subacromial area is prone to trauma during therapy and patient handling. The subacromial space includes the supraspinatus tendon, long head of the biceps, and subacromial bursa[40] (Fig. 10-21). All of these structures are prone to impingement and inflammation. Structure impingement can develop easily in hemiplegic patients during ROM activities because the normal scapulohumeral rhythm becomes impaired. If the scapula is not rotated upward (by therapist's manipulation or active control), the humerus becomes blocked by the acromion and causes impingement, inflammation, and pain (see Fig. 10-20). Combined motions of scapula retraction with forward flexion should be avoided to prevent impingement. Instead, the scapula should glide freely and be protracted and upwardly rotated during upper extremity activities. Objects for reaching activities should be placed in front or below waist level of the patient to encourage humeral forward flexion with scapular protraction. Indeed, Dromerick and colleagues[64] designed a study to clarify the pathophysiology of hemiplegic shoulder pain by determining the frequency of abnormal shoulder physical diagnosis signs and the accuracy of self-report. They found:

- Weakness of shoulder flexion, extension, or abduction was present in 94% of subjects.
- Neglect was found in 29%.
- Pain was present by self-report in 37%.

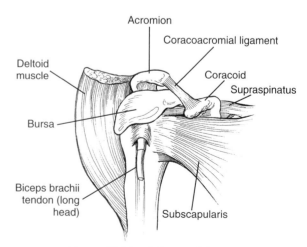

Figure 10-21 Subacromial space.

- The most common findings on physical examination (proactive tests and palpation) was bicipital tendon tenderness (54%), followed by supraspinatus tenderness (48%).
- The Neer sign was positive in 30%.
- 28% had the triad of bicipital tenderness, supraspinatus tenderness, and the Neer sign.
- Self-reported pain was a poor predictor of abnormalities elicited on the examination maneuvers, even in those without neglect.

Some patients may develop inflammation around the biceps tendon and supraspinatus insertion because of impingements. Palpation skills are important for determining which structures are involved (Fig. 10-22). To palpate the biceps tendon, the therapist palpates the acromion and drops one finger to the anterior shoulder; the biceps tendon lies in the groove between the greater and lesser tuberosities of the humerus. If the patient feels pain on application of pressure, the biceps tendon probably has been affected. (Passively rotating the humerus while palpating assists the therapist with locating the tuberosities.)

To palpate the supraspinatus tendon, the therapist palpates the acromion, but this time drops one finger to the lateral shoulder right below the center of the acromion. If pressure or slight friction elicits pain, the supraspinatus most likely has been affected.

Bohannon and colleagues[22] studied the relationship of five variables (age, time since onset of hemiplegia, range

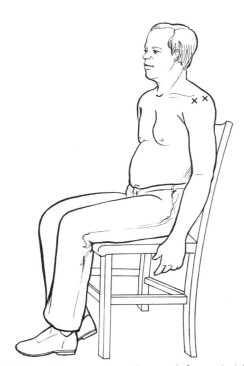

Figure 10-22 Palpation point. The *x* on left anterior) is palpation point for long head of biceps. The *x* on right (more lateral) is palpation point for supraspinatus tendon.

of external rotation of the hemiplegic shoulder, spasticity, and weakness) to shoulder pain. In their study of 50 patients, 36 had shoulder pain. Range of shoulder external rotation was considered the factor related most significantly to shoulder pain. They hypothesized that hemiplegic shoulder pain was in part a manifestation of adhesive capsulitis. In this study, only patients with full external rotation were free of pain. The suggested treatment was elimination of inflammation and maintenance of ROM.

Hecht[86] treated 13 patients with limited ROM and shoulder pain with percutaneous phenol blocks to the nerves of the subscapularis (a major shoulder internal rotator). Immediate and significant improvements were observed in the flexion, abduction, and external rotation ROMs; pain relief also was noted. This study indicates that the subscapularis is a key muscle and should be addressed during treatment focusing on maintaining soft-tissue length. The subscapularis muscle may tighten in patients with the previously mentioned pain syndrome. If the humerus resists external rotation with the arm at the side during evaluation, the therapist can presume the subscapularis to be a factor contributing to the deformity. Similarly, subscapularis injection of botulinum toxin A appears to be of value in the management of shoulder pain in spastic hemiplegic patients.[200] These studies adds more support to the concept of focusing on maintaining the range of humeral external rotation to prevent resulting complications.

Bohannon and Andrews[20] studied 24 patients in an effort to establish a relationship between subluxation and pain. Despite the emphasis placed on reduction of subluxation, the relationship between shoulder pain and subluxation has not been established. Their study did not find an association between shoulder pain and subluxation (which was defined in this study as the separation between the acromion and the humeral head). A study by Arsenault and colleagues[8] also found no significant relationship between subluxation and shoulder pain.

A more recent study by Zorowitz and colleagues[203] also focused on the correlation between subluxation and pain. Results showed that shoulder pain did not correlate with age, vertical or horizontal subluxation, shoulder flexion, abduction, or Fugl-Meyer Assessment scores, but it did correlate with the degree of shoulder external rotation. Wanklyn, Forster, and Young[186] also found an association between reduced external rotation and hemiplegic shoulder pain, with an incidence as high as 66%. This association was believed to be due to abnormal muscle tone or structural changes, namely adhesions. Similarly, Ikai and others[93] evaluated 75 subjects and found no correlation between subluxation and pain.

Kumar and colleagues[104] demonstrated a positive correlation between shoulder pain and therapy programs that did not consider biomechanical shoulder alignment during treatment. Patients were assigned to one of three exercise groups: ROM initiated by the therapist, skateboard treatment, and overhead pulley treatment. Of the patients who developed pain during the treatment programs, 8% were in the ROM group, 12% in the skateboard group, and 62% in the overhead pulley group. The probable cause of this discrepancy was soft-tissue damage resulting from forced abduction without external rotation. This study showed that poorly prescribed activities by the therapist could be the cause of pain syndromes. This study found no significant relationship between subluxation and pain.

In a three-year study of 219 hemiplegic patients, Van Ouwenaller, Laplace, and Chantraine[184] found that 85% of the patients who developed pain had spasticity (an increased myotactic reflex) compared with 18% of flaccid patients. They also found that 50% of the patients who developed pain had anteroinferior subluxations (which were not defined). The authors advocated use of muscle relaxation techniques for the shoulder girdle.

Jensen[98] attributed shoulder pain to traumatic tendinitis resulting from unskilled and strenuous joint treatment during ADL (e.g., bathing, dressing, and bed mobility) and bilateral ROM activities of more than 90 degrees resulting in "jamming [of] soft-tissue against the acromion resulting in lesions" (see Fig. 10-20). Jensen suggested the following precautions: educating all staff members, placing signs over patients' beds to warn staff of the shoulder instability, supporting the arm during the acute stage, avoiding treatment that may cause soft-tissue impingement, having a thorough understanding of shoulder anatomy, and dissuading use of pulley exercises and self-ROM activities.

Lastly, Wanklyn, Forster, and Young[186] found a 27% increased incidence of shoulder pain in dependent patients after discharge, which may reflect improper handling at home by caregivers. They suggested a greater emphasis on patient and caregiver education regarding proper transfer techniques and correct handling of the hemiplegic arm (Box 10-14).

Loss of Biomechanical Alignment

Immediately after a stroke, patients lose their ability to maintain upright control and become malaligned because of the effects of gravity, weakness, and muscle imbalance.

Occupational therapists must be able to identify malalignments to treat upper extremity dysfunction effectively. The following section discusses common trunk and upper extremity alignment problems and reviews activities to counteract the adverse effects of malalignment.

Loss of Pelvic/Trunk Alignment. After a stroke, patients commonly lose their ability to perform postural adjustments and maintain postural alignment because of weakness, a loss of equilibrium, and righting reactions; the trunk assumes an asymmetrical posture.[18,19,55]

Box 10-14

Hemiplegic Shoulder Pain Prevention

- Maintain and/or increase passive glenohumeral joint external rotation.
- Maintain scapula mobility on the thorax.
- Avoid passive or active shoulder movements beyond 90 degrees (flexion and abduction) unless the scapula is gliding toward upward rotation and sufficient external rotation is available. These two movements are necessary to prevent shoulder impingement.
- Educate the patient, family, and staff about potential complications related to an unstable shoulder.
- Teach patients and caregivers proper management during activities of daily living to avoid shoulder traction and forced overhead movements. Specific activities that should be addressed include applying deodorant, transfers, guarding during ambulation, bathing the axilla, and upper body dressing.
- Educate patients regarding different types (e.g., stretch versus sharp) of pain. Avoid sharp pain during any shoulder movements or activities.
- Provide positioning to prevent a dangling upper extremity. Assess shoulder positions in bed, in wheelchair, and during upright function.
- Avoid activities that may cause impingements such as use of overhead pulleys, forced overhead self range of motion, or overaggressive passive range of motion by the therapist.

The first area to observe is the patient's pelvis and its effect on spinal alignment. Patients typically bear weight asymmetrically through their pelvis (by one ischial tuberosity accepting more weight than the other), which results in lateral spine flexion. This lateral flexion causes the trunk musculature to become shortened on the nonweight-bearing side and lengthened on the weight-bearing side[55] (Fig. 10-23). At the same time, patients tend to assume a posterior pelvic tilt, which results in spinal flexion. Again the result is a muscle imbalance, with the anterior musculature (abdominals) becoming shortened and the posterior muscles (extensors) becoming elongated. Davies[55] hypothesized that patients sit with posterior pelvic tilt to compensate for weak abdominals. Patients assume this "safe" posture to prevent themselves from falling backward. The spinal flexion that results from the posterior tilt leads to loss of natural lumbar spine lordosis and accentuated thoracic spine kyphosis.

Abdominal weakness (especially the obliques) results in a destabilization of the rib cage. A lack of balance between the obliques results in trunk and rib cage rotation.[100] See Chapter 7.

Loss of Scapula Alignment. Upper extremity malalignment commonly results from pelvic and trunk malalignments. When in a resting position, the scapula is flush on

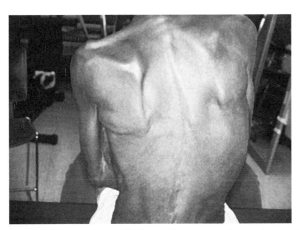

Figure 10-23 Asymmetrical trunk posture in patient with left hemiplegia. Note the left trunk shortening, right trunk elongation/overstretching, rib cage shift, loss of scapula stability on rib cage, relative downward rotation of scapula, increased weight-bearing on right ischial tuberosity, and shoulder asymmetry (left hemiplegia).

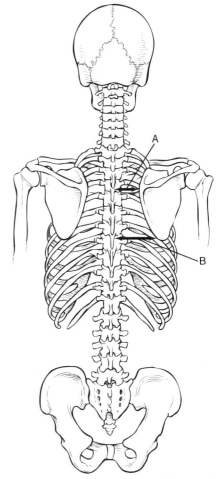

Figure 10-24 Normal resting posture of the scapula in upward rotation. *A* is the distance (in finger breadths or centimeters) from the medial border of the spine of the scapula to the vertebral column. *B* is the distance from the inferior angle of the scapula to the vertebral column. Distance *B* should be greater than distance *A* if the scapula is aligned appropriately. If *A* equals *B* or *A* is greater than *B*, then the scapula has assumed a position of relative downward rotation.

the rib cage (the scapulothoracic joint) and upwardly rotated. When one palpates the scapula, the distance between the inferior angle and the vertebral column should be greater than the distance between the medial border of the scapular spine and the vertebral column[100] (Fig. 10-24). In the resting position the glenoid fossa of the scapula faces upward, forward, and outward. Therefore, the trunk and rib cage must be stable to support the scapula properly. In hemiplegic patients, the scapula loses its orientation on the thoracic wall and assumes a position of relative downward rotation.[40]

Cailliet[40] described several events that result in a downwardly rotated scapula (Fig. 10-25), such as lateral flexion toward the hemiparetic side. The lateral flexion may be due to trunk weakness, perceptual dysfunction that results in an inability to perceive midline, or excess activity in unilateral trunk flexors (i.e., latissimus dorsi). Downward rotation also can be caused by unopposed muscle activity that depresses and downwardly rotates the scapula (i.e., rhomboids, levator scapulae, and latissimus dorsi) or by generalized weakness in the muscles that orient the scapula in a position of upward rotation (i.e., serratus anterior, upper and lower trapezius).

Loss of Glenohumeral Joint Alignment. Thus far the loss of pelvic/trunk, rib cage, and scapula control have been reviewed. All of the aforementioned alignment changes have an effect on the stability and alignment of the glenohumeral joint. The mechanisms of glenohumeral joint subluxation remains controversial. As reviewed by Cailliet[40] and Basmajian,[14] the following factors assist in maintaining glenohumeral joint stability: the angle of the glenoid fossa when facing forward, upward, and outward; the support of

the scapula on the rib cage; the seating of the humeral head in the fossa by the supraspinatus; possible support from the superior capsule; and contraction of the deltoid and cuff muscles when passive support is eliminated by slight abduction of the humerus.[40] Cailliet stated that any change in these factors may play a role in causing subluxation (Fig. 10-26).

Basmajian's EMG studies[14] confirmed that the supraspinatus prevents downward migration of the humeral head when a downward load is applied to the upper extremity (e.g., when a person holds a briefcase). Authors previously believed that the deltoid performed this function, but the deltoid actually shows no activity during this function. The author pointed out that the supraspinatus is a horizontally positioned muscle that runs through the

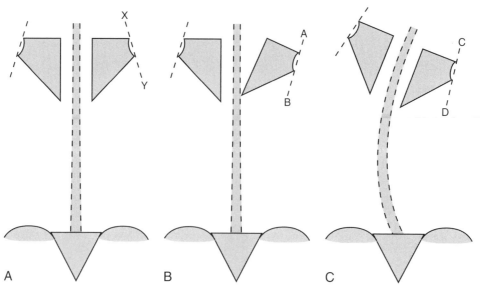

Figure 10-25   **A,** Scapular alignment with a straight spine (*xy* glenoid angle). **B,** Paresis with downward rotation of scapula (*AB* glenoid angle). **C,** Relative downward rotation of scapula with functional scoliosis (*CD* glenoid angle). (From Cailliet R: *The shoulder in hemiplegia,* Philadelphia, 1980, FA Davis.)

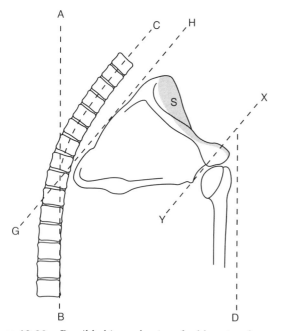

Figure 10-26   Possible biomechanics of subluxation from malalignment. Line *AB* indicates an aligned spine (the goal of treatment). Instead the spine assumes a position of lateral flexion (curve *CB*). The scapula downwardly rotates (*GH*), resulting in a downward angulation of the glenoid fossa (*XY*). Because of the scapula position, the supraspinatus (*S*) loses its mechanical line of pull, making it ineffective and prone to overstretching. The result is a subluxation of the glenohumeral joint. (Modified from Cailliet R: *Shoulder pain,* Philadelphia, 1990, FA Davis.)

supraspinous fossa and can be effective only if the scapula is oriented correctly on the thorax.

The upward orientation of the glenoid fossa creates a "cradle" for the humeral head. As the humerus is pulled downward, it is forced to move laterally by the slope of the fossa.[14] The supraspinatus (and superior portion of the capsule) prevents this lateral movement and therefore downward migration. Basmajian[14] also pointed out that this mechanism is not effective if the humerus is abducted. This position predisposes patients to subluxation by eliminating the described mechanism. Many patients are positioned so that their humerus is abducted slightly because of the lateral trunk flexion toward the more affected side or due to passive positioning.

The relationship between scapula rotation and inferior subluxation has been challenged. Prevost and colleagues[148] evaluated both shoulders of 50 stroke survivors with inferior subluxations using tridimensional radiograph. Results included the following:

- The affected and nonaffected shoulders were different in terms of the vertical position of the humerus vis-a-vis the scapula.
- The orientation of the glenoid cavities was also different; the subluxed one faced less downward.
- The angle of abduction of the arm of the affected side was significantly greater than on the nonaffected side, but the relative abduction of the arm was on the same order of magnitude for both sides.
- No significant relationship existed between the orientation of the scapula and the severity of the subluxation.

- The abduction of the humerus was weakly ($r = 0.24$) related to the subluxation, which partly explained the weak association found between the relative abduction of the arm and the subluxation.

Overall, the authors concluded that the position of the scapula and the relative abduction of the arm cannot be considered important factors in the occurrence of inferior subluxation in hemiplegia.

Similarly, Culham, Noce, and Bagg[54] examined 17 subjects with high tone and 17 subjects with low tone based on the Ashworth Scale. Linear and angular measures of scapular and humeral orientation were calculated from tridimensional coordinates of bony landmarks collected using an electromagnetic device with subjects in a seated position with arms relaxed by their sides. Glenohumeral subluxation was measured from radiographs. They found the following:

- The scapula was farther from the midline and lower on the thorax on the affected side in the low-tone group.
- Glenohumeral subluxation was greater in the low-tone group.
- The scapular abduction angle was significantly greater on the nonaffected side in the low-tone group compared with the affected side in this group and with the nonaffected side in the high-tone group.
- In the high-tone group, no differences were found between the affected and nonaffected sides in the angular or linear measures.

- No significant correlation was found between scapular or humeral orientation and glenohumeral subluxation in either group.

Chaco and Wolf[45] confirmed that the supraspinatus did not respond to loading in the hemiplegic patients they studied. Although not immediate, subluxation developed later in the study in the patients who remained flaccid. They inferred that the joint capsule holds the head of the humerus in relation to the glenoid fossa, but unless the supraspinatus starts responding, it cannot prevent subluxation indefinitely. Therefore, subluxation appears to be caused by the weight of the arm and mechanical stretch to the joint capsule and traction to unresponsive shoulder musculature.

Ryerson and Levit[156,157] described three patterns of subluxation in the glenohumeral joint. They emphasized that the therapist must assess trunk posture, determine the position of the scapula on the trunk, evaluate scapular mobility and rhythm, and examine the alignment and mobility of the glenohumeral joint before setting treatment goals for the shoulder. Table 10-7 reviews Ryerson and Levit's subluxation classifications, including inferior, anterior, and superior subluxations.

Hall, Dudgeon, and Guthrie[83] assessed the validity of three clinical measures (palpation, arm length discrepancy, and thermoplastic jig measurement) for evaluating shoulder subluxation in adults with hemiplegia resulting from a stroke. These measures were combined with anterior/posterior radiographic examinations of the hemiplegic shoulder; results indicated that palpation had the

Table 10-7

Subluxation/Malalignment Patterns in the Upper Extremity after Stroke

	TRUNK ALIGNMENT	SCAPULA ALIGNMENT	HUMERAL ALIGNMENT	DISTAL EXTREMITY ALIGNMENT	MOVEMENT AVAILABLE
Inferior subluxation	Lateral flexion to weak side	Downwardly rotated	Relative abduction and internal rotation; humeral head below inferior lip of fossa	Elbow extension and pronation	Scapula elevation and internal rotation
Anterior subluxation	Increased extension, lateral flaring, or rotation of rib cage	Downwardly rotated and elevated, winging	Hyperextension and internal rotation; humeral head inferior and forward relative to fossa	Elbow flexion and pronation or supination	Shoulder elevation, humeral internal rotation and hyperextension, and elbow flexion
Superior subluxation	Elements of flexion and extension; rib cage flaring	Elevated and abducted	Internal rotation and abduction; humeral head lodged under coracoid	Supination and wrist flexion	Shoulder elevation, abduction, and internal rotation; elbow/wrist flexion

Data from Ryerson S, Levit K: Glenohumeral joint subluxations in CNS dysfunction. *NDTA Newsletter* Nov 1988; and Ryerson S, Levit K: The shoulder in hemiplegia. In Donatelli RA, editor: *Physical therapy of the shoulder*, ed 2, New York, 1991, Churchill Livingstone.

highest correlation with successful subluxation evaluation. In their technique for palpating subluxation, the patient is seated with the upper extremity unsupported at the side in neutral rotation; trunk stability was maintained during the evaluation. During palpation, the therapist measured subluxation by palpating the subacromial space (the distance between the acromion and the superior aspect of the humeral head) with the index and middle fingers. The authors concluded that their findings provided cautious optimism in terms of measuring and identifying subluxation. Prevost and colleagues[149] also validated that palpation is a reliable measurement tool in the evaluation of subluxation. One should note that the evaluator should palpate both shoulders for comparison.

Hall, Dudgeon, and Guthrie[83] used a 0 (no subluxation) to 5 (2½ finger widths of subluxation) scale during their study. Bohannon and Andrews[20] used a 3-point scale to demonstrate interrater reliability for measuring subluxation: none, 0; minimal, 1; and substantial, 2.

Loss of Distal Alignment. Shoulder alignment problems directly effect the alignment and control of the distal extremity. Boehme[19] states that rotational movements of the forearm "occur at the proximal end with the radius rotating on a vertical axis . . . the ulnar head is displaced, . . . the mechanics are made possible by concurrent external rotation of the humerus." The typical alignment of the humerus after stroke is one of internal rotation, which blocks forearm rotation.

Kapandji[100] states that when the elbow is flexed (a typical posture), pronation is reduced to 45 degrees. Boehme[19] points out that when the wrist is bound by flexion and ulnar deviation (the typical posture of the CVA patient), control of forearm rotation also is blocked.

Wrist motion can become limited by virtue of its own alignment. The range of deviation is at its minimum when the wrist is in flexion and at its maximum when the wrist is in a neutral position or slight flexion. Flexion and extension ranges of the wrist are at a minimum when the hand has an ulnar deviation and at a maximum when the hand has a neutral deviation.[100]

A loss of palmar arches in the hand results in an inferior movement of the metacarpals followed by a distal hyperextension of the metacarpophalangeals and flexion of the proximal interphalangeal joints and distal interphalangeal joints, the typical claw-hand posture. See Chapter 13.

Interdependence of Trunk and Limb Alignment. Anatomically, therapists must remember that only one bony attachment connects the entire limb to the axial skeleton, the sternoclavicular joint. (The scapulothoracic joint is not a true joint; the scapula rides on the thoracic cage and is maintained by muscular attachments only.) Therefore, the clavicle serves as an anatomical link between the shoulder complex and trunk. This point should solidify the interdependence between the trunk and upper extremity. Any malalignments in the proximal segments have deleterious effects on the upper extremity (Fig. 10-27).

The musculature acting on the shoulder has proximal points of attachment. A group of upper extremity muscles (the trapezius, rhomboids, serratus anterior, and levator scapulae) runs between the trunk and scapula, and another (the pectoralis and latissimus dorsi) runs between the trunk and humerus. Another group of muscles (the deltoid, rotator cuff, and coracobrachialis) attaches from the humerus to the scapula. These attachments emphasize the interdependence of trunk alignment and extremity control.

Mohr[127] pointed out that biomechanical malalignment produces a pattern of movement that looks like stereotypical patterns used by patients with spasticity. For example, patients who gain early control of scapula elevation and humeral abduction continue to use this pattern and also flex the trunk, resulting in more elevation and abduction. As the scapula tips forward, it predisposes the humerus to internal rotation and extension because of its position in the fossa. The distal arm follows into elbow flexion, pronation, and wrist and digit flexion. The author stated that if a normal individual only activates the scapula elevators with humeral abductors, the resulting pattern looks similar to the patterns used by stroke survivors.

These alignment problems need to be addressed before and throughout the treatment session. Therapists should correct them by mobilization techniques, positioning, and appropriate activity choices. The therapist needs to ensure alignment during ROM activities and maintain appropriate alignment during functional activities. For example, the alignment of the trunk and pelvis of patients who are trying to feed themselves has a direct effect on the quality of the extremity movement pattern. Even in persons without a known neuropathological condition, the quality of the eating activity clearly is compromised if they assume a forward flexed and laterally flexed static posture rather than an aligned and active trunk posture.

Ryerson and Levit[156] suggest patients perform activities that maintain enhanced trunk alignment and simultaneously coordinate movements of the scapula, trunk, and humerus.

Shoulder Supports

Shoulder supports include any devices used to align, protect, or support an affected proximal limb. Shoulder supports include bed-positioning devices, adaptations to seating systems, and slings. The use of shoulder supports, especially slings, has been debated in the literature for at least 30 years. A recent review concluded that "There is insufficient evidence to conclude whether slings and wheelchair attachments prevent subluxation, decrease pain, increase function or adversely increase contracture in the shoulder after stroke."[4]

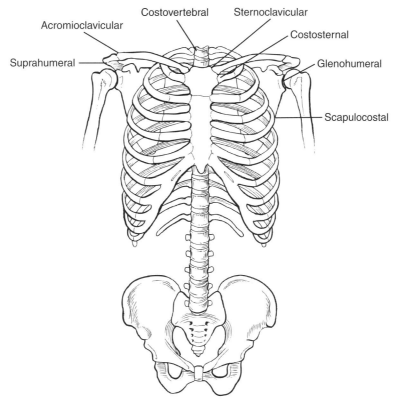

Figure 10-27 Shoulder anatomy. Seven joints make up the shoulder complex. The sterno-clavicular joint is the only bony attachment of the shoulder to the trunk, with the clavicle serving as a bridge between the trunk and shoulder. Skeletal alignment of the shoulder joint depends on trunk alignment and stability. For example, if the pelvis becomes malaligned (pelvic obliquity), the vertebral column, the rib cage, and other components lose their alignment (see Fig. 10-23).

Much of the debate is fueled by the variety of available slings, the controversy regarding their effectiveness, when and how they should be used, and whether they add to the already numerous complications resulting from an extremity affected by stroke.

Boyd and Gaylard[32] published the results of their survey of Canadian occupational therapists who prescribe slings. The respondents most frequently indicated that the goals of using a sling were to decrease and prevent subluxation and pain. The respondents frequently measured the effectiveness of their interventions by the level of resulting pain relief, subluxation assessments, and the amount of hand swelling. Less frequent measures of effectiveness included ROM, spasticity, and body awareness.

In light of the previously proposed cause of subluxation (see Loss of Biomechanical Alignment), Cailliet[40] suggested that if the goal of treatment is to provide glenohumeral joint stability, then the device must support the scapula on the rib cage with the glenoid fossa facing upward, forward, and outward and must compensate for a lack of support by the rotator cuff and possibly the superior capsule. At this point, no slings are available on the market that assist in realigning the scapula on the rib cage. Therefore, slings cannot be prescribed to "reduce a subluxation." They may lift the head of the humerus to the level of the glenoid fossa, but the scapular and trunk alignments (the key to correcting shoulder malalignment) remain impaired. This reduction may be seen as treating a symptom of a larger problem. The therapist must realize that they may find cases in which treating this symptom is appropriate. Analysis is critical for determining which goals certain interventions are achieving. Palpating the subluxation before and after the sling is donned is not sufficient. The therapist must evaluate the effect (if any) of the sling on the more proximal segments.

In their review of the literature, Smith and Okamoto[165] identified desirable and undesirable features of slings. Proper positioning of the humeral head in addition to humeral abduction, external rotation, and elbow extension are cited as desirable positions as opposed to humeral adduction, internal rotation, and elbow flexion. The latter positions typically cause problems in the maintenance of tissue length in the stroke population. The sling also should permit the impaired extremity to provide postural support when the patient is seated and should allow self-ROM. In terms of positioning, the sling should provide neutral wrist support, unobstructed hand function, finger abduction, and scapula protraction and elevation.

Smith and Okamoto[165] emphasized that if a therapist expects compliance with sling use, comfort, cosmetic appeal, and easy donning and doffing are crucial. The authors published a checklist to assist therapists in analyzing the slings they provide. The percentage of therapists using slings has been reported to be as high as 94%,[32] despite the fact no definitive studies support or reject the use of slings. Several studies have compared and contrasted the effectiveness of various supports. Zorowitz and colleagues[204] compared the following four supports:

1. The single-strap hemisling: The strap has two cuffs that support the elbow and wrist. The arm is held in a position of adduction, internal rotation, and elbow flexion.
2. The Bobath roll: This strap includes a foam roll that is placed in the affected axilla beneath the proximal humerus. The shoulder is maintained in a position of abduction and external rotation with elbow extension.
3. The Rolyan humeral cuff sling: This figure-of-eight strap system has an arm cuff that is sized to fit distally on the humerus of the affected arm. The shoulder is positioned in slight external rotation.
4. The Cavalier shoulder support: This type of support provides bilateral axillary support and consists of bilateral straps that are positioned along the humeral head and integrated posteriorly into a brace that rests between the scapula.

In this study, 20 patients were evaluated in the listed supports with anteroposterior shoulder radiography. The authors evaluated the vertical, horizontal, and total asymmetries of glenohumeral joint subluxation compared with the opposite shoulder. In terms of vertical asymmetry, the single-strap hemisling corrected the vertical displacement, the Cavalier support did not alter vertical displacement, and the remaining supports significantly reduced but did not correct vertical displacement.

Although as a group, the subjects had no significant horizontal asymmetry when no supports were used, the Bobath roll and the Cavalier support produced a significant lateral displacement of the humeral head of the more affected shoulder. This fact is of interest because one proposed goal of a sling is to decrease or prevent subluxation; this study demonstrated that equipment not well-researched actually may cause shoulder asymmetry in patients who previously had none.

In terms of total asymmetry, the Rolyan humeral cuff sling was the only support that significantly decreased (although it did not eliminate) total subluxation asymmetry.

Moodie, Brisbin, and Morgan[128] evaluated the effectiveness of five shoulder supports: the Bobath roll, an acrylic plastic lap tray on a wheelchair, a wheelchair-mounted arm trough, a conventional triangular sling (which is much like an arm cast support), and the Hook Hemi Harness (which has two adjustable shoulder cuffs with a suspension strap that are tightened while the affected arm is lifted, resulting in shoulders of equal height). Anteroposterior radiographs of 10 subjects demonstrated that the conventional sling, lap tray, and arm trough were effective in decreasing the width of the glenohumeral space to normal. The Bobath roll and the Hook Hemi Harness were not effective in reducing the subluxation. The authors pointed out that although the conventional sling decreased the subluxation, it reinforced the flexor pattern found in the upper extremity.

Brook and colleagues[36] compared the effects of three supports: the Bobath sling, an arm trough/lap board, and the Harris hemisling (which has two straps and cuffs that cradle the elbow and wrist, holding the arm in a position of adduction, internal rotation, and elbow flexion). The Harris hemisling resulted in good vertical correction; in comparison the Bobath sling did not correct the subluxation as well, the arm trough/lap board was less effective and tended to overcorrect, and the Bobath sling tended to distract the joint horizontally.

An important note is that none of the mentioned studies discussed scapular or trunk alignment; they only addressed the glenohumeral joint.

Hurd, Farrell, and Waylonis[92] alternately placed 14 patients into a control group (which used no sling) or treatment group (which used a sling). These patients were treated identically in all other respects. The patients were evaluated initially and again two to three weeks later and three to seven months later. No appreciable difference in shoulder ROM, shoulder pain, or subluxation was found between the treated or control groups. No evidence of increased incidence of peripheral nerve or plexus injury was noted in the control group. The authors concluded that the hemisling does not need to be used uniformly by all patients with a flaccid limb after a stroke. They suggested that a sling might be useful when used with discrimination but did not elaborate on this point.

Some authors have suggested that slings be prescribed to prevent overstretching of soft tissue. Chaco and Wolf[45] proposed that permanent subluxation of the glenohumeral joint could be prevented by avoiding loading on the joint when the limb is flaccid. They concluded that the joint capsule holds the head of the humerus in relation to the fossa when the supraspinatus is not responding but cannot prevent subluxation for an unlimited time unless the cuff responds.

If the joint capsule is prevented from stretching during the stage in which the limb is flaccid, patients may have a better opportunity to develop adequate muscle function to maintain joint alignment. Kaplan and colleagues[101] advised using a sling during the flaccid stage to prevent distraction of the joint resulting in a possible brachial plexus injury.

Some therapists have suggested that sling use may increase body neglect and interfere with body image, although this hypothesis has not been researched. Although they have not been specifically related to sling use, the learned nonuse studies of Taub, Uswatte, and Pidikiti[173] may influence therapists' decisions about whether to prescribe a sling, especially for a patient in the acute phase.

Zorowitz[204] stated that "although supports are commonly used during the rehabilitation of stroke survivors, there is no absolute evidence that supports prevent or reduce long-term shoulder subluxation when spontaneous recovery of motor function occurs, or that a support will prevent supposed complications of shoulder subluxation. Without proper training in the use of a support, stroke survivors may face potential complications such as pain and contracture." Although the literature does not give definitive answers about when or whether to use slings, one can infer the following guidelines:

- Therapists should minimize sling use during the rehabilitation process.
- Slings may be useful for supporting the more affected extremity during initial transfer and gait training.
- Slings that position the extremity in a flexor pattern should never be worn unless the patient is in an upright posture; in these cases, they should be worn only for select activities (initial mobility training) and short periods. This type of sling should never be worn by patients in recumbent postures.

- Therapists must evaluate each patient's clinical picture. Therapists need to weigh the pros and cons of slings and clarify the goal of sling use (Box 10-15). Following prescription of the sling, the therapist must reevaluate the effectiveness of the sling (i.e., determine whether the sling truly is meeting the predetermined goal).
- Therapists must become familiar with a variety of slings. One particular sling will not meet the needs of every patient (Fig. 10-28).
- Therapists should continue to investigate the use of alternative means to support the more affected extremity during activities performed in the upright position, such as putting the hand in a pocket, receiving support from an over-the-shoulder bag, using functional electrical stimulation, and adding scapular or humeral taping/strapping protocols to present treatment plans. A recent review concluded that "There is some evidence that strapping the shoulder delays the onset of pain but does not decrease it, nor does it increase function or adversely increase contracture."[4] There are a variety of taping/strapping techniques suggested. Optimal protocols require further analysis. (Fig. 10-29).

One may infer from the literature that the most effective way to reduce the level of subluxation is to provide the patient with activities that enhance trunk and scapula alignment, activate the rotator cuff, and enhance functional use of the extremity during weight-bearing and reach patterns.

Box 10-15

Considerations when Prescribing a Sling

PROS	CONS
■ Protects patient from injury during transfers.	■ May contribute to neglect of body scheme disorders.
■ Allows therapist freedom to control trunk and lower extremities during initial gait, transfer, and upright function training.	■ May contribute to learned nonuse.
■ May prevent soft-tissue stretching (e.g., supraspinatus and capsular stretching).	■ May hold upper extremity in a shortened position (e.g., internal rotators, adductors, and elbow flexors).
■ Prevents prolonged dangling of extremity.	■ Fosters dependence on passive positioning.
■ May relieve pressure on neurovascular bundle (brachial plexus/brachial artery).	■ May initiate shoulder-hand syndrome development (i.e., immobility leading to swelling, shortening, and pain)
■ Supports weight of arm.	■ May predispose patient to shoulder pain from shortened internal rotators.
	■ Does not reduce the amount of subluxation because the alignment of the scapula and trunk are not affected.
	■ Approximates head of humerus to malaligned scapula.
	■ Prevents reciprocal arm swing while walking.
	■ Prevents arm function (e.g., postural support and carrying) in upright postures.
	■ Blocks sensory input.
	■ Prevents balance reactions of the upper extremity.
	■ May block spontaneous use of the upper extremity.
	■ Places no motor demands on the upper extremity.

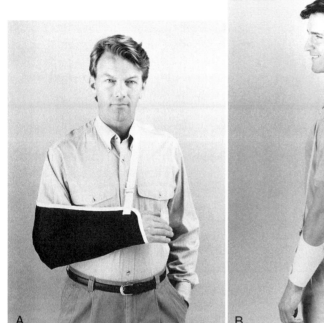
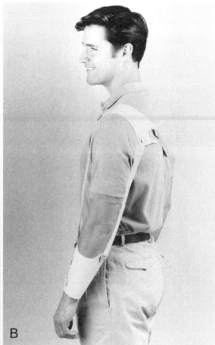
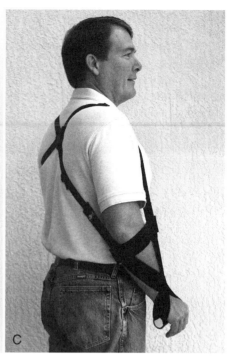

Figure 10-28 **A,** Pouch sling. Sling is only to be used for short periods with patients in upright postures and frees therapist's hands to control trunk and lower extremities. This sling may be appropriate for initial phases of walking, transfer, and upright function training. **B,** Shoulder saddle sling. Sling supports distal weight of extremity and can be worn under clothing. This style of sling can be worn all day because it does not block distal function or hold extremity in a flexor pattern. **C,** The GivMohr Sling (www.givmohrsling.com, 505-292-1144). (**A** and **B** courtesy of Sammons Preston Rolyan, Inc, Bolingbrook, Ill.)

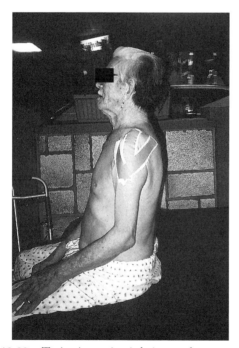

Figure 10-29 Taping/strapping is being used more commonly to treat shoulder instability. Further research is required to determine its effectiveness.

GENERAL TREATMENT PRINCIPLES

Therapists should consider the following treatment principles:

- Maintain a client-centered approach to the treatment of upper extremity dysfunction.
- Evaluate and plan treatments that focus on improving occupational performance.
- Focus treatment on task-specific training.
- Incorporate resistance training into treatment plans.
- Maintain mobility (upward rotation and protraction) of the scapula and humeral external rotation to prevent pain syndromes and prepare for return of function.
- Maintain soft-tissue length and joint mobility in the trunk, head, and neck, and more affected upper extremity.
- Provide appropriate positioning strategies for times when patients are not involved in activities and are in recumbent postures.
- Provide opportunities for patients to use the upper extremity outside of structured therapy time.

- Train all caregivers (staff and family) in the appropriate handling of the more affected upper extremity during ADL and mobility.
- Evaluate and treat any pain syndrome immediately and consistently until symptoms are alleviated.
- Guide appropriate usage of available motor control by providing functional activities that correspond to the patient's level of recovery. Discourage participation in activities that require extra effort.
- Grade activities systematically and with control to increase level of control and functional use.
- Prevent learned nonuse by incorporating the upper extremity into daily life immediately after the stroke.
- Encourage patients to take responsibility for the protection, maintenance, and improvement of their more affected upper extremity.
- Avoid the use of aggressive passive range of motion (PROM) and overhead pulleys.

CASE STUDY

Upper Extremity Function after Stroke

J.C. is a 60-year-old male who suffered a right middle cerebral artery stroke one week before referral. J.C. was in his usual state of good health until he experienced a sudden onset of left-sided weakness. Before this incident, J.C. had just sold his antique store to enjoy retirement. J.C. lives alone, and his interests include reading, gardening, watching movies, wine tasting, and restoring furniture. J.C.'s evaluation and occupational therapy treatment plan (focusing on improved upper extremity function for this study) were as follows.

Initial Evaluation

J.C. was alert and oriented, followed complex commands, had no evidence of cognitive-perceptual deficits with the exception of questionable difficulty with activities incorporating spatial relations components, and had intact sensation. His resting sitting posture consisted of a posteriorly tilted pelvis with minimal functional kyphosis, increased weight-bearing on the left ischial tuberosity, right trunk shortening, and a posteriorly rotated left rib cage. J.C. required minimal assistance with postural adjustments while performing reaching tasks with the right upper extremity. At rest, his left scapula was rotated downward and had minimal winging. The left glenohumeral joint had an anterior-inferior subluxation.

When asked to demonstrate any arm function, J.C. attempted to lift his arm against gravity with a resulting pattern of active lateral trunk flexion to the right, active scapula retraction and elevation, and active humeral abduction; during this attempted movement, the distal extremity fell passively into gravity with a resulting pattern of humeral internal rotation, pronation, and wrist flexion.

Passive range of motion was within normal limits after the scapula was mobilized and gliding with the exception of lacking 20 degrees of external rotation. No evidence of spasticity was found on quick stretch. J.C.'s muscle grades were grossly 2 out of 5; scapula and humerus (except external rotation), 0 out of 5; elbow, 3 out of 5; forearm, 2 out of 5; wrist, 1 out of 5; finger flexion, 3+ out of 5; finger extension, 2 out of 5; and finger abduction/adduction, 1 out of 5. J.C. did not have selective control of his extremity; instead he moved in gross patterns. He was not able to incorporate his left upper extremity into his ADL on initial evaluation. Limitations to J.C.'s ability to use his upper extremity were identified as inefficient movement patterns ("stereotypical") due to loss of postural control, weakness, and trunk and upper extremity malalignments.

Week 1 Goals and Treatments

Treatment goals for the first week were as follows:

1. Roll independently while protecting the left upper extremity.
2. Stretch independently (using the towel-on-table program).
3. Independently position the left upper extremity on a table while eating and performing leisure activities.
4. Independently relieve pressure by lateral weight shifting in the wheelchair. (J.C. was instructed to perform this in front of the dining table with both forearms supported on the table.)

At this stage, J.C. also was provided with a half swing-away lap tray and bed positioning items, including a pillow for under his left scapula and left elbow.

Treatment focused on left upper extremity protection during transitional movements and reaching activities using the right upper extremity in all directions, with a focus on trunk responses and inclusion of rotational activities to recruit abdominal muscle activity. Activities such as repotting plants were used because they required a variety of reach patterns and were previously enjoyed by J.C. At this point the left upper extremity was used to stabilize objects (e.g., the bag of soil).

J.C. was given a polystyrene plastic cup and asked to support his forearm on his lap tray, place the cup upside down into his left hand, and practice releasing it. As the task became easier, he turned the cup right side up to increase the difficulty level. During therapy, treatment focused on controlling the distal arm from the mouth to the table (eccentrically) with his elbow supported on the table and the therapist supporting the humerus with J.C.'s hand empty.

Continued

CASE STUDY

Upper Extremity Function after Stroke—cont'd

Weeks 2 and 3 Goals and Treatments

Treatment goals for the second and third weeks were as follows:

1. Independently hold a toothpaste tube in the left hand while unscrewing the cap with the right hand.
2. Lift the arm from the lap to the lap tray without the right upper extremity assisting.
3. Independently stretch the left wrist and digits into extension.

At this stage, J.C. progressed to assuming standing postures in front of a work surface. Activities included buffing tables and sliding papers across the table past arm's length with the left upper extremity to encourage scapula protraction. Wiping the table (hand-over-hand) and focusing on patterns to the far left were used to maintain soft-tissue length and encourage external rotation. As the task became easier, J.C. held the towel in his left hand and wiped the table using only his left upper extremity.

Weeks 3 and 4 Goals and Treatments

Treatment goals for the third, fourth, and fifth weeks were as follows:

1. Locking wheelchair brakes independently with the left upper extremity.
2. Use both upper extremities to pull pants up from midthigh to waist while standing with close supervision.
3. Independently support the left upper extremity in the pants pocket while walking.

Week 4 (the final week of inpatient treatment) goals and treatment activities included the following:

1. Independently opening a kitchen drawer with the left upper extremity while standing.
2. Holding an over-the-shoulder bag with the left upper extremity while walking.
3. Using both hands to don a sock.
4. Turning sink faucets on and off with the left upper extremity while standing.

The goals and treatment activities were not considered different entities. Treatment was task- and goal-specific.

When discharged from inpatient rehabilitation, J.C. was able to use his left upper extremity as a postural support during forearm and extended arm weight-bearing activities, integrate use of his left upper extremity during self-care activities (but limited to movement patterns below chest level [e.g., in lap activities and reaching below the hips]), integrate use of his left hand into fine motor activities, and carry items in his left hand while walking. Movement patterns that required further antigravity shoulder patterns, increased hand control, and strengthening with resistance were the focus of outpatient occupational therapy.

REVIEW QUESTIONS

1. Which factors contribute to glenohumeral joint subluxation?
2. Which factors contribute to a painful shoulder condition after a stroke?
3. In what way does biomechanical malalignment of the trunk and upper extremity contribute to ineffective and inefficient movement patterns?
4. Describe the learned nonuse phenomenon and treatments aimed at its prevention or reversal.
5. Which factors contribute to a malaligned scapula?
6. Describe a treatment progression aimed at increasing manipulation patterns.
7. What are the components of a task-oriented approach to improving upper limb function?

REFERENCES

1. Ada L, Canning CG, Call JH, et al: Task-specific training of reaching and manipulation. In Bennett KMB, Castiello U, editors: *Insights into the reach to grasp movements*, Amsterdam, 1994, Elsevier Science.
2. Ada L, Dorsch S, Canning CG: Strengthening interventions increase strength and improve activity after stroke: a systematic review. *Aust J Physiother* 52(4):241–248, 2006.
3. Ada L, Foongchomcheay A: Efficacy of electrical stimulation in preventing or reducing subluxation of the shoulder after stroke: a meta-analysis. *Aust J Physiother* 48(4):257–267, 2002.
4. Ada L, Foongchomcheay A, Canning CG: Supportive devices for preventing and treating subluxation of the shoulder after stroke. *Cochrane Database Syst Rev*, 1:1–25, 2009.
5. Ada L, Goddard E, McCully J et al: Thirty minutes of positioning reduces the development of shoulder external rotation contracture after stroke: a randomized controlled trial. *Arch Phys Med Rehabil* 86(2):230–234, 2005.
6. Ada L, O'Dwyer N, O'Neill E: Relation between spasticity, weakness and contracture of the elbow flexors and upper limb activity after stroke: an observational study. *Disabil Rehabil* 28(13–14): 891–897, 2006.
7. Armagan O, Tascioglu F, Oner C: Electromyographic biofeedback in the treatment of the hemiplegic hand: A placebo-controlled study. *Am J Phys Med Rehabil* 82(11):856–861, 2003.
8. AB Arsenault, M Bilodeau, E Dutil, et al: Clinical significance of the V-shaped space in the subluxed shoulder of hemiplegics. *Stroke* 22(7):867–871, 1991.
9. Ashworth B: Carisoprodol in multiple sclerosis. *Practitioner* 192:540, 1964.
10. Badics E, Wittmann A, Rupp M, et al: Systematic muscle building exercises in the rehabilitation of stroke patients. *NeuroRehabilitation* 17(3):211–214, 2002.
11. Bakheit AM, Thilman AF, Ward AB, et al: A randomized, double blind, placebo-controlled study of the efficacy and safety of botulinum toxin type A in upper limb spasticity in patients with stroke. *Eur J Neurol* 8(6):559, 2001.
12. Barreca S, Gowland C, Stratford P, et al: Development of the Chedoke Arm and Hand Activity Inventory: theoretical constructs, item generation, and selection. *Top Stroke Rehabil* 11(4): 31–42, 2004.
13. Barreca SR, Stratford PW, Lambert CL, et al: Test-retest reliability, validity, and sensitivity of the Chedoke arm and hand activity inventory: a new measure of upper-limb function for survivors of stroke. *Arch Phys Med Rehabil* 86(8):1616–1622, 2005.

14. Basmajian JV: The surgical anatomy and function of the arm-trunk mechanism. *Surg Clin North Am* 43:1471, 1963.

15. Bear-Lehman J, Bassile CC, Gillen G: A comparison of time-use on an acute rehabilitation unit: subjects with and without stroke. *Phys Occup Ther Geriatr* 20(1):17, 2001.

16. Belenkii VY, Gurfinkle VS, Paltsev YI: Elements of control of voluntary movements. *Biophysics* 12:135, 1967.

17. Blennerhassett J, Dite W: Additional task-related practice improves mobility and upper limb function early after stroke: a randomised controlled trial. *Austral J Physiother* 50(4):219–24, 2004.

18. Bobath B: *Adult hemiplegia: evaluation and treatment*, ed 3, Oxford, 1990, Butterworth-Heinemann.

19. Boehme R: In *Improving upper body control: an approach to assessment and treatment of tonal dysfunction*, Tucson AZ, 1988, Therapy Skill Builders.

20. Bohannon RW, Andrews AW: Shoulder subluxation and pain in stroke patients. *Am J Occup Ther* 44(6):507–509, 1990.

21. Bohannon RW, Larkin PA, Smith MB, et al: Relationship between static muscle strength deficits and spasticity in stroke patients with hemiparesis. *Phys Ther* 67(7):1068–1071, 1987.

22. Bohannon RW, Larkin PA, Smith MB, et al: Shoulder pain in hemiplegia: a statistical relationship with five variables. *Arch Phys Med Rehabil* 67(8):514–516, 1986.

23. Bohannon RW, Smith MB: Assessment of strength deficits in eight paretic upper extremity muscle groups of stroke patients with hemiplegia. *Phys Ther* 67(4):552–555, 1987.

24. Bohannon RW, Smith MB: Interrater reliability of a modified Ashworth scale of muscle spasticity. *Phys Ther* 67(2):206–207, 1987.

25. Bolton DA, Cauraugh JH, Hausenblas HA: Electromyogram-triggered neuromuscular stimulation and stroke motor recovery of arm/hand functions: a meta-analysis. *J Neurol Sci* 223(2):121–127, 2004.

26. Bonaiuti D, Rebasti L, Sioli P: The constraint induced movement therapy: a systematic review of randomised controlled trials on the adult stroke patients. *Eura Medicophys* 43(2):139–146, 2007.

27. Booth FW: Physiologic and biochemical effects of immobilization on muscle. *Clin Orthop* 219:15–20, 1987.

28. Botte MJ, Nickel VL, Akeson WH: Spasticity and contracture: physiologic aspects of formation. *Clin Orthop* 233:7–18, 1988.

29. Bouisset S, Zattara M: A sequence of postural movements precedes voluntary movement. *Neurosci Lett* 22(3):263, 1981.

30. Bourbonnais D, Vanden Noven S: Weakness in patients with hemiparesis. *Am J Occup Ther* 43(5):313–319, 1989.

31. Bourbonnais D, Vanden Noven S, Carey KM, et al: Abnormal spatial patterns of elbow muscle activation in hemiparetic human subjects. *Brain* 112(1):85–102, 1989.

32. Boyd E, Gaylard A: Shoulder supports with stroke patients: a Canadian survey. *Can J Occup Ther* 53(2):61, 1986.

33. Braun SM, Beurskens AJ, Borm PJ, et al: The effects of mental practice in stroke rehabilitation: a systematic review. *Arch Phys Med Rehabil* 87(6):842–852, 2006.

34. Braus DF, Krauss JK, Strobel JS: The shoulder-hand syndrome after stroke: a prospective clinical trial. *Ann Neurol* 36(5):728–733, 1994.

35. Brodal A: Self-observations and neuro-anatomical considerations after a stroke. *Brain* 96(4):675–694, 1973.

36. Brooke MM, de Lateur BJ, Diana-Rigby GC, et al: Shoulder subluxation in hemiplegia: effects of three different supports. *Arch Phys Med Rehabil* 72(8):582–586, 1991.

37. Brouwer BJ, Ambury P: Upper extremity weightbearing effect on corticospinal excitability following stroke. *Arch Phys Med Rehabil* 75(8):861–866, 1994.

38. Burgess MK: Motor control and the role of occupational therapy: past, present, and the future. *Am J Occup Ther* 43(5):345, 1989.

39. Butefisch C, Hummelsheim H, Denzler P, Mauritz KH: Repetitive training of isolated movements improves the outcome of motor rehabilitation of the centrally paretic hand. *J Neurol Sci* 130(1):59–68, 1995.

40. Cailliet R: *The shoulder in hemiplegia*, Philadelphia, 1980, FA Davis.

41. Carr EK, Kenney FD: Positioning of the stroke patients: a review of the literature. *Int J Nurs Stud* 29(4):355–369, 1992.

42. Carr JH, Shepherd RB: In *A motor relearning programme for stroke*, ed 2, Rockville, MD, 1982, Aspen.

43. Carr JH, Shepherd RB, Ada L: Spasticity: research findings and implications for intervention. *Physiotherapy* 81(8):421, 1995.

44. Carr JH, Shepherd RB, Nordholm L, et al: Investigation of a new motor assessment scale for stroke patients. *Phys Ther* 65(2):175–180, 1985.

45. Chaco J, Wolf E: Subluxation of the glenohumeral joint in hemiplegia. *Am J Phys Med* 50(3):139–143, 1971.

46. Chae J, Yang G, Park BK, Labatia I: Muscle weakness and cocontraction in upper limb hemiparesis: relationship to motor impairment and physical disability. *Neurorehabil Neural Repair* 16(3):241–248, 2002.

47. Chae J, Bethoux F, Bohine T, et al: Neuromuscular stimulation for upper extremity motor and functional recovery in acute hemiplegia. *Stroke* 29(5):975–9, 1998.

48. Chen CC, Bode RK: MAM-36: *Psychometric properties and differential item functioning in neurologic and orthopedic patients*. Paper presented at the AOTA 88th Annual Conference, Long Beach, CA, April 10, 2008.

49. Chen CC, Kasven N, Karpatkin HI, Sylvester A: Hand strength and perceived manual ability among patients with multiple sclerosis. *Arch Phys Med Rehabil* 88(6):794–797, 2007.

50. Chu DS, Petrillo C, Davis SW, et al: Shoulder-hand syndrome: importance of early diagnosis and treatment. *J Am Geriatr Soc* 29(2):58–60, 1981.

51. Collin C, Wade D: Assessing motor impairment after stroke: a pilot reliability study. *J Neurol Neurosurg Psychiatry* 53(7):576–9, 1990.

52. Cordo PJ, Nashner LM: Properties of postural adjustments associated with rapid arm movements. *J Neurophysiol* 47(2):287–302, 1982.

53. Crow L, Lincoln NB, Nouri FM, et al: The effectiveness of EMG biofeedback in the treatment of arm function after stroke. *Int Disabil Stud* 11(4):155–160, 1989.

54. Culham EG, Noce RR, Bagg SD: Shoulder complex position and glenohumeral subluxation in hemiplegia. *Arch Phys Med Rehabil* 76(9):857–864, 1995.

55. Davies PM: *Steps to follow: the comprehensive treatment of patients with hemiplegia*, New York, 2000, Springer-Verlag.

56. Daviet JC, Preux PM, Salle JY, et al: Clinical factors in the prognosis of complex regional pain syndrome type I after stroke. *Am J Phys Med Rehabil* 81(1):34–39, 2002.

57. Davis J: The role of the occupational therapist in the treatment of shoulder-hand syndrome. *Occup Ther Pract* 1(3):30, 1990.

58. Davis SW, Petrillo CR, Eichberg RD, et al: Shoulder-hand syndrome in a hemiplegic population: a five year retrospective study. *Arch Phys Med Rehabil* 58(8):353–356, 1977.

59. de Kroon J, Ijzerman M, Chae J, et al: Relation between stimulation characteristics and clinical outcome in studies using electrical stimulation to improve motor control of the upper extremity in stroke. *J Rehabil Med* 7(2):65–74, 2005.

60. Desrosiers J, Hebert R, Bravo G, et al: Upper extremity performance Test for the Elderly (TEMPA): Normative data and correlates with sensorimotor parameters. *Arch Phys Med Rehabil* 76:1125–1129, 1995.

61. Dietz V, Quintern J, Berger W: Electrophysiological studies of gait in spasticity and rigidity: evidence that altered mechanical properties of muscle contribute to hypertonia. *Brain* 104(3):431–449, 1981.

62. Dohle C, Pullen J, Nakaten A, et al: Mirror Therapy Promotes Recovery From Severe Hemiparesis: A Randomized Controlled Trial. *Neurorehabil Neural Repair* 3(3):209–217, 2009.

63. Dromerick A, Edwards DF, Hahn M: Does the application of constraint-induced movement therapy during acute rehabilitation reduce arm impairment after ischemic stroke? *Stroke* 31(12):2984–2988, 2000.

64. Dromerick AW, Edwards DF, Kumar A: Hemiplegic shoulder pain syndrome: frequency and characteristics during inpatient stroke rehabilitation. *Arch Phys Med Rehabil* 89(8):1589–1593, 2008.

65. Engardt M, Knutsson E, Jonsson M, et al: Dynamic muscle strength training in stroke patients: effects on knee extension torque, electromyographic activity, and motor function. *Arch Phys Med Rehabil* 76(5):419–425, 1995.

66. Exner CE: In-hand manipulation skills. In Case-Smith J, Pehoski C, editors: *Development of hand skills in the child*, Rockville, MD, 1992, American Occupational Therapy Association.

67. Fellows SJ, Kaus C, Thilmann AF: Voluntary movement at the elbow in spastic hemiparesis. *Ann Neurol* 36(3):397–407, 1994.

68. Fisher AG: *Assessment of motor and process skills*, ed 4, Fort Collins, CO, 2001, Three Star Press.

69. Fisher AG: The assessment of IADL motor skills: an application of many-faceted Rasch analysis. *Am J Occup Ther* 47(4):319–329, 1993.

70. Flinn N: A task-oriented approach to the treatment of a client with hemiplegia. *Am J Occup Ther* 49(6):560–569, 1995.

71. Francisco G, Chae J, Chawla H, et al: Electromyogram-triggered neuromuscular stimulation for improving the arm function of acute stroke survivors: a randomized pilot study. *Arch Phys Med Rehabil* 79(5):570–575, 1998.

72. Fugl-Meyer AR, Jaasko L, Leyman I, et al: The post stroke hemiplegic patient: a method for evaluation of physical performance. *Scand J Rehabil Med* 7(1):13–31, 1975.

73. Ghez C: Posture. In Kandel ER, Schwartz JH, Jessel TM, editors: *Principles of neural science*, ed 3, New York, 1991, Elsevier.

74. Ghez C: Voluntary movements. In Kandel ER, Schwartz JH, Jessell TM, editors: *Principles of neural science*, ed 3, New York, 1991, Elsevier.

75. Glenn MB, Whyte J: *The practical management of spasticity in children and adults*, Philadelphia, 1990, Lea & Febiger.

76. Gillen G: Improving mobility and community access in an adult with ataxia: a case study. *Am J Occup Ther* 56(4):462–466, 2002.

77. Gillen G: Improving activities of daily living performance in an adult with ataxia. *Am J Occup Ther* 54(1):89–96, 2000.

78. Gillen G: Managing abnormal tone after brain injury. *Occup Ther Pract* 8:18–24, 1998.

79. Gowland C, de Bruin H, Basmajian JV, et al: Agonist and antagonist activity during voluntary upper-limb movement in patients with stroke. *Phys Ther* 72(9):624–633, 1992.

80. Greenberg S, Fowler RS: Kinesthetic biofeedback: a treatment modality for elbow range of motion in hemiplegia. *Am J Occup Ther* 34(11):738–743, 1980.

81. Hakuno A, Sashika H, Ohkawa T, et al: Arthrographic findings in hemiplegic shoulders. *Arch Phys Med Rehabil* 65(11):706–711, 1984.

82. Halar EM, Bell KR: Contracture and other deleterious effects of immobility. In JB DeLisa, editor: *Rehabilitation medicine: principles and practice*, 1993, JB Lippincott, Philadelphia.

83. Hall J, Dudgeon B, Guthrie M: Validity of clinical measures of shoulder subluxation in adults with poststroke hemiplegia. *Am J Occup Ther* 49(6):526–533, 1995.

84. Hardy J, Salinas S, Blanchard SA, et al: Meta-analysis examining the effectiveness of electrical stimulation in improving functional use of the upper limb in stroke patients. *Phys Occup Ther Geratrics* 21(4):67–78, 2003.

85. Harris JE, Eng JJ: Paretic upper-limb strength best explains arm activity in people with stroke. *Physical Therapy* 87(1):88–97, 2007.

86. Hecht JS: Subscapular nerve block in the painful hemiplegic shoulder. *Arch Phys Med Rehabil* 73(11):1036–1039, 1992.

87. Heller A, Wade D, Wood V, et al: Arm functions after stroke: measurement and recovery over the first three months. *J Neurol Neurosurg Psychiatry* 50(6):714–719, 1987.

88. Horak FB, Esselman P, Anderson ME, et al: The effects of movement velocity, mass displaced, and task certainty on associated postural adjustments made by normal and hemiplegic individuals. *J Neurol Neurosurg Psychiatry* 47(9):1020–1028, 1984.

89. Hubbard IJ, Parsons MW, Neilson C, Carey LM. Task-specific training: evidence for and translation to clinical practice. *Occup Ther Int* 16(3–4):175–89, 2009.

90. Hufschmidt A, Mauritz KH: Chronic transformation of muscle in spasticity: a peripheral contribution to increased tone. *J Neurol Neurosurg Psychiatry* 48(7):676–685, 1985.

91. Hummelsheim H, Munch B, Butefisch C, et al: Influence of sustained stretch on late muscular responses to magnetic brain stimulation in patients with upper motor neuron lesions. *Scand J Rehabil Med* 26(1):3–9, 1994.

92. Hurd MM, Farrell KH, Waylonis GW: Shoulder sling for hemiplegia: friend or foe? *Arch Phys Med Rehabil* 55(11):519–522, 1974.

93. Ikai T, Tei K, Yoshida K, et al: Evaluation and treatment of shoulder subluxation in hemiplegia: relationship between subluxation and pain. *Am J Phys Med Rehabil* 77(5):421–426, 1998.

94. Jackson PL, Lafleur MF, Malouin F, et al: Potential role of mental practice using motor imagery in neurologic rehabilitation. *Arch Phys Med Rehabil* 82(8):1133–1341, 2001.

95. Jeannerod M: The formation of finger grip during prehension: a cortically mediated visuomotor pattern. *Behav Brain Res* 19(2):99–116, 1986.

96. Jeannerod M: The timing of natural prehension movements. *J Motor Behav* 16:235, 1984.

97. Jebsen RH, Taylor N, Trieschmann RB, et al: An objective and standardized test of hand function. *Arch Phys Med Rehabil* 50(6):311–319, 1969.

98. Jensen EM: The hemiplegic shoulder. *Scand J Rehabil Med* 7(suppl):113–119, 1980.

99. Joynt RL: The source of shoulder pain in hemiplegia. *Arch Phys Med Rehabil* 73(5):409–413, 1992.

100. Kapandji IA: *The physiology of the joints. The upper limb*, vol 1, New York, 1982, Churchill Livingstone.

101. Kaplan PE, Meridith J, Taft G, et al: Stroke and brachial plexus injury: a difficult problem. *Arch Phys Med Rehabil* 58(9):415–418, 1977.

102. Kopp B, Kunkel A, Flor H, et al: The arm motor ability test: reliability, validity, and sensitivity to change of an instrument for assessing disabilities in activities of daily living. *Arch Phys Med Rehabil* 78(6):615–620, 1997.

103. Kondo I, Hosokawa K, Soma M, et al: Protocol to prevent shoulder-hand syndrome after stroke. *Arch Phys Med Rehabil* 82(11):1619–1623, 2001.

104. Kumar R, Metter EJ, Mehta AJ, et al: Shoulder pain in hemiplegia: the role of exercise. *Am J Phys Med Rehabil* 69(4):205–208, 1990.

105. Kwakkel G, Wagenaar RC, Twisk JW, et al: Intensity of leg and arm training after primary middle-cerebral-artery stroke: a randomised trial. *Lancet* 354(9174):191–196, 1999.

106. Lankford LL: Reflex sympathetic dystrophy. In Hunter JM, Schneider L, Mackin E, et al, editors: *Rehabilitation of the hand: surgery and therapy*, ed 3, St Louis, 1990, Mosby.

107. Landau WM: Spasticity: what is it? what is it not? In Feldman RG, Young RR, Koella WP, editors: *Spasticity: disordered motor control*, Chicago, 1980, Year Book.

108. Landau WM: Spasticity: the fable of a neurological demon and the emperor's new therapy. *Arch Neurol* 31(4):217, 1974.

109. Lee WA: A control systems framework for understanding normal and abnormal posture. *Am J Occup Ther* 43(5):291–301, 1989.

110. Liepert J, Bauder H, Wolfgang HR, et al: Treatment-induced cortical reorganization after stroke in humans. *Stroke* 31(6):1210–1216, 2000.

111. Lin K: Enhancing occupational performance through occupationally embedded exercise: a meta-analysis. *Occup Ther J Res* 17(1):25, 1997.

112. Lin KC, Wu CY, Wei TH, et al: Effects of modified constraint-induced movement therapy on reach-to-grasp movements and functional performance after chronic stroke: a randomized controlled study. *Clin Rehabil* 21(12):1075–1086, 2007.

113. Lin KC, Wu CY, Liu JS, et al: Constraint-induced therapy versus dose-matched control intervention to improve motor ability, basic/extended daily functions, and quality of life in stroke. *Neurorehabil Neural Repair* 23(2):160–165, 2009.

114. Lin KC, Chang YF, Wu CY, Chen YA: Effects of constraint-induced therapy versus bilateral arm training on motor performance, daily functions, and quality of life in stroke survivors. *Neurorehabil Neural Repair* 23(5):441–448, 2009.

115. Lincoln N, Leadbitter D: Assessment of motor function in stroke patients. *Physiotherapy* 65:48–51, 1979.

116. Little JW, Massagli TL: Spasticity and associated abnormalities of muscle tone. In JA DeLisa, editor: *Rehabilitation medicine: principles and practice*, ed 2, Philadelphia, 1993, JB Lippincott.

117. Lyle R: A performance test for assessment of upper limb function in physical rehabilitation treatment and research. *Int J Rehabil Res* 4(4):483–492, 1981.

118. Marsden CD, Merton PA, Morton HB: Human postural responses. *Brain* 104(3):513–534, 1981.

119. Massion J: Postural changes accompanying voluntary movements: normal and pathological aspects. *Hum Neurobiol* 2(4):261–267, 1984.

120. Mathiowetz V, Volland G, Kashmanin N. et al: Adult norms for the Box and Block Test of manual dexterity. *Am J Occup Ther* 39(6):386–391, 1985.

121. Mathiowetz V, Bass-Haugen J: Motor behavior research: implications for therapeutic approaches to central nervous system dysfunction. *Am J Occup Ther* 48(8):733–745, 1994.

122. McIllroy WE, Maki BE: Early activation of arm muscles follows external perturbation of upright stance. *Neurosci Lett* 148(3):177–180, 1995.

123. Mercier C, Bourbonnais D: Relative shoulder flexor and handgrip strength is related to upper limb function after stroke. *Clin Rehabil* 18(2):215–221, 2004.

124. Merideth J, Taft G, Kaplan P: Diagnosis and treatment of the hemiplegic patient with brachial plexus injury. *Am J Occup Ther* 35(10):656–660, 1981.

125. Meyer AZ: The philosophy of occupational therapy. *Am J Occup Ther* 31(10):639–642, 1977.

126. Michaelsen SM, Dannenbaum R, Levin MF: Task-specific training with trunk restraint on arm recovery in stroke: randomized control trial. *Stroke* 37(1):186–192, 2006.

127. Mohr JD: Management of the trunk in adult hemiplegia: the Bobath concept. *Top Neurol* 1(1):1–12, 1990.

128. Moodie NB, Brisbin J, Grace Morgan AM: Subluxation of the glenohumeral joint in hemiplegia: evaluation of supportive devices. *Physiother Can* 38:151, 1986.

129. Morris JH, van Wijck F, Joice S, et al: A comparison of bilateral and unilateral upper-limb task training in early poststroke rehabilitation: a randomized controlled trial. *Arch Phys Med Rehabil* 89(7):1237–1245, 2008.

130. Moskowitz E, Porter JI: Peripheral nerve lesions in the upper extremity in the hemiplegic patient. *New Engl J Med* 269:776, 1963.

130a. Mudie M, Matyas T: Upper extremity retraining following stroke: effects of bilateral practice. *J Neurol Rehabil* 10:167–184, 1966.

131. Najenson T, Yacubovic E, Pikielni SS: Rotator cuff injury in shoulder joints of hemiplegic patients. *Scand J Rehabil Med* 3(3):131–137, 1971.

132. Nakayama H, Jorgensen HS, Raaschou HO, et al: Recovery of upper extremity function in stroke patients: the Copenhagen stroke study. *Arch Phys Med Rehabil* 75(4):394–398, 1994.

133. Neistadt ME: The effect of different treatment activities on functional fine motor coordination in adults with brain injury. *Am J Occup Ther* 48(10):877, 1994.

134. Nepomuceno CS, Miller JM: Shoulder arthrography in hemiplegic patients. *Arch Phys Med Rehabil* 55(2):49–51, 1974.

135. Nilsen D, Gillen G, Gordon A: The use of mental practice to improve upper limb recovery post-stroke: a systematic review. *Am J Occup Ther* 64(5): 2010.

136. Oxford Grice K, Vogel KA, Le V, et al: Adult norms for a commercially available Nine Hole Peg Test for finger dexterity. *Am J Occup Ther* 57(5):570–573, 2003.

137. Page SJ, Levine P, Leonard A, et al: Modified constraint-induced therapy in chronic stroke: results of a single-blinded randomized controlled trial. *Phys Ther* 88(3):333–340, 2008.

138. Page SJ, Levine P, Khoury JC: Modified constraint-induced therapy combined with mental practice: thinking through better motor outcomes. *Stroke* 40(2):551–554, 2009.

139. Page SJ: Imagery improves upper extremity motor function in chronic stroke patients: a pilot study. *Occup Ther J Res* 20(3):201, 2000.

140. Page SJ, Sisto SA, Levine P, et al: Modified constraint induced therapy: a randomized feasibility and efficacy study. *J Rehabil Res Dev* 38(5):583–590, 2001.

141. Patten C, Lexell J, Brown HE: Weakness and strength training in persons with poststroke hemiplegia: rationale, method, and efficacy. *J Rehabil Res Dev* 41(3A):293–312, 2004.

142. Perry J: Rehabilitation of spasticity. In Feldman RG, Young RR, Koella WP, editors: *Spasticity: disordered motor control*, Chicago, 1980, Year Book.

143. Petchkrua W, Weiss DJ, Patel RR: Reassessment of the incidence of complex regional pain syndrome type 1 following stroke. *Neurorehabil Neural Repair* 14(1):59–63, 2000.

144. Penta M, Tesio L, Arnould C, et al: The ABILHAND questionnaire as a measure of manual ability in chronic stroke patients: Rasch-based validation and relationship to upper limb impairment. *Stroke* 32(7):1627–1634, 2001.

145. Platz T, Pinkowski C, van Wijck F et al: Reliability and validity of arm function assessment with standardized guidelines for the Fugl-Meyer Test, Action Research Arm Test and Box and Block Test: a multicentre study. *Clin Rehabil* 19(4):404–411, 2005.

146. Poole, JL, Whitney, SL: Assessments of motor function post stroke: A review. *Phys Occup Ther Geriatr* 19(2):1–22, 2001.

147. Preston LA, Hecht JS: *Spasticity management: rehabilitation strategies*, Bethesda, MD, 1999, American Occupational Therapy Association.

148. Prevost R, Arsenault AB, Drouin G, et al: Rotation of the scapula and shoulder subluxation in hemiplegia. *Arch Phys Med Rehabil* 68(11):786–790, 1987.

149. Prevost R, Arsenault AB, Drouin G, et al: Shoulder subluxation in hemiplegia: a radiologic correlational study. *Arch Phys Med Rehabil* 68(11):782–785, 1987.

150. Price C, Pandyan A: Electrical stimulation for preventing and treating post-stroke shoulder pain: a systematic Cochrane review. *Clin Rehabil* 15:1–19, 2001.

151. Rensink M, Schuurmans M, Lindeman E, Hafsteinsdottir T: Task-oriented training in rehabilitation after stroke: systematic review. *J Adv Nurs* 65(4):737–754, 2009.

152. Rizk TE, Christopher RP, Pinals RS, et al: Arthrographic studies in painful hemiplegic shoulders. *Arch Phys Med Rehabil* 65(5):254–256, 1984.

153. Rosenbaum DR, Jorgensen MJ: Planning macroscopic aspects of manual control. *Hum Mov Sci* 11(1-2):61, 1992.

154. Rousseaux M, Kozlowski O, Froger J: Efficacy of botulinum toxin A in upper limb function of hemiplegic patients. *J Neurol* 249(1):76–84, 2002.

155. Roy CW, Sands MR, Hill LD: Shoulder pain in acutely admitted hemiplegics. *Clin Rehabil* 8(4):334, 1994.

156. Ryerson S, Levit K: The shoulder in hemiplegia. In RA Donatelli, editor: *Physical therapy of the shoulder*, ed 2, New York, 1991, Churchill Livingstone.

157. Ryerson S, Levit K: Glenohumeral joint subluxations in CNS dysfunction. *NDTA Newsletter*, 115–117, Nov 1988.

158. Sabari JS: Motor learning concepts applied to activity-based intervention with adults with hemiplegia. *Am J Occup Ther* 45(6):523–530, 1991.

159. Sahrmann SA, Norton BJ: The relationship of voluntary movement to spasticity in the upper motor neuron syndrome. *Ann Neurol* 2(6):460–465, 1977.

160. Savage R, Robertson L: Shoulder pain in hemiplegia: a literature review. *Clin Rehabil* 2(1):35–44, 1988.

161. Schleenbaker RE, Mainous AG: Electromyographic biofeedback for neuromuscular reeducation in the hemiplegic stroke patient: a meta-analysis. *Arch Phys Med Rehabil* 74(12):1301–1304, 1993.

162. Shah RR, Haghpanah S, Elovic EP, et al: MRI findings in the painful poststroke shoulder. *Stroke* 39(6):1808–1813, 2008.

163. Sietsema JM, Nelson DL, Mulder RM, et al: The use of a game to promote arm reach in persons with traumatic brain injury. *Am J Occup Ther* 47(1):19–24, 1993.

164. Simpson DM, Gracies JM, Graham HK et al: Therapeutics and Technology Assessment Subcommittee of the American Academy of Neurology. Assessment: Botulinum neurotoxin for the treatment of spasticity (an evidence-based review): report of the Therapeutics and Technology Assessment Subcommittee of the American Academy of Neurology. *Neurology* 70(19):1691–1698, 2008.

165. Smith RO, Okamoto G: Checklist for the prescription of slings for the hemiplegic patient. *Am J Occup Ther* 35(2):91–95, 1981.

166. Sterr A, Freivogel S: Intensive training in chronic upper limb hemiparesis does not increase spasticity or synergies. *Neurology* 63(11):2176–2177, 2004.

167. Sterr A, Elbert T, Berthold I, et al: Longer versus shorter daily constraint-induced movement therapy of chronic hemiparesis: an exploratory study. *Arch Phys Med Rehabil* 83(10):1374–1377, 2002.

168. Stewart KC, Cauraugh JH, Summers JJ: Bilateral movement training and stroke rehabilitation: a systematic review and meta-analysis. *J Neurol Sci* 244(1–2):89–95, 2006.

169. Stoykov ME, Corcos DM: A review of bilateral training for upper extremity hemiparesis. *Occup Ther Int* 16(3–4):190–203, 2009.

170. Stoykov ME, Lewis GN, Corcos DM: Comparison of bilateral and unilateral training for upper extremity hemiparesis in stroke. *Neurorehabil Neural Repair* 23(9):945–953, 2009.

171. Taub E, Miller NE, Novack TA, et al: Technique to improve chronic motor deficit after stroke. *Arch Phys Med Rehabil* 74(4):347–354, 1993.

172. Taub E, Uswatte G, King DK, et al: A placebo-controlled trial of constraint-induced movement therapy for upper extremity after stroke. *Stroke* 37(4):1045–1049, 2006.

173. Taub E, Uswatte G, Pidikiti R: Constraint-induced movement therapy: a new family of techniques with broad application to physical rehabilitation. *J Rehabil Res Dev* 6(3):237–251, 1999.

174. Tepperman PS, Greyson ND, Hilbert L, et al: Reflex sympathetic dystrophy in hemiplegia. *Arch Phys Med Rehabil* 65(8):442–447, 1984.

175. Tries J: EMG feedback for the treatment of upper extremity dysfunction: can it be effective? *Biofeedback Self Regul* 14(1):21–53, 1989.

176. Trombly CA: Observations of improvements of reaching in five subjects with left hemiparesis. *J Neurol Neurosurg Psychiatry* 56(1):40, 1993.

177. Trombly CA: Deficits of reaching in subjects with left hemiparesis: a pilot study. *Am J Occup Ther* 46(10):887–897, 1992.

178. Trombly CA, Wu CY: Effect of rehabilitation tasks on organization of movement after stroke. *Am J Occup Ther* 53(4):333–344, 1999.

179. Uswatte G, Taub E: Constraint-induced movement therapy: new approaches to outcome measurement in rehabilitation. In Stuss DT, Winocur G, Robertson IH, editors: *Cognitive neurorehabilitation: a comprehensive approach*, Cambridge, UK, 1999, Cambridge University Press.

180. Uswatte G, Taub E, Morris D et al: The Motor Activity Log-28: assessing daily use of the hemiparetic arm after stroke. *Neurology* 67(7):1189–1194, 2006.

181. Uswatte G, Taub E, Morris D et al: Reliability and validity of the upper-extremity Motor Activity Log-14 for measuring real-world arm use. *Stroke* 36(11):2493–2496, 2005.

182. van der Lee JH, Wagenaar RC, Lankhorst GJ, et al: Forced use of the upper extremity in chronic stroke patients: results from a single-blind randomized clinical trial. *Stroke* 30(11):2369–2375, 1999.

183. van Kuijk AA, Geurts AC, Bevaart BJ, van Limbeek J: Treatment of upper extremity spasticity in stroke patients by focal neuronal or neuromuscular blockade: a systematic review of the literature. *J Rehabil Med* 34(2):51–61, 2002.

184. Van Ouwenaller C, Laplace PM, Chantraine A: Painful shoulder in hemiplegia. *Arch Phys Med Rehabil* 67(1):23–26, 1986.

185. Van Vliet P, Sheridan MR, Fentem P, et al: The influence of functional goals on the kinematics of reaching following stroke. *Neurol Rep* 19(1):11, 1995.

186. Wanklyn P, Forster A, Young J: Hemiplegic shoulder pain (HSP): natural history and investigation of associated features. *Disabil Rehabil* 18(10):497–501, 1996.

187. Waylett-Rendall J: Therapist's management of reflex sympathetic dystrophy. In Hunter JM, Schneider L, Mackin E, et al, editors: *Rehabilitation of the hand: surgery and therapy*, ed 3, St Louis, 1990, Mosby.

188. Wilson DJ, Baker LL, Craddock JA: Functional test for the hemiparetic upper extremity. *Am J Occup Ther* 38(3):159–164, 1984.

189. Winstein CJ, Rose DK, Tan SM, Lewthwaite et al: A randomized controlled comparison of upper-extremity rehabilitation strategies in acute stroke: A pilot study of immediate and long-term outcomes. *Arch Phys Med Rehabil* 85(4):620–628, 2004.

190. Wolf SL, Catlin PA, Blanton S, et al: Overcoming limitations in elbow movement in the presence of antagonist hyperactivity. *Phys Ther* 74(9):826–835, 1994.

191. Wolf SL, Catlin PA, Ellis M, et al: Assessing Wolf motor function test as outcome measure for research in patients after stroke. *Stroke* 32(7):1635–1639, 2001.

192. Wolf SL, Lecraw DE, Barton LA, et al: Forced use of hemiplegic upper extremities to reverse the effect of learned nonuse among chronic stroke and head-injured patients. *Exp Neurol* 104(2):125–132, 1989.

193. Wolf SL, Winstein CJ, Miller JP et al: Effect of constraint-induced movement therapy on upper extremity function 3 to 9 months after stroke: the EXCITE randomized clinical trial. *JAMA* 296(17):2095–2104, 2006.

194. Woollacott MH, Bonnet M, Yabe K: Preparatory process for anticipatory postural adjustments: modulation of leg muscles reflex pathways during preparation for arm movements in standing man. *Exp Brain Res* 55(2):263–271, 1984.

195. World Health Organization: *International classification of function*, Geneva, 2002, The Organization.

196. Wu CY, Chen CL, Tsai WC, et al: A randomized controlled trial of modified constraint-induced movement therapy for elderly stroke survivors: changes in motor impairment, daily functioning, and quality of life. *Arch Phys Med Rehabil* 88(3):273–278, 2007.

197. Wu CY, Trombly CA, Lin KC: The relationship between occupational form and occupational performance: a kinematic perspective. *Am J Occup Ther* 48(8):679–687, 1994.

198. Wu S, Trombly CA, Lin K, et al: Effects of object affordances on movement performance: a meta-analysis. *Scand J Occup Ther* 5(2):83–92, 1998.

199. Yavuzer G, Selles R, Sezer N, et al: Mirror therapy improves hand function in subacute stroke: a randomized controlled trial. *Arch Phys Med Rehabil* 89(3):393–398, 2008.

200. Yelnik AP, Colle FM, Bonan IV, Vicaut E: Treatment of shoulder pain in spastic hemiplegia by reducing spasticity of the subscapular muscle: a randomised, double blind, placebo controlled study of botulinum toxin A. *J Neurol Neurosurg Psychiatry* 78(8):845–848, 2007.

201. Yen JG, Wang RY, Chen HH, Hong CT: Effectiveness of modified constraint-induced movement therapy on upper limb function in stroke subjects. *Acta Neurol Taiwan* 14(1):16–20, 2005.

202. Yue G, Cole KJ: Strength increases from the motor program: comparison of training with maximal voluntary and imagined muscle contractions. *J Neurophysiol* 67(5):1114–1123, 1992.

203. Zorowitz RD, Hughes MB, Idank D, et al: Shoulder pain and subluxation after stroke: correlation or coincidence? *Am J Occup Ther* 50(3):194–201, 1996.

204. Zorowitz RD, Idank D, Ikai T, et al: Shoulder subluxation after stroke: a comparison of four supports. *Arch Phys Med Rehabil* 76(8):763–771, 1995.

susan e. fasoli

chapter 11

Rehabilitation Technologies to Promote Upper Limb Recovery after Stroke

key terms

adjunctive interventions	haptics	robot assisted therapy
backdrivability	impedance	technology
degrees of freedom		

chapter objectives

After completing this chapter, the reader will be able to:

1. Discuss the rationale for using rehabilitation technologies and theories that have guided their development.
2. Describe similarities and differences among different technology devices, specifically how they work and what they might add to the therapist's repertoire of treatment tools.
3. Evaluate results of empirical studies on the use of rehabilitation technologies for the paretic upper limb after stroke.
4. Identify considerations for choosing rehabilitation technologies for clinical use, including their potential benefits and limitations.

Rehabilitation technologies to improve motor control after neurological injury have undergone tremendous growth during the past 15 years. Two forces in rehabilitation medicine have provided impetus for this technology development. The first is evidence of cortical reorganization in response to movement therapy after stroke. The second is the high cost of health care and significant reductions in rehabilitation services that have occurred in recent years.[38] This chapter provides an overview of rehabilitation technologies, ranging from complex robotic devices to relatively simple spring-driven wrist/hand orthoses. Theories guiding technology development, research findings, and considerations for technology use in clinical practice are discussed.

RATIONALE FOR DEVELOPMENT

Rehabilitation scientists are concerned about the lack of empirical evidence on treatment efficacy and its impact on motor recovery and functional outcomes after stroke.

At present, they do not have the knowledge needed to predict which treatment interventions, dose, or intensity elicit the best functional outcomes for a particular patient. Rehabilitation scientists are working diligently to quantify the "active ingredients" of various treatments, so they can make use of the most effective and efficient therapy methods when delivering clinical care to patients.

Rehabilitation technologies can provide quantifiable and repeatable treatment interventions and allow us to better measure the import of our interventions on impairments of motor function.[18] For example, robotic devices can quantify changes in motor functions during stroke rehabilitation by gathering kinematic and kinetic data related to variables such as speed and accuracy of task completion, smoothness of reach, or forces exerted during training. Movement scientists continue to explore these data to further the understanding of how changes in motor control may contribute to increased functional use of a paretic limb after stroke.

Rehabilitation technologies are not expected to replace occupational or physical therapists, but they will become part of their treatment arsenal to optimize functional performance after a disabling event. Although the present cost of these novel technologies is high, larger scale production is expected to lower costs for clinical use in the future. Proponents of rehabilitation technologies predict that these tools will help to reduce or control rehabilitation costs by providing intensive movement therapies with minimal supervision by a therapist, which is important at a time when patients receive less therapy after neurological injuries, such as stroke, despite research evidence that more therapy is better.[38] The use of this technology may help to shorten inpatient hospitalizations and enhance outpatient services, which hopefully will lead to improved long-term functional outcomes.

THEORIES GUIDING TECHNOLOGY DEVELOPMENT

Rehabilitation technology is a new and growing field, experiencing some of the same developmental challenges seen during the history of conventional rehabilitation practice. Its development has been strongly influenced by motor learning principles, in particular massed practice and explicit learning paradigms.[6] For example, rehabilitation robotics are designed to produce highly intensive upper limb training that is quantifiable, easily graded, cognitively challenging, and goal-directed. Motor learning principles guide their delivery of feedback with regard to knowledge of performance (e.g., via haptics), and knowledge of results, via graphs, changes in the virtual tasks and environment, and other forms of feedback. To date, robotic therapy trials have focused on improving motor performance at the International Classification of Functioning, Disability, and Health (ICF) level aimed at body structures and functions,

rather than the activity level, aimed at task execution and functional performance. The state of robotic development has dictated this focus, as robots used in clinical trials have primarily exercised the paretic shoulder and elbow during reaching movements while the wrist and hand are supported by the device.

Motor learning approaches to conventional stroke rehabilitation have evolved to emphasize task-oriented training aimed at increasing upper limb function and patient participation in valued roles and routines.[48] This task-oriented approach, in which skill-related tasks are practiced in natural contexts, has resulted in faster and better treatment outcomes than traditional methods, such as Bobath's neurodevelopmental therapy.[27] See Chapters 4 and 6. Recent trials of robot-assisted therapies have incorporated a task-oriented training approach in conjunction with other motor learning principles. For example, the Armeo and HOWARD devices provide task-oriented training via virtual games during upper limb therapy, and can allow interaction with real and virtual objects during repetitive, robot-assisted therapy. Studies have shown that the training of virtual tasks can lead to significant gains in motor performance during real world activities (see Brewer and colleagues[6] for review). As technological advances continue, rehabilitation technologies will be better equipped to deliver task-oriented therapies more aligned with current rehabilitation practice and directed toward the ICF activity level of performance.

ROBOT ASSISTED THERAPY

Two main classes of rehabilitation robots have been developed. Robots such as the Assistive Robotic Manipulator (ARM) (www.exactdynamics.nl) allow the user to compensate for lost skills when the potential for motor recovery is poor. The purpose of this chapter is to review a second class of robots, which provide repetitive, task-specific training to help restore lost motor function. Unlike constraint-induced movement therapy (CIMT), robot-assisted technologies are appropriate for persons with moderate to severe motor impairments.

Rehabilitation robots to restore lost motor function can be categorized by how the device is controlled or activated and how the user interface is designed. Robots for the upper limb can be broadly classified into three types: active systems, with actuators that provide movement assistance along a defined trajectory; passive systems that support the limb during movement attempts; and interactive systems in which actuators or motors are combined with impedance and control strategies that allow the robot to react to the patient's movement attempts.

The way in which the robot assists with movement affects how the robot "feels" to the user during therapy. Low impedance interactive robots such as the MIT-MANUS are highly "back-drivable" and compliant to a client's attempts to move, allowing precise and objective measures of motor performance. Active robots that use pneumatic actuators or "muscles" to power the device (e.g., Hand Mentor) are not as responsive to the patient's movement attempts, because the mechanics of the robot create a more viscous response, similar to moving through honey. Passive robotic systems offer varied forms of nonpowered assistance with elastic bands or springs that support the limb against gravity during movement attempts. Examples include the Therapy Wilmington Robotic Exoskeleton (T-WREX) and Armeo devices described later.

The user/robot interface is another consideration when selecting rehabilitation robots for clinical use. End-effector robots, such as the MIT-MANUS and Mirror Image Motion Enabler (MIME), are typically attached to the person's hand or forearm at a single point of contact. These robots are easily adjusted to different arm lengths, but do not control movement torques at individual joints. In contrast, the structure of exoskeletal robots more closely resembles human anatomy and allows separate control of torques applied to each joint. Exoskeletal robots, such as the interactive ARMin, require more effort when adapting them to different body sizes because each robot link must be adjusted to match the length of the user's upper and lower arm.[34] The therapeutic games used to visually direct the patient's movement attempts during robot-assisted therapy also vary in their degree of complexity, ranging from simple stimuli to virtual environments designed to simulate functional task performance.

The discussion that follows is arranged from high to low tech, starting with more complex, low impedance robots to simpler wrist hand orthoses. Proximal devices are presented before distal technologies. During this review, readers are encouraged to consider needs specific to their patient mix and clinical setting, and potential goals for intervention. Controlled studies that compare rehabilitation technologies to other forms of therapy are highlighted in Table 11-1.

MIT MANUS and InMotion2 Robots

The most widely studied rehabilitation robot is the MIT-MANUS and its successor the InMotion2 (Interactive Motion Technologies, Watertown, MA). During therapy, the client is seated at the robot workstation and the paretic hand is positioned in a customized arm support attached to the end-effector (i.e., handle) of the robot arm. Therapy involves repetitive goal-directed, planar reaching tasks that emphasize shoulder and elbow movements. As clients attempt to move the robot's handle toward designated targets, the computer screen in front of them gives visual feedback of the target location and movement of the robot handle (Fig. 11-1).

The low impedance controller of the MIT-MANUS is highly compliant when interacting with the client's arm, similar to hand-over-hand assistance from a therapist

during conventional therapy. Although MIT-MANUS is capable of providing passive, active-assistive, and active and resistive modes of therapy, the majority of studies have investigated the effects of active-assistive robotic therapy on motor recovery after stroke. The adaptive algorithm used in recent studies allows the robot to adjust the amount of guidance or assist provided to the patient based on his/her individual needs.

Proof of concept studies began in the mid-1990s, with a focus on the effects of intensive robot-assisted sensorimotor therapy for individuals in inpatient rehabilitation during the first weeks poststroke.[1] Since then, investigations have primarily included persons with chronic and moderate to severe motor impairments more than six months after stroke. In this research, participants typically received one hour of robotic therapy three times per week for six weeks, performing approximately 18,000 repetitive reaching movements over the course of therapy.

As a whole, these studies indicate that treatment intensity and task specificity play a critical role in upper limb robot-assisted therapy. Reductions in motor impairment after MIT-MANUS training were task-specific in that the largest gains were observed in the exercised shoulder and elbow vs. the unexercised wrist and hand.[12,50] Comparisons of robot vs. therapist directed therapy of equal intensity by Volpe and colleagues[51] revealed no significant group differences in motor outcomes (see Table 11-1).

Stein and colleagues[44] revealed that patients engaged in active-assistive or progressive-resistive training with the MIT-MANUS robot had similar gains in motor performance over the course of treatment (see Table 11-1). In this study, the level of initial severity vs. type of robotic therapy had a differential effect on motor outcomes. Individuals who were better able to reach the robotic therapy targets at study admission had larger gains in motor control on the Fugl-Meyer Assessment (FMA), regardless of treatment

Text continued on p.296

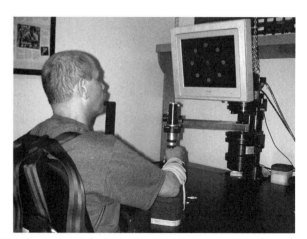

Figure 11-1 InMotion2 planar robot to exercise the paretic shoulder and elbow with wrist and hand supported. (Courtesy of Hermano Igo Krebs.)

Table 11-1

Post-Stroke Upper Limb Technology: Evidence Summary

AUTHORS AND YEAR	STUDY AIM/HYPOTHESIS	DESIGN AND SUBJECTS	INTERVENTION	PRIMARY OUTCOME MEASURES AND RESULTS	COMMENTS	RATING
Aisen and colleagues, 1997	Does intensive supplemental robotic therapy improve motor outcomes after stroke?	Controlled trial N = 20 Subacute inpatients in rehabilitation hospital.	Exp: 4–5 hrs of goal-directed movement therapy with MIT-MANUS. Control: Weekly or biweekly contact with MIT-MANUS: no active assist from robot. Both received conventional rehabilitation.	Functional Independence Measure (FIM), Fugl-Meyer Assessment (FMA), Motor Status Scale (MSS), Motor Power (MP) (shoulder and elbow) FIM: no significant group differences. All subjects showed improved motor scores. Non-significant (NS) group differences on MP and FMA although change scores greater in exp group. Exp group gains were significantly better on MSS shoulder and elbow subscore (p = 0.002). No change on wrist and hand items.	Focused robotic therapy had task-specific training effects on shoulder and elbow motor recovery. Additional therapy provided by robot yielded higher trends in motor scores. Separate study (Volpe and colleagues, 1999) showed that robot group participants continued to show significant gains in motor scores as compared to control at 3 years (n = 12 of original 20 subjects).	III

Continued

Table 11-1

Post-Stroke Upper Limb Technology: Evidence Summary—cont'd

AUTHORS AND YEAR	STUDY AIM/HYPOTHESIS	DESIGN AND SUBJECTS	INTERVENTION	PRIMARY OUTCOME MEASURES AND RESULTS	COMMENTS	RATING
Alon, Levitt, and McCarthy, 2007	H: Functional Electrical Stimulation (FES) with task-specific training can enhance recovery of upper limb function when begun during inpatient rehabilitation and continued for 12 wks.	Controlled trial N = 15 Subacute rehabilitation inpatients who continued program at home post d/c	Control: standardized task-specific occupational and physical therapy program (OT/PT) Exp: same standardized tasks as control synchronized with NESS H-200 e-stim for activation of wrist/finger flexors and extensors Two 30 min sessions/5 days/wk for 12 wks. FES group received additional e-stim without concurrent exercises	Box and Block test, light object subtest of Jebsen Taylor Test, Modified Fugl-Meyer Test (excluding reflex items and coordination/speed — max score = 54 points) Statistically significant and large effects seen on all measures favoring FES group Mean scores on modified FMA after 12 wks of treatment were 49.3 ($\pm$ 5.1) for FES, 40.6 ($\pm$ 8.2) for control group.	Length of time exercising and compliance at home not monitored No follow-up evaluations completed to test for sustained effects Total time of intervention differed across groups, as FES group received additional e-stim without exercise for about 2 hrs daily	II
Coote, Murphy, Harwin, and Stokes, 2008	To compare effects of robot mediated therapy with Haptic Master to sling suspension exercises for persons with hemiparesis poststroke	Series of single case studies using randomized multiple baseline design with ABC or ACB order N = 20 Time poststroke ranged from 3 mos to 75 mos.	Robot mediated therapy delivered 30 mins 3×/wk for 3 wks Haptic Master delivered virtual training with visual and haptic feedback Suspension sling group practiced single plane reaching exercises for same dose and frequency	FMA, Motor Assessment Scale, and active range of motion (AROM) at shoulder Modest recovery trends were seen across measures. Overall, rate of recovery was greater during robot-mediated therapy.	Different response to treatment was seen across the 20 subjects and can be attributed to group heterogeneity (time poststroke, baseline impairment). Intervention was more beneficial to subjects who scored >20 on baseline FMA. Optimal duration of intervention is likely higher than that delivered during this trial; further research needed to examine best dose and timing.	III

| Hesse and colleagues, 2005 | To compare effects of repetitive exercises with Bi-Manu-Track robotic arm trainer to repetitive EMG initiated electrical stimulation (ES) of paretic wrist extensors. | Randomized controlled trial N = 44 participants with severe UE paresis (initial FMA score <18) 4 to 8 wks poststroke (subacute) | Robot group performed 800 repetitions/session of unilateral and bilateral forearm and wrist exercises. ES group performed 60 to 80 repetitions wrist/extension exercises/session. Both groups received these interventions 20 min/5 days/wk for 6 wks. All subjects received conventional OT/PT based on neurodevelopmental principles 4 to 5 days/wk. | FMA Secondary Medical Research Council (MRC) motor power and Modified Ashworth Scale. FMA and MRC were significantly better at d/c in robot trained group. Gains were maintained at 3 mo follow-up. | Bilateral training and higher number of repetitions may have contributed to larger gains in robot group. | II |

Continued

Table 11-1

Post-Stroke Upper Limb Technology: Evidence Summary—cont'd

AUTHORS AND YEAR	STUDY AIM/HYPOTHESIS	DESIGN AND SUBJECTS	INTERVENTION	PRIMARY OUTCOME MEASURES AND RESULTS	COMMENTS	RATING
Housman and colleagues, 2009	To compare motor training with Therapy Wilmington Robotic Exoskeletor (T-WREX) to conventional table-top home exercise program	RCT N = 34 participants >6 mos poststroke with moderate to severe hemiparesis (FMA score ≥10 and ≤30)	All participated in 24 1-hour sessions 3×/wk for 8 to 9 wks. T-WREX group: completed 3 reps of 10 computer generated therapy games each session. Gravity support was decreased as tolerated every 3rd session. Control group received conventional self-ROM exercises, active assistive ROM, and AROM with towel exercises during table-top and prescribed ADL activities.	FMA: upper limb subtest, Rancho Functional Test for the Hemiplegic Upper Extremity, Motor Activities Log (quality and amount of use), Flock of Birds motion system to assess free reach No significant between group differences except greater 6-mo gain on FMA favored T-WREX group Satisfaction survey revealed that subjects in both groups found T-WREX less boring and more beneficial than conventional table-top exercises.	T-WREX computer generated games enabled repetitive task-specific practice. Tasks included simulated grocery shopping, cleaning a stove-top, and playing basketball. Feedback of task performance from T-WREX games enhanced motivation and awareness of progress.	II

						II
Kahn and colleagues, 2006	To compare effects of active assistive exercise delivered via ARM Guide to free reaching voluntary exercise with paretic arm	RCT N = 19 persons at least 1 year poststroke	Robot group performed active assistive range of motion (AAROM) reaching exercises with ARM Guide to targets located at limits of subject's reach. Free-reach group performed matched number of reaches to same targets as robot group. All movements were measured with Flock of Birds. Subjects in both groups were instructed to reach as fast as possible toward targets.	Chedoke-McMaster Stroke Assessment Scale Rancho Los Amigos Functional Test for Hemiparetic UE. Biomechanical assessment of limb stiffness and supported reach. Flock of Birds to measure unsupported free reach	No significant group differences. Both groups improved in ROM and velocity of supported arm movements and decreased time to complete functional tasks. Free reach group improved significantly more in movement smoothness. Gains were sustained at 6-mo follow-up.	Significant gains in both groups suggest that repetitive task-specific practice was key to improved motor recovery. ARM Guide therapy did not provide detectable benefit beyond that achieved with unassisted practice. Authors question whether type of assist provided by ARM Guide was optimal. Unclear whether individuals not involved in clinical research would perform high number of unassisted movements during independent home program.

Continued

Table 11-1

Post-Stroke Upper Limb Technology: Evidence Summary—cont'd

AUTHORS AND YEAR	STUDY AIM/HYPOTHESIS	DESIGN AND SUBJECTS	INTERVENTION	PRIMARY OUTCOME MEASURES AND RESULTS	COMMENTS	RATING
Luft and colleagues, 2004	To compare effects of bilateral arm training with bilateral arm training with rhythmic auditory cveing (BATRAC) to dose-matched therapeutic exercises based on neurodevelopmental treatment (NDT) approach. Authors hypothesized that BATRAC would be associated with cortical reorganization of sensorimotor cortex.	RCT. N = 21 participants with chronic motor impairments.	Both groups received 1-hour therapy sessions 3×/wk for 6 wks. BATRAC training involved repetitive bilateral pushing/pulling motion (symmetrical and asymmetrical) in response to auditory cues. Control group received dose matched therapeutic exercises (DMTE) based on NDT principles.	FMA upper limb subtest, Wolf Motor Function Test, University of Maryland Arm Questionnaire for Stroke (UMAQS). Functional Magnetic Resonance Imaging (fMRI). No significant group differences on clinical measures. Movement of paretic arm in BATRAC group led to significant increase in contralesional hemisphere activation, but no change in ipsilesional cortex.	Changes in brain activation were found in BATRAC group, but not DMTE group. Authors also report that BATRAC group had significantly greater gains on FMA when 3 BATRAC subjects with no change in cortical activation were eliminated from analysis. However, this assertion compares patients who experienced cortical changes (BATRAC n=9) to those who did not (DMTE n = 12).	II

Study	Purpose	Design/Subjects	Intervention	Results	Conclusions	
Lum and colleagues, 2002	To compare effects of robot-assisted therapy with Mirror Image Motion Enabler (MIME) robot to conventional therapy based on NDT principles	RCT N=27 subjects with motor impairments >6 mos poststroke	All subjects received 24 1-hr therapy sessions over 2 months. Robot group practiced 12 point-to-point reaching movements focused on shoulder and elbow movements. Four modes of robot-assisted movement: PROM, AAROM, active-constrained (against robot resistance) viscous, and bimanual (robot assists paretic arm to mirror unaffected). Control group: conventional NDT approach emphasizing muscle reeducation based on sensorimotor approach to control motor output. Time was spent on UE use during graded functional asks.	FMA upper limb and sensory subtests, Barthel Index and FIM transfers, shoulder and elbow strength, free reach kinematics. Robot group had larger gains in proximal items on FMA, strength, and reach extent. At 6-mo follow-up, no significant group differences remained on FMA, but robot group had higher FIM improvements.	Although time in therapy was equal across groups, movement repetition was greater in robot group. Faster rate of motor improvement was observed in robot group, which may be important clinical benefit if replicated in other studies.	II

Continued

Table 11-1

Post-Stroke Upper Limb Technology: Evidence Summary—cont'd

AUTHORS AND YEAR	STUDY AIM/HYPOTHESIS	DESIGN AND SUBJECTS	INTERVENTION	PRIMARY OUTCOME MEASURES AND RESULTS	COMMENTS	RATING
Lum and colleagues, 2006	To confirm results of clinical trial with chronically impaired subjects to those in subacute stage of motor recovery and to identify essential therapeutic features of MIME therapy. Authors hypothesized that bilateral mode would produce greater gains than unilateral mode.	RCT N = 30 Subacute stroke (1 to 5 mos. post onset):	All subjects received 15 1-hour sessions over 4 wks. 4 Exp Groups: Robot Unilateral Robot Bilateral Robot Combined (unilateral and bilateral) Conventional Therapy (NDT)	Measures: FMA, Motor Status Score, Motor Power, FIM At discharge: Robot Combined performed better than NDT control on FMA Significant gains in both unilateral and combined groups but no significant group differences on FMA, Motor Power, or FIM Smallest change in FMA, motor power, and FIM seen in bilateral only group At 6-mo follow-up, no group differences remained.	Gains on FMA were task-specific, in that proximal scores (not distal) improved with therapy Using an MCID of 10%, gains at d/c on impairment measures were clinically significant in unilateral and combined modes. Patients with moderate impairments benefitted most from robotic training.	II

Continued

| Stein and colleagues, 2004 | To examine whether progressive resistive training provides incremental benefits over active assistive robot-aided upper limb therapy after stroke | Controlled study N = 47 individual 1 to 5 years poststroke Subjects qualified for resistance training if able to reach all robot targets unassisted at baseline and 3 wk interim assessments. Qualifying subjects were randomly assigned to either the progressive resistive or active-assistive robot groups. | All subjects received therapy 3×/wk for 6 wks with InMotion2 robot. Both groups: arm was supported in wrist hand orthosis attached to robot handle. The same training tasks were used by both groups. Active-assistive training group: robot provided assist to reach targets as needed. Resistance group: reaching movements were performed against robot resistance. Amount of resistance was based on robotic measures of subject's strength. Participants in each group completed approximately 18,000 movement repetitions over course of therapy. | FMA Modified Ashworth Scale Robot measures of force generation in paretic arm. Subjects in all groups showed gains on FMA and maximal force generated. No group differences in outcome measures. Participants with better motor control at baseline showed greater gains on FMA, regardless of treatment group. | Contrary to traditional theories of motor recovery, resistance training did not exacerbate spasticity in the paretic arm. Limitation: functional use of limb during daily activities was not directly measured. | III |

Table 11-1

Post-Stroke Upper Limb Technology: Evidence Summary—cont'd

AUTHORS AND YEAR	STUDY AIM/HYPOTHESIS	DESIGN AND SUBJECTS	INTERVENTION	PRIMARY OUTCOME MEASURES AND RESULTS	COMMENTS	RATING
Takahashi and colleagues, 2008	Robotic therapy would improve motor function in patients with chronic motor deficits after stroke. A higher dose of active assist therapy mode would lead to greater behavioral gains. A movement performed by the paretic upper limb during therapy would show increased representation in the stroke affected primary sensorimotor cortex, while movement not performed would not.	Controlled trial N = 13 adults with stroke at least 3 mos prior to enrollment with resulting right upper extremity (RUE) weakness	ANA-A group: trained with robot in active nonassist mode for first 7.5 days and active assist mode in last 7.5 days of treatment AA group: used robot in active assist mode for all 15 days Each subject received 15 daily sessions over 3 wks, each ~1.5 hrs long. Practice of various open/close tasks with real or virtual objects displayed on computer monitor	Action Research Arm Test (ARAT), Box and Blocks Test, Fugl-Meyer arm motor scale fMRI and EMG Both groups showed significant gains on all measures: those in AA group improved significantly more than ANA-A group. fMRI showed increased sensorimotor cortex activation for practiced grasp/release task, but not for nonpracticed supination/pronation.	Findings indicate dose dependent benefit for active assist robotic therapy. ANA-A group showed some significant gains on primary measures during treatment in active nonassist mode (robot motors not active). Supports importance of challenging, repetitive task practice fMRI findings indicate task-specific cortical reorganization: impact on generalization of training needs further study	II

Continued

| Taub and colleagues, 2005 | To test the effectiveness of the AutoCITE device that automates CIMT when only partially supervised by therapists. Participants in 3 groups received supervision from a therapist 100%, 50%, or 25% of training time. | Controlled trial. N = 27 persons with chronic motor impairments after stroke (>1 year postonset) Subjects were assigned to 1 of 3 groups in alternating blocks. All subjects had minimum of 20-degree wrist extension and 10-degree finger extension in paretic hand with impaired functional use for ADL Subjects who received 100% supervision were treated during prior study (see Lum and colleagues, 2004). | All subjects wore padded safety mitt on less affected hand 90% of waking hours over 2-wk period. Subjects received training with AutoCITE 3 hrs/day on each weekday. Subjects in reduced supervision groups received therapist guided shaping, encouragement, or feedback to supplement computer monitor for either 25% or 50% of treatment time. | Wolf Motor Function Test; Motor Activity Log Large and significant gains on both outcome measures observed for all 3 groups with no between group differences. Gains on MAL at 1 mo and long-term follow-up were also significant (p <0.001) | Amount of therapist supervision did not affect outcomes: partial supervision with AutoCITE was as effective as nonautomated, therapist delivered intervention. This technology has potential to increase therapist efficiency by allowing partially supervised treatment of more than one patient simultaneously. No control group receiving only mitt constraint on less affected hand | III |

Table 11-1

Post-Stroke Upper Limb Technology: Evidence Summary—cont'd

AUTHORS AND YEAR	STUDY AIM/HYPOTHESIS	DESIGN AND SUBJECTS	INTERVENTION	PRIMARY OUTCOME MEASURES AND RESULTS	COMMENTS	RATING
Volpe and colleagues, 2000	Examined whether additional sensorimotor training with robotic device enhanced upper limb motor outcome	RCT N = 56 persons admitted to inpatient rehabilitation on average 2 wks poststroke (subacute)	All subjects received standard OT and PT. Robot group: 1 hr/day, 5 days/wk for minimum of 25 sessions. InMotion2 robot provided repetitive active-assistive exercises focused on shoulder and elbow reaching movements. Control group: Exposure to robot 1×/week. Half of trials were performed with unimpaired arm. Robot motors were not active: patient used unimpaired arm to assist when paretic limb could not complete task.	FMA Motor Status Score Motor Power FIM As a whole, subjects in both groups showed significant gains on all measures, except FMA for wrist and hand. Robot trained group had significantly greater gains in shoulder and elbow items on the Motor Status Score and in Motor Power, and significantly greater gains on FIM.	Task-specific effects of training were observed without generalization to wrist and hand (untrained in robot therapy). Duration of inpatient rehabilitation was longer than current practice.	II

Study	Purpose	Design	Intervention	Outcomes/Results	Level
Volpe and colleagues, 2008	To compare effects of a standardized therapist-delivered intensive physical therapy program with robotic-driven protocol	RCT N= 21 participants with upper limb motor impairments 6 or more mos poststroke	Matched session duration, number and timing of treatments: 1 hr sessions, 3×/wk for 6 wks Therapist-delivered treatment included static stretching, active assisted exercise, goal directed planar reaching tasks based on Carr and Shepherd principles; incorporating NDT techniques. Robot group: Adaptive active-assistive treatment using InMotion2 robot. Treatment involved repetitive planar reaching tasks focusing on shoulder and elbow control.	FMA (separated into proximal and distal subtests), Motor Power of shoulder and elbow, Modified Ashworth Scale. Disability scales included Stroke Impact Scale, Action Research Arm Test (ARAT). No significant group differences: statistically significant changes observed in both groups on FMA for shoulder and elbow and Motor Power that was sustained at 3 mo follow-up. No change in distal FMA scores for wrist and hand. No significant improvements on disability measures or group differences on Modified Ashworth Scale.	Intensity of therapist-delivered in this study was greater than traditional outpatient therapy.	II

CIMT, Constraint-induced movement therapy; *DMTE*, dose-matched therapeutic exercise; *MCID*, minimum clinically important difference; *RCT*, randomized controlled trial.

group. Although prior investigations have supported the use of compensatory strategies for persons with severe motor impairments after stroke,[4] gains observed across robotic therapy studies indicate a potential for improvement in persons with moderate to severe motor impairments.

A report of two pilot studies with the MIT-MANUS compared robot-assisted therapy (as described previously) to "functionally-based" robotic therapy in persons with moderate to severe motor impairments. This functionally-based therapy trained both reach and grasp/release during virtual or object present tasks. Although greater gains were reported for the robot-assisted therapy group, participants who received "functionally-based" therapy improved more on wrist and hand items of the Fugl-Meyer Assessment.[24] Study limitations include fewer movement repetitions and the treatment context during "functionally-based" robotic therapy (i.e., training occurred within the confines of the robot's workspace). The authors proposed that persons with moderate to severe motor impairments after stroke may benefit more from robotic therapy focused on motor functions vs. activity-based skills training. Future studies on the relationship between stroke severity, focus of robot-assisted therapy (e.g., ICF impairment vs. activity level), and functional outcomes will both inform clinical practice patterns and guide insurance resource allocation for therapy practice.

Finally, a comparison of proximal robot-assisted therapy with the MIT-MANUS to distal training via a three degree of freedom (DOF) forearm and wrist robot showed that distal robot assisted therapy led to a greater transfer of skill to proximal limb segments than vice-versa.[25] This small study implies that the sequence of treatment tasks may also be important, a finding that challenges conventional theories that support proximal to distal training after stroke.

Mirror Image Motion Enabler

The MIME is an industrial PUMA robot reconfigured for rehabilitation that provides passive, active-assistive, active-resisted, and bimanual training of the upper limb. Its controller is not as compliant to a patient's weak attempts to move as the MIT-MANUS described previously, so the MIME is not as sensitive for recording changes in motor performance over the course of treatment. During MIME therapy, the patient sits at the robot workstation, and his or her forearm and hand are supported in a splint attached to the robot manipulator (Fig. 11-2). The training exercises include a core set of 12 targeted reaching motions that emphasize shoulder and elbow movements in three-dimensional space.

In two influential studies, Lum and colleagues[29,30] compared the effects of MIME upper limb robotic therapy to conventional treatment based on Bobath's neuro-developmental approach. Persons in both chronic and subacute stages of motor recovery after stroke were examined (see Table 11-1). Lum found that subjects who received robotic therapy had statistically greater gains on

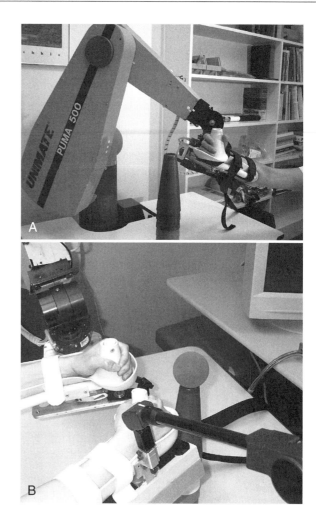

Figure 11-2   The Mirror Image Motion Enabler (MIME) robot can be used for unilateral or bilateral movement therapy. (From Kahn LE, Lum PS, Rymer WZ, et al: Robot-assisted movement training for the stroke-imparied arm: does it matter what the robot does? *J Rehabil Res Dev* 43(5) 631–642, Aug/Sept 2006.)

shoulder and elbow items of the FMA during the two month treatment period. However, no between-group differences were found in FMA scores for the unexercised wrist and hand during this time. In both studies, gains in the robot and conventional therapy groups were equivalent at the six month follow-up. The authors proposed that conventional therapy led to greater carryover of home exercise programs, which resulted in continued gains in this group after the intervention trial.

In those who received robot assisted therapy, the type of robot intervention produced different motor outcomes. Subacute patients who received bilateral training did not improve as much as those who had unilateral or combined unilateral and bilateral training. Persons who received this combined robot training in the subacute and chronic studies showed an accelerated rate of motor recovery on clinical scales. The increased effort required during the combined treatment likely contributed to these gains.

Although further research is needed to verify this effect, the accelerated motor recovery is an important consideration during clinical practice.

ARM Guide

The Assisted Rehabilitation and Measurement (ARM) Guide is a robotic device that applies and measures assistive or resistive forces while the user performs reaching movements along a linear track.[39] The patient's paretic arm is supported in a forearm trough that is attached to the track and actuated or controlled by the robot motors. The patient is asked to initiate reaching movements with the paretic arm, and the robot motors provide assistance when the person is unable to move along the desired trajectory. The device is statically counterbalanced, so it reduces gravitational forces on the arm during movement attempts, and a small margin of error is allowed before the robot provides assistance. The track can be oriented at various angles to allow reaching into different regions of the workspace. Targets are located at the limit of the patient's reach with elbow extended and shoulder flexed as much as possible without pain.[22]

Kahn and colleagues compared active assistive reaching exercises with the ARM Guide to free, unsupported reach to the same target locations.[22] The research aimed to compare the effects of robot-assisted movement therapy with the ARM Guide to free reaching voluntary exercises in persons with chronic upper limb paresis after stroke (see Table 11-1). The frequency, dose, and duration of practice were identical across treatment groups. Participants in both groups showed similar gains in range of motion (ROM) and speed of supported reaching and in the time needed to complete functional tasks on the Rancho Los Amigos Functional Test of Upper Extremity Function. This indicated that repetitive movement training, regardless of how it was administered, was a key stimulus for the observed motor recovery. The only significant group difference in this experiment was that greater improvement in the smoothness of unsupported reaching movements occurred in free reaching group. One possible explanation is that the unsupported reaching exercise involved a greater degree of error correction as subjects practiced moving toward targets, supporting motor learning principles that emphasize the importance of error detection and recognition.

The authors proposed that the type of assistance provided by the ARM Guide may not have been optimal and have since begun testing a novel guided-force training program. When this training program detects misdirected forces during reach (e.g., from a strong flexor synergy), it stops the movement, provides visual feedback of the misdirection, and guides the person to activate muscle groups in appropriate combinations to reach the desired target.[21] This guided-force training is also capable of adapting the amount of assistance or resistance offered, based on the person's performance. Testing is underway to compare motor outcomes of subjects who participate in free reaching tasks vs. guided-force training with the ARM Guide. As rehabilitation technologies continue to develop, scientists expect to learn much more about the types of training that best meet an individual's needs for motor recovery.

When thinking about clinical use of robotic devices, it is important to consider the degree to which successful practice of arm exercises influences adherence to exercise programs and contributes to gains in functional use. A home exercise program in which the patient is asked to repeatedly reach toward challenging target locations is likely to be met with frustration and limited engagement. Rehabilitation technologies can offer exercise programs that motivate, offer a relatively high degree of success and reinforcement, and give feedback concerning gains in motor performance.

Haptic Master

The Haptic Master is a three DOF robot that provides gravity assistance for the paretic arm while the user sits at a workstation. A free moving elbow splint attached to an overhead frame supports the arm, and a passive mechanism supports the hand and allows for supination and pronation and wrist flexion and extension. All exercises occur in a virtual environment while force and position sensors enable interaction with virtual tasks such as reaching to a supermarket shelf or pouring a drink. The Haptic Master has been used for task-oriented training in a three dimensional virtual environment as in the GENTLE/S project[3,10] or with real object manipulation as done with the Activity of Daily Living Exercise Robot (ADLER).[20] Depending on the user's movement abilities, three different therapy modes can be selected: passive, active assisted, or active. In addition to visual feedback, haptic feedback from the robot provides the user with the feeling of increased resistance when movements stray from the programmed trajectory.

Two clinical trials with the Haptic Master have shown modest reductions in upper limb impairment on the FMA following 30 minutes of therapy three times a week.[10,42] The authors attributed greater gains following robotic therapy to the repetitive practice of task-oriented movements with performance feedback from the Haptic Master (see Coote and colleagues[10] and Table 11-1). Their assertion that cortical reorganization and movement kinematics are optimized when persons are engaged in challenging and meaningful tasks is supported by prior research and is an important consideration when using rehabilitation technologies during clinical practice. The use of individualized task-oriented training in natural environments, as emphasized in occupational therapy practice, is gaining greater attention in the rehabilitation technology literature.[48]

REO

The Reo Therapy System (Motorika Ltd., Israel) is a widely marketed upper limb robot with little supporting research evidence published in peer reviewed journals. During Reo therapy the user performs computer generated games with the paretic hand attached to the robot arm. The robot provides upper limb assistance and feedback while the user performs reaching movements from a seated position at the work station. Patients have reported satisfaction with the Reo therapy program[49] when combined with conventional inpatient therapies. A pilot study with 10 outpatient participants reported gains in Fugl-Meyer scores between 2 to 11 points following two to three one-hour sessions a week, with decreased perceived exertion and reductions in shoulder pain and upper limb spasticity as measured by the Modified Ashworth Score.[35] Time poststroke and initial level of severity were not reported. Although additional studies are needed, initial work indicates that the Reo is well tolerated and may contribute to positive motor outcomes poststroke.

ARMin

The ARMin is an exoskeletal, low impedance robot designed for repetitive, task-oriented upper limb therapy after stroke. The interactive assistance it provides is based on "patient-cooperative" control strategies that allow patient-driven movements while the robot gives support only as needed (vs. preprogrammed levels of assistance). This form of control is expected to increase the intensity of practice while gamelike training scenarios enhance patient motivation to engage in repetitive training. Haptic, visual, and auditory feedbacks are provided during patient use.

The increased DOFs afforded by the ARMin and other exoskeletal devices (e.g., the T-WREX and Armeo discussed later) more closely mimic task-oriented therapy provided by rehabilitation clinicians.[34] Although passive nonmotorized devices (e.g., T-WREX, Armeo) support the arm against gravity and are intrinsically safer and less expensive, they cannot assist movements that the patient is unable to perform (e.g., elbow extension). However, the exoskeletal ARMin can apply and control torques at each joint individually when assistance is needed due to increased muscle tone or poor isolated movement.[34]

Clinical testing of the ARMin robot with patients after stroke has been reported for three individuals with moderate to severe motor impairments.[33] This pilot study by Nef and colleagues found that ARMin exoskeletal therapy led to modest but significant gains in motor function as evident on the FMA, with no change on the Barthel Index or Action Research Arm Test. Nef and colleagues[33] proposed that the threes DOFs allowed by the ARMin I device may have limited task-oriented training and functional outcomes. A newer model, the ARMin III (Fig. 11-3), allows six to seven DOFs during upper limb training and

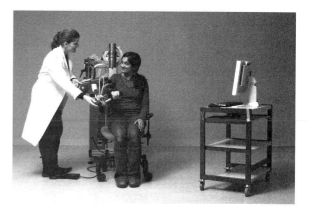

Figure 11-3 ARMin III exoskeletal robot with a healthy test subject. (Courtesy of the National Rehabilitation Hospital.)

is presently undergoing clinical investigations. Although the evidence is pending, this robot holds promise for providing high quality, task-oriented stroke rehabilitation in the future.

T-WREX and ARMeo

The T-WREX is a passive, body powered orthosis for the upper limb that was based on an earlier device developed for persons with muscular dystrophy.[37] It was adapted for individuals with stroke-induced motor impairments to allow a lower cost, safe option for semiautonomous upper limb training. Easily adjusted elastic bands provide a safe method of passively supporting the limb to allow greater active ROM and reach. The T-WREX enables naturalistic movement across two thirds or more of a normal workspace while the user engages in task-oriented virtual games, such as moving apples from a produce shelf to a shopping cart. Electronic sensors detect arm movement and hand grasp, allow the user to interact with the therapeutic games, and provide quantitative feedback about reach and grasp performance. A modified version of the T-WREX, the Armeo (Hocoma A.G., Switzerland) is commercially available for clinic use (Fig. 11-4).

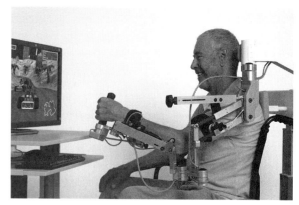

Figure 11-4 Armeo body powered orthosis with virtual training task. (Courtesy Hocoma AG, Switzerland.)

Housman and colleagues[17] reported results of a randomized control trial in which conventional table-top exercises were compared to T-WREX training in persons with chronic, moderate to severe upper limb paresis (see Table 11-1). In this study, the amount of weight support provided by the T-WREX orthosis was rarely decreased to less than 50% of the weight of the arm. Despite the high degree of gravity assist during training, effects did generalize to upper limb movements in nonweight-supported conditions, as seen by significant improvements in the FMA and Motor Activity Log scores. The amount of change measured on the FMA was comparable to that seen in studies of active devices, including the MIT-MANUS and MIME robots. This further suggests that highly repetitive movement therapy is a key stimulus to neuromotor recovery after stroke.[17]

The study also found that subjects could perform T-WREX exercises with only brief direct supervision from a therapist (four minutes for each hour of therapy),[17] so the T-WREX has good potential for cost effective, semiautonomous practice of upper limb motor tasks within clinical and home settings. Participants in both treatment groups found the novel T-WREX intervention more enjoyable and motivating than conventional table-top exercises typically prescribed as a home program after stroke.

HAND ROBOTS

Development of robots to assist with wrist and hand retraining has lagged behind that of shoulder and elbow devices, largely due to the complexity of control needed to assist with grasp and release. Two robots that have been empirically tested are the Hand Mentor (Kinetic Muscles Inc., Tempe, AZ) and the Hand Wrist Assistive Rehabilitation Device (HOWARD) developed at the University of California, Irvine.

The Hand Mentor is a repetitive motion device designed for home and clinical use (Fig. 11-5). It uses a pneumatic artificial muscle to extend the wrist and fingers and provides electromyographic (EMG) biofeedback of muscle activation via light emitting diodes displayed on a small screen. Its purpose is to inhibit flexor tone of the wrist and fingers, provide neuromuscular reeducation, and increase ROM and strength of the paretic wrist and fingers.

In two single case studies, Hand Mentor training was combined with repetitive task practice to improve upper limb function in persons seven and 11 months poststroke.[14,41] Intervention occurred four hours per day, either three or five days a week, over a three-week period. During two hours of each session, Hand Mentor training included use of EMG biofeedback to reduce abnormal muscle tone in the wrist and fingers, and two active motor control modes to elicit wrist flexion and extension. If the

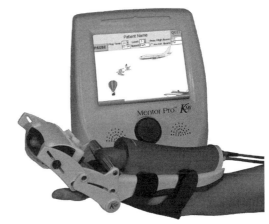

Figure 11-5 Hand Mentor device combines pneumatic "muscle" activation with electromyography to provide active assistive therapy for wrist and fingers. (Courtesy of Kinetic Muscles, Inc.)

user could not reach the target position during the active training mode, the pneumatic muscle inflated to assist wrist movements. Study participants spent up to two additional hours doing repetitive task practice of functionally oriented tasks with the paretic arm. The level of difficulty increased gradually, and participants selected activities for training. Gains reported at the end of intervention included faster speed of performance on some Wolf Motor Function Test items; increased active ROM in the shoulder, wrist, and thumb; better isolation of upper limb motions; and a slight decrease in maximum grip force.[14,41] Despite limited evidence of efficacy, the Hand Mentor has been used more frequently in rehabilitation clinics in recent years. Certainly, empirical studies are needed to more closely examine the potential uses and benefits of this technology.

The Hand Wrist Assistive Rehabilitation Device ("HOWARD") is another pneumatically actuated robot that assists with repetitive grasp and release movements.[46] While seated at a computer monitor, the subject's paretic hand is secured to the robotic device, and the forearm is supported in a padded splint. HOWARD controls flexion/extension of the four fingers about the metacarpophalangeal (MCP) joint; flexion/extension of the thumb at the MCP joint; and flexion/extension of the wrist (Fig. 11-6). Joint angle sensors allow for real time control of virtual hand movements displayed on the monitor, and the back-driveable control allows the patient to move freely when the robot is not engaged in active assistance. The palmar surface of the hand is left unobstructed to allow for grasping practice of both virtual and real objects. Takahashi and colleagues demonstrated HOWARD's effectiveness in promoting motor recovery and cortical reorganization in persons with chronic motor impairments after stroke[46] (see Table 11-1). HOWARD's unique capability to combine

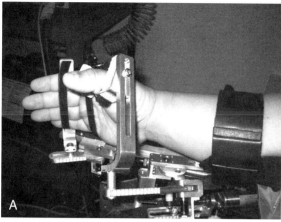

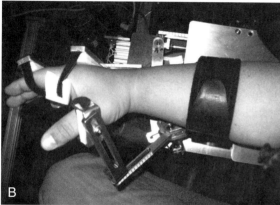

Figure 11-6 Hand Wrist Assistive Rehabilitation Device (HOWARD) can be used with virtual and actual training tasks. (Courtesy of Steven C. Cramer, MD.)

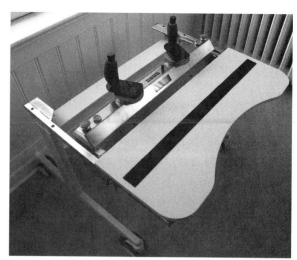

Figure 11-7 Bi-Manu-Track bilateral arm training device. (Courtesy of Dr. Stefan Hesse.)

repetitive robot-assisted training with the rich sensory experience of grasping and holding real objects represents another step toward more closely aligning robotic technology with current rehabilitation theories that emphasize task-oriented training.

BILATERAL ARM TRAINING

A number of studies have examined the effects of repetitive bilateral training on upper limb motor recovery. This research has shown that bimanual practice can have a facilitating effect on the paretic arm after stroke, with movement of the nonaffected upper limb stimulating ipsilateral corticospinal projections to the paretic arm. Two rehabilitation devices, the BI-MANU-TRACK and Bilateral Arm Training with Rhythmic Auditory Cuing (BATRAC) trainers, have undergone a fair amount of study.

The BI-MANU-TRACK is a one DOF computer-assisted arm trainer that allows bimanual practice of supination and pronation and wrist flexion and extension (Fig. 11-7).[15] Exercises can be performed passively or actively, and isometric resistance can be added at the start of active exercise, based patient's ability level and needs. When compared to a control group that received electrical stimulation, Hesse and colleagues[16] found that subjects who performed BI-MANU-TRACK training four to eight weeks poststroke had significant improvements on the FMA and in muscle power scores for the paretic arm (see Table 11-1). However, persons in the bilateral training group engaged in 10 times more movement repetitions than did those who received electrical stimulation. Follow-up research needs to examine whether the significant group differences were due to the greater number of movement repetitions or to the bilateral nature of the training. A similar BI-MANU-TRACK protocol for persons with chronic motor impairments[15] revealed less change in motor performance of the paretic arm than was seen in the subacute group. This suggests that the timing of intervention is important for this form of therapy.

The Bilateral Arm Training with Rhythmic Auditory Cuing (BATRAC) trainer is another device used for repetitive bilateral upper limb therapy. BATRAC therapy involves moving two unyoked handles forward and backward in a reaching motion, both symmetrically and asymmetrically in response to auditory cues set at individually determined rates. A single group pilot study by Whitall and colleagues[52] showed gains in Fugl-Meyer scores, speed of arm movements, and use of the paretic arm for supportive roles during bilateral tasks after 18 sessions of therapy over a six-week period. These improvements were largely sustained eight weeks posttraining. However, when Luft and colleagues[28] compared subjects who received NDT-based exercises to those treated by BATRAC, they found no significant group differences on clinical measures but did see changes in brain activation in the BATRAC group (see Table 11-1).

Other BATRAC research by Richards and colleagues[40] examined effects of a condensed BATRAC protocol, in which treatment was delivered to persons with mild chronic impairments during two-hour and 15-minute sessions, four times a week for two weeks. The condensed protocol led to small gains on the Motor Activity Log but no change in motor impairment or speed, as measured by the FMA and Wolf Motor Function Test. It appears that persons with severe motor impairments may benefit more from BATRAC training than those with milder impairments, and that the distribution of training sessions is an important consideration when using this device. Other studies also have reported smaller gains in motor recovery when patients engaged in a compressed treatment schedule.[13] This is an important consideration for clinicians faced with limited insurance coverage for patients following stroke. Evidence concerning optimal timing and distribution of treatment is sorely needed.

Although this bilateral training research may contribute to the knowledge of neuromotor recovery mechanisms poststroke, clinically relevant limitations of these devices include the lack of patient feedback and focus on impairment (not activity level) changes in performance. The effect of this bilateral training on functional use of the paretic arm and real life outcomes is unknown. McCombe Waller and colleagues[32] recommended that specific bilateral training exercises be matched to the patient's baseline characteristics, and that the contribution of supportive role functions by the paretic arm be further examined during unilateral and bilateral tasks. Research studies that include bilateral task analysis and assessment of interlimb coordination could play an important role in clarifying ways in which motor function of the paretic arm changes during the course of intervention.[32]

FUNCTIONAL ELECTRICAL STIMULATION

Functional electrical stimulation (FES) is another technological advancement designed to facilitate motor recovery after neurological insult. A number of studies have been published on neuromuscular electrical stimulation (NMES) and FES. FES is actually a subcategory of NMES and refers to the use of NMES to substitute for an orthosis while assisting with a functional activity, such as holding a glass to drink.[5] See Chapter 10.

MYOMO

The Myomo e100 NeuroRobotic system (Myomo, Inc., Boston, MA) is a wearable device that assists with elbow flexion and extension of the paretic arm. It uses a novel surface EMG control mechanism to detect and amplify signals generated by a stroke survivor's muscles. The Myomo device includes a surface electrode that is placed over the biceps or triceps muscle and a motorized elbow brace that is powered by rechargeable batteries in a portable control pack. The treating therapist selects the appropriate location for the sensing electrode and sets a virtual spring that counterbalances the powered assistance of the device, which allows the device to assist with the desired movement (e.g., elbow flexion) and aids return to the starting position when the EMG stimulus subsides and the person relaxes. The Myomo device controls the amount of force generated based on the amplitude of the EMG signal, which results in movement assistance that is proportional to the patient's effort.[43]

The Myomo e100 is a portable, exoskeletal device that can be used in different settings, unlike robotic devices limited to a fixed work station. It allows for the training of basic functional tasks, such as pushing up from an arm chair or reaching for a light switch. However, it only assists elbow motions and does not directly address impaired supination/pronation or distal function. At this time, its weight makes it inappropriate for use by persons with glenohumeral subluxation and weak shoulder control. Data from a small pilot study for patients with severe chronic upper limb paresis after stroke showed modest, but statistically significant gains in upper limb scores on the FMA.[45]

HANDMASTER

The Handmaster, marketed as the NESS H200 Hand Rehabilitation System (Bioness, Valencia, CA) is a noninvasive, advanced neuroprosthesis used for the treatment of upper limb paresis following stroke, traumatic brain injury, or C5-C6 spinal cord injury. It contains a custom-fit orthosis that uses functional electrical stimulation (FES) to provide neuromuscular reeducation, to sequentially activate muscle groups in the forearm, and to elicit active grasp and release in the paretic hand.

Research studies indicate that FES has the potential to benefit persons with subacute and chronic upper limb paresis after stroke. An evidence-based review by Chan[8] revealed that patients who performed FES in conjunction with active practice of functional tasks outperformed those involved with task-oriented training alone or sham stimulation. This outcome was reinforced by Alon and colleagues[2] in a study of the NESS H200 during subacute inpatient rehabilitation (see Table 11-1). Chan's review[8] also discovered that treatment protocols varied across studies, but the stimulation parameters did not appear crucial in determining motor outcomes. This is likely related to variations in residual motor abilities, degree of spasticity, and the duration and frequency of treatment across study samples. Cauraugh and Kim[7] proposed that FES works to improve voluntary initiation of movements in the impaired limb by decreasing the processing time needed for stimulus identification and response initiation. FES with the NESS H200 was suitable for persons with mild to moderate upper limb dysfunction after stroke, and was reported to be well tolerated by those engaged in home programs. As with all present rehabilitation technologies, the high cost of the NESS H200 may present a barrier to its widespread use after stroke.

OTHER DEVICES FOR REPETITIVE TASK PRACTICE

SAEBO

The SaeboFlex is a high-tech, dynamic orthosis developed to address the difficulty that many stroke survivors have in opening their paretic hand after stroke. This orthosis consists of a forearm cuff attached to a dorsal hand platform that anchors two spring attachments. Individual finger sleeves are placed over the distal phalanges and then are attached to the spring attachments via a high tensile line to provide assistance with finger and thumb extension (Fig. 11-8). A small phase 1 trial tested the feasibility of using this orthosis in 13 individuals with chronic upper limb motor impairments.[11] The training protocol, based on systems theory and motor learning principles, emphasized repetitive practice, active problem solving and use of the hand to promote motor recovery of the upper limb. Other interventions provided during the SaeboFlex training period included strengthening exercises, ROM, and electrical stimulation to wrist and finger extensors. Significant gains in upper limb measures were found after five days of intensive treatment. Although further research on its efficacy is indicated, this trial

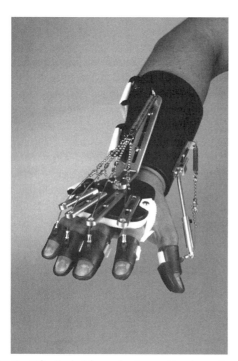

Figure 11-8   The SaeboFlex orthosis provides dynamic assistance during gross grasp and release activities. (Courtesy of Saebo, Inc.)

suggests that the SaeboFlex orthosis has good potential to provide low-cost, repetitive motor training to persons with moderate motor impairments after stroke.

AUTOCITE

The AutoCITE was developed to automate CIMT for individuals with mild to moderate motor impairments after stroke.[31] It is comprised of a computer, chair, and eight task devices arranged on four work surfaces in a modified cabinet. The training tasks are derived from those used in therapist-mediated CIMT and include reaching, tracing, peg board use, supination/pronation, threading, arc and rings, finger tapping and object flipping (Fig. 11-9). While the user sits at the workspace, instructions are given via a computer monitor, and device sensors monitor performance. Several types of feedback and encouragement are provided, including the number of successful repetitions and time for task completion.

The AutoCITE is another technological device designed to provide semiautonomous, repetitive task practice and reduce health care costs. Taub and colleagues[47] reported that patients with chronic mild to moderate upper limb paresis who trained with the AutoCITE had significant gains in motor ability and real world use, as indicated by improved scores on the Wolf Motor Function Test and Motor Activity Log. The authors found no significant difference in treatment outcome among subjects who received therapist supervision for 25%, 50%, or 100% of the AutoCITE treatment time (see Table 11-1). Taub and colleagues concluded that AutoCITE training with limited therapist supervision was as effective as one-on-one CIMT.

In addition to three hours of AutoCITE training five days a week, all participants were asked to wear a padded safety mitt on their less-affected hand for 90% of waking hours during the two-week trial period. This study did not include a control group that received only the mitt constraint. It is possible that these participants improved merely because of increased hand use during waking hours vs. the time spent on AutoCITE training (supervised or unsupervised). Future research may well address this question.

CLINICAL USE OF REHABILITATION TECHNOLOGIES

The rehabilitation technologies discussed previously offer a wide range of treatment options for persons with upper limb paresis after stroke. Choosing the "right" technology for a particular patient during clinical practice involves an appreciation for key features of the device, the patient's level of function, and therapeutic goals.

Key Features to Consider

Key considerations when choosing technologies for patient treatment after stroke include the type of assistance and DOFs afforded by the device, whether it is portable

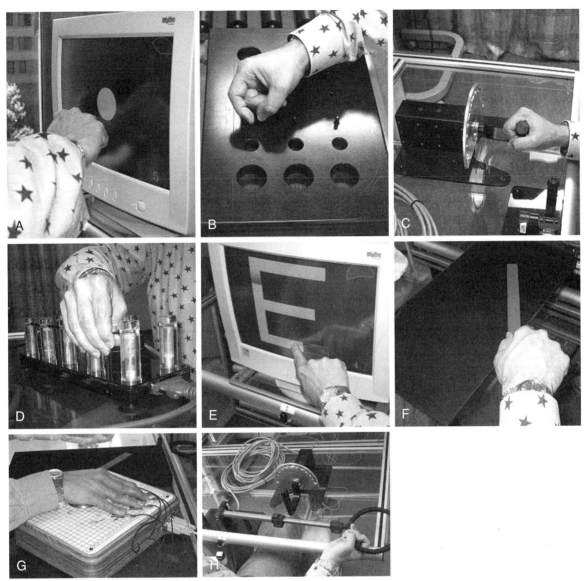

Figure 11-9 AutoCITE activities for persons with mild to moderate impairments after stroke. (From Taub E, Lum PS, Hardin P, et al: Automated delivery of CI therapy with reduced effort by therapists. *Stroke* 36(9):1301-1304, 2005.)

or stationary (e.g., requires treatment space for a workstation), and the amount of training needed to safely and effectively administer movement therapy. The device should be easily programmed to meet the patient's needs as motor recovery occurs and allow for semiautonomous training, which can enhance therapist productivity while the patient engages in CIMT. Many robotic devices provide quantitative measures of motor functions such as movement speed, accuracy, and forces generated. These objective measures can complement activity and participation level evaluation findings, and can be used when documenting treatment plans and progress toward goals. Ease and time for treatment set-up are other important considerations when selecting these tools for the clinic.

The present rehabilitation devices are most appropriately used as an adjunct to therapist-rendered intervention. Technologies are best at providing intensive practice while the therapist emphasizes use of the paretic arm during valued everyday tasks. Because individual devices are not currently able to assist with of all DOFs needed for task-oriented training, some researchers have advocated for the use of robotic "gyms"[23] or an "integrated suite of low cost robotic and computer assistive technologies."[19] The therapist's expertise in upper limb function and task analysis is essential when selecting rehabilitation technologies and establishing treatment plans that effectively combine technology-driven and therapist-rendered interventions.

Certainly the organization's rehabilitation agenda, patient caseload, and cost strongly influence decisions to purchase rehabilitation technologies for clinical use. In addition, barriers to therapist and physician acceptance deserve attention: specific concerns include treatment efficacy, equipment expense, and lack of time to evaluate technology options for stroke rehabilitation.[6] In terms of efficacy, research studies have begun to show that rehabilitation technologies can offer benefits not easily achieved by additional conventional therapy. For example, patients who had robot-assisted therapy early after stroke showed an accelerated rate of motor recovery when compared to a control group that received conventional therapy.[29] Although this study showed no group differences after six months, it is likely that accelerated motor recovery during inpatient rehabilitation could contribute to improved functional use of the upper limb and positively impact self-care performance and patient satisfaction at hospital discharge.

Level of Function and Therapeutic Goals

Many factors influence a patient's ability to benefit from rehabilitation of the paretic arm after stroke. Critical factors include the level of neurological damage and resulting motor impairment, and the individual's ability to engage successfully in therapeutic activities aimed at improving motor function. Rehabilitation technologies can be easily programmed to ensure a certain level of success for patients with a wide range motor abilities. This feature can enhance patient motivation and independent carryover of exercise programs. Although researchers are working to identify "active ingredients" needed for the learning and acquisition of motor functions after stroke, the "best" rehabilitation and technology choice for a given level of motor function is not well-established. It is not safe to assume that one treatment approach, or one form of rehabilitation technology, is optimal for all patients with hemiparesis.

Clinical practice illustrates the need for different techniques and treatment strategies for patients with minimal vs. moderate to severe levels of motor impairment. Unfortunately, therapist-rendered interventions are difficult to quantify or reproduce across treatment sessions. Rehabilitation robots are able to objectively measure the amount and type of assistance provided during therapy, and to track changes in motor functions that occur during the course of treatment. Clinicians can use these measures to judge the effectiveness of treatment, and to learn more about how changes in motor functions might translate to activity level performance.

Although many advocate for rehabilitation technologies able to deliver task-oriented training across multiple DOFs,[48] it is not known whether this approach would be as effective for persons with mild or with moderate to severe motor impairments after stroke. Krebs and colleagues[23] proposed that modular robotic systems may be particularly well-suited for addressing this question. Modular systems can deliver training to individual limb segments or can combine robot components to allow practice of tasks that involve greater DOFs. However, current modular systems are limited in their ability to provide true "task-oriented" training because they do not allow the practice of contextually-rich virtual or actual tasks. While these modular tools may be key to identifying what form of movement therapy is best for which patient, clinicians should use a combination of empirical evidence, clinical experience, and practice theory when deciding which technology features are best suited for their rehabilitation patients.

When selecting rehabilitation technologies, the therapist also should assure that the feedback provided by the device is clear, easily interpreted by the patient and clinician, and pertinent to the patient's goals for improved motor function. The therapeutic device should offer a variety of metrics relevant to functional task performance. Colombo[9] asserted that patients with greater motor impairments could benefit more from feedback regarding the efficacy of movement attempts. Conversely, patients with higher level motor functioning could expect to benefit more from feedback concerning movement accuracy or force control.[9] A patient's therapeutic goals may be better addressed when the clinician has a clear understanding of the types of feedback and forms of intervention that best promote functional motor recovery.

As research unfolds, specific treatment protocols to more efficiently and effectively address patient needs across levels of function will help to guide the integration of technology-driven and therapist-rendered rehabilitation. Thoughtful treatment planning for technology driven rehabilitation is no different from that of conventional therapies. It just requires an understanding of the therapy options made available by these technologies.

SUMMARY

The focus of conventional therapies during recent years has shifted from analytical training methods directed at impairments in motor function to an emphasis on task-oriented training for the upper limb.[48] The development of rehabilitation technologies, although still in its infancy, is following a similar trend. Potential benefits include controllable treatment intensity, repetition, task-specific practice, and sensory-motor feedback to enhance knowledge of performance and results.

The research presented in this chapter generally supports the use of rehabilitation technologies to improve upper limb motor functions after stroke. Although systematic reviews of robot-assisted therapies have substantiated task-specific training effects at the ICF impairment level, these have not generalized to arm and hand use during activities of daily living.[26-36] As technology-aided distal training and task-oriented interventions are further developed and therapists become more experienced with integrating technology-driven and therapist-rendered interventions, the effects of the activity and participation level functions are expected to improve. Ultimately, rehabilitation technologies are anticipated to provide cost effective treatment options and to help to inform clinicians about the "active ingredients" key to effective and efficient rehabilitation for persons after stroke.

REVIEW QUESTIONS

1. Describe the difference between active and passive rehabilitation robots and provide an example of each.
2. List the hand robots reviewed in this chapter and discuss research findings. Why has the development of shoulder/elbow robots exceeded that of distal robots for the wrist and hand?
3. Which rehabilitation technology would you choose for a patient with mild motor impairments after stroke? Explain the therapy approach you would take and why.
4. The studies in Table 11-1 compared the effectiveness of rehabilitation technologies with conventional therapy methods. Discuss one or two ways that you might use this evidence to guide your therapy for persons with moderate upper limb impairments after stroke.
5. There are many factors to consider when choosing rehabilitation technologies for use in the clinic. What considerations are especially important for your setting and what device(s) would you select based on these factors?

REFERENCES

1. Aisen ML, Krebs HI, Hogan N, et al: The effect of robot assisted therapy and rehabilitative training on motor recovery following stroke. *Arch Neurol* 54(4):443–6, 1997.
2. Alon G, Levitt AF, McCarthy PA: Functional electrical stimulation enhancement of upper extremity functional recovery during stroke rehabilitation: A pilot study. *Neurorehabil Neural Repair* 21(3):207–215, 2007.
3. Amirabdollahian F, Loureiro R, Gradwell E, et al: Multivariate analysis of the Fugl-Meyer outcome measures assessing the effectiveness of GENTLE/S robot-mediated stroke therapy. *J Neuroeng Rehabil* 4(4): Published online 19 February 2007.
4. Barreca S, Wolf S, Fasoli, S, et al: Treatment interventions for the paretic upper limb of stroke survivors: a critical review. *Neurorehabil Neural Repair* 17(4): 220–226, 2003.
5. Bracciano AG: Physical Agent Modalities. In Radomski MV, Latham CAT, editors: *Occupational therapy for physical dysfunction*, ed. 6, Baltimore, 2008, Lippincott Williams & Wilkins.
6. Brewer BR, McDowell SK, Worthen-Chaudhari LC: Poststroke upper extremity rehabilitation: A review of robotic systems and clinical results. *Top Stroke Rehabil* 14(6): 22–44, 2007.
7. Cauraugh JH, Kim SB: Stroke motor recovery: Active neuromuscular stimulation and repetitive practice schedules. *J Neurol Neurosurg Psychiatry* 74(11): 1562–1566, 2003.
8. Chan CKL: A preliminary study of functional electrical stimulation in the upper limb rehabilitation after stroke: An evidence-based review. *HKJOT* 18(2): 52–58, 2008.
9. Colombo R, Pisano FM Micera S, et al: Assessing mechanisms of recovery during robot-aided neurorehabilitation of the upper limb. *Neurorehabil Neural Repair* 22(1): 50–63, 2008.
10. Coote S, Murphy B, Harwin W, et al: The effect of the GENTLE/S robot-mediated therapy system in arm function after stroke. *Clin Rehabil* 22(5): 395–405, 2008.
11. Farrell JF, Hoffman HB, Snyder JL, et al: Orthotic aided training of the paretic upper limb in chronic stroke: Results of a phase I trial. *NeuroRehabilitation* 22(2): 99–103, 2007.
12. Fasoli SE, Krebs HI, Stein J, et al: Robotic therapy for chronic motor impairments after stroke: follow-up results. *Arch Phys Med Rehabil* 85(7):1106–11, 2004.
13. Finley, MA, Fasoli, SE, Dipietro, L, et al: Short duration upper extremity robotic therapy in stroke patients with severe upper extremity motor impairment. *J Rehabil Res Dev* 42(5):683–692, 2005.
14. Frick EM, Alberts JL: Combined use of repetitive task practice and an assistive robotic device in a patient with subacute stroke. *Phys Ther* 86(10):1378–1386, 2006.
15. Hesse S, Schulte-Tigges G, Konrad M, et al: Robot-assisted arm trainer for the passive and active practice of bilateral forearm and wrist movements in hemiparetic stroke. *Arch Phys Med Rehabil* 84(6):915–920, 2003.
16. Hesse S, Werner C, Pohl M, et al: Computerized arm training improves the motor control of the severely affected arm after stroke. *Stroke* 36(9):1960–1966, 2005.
17. Housman SJ, Scott KM, Reinkensmeyer DJ: A randomized controlled trial of gravity-supported, computer-enhanced arm exercise for individuals with severe hemiparesis. *Neurorehabil Neural Repair* 23(5):505–514, 2009.
18. International classification of functioning, disability and health: ICF, Geneva, 2001, World Health Organization.
19. Johnson MJ, Feng X, Johnson LM, et al: Potential of a suite of robot/computer-assisted motivating systems for personalized, home based stroke rehabilitation. *J Neuroeng Rehabil* 4:6, 2007.
20. Johnson MJ, Wisneski KJ, Anderson J, et al: Development of ADLER: The activities of daily living exercise robot, BioRob 2006. The First IEEE/RAS-EMBS International Conference on Biomedical Robotics & Biomechatronics, IEEE NY, NY, 2006.
21. Kahn LE, Lum PS, Rymer WZ, et al: Robot-assisted movement training for the stroke-impaired arm: Does it matter what the robot does? *J Rehabil Res Dev* 43(5):619–630, 2006.
22. Kahn LE, Zygman ML, Rymer WZ, et al: Robot-assisted reaching exercise promotes arm movement recovery in chronic hemiparetic stroke: a randomized controlled pilot study. *J Neuroeng Rehabil* 3:12, 2006.
23. Krebs HI, DiPietro L, Levy-Tzedek S, et al: A paradigm shift for rehabilitation robotics. *Engineering in Medicine & Biology Magazine, IEEE* 27(4):61–70, 2008.
24. Krebs HI, Mernoff S, Fasoli, SE, et al: A Comparison of Functional and Impairment-Based Robotic Training in Severe to Moderate Chronic Stroke: A Pilot Study. *NeuroRehabilitation* 23(1):81–87, 2008.
25. Krebs HI, Volpe BT, Williams D, et al: Robot-aided neurorehabilitation: A robot for wrist rehabilitation. *IEEE Trans Neural Syst Rehabil Eng* 15(3):327–335, 2007.
26. Kwakkel G, Kollen BJ, Krebs BI: Effects of robot-assisted therapy on upper limb recovery after stroke: A systematic review, of gravity-supported, computer-enhanced arm exercise for individuals with severe hemiparesis. *Neurorehabil Neural Repair* 22(2):111–121, 2008.

27. Langhammer B, Stanghelle JK: Bobath or motor relearning programme? A comparison of two different approaches of physiotherapy in stroke rehabilitation: a randomized controlled study. *Clin Rehabil* 12 (4):361–369, 2000.

28. Luft AR, McCombe-Waller S, Whitall J, et al: Repetitive bilateral arm training and motor cortex activation in chronic stroke. *JAMA* 292(15):1853–1861, 2004.

29. Lum PS, Burgar CG, van der Loos M, et al: MIME robotic device for the upper-limb neurorehabilitation in subacute stroke subjects: A follow up study. *J Rehabil Res Dev* 43(5):631–642, 2006.

30. Lum PS, Burgar CG, Shor PC, et al: Robot-assisted movement training compared with conventional therapy techniques for the rehabilitation of upper-limb motor function after stroke. *Arch Phys Med Rehabil* 83(7):952–959, 2002.

31. Lum PS, Taub E, Schwandt D, et al: Automated constraint-induced therapy extension (AutoCITE) for movement deficits after stroke. *J Rehabil Res Dev* 41 (3A):249–258, 2004.

32. McCombe Waller S, Whitall J: Bilateral arm training: Why and who benefits? *NeuroRehabilitation* 23(1):29–41, 2008.

33. Nef T, Quinter G, Muller R, et al: Effects of arm training with the robotic device ARMin I in chronic stroke: Three single cases. *Neurodegener Dis* 6(5–6):240–251, 2009.

34. Nef T, Guidali M, Riener R: ARMin III – arm therapy exoskeleton with an ergonomic shoulder actuation. *Appl Bionics Biomech* 6(2):127–142, 2009.

35. Padova J, Werner L, Mahoney R: Pilot trial of a robot-assisted upper limb therapy system. *Arch Phys Med Rehabil* 88(9): E106, 2007.

36. Prange GB, Jannink MJA, Groothuis-Oudshoorn CGM, et al: Systematic review of the effect of robot-aided therapy on recovery of the hemiparetic arm after stroke. *J Rehabil Res Dev* 43(2):171–184, 2006.

37. Rahman T, Sample W, Selliktar R, et al: A body-powered functional upper limb orthosis. *J Rehabil Res Dev* 37(6):675–680, 2000.

38. Reinkensmeyer DJ, Emken JL, Cramer SC: Robotics, motor learning and neurologic recovery. *Annu Rev Biomed Eng* 6:497–525, 2004.

39. Reinkensmeyer DJ, Kahn LE, Averbuch M, et al: Understanding and treating arm movement impairment after chronic brain injury: Progress with the ARM guide. *J Rehabil Res Dev* 37(6):653–662, 2000.

40. Richards LG, Senesac CR, Davis SB, et al: Bilateral arm training with rhythmic auditory cueing in chronic stroke: Not always efficacious. *Neurorehabil Neural Repair* 22(2):180–184, 2008.

41. Rosenstein L, Ridgel AL, Thota A, et al: Effects of combined robotic therapy and repetitive task practice on upper extremity function in a patient with chronic stroke. *Am J Occup Ther* 62(1):28–35, 2008.

42. Seelen, HAM, Geers RPJ, Soede, M, et al: Training of arm-hand kinaesthetics in subacute stroke patients using robotics. *J Biomech* 40 (Supplement 2):S645, 2007.

43. Stein J : e100 NeuroRobotic system. *Expert Rev Med Devices* 6(1):15–19, 2009.

44. Stein J, Krebs HI, Frontera WR, et al: Comparison of two techniques of robot-aided upper limb exercise training after stroke. *Am J Phys Med Rehabil* 83(9):720–728, 2004.

45. Stein J, Narendran K, McBean J, et al: Electromyography controlled exoskeletal upper-limb–powered orthosis for exercise training after stroke. *Am J Phys Med Rehabil* 86(4):255–261, 2007.

46. Takahashi CD, Der-Yeghiaian L, Le V, et al: Robot-based hand motor therapy after stroke. *Brain* 131(Pt 2):425–437, 2008.

47. Taub E, Lum PS, Hardin P, et al: AutoCITE Automated delivery of CI therapy with reduced effort by therapists. *Stroke* 36(6):1301–1304, 2005.

48. Timmermans AAA, Seelen HAM, Willmann RD, et al: Technology assisted training of arm-hand skills in stroke: concepts on reacquisition of motor control and therapist guidelines for rehabilitation technology design. *J Neuroeng Rehabil* 6:1, 2009.

49. Treger I, Faran S, Ring H: Robot-assisted therapy for neuromuscular training of sub-acute stroke patients. A feasibility study. *Eur J Phys Rehabil Med* 44(4):431–435, 2008.

50. Volpe, BT, Krebs, HI, Hogan, N, et al: A novel approach to stroke rehabilitation: Robot-aided sensorimotor stimulation. *Neurology* 54(10):1938–1944, 2000.

51. Volpe BT, Lynch D, Rykman-Berland A, et al: Intensive sensorimotor arm training mediated by therapist or robot improves hemiparesis in patients with chronic stroke. *Neurorehabil Neural Repair* 22(3):305–310, 2008.

52. Whitall J, McCombe Waller S, Silver KHC: Repetitive bilateral arm training with rhythmic auditory cueing improves motor function in chronic stroke. *Stroke* 31(10):2390–2395, 2000.

sandra m. artzberger
jocelyn white

chapter 12

Edema Control

key terms

complex edema	thoracic duct	neuroprosthesis
venous and lymphatic congestion	diaphragmatic breathing	terminus
dependency theory	complex regional pain syndrome type I	

chapter objectives

After completing this chapter, the reader will be able to accomplish the following:

1. Describe the proposed three theories of types of stroke hand edema and relate them to appropriate criteria for clinical treatment technique selection.
2. Provide neurological and anatomical rationales for treatment selection.
3. Be familiar with current research outcomes of treatment techniques for stroke hand edema reduction and be able to implement and expand data for clinical application problem-solving
4. Integrate realistic edema reduction expectations into treatment planning from material read in the case studies.

Research indicates that poststroke hand edema can range from 16%[21] to 82.8%[49] depending on the definition of edema, length of time since stroke occurred, and study design and methodology. Research also reports a broad range of time during which edema may develop, often from two weeks to two months poststroke.[43] There are numerous theories regarding the development of edema. Boomkamp-Koppen and colleagues[7] found that the loss of muscle activity, hyposensibility, and hypertonia link to edema, with hypertonia being the most significant predictor of hand edema.

There is no consensus on the etiology of poststroke hand edema[38] or on the most effective management technique.[7,23] Therefore, there are few guidelines for occupational therapists to employ with their clients. It is widely acknowledged that edema, particularly in the subacute and chronic stages, affects a client's range of movement, sensation, dexterity, and function. There are also correlations between edema and joint fibrosis and, in stroke, there is increasing evidence on the relationship between edema and Chronic Regional Pain Syndrome (CRPS).[30] Occupational therapists need to maximize their input into the multidisciplinary team to prevent CRPS and to minimize these barriers to rehabilitation.[43] It is also imperative to consider the impact of stroke on movement, cognition, perception, communication, and psychological aspects of individuals. These areas form the basis for most rehabilitation poststroke, with edema and sensation often being lower priorities. However, given the limitations imposed by stroke on the above areas, one must consider how these impairments may interplay with edema management and functional outcomes, such as neglect, strength, and learned nonuse (Fig. 12-1).

This chapter will focus on exploring available research regarding the etiology and treatment of poststroke hand edema and will present it in a format to enable the therapist to apply research data to clinical problem solving.

ETIOLOGY OF STROKE HAND EDEMA

The edema that therapists treat is defined as an excess accumulation of fluid in the interstitium. It occurs on the capillary level (microcirculation level) when there is an imbalance of pressure between the arterioles, venules, and interstitium, or an obstruction of the lymphatic system.[17,50] This is also known as an imbalance in Starlings Equilibrium. It is important to note that the vascular system refers not only to the venous and arterial capillaries but also to the lymphatic capillaries. All these structures influence poststroke arm edema.

A review of the literature has resulted in two major theories of poststroke hand edema: sympathetic vasomotor dysfunction due to the stroke, and venous congestion. The concept of vasomotor dysfunction as part of the stroke autonomic disturbance theory was proposed as early as 1930.[55] This theory has been expanded on in light of more recent research,[34] though, the role of the sympathetic vasomotor dysfunction deletion of post stroke hand edema formation remains unclear.[38] The second theory proposes that poststroke hand edema results from venous congestion due to lack of, or decreased, limb motor function and dependency positioning.[38] Aspects of both of these theories will be presented in the chapter when relative to a specific treatment technique.

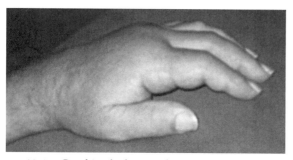

Figure 12-1   Combined edema eight weeks post cerebrovascular accident.

Anatomical Overview of the Venous and Lymphatic Systems Related to Stroke Hand Edema and its Etiology

The venous congestion and limb dependency theory is most relevant to the treatment techniques this chapter will present. Thus, it is important to take an anatomical look at the vascular system, which consists of both arterial and venous structures and the lymphatics. Both vascular structures, the venule and lymphatic capillaries, remove excess fluid from the interstitium and can be simultaneously activated in specific instances. Yet depending on the type of edema, in certain instances, each system must activate in its own unique way in order to reduce edema. Both the venous and lymphatic systems neurologically are controlled by the autonomic nervous system.[17,35] However, both systems rely on the muscle motor pump to remove tissue fluid from the interstitium.[17,35] Thus, with total or partial lack of motor function to an arm poststroke, swelling occurs.

Venous and lymphatic absorption of tissue fluid occurs on the microcirculation level. In the interstitium (interstitial spaces), the arterial and venule histologically join in an arc. The initial lymphatic (also called a lymphatic capillary or lymphatic net) is independent from the venule arterial arc, it is a "netlike" structure in the interstitium and is much larger than the venule.[17,28] On this microcirculation level, plasma proteins, fluid, electrolytes, nutrients, and a few other elements are excreted from the arteriole, because it has a pressure of 35 mm Hg.[6] These are the substances needed for surrounding cell metabolism. Ninety percent of what remain from the metabolism are small molecules that enter the venule via the process of osmosis and diffusion.[27,28] The remaining 10% of the molecules, such as plasma proteins, are too large to be absorbed by the venule and must be absorbed by the lymphatic capillaries. The artery system via arteriole filtration and diffusion excretes tissue fluid into the interstitium.[28] From the interstitium there are two structures, venules and lymphatic capillaries, that join with larger veins and lymphatic structures to bring fluid back to the heart (Fig. 12-2).[17]

The absorption process by the venule and lymphatic capillaries differ from each other. The wall of a venule is thin and absorbs small molecules via osmosis and diffusion.[17] Thus, elevation, light retrograde massage, muscle contraction, and compression will facilitate this absorption.

Lymphatic molecule absorption in the interstitium begins in the one cell initial lymphatic capillary that, most superficially, is part of a netlike structure located in the dermis layer of tissue. This initial lymphatic capillary is pencil shaped (tube closed on one end) and lined with one layer of overlapping endothelia cells (Fig. 12-3).[28] Anatomically, fluid cannot be physically "pushed" into the lymphatic

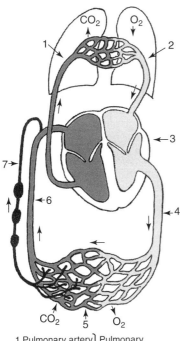

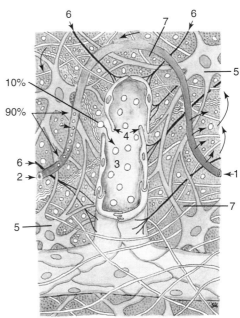

Figure 12-2 Blood and lymph circulatory systems space. (From Foldi M, Foldi E, Kubil S: *Textbook of lymphology for physicians and lymphedema therapists*, Munich, 2003, Urban & Fischer Verlag.)

1 Pulmonary artery ⎤ Pulmonary
2 Pulmonary veins ⎦ circulation
3 Heart
4 Aorta - arterial system ⎤ Systemic
5 Capillaries ⎦ circulation
6 Venous system
7 Lymph vessels and lymph nodes

Figure 12-3 Incorporation of the lymph capillary into the interstitium: *1*, Arterial section of the blood capillary. *2*, Venous section of the blood capillary. *3*, Lymph capillary. *4*, Open intercellular groove-swinging tip. *5*, Fibrocyte. *6*, Anchor filaments. *7*, Intercellular space. (From Foldi M, Foldi E, Kubil S: *Textbook of lymphology for physicians and lymphedema therapists*, Munich, 2003, Urban & Fischer Verlag).

capillaries, nor does it move from the interstitium by osmosis into the lymphatic capillary. Tissue fluid and large molecules can only be absorbed by the lymphatic capillary when changes occur in interstitial fluid pressure or by movement of the elastic anchor filaments that extend from an endothelial cell to connective tissue.[28,35] Then the junctions of these over lapping endothelial cells open like a trap door admitting large molecules from the interstitium into the pencil shaped lymphatic capillary.[28,35] These pressure changes occur with movement of skin, light compression, muscle contraction, and respiration.[14,28] The elastic anchor filaments extending from connective tissue to the endothelial junctions will open the junction flaps when pressure is put on their elastic filaments, such as from fluid congestion in the interstitium.[17]

Lymphatic absorption is stimulated by respiration. The deepest and largest lymphatic structure is the thoracic duct. It lies anterior to, and parallels, the spinal column running from L2 to T4.[56] Changes in thoracic pressure cause a proximal negative pressure vacuum and draws fluid proximally from the periphery. This is also called the *pulmonary pump*.[17] The thoracic duct operates according to hydrodynamic laws.[35] Therefore, inhalation and exhalation from diaphragmatic breathing cause changes in the thoracic duct pressure drawing the lymph within the duct

toward the subclavian veins. These pressure changes in the thoracic duct then create a vacuum (suction), pulling lymph from peripheral structures centrally.[14,35,36] The result is fluid from the periphery moves out of the area, and edema is reduced distally in a domino effect. Once the lymph enters the subclavian veins, it then becomes part of the venous system and continues on to lungs, heart, and other parts of the body.

The differences and similarities of the venous and lymphatic system of fluid absorption from the interstitium should be considered when choosing the appropriate edema reduction technique for poststroke arm and hand edema.

Three Proposed Theories of Etiology and Types of Stroke Hand Edema

An in-depth exploration of the types of Complex Stroke Hand Edema theories is necessary in order to make treatment choices.

Dependency Edema Theory

Dependency edema is due to a combination of the involved flaccid or hemiparetic upper extremity hanging in a dependent position, plus potentially the impairment of sympathetic controlled muscle function.[38,55] Thus tissue fluid pools distally. Often consistent elevation, daily light retrograde massage, and a light compression glove and/or elastic stockinette tube on the arm will reduce this edema. However, even after diligently following these methods, edema can persist. How much does this persistent edema relate to prolonged trunk immobility, lack of scapular movement, and lack of thoracic pressure changes?

This initial edema consists of small molecules that are readily absorbed by the venous system. However, the venous system has a maximum volume capacity. When this capacity is reached, the lymphatic system will carry off the excess. Often, the lymphatic system is referred to as the overflow system. Dependent venous edema has a soft "spongy feel" when pitted, rebounds quickly; and often reduces easily with elevation. This type of edema is often seen when poststroke edema first becomes evident.

Combined Edema Theory

When the lymphatic system acts as a *safety valve* or overflow system for the venous system, it carries out of the interstitium both the small molecule products that the venous system usually absorbs and the large molecules only removed by the lymphatic system. The lymphatic system also has a maximum load capacity. When the system reaches this capacity, there will be lymphatic congestion. Clinically, lymphatic congestion presents as viscous and has a very slow rebound time from being pitted of 20 to 30 seconds or more. At this point, the stroke edema is a combined venous and lymphatic edema that minimally reduces with elevation. Elevation alone will not reduce lymphatic congestion, because the large molecules do not go into the lymphatic capillary via osmosis and the overlapping endothelia cells surrounding the lymphatic capillary have to be stimulated to open and close. With combined edema, the reduction treatment has to be a combination of lymphatic proximal trunk stimulation (muscle contraction, diaphragmatic breathing), superficial tissue stimulation (creating absorption into the initial lymphatics), and elevation to aid in venous (low protein) return.

Minor Trauma Edema (Inflammatory Subacute Edema) Theory

Minor trauma to tissue is often caused by the arm or hand being bumped, getting caught on something, or from overzealous and improper exercise by the client or caregiver.[8,18,30,33] This accidental trauma often occurs due to an impaired visual field or perception, neglect, lack of limb position in space awareness, decreased sensation, and from learned nonuse once motor function returns. Inflammation from trauma becomes a third component to persistent edema. On a microvascular level, trauma causes high capillary permeability leading to a wound healing sequence in the involved joints and tissue. If the limb is already congested due to a dependency and/or a combined venous and lymphatic overload, there is an increase

in the colloidal osmotic pressure in the interstitium. This causes an imbalance in Starling equilibrium resulting in an excess of plasma proteins trapped in the interstitium for a prolonged period. Casley-Smith and Gaffney[16] found that when excess plasma proteins stayed in the interstitium 64 days or longer, they caused chronic inflammation. Fibroblasts are activated by the proteins trapped in the tissue and produce collagenous tissue.[32] This in turn can lead to the eventual shortening, scarring, and possible fibrosing of soft tissue and joints.[12,15] Only the lymphatic system can remove the excess plasma proteins. Thus, the lymphatic system has to be specifically activated to reduce the trapped plasma proteins and break the cycle to pain, scarring, and possible fibrosis of tissue.

Chronic Regional Pain Syndrome Edema*

Reflex Sympathetic Dystrophy (RSD), the original term used in literature and is now known as Chronic Regional Pain Syndrome (CRPS) Type I, may be seen post stroke (central lesion damage).[41,52] In the literature, Shoulder Hand-Syndrome (SHS) is used synonymously with CRPS Type I.[41] CRPS Type II has the same clinical symptoms but occurs because of peripheral nerve involvement.[41] It is defined as an exaggerated pain response to injury characterized by intense pain, trophic changes, and vasomotor changes in the involved limb.[52] CRPS progresses through three phases, each causing increased hand dysfunction. Clinically, in the first phase the hand presents as edematous, hyperesthetic, warm, perspiring, having burning pain, tenderness at the wrist and finger joints, and an increased blood flow to the extremity.[30,52] Poststroke edema occurs most frequently between two and four months after the stroke, as does the occurrence of RSD (CRPS Type I).[30,31] However, clients who developed RSD during this period showed a greater degree of edema than the non-RSD edematous stroke hands.[30] Another possible predictor of RSD researchers found was hand swelling occurring during the first month poststroke.[30]

The statistics for development of CRPS poststroke range anywhere from 1.56 %[52] to 25 %[49] of stroke hand edema cases, using both clinical evidence and a three-phase triple bone scan. This great range of statistics occurs because of timing of inclusion factors, methods of evaluation, when treatment began, and the type of treatment received. The researchers documenting the 1.56% incidence concluded that their incidence of CRPS was low because rehabilitation poststroke began early at 16 days after the first stroke, and treatment included proper positioning, early mobilization, and sensory stimulation.[52]

---

*The most current term for the syndrome discussed here is Complex Regional Pain Syndrome. In the recent past, this syndrome was referred to as Reflex Sympathetic Dystrophy (RSD) and Shoulder Hand Syndrome (SHS). The terms are synonymous here. The terms that were used in the original cited papers are being maintained.

Therapists can play a critical role in early identification and possible prevention or reversing of CRPS Type I. When evaluating and treating clients, occupational therapists should scan for neglect, sensory impairments, shoulder subluxation, and decreased visual field awareness. Pertoldi and colleagues[41] found that the presence of these increased the risk of CRPS. Also, early initiation of a treatment program to prevent trauma (proper positioning, functional use, and mobilization) to the involved shoulder and extremity is critical to preventing CRPS I. See Chapter 10.

In a detailed review of research from 1973 to 1998 on the etiology and treatment of poststroke hand edema and SHS, it was found that the shoulder was only involved in half the cases with a swollen painful hand.[23] Thus, a new term of *wrist-hand syndrome* has been coined.[23] This same study found that in SHS, trauma causes aseptic joint inflammation.[23]

EDEMA EVALUATION METHODS

Volumetric Measurement

Volumetric measurement is a water displacement method measuring hand and lower arm composite mass. The container called a volumeter is filled with enough room temperature water to flow out the container spout. When the water stops dripping out the spout, the client submerges his or her arm into the volumeter with the palm facing him or her, thumb facing the spout, and the web between the middle and ring fingers resting on the plastic stop bar. The therapist holds a beaker to catch the flowing water from the spout and then measures it in a graduated cylinder (Fig. 12-4). Care must be taken that the client does not lean his or her arm against the side of the volumeter or move the arm while water displacement is taking place, the container and cylinder sit on flat level surfaces, and measurements are consistently taken seated or standing and at same time of day and after same amount of activity. Tests have shown the volumeter measurements to be accurate within 10 mL, or 1% of the volume of the hand, when following the manufacturers' directions.[53] Measurements are then taken of the uninvolved hand for comparison sake. This method shows generalized, not site specific, changes in edema. A 12-mL change over time is considered clinically significant.[48] Volumetric measuring has shown to be more accurate than visual inspection for determining presence of edema because it shows small increments of change.[43] Clinically, it can be difficult to consistently position the client with a flaccid or spastic hand.

Circumferential Measurement

Results from using a nonweighted or spring loaded tape measure can vacillate greatly because of the inconsistency of tension put on the tape. The preference is to use a measuring tape with a weight on one end, or one having

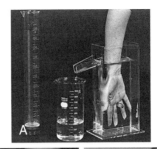
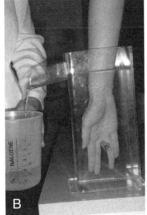
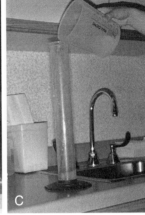

Figure 12-4 Volumeter, collection beaker, and graduated cylinder used to perform volumetric hand edema assessments. (From Fess, E: Documentation: essential elements of an upper extremity assessment battery. In Mackin EJ, Callahan AD, Osterman AL, et al, editors: *Rehabilitation of the hand and upper extremity*, ed 5, St Louis, 2002, Mosby.)

a spring loaded device. These devices will give a more consistent pull on the tape and therefore provide a more reliable, repeatable measurement. Circumferential measurements have the advantage of showing site specific changes in edema. Jeweler's rings can also be used to circumferentially measure digits

Cognitive and Perceptual Assessments

Occupational therapists are skilled in prioritizing person-centered goals and addressing the many personal and environmental factors that alter function poststroke. Cognition and perception may affect a client's ability to integrate the affected limb into normal tasks and to understand their role in preventing or managing edema (see Chapters 18 and 19). The caregiver may need education on how these areas influence function and a person's ability to follow an edema management program, such as the importance of positioning, safe ranging, and gentle edema massage.

Upper Limb Assessments

Many clinics use an upper limb or neurophysical screen to comment on range, strength, shoulder integrity, coordination, pain, and edema, among other things. When conducting a standardized assessment of upper limb quality of movement or function, it is important to consider not only how motor recovery may affect the outcome, but also how edema may influence the results. Further discussion of upper limb assessments can be found in Chapter 10.

Sensibility Testing

There is an old saying, "an insensitive hand is a blind hand." Hand insensitivity or decreased sensation facilitates decreased use and possible injury to the extremity, which can be further complicated by a unilateral neglect. The monofilament method tests for the degree of sensibility present and can indicate a sensory deficit ranging from decreased light touch to loss of protective sensation and to loss of deep touch. Various size monofilaments on individual rods are slowly pressed against the tissue until the monofilament bends, and then the monofilament is slowly lifted from the skin. Once the monofilament bends, no further pressure can be exerted. If the client doesn't detect "touch" from the monofilament, the therapist then uses a larger size monofilament for the next test. The client's vision is occluded during the test.

Testing is important because edema puts pressure on nerve endings decreasing sensibility. As edema decreases sensitivity should improve. Results can be related to safety and activity of daily living (ADL) function. It is imperative to follow directions for accurate, reliable, and repeatable testing. Checking for sensibility can be an important predictor of edema. Boomkamp-Koppen and colleagues[7] found that poststroke clients with hyposensibility, hypertonia, and motor impairment were 50% more likely to develop edema.

Rebound Test

This is a subjective test, but gives an indication if congested edema is softening and decreasing from an area. The therapist places a one ounce weight or the weight of his or her thumb (enough weight to begin blanching the therapist's finger nail) on the edematous area and counts to 10. This light pressure creates a pit in the edema. Then the therapist counts the time the tissue takes to rebound to the height of the adjacent tissue. Lymph congested tissue presents as slow to rebound and is clinically seen as significant with a 20- to 30- second rebound or slower. After doing edema reduction treatment, the test is repeated. If the rebound time is faster, then it is assumed that there has been some lymph decongestion in the area.

This is a quick easy test to do between more objective circumferential or volumetric measurements. It must be noted that tissue that does not pit is usually fibrotic.

Edematous Tissue Visual and Tactile Evaluation

■ Check for early signs of CRPS type I swelling

Edema present one month poststroke should be watched closely for early signs of CRPS Type 1. Most hand edema begins two to four months poststroke, and CRPS has been observed to start at the same time but tends to be more extensive.[30]

Tissue in early stages of CRPS Type I presents as edematous, hyperesthetic, warm, perspiring, red and white blotching of skin, pain and tenderness of the wrist and finger joints, having a constant burning pain, and having an increased in blood flow to the extremity.[30]

■ Swelling from a blood clot

This is rare in the upper extremity, but a therapist must be suspicious of any sudden onset of swelling that is accompanied by pain with a specific muscle movement, including tenderness and warmth. Do not treat the client; seek physician advice immediately.

■ Swelling from an infection

Infected tissue acutely presents as red, warm, swollen, and painful to touch or movement, and often the client has a fever. If there is an infected open wound, the drainage may be opaque and have a pungent odor, in addition to the proceeding symptoms. Seek physician help immediately. Do not treat the limb until the physician has given the approval to resume treatment.

Routinely check for excessively dry skin from sensory impairment. Dry skin cracks and can be a source for bacterial infections.

■ Swelling from a mastectomy

Check client's history regarding having had a mastectomy in the past. Approximately 15% to 20% of clients develop lymphedema postmastectomy node removal.[42] However, because there is a decrease in the number of lymphatic structures, clients are always at risk to develop lymphedema. A stroke survivor with dependent edema involving the arm on the mastectomy side could potentially compromise the deficient lymphatic system and cause lymphedema. If this occurs, a therapist certified in manual lymphatic drainage techniques must be sought out to treat the lymphedema.

■ Swelling from cardiac problems or from low protein edemas such as renal dysfunction, malnutrition, and liver disease

Swelling from cardiac problems, such as chronic heart disease or congestive heart failure (CHF), can be characterized by bilateral ankle swelling, and the tissue is often slightly pinkish. Therapists should check the client's chart regarding a possible cardiac condition. Edema reduction massage should not be performed because of the potential to send too much fluid back to the heart and further compromising the heart. This type of edema has to be controlled medically. Edema from renal disease, liver disease, and malnutrition is a low protein edema.[27] This too has to be reduced by medication. Edema reduction massage can potentially overload and decrease the function of the already compromised organs in this case.

CURRENT POSTSTROKE HAND EDEMA TREATMENT METHODS

Manual Lymphatic and Venous Absorption Stimulation Methods

Elevation and Retrograde Massage

In the early stages of poststroke edema, elevation and light retrograde massage followed by use of an elastic glove on the hand and cotton/elastic stockinette tube on the arm, if needed, can be effective for reducing hand/arm edema. The rationale is that elevation decreases arterial hydrostatic pressure and thus reduces the flowing of fluid into the interstitial spaces.[14,50] The elastic glove and stockinette give light pressure to prevent or lessen refilling of tissue. An active muscle pump is needed to intermittently compress venous and lymphatic structures to return fluid back toward the heart. Without an active or fully functioning muscle pump, dependent limb edema results. Furthermore, over time the volume of fluid increases distally and less edema reduces with elevation and compression. At this point, it is theorized that both the venous and lymphatic systems have reached their maximum capacity, and a combined edema situation exists.

Clinical Treatment Considerations. Avoid having the elastic glove or elastic/cotton stockinette tube being too tight and collapsing the initial lymphatics. This would prevent absorption of fluid from the interstitium. One clinical guideline is to be able to stretch the glove one eighth of an inch out from either side of a digit. The elastic/cotton stockinette tube should be firm but still allow a therapist's hands to fit under the stockinette at the tightest point. The goals are to provide compression, not to collapse the initial lymphatic net along without causing tissue trauma with application and removal. Both the venous and lymphatic systems take fluid out of the interstitium, but lymphatic absorption is stimulated in ways previously discussed. If sensory or vascular insufficiencies exist in the involved arm and hand, the therapist must take appropriate precautions.

Anecdotally, therapists have seen distal hand edema reduction while doing extensive active, active-assistive trunk and scapular work. Anatomically, this is logical because trunk and scapular movement activates changes in thoracic pressures and thus activates the thoracic duct pump of the lymph system. Thus, applying the elastic glove and cotton/elastic stockinette tube on the extremity immediately following active trunk and scapular exercise prevents or lessens refill after an edema reduction has been achieved.

When elevating the arm, precautions should be taken if the client has medical conditions such as right-sided heart weakness or Raynaud disease. The latter diagnosis involves arterial vascular insufficiency, so elevation of the extremity further decreases the blood flow to the extremity and

quickly increases the symptoms such as dysesthesia and further blanching of the finger tips.[10] Also, extreme elevation of the right upper extremity, especially in supine, to reduce edema would not be advisable if the client had a comorbidity of right-sided heart weakness.[10] This could potentially send fluid faster into the right side of the heart than it can be pumped into the left side to be reoxygenated, thus further compromising the heart.

Manual Edema Mobilization

Manual Edema Mobilization (MEM) was first introduced by Artzberger in 1995 with subsequent publications.[1-5,29,44] It recognizes that swelling that lasts longer than one week and presents as slow to rebound, i.e., 20 to 30 seconds or more to reach surrounding tissue height when pitted, indicates a lymphatic congested system. MEM teaches specific concepts to stimulate and quickly decongest the lymphatic system for postorthopedic trauma and poststroke extremity edema. Treatment begins in the trunk, creating a vacuum drawing peripheral lymph proximally, toward the trunk. Treatment for the sedentary patient begins with pretreatment exercises of stretching for the trunk and shoulders to facilitate proximal decongestion. The MEM program is initiated with diaphragmatic breathing, trunk exercise, and light trunk massage, and then proceeds distally in sections toward the hand. Active or passive exercise of muscles in each section just massaged is essential to pump the lymph proximally. At the end, along with distal to proximal exercise, light flow massage from hand to arm to the trunk is completed. Keys to success include diaphragmatic breathing, starting treatment at the trunk, exercise at specific intervals, use of a technique called *MEM Pump Points*, light massage strokes, a home self-massage and exercise program, and low stretch bandaging and/or chip bags as needed. This is designed exclusively for the patient with an intact lymph system (not status post mastectomy where nodes have been removed). Treatment usually takes 20 minutes and is incorporated into a patient's regular treatment program. The MEM technique includes specific guidelines and precautions, especially for the stroke survivor who often has many comorbidities, so taking a formal two-day MEM course is necessary.

When poststroke edema no longer reduces with elevation, light retrograde massage, and compression, it is theorized that both the venous and lymphatic systems are overloaded, and a combined edema exists. Thus, there has to be a specific activation of the lymphatic system to help reduce this type of edema. MEM is an appropriate treatment providing there are no medical contraindications relative to the technique. The following paragraphs will elaborate the key elements of MEM.

Manual Edema Mobilization Begins at the Trunk. This follows the previously discussed hydraulic, vacuum principle of first moving lymph centrally into the venous system (subclavian veins), which then draws lymph proximally from the periphery. Diaphragmatic breathing facilitates this process through changes in thoracic duct pressure that then moves lymph proximally.[14] Diaphragmatic breathing entails breathing air through the nose into the lower abdomen that pushes the naval area outward, and then slowly exhaling through pursed lips, bringing the lower abdomen inward.

Exercise Muscles in Area Just Massaged. According to Guyton and Hall,[27] the collector lymphatics move lymph ten to thirty times faster with exercise. MEM light massage techniques facilitate absorption of large molecules, permeable only to the lymph system, into the initial lymphatic net by exercising muscles under the tissue just massaged. This muscle pumping moves lymph faster through the system, and theoretically space is created for more absorption.

Light Massage Strokes. Since 65 mm Hg pressure[39] has been shown to begin collapsing the initial lymphatic net where absorption begins in the dermis layer of tissue, therapists are instructed to use a pressure no greater than half the weight of their hand. To quote a stroke survivor being taught a home program, "light is right." Strokes are "U" shaped beginning proximally (top of the "U"), moving the skin distally, and then back upward to where begun. It is emphasized that the hand does not slide on the skin but remains in place moving the skin over underlying structures. Terms used in the massage performed by the therapist are *clear* and *flow*.

Clearing "U"s consist of five "U"s done in each of three segments of a section of an extremity, i.e., volar forearm. In this case, the "U"s start proximal at the elbow and end at the wrist (Fig. 12-5) These stimulate absorption into the initial and collector lymphatics.

Flow "U"s begin at the distal end of the segment just cleared and end proximal to where clearing started, hopefully at a set of nodes. Only one, not five, "U"s are done in each section of the segment. These are repeated five times from the distal end of the segment and ending proximal to where clearing started. This action is believed to stimulate absorption, help to prevent refluxing of lymph, and create a proximal flow.

Because the "flowing" concept can be difficult to teach a patient for his or her home program, the term *sweep* is used. The patient is instructed to very lightly slide his or her fingers and palm over the involved extremity, starting distally and moving proximally (Fig. 12-6).

Manual Edema Mobilization Pump Points. The upper extremity has five specific pump point locations, which are sites of lymph nodes or bundles of lymphatic structures (initial and collector lymphatics). A therapist uses both hands to simultaneously massage a set of nodes and lymphatic bundles in a "U" shaped pump pattern (see Figs. 12-7 and 12-8). Clinically, these seem to provide a faster flow of lymph versus the usual "clear" and "flow" technique, especially for patients with the combined type of edema. Because of the effect, an increased volume of lymph flow could have another existing medical conditions, such as cardiac and pulmonary. It is necessary to complete a MEM course because pump point application is thoroughly discussed for the stroke survivor. Box 12-1 lists the upper extremity pump points.

Manual Edema Mobilization Home Self-Management Program. A home MEM program is essential to keep lymphatic structures open, and lymph

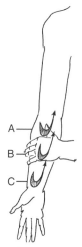

Figure 12-5 Manual Edema Mobilization forearm "clear" (*A* through *C*) and "flow." (*C* through *A*).

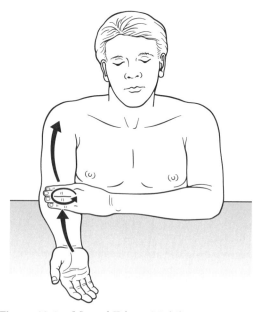

Figure 12-6 Manual Edema Mobilization "sweep."

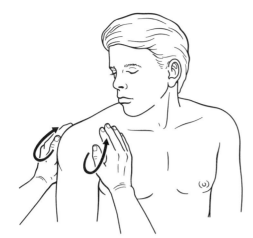

Figure 12-7 Manual Edema Mobilization Pump Point 1.

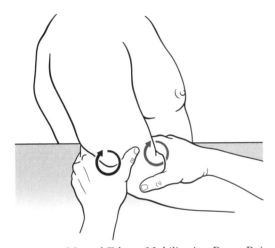

Figure 12-8 Manual Edema Mobilization Pump Point 3.

flowing for long-term edema reduction. Patients are given a simplified version of the program the therapist used in the clinic. Often simple proximal to distal node massage from trunk to elbow, "sweeping" from hand to uninvolved axilla, and exercise of the arm and trunk is enough. These can easily be incorporated into the patient's ADL tasks, such as daily hygiene and functional upper limb retraining, e.g., wiping the table.

Low Stretch Bandages. Low stretch bandages look like the high stretch bandages often used postsports injury, frequently called ACE bandages; however, low stretch bandages have no elastic fibers and are 100% cotton. Because they have minimal stretch, they facilitate a "pumping" action on the initial lymphatic net with muscle contraction and relaxation.[14] For more details, see the Bandaging Methods section.

Chip Bags. Chip bags are often placed under low stretch bandages or an elastic/cotton stockinette tube on

The Five MEM Upper Extremity Pump Point Hand Placement Areas

1. First hand is placed on deltoid pectoral node area of trunk and anterior deltoid of upper arm. Second hand is placed on teres minor, posterior axilla, and posterior deltoid of upper arm. A praying hands position (Fig. 12-7).
2. First hand is placed on teres minor, posterior axilla, and posterior deltoid of upper arm, as in Pump Point One. Second hand is placed on medial side of antecubital crease of elbow—elbow node location. Middle finger lies across antecubital crease and thumb on back of arm above elbow.
3. First hand is placed on medial antecubital crease as in Pump Point Two. Second hand is placed on the posterior of the upper arm just above the back of the elbow (Fig. 12-8).
4. First hand is placed on antecubital crease as in Pump Points two and three. Second hand is placed on the volar forearm at wrist.
5. First hand is placed at the volar forearm at the wrist. Second hand is on the dorsum of the hand.

areas of excessive swelling, especially areas of hard tissue. They consist of various densities of foam pieces one inch in size placed in a cotton stockinette with the ends sewn shut (Fig. 12-9). It is theorized that hard tissue is softened due to the neutral warmth that builds up under the foam pieces.[4] See Bandaging Methods Section for ideal lymph flow temperatures. It appears that the various densities of the foam further help to soften and stimulate lymphatic uptake because of the tissue pressure differentiation they cause.

Clinical Treatment Considerations. MEM techniques have been shown to reduce edema.[44] However, for the flaccid extremity, this reduction will not last because the lymphatic system, like the venous system, needs an active muscle pump system to continually move the lymph.[22] Light massage and passive exercise both put a stretch on the anchor filaments of the initial lymphatics (lymphatic net) and alter interstitial pressure, which will open the junctions of the endothelial cells, admitting molecules into the initial lymphatic. From there the collector lymphatics have a peristaltic pumping action that is controlled by the sympathetic and parasympathetic systems to conduct the lymph proximally.[17] However, some authors believe that the autonomic system can be neurologically impaired by the stroke.[55] This combined with lack of an active muscle pump causes lymph congestion. Proximal trunk exercise and diaphragmatic breathing stimulate the lymphatic system and will draw lymph

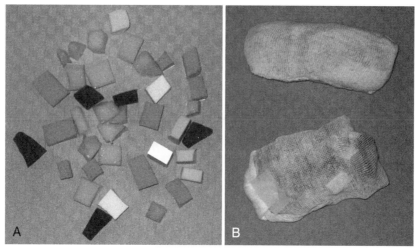

Figure 12-9 Foam "chips" and chip bag.

proximally.[14] Thus, even without knowing MEM techniques, a therapist can reduce the lymphatic congestion with diaphragmatic breathing, extensive trunk and scapular exercise and activation of the proximal noninvolved musculature. The decongestion then facilitates peripheral lymph absorption. By reducing edema, the occupational therapist may improve the patient's perception and awareness of the affected upper limb and increase the functional dexterity of the hand. Providing a clear and meaningful home program may increase the patient's ownership of his or her occupational therapy program.

Bandaging Methods
There are two types of bandaging systems: elastic (high stretch) and low elastic (low stretch).[14] Both look alike in thickness and color, but the low elastic (low stretch) bandages are usually 100% cotton and have no elastic fibers.[14] The Casley-Smiths[14] point out that the initial lymphatic net will only pump when compressed against something solid such between a contracting muscle and a solid counter-force (low elastic bandage). A tissue pressure differentiation, or pumping action, is created facilitating lymphatic absorption with muscle contraction against a counter-force (the lymphatic net is caught between the contracting muscle and the resistive bandage) and then relaxation of the muscle. The Casley-Smiths[14] refer to low stretch bandages as having "high-working and low resting pressures." An elastic bandage stretches and does not produce this counter-force.

Low stretch bandages are "rolled on," not pulled tight, in order not to collapse the initial lymphatic net. Miller and Seale[39] found that the initial lymphatic net begins to close as 60 mm Hg pressure and is completely closed at 75 mm Hg pressure. Graduated pressure with low stretch bandages is thus obtained not by pulling tightly, but by layers of bandages in an area.

Clinical Treatment Considerations. Low stretch bandages create a pump action facilitating lymphatic absorption and prevent tissue refill.[14] The neutral warmth (body temperature) that builds up under bandages softens indurated (hard) tissue facilitating fluid absorption. Kurz[36] states that the ideal temperatures to facilitate lymph flow is between 22 degrees and 41 degrees C (71.6 F and 105.8 F). Please note that temperatures above 98.6 F or 37 degrees C will increase blood flow to the area and increase edema, so a therapist would not use these high temperatures when trying to reduce edema. Most importantly, when applied properly, the short stretch bandages do not collapse the lymphatic net, which prevents excess tissue fluid absorption, and they can be worn during periods of rest. Unfortunately, low stretch bandages are not often practical and have limitations for poststroke hand and arm edema, because they can potentially cause neurovascular problems or can limit function when applied too tightly by an untrained person; if an active muscle movement causes the desired excess tissue fluid absorption, the extremity loses girth, the bandages have to be reapplied, and most stroke survivors require assistance to reapply bandages due to their cognitive, perceptual, or motor limitations; and bandages may limit sensory retraining.

When there is minimal to no active muscle contraction, a cotton/elastic stockinette tube is more practical for stroke edema. Because the cotton stockinette tube is elastic, it only prevents or lessens tissue fluid refill, and, if loose enough, it will not collapse the initial lymphatic net. To ensure that an elastic/cotton stockinette tube is not too tight, the therapist should be able to get both hands in the tube on either side of the patient's arm.

Rolling down of the elastic/stockinette tube can be a problem. Suggested ways to prevent this include: (1) Double the elastic stockinette tube, but make sure that the pressure is not too tight; (2) Loosely place a to-tally stretched out 3 inch-wide piece of Coban circumfer-entially 1 inch below the proximal end of the elastic stockinette tube and "cuff" the 1 inch proximal end over the Coban (Fig. 12-10). This can also be done with a loosely placed one inch foam splinting strap instead of the Coban. To achieve graded compression, place one piece of the cotton/elastic stockinette tube, for instance, from palm to elbow and a second smaller piece from palm to mid-forearm. Then stitch the two pieces to-gether enabling the patient or caregiver to pull it on in one piece. When introducing bandaging, therapists must educate and closely monitor the patient and caregiver for appropriate application to prevent rolling down of the elastic/cotton stockinette tube that would then increase distal swelling. Chip bags can be placed under the elastic/cotton stockinette tube to soften hard edema or to pre-vent refill at a specific site.

Continuous Passive Motion

In 1990 Giudice[25] published an article reporting hand edema reduction outcomes comparing 30 minutes of hand elevation and 30 minutes of hand elevation with continu-ous passive motion (CPM). Eleven of the 16 subjects had hemiplegia. Edema reduction was significantly greater with the combination of elevation and the use of the CPM machine. However, when the CPM was discontinued, the edema returned to its former rate.[25]

More extensive use and evaluation of use of the CPM machine was reported by Dirette and Hinojosa in 1994.[20] In their ABA single subject design study, two clients one month poststroke received CPM treatment for two hours daily for one week. Results showed a continuous significant reduction of edema during the treatment week. During the withdrawal week, the edema increased, leveled off, but did not return to evaluation week edema volume.

Clinical Treatment Considerations and Rationale.

The CPM provides gentle and nonexcessive motion to the hand, thus eliminating microscopic tearing of tissue that can lead to edema and potential fibrosis of tissue and joints. The passive movement stretches the elastic anchor fila-ments of the initial lymphatic net and causes changes of

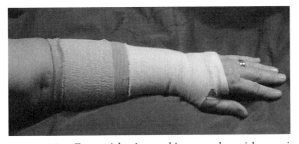

Figure 12-10 Cotton/elastic stockinette tube with proximal Coban.

interstitial pressure, all facilitating opening of the endothe-lial cell junctions and absorption of fluid into the lymphatic net. It has been suggested that the CPM might have more pumping and drainage action on the dorsal hand lymphat-ics if it was set to flex metacarpophalangeal (MCP) joints to near normal flexion range.[22] Because the CPM is on the hand, increased attention the involved limb may be noted during that period of usage.

Pneumatic Pump and Air Splints

Pneumatic intermittent compression pumps were first introduced to reduce venous leg edema, such as from varicose veins, and were then expanded to usage with the lymphedematous extremity. Leduc[37] reported that pneu-matic pumps only force water back into blood and do not remove excessive protein from tissues. In 1999 Roper and colleagues[47] reported on their study of 37 clients with stroke hand edema who received a two two-hour session two times a day of intermittent pneumatic compression for one month. Compression was 50 mm Hg. They found no change in hand volume in the treated group.[47]

Clinical Treatment Considerations, Rationale, and Potential Future Research Ideas.

1. A Casley-Smith and Bjorlin[13] research study con-cluded that 45 mm Hg pump pressure would not col-lapse the initial lymphatics. Would a graded sequential pump, meaning progressive chamber pressures from 40 mm Hg at the hand to 10 mm Hg at the axilla, be more effective versus 50 mm Hg pressure up the en-tire arm?
2. Did the Roper and colleagues[47] study include early or combined edema?
3. If it were combined edema, would central trunk clear-ing performed before pumping positively affect the results? Recently new pumps have been developed that use lower pressures and begin massage at the trunk. Would these be more effective because they start drainage centrally, massage in a proximal to distal seg-ment sequence, and then distal to proximal? Raines and colleagues[45] found that the pneumatic pumps could only reduce edema, even temporarily, only if the venous drainage is normal. According to the vasomo-tor dysfunction theory of stroke edema development, venous drainage is impaired.[55]

If a pneumatic pump is used, precautions should be ob-served. It should not be used if there is a blood clot or any suspicion of a clot, infection, cellulitis, symptoms of CHF or chronic obstructive pulmonary disease, dizzi-ness, lightheadedness, or headaches.[14] Beta blockers in combination with pumping have been known to cause hypotension.[11] The pneumatic pump or air splints should not be used on stroke clients who are on anticoagulant medications that can drop their platelet level below 120,000 mm.[19]

Clinically, the rationale of using air splints to reduce edema should be evaluated and appropriately applied. They provide single chamber circumferential compression that can push fluid both distal and proximal because there is no grading of compression. The air splint compression pushes tissue fluid back into the interstitium, which may work to reduce edema in the early stages when it is a low protein edema. Also, the neutral warmth that builds up under the plastic splint could soften indurated tissue. However, when the edema becomes a combined edema, this method will only push fluid out of the interstitium temporarily. The hydrophilic plasma proteins remain in the lymph, because anatomically they cannot be physically "pushed out." They will reattract the water molecule, and swelling will return. In fact, if the pressure is above 40 mm Hg, it could collapse the lymphatic net.

Splinting

There is some evidence that splinting reduces edema. Garcies and colleagues[26] found that a custom-made lycra garment with flexible plastic inserts when worn three hours a day provided a continuous stretch of spastic muscles and reduced edema. There are some clinical arguments for the use of a wrist cock up splint to reduce edema, to protect joints, and to minimize pain.[24] Burge and colleagues[9] conducted a randomized trial of a neutral functional realignment orthosis on 30 clients with subacute hemiplegia, with the orthosis group wearing it for six hours a day. They found the orthoses prevented pain but had little effect on edema or mobility. They also stated that they used circumferential measurements as directed by Leibovitz.[9]

Clinical Treatment Considerations and Rationale.
The splint used by Gracies[26] allowed for restricted movement, thus preventing overzealous passive movement of the hand and arm to cause trauma edema. Also, the ability to move the hand while it is in the splint helps to increase attention to the affected limb. Consideration should also be given to the role the combination of the elastic lycra and muscle contraction play to move low protein edema from the periphery centrally or in preventing further filling of tissue. See Chapter 13.

Exercise and Positioning

Research regarding poststroke development of SHS, CRPS, and elbow-hand syndrome repeatedly show that the incidence can be reduced by half or more if inflammation of tissue can be avoided.[7,8,30,33] Braus and colleagues[8] reduced the frequency of SHS from 27% to 8% in their study by extensively educating everyone involved in client care on how to prevent trauma to the involved shoulder and extremity. Their regimen included immediately repositioning the hand/arm/shoulder if pain occurred; performing passive humeral motions of abduction and external rotation only after fully mobilizing the scapula; having not only the therapist perform the motion during treatment, but having other hospital services do so when handling the involved limb as part of their treatment, such as computerized tomography, electroencephalography, or when relatives assist with care; and avoiding needle sticks in the involved hand/arm.[8]

In their research article, Kondo and colleague[33] included a passive exercise protocol for both the therapist and client to follow to prevent SHS. This article detailed a controlled passive movement regimen by a trained therapist and restriction of passive movement by the client for a minimum of four months poststroke. Restricted passive motion not only included shoulder-scapula protective ROM, but also included preventing the client from repeatedly hyperextending his fingers, which causes trauma to the finger joints. Clients with impaired sensation were more likely to excessively range or hyperextend their fingers.[33] Another study also showed that the hand stayed edematous, even if the client had active motor return and did not use it.[7] Furthermore, studies have shown that prolonged positioning of the wrist and fingers in flexion will exacerbate swelling, because it impedes venous and lymphatic flow at the wrist.[7]

Avoiding microtrauma to tissue is difficult if the client also has unilateral neglect and/or visual field deficits. Wee and colleagues[54] found that 80% of those with shoulder-hand problems had unilateral neglect. They concluded that the neglect predisposed the client to shoulder-hand problems.[54]

Microscopic tearing of tissue that occurs from repeated mishandling and mispositioning of a nonfunctioning to a minimum functioning arm causes trauma to tissue. This will cause a wound healing sequence to occur to the involved joints and tissue. With the invasion of excess plasma proteins into tissue from trauma to a hand or arm with a preexisting diminished motor function and/or dependency edema, the cycle to possible fibrosis is established. Only the lymphatic system can remove these excess plasma proteins and thus has to be specifically stimulated.

Clinical Treatment Considerations and Rationale.
Diligence is recommended to avoid causing tissue inflammation during all aspects of client care and rehabilitation. The client, family, nursing, nursing assistants, and even x-ray and lab technicians from the facility have to be trained in proper handling and positioning of the arm at all times during treatment and care, including bed mobility and walking. Pain to the involved limb has to be avoided or immediately corrected, such pain as from improper positioning. Education and repeated use of educational material is essential. Suggestions include: wheelchair lap tables should be at the appropriate height or include an

arm wedge to support the affected limb in neutral; when moving the flaccid arm, even for bed positioning, support and glide the scapula at the same time; do not pull the affected arm during transfers and bed mobility; begin proper scapular and shoulder ROM glides as soon as possible after the stroke; position on pillows to support the shoulder complex; support the arm and shoulder during transfers and ambulation to prevent stretching on the shoulder capsule or dependent arm positioning; thoroughly and repeatedly educate the client and family not to exuberantly exercise the shoulder, wrist, and fingers, and to force extremes of range; all personnel involved with client care must glide the scapula concurrently while the humerus is moved when working with the client; and prevent wrist and fingers from assuming a flexed position for a prolonged period of time.

Diligently avoid head, arm, and trunk positioning or exercise that can cause tissue inflammation of the brachial plexus. CRPS Type II involves peripheral nerve lesions. Overzealous shoulder capsule stretching or prolonged subluxation of the glenohumeral joint can cause brachial plexus inflammation and potential nerve damage that could potentially lead to CRPS Type II.[41] See Chapter 10.

Scalenus anticus syndrome is a cervical neurovascular (brachial plexus and subclavian artery) impingement syndrome involving the scalenus anticus muscle. It is facilitated by prolonged sitting with a forward head position, inwardly rolled shoulders, and flexion of the spine causing cervical and brachial plexus inflammation.[10] Clients present with mild neck and shoulder pain including tingling sensation in the fingers.[51] A corrective position is achieved by positioning the clients pelvis into a neutral tilt, placing a small rolled pillow or towel at the lower back to get a lumbar curve, which will then facilitate a normal shoulder external rotation position and head alignment above the trunk.

Clients who complain of bilateral arm pain, paraesthesia, and arm weakness with activities that require overhead reaching should be evaluated for thoracic outlet syndrome (TOS). For the client who has decreased proprioceptive or kinesthetic sensation in the involved arm, an activity such as weight-bearing on that arm with an unsupported shoulder girdle having poor scapula stability could cause or exacerbate a TOS.[10] Furthermore, a client who repeatedly over stretches the arm above the shoulder without scapular gliding not only can cause microscopic tearing of the shoulder capsule soft-tissue structures, but could cause an impingement and inflammation at the thoracic outlet as well.

Begin treatment sessions with diaphragmatic breathing (or activities that cause changes in thoracic pressure such as laughing) and extensive trunk and scapular exercise to activate the lymphatic pump centrally drawing venous and lymphatic fluid forward. Remember that even passive exercise anatomically stimulates lymphatic absorption in the extremity, but absorption begins with central clearing as described previously.

For the client who has some motor return, emphasize the importance of frequent short hand exercise sessions and functional usage throughout the day to reduce hand edema. Relate exercise to functional tasks. Boomkamp-Koppen and colleagues[7] found hand edema in 17.6% of their clients who had good hand function. They concluded that these clients were unwilling to perform active exercises with the hemiparetic hand as much as the noninvolved hand. Hemi neglect, visual field limitations, sensory limitations, and "learned" neglect all contribute to nonuse.

Clients with unilateral neglect have to be taught various compensation methods or use of safety devices to prevent microtrauma to the involved arm. Suggested methodologies have included modifications of the home and work environments to enable safe functional task performance; position in space awareness cuing and sensory cuing; auditory warning signals; and proprioceptive and visual correction techniques (see Chapter 19).

Electrical Stimulation

Over the last 25 years, there has been considerable interest in and evolving research and clinical usage of Short Term Electrical Stimulation for neurological stimulation poststroke for pain reduction, muscular stimulation, muscle strengthening, and tone reduction. Recognizing the role the venous and lymphatic systems play for reducing edema and the effect the muscle pump has on these two systems to reduce edema, Faghri[22] designed a research study using neuromuscular stimulation (NMES) to facilitate the muscle pump for edema reduction in the flaccid/paralyzed edematous poststroke hand. His study showed that edema reduction with 30 minutes of NMES of the flaccid/paralyzed wrist and finger flexors and extensors was significantly greater than 30 minutes of limb elevation alone. However, when the NMES was discontinued, the edema returned to its former volume in the limb. This study is very significant because it addresses the two theories of stoke edema: neurological impairment and dependency edema due to lack of an active muscle motor pump.

Neuroprosthetic Functional Electrical Stimulation.

Faghri's[22] study involved only 30 minutes of treatment daily, and edema reduction occurred with electrically induced muscle contraction. A study done by Ring and Rosenthal also showed a result of edema reduction.[46] This study involved clients six months poststroke, using one group with a flaccid hand and a second group with some motor return in the involved hand. In addition to their regular therapy, the subjects wore a neuroprosthesis on their involved forearm/palm for 50 minutes three times daily for six weeks. This neuromuscular stimulator stimulated five forearm muscles, activating the wrist and fingers, and the stimulation modes alternated finger flexion and extension. Those with some motor return were encouraged to actively carry out movement during stimulation, such as grasp and release. Results for the flaccid extremity group showed greater decrease in spasticity and greater improvement in proximal limb active ROM, compared to the control group. The group with some motor return demonstrated significant gains in hand function, a decrease in spasticity, and increased voluntary motion, as compared to the control group. Outcomes also showed that existing hand edema reduced in the neuroprosthesis study group but not in the control group. Long-term continuance of the gains made by usage of the neuroprosthesis unit was not assessed in this study. The authors cite a similar study[40] of clients in the flaccid hand category that showed all gains made were lost within two weeks once the stimulation was removed.

Clinical Treatment Considerations and Rationale. Neurologically, usage of a multihour electrical stimulation device shows much promise for the clients with hand spasticity, a hemiparetic hand, or flaccid hand. More research is needed to determine the optimum lengths for daily and total usage to get the longest carry over when the treatment is discontinued. This will help the treating therapist decide if this treatment is applicable for their particular poststroke clients with hand edema.

Use of neuroprosthesis devices promotes gentle active and passive motion and does not cause microtrauma to tissue. Potentially multihour usage of the device helps to lessen hemineglect if the client uses it for functional tasks.

Functional Activities

Edema and the associated deficits it causes, such as reduced sensation and range of movement, may limit a person's integration of the affected limb into normal tasks and may reinforce learned nonuse. Occupational therapists can grade and provide cuing in daily functional tasks to address the cognitive, perceptual, sensory, and motor aspects of performance, and can facilitate use of the affected limb. Through task analysis, occupational therapists can highlight to a client what the client can do to maximize independence and reduce the impact of edema. Boomkamp-Koppen and colleagues[7] found a significant relationship between edema and hand function when paresis was controlled in a statistical analysis. Clinically, edema may mask the motor and sensory potential of the upper limb may and limit progress of a client's goals. Gilmore and colleagues[24] advocated the use of purposeful activities that

position the shoulder complex in normal alignment or facilitated scapulohumeral rhythm to minimize pain and trauma.

Clinical Treatment Considerations and Rationale. Occupational therapists are in the position to select meaningful tasks with their clients for therapy and to set specific functional goals. As the lymphatic system is activated by muscle pumping, the use of the affected upper limb in normal tasks within a safe range of movement will facilitate lymphatic flow. Reinforcing to the client and caregivers what activities, or parts of activities, a client can undertake with the affected upper limb can assist in this process.

SUMMARY

It is essential to screen for and address poststroke upper limb edema as soon as possible. By effectively managing edema the incidence of CRPS Type I, pain, stiffness, and possible joint contractures can be reduced. However, most important, edema must decrease in order to facilitate functional arm and hand usage for occupation, especially as motor function return occurs. Unfortunately, there is no specific consensus on which of the discussed treatment technique is most effective for reducing poststroke hand edema.[7,23,38] However, it is hoped that this chapter will give therapists a foundation for client treatment planning, critical problem-solving, and a basis to do further research of techniques.

CASE STUDIES

In this Australian setting, clients receive intensive neurological rehabilitation as directed by a multidisciplinary team. The occupational therapist's role is to evaluate and maximize performance in activities of daily living, domestic roles, community safety, driving, work, and leisure. Numerous treatment frameworks are used. In these three case studies, the author provided intensive edema treatment to address functional goals.

Evaluation Criteria

All edema measurements were conducted by the same occupational therapist to increase intrarater reliability. It was clinically reasoned that a volumeter was not a reliable way of measuring edema given the limitations of consistently positioning the stroke upper limb. Circumferential measurements were chosen to increase consistency of measurement and to identify change in anatomical regions. Measurements of the affected limb were taken at consistent landmarks with the client's limb in the same position.

Subacute Stroke with Hemiplegia and Motivation

S.O. was 56-years-old when he suffered a left basal ganglia and corona radiata stroke. Two weeks after his stroke, he was transferred from an acute hospital to a specialized neurological rehabilitation setting. His main deficits were right hemiplegia, mild dysarthria, mild expressive aphasia, and mild memory impairment. He was right dominant. Prior to the stroke, S.O. lived independently in a country town and worked in the mining industry operating machinery. He enjoyed dancing and socializing and was motivated to return to independent living and driving.

Approximately two months poststroke, S.O. developed edema in his right arm that did not respond to elevation and massage alone. The primary occupational therapist identified S.O. as a good candidate for MEM because his edema was limiting grasp and manipulation and release of objects, he had no medical contraindications limiting participation in MEM, and he had the cognitive ability to complete a self-MEM program. He was motivated to participate in all aspects of therapy and hospital life. S.O. was concerned that his edema was "holding him back" from using his arm; for example, he felt that he could not grasp a flannel shirt as his fingers felt ". . . like sausages." At initial assessment, S.O. had nonpitting edema over his hand and upper limb, and his hand was hot to touch (an indication of tissue fluid congestion as no infection was present). Sensation was grossly intact, and he had some minor shoulder pain. Elbow extension was normal, but his wrist and finger extension were limited by his edema and increased flexor skeletal muscle activity. He was independent in self-care in the ward and used an electric wheelchair for mobility.

During the first session, S.O. was educated regarding the theoretical background of MEM and treatment progressed through Pump Point Two. The importance of light and "U" shaped strokes were emphasized, rather than the rough massaging of "up and down" the dorsum of the hand that he had been doing in an effort to reduce his swelling. S.O. was advised to complete a basic home program three times a day, which consisted of diaphragmatic breathing, exercises, axilla and terminus massage (supraclavicular area), and sweeping, in addition to his standard occupational therapy and physiotherapy sessions. An edema glove was tried, but S.O. did not tolerate it, saying it was uncomfortable. Instead, he used a foam wedge on his wheelchair arm trough to elevate his arm as much as possible.

In the second session, the therapist noted that there was increased flexor skeletal muscle activity in the forearm. MEM was used on all five Pump Points, and traditional retrograde massage was used on the hands and fingers to facilitate further clearance. S.O. could use the technique on his fingers himself, and he reported that his arm felt "lighter" by the end of the second session. The therapist noted post-MEM a decrease in flexor skeletal muscle activity, improved supination to wash his face, and an increase in wrist skin folds.

By the final two sessions, S.O.'s right hand was the same temperature as his left (fluid decongestion had occurred as the edema reduced), the circumference of his elbow and axilla had reduced by 1.3 and 5.4 cm respectively, and there was a reduction in flexor activity. S.O. had increased range of finger abduction and adduction, thumb extension, and composite flexion, which he could use in grooming tasks. S.O.'s primary occupational therapist was aware of MEM treatment principles and continued to use these when working with S.O. As he noted improvements, S.O. began to complete his self-MEM program three times a day without prompting by his occupational therapist.

MEM was a technique that S.O. could independently use and what he preferred when compared to the medical suggestion of bandaging, which was likely to restrict his progress in grooming. It appeared that the combination of diaphragmatic breathing, stretches, flowing ("sweeping") up the arm, and elevation contributed greatly to the reduction of edema and subsequent functional goals. There were reductions of over 1 cm at the wrist and MCP joints and small changes over the digits. At the time of writing, S.O. had returned to independent living and was beginning to have the dexterity to write with his dominant hand.

Chronic Stroke with Minimal Hand Movement and Increased Skeletal Muscle Activity

K.P. was 55-years-old when he had a left middle cerebral watershed infarct at home. After acute and rehabilitation inpatient stays, K.P. could walk independently and was discharged home to live with his supportive long-term partner, who supervised him with ADL. Prior to his stroke, K.P. worked as a bus driver and enjoyed visiting his young granddaughter, woodworking, and sailing. K.P. received home-based occupational therapy and was then referred for outpatient occupational therapy. K.P. was then four months poststroke and was beginning to achieve active upper limb movement in his affected right arm. He was left dominant.

K.P. was driven by his partner for an hour each way, twice a week to attend occupational therapy and physiotherapy. K.P. had memory deficits and reduced attention.

Continued

CASE STUDY 2

Chronic Stroke with Minimal Hand Movement and Increased Skeletal Muscle Activity—cont'd

His partner used prompting with K.P. at home and had set up cue cards to assist in routine tasks around the house. His primary occupational therapy goal was to use his right hand in leisure activities. K.P. presented with poor trunk, shoulder, and head symmetry, both with standing and sitting. His rehabilitation had been limited by his lack of awareness, body positioning, and attention. As K.P. developed elbow extension and finger extension, a short thumb postsplint was fabricated for him to use for functional grasp.

It was noted that K.P. had significant pitting edema at his hand and wrist, which would fluctuate and appeared to restrict wrist extension and contributed to poor upper limb, head, and trunk dissociation and clonus in his upper arm. By this stage, K.P. was six months poststroke. Five MEM sessions were provided by the author to assist the primary occupational therapist. At the first session, subluxations were noted at the shoulder and wrist, and there was pitting edema over the dorsum of the hand. The first MEM session focused on treatment to Pump Point 3 and education for K.P.'s partner on the importance of light massage strokes. See Figs. 12-7 and 12-8 in Box 12-1. K.P. and his partner were motivated to continue therapy at home and were taught a basic MEM home program to do at least twice a day.

At the second session, MEM was expanded to include all pump points and the hand. Wrist and elbow extension range increased after the second session to enable reaching to furniture and large objects, and an increase in skin folds was noted. After the third session, there was no pitting edema. His partner reported that they were doing the home program at least once a day and that she was encouraging K.P. to use his hand in activities.

On the fourth session, slight pitting at the MCP joints was noted, and K.P.'s partner reported that they had done less of the home program, so treatment focused on Pump Points 4 and 5, rather than the fingers. Particular emphasis was placed on wrist and hand pump points and treatment of his fingers to facilitate grasp. See Figs. 12-11 and 12-12 for pre- and post-MEM views of K.P.'s hand and body position. These sessions were complemented by facilitated reaching to objects, sliding items, and separation of the forearm flexor and extensor muscle bodies.

By the final session, it was noted that most gains were maintained, and there was no pitting edema. Other benefits included a reduction of overactive skeletal muscle activity at the wrist, and K.P.'s elbow

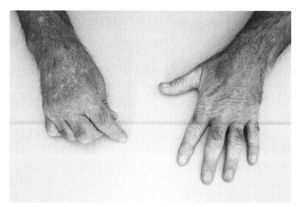

Figure 12-11   KP's right hand before treatment.

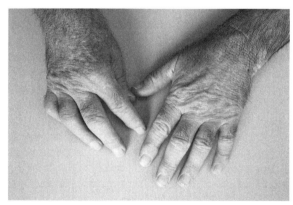

Figure 12-12   KP's right hand edema after four Manual Edema Mobilization treatment sessions.

extension lag had improved by 10 degrees. K.P. also reported some improvement in sensation in his hand. Overall, the greatest edema changes were evident at the thumb and index finger. It appeared that the exercises and caregiver education on MEM were of great benefit to K.P. At time of writing, K.P. had achieved a lateral pinch grasp and was working on leisure goals. He and his partner still did MEM at home if his edema increased.

CASE STUDY 3

Chronic Stroke with Neuropathic Pain

T.W. was 56-years-old when he had a left middle cerebral artery stroke, nine months prior to receiving intensive edema treatment. After acute rehabilitation, T.W. was transferred to a specialist neurological rehabilitation ward for one month, primarily to address his expressive and receptive aphasia and apraxia. At discharge, he was independent in ADL, mobility and had developed some communicative skills. The ward multidisciplinary team then referred T.W. for home-based therapy for four weeks, followed by further outpatient occupational therapy.

T.W.'s goals included using cutlery bilaterally, increased ease of bed mobility, to shop and cook independently, and use a computer mouse. T.W. presented with severe expressive aphasia, moderate receptive aphasia, ideational apraxia, and gross upper limb movement, but also poor strength and dexterity, reduced sensation, right sided neuropathic pain, and chronic edema. Formal cognitive assessment was limited due to T.W.'s aphasia; however, reduced speed of processing and reduced scanning efficiency were evident in functional tasks. T.W. also attended outpatient physiotherapy, speech pathology, and an education center.

Prior to his stroke, T.W. lived independently in another state and had retired. He was involved in darts and enjoyed fishing and sports. Poststroke, T.W. decided to move back to the same state as his family and live with his mother. His mother completed the majority of the domestic ADL. T.W. was not motivated to resume any domestic or household maintenance roles himself and was socially isolated. He reported little community involvement and tended to stay home to watch TV or go on the computer. The outpatient team was concerned regarding his loss of roles.

T.W.'s pain and edema continued to limit his rehabilitation, and he was identified as a candidate for intensive MEM at five months poststroke. At initial assessment, T.W. presented with chronic neuropathic pain and dystrophic changes. His mobility and overall task efficiency were limited by his guarded pain postures. Brawny, pitting edema was evident throughout the hand, restricting his function to gross grasp. T.W. reported neuropathic pain down his entire right side and was initially tense during therapist's contact. He reported less pain as each session progressed and always tolerated light touch.

Treatment on the first session was MEM up to Pump Point 2 and the posterior Big "V" (Fig. 12-13). T.W. was provided with an off-the-shelf Isotoner glove to wear at night and a basic home program of exercises, deep breathing, terminus and axilla massage, and sweeping. Between the first and second sessions, T.W.'s primary occupational therapist used MEM with him and reported reduction of nearly 1 cm at the wrist and MCP joints. On the second session, T.W. reported that he had done his home program once in the four days between sessions and had not used his affected arm in many bilateral tasks. T.W. had significant edema pooling behind his scapula and poor scapula stability during reaching tasks. MEM was conducted to Pump Point 4,

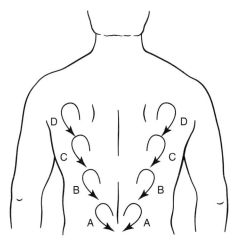

Figure 12-13 Manual Edema Mobilization Posterior "V" "clear" (*A* through *D*) and "flow" (*D* through *A*).

and emphasis was placed on low functional reach and shoulder movements. He was also provided with a elastic/cotton stockinette tube to wear with the glove and ideas to increase his hand use.

By the third session and reported daily following of his home program, T.W. no longer had brawny edema, and there was an increase in skin folds, particularly over the dorsal web spaces. MEM was done at all pump points and the posterior Big "V" (see Fig. 12-13). Functional activities were used at the end of treatment, including grasp and release of a cup and practice of a computer mouse. On the fourth session, there was an increase in pretreatment measurements, but this may have been due to the hot weather on that day and an apparent increase in T.W.'s neuropathic pain. The increase in pain only occurred once and reduced with MEM. Light bandaging was also tried overnight to reduce distal edema. On the final session for the case study, T.W. indicated that the bandaging was tolerable, but it did not result in significant measurable change.

After five intensive edema treatment sessions, T.W. had maintained reduction of his wrist and MCP joints edema. Edema at his axilla continued to respond well to treatment, but gains were not maintained between sessions. Treatment involved MEM to all pump points, the hand, the posterior Big "V," and the neck. Sternal nodes were not treated due to an extensive scar. MEM was progressed gradually due to medical contraindications, although his consultant approved of the intervention. Progress was enhanced by trunk stretches and functional movement within pain, and was limited by aphasia, pain, and learned nonuse. T.W. reported doing his home exercise and MEM program, but only once every few days. Edema changed from brawny to only

Continued

CASE STUDY 3

Chronic Stroke with Neuropathic Pain—cont'd

pitted on the ulnar side of the hand, and the skin at the upper arm had improved color and temperature. There was a slight functional increase in T.W.'s right grip strength, and his elbow extension lag had decreased from 10 degrees to neutral, without any passive ranging or facilitation at the elbow joint. T.W.'s primary occupational therapist continued with once to twice weekly sessions focusing on the above and functional hand use.

T.W. was discharged three months later from all outpatient services, given his limited involvement with home programs and limited progress. However, his pincer grip had improved, and he was able to pick up a glass and use a computer. T.W. was referred to a community-based acquired brain injury service for long-term follow-up, with goals of commencing volunteer work and resuming leisure interests. The occupational therapist recommended that T.W. be referred to a pain specialist as his neuropathic pain contributed to learned nonuse.

REVIEW QUESTIONS

1. Describe two key points unique to each of the three proposed theories of types of poststroke hand edema.
2. Treatment of poststroke hand edema is often impeded by what other neurological and sensory conditions?
3. Since trauma to the arm or hand poststroke could lead to edema and/or CRPS, list five ways that caregivers and treating staff can prevent trauma to the involved arm.
4. Describe how a functional treatment approach can decrease edema.

REFERENCES

1. Artzberger S: Edema reduction techniques: a biological rationale for selection. In Cooper C, editor: *Fundamentals of hand therapy: clinical reasoning and treatment guidelines for common diagnoses of the upper extremity*, St Louis, 2006, Mosby/Elsevier.
2. Artzberger S: A critical analysis of edema control techniques. *American Occupational Therapy Association Physical Disabilities Special Interest Section Quarterly* 28(2):1–3, 2005.
3. Artzberger S: Hand manual edema mobilization: overview of a new concept. *SAJHT* 1:1(edoc) 2003.
4. Artzberger S: Manual edema mobilization: treatment for edema in the subacute hand. In Mackin E, Callahan A, Skirven T, et al, editors: *Rehabilitation of the hand and upper extremity*, ed 5, St Louis, 2002, Mosby.
5. Artzberger S: Edema control: new perspectives. *American Occupational Therapy Association Physical Disabilities Special Interest Section Quarterly* 20:1, 1997.
6. Berne R, Levy M: *Physiology*, ed 4, St Louis, 1998, Mosby.
7. Boomkamp-Koppen H, Visser-Meily J, Post M, et al: Poststroke hand swelling and oedema: prevalence and relationship with impairment and disability. *Clin Rehabil* 19(5):552–559, 2005.
8. Braus D, Krauss J, Strobel J: The shoulder-hand syndrome after stroke: a prospective clinical trial. *Ann Neurol* 36(5):728–733, 1994.
9. Burge E, Kupper D, Finckh A, et al: Neutral functional realignment orthosis prevents hand pain in clients with subacute stroke: a randomized trial. *Arch Phys Med Rehabil* 89(10):1857–1862, 2008.
10. Burkhardt, A: Edema control. In Gillen G, Burkhardt A editors: *Stroke rehabilitation: a function-based approach*, ed 2, St Louis, 2004, Mosby.
11. Burkhardt, A: High stakes from the clinical horizons in the treatment of lymphedema —to Pump or not pump. *Occupational Therapy Forum* 44:1–5, 1990.
12. Casley-Smith JR: Modern treatment of lymphoedema. *Modern Medicine of Australia* 35(5):70-83, 1992.
13. Casley-Smith JR, Bjorlin M: Some parameters affecting the removal of oedema by massage—mechanical or manual. In Calsey-Smith JR, Piller NB, editors: *Progress in Lymphology X*, Adelaide, 1985, Univ Adelaide Press.
14. Casley-Smith JR, Casley-Smith JR: *Modern treatment for lymphoedema*, ed 5, Adelaide, 1997, Lymphoedema Association of Australia.
15. Casley-Smith JR, Casley-Smith JR: The pathophysiology of lymphoedema and the action of benzo-pyrones in reducing it. *Lymphology* 21(3):190: 190–194, 1988.
16. Casley-Smith JR, Gaffney RM: Excess plasma proteins as a cause of chronic inflammation and lymphodema: quantitative electron microscopy. *J Pathol* 133(3):243–272, 1981.
17. Chikly, B: *Silent waves: theory and practice of lymph drainage therapy*, Scottsdale, AZ, 2001, I.H.H.
18. Davis PM: *Steps to follow with hemiplegia*, ed, 2, Berlin, 2000, Springer.
19. Davis PM: *Steps to follow: a guide to the treatment of hemiplegia*, Heidelberg, 1985, Springer-Verlag.
20. Dirette D, Hinojosa J: Effects of continuous passive motion on the edematous hands of two persons with flaccid hemiplegia. *Am J Occup Ther* 48(5):403–409, 1994.
21. Exton-Smith A, Crockett D: Nature of oedema in paralysed limbs of hemiplegic patients. *BMJ* 2(5056):1280–83, 1957.
22. Faghri P: The effect of neuromuscular stimulation-induced muscle contraction versus elevation on hand edema in CVA patients. *J Hand Ther* 10(1):29–34, 1997.
23. Geurts A, Visschers B, van Limbeek J, Ribbers G: Systematic review of aetiology and treatment of post-stroke hand oedema and shoulder-hand syndrome. *Scand J Rehab Med* 32(1):4–10, 2000.
24. Gilmore P, Spaulding S, Vandervoort, A: Hemiplegic shoulder pain: implications for occupational therapy treatment. *Can J Occup Ther* 71(1):36–46, 2004.
25. Giudice, ML: Effects of continuous passive motion and elevation on hand edema. *Am J Occup Ther* 44(10):914–921, 1990.
26. Gracies JM, Marosszeky J, Renton R, et al: Short-term effects of dynamic lycra splints on upper limb in hemiplegic patients. *Arch Phys Med Rehabil* 81(12):1547–1555, 2000.
27. Guyton A, Hall J: *Textbook of medical physiology*, ed 9, Philadelphia, 1996, Saunders.
28. Hole JW: *Human anatomy and physiology*, ed 4, Dubuque, Iowa, 1987, William C Brown.
29. Howard S, Krishnagiri S: The use of manual edema mobilization for the reduction of persistent edema in the upper limb. *J Hand Ther* 14: (4):291–301, 2001.
30. Iwata M, Kondo I, Sato Y, et al: Prediction of reflex sympathetic dystrophy in hemiplegia by evaluation of hand edema. *Arch Phys Med Rehabil* 83(10):1428–1431, 2002.
31. Iwata M, Kondo I, Sato Y: Considerations on hand edema in hemiplegia. *Arch Orthop Surg Trauma* 34: 401–4, 1990.
32. Kasseroller R: *Compendium of Dr. Vodder's manual lymph drainage*, Heidelberg, Germany 1997, Haug.
33. Kondo I, Hosokawa K, Soma M, et al: Protocol to prevent shoulder-hand syndrome after stroke. *Arch Phys Med Rehabil* 82(11):1619–1623, 2001.

34. Korpelainen J, Sotaniemi K., Myllyla U: Autonomic nervous system disorders in stroke. *Clin Autonom Res* 9(6):325–333, 1999.

35. Kubik, S: Anatomy of the lymphatic system. In Foldi M, Foldi E, Kubik, S, editors: *Textbook of lymphology for physicians and lymphedema therapists*, Munich, 2003, Urban & Fischer.

36. Kurz I: *Textbook of Dr. Vodder's manual lymph drainage*, vol 2, ed 4, Heidelberg, Germany 1997, Haug.

37. Leduc A, Bastin R, Bourgeois P: Lymphatic reabsorption of proteins and pressotherapies. In Partsch H, editor: *Progress in Lymphology-XI*, Amsterdam, 1988b, Elsevier, *Excerpta Med Int Cong Ser* 779:591–592.

38. Leibovitz, A, Baumoehl Y, Roginsky Y, et al: Edema of the paretic hand in elderly post-stroke nursing patients. *Arch Gerontol Geriatr* 44(1):37–42, 2007.

39. Miller GE, Seale J: Lymphatic clearance during compression loading. *Lymphology* 12(161):161–168, 1981.

40. Pandyan A, Granat M, Stott D: Effects of electrical stimulation on flexion contractures in the hemiplegic wrist. *Clin Rehabil* 11(2):123–130, 1997.

41. Pertoldi S, Benedetto P: Shoulder-hand syndrome after stroke: a complex regional pain syndrome. *Eura Medicophys* 41(4):283–292, 2005.

42. Petrek JA, Pressman PI, Smith RA: Lymphedema: current issues in research and management. *CA Cancer J Clin* 50(5):292, 2001.

43. Post M, Visser-Meily J, Boomkamp-Koppen H, et al: Assessment of oedema in stroke patients: comparison of visual inspection by therapists and volumetric assessment. *Disabil Rehabil* 25(22):1265–1270, 2003.

44. Priganc V, Ito M: Changes in edema, pain, or range of motion following manual edema mobilization: a single-case design study. *J Hand Ther* 21(4):326–334, 2008.

45. Raines J, O'Donnell T, Kalisher L, et al: Selection of patients with lymphedema for compression therapy. *Am J Surg* 133(4):430–437, 1977.

46. Ring H, Rosenthal N: Controlled study of neuroprosthetic functional electrical stimulation in sub-acute post-stroke rehabilitation. *J Rehabil Med* 37(1):32–36, 2005.

47. Roper TA, Redford S, Raymond CT: Intermittent compression for the treatment of the oedematous hand in hemiplegic stroke: a randomized controlled trial. *Age and Aging* 28(1):9–13, 1999.

48. Stanley BG, Tribuzi SM: *Concepts in hand rehabilitation*, Philadelphia, 1992, FA Davis.

49. Tepperman PS, Greyson ND, Hilbert L, et al: Reflex sympathetic dystrophy in hemiplegia. *Arch Phys Med Rehabil* 65(8): 442–447, 1984.

50. Vasudevan S, Melvin J: Upper extremity edema control: rationale of the techniques. *Am J Occup Ther* 33(8):520–524, 1979.

51. Wang J, Yang C, Liaw M, et al: Suppressed cutaneous endothelial vascular control and hemodynamic changes in paretic extremities with edema in the extremities of patients with hemiplegia. *Arch Phys Med Rehabil* 83(7):1017–1023, 2002.

52. Wannapha P, Weiss D, Patel R: Reassessment of the incidence of complex regional pain syndrome type 1 following stroke. *Neurorehabil Neural Repair* 14(1):59–63, 2000.

53. Waylett-Rendal J, Seibly G: A study of the accuracy of a commercially available volumeter. *J Hand Ther* 4(10):10–13, 1991.

54. Wee J, Hopman W: Comparing consequences of right and left unilateral neglect in a stroke rehabilitation population. *Am J Phys Med Rehabil* 87: (11) 910–920, 2008.

55. Weiss S, Ellis LB: The circulation and unilateral edema in cerebral hemiplegia. *J Clin Invest* 9: 17–18, 1930.

56. Weissleder H, Schuchhardt C: *Lymphedema diagnosis and therapy*, ed 2, Bonn, 1997, Kagerer Kommunikation.

stephanie milazzo
glen gillen

chapter 13

Splinting Applications

key terms

alignment	function	prevention
biomechanics	low-load prolonged stress	splinting
clinical reasoning	neurophysiological approach	thermoplastics
contracture	orthotics	

chapter objectives

After completing this chapter, the reader will be able to accomplish the following:

1. Identify a variety of splinting options.
2. Review positive and negative aspects of commonly used splints.
3. Summarize the published research for splinting and persons who have had strokes.
4. Present rationales for splinting that consider current concepts of motor control, including biomechanical principles.
5. Critically analyze and reconsider the present approach to splinting, evaluating, and developing interventions for each extremity based on individual findings.

Any discussion of splinting of the upper extremity after stroke produces debate among occupational therapists. The use of splints after stroke can be traced as far back as 1911.[37] Since then the debate about whether to splint and about the rationales for splinting has continued.

The following principles guide splinting decisions for patients after stroke:

■ Splints are used to maintain or increase the length of soft tissues (e.g., muscles, tendons, and ligaments) by preventing or lengthening shortened tissues and preventing overstretching of antagonist soft tissue.

■ Splints are used to correct biomechanical malalignment, restoring muscles to normal resting length and protecting joint integrity. This biomechanical correction may result in a decrease in excessive skeletal muscle activity.

■ Splints are used to position the hand to assist in functional activities.

■ Splints may be used to promote independence in specific areas of occupation.

■ Splints compensate for weakness by providing external support, blocking the pull of muscle groups that have lost a balanced agonist-antagonist relationship, and altering the resting alignment of the joints to enhance functional postures.

The use of one splinting rationale (i.e., never splinting, always splinting, only using resting splints, etc.) for those after stroke is not effective because of the variety of patterns of impairments that occur after stroke. Each individual must be evaluated separately to determine if there are splinting needs. The sequelae of stroke are multilayered, encompassing a variety of symptoms and problem areas. The complexity of these problems has served as fuel for the splinting debate and the controversies surrounding splinting.

HISTORICAL PERSPECTIVE

Neuhaus and colleagues[37] have published a review of the splinting literature covering a 100-year period. Their review has documented two different approaches to splinting: the biomechanical approach and the neurophysiological approach.

The biomechanical perspective considers issues such as soft-tissue lengthening, prevention of contracture and deformity, maintenance of biomechanical alignment, and effects on the nonneural components of spasticity. In contrast, the neurophysiological perspective considers reflex inhibition, effects on the neural basis of spasticity, facilitation through sensory input, and inhibition through positioning and sensory input.

Earlier publications (from the early 1900s to the 1950s) emphasized a biomechanical approach, whereas literature after World War II emphasized a shift toward the neurophysiological frame of reference. During this time, therapists (Rood, Bobath, Knott, and Voss) developed theories based on neurophysiological principles. Many of the neurophysiological theorists clearly were opposed to splinting; others did not mention splinting at all as part of their treatment regimens. Rood (as cited by Stockmeyer[46]) stated that spasticity may be increased "by activating sensory stimuli of touch, pressure, and stretch, which result in undesirable contraction of muscle."

The neurophysiological perspective is currently being seriously questioned because of a lack of research support, and a shift is occurring toward a more comprehensive and current understanding of motor behavior. Nevertheless, many styles of splints and rationales are still based on neurophysiological principles.

To date, research does not support one style of splint as superior to another. Many of the statements and principles documented by the originators of the neurophysiological theories have been accepted as fact. In light of current understanding of motor control, these statements need to be analyzed and researched critically before further splinting interventions are based on these concepts. See Chapter 6 for a comprehensive review of these issues.

In general, a current review of the empirical literature related to stroke cannot support or refute the use of splints. There are few well-designed studies, and most have methodological flaws. Nonetheless, conclusions from current reviews include:

- Steultjens and colleagues[43] systematically reviewed five studies (two randomized controlled trials, two case control trials, and one crossover trial) that evaluated the effect of splinting on muscle tone. They found that all studies were of low methodological quality and that none of the studies presented significant results of the measures used. They concluded that there is insufficient evidence that splinting is effective for decreasing muscle tone.

- In their review of studies aimed at testing the effects of splinting on reducing tone, Ma and Trombly[27] concluded that "In summary, based on study of a total of only 35 participants with stroke, we can make no conclusive statement about splinting and its effect on spasticity. However, it appears that splinting for less time is the most beneficial. Research using much larger samples is needed." They also stated that "best evidence" indicates that, although commonly used, treatments using splints to decrease spasticity may be ineffective, and recommend that the treatment not be used.

- Based on a review of three studies, Tyson and Kent[49] concluded that "An upper limb orthosis does not affect on upper limb function, range of movement at the wrist, fingers or thumb, nor pain." It should be noted that these three studies involved a mixed group of participants, and none of the studies recruited participants who had functioning upper limbs.

- Lannin and Herbert[23] assessed the effectiveness of hand splinting on the hemiplegic upper extremity following stroke via a systematic review. They appraised 19 studies for content. Sixty-three percent were reports of case series, and 21% were randomized controlled trials. They concluded that there is insufficient evidence to either support or refute the effectiveness of hand splinting for adults following stroke. They also stated that the "limited research and a lack of a no-splint control group in all trials to date limit the usefulness of these results."

Clearly well-designed studies are critical to help therapists make informed decisions about this intervention. At this point, each patient/client must be evaluated individually based on their clinical presentation. Clinical reasoning suggestions follow.

DORSAL VERSUS VOLAR SPLINTING

Splint fabrication and points of contact are areas of continuing debate. The following studies have investigated this controversy.

Zislis[53] compared the effects of two different wrist-hand splints on a patient with spastic hemiplegia. The author used simultaneous electromyographic (EMG) recordings of the flexors and extensors in the forearm to provide an objective measure of muscle activity. EMG readings were taken with no splint, with a dorsal-based splint (which kept the wrist neutral, fingers adducted and extended, and thumb free) used in hopes of facilitating the extensors, and with a volar-based splint (which kept the wrist neutral, fingers extended and abducted, and thumb free).

Zislis' results[53] indicated that extensor muscle activity was not altered in any of the three situations, although flexor activity was varied. With no splint, flexor activity was exaggerated compared with extensor activity. The dorsal splint greatly increased the flexor activity, even more so than when no splint was worn. Finally, the volar-based splint diminished flexor activity and achieved a state of "balanced physiological activity between flexor and extensor muscle groups."

Zislis[53] drew the following conclusions from the patient he studied:

- Dorsal facilitation of the extensor was not evident, although dorsal facilitation of the flexors did occur.
- Flexor inhibition from volar cutaneous receptors may occur.
- Abduction and extension of the fingers may produce flexor inhibition.

Therefore, Zislis[53] recommended the use of volar-based splints with extension and abduction of the fingers.

Charait[7] observed 20 patients in her study of dorsal versus volar "functional position splints." In the splinted position, the wrist varied from less than neutral to 30 degrees, the thumb was abducted and opposed, and the fingers were positioned at 45 degrees of finger flexion at the metacarpophalangeal (MCP) and proximal interphalangeal (PIP) joints.

Charait[7] observed the amount of spasticity and voluntary movement in both groups. In the group wearing volar splints, four patients showed no change in spasticity or voluntary motion, and six experienced increased spasticity. In the group wearing dorsal splints, one patient showed no change, one experienced a considerable increase in spasticity, and eight had decreased spasticity (four of these also exhibited increased active finger and wrist extension). The author drew the following conclusions from her observations:

- Volar pressure facilitates flexor muscles.
- Dorsal pressure with decreased volar contact facilitates the extensors.
- Prolonged stretch enhances inhibition.

Charait[7] recommended splinting using dorsal-based appliances.

McPherson and colleagues[32] compared dorsal and volar resting splints for the reduction of hypertonus. They assigned 10 subjects with hypertonic wrist flexors to the dorsal or volar group. For the purposes of the study, the authors defined hypertonus as "the plastic, viscous, and elastic properties of the muscle resistant to stretch and with a tendency to return a limb to a particular abnormal resting posture." They used a spring-weighted scale to take measurements to assess the effectiveness of the splints in reducing hypertonicity. The results indicated no significant difference between the volar and dorsal splints in the reduction of hypertonus. As an aside, the authors found a correlation between age and reduction in hypertonus. The older subjects in the study demonstrated gradual but not statistically significant decline in hypertonus, whereas the younger adults demonstrated significant decline in hypertonus over 6 weeks.

Other studies have not compared dorsal and volar splinting specifically but instead have evaluated the effects of one or the other. Kaplan[21] evaluated 10 patients who wore dorsal wrist splints. His study set out to "determine whether prolonged therapy with a dorsal splint will inhibit or diminish hyperreflexia or stretch reflex and at the same time increase muscular power by sensorimotor stimulation." The splint used in this study positioned the wrist and fingers in extension and supported the thumb in abduction. Most of the subjects wore the splints at least eight hours per day, and Kaplan noted that many patients required several serial splints to increase the stretch on the flexors gradually. Patients were evaluated with EMG, strength testing, and hand function evaluation before and after splint application. The subjects in this study demonstrated "improvement in strength and function of muscle, with a decrease in the stretch reflex and spasticity . . . when a dorsal splint was properly applied in treatment of hemiplegia involving an upper extremity."

Brennan[5] studied the effects of volar-based splints on his subjects. At the end of his study the patients who wore the volar-based wrist and hand splints demonstrated increased range of passive movement in which no resistance to stretch could be felt.

In their study of positioning devices on normal and spastic hands, Mathiowetz, Bolding, and Trombly[30] demonstrated that a volar-based resting splint increased EMG activity as the subjects performed a grasping activity on the contralateral side. They noted that the volar splint "is the least desirable positioning device while the hemiplegic subject is doing any activity that requires a comparable effort to squeezing 50% maximal voluntary contraction of grip."

The variability in the aforementioned studies makes decisions regarding dorsal-versus volar-based treatment difficult to reach based on available research. Therapists must still evaluate each patient individually to determine the effect of variables on splinting outcomes. Moreover, the studies discussed in this chapter used a variety of outcome measures, varied in their methodologies, and implemented variable definitions and styles of splints.

REVIEW OF SPLINTS COMMONLY USED FOR PATIENTS AFTER STROKE

This section reviews positive and negative aspects of splints frequently used by occupational therapists; available research is discussed. Several of the following splints were developed based on a now outdated understanding of motor function. Some of the splints still may be useful and effective, although the rationale for their use may no longer be based on the original purpose of the splint.

Finger Spreader (Finger Abduction Splint)

The finger spreader (finger abduction splint) is fabricated of foam rubber and positions the fingers and thumb in abduction. According to Bobath,[3] the purpose of the splint is to "obtain extension of wrist and fingers.... Abduction not only facilitates extension of the fingers, but also reduces flexor spasticity throughout the whole arm.... It has a better and more dynamic effect than the use of a (standard) splint and reduces the possibility of edema." One should note that Bobath's rationale is not consistent with the current understanding of motor control and related neurological principles.

A sturdier version of this splint (fabricated of low-temperature plastic) was proposed by Doubilet and Polkow.[9] They recommended wearing the splint only during the day. Their paper includes anecdotal evidence of the effectiveness of the splint.

The finger abduction splint was worn by fifteen patients who were two to six months post stroke, these patients exhibited moderate to severe spasticity of the fingers and wrist, decreased range of motion, and edema in the wrist and hand. After one week of using the splint plus standard treatment in the therapy sessions a moderate reduction of spasticity was seen in these patients.

Doubilet and Polkow[9] concluded that the splint results are promising and warrant continued trial and experimentation.

Mathiowetz, Bolding, and Trombly[30] objectively evaluated the finger abduction splint in a study investigating the effects of a variety of splints on the distal muscle activity of normal and hemiplegic subjects. Subjects wore the splints while performing resistive activities with the opposite hand. The results indicated "significantly greater EMG activity for the finger spreader compared to no device in the flexor carpi radialis of normal subjects during grasping" with the contralateral hand. In hemiplegic subjects, the finger spreader did not

evoke less EMG activity than no device. According to the authors, the belief that this splint decreases spasticity shortly after application needs to be questioned seriously.

The finger spreader may be useful in maintaining the length of the flexors; however, wrist position is not considered with this splint, and the therapist must be aware of the wrist position. To control this problem, the therapist may combine the finger spreader with a standard wrist extension splint. Because the splint is subtle in terms of corrective forces, it may be indicated for patients with low tolerance for other, more cumbersome devices and for patients with low pain thresholds. Donning and doffing procedures are straightforward for the confused patient (Fig. 13-1).

Firm Cone

The firm cone can be fabricated of low-temperature plastic or purchased commercially; it is based on the traditional theories of Rood. Rood's theory (as interpreted by Stockmeyer[46]) states that firm and prolonged pressure over the flexor surface of the palm and fingers results in an inhibition of the long flexors. A more current understanding of the mechanism of this splint from a biomechanical and functional perspective is that the cone is positioned to place stretch on the shortened long flexors and is graded progressively to increase stress to the soft tissues to promote a more normal resting length. The cone initially is positioned with the narrow end of the cone toward the radial side of the hand in the web space if the hand is excessively tight. As the hand begins to relax from the directed stress, the ideal *biomechanical* position is for the cone to be positioned opposite to the initial position; that is, the wide end of the cone is placed in the radial side of the hand in the web space, and the narrow end is placed in the ulnar side of the hand (Fig. 13-2). The therapist can use strapping material to hold the cone in place. This device was included in the study by Mathiowetz, Bolding, and Trombly;[30] the researchers found that the cone did not evoke significantly less EMG activity during contralateral resisted function.

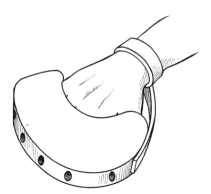

Figure 13-1   Bobath finger spreader (finger abduction splint).

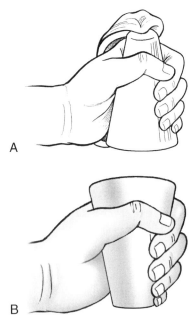

Figure 13-2   **A** and **B**, Firm cone.

Neurophysiological principles aside, the cone may be an effective positioning device for patients who have developed contracture in the long flexors. Combined applications of the cone with a standard wrist-extension splint, controlling the stretch on the wrist and digit flexors separately, are feasible. The size of the cone and the angle of wrist extension can be graded as the patient's status improves.

Another practical use of the cone is in the prevention of maceration of tissue in patients with moderate to severe flexion of the digits. The maintenance of flexor length is required for hygiene and cosmesis. Similar to the use of the finger abduction splint, the use of the cone in isolation does not provide wrist support, thus predisposing the wrist to a flexed posture. Donning and doffing procedures are straightforward.

Orthokinetic Orthotics

According to Neeman and Neeman,[34] the term *orthokinetic orthosis* "describes a cuff-shaped dynamic orthopaedic appliance which does not include rigid polymer or metal components. It does not apply any extraneous modulating force or constraint, in contrast to the typical splint." The orthokinetic cuffs designed by Blashy and Fuchs-Neeman[1] have been used for almost 40 years for patients with muscle weakness, muscle paresis, and resulting agonist-antagonist imbalance. The action of these orthoses is "exerted through internal restoration of neuromuscular balance between agonist and antagonist musculatures, by input of mild neural stimuli to mechanoreceptors in specifically targeted skin areas."[1] The designers state that the neurophysiological mechanism involves activation of paretic agonist muscles and reciprocal inhibition of antagonist musculature.

The orthokinetic cuffs are fabricated of ribbed elastic bandage material applied circumferentially around various aspects of the patient's upper extremity and are held on the arm by fasteners. Half of the cuff is designed to be elastic (the active field), and the other half of the cuff is sewn to reduce the stretch (the inactive field). The active field is worn over the muscle belly to be activated, and the inactive field is placed over the antagonist.

Neeman and Neeman have published several studies[33-36] on the effectiveness of these cuffs in the rehabilitation of the upper extremity after stroke. They concluded that use of the cuffs results in pronounced restoration of agonist-antagonist muscle balance, increased active range of motion (ROM) throughout the extremity, and increased ability to participate in functional tasks.

The orthokinetic cuffs have been subjected to the greatest number of efficacy studies, all showing positive results. Fabrication guidelines are stated clearly in the cited studies, and the cuffs are applied easily and are comfortable.

The neurophysiological rationale for the orthokinetic cuff has not been established fully. The active field may produce cutaneous stimulation and activate the exteroceptors of the skin and Ia afferent neurons of the muscle spindle. The inactive field seems to provide sustained deep pressure, which may produce an inhibitory response (Fig. 13-3).

Orthokinetic Wrist Splint

The dynamic design of the orthokinetic wrist splint is based on the concepts of Rood (as cited in Stockmeyer[46]). Components of the splint include a firm cone in the palm of the hand, a volar-based forearm support, elastic straps to secure the forearm support by acting as orthokinetic cuffs, and a wrist hinge.[22] This splint has been recommended for patients with flexor hypertonicity who have at least minimal voluntary extensor activity. However, no data support the effectiveness of this splint (Fig. 13-4).

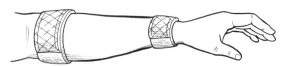

Figure 13-3   Orthokinetic orthotics.

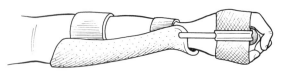

Figure 13-4   Orthokinetic wrist splint.

Spasticity Reduction Splint

The spasticity reduction splint was developed by Snook[44] and is based on the Bobath[3] principle of reflex-inhibiting patterns that has not been supported by current research. The splint is fabricated of low-temperature plastic. The forearm support is dorsal based and continues into a volar-based finger support. The wrist is positioned in 30 degrees of wrist extension; the MCP joints are at 45 degrees of flexion. The interphalangeal (IP) joints are extended fully, the fingers are abducted with separators, and the thumb is positioned in abduction and extension. Snook[44] notes that if a flexion contracture is present, the wrist may be positioned at neutral or slightly less than neutral without producing a significant effect on the effectiveness of the splint.

Snook[44] recommended an intermittent wearing schedule, observing that "a decrease in tone is usually seen almost immediately upon splint application; however, after an extended period of wearing time, tone tends to gradually increase."

Snook's original article described fabrication and provided clinical observations and case studies. Research was not included in this article. Snook[44] concluded that based on preliminary findings, the spasticity reduction splint has an effect "on the reduction and normalization of tone" and should be considered as a therapeutic tool when the therapist is dealing with a spastic hand.

McPherson[31] evaluated the effect of this splint on five severely and profoundly handicapped subjects (no patients who had strokes were included in this study). His results demonstrated a significant reduction in hypertonicity after four weeks of splint use. He further stated that the effects of the splint were not permanent; after the splints were removed, hypertonicity increased. The author measured "the force of spastic wrist flexors in pounds of pull on a spring weighted scale."

The fabrication guidelines for this splint are outlined in Snook's article.[44] Compliance in wearing schedules may be problematic because the splint is bulky and the wrist and hand are held in an extreme range. Many patients require assistance donning the splint, depending on the level of flexion posturing in their hands.

Although the principles that this splint was based on originally are out of date, this splint maintains a stretch to the musculature that traditionally becomes shortened in patients after stroke. It may be useful as an adjunct to treatment focusing on the maintenance of soft-tissue length. Further research is required on patients after cerebrovascular accident (CVA) to document this splint's effectiveness (Fig. 13-5).

Pressure Splints (Air Splints)

The use of inflatable pressure splints as adjuncts to therapy was first advocated by Johnstone.[19] These splints are commercially available and exert continuous or intermittent

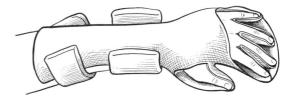

Figure 13-5 Spasticity reduction splint.

pressure to the area to which they are applied. The pressure of the splints should not exceed 40 mm Hg.[42] According to Poole and colleagues,[42] "inflatable splints have been used with patients who have had a stroke to reduce tone, facilitate muscle activity around a joint, facilitate sensory input, control edema, and reduce pain." Their article includes a review of the neurophysiological rationales for the use of inflatable splints.

Three studies have been published of investigations of the effectiveness of inflatable splints on patients who have had strokes. The earliest was a case study by Bloch and Evans;[2] its results indicated a reduction in spasticity and an increase in hand ROM.

Nicholson[38] (as cited by Poole and Whitney[41]) treated patients for one week with inflatable splints along with weight-bearing patterns. At the end of the treatment protocol, no improvements had occurred in sensation, strength, and ROM.

Likewise, Poole and colleagues[42] treated 18 persons and assigned them to splint or nonsplint treatment protocols. The splinted group wore the splint for 30 minutes five days a week for three weeks. The splinted patients did not perform activities with the splinted extremity. The authors' results indicated no statistically significant differences in mean change in upper extremity sensation, pain, and motor function between the splinted and nonsplinted groups.

Although inflatable pressure splints do not seem to elicit the effects originally proposed, some therapists may consider using this style of splint to enhance functional performance during weight-bearing activities (Fig. 13-6). In essence, this splint can be used to control the degrees of freedom in the upper extremity, thereby promoting functional use during daily activities.

Wrist Extension Splints

Wrist splints are commonly used in stroke populations to prevent wrist contracture and to stabilize the wrist to provide the fingers a steady base from which they can function. Lannin and colleagues[25] aimed to determine whether wearing a hand splint, which positions the wrist in either a neutral or an extended position, reduces wrist contracture in adults with hemiplegia after stroke (N=63). The subjects were randomized to either a control group (routine therapy) or one of two intervention groups (routine therapy and splint in either a neutral or an extended wrist

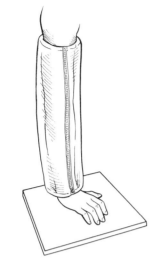

Figure 13-6   Inflatable pressure splint.

position). Participants in the neutral splint group wore a hand splint, which positioned the wrist in zero degrees to 10 degrees extension, and those in the extension splint group wore a hand splint, which positioned the wrist in a comfortable end-of-range position (greater than 45 degrees wrist extension) with the MCP and IP joints extended. The splints were worn overnight for, on average, between nine and 12 hours, for four weeks. The outcome was extensibility of the wrist and long finger flexor muscles (angle of wrist extension at a standardized torque). The authors concluded that splinting the wrist in either the neutral or extended wrist position for four weeks did not reduce wrist contracture after stroke.

Resting Splints

The resting splint can be dorsal or volar based. The suggested position is 20 to 30 degrees of wrist extension, MCP joints at 40 to 45 degrees of flexion, IP joints in 10 to 20 degrees of flexion, and thumb in opposition to the index finger.[29]

One of the most important aspects of clinical reasoning is that each patient must be evaluated and treated individually, and these goniometrics should be used as a guideline only. The goal is to adjust the splint to promote a low-load prolonged stress (LLPS) to achieve a more advantageous biomechanical position as necessary.

Lannin and colleagues[24] evaluated the effects of four weeks of hand splinting on the length of finger and wrist flexor muscles, hand function, and pain in people with acquired brain damage via randomized, assessor-blinded trial. They examined 28 adults, all within six months of injury. Subjects in both experimental (n=17) and control (n=11) groups participated in routine therapy-motor training for upper limb use and upper limb stretches five days a week. The experimental group also wore an immobilizing hand splint in the functional position (10 to 30 degrees wrist extension) for a maximum of 12 hours each night for the duration of the four-week intervention period. Outcomes included length of the wrist and extrinsic finger flexor muscles measured via torque-controlled range of wrist extension with the fingers extended, the Motor Assessment Scale, and pain via a visual analog scale. The authors found that the effects of splinting were statistically nonsignificant and clinically unimportant, and they concluded that "an overnight splint-wearing regimen with the affected hand in the functional position does not produce clinically beneficial effects in adults with acquired brain impairment."

The resting splint is used commonly in clinics. Although the splint may be effective in the long-term for patients after stroke, therapists must analyze critically the effects of this splint on the patient with acute and subacute impairments. This splint blocks any automatic and voluntary attempts at movement, thereby promoting learned nonuse. It completely covers the surface of the hand (thus preventing sensory input) and gives full passive support to the wrist and digits, which may be contrary to treatment programs attempting to train patients to be responsible for the positioning and ranging of their hands. Therapists need to consider alternatives to this splint.

Mathiowetz, Bolding, and Trombly[30] demonstrated that the use of a volar-based resting splint increased EMG activity in hemiplegic subjects who were performing grasping tasks with the opposite extremity. They concluded that this type of volar splint "is the least desirable positioning device while the hemiplegic subject is doing any activity that requires a comparable effort to squeezing fifty percent maximal voluntary contraction of grip."

Resting splints can be custom fabricated; they also are available commercially. The therapist may consider nighttime use of the resting splint for prevention of soft-tissue contracture, but this style of splint should not be worn during daytime because it completely blocks spontaneous function, sensory input, and self-management of the hand and may promote learned nonuse (Fig. 13-7).

Tone and Positioning Splint

The tone and positioning splint is semidynamic and is commercially available from Smith & Nephew Rolyan. The splint supports the thumb in abduction and extension with a neoprene glove. The tone and positioning splint includes an elastic strap that is wrapped spirally up the forearm, providing a dynamic assist into pronation and supination. Data supporting the effectiveness of this splint are not available.

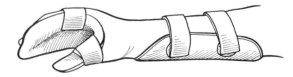

Figure 13-7   Resting pan splint and submaximal range splint.

Casey and Kratz[6] have published a paper on the thumb abduction supinator splint. This splint is similar in design to the commercially available tone and positioning splint. Their paper included fabrication guidelines and recommended a wearing schedule of three to four hours on, and then 30 minutes to one hour off to allow the skin to be exposed to the air. They recommended using the splints on patients with mild to moderate spasticity without severe contractures: those who posture in a pattern of forearm pronation, with a fisted hand, and with the thumb in the palm.

The tone and positioning splint and thumb abduction supinator splint may present difficulties to patients learning to don and doff splints independently. These splints are designed to be used to enhance positioning and to be worn during functional activities. They may be particularly effective if worn during activities that result in stereotypical posturing of the limb (e.g., gait and transfers). They also may be effective during upper extremity activities because the digits are free to move (Fig. 13-8).

Thumb Loop and Thumb Abduction Splint

Variations of the thumb abduction splint have been proposed by several authors.[8,16,45] The papers cited in the references include fabrication guidelines; the splint is commercially available. The thumb abduction splint is considered a semidynamic splint, and the focus of positioning is on thumb and wrist alignment. The strapping material used in the fabrication of this splint positions the thumb in abduction and aligns the wrist in a position of slight radial wrist extension. The hand is placed in a position that enhances prehension, manipulation, and release of objects, and provides the freedom of movement needed for bilateral coordination.[16]

Stern[45] stated that another indication for use is during any activity involving effort, particularly when performing fine activities with the unaffected limb results in increased thumb adduction on the affected side. Therefore, this splint has been suggested for positioning and enhancement of functional performance.

Stern[45] cautioned that, "For this splint to be of any value, the patients must be able to use the affected hand for grasp and release, their main problem being adduction of the thumb, which prevents sufficient opening of the hand to allow for palmar grasp." Patients with fixed adductor contracture are less likely to benefit.

Research evaluating the effectiveness of this splint in the adult population is lacking. Currie and Mendiola[8] evaluated the effectiveness of a variation of this type of splint on five children with "mild to moderate spastic hemiplegic cerebral palsy." These children exhibited a cortical thumb (adducted thumb) at rest, and their hand functions were limited to a "raking" ulnar type of prehension pattern.

With the use of this splint, all five children's resting thumb patterns were enhanced, and their prehension patterns improved to a radial grasp, usually in a three jaw chuck or large cylindrical prehension pattern, depending on the size of the object being manipulated (Fig. 13-9).

Hand-Based Thumb Abduction Splint

If the patient has controlled wrist movement in flexion and extension (not necessarily full wrist ROM, but some isolated control) but continues to have flexor activity influencing the digits, a hand-based thumb abduction C-spacer splint may be useful during functional activities. The splint is custom fabricated from thermoplastic material. The thumb abduction splint positions the thumb in an enhanced prehension pattern for manipulation of objects during grasp and release activities (Fig. 13-10).

MacKinnon Splint

Although the MacKinnon splint was developed for the pediatric population, it may be indicated at times for the adult population. The splint includes a dorsal-based forearm support that wraps three fourths of the distal half of the forearm, a dowel placed in the palm of the hand to provide pressure on the MCP heads, and rubber tubing

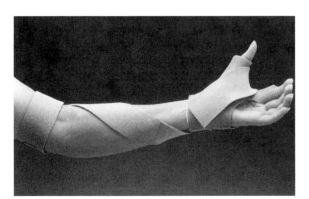

Figure 13-8 Rolyan tone and positioning splint. (Courtesy Smith & Nephew Rolyan, Germantown, WI.)

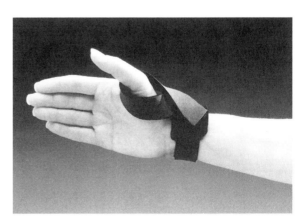

Figure 13-9 Rolyan thumb loop and thumb abduction splint. (Courtesy of Smith & Nephew Rolyan, Germantown, WI.)

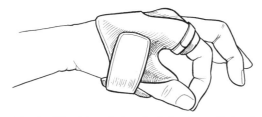

Figure 13-10 Hand-based thumb abduction splint to be used when wrist control returns; thumb requires abduction assistance for functional opposition activities.

attaching the dowel to the dorsal forearm support; the fingers are left free to assume functional patterns.

The goal of this splint is to release the overactive finger flexors and adductor pollicis to gain balanced muscle action of the wrist. The paper by MacKinnon, Sanderson, and Buchanan[28] included fabrication guidelines and observations of approximately 30 children who used the splint and gained improved hand awareness, increased use, and decreased spasticity when the splint was removed. Research regarding the effectiveness of this splint is not available, and it has not been documented for use with the adult patient recovering from CVA (Fig. 13-11).

Submaximal Range Splint

The submaximal range splint was described by Peterson;[40] its design is based on the clinical observation that muscles splinted on full stretch or maximal ROM increased in tightness.

The splint is fabricated in the fashion of a resting hand splint. The splint should position the distal extremity with the thumb in partial opposition to the index finger, the MCP and PIP joints in 45 degrees of flexion, with distal interphalangeal (DIP) joint extension, and the wrist in 10 to 20 degrees of extension; the splint should provide pressure to the palmar arch. If the patient cannot achieve this ideal range, each joint should be positioned in five to 10 degrees less than the available range.[10] Fabrication guidelines are the same as those for a resting hand splint.

No research is available that evaluates the effectiveness of this splint, but the precautionary statements about the resting hand splint are similar to those for this splint design (see Fig. 13-7).

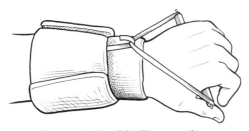

Figure 13-11 MacKinnon splint.

Serpentine Splint

The serpentine splint must be custom fabricated from thermoplastic materials. The splint was originally designed for use with pediatric patients with cerebral palsy who had difficulty grasping objects. The splint is adapted easily to the adult with neurological impairments. The serpentine splint provides sufficient thumb abduction support, positions the hand and wrist in a more optimal position for function, and allows "active wrist function in the child with moderately increased tone."[47] The designers of the splint feel that the serpentine splint inhibits the thumb-in-palm reflex by using the thumb abduction position.

The authors have used an adaptation of the serpentine splint with several patients after CVA, with positive outcomes. The serpentine splint can be used for patients with mild to moderate increased skeletal muscle activity (it is not recommended for the flaccid hand). This splint is never recommended for hands that exhibit severe increases in skeletal muscle activity for the reasons outlined previously in this chapter.

The wrist is positioned in 20 to 30 degrees of extension, the thumb is positioned in 30 to 40 degrees of abduction, and the material continues two thirds of the length proximally up the forearm. The splint positions the hand in a more functional position for grasping exercises and activities.[47] The splint is worn during the day for activities and wrist support and is removed at night. The serpentine splint requires maximal assistance for application and moderate assistance for removal and is a practical alternative to more conventional static splints. Because the splint is an open splint, it is less confining; it also is lightweight and allows for air circulation, which results in decreased perspiration, decreased skin maceration, and reduced potential for skin breakdown. When fabricating this splint, the therapist places the roll in the palm, then wraps it around the ulnar aspect of the hand, forms it over the dorsum of the hand through the web space, brings the roll over the thenar eminence and under the base of the thumb, and continues wrapping the material two thirds of the way up the forearm. The seam made by rolling the splint material should face away from the skin to prevent skin irritation and breakdown (Fig. 13-12).

Drop-Out Splint

The drop-out splint is a custom-fabricated splint designed to decrease elbow contractures that may be common in the patient after stroke. The splint is designed from thermoplastic material positioned volarly on the humerus, distal to the axilla; it extends into the palm of the hand proximal to the distal palmar crease. The splint is fabricated with the shoulder and humerus externally rotated and the forearm in as much supination as possible. It is customized with a gentle stretch to the contracted elbow

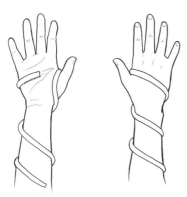

Figure 13-12 Serpentine splint.

joint (not to the point of discomfort) using the LLPS principles in the section Treatment of Joint Contractures with Low-Load Prolonged Stress. The splint is used during rest periods to maximize the low-load prolonged stretch to the elbow. The elbow contracture is measured with a goniometer before application of the splint and checked weekly to allow appropriate adjustments of the splint for increased extension as needed. As with all splints used in the patient who has had a stroke, but especially for splints using the low-load prolonged stretching principles, the therapist must monitor the upper extremity frequently for skin maceration and breakdown (Fig. 13-13).

Belly Gutter Splint for Proximal Interphalangeal Joint Flexion Contractures

The belly gutter splint is a static PIP extension splint custom fabricated from thermoplastic material. Many PIP extension splints are commercially available. Joint Jack, LMB Wire-foam, and safety-pin splints, which apply two points of volar pressure to make a perpendicular pull on the involved segments, are a few. If the flexion contracture is greater than 35 degrees, these splints are not effective. Dynamic extension splints and the belly gutter splint provide traction tension at a 90-degree angle to the phalanx. The belly gutter splint provides the 90-degree angle pull by incorporating a convex belly in the middle of the gutter.[52] When fabricating and applying this splint, the therapist must place the Velcro strap directly over the PIP joint; the

belly of the splint must be directly under the PIP joint axis for the splint to be effective. The authors have found this splint to be effective for flexion contractures of the PIP joint from approximately 15 degrees of contracture to 35 degrees of contracture. A PIP joint contracture of more than 35 degrees requires dynamic splinting.[11] The belly gutter splint is used at the beginning of treatment for one hour on and one hour off. Gradually, as the contracture decreases, the time may be extended to as much as four hours, but as always, close monitoring of the splint is mandatory (Fig. 13-14).

Inflatable Hand Splint

The inflatable hand splint, which is commercially available, is marketed for contracture management of the population in the chronic stages of stroke rehabilitation. The splint consists of an adjustable volar-based wrist support that is easily adjusted to achieve the desired range of extension. The palmar aspect of the splint is an air bladder that can be inflated or deflated easily, depending on the desired stretch and level of contracture. The splint is easily donned and is comfortable (Fig. 13-15).

The therapist must consider many issues when prescribing or designing a splint for use on persons after stroke. The following section exposes therapists to the complexity of issues to be considered during the splinting evaluation.

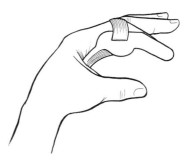

Figure 13-14 Belly gutter splint for proximal interphalangeal joint flexion contractures.

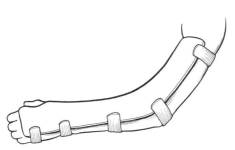

Figure 13-13 Drop-out splint.

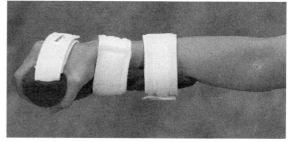

Figure 13-15 DeRoyal's Pucci Air-T Inflatable Hand Orthosis. (Manufactured and distributed by DeRoyal.)

CONSIDERATIONS IN PRESCRIBING AND DESIGNING A SPLINT FOR THE DISTAL EXTREMITY AFTER STROKE

Spasticity

Many commonly used splints are applied in the hope that they will inhibit spasticity with a result of improved function. As outlined in Chapter 10, the cause-and-effect relationship between spasticity and function has not been supported in available research.

The link between spasticity and contracture has been well-documented; see Chapter 10. Therefore, splinting of patients who are experiencing distal spasticity may be indicated to prevent painful contractures and loss of tissue length. This differentiation is important if therapists are to analyze objectively the effectiveness of the splints provided.

Hummelsheim and colleagues[17] have demonstrated that prolonged stretch resulted in "a significant reduction in the spastic hypertonus in elbow, hand and finger flexors" of the 15 patients they studied. Spasticity was measured by the Ashworth Scale. The EMG recordings included in their study objectively demonstrated that late EMG potentials are reduced or disappear after sustained muscle stretch. The authors hypothesized that "the beneficial effect resulting from sustained muscle stretch is due to stretch receptor fatigue or adaptation to the new extended position."

Although this study was based on manual stretching techniques, the same principles may be applied to splinting. Therefore, splinting may be used as an adjunct to interventions aimed at relaxing the distal extremity.

Feldman[10] recommended early splinting interventions for patients with spasticity; treatment should begin before the spasticity becomes severe. She stated that "the longer tonal influences are left to bear on the joints, the greater the risk for contractures and other complications." Feldman also warned that patients with severe spasticity should not be considered for splinting programs. These patients are at risk for skin breakdown, edema, and circulatory impairment. Instead, Feldman recommended interventions with spasticity medication and nerve blocks for these patients (see Chapter 10).

Soft-Tissue Shortening

Many of the wrists and hands that therapists evaluate are immobilized. This immobilization may be because of weakness, static splinting for prolonged periods, excessive skeletal muscle activity, or contracture. The deleterious effects of immobilization begin to occur soon after immobilization begins.

Consequences of prolonged positioning following immobilization include anatomical, biochemical, and physiological changes. Specific changes include the number of sarcomeres, protein content, loss of muscle weight, the amount of passive and active soft-tissue tension, decreased aerobic function, and type I and II fiber atrophy.[14]

From their review of the literature, Gossman, Sahrman, and Rose[14] concluded that "evidence from experimental studies and clinical observations clearly indicates that muscle is an extremely mutable (prone to change) tissue. Change is more pronounced when a muscle is shortened than when it is lengthened. The changes can be deleterious, but they are reversible, a condition that can be used in correcting movement dysfunction."

Halar and Bell[15] stated that if mild contractures have formed, prolonged stretches for 30 minutes are effective. More severe contractures may require longer sustained stretch through splinting. They recommended application of heat before splinting to decrease the viscous properties of connective tissue and maximize the effects of stretching.

During the splinting evaluation, the therapist must assess the differences between extrinsic and intrinsic tightness and joint contractures. Therapists must understand the biomechanical mechanism of the extrinsic flexors and extensors. To review, when the wrist and digits are in composite flexion (i.e., all joints are flexed), the extensors are stretched fully and the flexors are slack. In contrast, when the wrist and digits are in composite extension (i.e., all joints are extended), the flexors are stretched fully and the extensors are slack (Fig. 13-16).

Fess and Philips[11] suggested altering wrist posture to detect extrinsic soft-tissue involvement. If extrinsic tightness is evident, changing the wrist posture from slight extension to flexion results in an increase in the ROM of the digits (the tenodesis effect). In contrast, if ROM limitations are caused by a pathological condition of the joint, an altered wrist position does not affect the ROM. Evaluation procedures for assessing extrinsic tightness are as follows: (1) extend the wrist with the digits flexed, and (2) maintain the wrist in extension and attempt to extend the digits. If

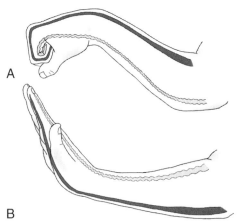

Figure 13-16 Normal excursion of the flexor and extensor muscles acting on the wrist and hand. **A**, Wrist and digits flexed: extensors are fully stretched (elongated) and the flexors are slack (shortened). **B**, Wrist and digits extended: flexors are fully stretched (elongated) and extensors are slack (shortened).

composite extension can be achieved, then the extrinsic flexors have full excursion. If the digits cannot be extended while the wrist is in extension, the evaluation must continue to determine whether the limitation is related to a pathological joint condition or extrinsic flexor tightness. The evaluation continues as follows: (3) flex the wrist and determine if the excursion of the digits toward extension (tenodesis) is increased. If so, the limitation is due to extrinsic flexor tightness. If no change in available digit extension occurs, the pathological condition of the joint is the limiting factor[48] (Fig. 13-17).

In terms of the biomechanics of the intrinsic mechanism, when the MCP joints are flexed and the IP joints are extended (intrinsic plus), the intrinsic muscles are shortened. In contrast, when the MCP joints are extended and IP joints are flexed, the intrinsic muscles are fully stretched (Fig.13-18).

Fess and Philips[11] suggested evaluating intrinsic tightness by holding the MCP joint in extension and

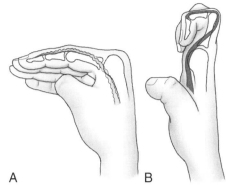

Figure 13-18 Normal excursion of the intrinsic muscles (lumbricales). **A,** When the metacarpophalangeal joints are flexed and the interphalangeal joints are extended ("intrinsic plus"), the intrinsic muscles are in a shortened position. **B,** When the metacarpophalangeal joints are extended and the interphalangeal joints are flexed ("intrinsic minus"), the intrinsic muscles are elongated.

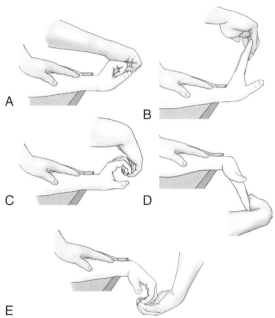

Figure 13-17 Testing for extrinsic shortening. **A,** The therapist extends the wrist with the digits flexed. This position partially elongates the long flexors. **B,** The therapist maintains the wrist in extension and extends the digits. If composite extension can be achieved, the extrinsic flexors have full excursion and the evaluation is complete. **C,** If the therapist cannot extend the wrist and digits fully simultaneously, the evaluation must continue to determine whether the limitation is related to a pathological joint condition or extrinsic flexor tightness. **D,** The therapist flexes the wrist to determine if excursion of the digits toward extension (tenodesis) is increased. If so, the limitation is due to extrinsic flexor tightness. **E,** If no change in available digit extension occurs while the wrist is flexed, the pathological joint condition (i.e., bony contracture) is the limiting factor.

attempting to flex the PIP joint; full passive flexion of the PIP joint is absent if the intrinsic muscles have become tight. With intrinsic tightness, however, one may possibly attain full passive PIP joint flexion with the MCP joint in flexion (Fig. 13-19).

Many patients also develop contracture of the extensor tendons. Therapists must determine whether the alteration of the position of the MCP joint affects the amount of flexion obtained at the PIP joint. If shortening or adhesion of the extensor has occurred, the therapist is able to flex the PIP joint further with the MCP joint extended than with it flexed.[48] This phenomenon occurs because extension relaxes the extensor system, whereas flexion builds up the passive tension.

Collateral ligament tightness of the PIP joint limits PIP joint motion regardless of the position of the MCP joint.[18] The testing is performed by flexing the PIP joint with the MCP joint extended and again with it flexed; if PIP joint motion is limited in both testing positions, the collateral ligaments of the PIP joint have shortened (Fig. 13-20) and splinting of the PIP joint is indicated. A dynamic PIP extension splint is used if the contracture is greater than 35 degrees; a static PIP extension splint is used if the contracture is less than 35 degrees.[11] A combination of both splints sometimes is used; the dynamic splint is applied for the more severe contracture, and a static extension splint is worn after the contracture is reduced to less than 35 degrees.

Loss of active flexion of the DIP joint may be caused by joint contracture or contracture of the oblique retinacular ligament. The therapist performs the oblique retinacular ligament tightness test by passively flexing the DIP joint with the PIP joint in extension and then repeating the test with the PIP joint in flexion. If more motion

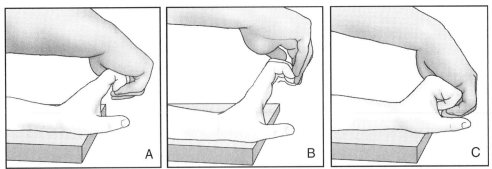

Figure 13-19 Testing for intrinsic shortening. **A,** The therapist holds the metacarpophalangeal joints in extension and attempts to flex the proximal interphalangeal joints. If the therapist can achieve this position, then full excursion of the intrinsic muscles is present. The evaluation is complete. **B,** If therapist cannot achieve full passive flexion of the proximal interphalangeal joint while the metacarpophalangeal joints are extended, the intrinsic muscles have become tight. **C,** With intrinsic tightness, however, the therapist possibly may attain full passive proximal interphalangeal flexion with the metacarpophalangeal joint in flexion.

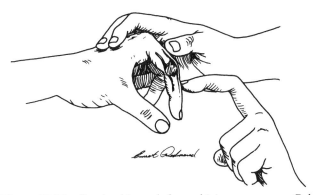

Figure 13-20 Proximal interphalangeal joint contracture. Collateral ligament tightness limits proximal phalangeal joint motion, regardless of the position of the metacarpophalangeal joint. (From Hunter JM, Mackin E, Callahan A: *Rehabilitation of the hand: surgery and therapy*, ed 4, St Louis, 1995, Mosby.)

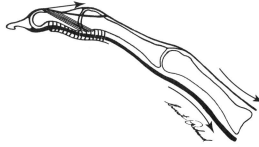

Figure 13-21 Oblique retinacular ligament. (Redrawn from Tubiana R: *The hand*, Philadelphia, 1981, Saunders.)

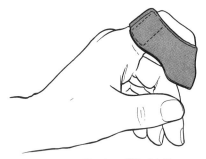

Figure 13-22 Flexion ("Buddy") strap.

occurs when the PIP joint is flexed than when it is extended, a shortening or contracture of this ligament has occurred (Fig. 13-21). If equal loss of flexion occurs with the PIP joint flexed or extended, a joint contracture is evident.[18] Contracture of the DIP joint with decreased DIP flexion can be treated with the use of a flexion strap with the MCP, PIP, and DIP joints in as much flexion as possible. This strap can be fabricated from Velcro strapping and is commercially available (Fig. 13-22). The patient can use the strap intermittently during the day for one hour on and one hour off.

Treatment of Joint Contractures with Low-Load Prolonged Stress

Neuromuscular dysfunction is a common cause of physiological joint restriction and contractures.[26] Splints are used to maintain or lengthen soft tissues and maintain joint integrity. If a joint has become contracted, the joint capsule becomes stiff, the synovial fluid becomes thickened from nonmovement, and the ligaments around one side of the joint become shortened, whereas the ligaments on the other side become lax. Soft-tissue involvement in contractures includes shortened tendons and skeletal muscle. High-load brief stretch manual therapy alone does not achieve plastic elongation of tissues over time.[12] LLPS involves holding the tissues in a low-lengthened position for a total end range time. A low-lengthened position is a passive position with a low-load stress (in which the patient feels a slight stress but one that he or she can tolerate for a significant amount of time, i.e., three to four hours total end range time). The total end range time increases over time to an ideal of six to eight hours. The soft tissue grows, not stretches, to the new lengthened position.[26]

Current literature supports LLPS as the preferred method of lengthening shortened tissues. The common clinical practice of stretching contractures manually with high brief-load periods for one to two minutes is contraindicated in the literature.[26] The elongation accomplished by manual stretch alone shortens when the force is relaxed. Manual therapy prepares tissues but must be followed with splinting and activities to affect permanent changes.[12]

A study by Light and colleagues[26] tested knee contractures using high-load brief stretch or LLPS on 11 geriatric patients. All subjects had bilateral knee contractures; high-load brief stretch was the treatment for one knee, and LLPS was the treatment for the other. The LLPS in this study was accomplished by traction. LLPS produced a greater overall increase in passive ROM than did the high-load brief stretch.

Splinting to provide an LLPS is a noninvasive, nonstressful, and ideally painless treatment.[26] The treatment for joint stiffness and contracture is stress, which involves intensity (amount of effort), duration (amount of time), and frequency (amount of repetition).[12] Although all these stress factors are important, duration is the most important for LLPS, the optimal time being six to eight hours. This optimal duration usually must be built up slowly, beginning with one to two hours. As the joint contracture decreases, the splint must be readjusted regularly (usually weekly) to increase prolonged stress. LLPS is the principle used in some of the splints mentioned previously in this chapter, including the elbow drop-out splint, the belly gutter splint, and any dynamic splinting. As with all splinting, but especially in using LLPS splinting for patients with sensory impairments, therapists must monitor patients using these splints for skin breakdown.

Injury to the Extremity

Because of decreased motor control and perceptual dysfunction (e.g., body neglect and somatoagnosia), many patients are at risk for injuries to the already compromised extremity. Many times these patients assume malaligned upper extremity patterns for prolonged periods. A common example may be observed during bed mobility training. Patients assume sitting postures from side lying and end up bearing their weight through the dorsum of their hands with the wrist flexed. This posture puts patients at risk of developing traumatic synovitis, increased edema, and pain. The patient, depending on the level of awareness, may maintain this maladaptive posture during the

next task (e.g., dressing) before noticing the problem, resulting in the potential for tissue damage.

Another common alignment problem that puts patients at risk for injury occurs if upper extremity positioning devices are ineffective. Many patients are prescribed half or full lap trays to provide upper extremity support while they are seated in their wheelchairs. In many cases, the supported extremity slides between the lapboard and the patient's trunk, pinning the wrist in extreme flexion. Depending on patient and staff awareness, this position unfortunately may be maintained for prolonged periods. Injury also can lead to pain and swelling, which in turn may trigger the initial symptoms of shoulder-hand syndrome.

Biomechanical Alignment

The position a hand assumes at rest (the resting posture) has been documented by several authors. A summary of this posture is as follows:

- Forearm midway between pronation and supination[29]
- Wrist at 10 to 15 degrees of extension[11]
- Thumb in slight extension and abduction with the MCP and IP joints flexed approximately 15 to 20 degrees
- Digits posture toward flexion, exhibiting greater composite flexion toward the ulnar side of the hand
- Second metacarpal aligned with the radius
- Palmar arches maintained (see the following section)
- Hand exhibiting "dual obliquity"

The therapist must consider the concept of dual obliquity when evaluating the alignment of the hand. Because of a successive decrease in the length of the metacarpals from the radial to the ulnar side, objects held in the hand assume two oblique angles.[39] For example, if a pencil is held in the palm across the metacarpal heads (eraser toward the ulnar side) and the forearm is held in pronation resting on the table, the examiner can identify two oblique angles. The first angle is observed with the pencil point angled upward in relation to the wrist joint axis. The second oblique angle is observed on examination of height of each end of the pencil. The radial side is held higher than the ulnar side, that is, the pencil is not parallel to the table (Fig. 13-23).

The obliquity of the palmar transverse arch follows a line from "the second to the fifth metacarpal head and forms an angle of seventy-five degrees with the axis of the third ray."[48] Therefore, from a biomechanical perspective, the firm cone splint discussed earlier for a moderately relaxed hand should be placed with the narrow end in the ulnar side and the wide end on the radial side, following the normal obliquity.

The therapist must note deviations from the resting posture; they assist in the design of the splint. Therapists must consider that patients may differ slightly from the normal resting posture because of heredity,

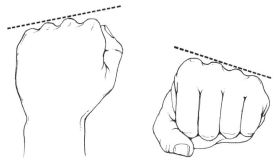

Figure 13-23   Dorsally, the consecutive metacarpal heads create an oblique angle to the longitudinal axis of the forearm. Distally, the fisted hand exhibits an ulnar metacarpal descent that creates an oblique angle in the transverse plane of the forearm. (From Fess EE, Philips CA: *Hand splinting: principles and methods*, ed 2, St Louis, 1987, Mosby.)

habits, and job descriptions; examining the opposite hand is helpful in determining the "normal" resting posture for each patient.[22]

The distal extremity assumes several typical alignment deviations after stroke. These deviations and their consequences include the following:

1. Wrist flexion following decreased skeletal muscle activity. This common posture (most often observed in the flaccid stage) produces a variety of pathological processes. A hand positioned in wrist flexion results in the following: flattening of the palmar arches, passive extension of the fingers due to tenodesis action, shortened collateral ligaments because of the extended digits, narrowing of the web space,[11] inability to perform the grasping function (flexor action of the thumb and digits reinforced by extension of the wrist),[48] blockage of ulnar and radial deviation of the wrist when it is in flexion,[20] overstretching of the wrist extensors and dorsal ligaments,[48] shortening of the long flexors, and a tendency to develop an edema syndrome.

2. Extreme ulnar deviation. The posture of ulnar deviation results in a variety of compounded problems. A wrist positioned in extreme ulnar deviation produces the following: effective blockage of wrist extension,[20] shortening of the ulnar deviators and overstretching of the radial deviators, and shifting of the proximal and distal rows of carpal bones.[48]

3. Wrist and digit flexion. This posture may occur following excessive skeletal muscle activity and soft-tissue shortening. This posture results in the following: loss of normal tenodesis function (wrist extension with digit flexion and adduction, wrist flexion with digit extension and abduction), shortening of the extrinsic flexors with resultant overstretching of the extensors, potential for skin maceration, and painful contracture and deformity.

Loss of Palmar Arches

A familiar alignment problem in patients after stroke is the loss of palmar arches, or the development of a "flattened hand." The maintenance of the palmar arches is crucial for hand function.[4] Kapandji[20] outlines the arches of the hand as follows (Fig. 13-24):

- Transverse arch: This structure consists of two arches and includes the carpal arch, which corresponds to the concavity of the wrist and is continuous with the distal metacarpal arch formed by the metacarpal heads. The carpal arch is rigid, whereas the metacarpal arch is mobile and adaptable. The long axis of the transverse arch crosses the lunate, capitate (the "keystone" of the carpal arch[11]), and the third metacarpal bones. Boehme[4] states that the functional significance of this arch stems from its forming the hand into a gutter, bringing together the radial and ulnar borders of the hand. This arch can widen or narrow the surface area of the hand.

- Longitudinal arch: This arch includes the carpometacarpophalangeal arches. These arches are formed for each finger by the corresponding metacarpal bones and phalanges. Kapandji[20] notes that the arches are

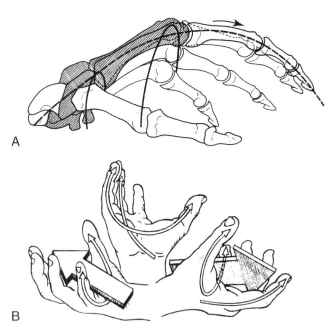

Figure 13-24   **A,** Side view of the longitudinal and transverse arches of the hand. The shaded areas show the fixed part of the skeleton. **B,** The thumb forms, along with the other digits, four oblique arches of opposition. The most useful and functionally important arch is between the thumb and index finger, used for precision grip. The farthest arch, between the thumb and little finger, ensures a locking mechanism on the ulnar side of the hand in power grips. (From Tubiana R, Thomine JM, Mackin E: *Examination of the hand and wrist*, St Louis, 1996, Mosby.)

concave on the palmar surface; the "keystone" of each arch lies at the level of the MCP joint. According to Boehme,[4] in its simplest form, this arch supports a basic cylindrical grasp. If the arches are expanded, the hand is longer. This arch allows the palm to flatten and cup itself around objects.[11]

■ Oblique arches: These arches are formed by the thumb during opposition with the other fingers. Kapandji[20] states that the most important of these arches is the one linking the thumb and index finger; the most extreme is the one linking the thumb and the little finger. These arches are obviously crucial in the opposition of the digits.

Patients lose their arches after stroke for a variety of reasons, including edema in the dorsum of the hand that biomechanically forces the metacarpals inferiorly, inactivity of the wrist and hand, prolonged and extreme wrist flexion (resulting in a flattening of the arches), and inappropriate support of the hand during weight-bearing activities.[4]

During evaluation of splinting, therapists should examine the arches of the hand and compare them with those of the unaffected hand. In the dorsal surface of a normal hand at rest, the MCP joints form an arch with the apex at the third metacarpal (i.e., the third metacarpal head is higher than the others are) (see Fig. 13-24). Many patients have a flattened arch (i.e., the MCP joints lose their arches), and in response the proximal phalanges hyperextend. This posture puts the patient at risk for developing a permanent claw-hand deformity and effectively blocks opposition of the thumb (Fig. 13-25).

In these cases, splinting may be indicated to give outside support to the arches through upward pressure on the palmar surface of the hand. To be effective and give full support to the metacarpals, the splint must conform to the arches and be contoured to the individual's hand. Commercially available splints are not effective for this type of intervention because they do not take into account the variability of arches.

For patients with hyperextended MCPs and flexed PIP joints (i.e., claw-hand deformity), a dorsal MCP extension restriction splint can be fabricated in thermoplastic material to eliminate deformity and increase function (Fig. 13-26).

Learned Nonuse

Current research (see Chapter 10) has demonstrated the existence of a component of upper extremity dysfunction resulting from a learned phenomenon of nonintegration of the hand into functional tasks. This process likely begins in the early stages after stroke, before any functional recovery has commenced. Patients learn to compensate with their unaffected sides, thereby repressing any return of function on the hemiplegic side.

Many CVA protocols call for splinting immediately after stroke. Some facilities have standing orders for splinting in their acute services. Current research indicates that early splinting in the early poststroke phase may be detrimental. The splint gives a message that an outside device is responsible for the maintenance and improvement of the affected hand. Because the hand is supported and aligned through outside means, the patient does not attend to the hand, stretch the wrist and hand, or attempt to integrate it into functional tasks. Early splinting may predispose patients to a learned nonuse phenomenon. A sign that a patient is predisposed to learned nonuse is the observation that a patient, after cueing, can integrate functional return during a therapy session but does not integrate this new function outside the sessions. The therapist must balance interventions for contracture prevention with activities that encourage functional use of the hand, thereby negating the effects of learned nonuse. Splinting for contractures can be used at night instead of during the day to prevent learned nonuse behavior patterns.

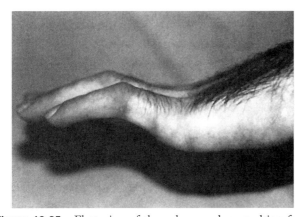

Figure 13-25 Flattening of the palmar arches resulting from hand paralysis. Hyperextension of the metacarpophalangeal joints and flexion of the proximal and distal interphalangeal joints occur because of an imbalance of the extrinsic flexor and extensor systems. (From Hunter JM, Mackin E, Callahan A: *Rehabilitation of the hand: surgery and therapy*, ed 4, St Louis, 1995, Mosby.)

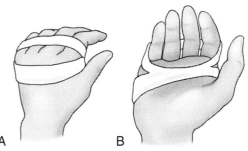

Figure 13-26 Anticlaw splint. **A,** Dorsal view. **B,** Palmar view.

DECISION-MAKING PROCESS

The therapist must evaluate all of the following areas when deciding whether to splint and choosing the type of splint to fabricate. This section is designed to help guide the therapist's clinical reasoning in making splinting decisions.

1. Evaluate cognitive and perceptual status: Does the patient attend to the extremity during the day (attending includes self-ranging, rubbing, positioning, and protecting)? Is the patient alert for the greater portion of the day?
   - If the answer is yes, the patient may be able to maintain ROM and alignment in the extremity without the use of splints; the therapist should consider not splinting.
   - If the answer is no, neglect, decreased attention, somatoagnosia, and decreased alertness and arousal may place the patient at risk for contracture and malalignment; splinting therefore may be indicated.
2. Evaluate soft tissue tightness: Does the patient have full composite flexion and extension? Can the patient be ranged into a full intrinsic minus/intrinsic plus position? Does the patient have full and pain-free range of wrist motion, especially extension and radial deviation?
   - If the answer is yes, the therapist should consider not splinting. Treatment should focus on teaching the patient and family techniques to maintain this range and prevent pain and contracture.
   - If the answer is no, splinting may be indicated to improve or at least maintain soft-tissue length. The splint should be designed to place the shortened soft tissues on prolonged stretch.
3. Evaluate joint contracture: Splinting is necessary to ameliorate joint contracture and prevent further deformity.
4. Evaluate learned nonuse: Does the patient integrate the extremity into functional tasks in the clinic without carryover into nontherapy hours?
   - If the answer is yes, the therapist should consider not splinting. In this situation, the patient does have distal function; this function should not be impeded by splinting. The splint may in fact feed into the learned nonuse cycle.
5. Evaluate function: Does the patient exhibit distal motor control (including gross patterns) that can be integrated into activities of daily living and instrumental activities of daily living?
   - If the answer is yes, the therapist should consider not splinting or should choose a splint that enhances the functional return (e.g., a basic wrist extension splint to provide a stable proximal segment for the digits to work from or a simple opponens splint to improve fine motor control).

- If the answer is no, splinting may be indicated, although the therapist must consider that splinting a hand without functional recovery may block the initial motor return (sometimes automatic reactions and protective responses) or the patient's initial attempts at function.
6. Evaluate potential for soft-tissue injury: Is evidence of skin maceration and laceration in the palm of the hand and lateral aspect of the thumb from extreme flexion apparent?
   - If the answer is yes, the therapist seriously must consider splinting to prevent further damage and enhance the healing process; wrist extension splints with distal cones or palm guards are recommended.
   - If the answer is no, the therapist should consider not splinting.
7. Evaluate biomechanical alignment: Are deviations from the standard resting position of the hand evident? Does realigning the hand result in increased relaxation?
   - If the answer is yes, the therapist should consider splinting to improve resting alignment of the extremity to prevent shortening and overstretching of soft tissue.
   - If the answer is no, the therapist should consider not splinting.
8. Evaluate sensation: Does the patient have sensory impairments?
   - If the answer is yes, the therapist should consider the amount of cutaneous surface area that is covered by splinting. The splint may end up blocking the little sensory input the hand is receiving. A general goal for the involved extremity is to maximize sensory input. If sensation is impaired, extra precautions are necessary for careful, custom splint fabrication and diligent, ongoing monitoring of the skin condition by the therapist, patient, and family for any breakdown or maceration, which the patient may not detect. This is especially important if cognitive deficits are present.
9. Evaluate edema: Does the patient have distal edema?
   - If the answer is yes, the therapist should consider whether a splint will support a flexed wrist with the goal of counteracting the dependent positioning of the hand, thereby decreasing or preventing further edema. Will the immobilization of the splint increase the edema by blocking the "pumping action" of muscles generated by active ROM? Patients with edema tend to lose digit flexion, thereby keeping the collateral ligaments in a shortened position. Will the splint block digit flexion, thereby exacerbating this problem? Will the splint impinge on neuromuscular structures and further limit hemodynamic function?

10. Evaluate posturing: Does the patient posture in persistent flexion?
    - If the answer is yes, the therapist should consider splinting to maintain stress on soft tissues. Rechecking of biomechanical alignment is essential; proximal realignment may relax the hand.
    - If the answer is no, the therapist should consider not splinting.

GENERAL SPLINTING GUIDELINES

Therapists should consider the following guidelines regarding splinting:

1. Check for abnormal pressure points, especially over bony prominences (e.g., ulnar head).
2. Decide during which activities and periods the patient will wear the splint. The splint must be evaluated or fabricated while the patient is in the most difficult posture and performing the most stressful activities if the effectiveness of the splint is to be evaluated. For example, fabricating a splint while the patient is seated and relaxed may result in a good fit with a relaxed hand. However, if the patient then leaves therapy to prepare a meal at home, the therapist may find the patient's hand "clawing" and flexing out of the splint. If the splint was fabricated with the patient standing and with the appropriate level of stretch, this phenomenon may not be a problem.
3. Splint for comfort. Pain and pressure responses may increase the patient's bias toward stereotypical posturing.
4. Patients need to experience full ROM. Use positioning splints only as adjuncts to a comprehensive upper extremity program.
5. Monitor full ROM. Many patients have been provided with resting hand splints to prevent flexion contractures only to end up with extension contractures, or "intrinsic lock."
6. Make wearing schedules practical to ensure patient compliance.
7. Therapists must have reasonable expectations for splints. An extremely tight hand may require several serial splints to achieve a desired position. Splints designed to provide correction at more than one joint can lead to added deformity if excessive skeletal muscle activity is present. For example, attempting to position the wrist and digits into extension may create a clawing effect in the digits as a result of the amount of stretch at the wrist and digits.[50] A severely malaligned hand may respond best if the therapist only focuses on one particular aspect of the malalignment (proximal first). For example, counteracting the extreme ulnar deviation in this type of extremity may be the goal of the first splint, followed by neutral deviation with slight wrist extension for the next splint. The therapist must remember that with an extremely tight or contracted hand, all deformities cannot be addressed simultaneously; if simultaneous correction is attempted, compliance with splinting may be jeopardized because of the discomfort level and skin breakdown.
8. Educate patients about the realistic goals and expectations of the use of a splint. Many patients wear their splints for prolonged periods with the hope that the splint will "make their hand better." Most patients interpret "better" as a return in function. However, this may not be the case for all patients; therefore, the patient should be aware of the reasons that the splint was prescribed. No splint should be worn continuously.

GENERAL FABRICATION GUIDELINES

Many splinting materials are commercially available today. They are thermoplastic materials; some have more rubber content base than others do. The rubber content base materials tend to have increased conformability and drape compared with pure thermoplastic materials, but they may be more difficult to handle because of their draping quality.

Thermoplastic materials generally have a greater memory capacity than do the rubber-based thermoplastics. Memory indicates the capability of the material to return to its original shape after the reheating that occurs during fabrication of the splint. Some therapists prefer the thermoplastics because of the memory capacity. The thermoplastics are available in perforated and solid forms. Perforated materials are recommended to allow for breathability and decrease the possibility of skin maceration (especially with patients with sympathetic nerve changes and sensory impairments). The therapist must take care when using maxiperforated thermoplastics to eliminate sharp edges after cutting the material. The edges must be heated with a heat gun and turned down to smooth the edging; the edges may also be covered with $\frac{1}{16}$-inch solid material cut into 1-inch wide but long pieces, heated in water, and then applied to the edging. The therapist also may use a thin layer of moleskin to smooth the edges of perforated material.

The thermoplastic materials and rubber-based thermoplastics are available in various thicknesses ranging from $\frac{1}{8}$-inch, $\frac{3}{32}$-inch, $\frac{1}{12}$-inch, and 1-inch; the most common width is $\frac{1}{8}$-inch. Some of the splinting materials are available in a wide range of colors; these may help draw attention to the involved limb and prevent the splint from being lost in hospital bedding. Color also may enhance compliance. Several vendors offer precut splint blanks and kits. These products can be cut to size for customization and to decrease the amount of splinting time required for fabrication. Prefabricated splints also are available for many splinting needs, but some may be difficult to customize. The authors do not recommend some of the commercially available spring wire splints for patients with sensory impairments because these splints may apply too much pressure that the patient will not be able to detect. Custom-fabricated splints are the splints of choice for patients with sensory impairments.

Velcro strapping materials are now available in multiple colors. Velfoam, a padded strapping material, is highly recommended for the patient with sensory impairments because it is a softer strapping material.

Splint padding does not compensate for a poorly fitted splint and increases the pressure within the splint. Splint padding is recommended to cushion fingers at the point of contact of the thermoplastic material in dynamic splints only. Splint padding is available under different trade names. Splint padding materials only increase the pressure of an ill-fitting splint, and when used in this way, may also be hot and uncomfortable for the patient and may increase the possibility of skin maceration because of the increased perspiration that the padding may cause in a patient.

Splinting the extremity of a patient with neurological involvement is sometimes difficult if severely increased skeletal muscle activity is evident in the upper extremity. Maintaining the desired alignment and molding the splinting material may be almost impossible. The assistance of another person for positioning usually is indicated for a proper fit. Pattern-making also may be difficult with this type of patient. The fabrication of a gross pattern on the unaffected hand and reversal of the pattern for transfer to the splinting material are helpful at times.

The therapist must make allowances for bony prominences by cutting around or flaring the splinting material over the prominence. A helpful hint for flaring out the material is to place a spot of dark lipstick over the bony prominence (on the patient's skin); place the cooled, already formed splint on the patient; and remove the splint. The lipstick now will be on the splint in the exact spot at which the splint requires flaring.

During the use of thermoplastic materials in splinting, the placement of curve in the material increases the tensile strength of the material to approximately 20 times that of straight material. This is helpful to remember in the fabrication of dynamic outriggers from thermoplastic material or the creation of an additional roll in the material as a spine or support.

SPECIFIC FABRICATION GUIDELINES

Forearm Support

If the splint prescribed for a patient includes a forearm trough, basic splinting principles call for the trough to cover two thirds of the forearm. To compensate for the weight of the hand and the excess force created by increased distal flexor activity, the forearm trough should be two thirds of the length of the forearm to provide a sufficient lever.

Palmar Support

Many patients with neurological involvement have flattened arches at the MCP joints, with resultant clawing of the digits. This malalignment usually occurs in patients with little or no skeletal muscle activity in the affected hand. In molding the splint into the palmar arch in these cases, the therapist can use the thumb to mold a letter T pattern over the palmar surface of the splint. The base of the T runs longitudinally through the center of the palm, whereas the top of the T runs across the metacarpal heads. The base of the T should connect to the top of the T at the third MCP head. The T shape is molded into the palm to enhance the arch. To ensure sturdy arch support, the splint must progress distal to the distal palmar crease and does not need to clear the thenar eminence in a hand without movement. The therapist should reevaluate the patient frequently for returning motor control and should adjust the splint as needed. If the patient exhibits controlled digit flexion, the distal end of the splint needs to be rolled back proximal to the distal palmar crease so that returning function is not blocked. If the patient begins to exhibit thumb function, the palmar support surface of the splint must again be rolled back to clear the thenar eminence and therefore not block active movement.

After splint fabrication, the therapist evaluates the palmar support section of the splint by checking that the dual obliquity of the hand is maintained, the third metacarpal head is the apex of the arch formed by the metacarpal heads, and the hand is not "flattened" in the splint (Figs. 13-27 and 13-28).

Wrist Support

When molding and evaluating the wrist component of a splint for the patient after stroke, the therapist must consider alignment:

- The third metacarpal should lie midway between the radius and ulna in a neutral deviated hand. Many hands with neurological involvement have a tendency to assume a position of ulnar deviation. Splint modifications to the wrist component include raising the border of the splint that lies lateral to the fifth metacarpal. This modification effectively blocks the ulnar deviation (Fig. 13-29).
- The wrist should be supported between zero and 20 degrees of extension. Gillen and colleagues[13] examined the effect of various wrist positions on upper extremity function in adults wearing a wrist immobilizing splint. The Jebsen Taylor Test of Hand Function was administered to 20 adults without upper extremity impairment to determine the

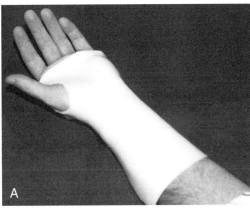

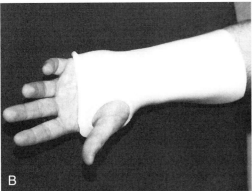

Figure 13-27 Variations on palmar support fabrication. **A,** Full palmar support (material progresses past the distal palmar crease and gives the thumb support over the first metacarpal). **B,** As function returns, the distal and thenar aspects of the splint are rolled back to allow for joint excursion during functional tasks. The T shape is molded into the palmar aspect of the splint.

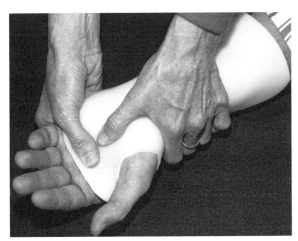

Figure 13-28 Molding the T support into the splint. The base of the T runs longitudinally through the palm, whereas the top of the T supports the metacarpal arch. The base of the T intersects the top of the T at the third metacarpal head. Palmar support is accurate if the arches of the hand are maintained, and the third metacarpal head is superior to the metacarpal heads of digits two and four.

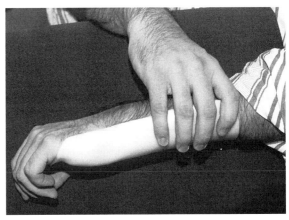

Figure 13-29 The lateral aspect of the splint is built up along the fifth metacarpal effectively to block ulnar deviation.

effects, if any. The test was administered three consecutive times. Each time the subject wore a commercially available wrist extension splint that positioned the wrist in zero degrees (neutral), 15 degrees, or 30 degrees of wrist extension. Wrist angles were confirmed via goniometry. The order in which the wrist angles were tested was randomized to control for fatigue and practice effects. The results of this study indicated that there was no significant difference between the tested wrist positions (0 degrees, 15 degrees, 30 degrees) when using the nondominant hand to perform activities while wearing a wrist splint. However, significant differences were found when wearing various angled wrist splints to perform functional activities with the dominant hand albeit only for select tasks (feeding and stacking checkers). During the feeding subtest, participants performed at a significantly faster rate when their dominant wrists were positioned in 15 degrees of extension as compared to performance with a neutral wrist. During the stacking checkers subtest, participants performed at a significantly faster rate when their wrists were positioned in neutral when compared with when they were positioned in 30 degrees of extension. Nonetheless, the final decision depends on which angle allows the maximal amount of function or (if the hand is not functional) which angle in this range decreases the usual abnormal flexor activity in the digits. (Many patients' digits relax if they are realigned proximally.) In some cases, the splint may be fabricated in some degree of flexion. This may be required if contracture of the extrinsic flexors is evident and the goal is systematically to lengthen the flexors with serial splinting. In these cases, each subsequent splint should be molded with an increased stretch on the flexors. For example, the first splint may be molded in 20 degrees of wrist flexion; the next in 10 degrees of flexion, neutral wrist; and finally in some degree of extension. Therapists must remember that if the goal is to lengthen the extrinsic flexors, wrist and digit support is required.

■ After molding the splint, the therapist should check that the hand is not in a position of medial or lateral rotation (neutral) compared with the forearm. Many patients who exhibit excessive skeletal muscle activity develop a tendency for the hand to rotate medially or laterally in relation to the forearm. The hand should be positioned in the splint so that the fifth metacarpal is aligned with the ulna instead of lying inferior to the ulna (the hand is laterally rotated in relation to the forearm) or lying superior to the ulna (the hand is medially rotated in relation to the forearm).

Digit Support

The therapist should use a digit support platform only as a last resort. The therapist must include a digit support platform in the splint if the patient exhibits excessive flexor activity in the digits that cannot be otherwise controlled and if the patient is being splinted for contracture management. If the splint includes a digit platform, daytime use of the splint is discouraged.

If a patient exhibits excessive flexor activity, the therapist first should try a forearm and wrist splint that enhances alignment. In many patients, a proximal realignment of the joints and a prolonged state of accommodation of muscles to their resting length relaxes the hand. Therapists can evaluate this phenomenon by manually realigning the joints with their hands and evaluating whether a relaxation response occurs.

If a digit support platform is necessary, the digits should not be overstretched to the point that a "clawing" of the hand or a "bottoming out" of the metacarpals occurs. The therapist must ensure that the palmar arch remains intact when the digits are stretched onto the platform (Fig. 13-30).

Thumb Support

In the nonfunctional hand, the thumb should be supported in a position midway between palmar and radial abduction. This position can be maintained by the previously described palmar support, which also supports the first metacarpal; if the splint is rolled back to clear the thenar eminence, the thumb cannot be supported in this position (see Fig. 13-27).

If the thumb is functional, the splinted position is dictated by evaluation of the position of thumb that is the most effective at enhancing function with the thumb in opposition. Fig. 13-31 describes the clinical reasoning process followed for deciding on the type and style of splint to fabricate.

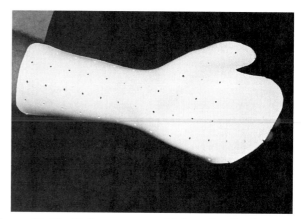

Figure 13-30 Full support provided to the distal extremity. This style of splint is recommended only if alternative attempts of proximal realignment do not relax the hand. This splint is recommended for night use only.

Prefabricated Splints

In cases in which prefabricated splints are indicated, therapists must take great care to ensure proper fitting. Patients should not be encouraged to purchase splints "off the shelf" without a therapist's input because of the potential complications. Examples of commonly used and useful prefabricated splints include air-assist splints for LLPS (see Fig. 13-15), a Multi Podus ankle/foot orthosis (Fig. 13-32), and elbow splints to provide stretch (Fig. 13-33).

SUMMARY

When designing or fabricating a splint for a patient after stroke, the therapist must consider each patient individually; no set of rules applies to all patients with neurological impairments. No definitive answers or protocols are available. The reader is encouraged to consider the questions in the decision-making section of this chapter to guide clinical reasoning, because the therapist must consider so many factors in treatment.

Any hand with a malalignment or deformity results in an overstretching of the soft tissues (muscles, ligaments) on one side of the joint and shortening of the soft tissues on the opposite side. All treatment, including splinting, should be instituted after consideration of this phenomenon and should aim to preserve the length and balance of soft tissue on either side of the joint. This treatment prepares the hand for possible future integration into functional activities and prevents permanent deformity.

All splints applied to patients after stroke, especially patients with increased skeletal muscle activity and decreased sensation who are being treated with the principles of LLPS, must be monitored continually by therapists, nursing staff, and family members to assess for skin

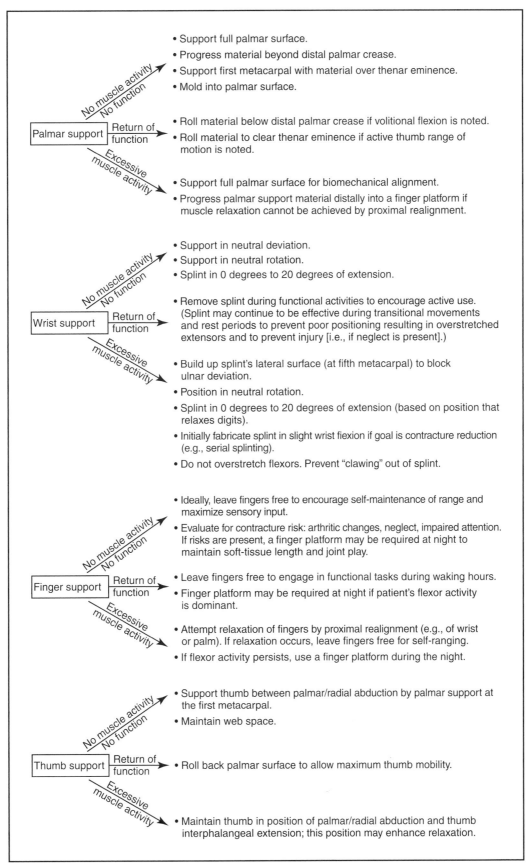

Palmar support

No muscle activity / No function
- Support full palmar surface.
- Progress material beyond distal palmar crease.
- Support first metacarpal with material over thenar eminence.
- Mold into palmar surface.

Return of function
- Roll material below distal palmar crease if volitional flexion is noted.
- Roll material to clear thenar eminence if active thumb range of motion is noted.

Excessive muscle activity
- Support full palmar surface for biomechanical alignment.
- Progress palmar support material distally into a finger platform if muscle relaxation cannot be achieved by proximal realignment.

Wrist support

No muscle activity / No function
- Support in neutral deviation.
- Support in neutral rotation.
- Splint in 0 degrees to 20 degrees of extension.

Return of function
- Remove splint during functional activities to encourage active use. (Splint may continue to be effective during transitional movements and rest periods to prevent poor positioning resulting in overstretched extensors and to prevent injury [i.e., if neglect is present].)

Excessive muscle activity
- Build up splint's lateral surface (at fifth metacarpal) to block ulnar deviation.
- Position in neutral rotation.
- Splint in 0 degrees to 20 degrees of extension (based on position that relaxes digits).
- Initially fabricate splint in slight wrist flexion if goal is contracture reduction (e.g., serial splinting).
- Do not overstretch flexors. Prevent "clawing" out of splint.

Finger support

No muscle activity / No function
- Ideally, leave fingers free to encourage self-maintenance of range and maximize sensory input.
- Evaluate for contracture risk: arthritic changes, neglect, impaired attention. If risks are present, a finger platform may be required at night to maintain soft-tissue length and joint play.

Return of function
- Leave fingers free to engage in functional tasks during waking hours.
- Finger platform may be required at night if patient's flexor activity is dominant.

Excessive muscle activity
- Attempt relaxation of fingers by proximal realignment (e.g., of wrist or palm). If relaxation occurs, leave fingers free for self-ranging.
- If flexor activity persists, use a finger platform during the night.

Thumb support

No muscle activity / No function
- Support thumb between palmar/radial abduction by palmar support at the first metacarpal.
- Maintain web space.

Return of function
- Roll back palmar surface to allow maximum thumb mobility.

Excessive muscle activity
- Maintain thumb in position of palmar/radial abduction and thumb interphalangeal extension; this position may enhance relaxation.

Figure 13-31 Fabrication decisions: clinical reasoning. A volar-based forearm trough that supports two thirds of the forearm with sides parallel to the radius and ulna serves as the base splint in this decision-making process.

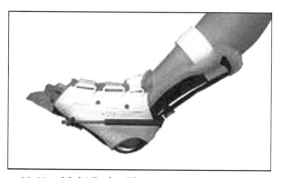

Figure 13-32 Multi Podus Phase II System (Restorative Care of America). This orthosis allows the ankle to be positioned incrementally towards neutral. The total range is from 40 degrees of plantar flexion to 10 degrees of dorsiflexion.

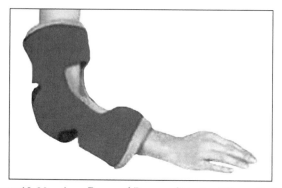

Figure 13-33 Arm-Respond Range of Motion Elbow Orthosis (Restorative Care of America). This orthosis allows the elbow to be positioned in 10-degree increments of flexion or extension.

integrity. This concept is particularly crucial for patients with cognitive and perceptual deficits. Factors in the monitoring of skin integrity include signs of skin discoloration, maceration, edema, and breakdown.

Splinting for patients after stroke that combines the principles of biomechanical positioning and the neurophysiological concepts of facilitation and inhibition may lead to the most favorable components of function.[51]

Realistic outcomes must be the guiding forces in the decision-making process in the fabrication of splints for patients after stroke. Clinicians working with this population who use splinting as an adjunct treatment should strive to gain a solid understanding of anatomy, biomechanics, and motor control theories.

Finally, therapists have a responsibility not only to stay current on research regarding this area of intervention but also to add to the literature through research, from single-subject case studies to qualitative trend analyses to large subject-sample qualitative studies. Until more definitive and well-designed research studies are available concerning this treatment, the splinting controversy for patients after stroke will continue, and therapists may be providing patients with less than optimal care.

REVIEW QUESTIONS

1. What is the normal resting posture of the hand? What are the common malalignments observed after a stroke?
2. What precautions should be followed when splinting a patient after stroke?
3. What is the recommended rationale for splinting the patient after stroke?
4. How does the therapist differentiate among intrinsic tightness, extrinsic tightness, and joint contracture when evaluating for a splint?
5. What are the advantages of LLPS versus high-load brief stretch?

REFERENCES

1. Blashy MRM, Fuchs-Neeman RL: Orthokinetics: a new receptor facilitation method. *Am J Occup Ther* 13(5):226–234, 1959.
2. Bloch R, Evans MG: An inflatable splint for the spastic hand. *Arch Phys Med Rehabil* 58(4):179–180, 1977.
3. Bobath B: *Adult hemiplegia: evaluation and treatment*, ed 3, Oxford, 1990, Butterworth-Heineman.
4. Boehme R: *Improving upper body control: an approach to assessment and treatment of tonal dysfunction*, Tucson, AZ, 1988, Therapy Skill Builders.
5. Brennan J: Response to stretch of hypertonic muscle groups in hemiplegia. *Br Med J* 1(5136):1504–1507, 1959.
6. Casey CA, Kratz EJ: Soft splinting with neoprene: the thumb abduction supinator splint. *Am J Occup Ther* 42(6):395–398, 1988.
7. Charait SE: A comparison of volar and dorsal splinting of the hemiplegic hand. *Am J Occup Ther* 22(4):319–321, 1968.
8. Currie DM, Mendiola A: Cortical thumb orthosis for children with spastic hemiplegic cerebral palsy. *Arch Phys Med Rehabil* 68(4):214–217, 1987.
9. Doubilet L, Polkow LS: Theory and design of a finger abduction splint for the spastic hand. *Am J Occup Ther* 21(5):320–322, 1977.
10. Feldman PA: Upper extremity casting and splinting. In Glenn MB, Whyte J, editors: *The practical management of spasticity in children and adults*, Philadelphia, 1990, Lea & Febiger.
11. Fess EE, Philips CA: *Hand splinting: principles and methods*, ed 2, St Louis, 1987, Mosby.
12. Flowers K: *Orthopaedic assessment and mobilization of the upper extremity, Scar Wars I & II.* Seminar conducted in New York City, 1992.
13. Gillen G, Goldberg R, Muller S, Straus J: The effect of wrist position on upper extremity function while wearing a wrist immobilizing splint. *J Prosthet Orthot* 20(1):19–23, 2008.
14. Gossman MR, Sahrman SA, Rose SJ: Review of length associated changes in muscles: experimental evidence and clinical implications. *Phys Ther* 62(12):1799–1808, 1982.
15. Halar EM, Bell KR: Contracture and other deleterious effects on immobility. In Delisa JA, editor: *Rehabilitation medicine: principles and practice*, ed 2, Philadelphia, 1993, JB Lippincott.
16. Hill SG: Current trends in upper extremity splinting. In Boehme R, editor: *Improving upper body control: an approach to assessment and treatment of tonal dysfunction*, Tucson, AZ, 1988, Therapy Skill Builders.
17. Hummelsheim H, Munch B, Butefisch C, et al: Influence of sustained stretch on late muscular responses to magnetic brain stimulation in patients with upper motor neuron lesions. *Scand J Rehabil Med* 26(1):3–9, 1994.
18. Hunter JM, Mackin E, Callahan A: *Rehabilitation of the hand: surgery and upper extremity*, ed 5, St Louis, 2002, Mosby.
19. Johnstone M: *Restoration of motor function in the stroke patient: a physiotherapist's approach*, New York, 1983, Churchill Livingstone.

20. Kapandji IA: In *The physiology of the joints*, ed 5, Upper limb, vol 1, New York, 1982, Churchill Livingstone.
21. Kaplan N: Effect of splinting on reflex inhibition and sensorimotor stimulation in treatment of spasticity. *Arch Phys Med Rehabil* 43:65–569, 1962.
22. Kiel JH: *Basic hand splinting: a pattern-designing approach*, Boston, 1983, Little, Brown.
23. Lannin NA, Herbert RD: Is hand splinting effective for adults following stroke? A systematic review and methodologic critique of published research. *Clinical Rehabilitation* 17(8):807–16, 2003.
24. Lannin NA, Horsley SA, Herbert R, et al: Splinting the hand in the functional position after brain impairment: a randomized, controlled trial. *Arch Phys Med Rehabil* 84(2):297–302, 2003.
25. Lannin NA, Cusick A, McCluskey A, Herbert RD: Effects of splinting on wrist contracture after stroke: a randomized controlled trial. *Stroke* 38(1):111–6, 2007.
26. Light KE, Nuzik S, Personius W, et al: Low-load prolonged stretch vs high-load brief stretching in treating knee contractures. *Phys Ther* 64(3):330–333, 1984.
27. Ma HI, Trombly CA: A synthesis of the effects of occupational therapy for persons with stroke, part II: remediation of impairments. *Am J Occup Ther* 56(3):260–74, 2002.
28. MacKinnon J, Sanderson E, Buchanan J: The MacKinnon splint: a functional hand splint. *Can J Occup Ther* 42(4):157–158, 1975.
29. Malick MH: *Manual on static hand splinting*, ed 5, Pittsburgh, 1985, Harmarvile Rehabilitation Center.
30. Mathiowetz V, Bolding DJ, Trombly CA: Immediate effects of positioning devices on the normal and spastic hand measured by electromyography. *Am J Occup Ther* 37(4):247–254, 1983.
31. McPherson JJ: Objective evaluation of a splint designed to reduce hypertonicity. *Am J Occup Ther* 35(3):189–194, 1981.
32. McPherson JJ, Kreimeyer D, Aalderks M, et al: A comparison of dorsal and volar resting hand splints in the reduction of hypertonus. *Am J Occup Ther* 36(10):664–670, 1982.
33. Neeman RL, Liederhouse JJ, Neeman M: A multidisciplinary efficacy study on orthokinetics treatment of a patient with post-CVA hemiparesis and pain. *Can J Rehabil* 2(1):41–52, 1988.
34. Neeman RL, Neeman M: Efficacy of orthokinetic orthotics for post-stroke upper extremity hemiparetic motor dysfunction. *Int J Rehabil Res* 16(4):302–307, 1993.
35. Neeman RL, Neeman M: Orthokinetic orthoses: clinical efficacy study of orthokinetics treatment for a patient with upper extremity movement dysfunction in late post-acute CVA. *J Rehabil Res Dev* 29(ann suppl):41–53, 1992.
36. Neeman RL, Neeman M: Rehabilitation of a post stroke patient with upper extremity hemiparetic movement dysfunction by orthokinetic orthoses. *J Hand Ther* 5:47–155, 1992.
37. Neuhaus BE, Ascher ER, Coullon BA, et al: A survey of rationales for and against hand splinting in hemiplegia. *Am J Occup Ther* 35(2):83–90, 1981.
38. Nicholson DE: *The effects of pressure splint treatment on the motor function of the involved limb in patients with hemiplegia*, master's thesis, Chapel Hill, 1984, University of North Carolina.
39. Pedretti LW: Hand splinting. In Pedretti LW, Zoltan B, editors: *Occupational therapy: practice skills for physical dysfunction*, ed 3, St Louis, 1990, Mosby.
40. Peterson LT: *Neurological consideration in splinting spastic extremities*, unpublished paper, 1980.
41. Poole JL, Whitney SL: Inflatable pressure splints (airsplints) as adjunct treatment for individual with strokes. *Phys Occup Ther Geriatr* 11(1):17–27, 1992.
42. Poole JL, Whitney SL, Hangeland N, et al: The effectiveness of inflatable pressure splints on motor function in stroke patients. *Occup Ther J Res* 10(6):360–366, 1990.
43. Steultjens EM, Dekker J, Bouter LM, et al: Occupational therapy for stroke patients: a systematic review. *Stroke* 34(3):676–87, 2003.
44. Snook JH: Spasticity reduction splint. *Am J Occup Ther* 33(10):648–651, 1979.
45. Stern GR: Thumb abduction splint. *Physiotherapy* 66(10):352, 1980.
46. Stockmeyer S: An interpretation of the approach of Rood to the treatment of neuromuscular dysfunction. *Am J Phys Med* 46(1):900–961, 1967.
47. Thompson-Rangel T: The mystery of the serpentine splints. *Occup Ther Forum* Sept 20:4–6, 1991.
48. Tubiana R, Thomine JM, Mackin E: *Examination of the hand and wrist*, St Louis, 1996, Mosby.
49. Tyson SF, Kent RM: Orthotic devices after stroke and other non-progressive brain lesions. *Cochrane Database of Syst Rev* (1):CD003694, 2009.
50. Wilson D, Caldwell C: Central control insufficiency. III. Disturbed motor control and sensation: a treatment approach emphasizing upper extremity orthoses. *Phys Ther* 58(3):313–320, 1978.
51. Woodson AM: Proposal for splinting the adult hemiplegic hand to promote function. In Cromwell FS, editor: *Hand rehabilitation in occupational therapy*, Redding, CA, 1988, Hawthorne Press.
52. Wu SH: A belly gutter splint for proximal interphalangeal joint flexion contracture. *Am J Occup Ther* 45(9):839–843, 1991.
53. Zislis JM: Splinting of hand in a spastic hemiplegic patient. *Arch Phys Med Rehabil* 45:41–43, 1964.

leslie a. kane
karen a. buckley

chapter 14

Functional Mobility

key terms

bed mobility	scooting	transitional movements
environmental conditions	task-specific training	trunk control
mobility	transfers	upright function

chapter objectives

After completing this chapter, the reader will be able to accomplish the following:

1. Recognize the impact of impairment on mobility tasks.
2. Analyze specific movement patterns observed during mobility tasks and common compensatory strategies.
3. Use a function-based approach to retraining mobility patterns.
4. Understand the impact of environmental changes on mobility tasks.
5. Understand how to structure the environment to promote learning of mobility tasks.
6. Understand how to use specific strategies to promote learning of mobility tasks.
7. Understand fall risks.

TERMINOLOGY

Many terms have been used in occupational therapy practice to describe an individual's ability to change the position of the body in space and move within the environment. *Mobility* broadly refers to movements that result in a change of body position or location. The term *bed mobility* has been used interchangeably with *gross mobility* within the rehabilitation setting and traditionally has included tasks such as rolling to both sides, rolling to side lying, moving from a sitting to a supine position and vice versa, and moving from sitting to standing. *Transfer* refers to movement from one surface to another such as from a bed to a wheelchair, from a wheelchair to a toilet, or from a wheelchair to a car, and involves varied methods of achievement.

OVERVIEW OF THE LITERATURE

Within the literature, numerous studies have carefully examined mobility functions of the adult in relation to gait and locomotion. Unfortunately, few studies have examined functional mobility tasks. The analysis of the normal sit-to-stand sequence of movement has received attention and is reviewed later in this chapter.[19,20,30,82,83] Rising from bed has been examined in relation to age differences and the most common movement strategies selected.[36] This research demonstrates that age-related trends occur across the life span, but great variety remains evident in the selection of specific movement strategies. A limitation of this study is that the oldest age group examined was the 50- to 59-year-old group; thus, information concerning older adults most at risk for stroke was not included. A study of normal adult rolling patterns also has shown that adults exhibit great variability in the selection of movement patterns. In addition, the authors of this study have noted indications that a developmental sequence of movement patterns exists but is not inclusive of all individuals. Clearly many aspects of functional mobility still warrant further investigation.[91]

FUNCTIONAL MOBILITY: RELATIONSHIP TO ACTIVITIES AND PARTICIPATION

Occupational therapists have always approached functional mobility from the perspective that individual elements involved in changing the position of the body were necessary to achieve competency in broad areas of occupation. Improvement in activities of daily living (ADL), instrumental activities of daily living (IADL), education, work, play, leisure, and social participation has always been the ultimate goal of occupational therapy. The American Occupational Therapy Association, in "Practice Framework: Domain and Process," describes functional mobility as "moving from one position or place to another (during performance of everyday activities), such as in-bed mobility, wheelchair mobility, transfers (wheelchair, bed, car, tub, toilet, tub/shower, chair, floor). Performing functional ambulation and transporting objects."[4]

Within the Practice Framework, functional mobility is presented as a separate activity category of basic ADL, in which mobility functions occur relative to taking care of one's own body.

Alternatively, in the *International Classification of Functioning, Disability and Health*, the World Health Organization presents mobility as a separate domain under the broader category of Activities and Participation. Mobility "is about moving by changing body position or location or by transferring from one place to another, by occupying, moving or manipulating objects, by walking, running or climbing, and by using various forms of transportation."[97]

In this more global perspective, mobility is presented as much more than a function of personal self-care. Mobility is viewed as essential to enabling an individual to engage in a full range of life areas and is central to enabling the individual to participate in life situations.

In planning comprehensive treatment programs, the occupational therapist should be mindful that functional mobility is not just relevant to performing self-care tasks but is necessary to permit engagement in education, work opportunities, community life, recreation, leisure, religious pursuits, and domestic life. In practice, the extent to which these areas are addressed may be limited by time constraints imposed by the venue of treatment. Clinicians working within an acute care setting often emphasize basic bed mobility tasks to prepare the patient for independence in grooming, bathing, and dressing activities (see Chapter 1). Within a rehabilitation setting, occupational therapists may have the opportunity to approach functional mobility more comprehensively in relation to more advanced tasks such as community mobility and tasks related to specific work and home-management requirements. The occupational therapist determines goals of treatment with the patient, contingent on imminent and future plans to resume responsibility for activities demanding advanced mobility.

The task-related approach of occupational therapy to intervention to improve functional mobility is consistent with present motor learning research emphasizing the important role environment plays in the organization of movement to solve motor problems (see Chapters 4 to 6).[10,39]

Impairments of body functions and structures and performance skills have been used to assess abilities in the patient with hemiplegia. Each patient has different strengths, abilities, and impairments that affect the performance of functional mobility. A patient may have strong neuromusculoskeletal and movement-related functions but demonstrate significant impairment in mental functions of sequencing complex movements (e.g., apraxia). Alternately, a patient may have several problems affecting the neuromusculoskeletal system, including decreased alignment and postural stability that interfere with the ability to roll efficiently toward the nonaffected side. Nevertheless, such a patient may demonstrate the ability to learn new strategies to sequence movement to accomplish the task.

INFLUENCE OF CONTEXTUAL FACTORS ON FUNCTIONAL MOBILITY

Contextual factors represent a variety of interrelated conditions and situations that may influence an individual's ability to become proficient in performing mobility tasks. Personal and environmental factors affect the patient with hemiplegia and may support or impede performance.

Personal factors are unique to the individual's life and living situation and influence the selection of mobility interventions. The occupational therapist considers factors such as age, gender, race, and social background.

When considering the age of an individual who has sustained a stroke and assessing expectations of the potential for functional mobility, the therapist must use caution. Many factors besides age contribute to the differences in the abilities older adults exhibit in functional mobility. The reader is encouraged to explore the literature examining the effect of aging on postural control and life span mobility.

Certainly the patient's stage in the life cycle more clearly guides assessment and interventions in the consideration of overall mobility needs. The young patient with hemiplegia who attends college has specific mobility needs. Sit-to-stand movements must be accomplished in changing environments and under varying conditions. For example, using public transportation, which may be moving or stationary; rising from a low seat at a football stadium; sitting down in a crowded and darkened movie theater; and getting into a truck present different challenges. These mobility tasks are not unique to young persons, however. The retired person who enjoys traveling frequently and visiting family members also has special mobility needs.

Social and cultural variations also have an effect on the success of functional mobility interventions. The therapist must consider culturally derived boundaries of interaction,[57] because the therapist must frequently work within an intimate distance during mobility retraining.[43] The physical environment in which interventions occur also affects the patient's willingness to participate actively. Some patients prefer treatment to occur in the privacy of their hospital rooms, whereas others are more comfortable with these "close encounters" occurring in the open space of a therapeutic gymnasium. The patient, family, significant individuals, and therapist have perceptions and beliefs founded on their cultural conditionings. Similarities and differences of belief may occur in three areas influencing the success of functional mobility retraining: the perceived state of health and illness, the perceived relevance of therapeutic interventions, and the belief that functional mobility is relevant to resuming previous occupations.[60]

The therapist's ability to listen to personal needs and appreciate individual values helps ensure success.[60] The degree of independence a patient finds acceptable must be self-determined. The therapist must remember that cultural variations influence patient participation and successful outcomes of home programs.[4,60,65]

Environmental factors are external to the individual and are considered at two levels, individual and societal. Individual environmental factors include the immediate environment of the individual, which can be viewed as the hospital or clinical venue, and the natural environments. Environment determines a patient's function. The patient with hemiplegia may be able to roll to either side and come to a seated position on a mat or plinth within the clinical setting and engage in donning and doffing of upper extremity clothing. However, in bed within a home setting, the patient may not be able to roll as efficiently or come to a seated position without some assistance. Grooming and dressing tasks may not be practical because of changes in the height and firmness of the supporting surface. These occurrences and the reasons underlying the performance deficits are well-represented in the current motor learning literature. The postural adjustments necessary to roll and come to a seated position to engage in self-care tasks can be learned only in the context of task performance[1,21] and in the expected environment.[39,40]

The treatment of a patient with hemiplegia often occurs on a continuum from acute care through community reintegration. Many treatment environments impose constraints that limit the therapist's interventions. For example, in intensive care unit settings, therapists must contend with multiple lines, monitors, and alarms (see Chapter 1). Ideally the relearning of motor skills and tasks should occur in the actual environment in which the task will be performed.[22,69]

Societal environmental factors directly influence the patient's ability to resume participation in IADL and include systems within the community or society that can assist the individual to resume an active lifestyle outside of one's immediate living situation.

FUNCTIONAL MOBILITY: THE OUTCOME OF MULTIPLE PROCESSES

Functional mobility requires the successful interaction of a number of systems. Carrying out skilled rolling, sitting, and standing does not depend solely on the integrity of the neuromusculoskeletal system. Occupational therapists must be mindful of the interdependence of various sensory, perceptual, and cognitive functions in the execution of these tasks and create evaluation tools that respect this relationship, such as the Árnadóttir Occupational Therapy Neurobehavioral Evaluation (see Chapter 18). This awareness ensures more comprehensive assessment than do evaluations that look at motor behaviors in isolation. Occupational therapists' knowledge and expertise in task analysis render them uniquely qualified to evaluate and plan treatment to improve functional mobility skills while keeping all the patient's needs in mind.

Individual differences and variations in movement strategies may be related to factors such as the patient's build (short, tall, obese, thin) and performance patterns before the stroke (i.e., the patient was a trained athlete, dancer, physically inactive, occasional exerciser, or physical laborer). Additionally, each patient presents with individual habits, routines, and roles that influence movement.[29] The psychological state may indeed be reflected in movement (e.g., inhibitions or lack thereof and reactive depression about the current situation). Pain from preexisting conditions or pain as secondary impairment to the stroke may affect movement patterns. These individual differences and their effects on functional mobility have been explored in the literature.[91] The occupational therapist must be cognizant of these factors and others in assessment and treatment planning.

IMPAIRMENT OF BODY FUNCTIONS AND STRUCTURES AND SKILLS

Many sequelae associated with a stroke impede performance of functional mobility tasks. The occupational therapist uses basic knowledge of body functions and structures, performance skills, and impairments as a means to organize assessment of an individual's capacity for functional mobility. The following table summarizes impairments resulting from stroke and their effects on performance of functional mobility skills (Table 14-1).

FUNCTIONAL MOBILITY TASKS

Functional mobility tasks occur throughout the daily routine under varying circumstances within changeable environments. Each task requires the individual to stabilize the body in space or exhibit dynamic postural control. Das and McCollum[27] identified three major requirements

for locomotion that can be applied to all functional mobility tasks:

1. Progression or movement in a desired direction
2. The ability to stabilize the body against the forces of gravity
3. The ability to make changes in movement in relation to specific tasks within different environments

This view of functional mobility is congruent to a systems approach for analyzing and explaining normal movement, which emphasizes the interaction of the individual, task, and environment.[84]

ACTIVITIES IN THE SUPINE POSITION

The performance of supine activities is often associated with the acute stages of the rehabilitation process. Bridging, rolling, and movement from side lying-to-sit are basic functional mobility tasks that are necessary to the provision of nursing care and movement of the client

Table 14-1

Managing Impairments that Affect Functional Mobility

IMPAIRMENTS OBSERVED DURING TREATMENT	SUGGESTED STRATEGIES/INSTRUCTIONS
Reduced visual field	Teach compensation by reinforcing head-turning during functional mobility tasks. See Chapter 16.
Reduced perceptual processing	Anticipate that patients may misperceive distance between themselves and supporting surfaces. Help the patient to reappraise distances prior to moving. See Chapter 16.
Reduced arousal	Arousal can vary over the course of the day. Monitor for optimal state of arousal to determine when treatment should be carried out. Observe for signs of diminishing arousal during therapy. See Chapter 19.
Reduced attention	Work in distraction-free environments. Use patient's room prior to using the therapy rooms. Gradually introduce stimuli into treatment as the patient tolerates. See Chapter 19.
Reduced awareness of impairments	Heighten awareness of impairments. Engage patients before they attempt the activity as to how they feel they can execute the activity; posttask ask the patients for feedback on performance; consider use of videotaped feedback. See Chapter 19.
Unilateral inattention	Increase attention to the affected side and engage extremities wherever possible. See Chapter 19.
Reduced learning	Use "Show" versus "Tell" when teaching functional mobility tasks.
Reduced problem-solving	May manifest in novel situations; offer varying practice conditions (i.e., rolling on a mat or in a bed with sheets and a blanket) to provide opportunities to develop strategies for solving movement challenges.
Reduced language/communication	Avoid speaking in a loud voice. Give the patient ample time to respond. Observe the patient for signs of fatigue or anxiety. Encourage self-expression through gestures, if necessary. If the patient has comprehension problems, ask simple, short questions and augment verbal with pantomime and gestures. Use tactile cueing. See Chapter 20.
Reduced pragmatics	Minimize distractions. Use demonstration and do not rely on self-report. Provide feedback on statements irrelevant to the situation.
Reduced motor planning	Use tactile-kinesthetic cues. Keep environment and context appropriate to task. See Chapter 19.

from a bed to a wheelchair. However, these mobility sequences are also important in enabling the client to participate in a wide range of life areas. For example, consider the individual who chooses to lie on a beach to enjoy the sun and surf. The soft surface of the sand may require the individual to assume a bridge position to shift his or her position if rolling is inadequate. Supine activities require the individual to gain control of flexor and extensor patterns of the trunk, which can be viewed as a prerequisite for more advanced trunk positions.

Bridging

Analysis of Movement. In the functional mobility task of bridging, the back and hip extensors support the body against the forces of gravity. The arch formed when the upper back and feet are in contact with the supporting surface is maintained by the activation of muscles located on the underside of the arch. Use of the arms or legs increases the demands placed on the trunk musculature. When an arm or leg is raised (as in attempts to dress), the muscles located above the arch (the oblique abdominal muscles) must become active to support the limb.[28]

Selected Problems. The mobility task of bridging is a challenge for patients with hemiplegia because of loss of activity in the extensors and the abdominal muscles. This problem, when combined with early return of extensor activity, results in ineffective and inefficient movement patterns.

Observations in supine indicating decreased abdominal activity include the following:

- Outward flaring of the ribcage (that is, the affected side rides higher in the cavity because the abdominal muscles do not tether the ribcage downward)
- Shortening of the neck resulting from unopposed elevation of the shoulder girdle
- Hypotonic appearance of the abdomen
- Shift of the umbilicus to the nonaffected side
- Reduced proximal stability effecting the lower extremities
- Difficulty moving or maintaining the position of the lower extremity due to reduced proximal stability

Treatment Strategies. Bridging is an important position that the patient should be instructed to assume early in the intervention process. Bridging is a mobility function necessary for the use of a bedpan, reduction of pressure on the buttocks, and movement within the bed (bed scooting).[53]

The patient with hemiplegia may have trouble in assuming the crook-lying position and forming a bridge because of a variety of underlying causes. The lack of selective muscle activity on the affected side, caused by the use of mass patterns, prevents the patient from combining the necessary hip components of flexion and adduction.[13]

Patient attempts to place the affected leg usually result in a mass pattern of movement characterized by hip flexion and external rotation and supination of the foot. The patient's inability to stabilize the pelvis while attempting this movement results in increased extension of the lumbar spine combined with forced extension of the nonaffected side into the supporting surface. Another possible reason for the increase in the extension of the lumbar spine is tightness of the hip flexors,[86] although this is unlikely in the early stages after stroke unless the patient exhibited tightness before sustaining the stroke.

The therapist can assist the patient to assume the crook-lying position. The therapist encourages the patient to assist with active flexion of the unaffected leg and may be required to assist and hold the required crook-lying position. Active flexion on the affected leg helps position the pelvis forward and may promote active holding of the affected leg in a flexed position.[53] The therapist may provide downward pressure on the flexed knee of the affected side to ensure appropriate foot placement.[13]

Active bridging can be used to improve selective extension of the hip and abdominal muscle activity. As the patient lifts the buttocks from the supporting surface, the therapist should make sure the patient does not use excessive extensor activity, which is characterized by extension of the hips, overarching of the back, and pushing of the head into the supporting surface. To improve selective movement, the therapist encourages the patient to initiate the movement by actively tilting the pelvis upward. The therapist may need to prepare the patient for this movement (Fig. 14-1). After tilting the pelvis forward, the patient lifts the buttocks off the surface while holding the pelvis level. The therapist may assist this movement by placing one hand under the hemiplegic hip and one hand on the abdominals. If the feet are

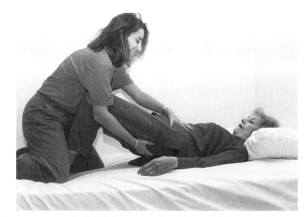

Figure 14-1   In bridging, one should avoid increased extensor activity that results in arching of the back. To assist with selective movement of the pelvis, the therapist cues the gluteal region and the lower abdominals. This sequence may be applied first to the unaffected side and then to the hemiplegic side.

positioned close to the body, the therapist also may guide the femoral condyles forward toward the feet while applying downward pressure (Fig. 14-2).

After the patient can maintain this position, the next step is to lift the unaffected foot off the surface while maintaining the pelvis level. The therapist should observe any asymmetries or rotation of the pelvis. The therapist must not permit the patient to drop the unaffected side to gain more stability. This task is difficult for the patient with hemiplegia because it places demands on the oblique abdominal muscles[22,29,86] and the other weakened core trunk muscles. Bridging can be graded according to the patient's ability to control movements selectively. Placement of the feet further away from the buttocks requires a greater degree of selective activity to maintain knee flexion with hip extension.[29] Alternate lifting of the feet off the supporting surface while maintaining the level of the pelvis requires increased muscular activity and greater coordination (Figs. 14-3 and 14-4).[86]

Bridging can be used to move up in bed and don pants while in a supine position. Therapists should instruct caregivers in the appropriate techniques to ensure that

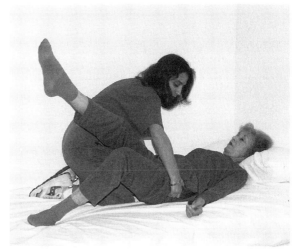

Figure 14-3 Lifting a leg off the supporting surface places increased demands on the abdominal muscles because the pelvis must be held up. The therapist asks the patient to lift the unaffected foot off the bed so that all the patient's weight is placed on the affected side. The patient must maintain the pelvis in a level position. This patient is experiencing difficulty maintaining the optimal pelvic position (left hemiplegia).

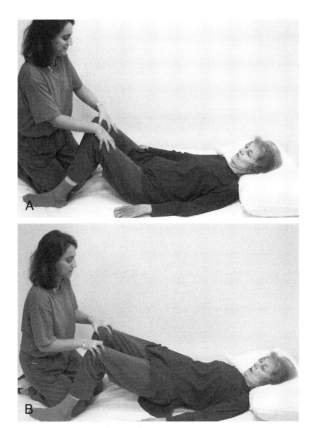

Figure 14-2 **A,** As the patient gains selective control over the pelvis, the therapist can provide downward pressure through the knees and guide the femoral condyles forward toward the feet. **B,** The therapist asks the patient to lift the buttocks off the bed. Physical assistance can be diminished as the patient gains control.

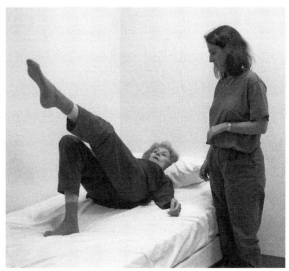

Figure 14-4 This patient has less difficulty in lifting the hemiplegic side (left hemiplegia).

these movements are transferred into the patient's daily life routine. The occupational therapist can incorporate these movement strategies while training the patient in self-care activities.

Rolling

Analysis of Movement. Rolling is an important part of bed mobility and an essential part of many other tasks. Research has demonstrated that normal adults use a variety of movement strategies to roll from supine to prone.[72]

One of the most common movement strategies used by young adults in rolling from supine to prone includes a lift-and-reach arm pattern. Movement of the head and trunk is initiated by the shoulder girdle; a unilateral lift of the leg also occurs. Rotation of the spine, which results in dissociation of the shoulder and pelvic girdles, is not observed (Fig. 14-5).[72] This rotation was once assumed a prerequisite to attaining the ability to roll in a normal pattern of movement.[13]

The most important finding of this study[72] is that normal adults have a repertoire of movements available to them, unlike patients after stroke, who are limited to stereotypical patterns of movement.[26] The environmental conditions of this study were limited to rolling on an exercise mat, and the subjects were asked to roll "as fast as you can." Thus, the variety of patterns observed may relate to the temporal demands and implied goal of the task. The strategies used to roll for speed may differ significantly from the strategies used to target a particular object in the environment. Therapists who work with patients with hemiplegia must consider the rolling surface (environment), the goal of changing the position of the body while supine, and future mobility goals such as attaining supine-to-sit. Thus, therapists must determine movement sequences most suitable for ensuring safety and achieving the goal of the movement. Rotation of the spine during rolling is just one strategy that may be useful in providing a greater variety of movement possibilities for the patient with hemiplegia.[22,28,29]

Rolling to the Hemiplegic Side: Selected Problems and Treatment Strategies. The patient with hemiplegia frequently rolls over using an extensor pattern to initiate the movement sequence because of lack of flexor control of the trunk and the early return of extensor activity. The patient relies on the unaffected side to push against the supporting surface, resulting in an arching of the axial spine as the body is thrust forward in the direction of the roll.

Davies[28] suggested that rolling activities can be used to promote active flexion of the trunk and achieve subsequent improvement in active control of the trunk musculature. The need exists balance the concentric and eccentric contractions of the trunk muscles in proportion to the change in force exerted by gravity as the patient changes position.

The hemiplegic arm requires protection before rolling to the affected side is practiced. The therapist can provide this protection by prepositioning the arm, assisting the patient in bringing the shoulder and arm forward, and giving physical support to the hemiplegic arm while standing on the affected side.

The patient is encouraged to lift the unaffected arm and leg up and forward across the body; this movement is consistent with the pattern identified by Richter, Van Sant, and Newton.[72] This movement should occur without the patient pushing against the supporting surface with the unaffected foot (Fig. 14-6). The patient may repeat this movement by returning to the supine position. A part of or the whole leg should be held in abduction and slowly lowered to the surface as the patient returns to the supine position.

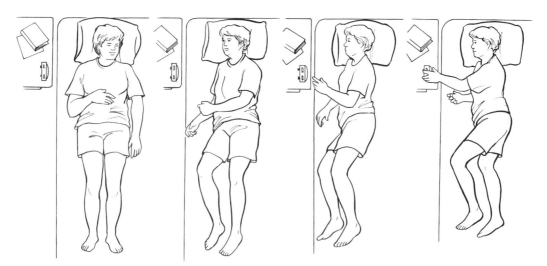

Figure 14-5 Research has determined that a common form of rolling observed in adults is initiated by a lift-and-reach above shoulder level; the shoulder girdle leads the movement, and a unilateral lift of the lower extremity follows. Many subjects also use a unilateral push of the lower extremity. A great variety of patterns is observed because of individual differences in build and strength and in the support surface.

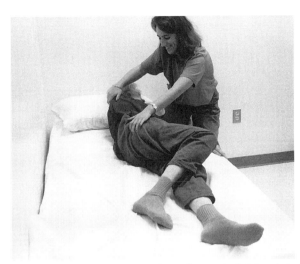

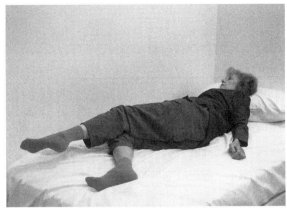

Figure 14-7 Rolling toward the unaffected side. The patient should avoid using the back extensors to bring the lower extremity forward while neglecting the hemiplegic arm (left hemiplegia).

Figure 14-6 Rolling toward the hemiplegic side (left hemiplegia) is accomplished by lifting the unaffected leg over the hemiplegic side without pushing off the bed surface. The therapist assists with movement of the shoulder and pelvic girdles.

As the patient gains control of this movement sequence, the next step is to lift the head from the surface to assist with initiation of movement. As the patient turns, the head is rotated toward the direction of the movement. Throughout the sequence, physical assistance should decrease as changes in the patient's ability to control movement occur.

Rolling to the Unaffected Side: Selected Problems and Treatment Strategies. Rolling to the unaffected side may be more difficult for the patient with hemiplegia. The movement is frequently initiated by an extensor pattern that includes extension of the head, neck, and back. The patient relies on extension of the back to bring the hemiplegic leg over the trunk in a pattern of extension that may be viewed as an inefficient compensatory strategy. The affected arm may be left behind as the patient rolls (Fig. 14-7).[29]

When teaching patients to roll to the unaffected side, the therapist's goals are to decrease maladaptive compensatory strategies contributing to inefficient movement and to enhance more effective and efficient patterns of movement. The patient may be instructed to use the stronger arm (Fig. 14-8) to bring the hemiplegic arm up and forward while the therapist attempts verbally or physically to cue the movement of the pelvis and lower extremity. The therapist supports the affected leg while assisting with anterior movement of the pelvis (Fig. 14-9).

Repetition of this sequence may assist with learning. The therapist encourages the patient to lift the affected leg off the supporting surface and lower it slowly after returning to the supine position. This strategy is used to assist the patient in maintaining a slight degree of hip and

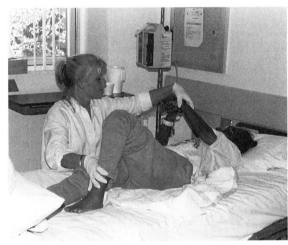

Figure 14-8 Early in the rehabilitation process, the therapists instructs the patient with left hemiplegia to use the stronger hand to assist in bringing the shoulder forward; the therapist positions the hemiplegic leg in hip and knee flexion to avoid an extensor pattern.

knee flexion, which decreases reliance on the extensor compensatory pattern. An alternative method is to flex both legs to roll.[13,29]

Supine-to-Sit

Analysis of Movement. The transitional movement from supine-to-sit may be achieved through a variety of movement strategies. Adults have a tendency to use a momentum strategy to achieve the goal (Fig. 14-10). Their movements are smooth and efficient as they "bound" out of bed, off the couch, or out of a chair. A momentum strategy requires forces within the trunk to be generated and transferred to the lower extremities to initiate the rolling sequence. Trunk muscles must contract concentrically to

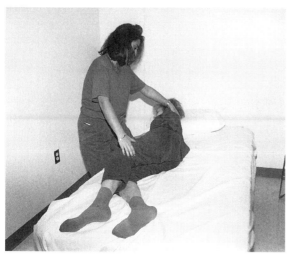

Figure 14-9 Assistance can be decreased as the patient gains control of the movement. The therapist assists with knee flexion and protraction of the shoulder (left hemiplegia).

initiate and propel the movement; eccentric muscle contractions provide control. The reciprocal shortening and lengthening of muscle contractions provide maintained stability.

Many older adults demonstrate a tendency to use a force control strategy (Fig. 14-11). The individual transfers forces from one body part to another as graduated changes in position occur. Rolling to side lying, then pushing up with the upper extremities, and swinging the lower extremities over the side of the bed is an example of

this strategy. This method provides increased stability because concentric and eccentric forces are required in increments. Increased effort (force) must be used if momentum is lacking.[20,22,29,72,81]

Evidence exists to support that older adults use their upper limbs to assist the trunk musculature when moving from supine-to-sit.[3] Thus, therapists need to consider the movement strategies and positioning of the arms when retraining the supine-to-sit sequence. A great variety of movement possibilities to achieve a supine-to-sit sequence remains. The described sequence often is used spontaneously by patients after stroke and by the therapists as a method of instruction.[22] This sequence is referred to as side lying-to-sit for the remainder of this chapter.

Selected Problems. Movement from the side lying to seated position becomes a challenge for the patient after stroke because of the combined effects of limited muscular activity and maladaptive compensatory strategies. Patients lack appropriate postural alignment and stability.[22,28] The lack of flexor control of the trunk and early return of extensor activity interfere with the patient's ability to grade concentric and eccentric muscle activity effectively relative to the changing forces of gravity.[28] If inadequate control of the trunk musculature is evident, the patient must rely on compensatory strategies that may include overuse of the unaffected arm or leg or exaggerated use of head movements. The patient applies these compensatory strategies instead of effective lateral movements of the neck and trunk. When side lying, the patient flexes the head forward instead of laterally and uses the unaffected arm to move

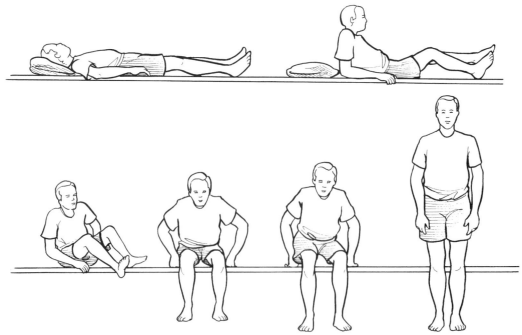

Figure 14-10 The most common movement strategy used by adults to get out of bed relies on momentum. Strategies vary greatly.

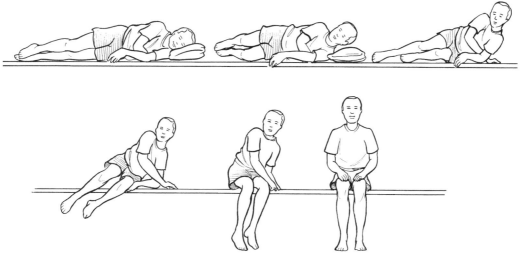

Figure 14-11 A force control strategy for getting out of bed has the individual performing the task in two parts: the patient moves from supine to side lying and then pushes to a seated position. This strategy is useful for patients who exhibit reduced stability functions.

the body away from the supporting surface. The forward movement of the head may be a compensatory strategy to shift the center of gravity forward. The patient may be unable to combine lateral flexion and extension of the trunk because of lack of selective muscle activity. Hooking of the unaffected leg under the affected leg to lift and lower the leg over the side of the bed is yet another compensatory strategy many patients are instructed to perform. This strategy prevents selective movement of the pelvis in an anterior and lateral direction.[22,28] The patient with hemiplegia experiences difficulty whether rising from the hemiplegic or the unaffected side because of the problems presented.

Additionally, while changing positions, the patient may not exhibit appropriate head-righting responses; this deficit requires the patient to flex the neck laterally while controlling eccentric muscle activity on the opposite side. Furthermore, the patient also may be unable to move or place the affected limbs appropriately in preparation for transitional movement or may neglect the affected limbs entirely.

Treatment Strategies. Many methods are suggested to retrain the patient in the supine-to-sit movement sequence. One method suggests that patients with hemiplegia be taught initially to roll toward the affected side to decrease the amount of effort required and to reduce maladaptive strategies such as pulling and pushing to achieve the seated position.[22] Others suggest that the patient with hemiplegia be instructed to rise from both sides early in treatment to prevent associated reactions.[12,28,29] Another option is for the patient to start the movement sitting upright and learn to lie down first. This method may decrease the force gravity exerts on the trunk musculature as

the patient first learns to control movement into gravity using eccentric muscle activity.[28] The physical environment and the patient's premorbid preferences for movement sequences also may influence the methods selected. Patients may benefit from learning more than one method to move more effectively in different environments.

Side Lying-to-Sit Toward the Affected Side. The therapist assists the patient in lifting the hemiplegic leg over the side of the bed; the head, neck, and upper thorax are brought forward, requiring the neck to flex laterally. Concurrently the nonaffected arm must be brought across the body and placed on the bed. The unaffected leg also must be lifted over the side of the bed as the patient pushes down with the hand. The movement of the unaffected leg as the patient simultaneously pushes with the hand adds a momentum strategy to this movement sequence; the weight of the leg assists the patient in attaining a seated posture. The therapist may need to assist with bringing the unaffected shoulder forward over the base of support of the body. The therapist may place hands on the shoulder and pelvic girdle to give support and to assist with movement of the unaffected leg (Fig. 14-12). As the patient gains some control over this movement, the therapist may provide support to just the unaffected shoulder and pelvis (Fig. 14-13). The therapist can use verbal cues or downward pressure on the shoulder physically to cue lateral flexion of the trunk and appropriate head righting. To reverse this sequence, the patient may require assistance with lifting the hemiplegic leg onto the bed. Care should be directed toward maintaining the hemiplegic shoulder in a forward position as the patient turns and lowers the body to the bed surface.[28]

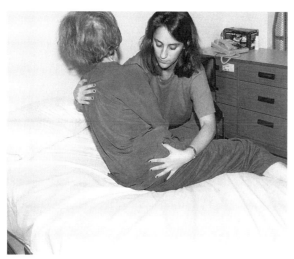

Figure 14-12 The therapist uses one arm around the patient's shoulders while the other hand provides downward pressure to the pelvis to assist with weight transfer in movement to a seated position (left hemiplegia).

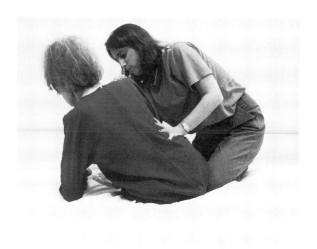

Figure 14-14 Propping of the affected upper extremity as the patient prepares to assume the seated position. The therapist is assisting with lateral flexion of the unaffected side while observing for appropriate head and trunk alignment on the affected side.

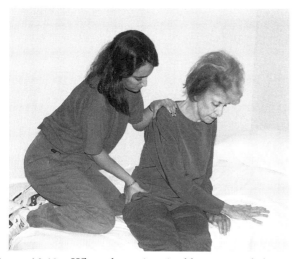

Figure 14-13 When the patient is able to control the trunk muscles actively, the therapist can decrease assistance. The therapist may cue lateral flexion of the head and trunk by providing downward pressure to the shoulder and pelvic girdles of the unaffected side.

When assuming a sitting position from the affected side, the patient is active in the trunk, particularly while bearing weight on the affected upper extremity; therapists should be mindful of this. Furthermore, the therapist may have to cue movement of the trunk on both sides to promote the correct sequence of lateral flexion and extension responses (Fig. 14-14).

Side Lying-to-Sit Toward the Unaffected Side. The sequence of movement in side lying-to-sit toward the unaffected side remains the same as that in the previous

example; however, the placement of the therapist's hands to assist movement changes. The therapist should instruct the patient to lift the affected arm while lifting the unaffected leg over the side of the bed. The therapist assists with movement of the affected leg forward and over the edge of the bed as the patient lifts the head, neck, and upper thorax over the sound arm (Fig. 14-15). The

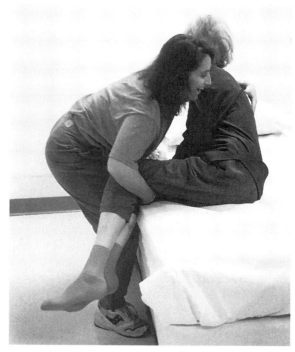

Figure 14-15 Rising from the unaffected side. For patients who require significant support, the therapist places one hand on the scapula while assisting with movement of the legs.

therapist needs to ensure that the hemiplegic shoulder remains in a forward position as the patient begins to push down with the unaffected side. A movement sequence that begins as a force control strategy can with increased motor control of the head, neck, and trunk become a momentum strategy.

Patients demonstrating a lack of lateral flexion of the neck require preparatory interventions. The patient should be positioned side lying on the unaffected side with the head on the bed (Fig. 14-16, *A*). The patient lifts the head with the therapist's assistance as needed (Fig. 14-16, *B*). The therapist then asks the patient to lower the head to the bed; this movement requires eccentric contraction of the lateral flexors. This maneuver is followed by active lifting of the head, which requires concentric muscle contractions. The therapist should not permit the patient to rotate or flex forward while performing this task. A visual target such as an alarm clock, television, or family picture may assist in establishing this task-related goal.[22]

Additional interventions to promote lateral flexion and extension of the trunk, which are necessary to perform side lying-to-sit, are described in the section on sitting.

ACTIVITIES IN SITTING

The ability to maintain a seated position and perform ADL safely and efficiently is a goal many occupational therapists seek with their patients (see Chapter 7). In the acute stages after stroke, the therapist should begin to work on control of sitting and standing with the patient as soon as possible to promote the ability to manage the upright position and increase overall visual input in functional positions.[22]

Analysis of Movement

For controlled movement in sitting the ability to bear and shift weight anteriorly, posteriorly, laterally, and in a rotary pattern must be present. This suggests that the concentric and eccentric abilities of the trunk flexors and extensors and the ability to activate these muscle groups selectively relative to the task demand must be present. For example, for controlled anterior weight shift through the pelvis, the need for concentric contraction of the low back extensors and an associated eccentric contraction of the trunk flexors (abdominals) is evident. In a posterior weight shift through the pelvis, the need for concentric contraction of the trunk flexors and an associated eccentric contraction of the trunk extensors is evident. With lateral weight shift through the pelvis the trunk extensors and flexors work together concentrically (shortening) on the nonweight-bearing side and eccentrically (lengthening) on the weight-bearing side.[13] During trunk rotation, the primary muscles involved are the oblique muscles.

Selected Problems

The trunk is crucial in postural control. Many patients display difficulty with voluntary trunk control in sitting following the stroke. Messier and colleagues[63] looked at trunk flexion in sitting poststroke and noted decreased displacement of the center of pressure and lower extremity weight-bearing through the feet. They felt that this was probably indicative of minimal anterior tilt of the pelvis, and most of the trunk motion initiating from the upper trunk.[63]

There is electromyography (EMG) evidence to support alterations in trunk muscle activity following stroke. Trunk velocity during flexion and extension is lower following stroke compared to normal subjects.[33] With the addition of

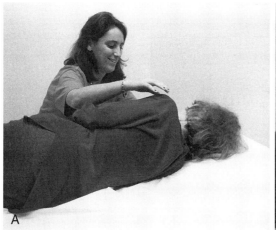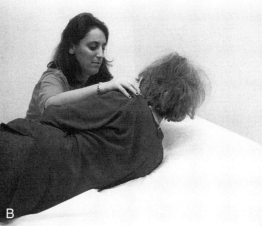

Figure 14-16   **A,** To encourage active control of the lateral neck muscles, the patient first learns to control eccentric contraction while lowering the head to the bed. **B,** This is followed by active lateral neck flexion while raising the head.

voluntary arm and leg movements, there is delayed onset of contraction and reduced activation of paretic trunk muscles.[33] In contrast to Dickstein and associates' findings, Winzeler-Mercay and Mudie[96] found that muscle activity in the paretic rectus abdominis and erector spinae following stroke were the same as normal subjects during forward and backward voluntary sway and reaching, but for the task of donning the shoes, the rectus abdominus showed reduced activity. The erector spinae activation was much higher in the stroke group during all postural activities.[96]

The therapist must begin an assessment on functional capabilities in this area by close examination of the patient's ability to control movements in sitting (see Chapter 7). A full appreciation of the normal ranges of motion (ROMs) within the spine is useful when comparing patients with hemiplegia and the patterns they use with the normal population. The therapist must be cognizant that these ranges decrease with age; ascertaining the baseline from which these patients were operating before the onset of hemiparesis is important. Mohr[64] emphasized the importance of establishing a patient's ROM in spinal extension and flexion, lateral flexion, and rotation before treatment is implemented. This provides the therapist with information needed to decide whether interventions should include increasing ranges in these areas with the goal of promoting activation by the patient in these patterns for function. Davies[28] also recommended this approach. For example, passive mobilization of the lumbar spine for lateral flexion may be an important preparatory treatment to working on increased trunk control in activities requiring a lateral weight shift such as side lying-to-sit. The therapist, having encouraged increased mobility in this plane, can progress to facilitation of the appropriate muscle contractions needed to hold and move into this position by placing the hand in the patient's axilla and assisting the side to lengthen while placing the other hand on the patient's opposite trunk to guide shortening on that side. Conversely, many clinicians with a motor learning perspective suggest that the therapist set up the environment to create a natural situation that places increased demand on trunk muscles for function.

A deeper look at the location of movement and the way it is initiated is necessary before proceeding in evaluation. Mohr[64] provided guidance by categorizing trunk movements in sitting by dividing them into movements initiated from the upper trunk versus the lower trunk. Mohr further analyzed anterior, lateral, and posterior weight shifts in each of these categories and then provided functional examples for each movement pattern.

Functional Activities in Sitting

Task-oriented functional practice must follow all "preparatory" trunk activity such as mobilization. Following hands-on treatment, one hopefully will see gains in passive mobility or the patient's ability to "find" the

muscle and activate it. However, the patients themselves must use these gains immediately particularly in the context of a functional activity; otherwise, carryover is doubtful (Figs. 14-17 and 14-18).

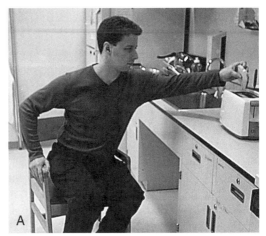
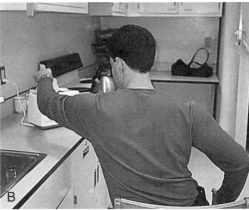

Figure 14-17 A, Reaching for toast combines patterns of trunk lateral flexion and extension. **B,** Using the right affected arm to bear weight on the armrest results in scapula depression, which contributes to the shortening of the trunk muscles on the right side.

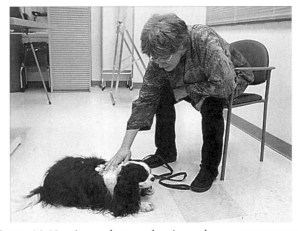

Figure 14-18 A pet therapy dog is used to encourage trunk flexion and weight-bearing on the affected left arm and leg.

Gentile[37] proposed two distinct processes that mediate skill learning: an explicit process and an implicit process. In the explicit process, patients consciously involve themselves with shaping the movements to achieve a specific goal. In the implicit process, the main concern is the dynamic of force generation, which is not under the conscious control of the patient. Implicit processes rely on the interplay of muscle contractions against the passive components affected by gravity and joint torques. Gentile suggested that for the explicit process to occur, therapists can use information consciously available to the patient and provide coaching such as around how a movement is organized and features in the environment. For implicit learning to occur, therapists must challenge themselves creatively to set up the environment to elicit a response from the patient that produces force generation as a byproduct of the functional activity in which they are engaged. Clearly, the therapist must set up opportunities for practice for the greatest benefit to occur to the learner.

Dean and Shepherd[30] designed a study specifically to look at the efficacy of task-related training, which proves to be an excellent example of using explicit and implicit learning processes in treatment. Their intent was to increase the distance stroke patients could perform forward reach in sitting and to note the contribution of the affected lower limb to support and balance in this activity. Twenty subjects were used in this study, and they had to be a minimum of one year poststroke. They were randomized into two groups—an experimental group that received treatment involving reaching forward for natural objects beyond arm's length (in a gradual progression) and a control group that received sham training with cognitive tasks within arm's length. EMG, videotaping, and two force plates (to evaluate the amount of lower extremity force generated during the activity and sit-to-stand) were used before and after training to gain objective measures. After training, subjects were capable of reaching farther and faster, suggesting that the affected lower limb was assisting more in support. Furthermore, the researchers noted that subjects demonstrated improved force generation of the affected lower limb in sit-to-stand. The explicit learning process subjects were engaged in was demonstrated by the problem-solving and practicing of forward reaching farther and farther. The implicit learning process was activating the lower extremity in the process.[30,37]

Scooting

Analysis of Movement. Scooting, or "butt walking," involves the transfer of weight over first one buttock and then the other, creating overall movement of the body anteriorly in a seated position.[12] Appropriate elongation of the trunk on the weight-bearing side and shortening on the nonweight-bearing side is required. This movement pattern is useful for a number of functional activities such as donning and doffing pants in a seated position. From a mobility perspective, it allows the individual to approach the edge of a supporting surface to transfer.

Selected Problems. As indicated previously, problems with passive restriction in the trunk and the inability to activate trunk muscles selectively are of primary concern with this activity and may preclude the appropriate balance reactions needed for success and safety. The patient must have intact skin on the buttocks to practice scooting.

Treatment Strategies. Verbal or physical cueing to assist patients with scooting can be accomplished in a variety of ways, depending on the level of involvement of the individual. The therapist may elicit the desired movement pattern through a series of contacts in which the therapist first cues a lateral weight shift and then places the hand on the patient's pelvis to cue forward advancing of the hip on the nonweight-bearing side.[12] The therapist then changes hands to cue forward movement of the opposite buttock (Fig. 14-19). Patients with more profound physical involvement may require added assistance by the therapist, particularly in advancing the buttock (Fig. 14-20).

Transfers

Analysis of Movement. The ability to move from a given surface to an adjacent surface safely and efficiently is a primary goal in treatment for many of the patients with whom occupational therapists work. This maneuver requires enough forward flexion of the trunk over the feet to allow the individual to pivot about the feet and sit on the nearby surface.

Selected Problems. Patients with neglect who attempt to transfer often succeed in transporting only half the body onto the supporting surface. Additionally, the left foot may be neglected, and the patient may be oblivious to proper left foot placement before transferring.

Many patients require considerable help to maintain a flat foot on the floor. This may be because of unilateral inattention, poor sensation on the affected side, shortened trunk muscles resulting in asymmetrical sitting, and shortening of the calf muscles on the affected side.

Treatment Strategies. Bobath[12] and Davies[29] described the anterior weight shift that can be facilitated through contact on the patient's pelvis or scapulae. Carr and Shepherd[22] recognized the same forward weight shift and encouraged patients to move the shoulders forward during active participation in transfers (Fig. 14-21). All four therapists described ways the therapist may use manual contact to the knee to draw the knee forward and encourage weight-bearing on the hemiplegic side.

Patients have varying degrees of motor control for this activity. The therapist needs to create an environment in

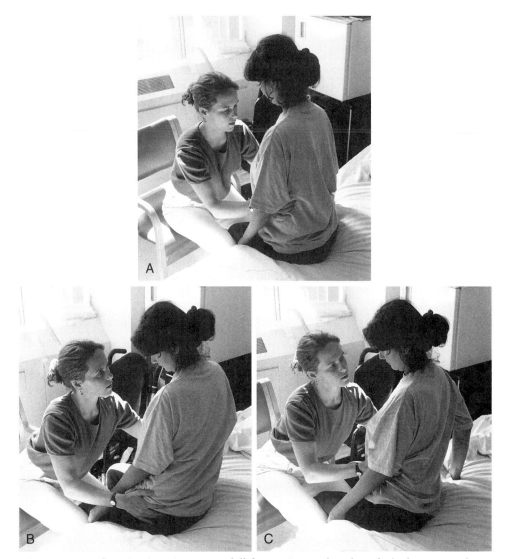

Figure 14-19   Scooting is an important skill for moving to the edge of a bed or seat and can be a useful movement pattern in activity of daily living tasks such as donning pants in a seated position. **A,** The patient begins in symmetrical sitting. **B,** The therapist can encourage scooting by first cueing a lateral weight shift and then advancing the nonweight-bearing buttock to move anteriorly **(C).**

which the patient has enough guarding by the therapist to make training safe and enough "room" to try to make the transfer with as little assistance as possible. This is not always easy to do, and some patients inevitably require much assistance to transfer. However, the more the patient can be encouraged to do, the more the patient learns during the session. Consistent grading of the level of assistance a patient requires (i.e., minimal, moderate, or maximal) is important in measuring progress and communicating to other staff members the amount of help required by the patient to carry out the task.

In the initial stages of transfer training, a patient may require maximal assistance, and the therapist may need to clasp both hands around the pelvis to pivot the patient

from one surface to another. As the patient gains greater strength and control over balance, the therapist may reduce this level of assistance to a lighter hold around the pelvis and then the scapula.

Patients tend to be taught stand-pivot or modified stand-pivot (sit-pivot) transfers. Many therapists train stand-pivot transfers for the presumed benefits they afford in getting the patient into an upright position and putting full weight on the involved lower extremity. However, these transfers do not resemble the maneuvers performed by normal subjects in moving from one surface to the other (i.e., coming to a full stand or turning and sitting down on an adjacent surface). As Shumway-Cook and Woollacott[84] pointed out, stand-pivot transfers may be more difficult

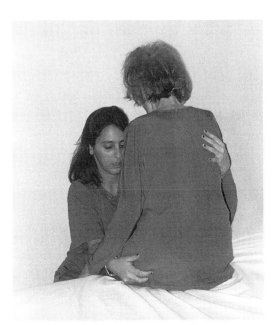

Figure 14-20 Patients requiring a more direct contact to scoot can be guided first by the therapist to advance the buttock.

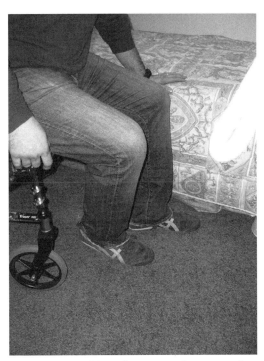

Figure 14-22 Foot placement prior to transfer.

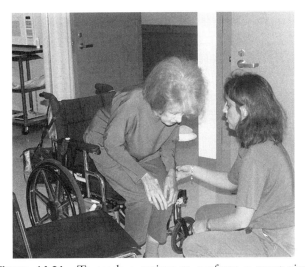

Figure 14-21 To teach a patient to perform a squat-pivot transfer, the therapist should encourage the appropriate amount of anterior weight shift by instructing the patient to move the shoulders forward.

because they do not allow the patient to use a momentum strategy; the need to come to a stand instead of pivoting blocks the benefits the momentum strategy provides. When training pivot transfers, foot placement is important. One foot is slightly in front of the other at the outset and is adjacent to the surface to which the patient is moving (Fig. 14-22). With environmental constraints or more advanced patients, a stand-and-step transfer may be used.

Promoting weight shift onto the affected lower extremity is important during transfers and sit-to-stand activities. The therapist may position both knees around the patient's affected knee physically to assist a forward weight shift onto the lower extremity and to guard against buckling at the patient's knee. For patients requiring less cueing and guarding, the therapist may assist the knee by placing a hand on the patient's distal femur and gently pulling anteriorly and then down toward the floor as the patient takes weight on the leg.

The role of the arms in this training process has become controversial. Bobath[12] and Davies[29] supported using clasped hands in front of the body to facilitate a forward weight shift, placing the arms on a stool, chair, or other supporting surface. However, a study by Carr and Gentile[19] examined the role of the upper extremities in sit-to-stand and determined that "fixing" the arms (by holding a rod as subjects in the study did) had a tendency to cause an increase in what was described as extension force (the force needed by the lower extremities to extend the body into an upright position) and a decrease in momentum of the body during sit-to-stand; this determination may have implications for transfers. The authors advocated that patients work on increasing strength in the lower extremities (particularly in extension) to enhance functioning in sit-to-stand. They contended that although patients tend to use the hands to push down on the armrests of a chair to stand or alternatively swing the arms forward to assist horizontal and vertical propulsion of the body mass, these strategies cannot be used in varying environmental conditions[19] (Figs. 14-23 to 14-27).

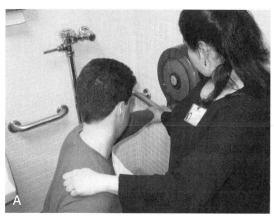

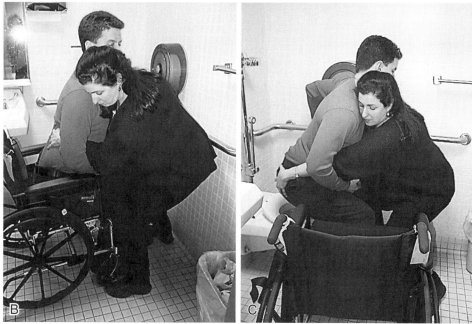

Figure 14-23 **A,** Use of a grab bar can encourage a forward weight shift in a transfer requiring greater physical assistance. **B,** Positioning and proper handling can be difficult with space constraints. This requires problem-solving for the therapist, patient, and caregiver. **C,** While this patient may require moderate physical assistance to perform the transfer, he is actively encouraged to use the movements he is capable of in the transfer, in this case, thoracic extension.

A study by Gillen and Wasserman[40] analyzed how altering the environmental context of a transfer activity affected mobility performance in patients receiving inpatient rehabilitation. They compared performance in transfers carried out in a traditional clinic setting and in a more naturalistic apartment-like setting. Twenty-five participants carried out four transfer tasks in each environment: two bedside commode transfers and two bed-to-chair transfers. The Functional Independence Measure (FIM) was used to provide the level of assistance required in transfers.

Their findings revealed that environment plays a role in mobility performance. Forty-four percent of the patients performed better in the traditional clinic setting. Twenty percent performed better in the simulated apartment.

Sixty-four percent of patients were inconsistent with the same transfer task between the two environments, while 36% of the patients transferred consistently in the two environments, as per the FIM data. Therapists asked to provide FIM data early in the inpatient rehabilitation stay must never assume that performance in the clinic equals performance in other environments.

Sit-to-Stand

Analysis of Movement. Sit-to-stand can be divided into different phases, depending on the description of the researcher (Fig. 14-28). Shepherd and Gentile[82] described sit-to-stand using the terms *preextension phase*, a phase characterized by the beginning of the movement to the position in which the thighs are off the surface; and *extension phase*,

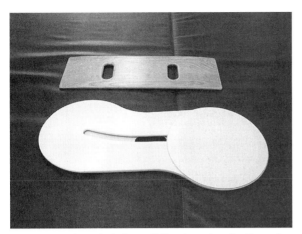

Figure 14-24 A typical short sliding board and a Beasy board. These devices can be used to assist patients who have greater physical needs.

the phase from the thighs-off position through the end of movement (full stand). Shenkman and colleagues[81] described four phases in sit-to-stand (Fig. 14-29). Phase 1 (Fig. 14-30, *A*) is referred to as the flexion momentum phase and is used to generate the initial momentum for rising. During this phase, the center of mass is within the base of support, and eccentric contractions of the erector spinae are required to control forward motion of the trunk. Phase 2 (Fig. 14-30, *B*) begins as the individual leaves the chair seat and ends at maximal ankle dorsiflexion. Forward momentum of the upper body is transferred to forward and upward momentum of the total body. The center of mass now moves from within the base of support of the chair to the feet. By definition, the phase is unstable and requires co-activation of hip and knee extensors. Phase 3 (Fig. 14-30, *C*) is an extension phase during which the body rises to its

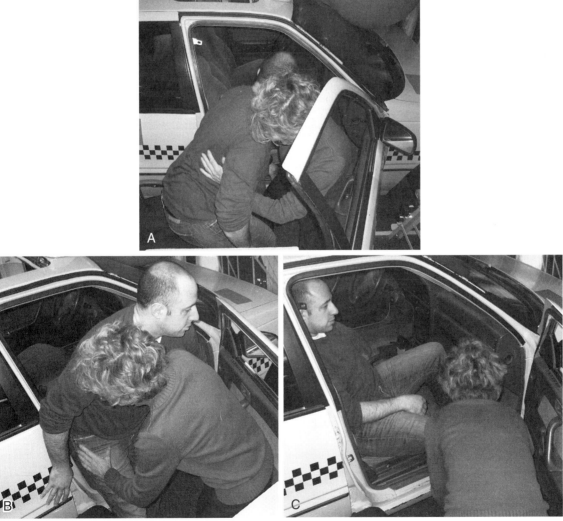

Figure 14-25 **A,** Early practice with car transfers may take place using a simulated car in the clinic and where possible should progress to an actual vehicle. **B,** Controlled descent into gravity requires coactivation of the abdominal muscles (flexors) and back extensors to avoid injury in a constrained space. **C,** The patient is shown how to manage the affected leg during the transfer.

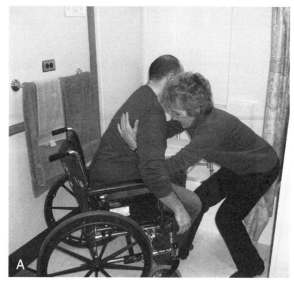

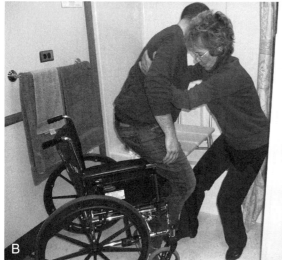

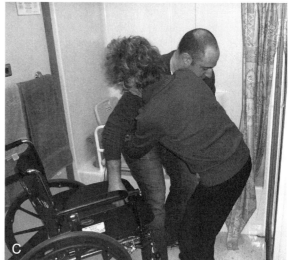

Figure 14-26   **A** to **C,** Sequence of transfer to tub bench.

full upright position by expansion of the hips and knees. The stability requirements are not as great as in phase 2 because the center of mass is well within the base of support of the feet. Phase 4 (Fig. 14-30, *D*) is a stabilization phase in which complete extension of the hips and knees occurs. Regardless of the way researchers divide the task, an appreciation of the biomechanics of this movement pattern is crucial in training and in understanding potential problems that occur in hemiplegia.

Carr and Shepherd[20] outlined key factors that influence the way sit-to-stand is executed in normal individuals. The therapist must consider the role of foot position, the starting position of the trunk, the speed of movement, and the role of the upper limbs in balance and propulsion. Carr and Shepherd stated that:

1. Sit-to-stand is accomplished most easily when the initial starting position of the foot is in a posterior position (with the ankle in approximately 75 degrees of dorsiflexion).

2. Initiating active trunk flexion from the erect position and encouraging the individual to swing the trunk forward at a reasonable speed allows for the greatest generation of extension force in the lower limbs to raise the body vertically.

3. Increased velocity of trunk flexion facilitates extensor force in the lower limbs.

4. Constraint of the arms (as in holding the hemiplegic arm forward while attempting sit-to-stand) results in increased time producing sufficient lower limb extensor forces to stand.

Janssen, Bussman, and Stam[51] reviewed key factors affecting sit-to-stand by searching the literature for the most frequently mentioned determinants, and they found that chair height, use of armrests, and foot position significantly

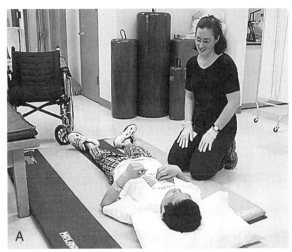

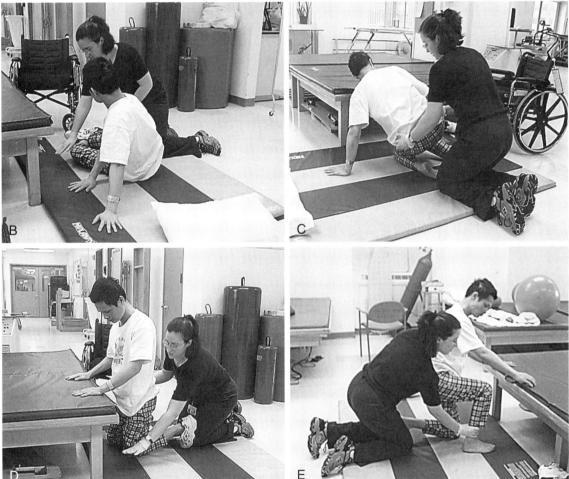

Figure 14-27 **A,** Teaching the patient and caregiver how to get up safely from the floor is important before discharge to the community. **B,** The therapist instructs this patient with right-sided weakness to assume a side-sitting position on the left arm and hip. **C,** The therapist or caregiver assists the patient at the pelvis to assume weight on his knees. She uses a surface immediately in front of the patient to allow for arm support. **D,** The patient now is supported fully on his hands and knees. She prepares him for the next stage by asking him to shift his weight to his left. **E,** When the patient shifts weight over to the left knee, he is able to move his weaker right leg into a half-kneeling position. *Continued*

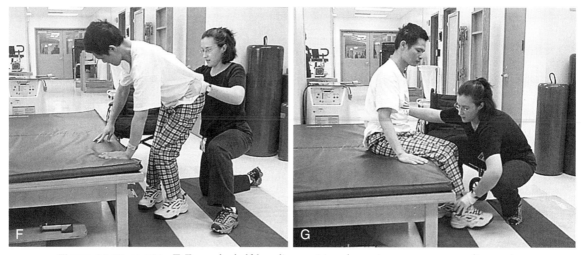

Figure 14-27, cont'd   F, From the half-kneeling position the patient assumes a standing position and begins to shift his weight to sit on the adjacent surface. **G,** The patient is seated safely.

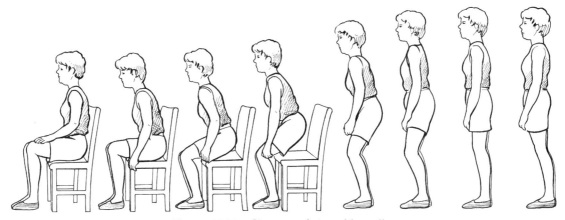

Figure 14-28   Sit-to-stand viewed laterally.

influence the ability to carry out sit-to-stand. Use of a higher chair resulted in decreased movements needed at the knee and hip, while using armrests reduced the movements needed at the hip. Repositioning the feet from anterior to posterior reduced the maximum mean extension movements at the hip.

Selected Problems. As mentioned in the previous section, patients may have difficulty maintaining their feet flat on the floor because of poor sensation, unilateral inattention, or shortening of the trunk and calf muscles.

Difficulties with spatial relations and praxis have been noted during transfer training, regardless of whether the therapist is training the patient for pivot transfers or sit-to-stand. Certain patients lean backward instead of forward while the therapist is attempting to transfer. These patients' actions are unpredictable and often run counter to those expected after instruction from the therapist.

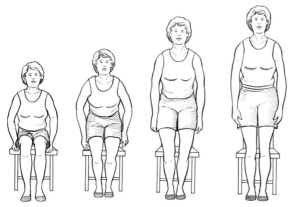

Figure 14-29   Sit-to-stand viewed anteriorly.

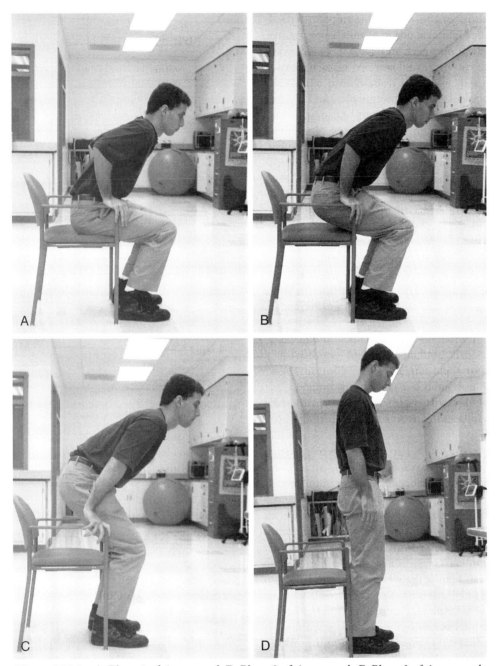

Figure 14-30   **A,** Phase 1 of sit-to-stand. **B,** Phase 2 of sit-to-stand. **C,** Phase 3 of sit-to-stand. **D,** Phase 4 of sit-to-stand.

As Arnadottir[6] noted, transfers also reveal problems with organizing and sequencing and conditions such as ideational apraxia. These problems may become evident when a patient attempting to rise from bed omits the appropriate steps of handling the bedclothes in preparation to transfer (see Chapter 18).

Motor impersistence, a term first introduced by Fisher[35] to describe failure to persist at various tasks such as eye closure, breath holding, conjugate gaze, and tongue protrusion may explain some patients' inabilities to persevere

with certain tasks such as transfers, sit-to-stand, and ambulation. These patients tend to collapse midway through the task, sometimes without warning, and reduced muscle strength, per se, does not appear to be the cause. Impersistence, in most studies, has been found to correlate more with right-hemisphere lesions than with left-hemisphere lesions.[35,54]

The manner in which the sit-to-stand movement pattern is executed may reveal who is at risk for falls. Cheng and colleagues[23] found that when comparing stroke survivors who had a history of falls against stroke survivors who had no history of falls, the differences were clear in measurable parameters such as body weight distribution. Stroke patients with a history of falls executed the task of sit-to-stand asymmetrically, taking much more weight on their sound side.[23] This suggests that, certainly from the point of view of safety concerns, stroke survivors need as many opportunities as possible to develop better control of their affected lower limbs in sit-to-stand.

Treatment Strategies. Bobath[12] described the need to begin training patients in sit-to-stand from a high seat (Fig. 14-31, *A*), progressing gradually to lower seats or a plinth (Fig. 14-31, *B*). Similarly, the environment can be used to change the demands required to transition from sit to stand (Fig. 14-32). Other studies have substantiated her assertion, including the conclusion that high-surface chairs can decrease significantly the joint ROMs needed at the hip and knee and the strength requirements to lift the body.[18,85]

Verbal or physical cues may be required to promote appropriate weight-bearing on the affected lower extremity as recommended for transfer training. In Fig. 14-33, the therapist's assistance provides much stability for the patient. In Fig. 14-34, the therapist needs only to cue the patient through the distal femur to get the desired response.

Because getting the feet back and under in sit-to-stand is so important, training patients to move to the edge of the supporting surface is necessary for optimal foot placement. This enables forward flexion of the trunk and movement of the center of mass over the base of support. A patient who attempts to stand without appropriate foot placement will encounter difficulty (Fig. 14-35).

Normal subjects frequently use a momentum strategy in mobility skills as a way to move with less energy requirements and hence with greater efficiency. Momentum strategy is used frequently in rising from bed, and no cessation of movement occurs. The momentum strategy can be used in a modified way with appropriate patients who have sustained a stroke, because it allows them to use the force generated by forward flexion to take them into an upright position. They then need adequate stability when their thighs are off the supporting surface to prevent them from falling forward. Momentum provides the patient with a strategy to move but by definition requires increased control of stability functions. Patients with poor trunk control or significant cognitive impairments are not candidates for using such a strategy. When introducing the momentum strategy in therapy, the therapist must adequately guard the patient to prevent a possible fall.

Practicing forward reach while sitting appears to improve the ability of the affected foot to accept weight and improves weight-bearing in sit-to-stand activities.[30] These were Dean and Shepherd's[30] conclusions from

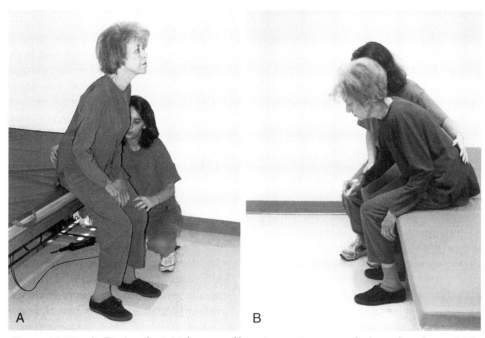

Figure 14-31   **A,** During the initial stages of learning, patients may find standing from a high surface easier. Among other things this provides the patient with a feeling of success. **B,** The patient can attempt lower surfaces after becoming more skillful. Varying the surfaces from which patients practice standing is important to promote learning and enables the patient to cope with varying situations that arise in the real world.

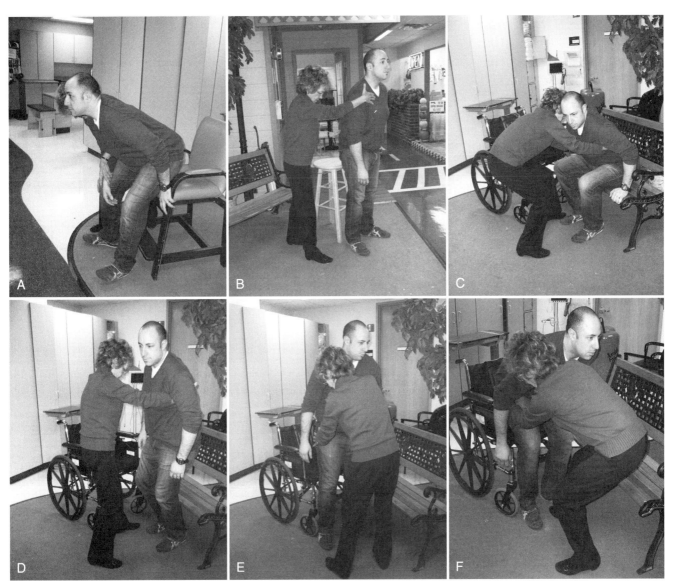

Figure 14-32   A-F, Training sit-to-stand and transfers using a variety of functional seating surfaces.

their study using individuals who were at least one year poststroke. Dean and colleagues[31] have since looked at the effects of sitting training in the acute stages following a stroke. In this study, the researchers provided a two-week sitting training protocol that improved sitting ability as measured by distances reached and quality as measured by reaching performance. They also explored whether the two-week sitting training protocol benefited patients' ability to stand up and walk, and they further examined if any gains were maintained six months following training. This study was set up as a randomized placebo-controlled clinical trial (CCT) involving six experimental and six control group subjects, all having sustained a stroke in under three months. Participants in the experimental group received the training protocol

designed by Dean and Shepherd.[30] Participants in the control group completed a sham sitting training protocol involving cognitive manipulative tasks.

Sitting ability, the main outcome measure, was significantly improved as measured by the average maximum reach distance during forward and across reaches, compared with the control group. In addition, the quality of reach improved in the experimental group, as evidenced by use of the standardized "reach to grasp and drink from a glass" task in forward and across directions. The carryover to standing up was evident, but not to walking, and there was some evidence of effectiveness of the interventions six months later.[31]

The operative word for improving sit-to-stand performance appears to be *practice*. A randomized controlled

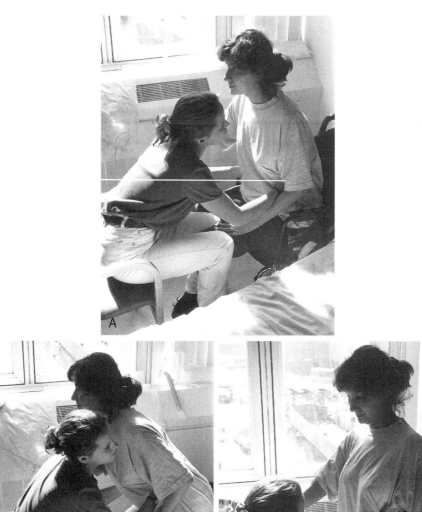

Figure 14-33   A, The therapist promotes weight bearing on the patient's affected lower extremity in sit-to-stand by placing the knees around the patient's affected knee, drawing the patient forward **(B),** and discouraging "buckling" when the patient achieves the standing position **(C).**

study by Britton and colleagues[16] looked at the amount of practice that could be carried out by a physical therapy assistant in 30 minutes a day over a two-week period in a stroke rehabilitation unit and its potential effects on sit-to-stand. Eighteen patients all requiring supervision in sit-to-stand were divided evenly into experimental and control groups. The experimental group practiced sit-to-stand and leg strengthening exercises for 30 minutes on

weekdays for two weeks (in addition to their rehabilitation program) while the members of the control group received upper extremity therapy.

Results showed that the provision of 30 minutes of practicing sit-to-stand resulted in a mean of 50 stands per day above what was practiced in the routine rehabilitation program. The researchers noted a significant mean difference of 10% body weight taken through the affected foot

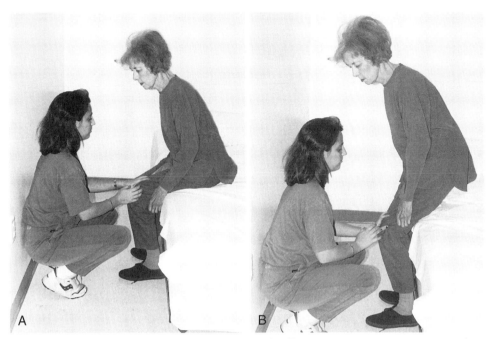

Figure 14-34 Patients with greater motor control still may require some cueing to equalize the weight-bearing between the lower extremities if they have a tendency to stand up using their unaffected side more than the other. **A,** The therapist places a hand on the distal femur of the affected lower extremity, draws the knee anteriorly, and then applies downward pressure as the patient comes to stand **(B).**

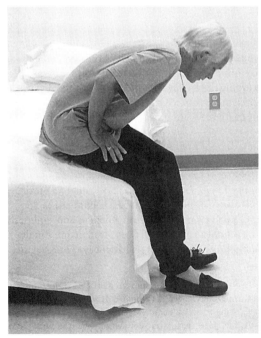

Figure 14-35 Foot placement is important in sit-to-stand. Note how far forward this individual's feet are as he attempts to stand.

after one week of the program. In addition, the control group showed reduced weight through the affected leg while the experimental group showed increased weight on the affected leg.[16] The findings of this study indicate that rehabilitation practitioners need to provide as many opportunities as possible for practicing newly acquired skills. This will require creative solutions and reassessment of current models of treatment delivery.

ACTIVITIES IN STANDING

Analysis of Movement

The ability to stand is a goal many patients with hemiplegia want to achieve because the drive to be upright is strong. Patients should be provided the opportunity to practice standing and shifting their centers of gravity in all directions and reaching for functional objects in the environment. The trunk responses needed for controlled sitting (i.e., selective lengthening and shortening depending on the requirements of the task) also are needed for controlled standing; however, these trunk responses are carried out over a much narrower base of support.

Selected Problems

Standing may prove challenging for patients with severe hemiplegia who have only one side of the body available to use for movement; moving with one half of the body is stressful work. The slow, laborious effort of standing and attempting to move in this position causes an increase in posturing and skeletal muscle activity. Movements often are lacking in spontaneity and must occur at a conscious level for the patient. Postural deviations noted in sitting in these patients become even more exaggerated in standing. For example, the patient who tends to "fix" the upper limb to stay upright while sitting will present with greater fixation of the upper limb when challenged in the standing position.

Studies have shown that the role of the paretic leg typically reflects its contribution in compensatory strategies, rather than in the restoration of support functions and equilibrium reactions.[32,73] This speaks to the need to train weight-bearing over the affected leg in reaching and sit-to-stand activities as mentioned previously in this chapter.

Postural control performance in individuals with stroke is affected by attentional tasks.[9,73] This implies a high degree of cognitive vigilance on the part of the patient to maintain balance, and whenever there is a demand on cognitive systems, there may be a risk for losing postural control.

Treatment Strategies

As stated previously, standing as early as possible if medical clearance is permitted is ideal for patients. Standing helps increase the patient's level of arousal and can be motivating. Bobath,[12] Davies,[29] and Carr and Shepherd[22] emphasized the need to help the patient stand so that body segments are aligned properly and weight is accepted through the affected lower extremity. For some patients, accomplishing this requires all of their attention and energy. Therefore, the therapist should be mindful of the need (at least initially) to train the patient to stand and take weight on the affected lower extremity in a quiet, minimally distracting environment. This may be even more critical for patients with attention disorders manifesting as distractibility, impulsivity, and irritability with increased stimulation. As noted earlier, the therapist must consider the need to incorporate competing stimuli into therapy gradually; otherwise, the therapist cannot assert that functional balance has been achieved.

Achieving weight shift in standing requires a substantial amount of cueing by the therapist, because patients often are fearful of standing on the affected leg due to reduced muscle strength, postural control, and sensation. Visual disturbances also may make standing a frightening activity for the patient.

Early in treatment, the use of a wall (Fig. 14-36) may be desirable to offer the patient substantial support; however, this should not be used to train functional reach in standing, because postural muscle activity in the legs is reduced (with the help of the wall) when the patient makes an arm movement. A manually guided approach is useful to help the patient learn the desired end of the movement pattern. Contact by the therapist directly on

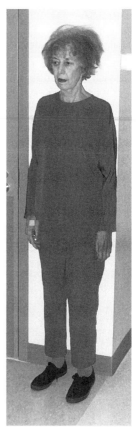

Figure 14-36   A wall can be a helpful starting place in teaching a patient to maintain a standing position. The wall can assist the patient to achieve alignment of body parts in what can be a frightening position to assume. However, the wall does not substitute for the need to learn to stand and function in open space.

the pelvis (with one hand on each side) offers optimal control to guide the weight shift, and the therapist gradually can taper the amount of guidance required as the patient begins to activate more.

Free-standing balance should be attempted as soon as possible (see Chapter 8). Standing while simultaneously scanning the environment or having a conversation with the therapist is challenging and meaningful (Fig. 14-37).

A progression to standing and reaching prepares the patient to be able to perform personal self-care and IADL safely and efficiently in a standing position. The patient needs to practice reaching in all directions in functional environments (Fig. 14-38). As Carr and Shepherd[22] outlined, this should include reaching overhead, to the side, backward, and down, progressing to unilateral and bilateral reaching to the floor. Task-specific training provides the patient with the opportunity to develop strategies to solve problems encountered in standing.

A commonly held view about asymmetrical hemiparetic gait is that it may be subject to amelioration by balance training emphasizing weight-bearing on the paretic lower extremity. However, a study by Winstein and colleagues,[93]

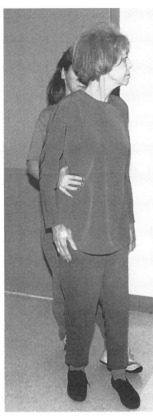

Figure 14-37 The therapist cues weight shifting in standing while encouraging the patient to scan the environment. Standing and looking around a room can prove challenging for patients in the initial stages of learning to stand.

in which hemiparetic subjects received specific balance training with a specially designed feedback device, revealed that balance in standing may be improved, but no carryover into a more symmetrical gait pattern occurs. This suggests that skill acquisition has a task-specific nature, and therapists cannot assume progress achieved in one skill area can be carried over or transferred to another. This finding calls into question many commonly held beliefs about the use of developmental progression to increase functional capabilities in upright positions.

Sit-to-stand and stand-to-sit may be the same in certain basic ways. However, the key differences have implications for treatment. First, movement duration has been found to be longer in stand-to-sit than in sit-to-stand.[56,83] In stand-to-sit, lower limb extensors are working in a flexed position and execute the task by eccentric (lengthening) rather than concentric (shortening) the way they do in sit-to-stand. Controlling the descent is a difficult task for muscles with compromised strength, and certainly in the initial stages following stroke, many patients with hemiplegia sit by letting go and almost collapsing into a seated position, rather than executing a smooth, controlled descent into a seat. Practicing stand-to-sit

with patients is important and should be practiced as often as sit-to-stand. Gaining control in sit-to-stand does not translate to stand-to-sit.

Falls Prevention

It has been identified that falls in the elderly have been associated with underlying precipitants, such as intrinsic factors (related to physiological changes, pathological conditions, and adverse medication effects) and situational factors (length of stay in institutional settings, time of falling, and availability of caretakers).[71] These factors apply similarly to the stroke population as well.

Falling can be a major complication during stroke rehabilitation. Nyberg and Gustafson[67] studied the incidences, characteristics, and consequences of falls in an inpatient rehabilitation setting. They sampled 161 patients consecutively admitted for geriatric stroke rehabilitation. They found that 62 patients (39%) sustained a fall, and 39 patients (24%) suffered more than one fall. Most of these falls occurred during transfers or from sitting in a wheelchair or some other type of furniture.

Nyberg and Gustafson[67] further noted that extrinsic factors (slips, trips, furniture moving, etc.) accounted for 17 falls (11%), while intrinsic factors were involved in 49 falls (32%). Intrinsic factors were specifically related to impaired balance, motor issues such as the legs giving way, and cognitive impairments such as perceptual issues and distraction or inattention. Six falls (4%) involved fractures or other serious injury. The authors concluded that falls constitute a significant problem in stroke rehabilitation, and fall prevention strategies must be developed and incorporated into rehabilitation programs.[67]

It appears that fear of falling in stroke patients has a relationship to a history of earlier falls and functional characteristics of these individuals, as noted by a study conducted by Andersson and colleagues.[5] The study included 140 patients who had been treated in a stroke unit during a 12-month period. The Falls Efficacy Scale, Swedish version (FES-S) and tests of motor ability, functional mobility, and balance were used to evaluate factors contributing to fear of falling. In univariate analysis, there was a significant association between increased age, female sex, previous falls, visual and cognitive impairment, low mood, and impaired physical functioning with low fall-related self-efficacy. In multivariate analysis, only a history of previous falls and physical function remained significant. Fear of falling was associated significantly with poor physical function and previous falls. The findings in this study support the importance of offering fall prevention programs to stroke survivors, whether they have sustained a fall or not.[5]

This study raises the important topic of *excess disability*. Excess disability is defined as the restriction of ADL beyond that which the person is physically and cognitively capable of performing. This concept has been gaining

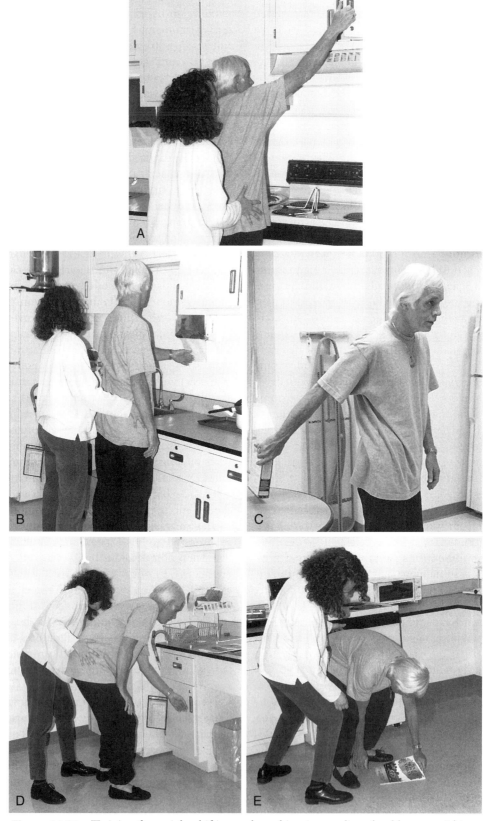

Figure 14-38 Training for weight shifting and reaching in standing should occur within a functional context because task-specific training is most beneficial to the learner. Reaching up **(A)**, forward **(B)**, backward **(C)**, reaching down **(D)**, and toward the floor **(E).** These patterns are among the many patterns of movement the patient should practice within functional activities. Occupational therapists are uniquely qualified with their expertise in task analysis to train patients to perform basic and instrumental activities of daily living.

increased attention in the public health literature over the past few decades.

Even among the general aging population, there is evidence of excess disability created by the fear of falling. Yardley and Smith[98] explored feared consequences of falling with over 200 community-living people over the age of 75 years. Their findings showed many individuals had a loss of functional independence and damage to their identities from the fear of falling. Fears were correlated with avoidance of activity (after adjusting for age, sex, and recent falling history) and predicted further avoidance in activity months later.[98]

Lach[58] reported that having two or more falls, feeling unsteady, and reporting fair or poor health status were independent risk factors for developing fear of falling. Bruce and colleagues[17] saw that fear of falling is common in healthy, high-functioning older women and is independently associated with reduced levels of participation in recreational physical activity.

It is clear that a program of falls prevention for stroke survivors, starting in the inpatient rehabilitation setting, is important to help these individuals develop strategies for dealing with changes in physical and cognitive functioning. These programs also have the potential to help address fear of falling that may exist whether or not the patients have actually fallen.

To date, there are no publicized randomized controlled trials (RCTs) researching the effectiveness of falls prevention strategies in stroke survivors. The Falls Prevention After Stroke Survivors Return Home (FLASSH) study[8] is an RCT seeking to evaluate stroke survivors now living at home, who have been discharged from inpatient rehabilitation. The patients present at a high risk for falling and will participate in a multifactorial prevention program. In the future, the results of this study will be important to contributing to the evidence-based practice in fall prevention programs.

As of the writing of this chapter, there are a number of web-based fall prevention resources available (Box 14-1).

Box 14-1

Fall Prevention Websites

National Center for Injury Prevention and Control, CDC: Preventing Falls: How to Develop Community-Based Fall Prevention Programs for Older Adults: www.cdc.gov/ncipc/preventingfalls/

National Council on Aging, Center for Healthy Aging: National Action Plan: www.healthyagingprograms.org/content/asp?sectionid=69

Creative Practices in Home Safety Assessment and Modification Study: www.healthyagingprograms.org/content.asp?sectionid=31&ElementID=568&FromSEarchResult=creative

ADJUNCT TECHNIQUES TO ENHANCE SKILL ACQUISITION

Feedback

Patients rely on feedback for performance of all mobility tasks. For example, before initiating a transfer, a patient uses visual information about the appropriate position of the limbs before movement begins. As the patient begins to rise from the seated position, the somatosensory system provides information about the forces exerted and the ongoing changes in limb position. On completion of this task, the results of the sequence provide additional feedback. The patient uses the feedback given to gain a sense of how it felt to rise to a standing position. Was it efficient? Was it difficult? This information gained during or after the mobility sequence is termed *movement-produced feedback*.[78]

As discussed in Chapter 5, feedback is divided into two broad categories: intrinsic and extrinsic (augmented). Intrinsic is information from the sensory systems while extrinsic (augmented) is information that supplements sensory information such as verbal directives provided by the therapist.[78] For example, the therapist tells the patient to "straighten your hips and stand tall," as the patient rises to stand at a sink for grooming.

Feedback is important to the rehabilitation process, and the therapist should carefully select the type of feedback provided, the amount, and the schedule. Feedback should be distinguished from encouragement, which facilitates continued participation of the patient in the mobility task. "Try more" or "Keep going!" are examples of encouragement that recognize the patient's effort. Forms of feedback for coming to the stand position would include: "Good job. You were able to stand at the sink" (knowledge of results [KR]) or "Next time you need to lean forward more before rising"(knowledge of performance [KP]). Gentile[38,39] described two kinds of augmented feedback that are illustrated in two examples:

1. Knowledge of results: defined as knowledge of information about the performer-environment interaction
2. Knowledge of performance: defined as knowledge of information about movement

Gentile suggested that the demands of the task best dictate the most effective form of feedback. Activities that can be characterized according to the taxonomy of tasks as closed and consistent motion tasks require information about the movement to be transmitted from the instructor to the learner. For example, when training a patient in rolling over in bed or achieving sit-to-stand from a wheelchair, the provision of feedback about placement of the extremities and maintenance of alignment is useful. Using Gentile's taxonomy, tasks that can be categorized as open and variable motionless tasks are performed under changing environmental conditions. These tasks require that feedback to the learner should focus on directing attention to environmental factors that may influence selection of movement strategies and patterns. For example, standing up while on a bus requires anticipation of the motion of the bus, movement of persons in the immediate environment, and consideration of changing space constraints. See Chapter 5.

Almost all of the research investigating the efficacy of feedback has emphasized knowledge of results focusing on the relative frequency and timing of delivery. Winstein and Schmidt[95] compared the performance of two groups and the frequency of feedback. In this study, one group received feedback on a fading schedule (50% of the trials) while the other group received feedback on 100% of the trials. The study found that during the acquisition phase, the group receiving 100% frequency had a slight advantage; however, it also found that the group receiving 50% frequency performed better on a delayed retention test. The investigators proposed that the decreased KR provided to the 50% group encouraged development of alternative strategies, while the group receiving 100% feedback may have come to rely too heavily on the KR.

In another study, Lavery and Suddon[59] compared summary and immediate feedback and the effects on transfer of skills. The study explored the results of the schedule of feedback and performance of three groups of subjects. One group received immediate feedback on every trial, a second group received summary (at the end of a block of 20 trials), and a third group received both types of feedback. At the end of the acquisition trials, the groups receiving feedback after each trial (groups 1 and 3) performed better than group 2. When groups were compared on a subsequent transfer test where no feedback was provided, group 2's (summary feedback) performance was significantly better than groups 1 or 3. At first glance, summary feedback appears more effective than immediate feedback. Schmidt and Lee[78] suggested that the results indicate that immediate KR is detrimental to learning, based on the findings that group 3, which received both immediate and summary, did not perform as well as group 2. They hypothesized that too much information and overreliance on the immediate KR were disadvantageous to learning information. Alternatively, summary KR encourages the subject to develop strategies that are flexible and suitable to transfer. The findings of these two studies give cause for reflection on the degree, frequency, and timing on when the therapist should provide feedback during mobility training. Winstein[92] posited that less information feedback creates an environment conducive to facilitating the learner to develop problem-solving strategies. Information about movement and performance of mobility tasks should be precise and should identify movements that are critical to efficiency and safety. At all times, a therapist should avoid "liberal" use of feedback and inaccurate or untruthful feedback. An example of

this would include the therapist who spontaneously says "great job" when a patient performs a transfer just because he or she made it to the transfer surface, even though the feet were not positioned correctly or the hips were not adequately extended. This feedback may negatively affect performance and learning. Patients may discount their own abilities to assess performance and to identify errors because of the powerful influence a therapist's feedback can have on shaping future efforts.

Many therapists videotape patients to provide information about performance and measure improvement in skill. This can prove useful, particularly with patients who may lack awareness about their performance (see Chapter 19). The use of videotape as a form of augmented feedback is not new to the rehabilitation process, but the increased ease in taping with a wide variety of commercially available products has increased the viability. A videotape captures the client's movement, features in the environment that are stable and do not change, and the everyday spontaneous occurrences that require immediate adaptations. Videotaping may be instrumental to assisting clients in developing flexible movement strategies that can solve the movement dilemmas encountered during participation in routine tasks.

Research supports that just showing a video tape does not influence performance; it must be supplemented with structured feedback by the clinician. Videotape has been used to improve awareness of performance and to assist patients in identifying behaviors that impede performance in clients exhibiting unilateral neglect. The therapist identifies salient features, provides verbal feedback during review of the videotapes, and focuses the patient's attention to details.[87] Hodges, Chua, and Franks[46] identified that videotape may be used to augment the learning of complex motor skills and may contribute to retention of these skills.

Mental Practice

A substantial body of research suggests that mental practice can improve learning of new motor skills in healthy individuals and, as a result, has been getting increased attention in the rehabilitation literature.[50] The past several years have seen an increase in research conducted on the efficacy of mental practice with a stroke population. Braun and colleagues[14] conducted a systematic literature search of studies published through August 2005. These included four RCTs, one CCT, two patient series, and three case reports. The studies examined the use of four different mental practice strategies with most tasks involving mental rehearsal of arm movements. They noted that studies were limited in size and determined that no definite conclusions could be made except that further research is needed for a clear definition of the content of mental practice and standardized measurements of outcomes.[14]

Braun and colleagues[15] set out to provide a framework for integrating mental practice into therapy by looking at the available evidence and theory. Drawing on sports literature and their own experiences, they described five steps to facilitate the patient's imagery capabilities: (1) assessing mental capacity to learn imagery technique, (2) establishing the nature of mental practice, (3) teaching imagery technique, (4) embedding and monitoring imagery technique, and (5) developing self-generated treatments.[15]

Manual Guidance

Manual guidance is a technique frequently used during the rehabilitation process, which is often described as assisting the patient to "feel" the appropriate movement pattern or to position the patient in a desired posture using physical handling techniques. The degree of manual guidance provided and when it is supplied remains a controversial subject. Two types of manual guidance have been identified in the literature: passive movement and spatiotemporal constraint (physical restriction); both forms are often incorporated during mobility training.[48,49,62] For example, during the mobility task of rolling toward the affected hemiplegic side, the paretic arm is often passively moved and placed in a safe position in preparation for the patient to move his or her body over the prepositioned arm. Another application of this strategy occurs when a patient attempts to roll toward the nonaffected side. The therapist passively moves the paretic arm up and across the body before the patient attempts to move the trunk. The passive movement of the arm is thought to serve as a "guide" for the patient to gain an understanding of what actions are necessary to effectively roll (e.g., scapular protraction or flexion of the humerus). Likewise, spatial constraint is also used during retraining of many mobility tasks such as sit-to-stand or transfer training. A therapist may stabilize a part of a limb while the patient attempts to control only part of the limb (limit the degrees of freedom). An example of spatial-restraint during the sit-to-stand sequence is when the therapist applies an external force to stabilize the foot on the floor, thus enabling the patient to optimally use any muscular activity generated by the quadriceps combined with the extensor forces of the hip, knee, and ankle to rise vertically to the standing position.

The use of manual guidance during intervention needs to occur with careful consideration of the research findings that have identified significant concerns about the benefits or efficacy of the techniques.[78,79] The literature supports that guidance may be most effective during the acquisition of motor skills, when the requirements and demands of the task are new to the learner. The literature also recommends that therapists attempt to integrate active practice trials with interspersed passive guidance.[94]

EVALUATION TOOLS

Many therapists perform a subjective assessment of functional mobility based on clinical observation. However, it is advantageous to use a recognized evaluation tool to support the need for services, to document progress, and to assess treatment efficacy. Table 14-2 includes a list of relevant tools for evaluating mobility functions. Currently the only standardized evaluation for mobility skills is Carr and Shepherd's Motor Assessment Scale for Stroke Patients.[20] This test assesses the following eight areas:

1. Supine to side lying
2. Supine to sitting over side of bed
3. Balanced sitting
4. Sitting to standing
5. Walking
6. Upper arm function
7. Hand movements
8. Advanced hand activities

The advantages of the Motor Assessment Scale include the following:

1. It tests recovery specific for the patient recovering from stroke.
2. It takes less time to administer and infringes little on treatment time.
3. It is simple to administer and has objective and clear descriptions of criteria for rating patients.
4. It is sensitive to changes in patients' motor recovery status and therefore is useful in describing patient progress over time.

The FIM was developed by the Uniform Data System at the State University of New York at Buffalo as a standardized way for professionals to evaluate patient progress regarding levels of assistance needed to perform personal self-care, functional mobility, communication, cognition, and social interaction. Each area is graded on a scale of 1 to 7, with a score of 1 indicating total dependence and 7 indicating complete independence. The areas of functional mobility covered in this test include transfers to bed, chair, toilet, tub, locomotion, and stairs. This test is used in rehabilitation centers across the United States and has been found to have good to excellent reliability.[41,42]

The Assessment of Motor and Process Skills is a standardized test created by occupational therapists that simultaneously evaluates motor and process skills to predict effect on the ability to perform IADL. Such an evaluation tool, if developed for functional mobility skills, would prove invaluable for occupational therapists (see Chapter 21).

ANTICIPATING CHANGING ENVIRONMENTS

The ultimate goal of functional mobility retraining is to have the patient resume the roles and activities associated with the lifestyle before the stroke. This goal presumes

Table 14-2

Tools for Evaluating Mobility Functions

ASSESSMENT/AUTHOR	POPULATION/PURPOSE	SOURCE/CONTACT
Activities-Specific Balance Confidence Scale (ABC)[70]	*Adults with balance deficits*: evaluate balance confidence in daily activities. A 16-item scale in a questionnaire format	Contact: Anita Myers Department of Health Studies and Gerontology, University of Waterloo, Waterloo, ON N2L 3G1
Falls Efficacy Scale (FES) (1990)[89]	*Elderly individuals in a community setting*: survey related to perceived self-confidence connected to daily activities	
Frenchay Activities Index[47]	*Adults*: to assess function in adults status poststroke: ADL and IADL	
Functional Independence Measure (FIM)[41]	*Adults with various impairments*: measures functional status; reflects the impact of disability on the individual and on human and economical resources in the community. 18 activities, 13 with a motor emphasis related to self-care, 5 with a cognitive emphasis involving communication	Uniform Data System for Medical Rehabilitation. 270 Northpointe Parkway, Suite 300, Amherst, NY 14228 (716) 817-7800
Home Falls and Accidents Screening Tool (HOME-FAST)[61] Environment Checklist	*Adults at risk of falling*: to identify environment and functional safety at home	
Melville-Nelson Self-Care Assessment (SCA)[66]	*Adults in subacute rehabilitation and nursing homes*: to assess self-care skills including bed mobility, transfers, toileting, personal hygiene, and bathing	http://hsc.utoledo.edu/allh/ot/melville.html
Morse Fall Scale (MFS)	*Adults with balance deficits*: rapid and simple method of assessing a patient's likelihood of falling. Acute care hospital and long-term inpatient settings	Contact: Janice M. Morse. Pennsylvania State University, School of Nursing, 201 Health and Human Development East, University Park, PA 16802-6508
Stroke Impact Scale (SIS), (SIS-16)[34]	*Adults*: measures stroke recovery in 8 domains: strength, hand function, mobility, ADL, emotion, memory, communication, and social participation	Langdon Center on Aging. University of Kansas Medical Center Mail Stop 1005, 3901 Rainbow Boulevard, Kansas City, KS 66160. (913) 588-1203 www2.kumc.edu/coa/SIS/Stroke-Impact-Scale.htm
Timed Get Up and Go (TGUG)[68]	*Adults with balance deficits*	
Tinnetti Balance Test of the Performance-Oriented Assessment of Mobility Problems (Tinnetti)[88]	*Adults with balance deficits*	
Trunk Control Test[25]	*Adults with stroke*: assess the motor impairment in a patient who has had a stroke. Rolling, balance in sitting, and sit up from lying down	
Westmead Home Safety Assessment[24]	*Older adults at risk of falling*: to identify fall hazards in the home	

that patients need to transfer reacquired mobility skills to environments unique to the individual lifestyle and participation patterns. The treatment setting presents a predictable environment in which the physical aspects of therapeutic equipment and furnishings remain unchanged from one treatment session to another. The patient's home environment also may be viewed as predictable because of the patient's familiarity with the surroundings. The physical layout and home furnishings change little over time, even if home modifications are introduced. Nevertheless, therapists frequently observe problems as the patient attempts to make the transition from the treatment setting to the home environment. Unexpected problems occur within the closed home environment, and community-based activities challenge the individual's ability to solve newly encountered problems. The occupational therapist is well-qualified to address these dilemmas through task analysis of occupations and careful consideration of the environmental contexts in which each task is performed.[75] The patient recovering from stroke is required to generalize and adapt mobility skills learned in the clinic setting to meet the changing environmental demands encountered on discharge. This generalization and adaptation occurs through the interaction among multiple systems: perceptual, cognitive, sensory, and motor. This chapter previously presented specific strategies for ameliorating performance impairments influencing functional mobility. These strategies should be incorporated throughout the intervention process as a means to attain generalization and encourage participation in life situations or IADL on discharge.

Strategy Development

The research examining normal movement sequences has found great variety in the movement patterns used to perform each mobility task. A single pattern may be identified as occurring more frequently during rolling, although many subjects use alternative patterns that are equally effective. Similarly, the methods described to retrain patients to roll over also vary. No single correct strategy is available to achieve this mobility task. Strategy development is more than learning to use a normal pattern of movement; it results from the patient's exploration of movement possibilities in relation to tasks occurring in different environments.[84] Thus, the occupational therapist may use several methods of instruction while assisting the patient in learning movement limitations and determining future mobility potentials.[75,84] The two primary strategies for functional mobility include a force control strategy and a momentum strategy.[26] Early in the intervention process, patients may benefit from instruction in a force control strategy to prevent secondary impairments of fixations and resultant development of inappropriate compensatory strategies.[12,20,22,28,29] This method of instruction also is preferred for patients who do not have

adequate stability of the trunk musculature because it may facilitate independent performance.[22] A momentum strategy or a combination of momentum and force control may be introduced if stability of the trunk is evident. Momentum is more efficient, requires less muscular activity, and approximates more normal-looking movement.

Not all patients can achieve a momentum strategy, but many patients may attempt to do their own in the home environment, particularly if it was their preferred method of movement before the stroke. Therapists need to anticipate this possibility and explore momentum as an alternative before discharge. Transition from a force control to a momentum strategy requires simple, concise instruction to move quickly without stopping the movement. The therapist may use manual cues at the shoulder girdle to ensure safety, and demonstration by the therapist is also helpful. The practice of momentum strategies also may prepare the patient to control movement during stressful life situations that occur unexpectedly and require quick transitional movements.

Practice Conditions

To prepare the patient to resume the previous lifestyle, the occupational therapist must consider carefully the conditions under which practice takes place. The goal of intervention is to maximize retention and transfer of acquired skills to everyday life situations the patient will encounter.[44] The therapist must increase the demands of the learning context during practice to prepare the patient to respond to unpredictable events. Chapter 5 presented an overview of factors the therapist considers when structuring the practice conditions in stroke rehabilitation. The following are considerations specific to functional mobility retraining.

Blocked and Random Practice. Blocked practice in functional mobility retraining is the rote practice of mobility functions in sequence. For example, the patient initially practices rolling to the unaffected side, then to the affected side, and then to the seated position. Repetition of experiences and a degree of mastery must occur at each level before the patient proceeds to the next level of skill. This method of structuring practice initially may assist the patient in gaining proficiency during the practice session but is not effective in preparing the patient to engage in self-care tasks in which changes in the position of the body occur randomly in response to task requirements. For example, the patient rolls to the left to reach for a brush on the table; it is just beyond reach. The patient rolls back to supine and assumes a bridge position, pushing upward in bed. The patient then rolls again and is able to grasp the brush. Random practice of mobility tasks improves learning, retention, and the ability to solve motor problems encountered in life situations.[80] Schmidt[76] recommended that randomized practice be incorporated throughout the intervention process. Mobility tasks should be interspersed with other tasks such as ADL training in which the patient must make transitional movements in a natural context. The trial-and-error exploration of functional mobility in this context initially may prove difficult for the patient. Progress may be slow, and the therapist may be tempted to instruct the patient in a single movement strategy to speed progress. Varying the practice conditions increases the contextual interference, facilitating generalization as the patient relies on multiple processes and promoting the development of versatile motor strategies.[52,90]

Schmidt noted one exception in which a part-to-whole method of practice may be beneficial. Early in the intervention process, when the patient is acquiring foundational skills, practicing of component movements may be necessary. For example, the patient initially may need to gain control of lateral flexion of neck and trunk muscles before these movements can be incorporated into the side lying-to-sit sequence. Schmidt suggested that as soon as patients are able to perform these component movements, they should be integrated immediately into programs emphasizing random practice.[76] This method of practice can be used only with mobility functions that are readily divided into natural component parts.[77,92]

Varying the Practice Conditions for Specific Tasks. Gentile's taxonomy of motor tasks[38,39] is useful for determining the most appropriate practice conditions for each mobility task. Objects, persons, and the spatial temporal characteristics of each task influence the motor strategies selected. Sabari[75] suggested that the occupational therapy process inherently considers the importance of the regulatory conditions to task performance. Occupational therapists frequently adapt and regulate the environment to facilitate mobility functions, as in adjusting the height of a bed in preparation for a transfer (Figs. 14-39 and 14-40). Similarly, the amount of verbal cues and physical assistance is adjusted to foster independent performance and skill development. Sabari also directed attention to the crucial role occupational therapists assume as regulators throughout mobility retraining.

Closed Tasks

Early in the treatment process, most functional mobility tasks may be considered closed, and the environmental features are regulated easily to improve performance. Rolling over and coming to a seated position in a hospital bed occurs on a stationary surface. The therapist can regulate the environment further by positioning pillows and bed linens appropriately, raising the bed guard rails, adjusting the height of the bed, limiting the number of persons moving around the patient's bed, and positioning the body in a fairly static position to assist the patient if needed. Another important characteristic of a closed task

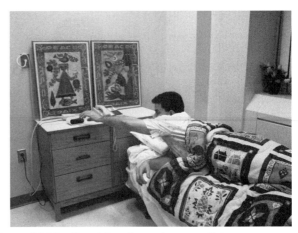

Figure 14-39 Requiring the patient to roll in response to the buzzer of an alarm clock while under a heavy quilt is an example of how a therapist regulates the spatial and temporal characteristics of the environment.

is that movement is self-paced and no temporal constraints are placed.

The therapist's role as a regulator can be equated with the degree of assistance or handling provided. The therapist initially may give significant physical assistance and use a variety of adjunct techniques to promote perceptual, cognitive, and sensory processing. As the patient regains control of movements in desired sequences, physical assistance and the amount of cueing is reduced gradually or eliminated.[75]

Variable Motionless Tasks

Bed mobility becomes a variable motionless task if the therapist is not present to regulate certain features of the environment. Patients preparing to get out of bed independently may find the pillows and bed linens in disarray, making movement difficult; the bed guard rails are lowered, the top of the bed remains slightly elevated, and the height of the bed may be too high. Simultaneously the patient may be receiving verbal encouragement to "hurry up." Without the therapist present to structure the environment, the patient may experience difficulty and may use compensatory strategies incompatible with the restoration of performance component deficits. The patient may hook the unaffected leg under the affected leg and use the hands to pull up to a seated position.

This comparison illustrates the way overstructuring the environment does not prepare the patient recovering from stroke to develop flexible motor strategies. The patient needs to have opportunities to process information and acquire the ability to solve future problems.[2,76] Abreu[1] studied the effects of environmental regulation on postural control and found that unpredictable environments elicited improved control. These findings are contrary to beliefs occupational therapists have held concerning the

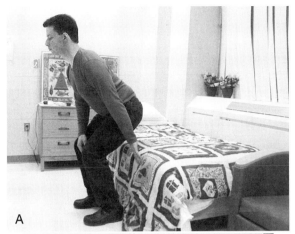

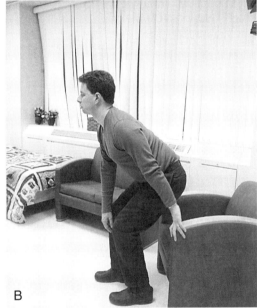

Figure 14-40 **A** and **B,** Varying the sitting surface when practicing sit-to-stand and stand-to-sit assists the patient to learn flexible strategies.

grading of tasks from simple to complex and the structuring of environments from predictable to unpredictable. Abreu[1] postulated that the results of this study indicate that both types of environments should be incorporated concurrently in the intervention process. The therapist may regulate the environment but not on all trials. Perhaps the height of the bed is adjusted and the guard rails are elevated on one trial, whereas the next session may require the patient to instruct the therapist verbally in the arrangement of the immediate surroundings in preparation for the mobility task.

Consistent Motion Tasks

During consistent motion tasks, the pace of the environment remains the same and the environment moves. These tasks are associated with mechanical devices such as conveyor belts. Most functional mobility tasks do not meet this criterion.

Open Tasks

Many advanced mobility skills meet the criterion of an open task in which the spatial and temporal parameters of movement are determined by events occurring in the environment. Open tasks require more precise timing of movement, and the patient is challenged to anticipate and react to unexpected events. Sit-to-stand on a moving train, plane, or bus are examples of open tasks. Practice of these tasks should occur in the actual environment whenever possible.[45,75] Patients who are physically capable of attempting these advanced skills should be engaged in them while in the rehabilitation setting whenever possible.

Patients who do not have adequate foundational skills while hospitalized can benefit from interventions to improve future potential for the acquisition of advanced mobility skills. Patients need to be introduced to unpredictable environments in which they have the opportunity to explore movement strategies and develop problem-solving abilities. Early in the intervention process, the therapist's handling techniques to prepare and assist the patient can be modulated using different degrees of tactile, proprioceptive, and kinesthetic input as the patient engages in functional mobility tasks. For example, as the patient learns to transfer, the therapist can vary the sensory cues and amount of assistance.[11] Responding to changes in sensory input may be helpful in the development of anticipatory postural adjustments.[84]

SUMMARY

The performance of functional mobility tasks should not occur in isolation, as in a gross mobility mat program. Practice of mobility skills while the patient is engaged in life tasks presents opportunities to solve unexpected problems that arise as the patient manipulates different objects and encounters changing support surfaces and changing temporal demands. The following are some suggestions for altering the regulatory features in the clinical environment.

Rolling

- Practice rolling on a narrow surface such as a sofa.
- Encourage abrupt change in direction, as in reversing the movement in midstream.
- Practice rolling under a heavy quilt.
- Try rolling with an object such as a newspaper in the hand.
- Attempt propping to side lying to adjust pillows.
- Practice rolling in a darkened room.
- Ask the patient to roll quickly.

Side Lying-to-Sit

- Attempt side lying-to-sit with an immediate reach pattern.
- Practice side lying-to-sit on a narrow surface.
- Try modifying the sequence to get out of a chaise lounge chair.
- Practice side lying-to-sit on a soft surface such as a sofa.
- Ask the patient to come to sitting as "fast as they can."

Sit-to-Stand

- Use varying seat surfaces:
  Chair with arms
  Chair without arms
  Reclining chair with a significant seat depth
  Aluminum patio chair
  Side of the sofa
  Middle of the sofa
  Chair with wheels such as a desk chair
  Stool
  Swivel chair
  Dentist's chair
  Chair in theater or stadium
  Seat on public transportation (such as a bus or subway)
- Incorporate varying standing surfaces:
  Different textures of carpet
  Linoleum
  Tile floor
  Grass
  Concrete
- Include varying speed of movement.
- Account for varying objects and pets in the environment.
- Incorporate changing lighting.
- Attempt holding of various objects:
  Coat
  Briefcase
  Shopping bag
- Relearn turning right and left.

REVIEW QUESTIONS

1. What effect does the patient's place in the life cycle have on planning relevant treatment in functional mobility retraining?
2. What are the impairments associated with stroke and how do they affect functional mobility tasks?
3. What is the force control strategy?
4. What are the three major task requirements for locomotion that can be applied to all functional mobility tasks?
5. What three possible interventions can be used to maximize a patient's ability to achieve lateral trunk flexion?
6. What implications for treatment may be derived from the research done by Carr, Shepherd, and Gentile on sit-to-stand?

7. What does the research show regarding the use of practice in rehabilitation?
8. How can the therapist structure the practice of functional mobility tasks, considering the venue of care?
9. What factors contribute to fall risk in stroke patients?

REFERENCES

1. Abreu BC: The effect of environmental regulations on postural control after stroke. *Am J Occup Ther* 49(6):517–525, 1995.
2. Abreu BC, Toglia JP: Cognitive rehabilitation: a model for occupational therapy. *Am J Occup Ther* 45(7):439–448, 1987.
3. Alexander NB, Grunawalt JC, Carles S, et al: Bed mobility task performance in older adults. *J Rehabil Res Dev* 37(5):633–638, 2000.
4. American Occupational Therapy Association: Practice framework: domain and process, 2nd ed. *Am J Occup Ther* 62(6):625, 2008.
5. Andersson AG, Kamwendo K, Appelro P: Fear of falling in stroke patients: relationship with previous falls and functional characteristics. *Int J Rehabil Res* 31(3): 261–264, 2008.
6. Árnadóttir G: *The brain and behavior: assessing cortical dysfunction through activities of daily living*, St Louis, 1990, Mosby.
7. Deleted.
8. Batchelor FA, Hill KD, Mackintosh SF, Said CM Whitehead CH: The FLASSH study: protocol for a randomized controlled trial evaluating falls prevention after stroke and two sub-studies. *BMC Neurol* 31: 9–14, 2009.
9. Benoussan L, Viton JM, Schieppati M, et al: Changes in postural control in hemiplegic patients after stroke performing a dual task. *Arch Phys Med Rehabil* 88(8): 1009–1015, 2007
10. Bernstein N: *The coordination and regulation of movement*, Elmsford, NY, 1967, Pergamon.
11. Bly L: What is the role of sensation in motor learning? What is the role of feedback and feedforward? *NDTA Network* 5:5, 1996.
12. Bobath B: *Adult hemiplegia: evaluation and treatment*, ed 3, Oxford, 1990, Butterworth-Heinemann.
13. Bobath B: *Adult hemiplegia: evaluation and treatment*, ed 2, London, 1978, Heinemann.
14. Braun SM, Beurskens AJ, Borm PJ, et al: The effects of mental practice in stroke rehabilitation: a systematic review. *Arch Phys Med Rehabil* 87(6): 842–852, 2006.
15. Braun S, Kleyman M, Schols J, et al: Using mental practice in stroke rehabilitation: a framework. *Clin Rehabil* 22(7):579–591, 2008.
16. Britton E, Harris N, Turton A: An exploratory randomized controlled trial of assisted practice for improving sit-to-stand in stroke patients in the hospital setting. *Clin Rehabil* 22(5):448–458, 2008.
17. Bruce DG, Devine A, Prince RL: Recreational activity levels in healthy older women: the importance of fear of falling. *J Am Geriatr Soc* 50(1):84–89, 2002.
18. Burdett RG, Habasevich R, Pisciotta J, et al: Biomechanical comparison of rising from two types of chairs. *Phys Ther* 65(8):1177–1183, 1985.
19. Carr JH, Gentile AM: The effect of arm movements on the biomechanics of standing up. *Hum Mov Sci* 13(2):175, 1994.
20. Carr JH, Shepherd RB: *Neurologic rehabilitation: optimizing motor performance*, Oxford, 1998, Butterworth-Heinemann.
21. Carr JH, Shepherd RB: A motor learning model for rehabilitation. In Carr JH, Shepherd RB: *Movement science: foundations for physical therapy in rehabilitation*, Rockville, MD, 1987, Aspen.
22. Carr JH, Shepherd RB: *A motor relearning programme for stroke*, Oxford, 1987, Butterworth-Heinemann.
23. Cheng PT, Wu SH, Liaw MY, et al: Symmetrical body weight distribution training in stroke patients and its effect on fall prevention. *Arch Phys Med Rehabil* 82(12):1650–1654, 2001.

24. Clemson L: *Home fall hazards: a guide to identifying fall hazards in the homes of elderly people and an accompaniment to the assessment tool, the Westmead Home Safety Assessment (WeHSA)*, West Brunswick, Victoria, 1997, Coordinates Publications.

25. Collin C, Wade D: Assessing motor impairment after stroke: a pilot reliability study. *J Neurol Neurosurg Psychiatry* 53(7):576–579, 1990.

26. Crutchfield CA, Barnes MR: *Motor control and motor learning in rehabilitation*, Atlanta, 1993, Stokesville.

27. Das P, McCollum G: Invariant structure in locomotion. *Neuroscience* 25(3):1023–1034, 1988.

28. Davies PM: *Right in the middle: selective trunk activity in the treatment of adult hemiplegia*, New York, 1990, Springer-Verlag.

29. Davies PM: *Steps to follow: a guide to treatment of adult hemiplegia*, New York, 1985, Springer-Verlag.

30. Dean CM, Shepherd RB: Task-related training improves performance of seated reaching tasks after stroke: a randomized controlled trial. *Stroke* 28(4):722–728, 1997.

31. Dean CM, Channon EF, Hall JM: Sitting training early after stroke improves sitting ability and quality and carries over to standing up but not to walking: a randomized controlled trial. *Aust J Physiother* 53(2):97–102, 2007.

32. De Haart M, Geurts AC, Huidekoper SC, et al: Recovery of standing balance in postacute stroke patients: a rehabilitation cohort study. *Arch Phys Med Rehabil* 85(6):886–895, 2004.

33. Dickstein R, Shefi S, Marcovitz E, Villa Y: Anticipatory postural adjustments in selected trunk muscles in post stroke hemiparetic patients. *Arch Phys Med Rehabil* 5(2):261–267, 2004.

34. Duncan PW, Wallace D, Lai SM, et al: The stroke impact scale version 2.0: evaluation of reliability, validity and sensitivity to change. *Stroke* 30(10):2131–2140, 1999.

35. Fisher CM: Left hemiplegia and motor impersistence. *J Nerv Ment Dis* 123(3):201, 1956.

36. Ford-Smith CD, Van Sant AF: Age differences in movement patterns used to rise from a bed in the third through fifth decades of age. *Phys Ther* 73(5):305, 1992.

37. Gentile AM: Implicit and explicit processes during acquisition of functional skills. *Scand J Occup Ther* 5(1):7–16, 1998.

38. Gentile AM: Skill acquisition: action, movement and neuromotor processes. In Carr JH, Shepherd RB: *Movement science: foundations for physical therapy in rehabilitation*, Rockville, MD, 1987, Aspen.

39. Gentile AM: A working model of skill acquisition with application to teaching. *Quest* 17:3–23, 1972.

40. Gillen G, Wasserman M: Mobility: examining the impact of the environment on transfer performance. *Phys Occup Ther Geriatr* 22(4):21–29, 2004.

41. Granger CV, Hamilton BB: The Uniform Data System for medical rehabilitation report of first admissions for 1990. *Am J Med Rehabil* 71(2):108–113, 1992.

42. Granger CV, Hamilton BB, Linacre JM, et al: Performance profiles of the Functional Independence Measure. *Am J Phys Med Rehabil* 72(2):84–89, 1993.

43. Hall ET: *The hidden dimension*, New York, 1966, Doubleday.

44. Hartman-Maeir A, Soroker N, Oman SD, et al: Awareness of disabilities in stroke rehabilitation: a clinical trial. *Disabil Rehabil* 25(1):35–44, 2003.

45. Higgins JR, Spaeth RK: Relationship between consistency of movement and environmental condition. *Quest* 17:61, 1972.

46. Hodges NJ, Chua R, Franks IM: The role of video in facilitating perception and action of a novel coordination movement. *J Mot Behav* 35(3):247–260, 2003.

47. Holbrook M, Skilbeck CE: An activities index for use with stroke patients. *Age Ageing*, 12(2):166–170, 1983.

48. Holding DH: Learning without errors. In Smith LE, editor: *Psychology of motor learning*, Chicago, 1970, Athletic Institute.

49. Holding DH, Macrae AW: Guidance restriction and knowledge of results. *Ergonomics* 7(3):289–295, 1964.

50. Jackson PL, Lafleur MF, Malouin F, et al: Potential role of mental practice using motor imagery in neurologic rehabilitation. *Arch Phys Med Rehabil* 82(8):1133–1141, 2001.

51. Janssen WG, Bussman HB, Stam HJ: Determinants of the sit-to-stand movement: a review. *Phys Ther* 82(9):866–879, 2002.

52. Jarus T: Motor learning and occupational therapy: the organization of practice. *Am J Occup Ther* 48(9):810–816, 1994.

53. Johnstone M: *Restoration of motor function in the stroke patient*, ed 2, New York, 1983, Churchill Livingstone.

54. Joynt RL, Benton AL, Fogel ML: Behavioral and pathological correlates of motor impersistence. *Neurology* 12:876, 1964.

55. Kernodle MW, Carlton LG: Information feedback and the learning of multiple-degree-of-freedom activities. *J Mot Behav* 24(2):187–196, 1992.

56. Kralj A, Jaeger RJ, Munih M: Analysis of standing up and sitting down in humans: definitions and normative data presentation. *J Biomech* 23(11):1123–1138, 1990.

57. Krefting LH, Krefting D: Cultural influences on performance. In Christiansen C, Baum C, editors: *Occupational therapy: overcoming human performance deficits*, Thorofare, NJ, 1991, Slack.

58. Lach HW: Incidence and risk for developing fear of falling in older adults. *Public Health Nursing* 22(1):45–52, 2005.

59. Lavery JJ, Suddon FH: Retention of simple motor skills as a function of the number of trials by which KR is delayed. *Percept Mot Skills* 15:231–237, 1962.

60. Levine RE: Culture: a factor influencing the outcomes of occupational therapy. *Occup Ther Health Care* 4(1):3, 1987.

61. Mackenzie L, Byles J, Higginbotham N: Designing the home falls and accidents screening tool (home fast); selecting the items. *Brit J Occup Ther* 63(6):260–269, 2000.

62. Macrae AW, Holding DH: Method and task in motor guidance. 8(3):315–320, 1965.

63. Messier S, Bourbonnais D, Desrosiers J, Roy Y: Dynamic analysis of trunk flexion after stroke. *Arch Phys Med Rehabil* 85(10):1619–1624, 2004.

64. Mohr JD: *Management of the trunk in adult hemiplegia: the Bobath concept, topics in neurology*, Alexandria, VA, 1990, American Physical Therapy Association.

65. Mosey AC: *Psychosocial components of occupational therapy*, New York, 1986, Raven.

66. Nelson DL, Melville LL, Wilkerson JD, et al: Interrater reliability, concurrent validity, responsiveness, and predictive validity of the Melville-Nelson Self-Care Assessment. *Am J Occup Ther* 56(1):51–59, 2002.

67. Nyberg L, Gustafson, MD: Patient falls in stroke rehabilitation: a challenge to rehabilitation strategies. *Stroke* 26(5):838–842, 1995.

68. Podsiadlo D, Richardson S: The timed "Up & Go": a test of basic functional mobility for frail elderly persons. *J Am Geriatr Soc* 39(2):142–148, 1991.

69. Poole JI: Application of motor learning principles in occupational therapy. *Am J Occup Ther* 45(6):531–537, 1991.

70. Powell LE, Myers AM: The activities-specific balance confidence (ABC) scale. *J Gerontol* 50A(1):M28–M34, 1995.

71. Rein Tideiksaar: *Falls in older persons: prevention and management* (2nd ed), Baltimore, Health Proffessions Press, 1998.

72. Richter RR, Van Sant AF, Newton RA: Description of adult rolling movements and hypothesis of developmental sequences. *Phys Ther* 69(1):63–71, 1989.

73. Roerdink M, Geurts AC, de Haart M, Beek PJ: On the relative contribution of the paretic leg to the control of posture after stroke. *Neurorehabil Neural Repair* 23(3):267–274, 2009.

74. Ryerson S, Levit K: *Functional movements reeducation*, New York, 1997, Churchill Livingstone.

75. Sabari JS: Motor learning concepts applied to activity-based interventions with adults with hemiplegia. *Am J Occup Ther* 45(6):523–530, 1991.

76. Schmidt RA: Motor learning principles for physical therapy. In Lister MJ, editor: *Contemporary management of motor control problems: proceedings of the Second STEP Conference*, Alexandria, VA, 1991, Foundation for Physical Therapy.

77. Schmidt RA, Lee TD: *Motor control and learning: a behavioral emphasis*, ed 2, Champaign, IL, 1999, Human Kinetics.

78. Schmidt RA, Lee TD , *Motor control and learning: a behavioral emphasis*, ed. 4, Champaign, IL, 2005, Human Kinetics.

79. Schmidt RA, Wulf G: Continuous concurrent feedback degrades skill learning: implications for training and simulation. *Hum Factors* 39:509–525, 1997.

80. Shea JB, Morgan RL: Contextual interference effects on the acquisition, retention, and transfer of a motor skill. *J Exp Psychol Learn Mem Cogn* 5:179, 1979.

81. Shenkman M, Berger RA, Riley PO, et al: Whole-body movements during rising to standing from sitting. *Phys Ther* 70(10):638–648, 1990.

82. Shepherd RB, Gentile AM: Sit-to-stand: functional relationship between upper body and lower limb segments. *Hum Move SCI* 13(6):817, 1994.

83. Shepherd RB, Hirschorn AD: *Standing up and sitting down at two different seat heights.* Proceedings of the sixteenth International Society of Biomechanics Congress, 1997, Tokyo.

84. Shumway-Cook A, Woollacott MH: *Motor control: theory and practical applications*, ed 2, Baltimore, 2001, Lippincott Williams & Wilkins.

85. Shumway-Cook A, Woollacott MH: *Motor control: translating research into clinical practice*, ed 3, Baltimore, 2007, Lippincott Williams & Wilkins.

86. Sullivan PE, Markos PD, Minor MD: *An integrated approach to therapeutic exercise: theory and clinical application*, Reston, VA, 1982, Reston.

87. Tham, K, Tegnér, R: Video feedback in the rehabilitation of patients with unilateral neglect. *Arch Phys Med Rehabil* 78(4):410–413, 1997.

88. Tinnetti, ME: Performance-oriented assessment of mobility in elderly patients. *J Am Geriatr Soc* 34(2):119–126, 1986.

89. Tinetti, M, Richman, D, Powell, L: Falls efficacy as a measure of fear of falling. *J Gerontol* 45(6):239, 1990.

90. Toglia J: Generalization of treatment: a multicontext approach to cognitive perceptual impairment in adults with brain injury. *Am J Occup Ther* 45(6):505–516, 1991.

91. VanSant A: Life-span development in functional tasks. *Phys Ther* 70(12):788–798, 1990.

92. Winstein CJ: Knowledge of results and motor learning-implications for physical therapy. *Phys Ther* 71(2):140–149, 1991.

93. Winstein CJ, Gardner ER, McNeal DR, et al: Standing balance training: effect on balance and locomotion in hemiparetic adults. *Arch Phys Med Rehabil* 70(10):755–762, 1989.

94. Winstein CJ, Pohl PS, Lewthwaite R: Effects of physical guidance and knowledge of results on motor learning: support for the guidance hypothesis. *Res Q Exerc Sport* 65(4):316–323, 1994.

95. Winstein CJ, Schmidt RA: Reduced frequency of knowledge of results enhances motor skill learning. *J Exp Psychol Learn Mem Cogn* 16(4):677–691, 1990.

96. Winzeler-Mercay J, Mudie H: The nature of the effects of stroke on trunk flexor and extensor muscles during work and rest. *Disabil Rehabil* 24(17):875–886, 2002.

97. World Health Organization: *International classification of functioning, disability and health (short version)*, Geneva, 2001, The Organization.

98. Yardley L, Smith H: A prospective study of the relationship between feared consequences of falling and avoidance of activity in community-living older adults. *Gerontologist* 42(1):17–23, 2002.

clare c. bassile
sheila m. hayes

chapter 15

Gait Awareness

key terms

assistive devices

cerebellar strokes

contraversive pushing

gait analysis

gait patterns

hemiplegic gaits

orthotic devices

perceptual deficits

proprioceptive deficits

visual impairments

chapter objectives

After completing this chapter, the reader will be able to accomplish the following:

1. Understand normal gait components.
2. Identify common gait deviations after a stroke.
3. Understand the basics of gait retraining.
4. Identify and describe commonly used orthoses and assistive devices.

In the management of a stroke survivor, gait analysis and gait training traditionally have been the responsibility of physical therapists. Because of the interdisciplinary approach used to rehabilitate the stroke survivor, much sharing of information occurs between team members regarding the patient's functional and mobility status. Occupational and physical therapists often "cotreat" to enhance problem-solving regarding specific barriers to independence in activities of daily living.

Just as physical therapists have much to gain by familiarizing themselves with terminology and treatments used by occupational therapists (e.g., in the area of perceptual motor deficits), occupational therapists should benefit from having a basic understanding of normal gait components, common gait deviations after a stroke, and gait retraining. An integrated approach to treatment of the stroke survivor necessitates a working knowledge of the terminology, evaluation techniques, and rationale for treatment of other disciplines.

The physical therapist should perform a thorough examination before gait analysis and retraining. This examination includes factors such as range of motion, posture and bony alignment, strength, motor control, coordination, sensation, and balance. The therapist notes any deficits in these areas and is then ready to observe and analyze gait and to speculate on which of the deficits may be contributing to a specific gait deviation. The therapist can address specific deficits with appropriate treatment interventions and modalities.

Gait analysis is the objective documentation of gait[71] and ranges in complexity from observational assessment to quantitative analysis using instrumented gait analysis systems. These systems can include tools such as videotaping, three-dimensional motion analysis, dynamic electromyograms, and force plates. A variety of such quantitative systems is available and differs widely in sophistication and price.[11,60]

Kinematic analysis evaluates movement patterns, including the movement of the body, and specific angles between body segments (joint angles) as the body moves through the gait cycle. Observational gait analysis is a qualitative method of kinematic analysis. When kinematics is measured by instrumented analysis, it is considered a quantitative gait analysis.[60] Observational gait analysis is the visual inspection of walking.[88] Although not as reliable as quantitative gait analysis, observational gait analysis is the method most often used by practitioners. Most physical therapists do not have access to highly technical evaluation equipment, although videotaping is now more commonly available. Perry developed a systematic method for observational gait analysis that helps standardize this evaluation.[77]

Observational gait analysis is an acquired skill that requires much practice and repetition. The physical therapist must learn how to look at nine different points on the body (head, shoulders, arms, trunk, pelvis, hips, knees, ankles, and feet) while simultaneously comparing the observed gait with normal gait features, in three body planes. When one is first learning gait analysis, observation of as many normal gaits as possible is necessary. When one is first performing observational gait analysis in the clinic, the recommendation is that the physical therapist choose patients who can tolerate walking for several minutes. This allows the therapist to apply Perry's approach to viewing trunk and limb excursions during the gait cycle.

Observational gait analysis should take place in the sagittal and frontal planes. The frontal or coronal view must include anterior and posterior vantage points. Certain motions such as leg rotation and foot abduction and adduction take place in the transverse or horizontal plane, although the therapist usually is not in a position to observe motion specifically in this plane. In normal gait, most movement occurs in the *sagittal* plane, whereas in abnormal gait, many of the deviations are observed as compensations in the *frontal* (coronal) and *transverse* (horizontal) planes[71] (Fig. 15-1).

TERMINOLOGY

Physical therapists must first familiarize themselves with the components of the normal gait cycle and with the terminology used to describe these components before they can analyze the gait of a person who has had a stroke. A cycle begins when the heel of one foot touches the ground and ends after the leg and body have advanced through space and time and the heel of that *same* foot hits the ground again.

The cycle includes a period when the leg is in contact with the ground, which is followed by a period when it is

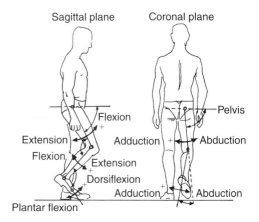

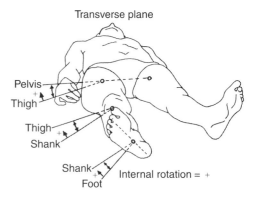

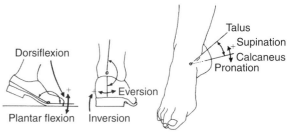

Figure 15-1 System of naming angular motion. (From Inman VT, Ralston HJ: *Human walking*, Philadelphia, 1981, Williams & Wilkins.)

advancing through space. Thus the gait cycle of one leg can be divided into two phases: the stance phase (in which the leg is in contact with the ground) and the swing phase (in which the leg is off the ground). The stance phase makes upto 60% of the gait cycle, and the swing phase makes upto 40% (Fig. 15-2). In a normal gait, the opposite leg also is going through a gait cycle simultaneously (i.e., has a stance phase and a swing phase). Each leg has two periods at the beginning and end of stance when the opposite leg is also in contact with the ground. These are called the periods of *double support*. Together they account for 10% of the initial stance phase and 10% of the end of stance for both legs.

The phases of swing and stance are further divided into substages. The language used to describe these subdivisions uses the traditional terms or the terms

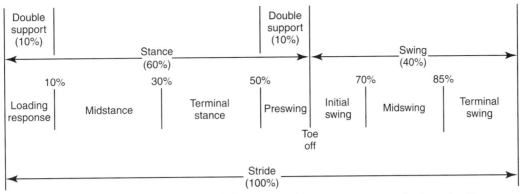

Figure 15-2 Phases of gait cycle and their proportions as percentages of gait cycle. (From Ounpuu S: *Evaluation and management of gait disorders*, New York, 1995, Marcel Dekker.)

developed at Rancho Los Amigos Medical Center (Table 15-1). Because the terms are similar, physical therapists often use a mixture of old and new terms unless the facility in which they work advocates strict adherence to one terminology. Most physical therapists are familiar with the Rancho Los Amigos terminology because of the abundance of research, literature, and gait assessment forms that have been produced by the pathokinesiology service and physical therapy department at that facility.[73]

The Rancho Los Amigos definition of swing phase is divided into the substages of initial swing, midswing, and terminal swing. The stance phase is divided into initial contact, loading response, midstance, terminal stance, and preswing (Fig. 15-3). Within these substages, the physical therapist observes the joint displacements and movements occurring at the trunk, pelvis, hip, knee, ankle, and toes. Fig. 15-4 illustrates the phases of the gait cycle and the corresponding normal joint displacements that occur as the body moves through the sagittal plane.

Other terms used in describing gait cycles are stride, step, cadence, and velocity. A *stride* is equal to a gait cycle (i.e., from heel strike of one leg to the next heel strike of the same leg). Stride can refer to distance (stride length) or time (stride time) in the gait cycle of one leg. A *step* is described as the distance (step length) or time (step time) from the heel strike of one leg to the heel strike of the opposite leg (Fig. 15-5).

RELIABLE GAIT PARAMETERS

Cadence is the number of steps or strides per unit of time. Walking velocity equals speed: the distance walked divided by time. Because time-distance variables are the components of gait that can be measured most reliably, therapists can use them in assessing improvement in stroke patients.[39,83,84] For example, persons who have had a stroke with a resulting hemiparesis typically walk with a slower than normal gait.[56,67] Routine recording of the cadence and velocity of these patients is an objective way of documenting change over time. Velocity measures are traditionally taken during a standard 10 minute walk test and show improvement for physical therapists that do not have access to the instrumented gait analysis systems mentioned previously.

It is important for therapists to have reference values from the healthy able-bodied population for cadence (100 to 120 steps/min) and velocity (1.2 to 1.5 m/sec) at their disposal, so a quick comparison with their patients' values can be made if one has the goal of recovery.[23] In addition, comparing an individual's cadence and velocity measure at two points in time may help to document improvement objectively.

Improvements in cadence and velocity also can be an indication of functional improvement and limb recovery. A study of hemiplegic patients by Harro and Giuliani[43] showed positive correlations between high scores (greater than 90) on the motor portion of the Fugl-Meyer motor assessment scale and the ability to increase walking speeds. Richards and colleagues[83] studied 18 hemiplegic subjects divided into three subgroups: slow, intermediate, and fast walkers. They found that the fast walkers had movements and muscle activations more like those of able-bodied subjects than the slow or intermediate speed walkers.

In recent years, the six-minute walk test has been used in the stroke population. While it was first used in the cardiopulmonary population to assess functional capacity,[6] its utility in the stroke population has been demonstrated. Dean and other separate investigators have consistently reported that this population's ambulation endurance is very limited.[26,58] The initial ambulation speed is not maintained throughout the six-minute walk test, and an individual's final walk distance is both lower than predicted from their 10-minute walk velocity and below the value used to identify heart transplant patients.[26] Thus, emphasizing the need to measure and train for both ambulation speed and endurance in this population.

Shaughnessy and colleagues have shown that monitoring step activity throughout the day using a portable microprocessor is another tool for demonstrating improvement

Table 15-1

Gait Terminology

	TRADITIONAL	RANCHO LOS AMIGOS
Stance phase	Heel strike: The beginning of the stance phase when the heel contacts the ground; the same as initial contact	Initial contact: The beginning of the stance phase when the heel or another part of the foot contacts the ground
	Foot flat: Occurs immediately following heel strike when the sole of the foot contacts the floor; occurs during loading response	Loading response: The portion of the first double support period of the stance phase from initial contact until the contralateral extremity leaves the ground
	Midstance: The point at which the body passes directly over the reference extremity	Midstance: The portion of the single limb support stance phase that begins when the contralateral extremity leaves the ground and ends when the body is directly over the supporting limb
	Heel off: The point following midstance when the heel of the reference extremity leaves the ground; occurs prior to terminal stance	Terminal stance: The last portion of the single limb support stance phase that begins with heel rise and continues until the contralateral extremity contacts the ground
	Toe off: The point following heel off when only the toe of the reference extremity is in contact with the ground	Preswing: The portion of stance that begins the second double support period from the initial contact of the contralateral extremity to lift off of the reference extremity
Swing phase	Acceleration: The portion of beginning swing from the moment the toe of the reference extremity leaves the ground to the point when the reference extremity is directly under the body	Initial swing: The portion of swing from the point when the reference extremity leaves the ground to maximum knee flexion of the same extremity
	Midswing: The portion of the swing phase when the reference extremity passes directly below the body: extends from the end of acceleration to the beginning of deceleration	Midswing: The portion of the swing phase from maximum knee flexion of the reference extremity to a vertical tibial position
	Deceleration: The swing portion of the swing phase when the reference extremity is decelerating in preparation for the heel strike	Terminal swing: The portion of the swing phase from a vertical position of the tibia of the reference extremity to just before initial contact

From O'Sullivan SB, Schmitz TJ, editors: *Physical rehabilitation assessment and treatment*, Philadelphia, 1994, FA Davis.

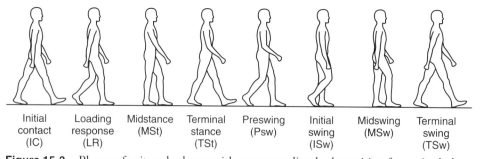

Initial contact (IC)	Loading response (LR)	Midstance (MSt)	Terminal stance (TSt)	Preswing (Psw)	Initial swing (ISw)	Midswing (MSw)	Terminal swing (TSw)

Figure 15-3 Phases of gait cycle shown with corresponding body position for sagittal plane motion. (From Ounpuu S: *Evaluation and management of gait disorders*, New York, 1995, Marcel Dekker.)

in ambulation tolerance.[87] They demonstrated an 80% improvement in step activity across a three-month outpatient rehabilitation period. Clinicians could monitor step activity during the course of a day by placing pedometers on their patients.

Perry has shown that ambulation speed differentiates level of ambulatory functioning and that individuals ambulatory in the community (0.58 m/sec) ambulate at speeds higher than independent household ambulators (0.4 m/sec) do. She has further classified levels within

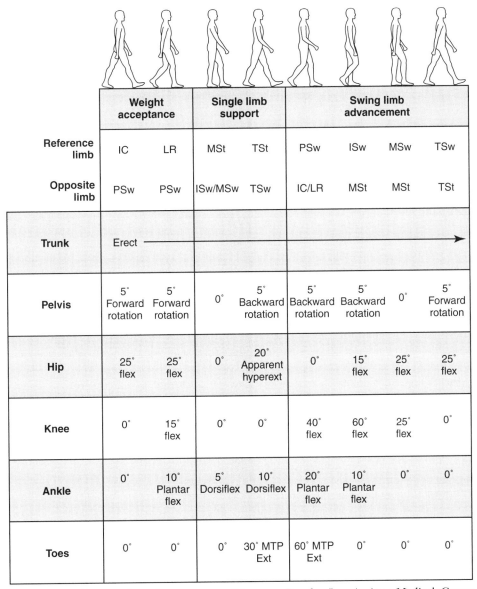

	Weight acceptance		Single limb support		Swing limb advancement			
Reference limb	IC	LR	MSt	TSt	PSw	ISw	MSw	TSw
Opposite limb	PSw	PSw	ISw/MSw	TSw	IC/LR	MSt	MSt	TSt
Trunk	Erect ⟶							
Pelvis	5° Forward rotation	5° Forward rotation	0°	5° Backward rotation	5° Backward rotation	5° Backward rotation	0°	5° Forward rotation
Hip	25° flex	25° flex	0°	20° Apparent hyperext	0°	15° flex	25° flex	25° flex
Knee	0°	15° flex	0°	0°	40° flex	60° flex	25° flex	0°
Ankle	0°	10° Plantar flex	5° Dorsiflex	10° Dorsiflex	20° Plantar flex	10° Plantar flex	0°	0°
Toes	0°	0°	0°	30° MTP Ext	60° MTP Ext	0°	0°	0°

Figure 15-4   Range of motion summary. (Courtesy Rancho Los Amigos Medical Center Physical Therapy Department and Pathokinesiology Laboratory, Downey, CA)

household (most and least limited) and community (most and least limited) ambulation based on speed and independence of ambulation while performing activities in the home and outside.[78] Common threads to community ambulation were increased ambulation distance/endurance, the ability to change level and terrain irregularity, obstacle avoidance, and the manual handling of loads. All these threads are essential for successful full access community ambulation. Thus, when they work on gait recovery in the stroke population, therapists must routinely take quantified measures of gait speed and endurance during a variety of ambulation tasks to assess household and community ambulation feasibility and reentry.

Hemiplegic Gaits

The type of gait of a person who has had a stroke depends on where in the brain the insult has occurred and which systems are affected, such as motor, sensory, balance, coordination, perceptual, and visual systems. If a motor area in the cortex or a motor track is involved, hemiplegia or hemiparesis is manifested in the contralateral limbs. The location of the infarction within these areas determines whether the arm or the leg is more impaired. Not all stroke patients are hemiplegic or hemiparetic, nor do all hemiparetic patients have the same degree of motor deficits. Unfortunately, the term *hemiplegic gait* frequently is applied to all individuals with hemiparesis, although many varieties and degrees of deficits exist.[39] Individuals who

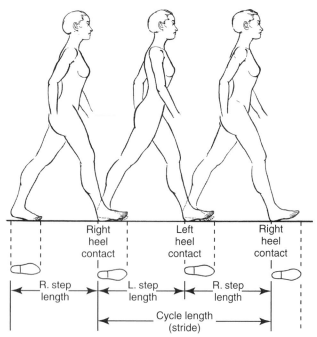

Figure 15-5 Distance dimensions in a gait cycle. *R.*, Right, *L.*, left. (From Inman VT, Ralston HJ: *Human walking*, Philadelphia, 1981, Williams & Wilkins.)

have suffered ischemia in areas of the brain supplied by the anterior cerebral artery usually have greater deficits in the leg. Those with ischemic lesions in areas supplied by the middle cerebral artery have greater arm involvement, although leg weakness is usually also present in varying degrees. Middle cerebral artery infarctions are the most common type of stroke.[16] The gait deviations seen with these lesions are those most often described by the generic term *hemiplegic gait*. Following are descriptions of some of the more common alterations.

During the stance phase of the hemiparetic leg, a patient may exhibit "foot flat" or even a "forefoot first" at the initial contact instead of a heel strike with adequate ankle dorsiflexion. The patient also may exhibit plantar flexion (forefoot first) *and* supination (in the frontal plane) at initial contact and then begin to bear weight precariously on the lateral border of the foot.[17,39,60,70]

During the loading response, while the patient is still in double limb support, weight is being "loaded," or accepted, onto the leg. Normally, 10 to 15 degrees of knee flexion is needed to absorb the forces of momentum and body weight. This flexion may be absent, in which case the knee remains extended or even hyperextends (genu recurvatum) during midstance, as the body moves forward. In this instance, no tibial advancement occurs over the foot because no dorsiflexion is occurring at the ankle (Fig. 15-6).

Midstance begins the period of single limb support. In addition to knee hyperextension, the therapist also may observe trunk and hip flexion as the body attempts to move its center of mass forward over a stiff knee. The

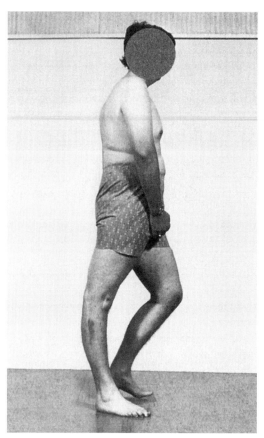

Figure 15-6 Genu recurvatum in midstance caused by a rigid plantar flexion contracture (greater than 15 degrees). Tibia is prevented from advancing forward, driving the knee posteriorly into recurvatum, impeding progression, and reducing momentum. (From Adams J, Perry J: *Human walking*, Philadelphia, 1994, Williams & Wilkins.)

problem may be compounded by pelvic retraction. Other patients may display the opposite scenario during midstance on the paretic leg; knee flexion may be excessive in the sagittal plane, with concurrent excessive dorsiflexion and hip flexion.[3,17,60,70]

In the *frontal* plane, lateral trunk lean may be excessive over the ipsilateral leg during midstance or a positive Trendelenburg sign may be evident, both of which indicate weak hip abductors of the stance leg. A positive Trendelenburg sign is present when excessive lateral displacement of the pelvis occurs over the stance leg, with an excessive lowering of the pelvis on the contralateral swing leg.[63,71]

During the terminal stance phase, which is still a period of single limb support, normal hip extension may be absent along with the ability to transfer weight onto the forefoot in preparation for push off. Dorsiflexion at the ankle joint may continue to be excessive or diminished. Lack of heel rise can occur in the *sagittal* plane, combined with excessive dorsiflexion, and the contralateral leg makes initial contact early.[3,39,60,71]

The preswing phase is the final stance stage and the second double support period. A lack of knee flexion (normally between 30 and 40 degrees) often occurs in the paretic leg, accompanied by a lack of ankle joint plantar flexion at the end of preswing.[3,17,70,73]

Many of the deviations observed in the hemiparetic limb during stance can contribute to a *decreased step length* by the *opposite* leg. The body is not able to complete its normal excursion forward because of lack of movement, or ineffective movement, of the pelvis, hip, knee, or ankle of the hemiparetic limb. The opposite limb may "step to" instead of stepping *past* the paretic limb. Step length also can be reduced in the hemiparetic leg.

The therapist sometimes can see the swing phase of the paretic limb as a mass flexion movement instead of a series of sequential flexion movements.[39,56] More often the swing phase is characterized by a stiff-legged swing, with a decrease in hip flexion and in the velocity and amount of reciprocal knee flexion and extension. The velocity of the entire paretic limb is often decreased.[39,66] The decrease in hip flexion, together with the lack of knee flexion and dorsiflexion, often results in *circumduction* to advance the stiff limb.[3,39,56,63,70,73] *Circumduction* occurs when the patient swings the leg through in a semicircle and is most noticeable when looking at the patient in the frontal plane (Fig. 15-7). The patient combines external rotation and abduction at the hip to lift the leg out to the side and then adducts and often internally rotates the leg to bring it back in.[63] In a normal gait pattern,

no abduction, adduction, or external or internal rotation occurs in the frontal plane during the swing phase.[73]

The limited knee flexion in the preswing phase persists into the initial swing phase and often throughout the entire swing phase. The toe drag first seen in the initial swing phase may continue because of the decreased knee swing but also may be a consequence of decreased hip flexion and decreased ankle dorsiflexion. The patient can initiate compensatory hip hiking at this stage to assist with clearing the toes as the leg advances.[3,39,60,66,70] Other compensations used to counteract toe drag are increased hip and knee flexion or vaulting by the opposite (stance) leg. Vaulting occurs when the person rises up on the toes of the stance foot for better clearance of the swing leg.[3]

In the midswing phase, the pelvis may remain retracted instead of rotating forward to neutral. Hip hiking and leg circumduction may continue, especially if knee flexion and dorsiflexion remain limited. Dorsiflexion may be decreased or absent, with the ankle assuming a plantarflexed (foot-drop) position. The foot may supinate during midswing because of an imbalance in ankle dorsiflexor muscle function[17,24,60,73] (see Fig. 15-7). Normally, the anterior tibialis and long toe extensors dorsiflex the foot symmetrically. Some stroke patients have overactive anterior tibialis muscles and weak long toe extensors, causing the medially placed anterior tibialis tendon to pull the foot into supination.[24]

As the limb progresses toward the terminal swing phase, many patients are unable to extend the knee while simultaneously flexing the hip and ankle. Instead, knee extension is decreased, and the foot initially contacts the ground with the knee flexed.[60,66] The pelvis still may be retracted or may not have rotated forward past neutral. This, in addition to the decrease in knee extension, results in a decreased step length by the paretic leg. Other subjects may exhibit knee extension with plantar flexion during the terminal swing phase, instead of the normal dorsiflexion seen in preparation for upcoming heel strike.[39,73] In other persons, adduction of the hip with knee extension can be so pronounced as to cause the swing leg to cross in front of the stance foot. Patients literally end up tripping over themselves.

CAUSES OF GAIT DEVIATIONS

One cannot overemphasize that the causes of the aforementioned *observed* gait deviations may vary from patient to patient. For example, a common deviation at initial contact is foot flat or forefoot first instead of heel strike. This abnormality could result from weak dorsiflexor muscles,[29,30,56,59,73] excessive activity of the plantar flexors,[3,55,56,73] a decreased ability to perform fast reciprocal movements,[39,53,56] disruption in the central generation of preprogrammed muscle activation,[45] noncontractile soft tissue tightness in the plantar flexors,[3,21,29,73] or a pathological condition of the

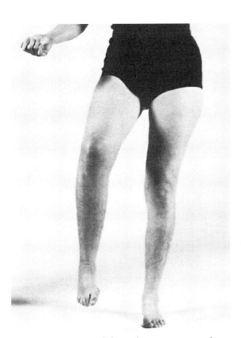

Figure 15-7 Supination of foot during swing phase resulting from uninhibited activity in the tibialis anterior. Circumduction of hip is also present during this swing phase. (From Davies P: *Steps to follow: the comprehensive treatment of patients with hemiplegia,* New York, 2000, Springer-Verlag.)

ankle joint. Even when soft tissue tightness and joint contractures are ruled out, hypotheses vary and often conflict about the precipitating factor. This is especially true when the issue of voluntary versus reflex skeletal muscle activation is addressed. A number of recent papers and publications provide an abbreviated review of the literature on this topic.[21,29,34,39,43,44,52,53,56]

OSTEOPOROSIS

Stroke survivors have a fourfold increased risk of falling compared to the healthy community dwelling population.[64] Falls in this population have an increased risk, from 1.2% to 6%, of resulting in fractures to the distal radius, humeral head, and hip.[15,81,100] Fractures occur predominantly on the paretic side and hip fractures in particular and accelerate the downward spiral toward increased morbidity and mortality.[80,81] Risk factors for fracture include reduced mobility, strength of the paretic leg, and reduced bone mineral density (BMD).[82] In Chapter 14, falls in the stroke population are explored; however, an analysis of the timeline for bone density demineralization is warranted so interventions to minimize this loss and possibly lessen the fracture risk can be developed.

In the spinal cord injury (SCI) population, bone demineralization occurs within the first three months postinjury and proceeds up to 16 months after injury. The demineralization has been attributed to prolonged bedrest, immobility, and lack of muscle contraction and gravitational loading below the level of SCI.[37,101] In the stroke population, investigations of BMD loss have been compared within a limb and between limbs (paretic vs. nonparetic) in longitudinal fashion for up to 12 months after stroke.[46,47,82] The rate of bone demineralization over the first year and the factors that might alter the loss are explored next.

As early as one month after stroke, significant BMD loss for the paretic upper limb (UL) compared to the nonparetic UL has been shown for the humerus (4%) and total arm (4%).[82] The paretic limb's distal radius loss reaches significance when compared to the other side at four months (3%). However, all three sites of the paretic UL continue to decline over the year (total arm 3%, humerus 14%, distal radius 3%), which puts the paretic UL at risk for fracture if used to break a fall. The nonparetic UL's distal radius demonstrates a 2% increase in BMD for the first year, which may be attributed to increased loading activity associated with the nonparetic UL during ambulation, although this hypothesis has not been tested.

Ranmnemark and colleagues[82] demonstrated that, at four months after stroke, a significant BMD loss for the proximal femur had already occurred in the paretic limb (6%), and loss continued throughout the remainder of the first year (12%). The nonparetic limb appeared to lose BMD as well, although at a slower rate compared to the other side (4% at 12 months). Studies reported that when BMD loss rate was analyzed across the first year, the most loss occurred within the first seven months in both the paretic (10%) and nonparetic legs (2%) of stroke survivors.[46,47,82]

Jorgensen[46,47] has demonstrated that ambulatory status and weight-bearing load on the paretic limb after stroke affect the rate of BMD loss. Using the 6 level ordinal scale for the Functional Ambulation Category (FAC) to qualify ambulation status, a linear relationship of ambulation assistance to BMD loss was demonstrated. Thus, if subjects ambulated independently or with assistance (FAC 2 to 6) within the first two weeks after stroke, subjects lost less BMD at one year (2%) compared to those who achieved ambulation by two months (7%) and to those still nonambulatory at two months (10%).[47] In addition, the amount of weight on the paretic limb during 30 seconds of static standing was linearly related to walking onset after stroke. Subjects who walked within two weeks of stroke had a higher percentage of body weight (51%) loaded through the paretic limb versus those who walked by seven months (43%) and those immobile at seven months (35%).[46]

BMD loss has been demonstrated for the paretic upper and lower limb throughout the first year after stroke. The upper extremity loss occurs sooner than the lower extremity loss, but both limbs show significant loss that could contribute to fracture risk during a fall. Early ambulation after stroke has been shown to modulate bone demineralization of the paretic limb during the first year. Therapists should use interventions that promote independent ambulation as early as possible after stroke with the knowledge that the sooner independent ambulation is achieved, the less bone loss occurs.

TREATMENT INTERVENTIONS

The physical therapist first addresses deficits identified during the physical assessment that are contributing to the abnormal gait, such as decreased range of motion and strength. Interventions can include basic modalities and therapeutic exercise and a variety of approaches to address the lack of movement and voluntary control. Many interventions are based on theories that advocate facilitation of normal movement and sensory stimulation of the patient by the therapist. In this context, the patient is a passive recipient of the therapist's efforts. However, during the past 20 years, therapists gradually have shifted away from using these more traditional therapeutic approaches to using the motor control perspective. The motor control approach also is based on a theoretical model, but it does not advocate specific treatment techniques that are done by the therapist to the patient. In the motor control model the main task of the therapist is not to facilitate normal movement but to structure the environment in such a way that the patient actively will relearn to use the affected limbs functionally. The motor control relearning theory is based on research from a variety of fields: neurophysiology, muscle physiology, biomechanics, and psychology.[20,42] Patients are believed to learn by actively trying to solve problems (see Chapter 6). Therefore, therapists should structure tasks to promote acquisition of the movements needed to solve specific motor control problems in a variety of situations (see Chapters 4 and 5). This pertains not only to patients with a hemiplegic gait but also to patients with motor control deficits described in the following sections.

In the last ten years, the research directed at improving gait function in patients after stroke have supported a basic tenet of motor skill acquisition. In order to improve gait functioning, the individual must practice the task of gait. The part practice intervention of weight shifting activities in standing with two feet in contact with the ground was not superior to the conventional neurodevelopmental treatment (NDT) based physical therapy intervention at improving gait.[102] Thus, suggesting that improvements in gait may not be amenable to part practice in standing positions where 2 feet are always in contact with the ground.

The question becomes if ambulation practice is required to improve ambulation, then how much practice does a patient require to improve gait? The recent literature shows that at least twenty minutes of ambulation practice is the minimum amount of time per session needed to note improved ambulation. Table 15-2 shows that the amount of practice for any of the ambulatory intervention groups is a considerable increase from what is presently observed in the rehabilitation clinic. This increase in time on task results in significant gains in overground walking speed and endurance.

Recent ambulatory intervention advancements have been the use of body weight support treadmill training (BWSTT), task-related circuit training, BWS + electric stimulation, overground walking practice, obstacle training, and home-based exercise programs (see Table 15-2). Visitin and Barbeau[96] first demonstrated that BWSTT was better than non-BWS walking for recent stroke survivors. At the end of a six week inpatient rehabilitation unit stay, those individuals who received BWSTT ambulated at a faster overground speed (0.34 m/sec) than individuals who received the non-BWS (0.25 m/sec) (control group). At the three-month retention, while both groups continued to improve, the BWSTT group was clearly superior (0.52 m/sec) to the control group (0.30 m/sec) (Fig. 15-8).

Sullivan's group[91] demonstrated that the speed which therapists train ambulation may be a critical factor in enhancing ambulation recovery. While BWSTT was performed for all groups, the training speeds for each group was different (fast vs. slow vs. variable). While all groups

improved, the fast group (2.0 m/hr) made the most gains in overground walking speed. This speaks to the specificity of speed training and suggests that training should occur at the speed to with the therapist wants the patient ultimately ambulate.

An additional innovation to the BWS device is the incorporation of an electric stimulation component during gait training. However, when compared to overground ambulation training, both groups of chronic stroke survivors made similar gains in walking velocity and endurance.[75] Ada's group[2] in their study of treadmill vs. overground walking programs found similar results in a community dwelling population of stroke survivors, and Nilsson's group[62] corroborated these results in acute stroke survivors, which suggests that the practice of ambulation is the common critical element for patients already somewhat ambulatory.

Dean[25] in her pilot study and Salbach[85] in a larger study found that training individuals in upright dynamic activities through a circuit system was more beneficial than no treatment or conventional treatment. The circuit included stations for walking overground at comfortable and fast speeds, walking over obstacles, transitions of sit-to-stand from varying height chairs, dynamic upright balance activities, and lower extremity strengthening activities performed in standing. Bassile[9] demonstrated that an obstacle ambulation training program was feasible and improved the gait and quality of life in chronic stroke survivors. Lastly, Duncan's specific home-based therapy program for acute stroke survivors that incorporated dynamic balance and LE strengthening performed in upright along with ambulation and aerobic training was found to be better than standard of care.[31]

In conclusion to this section, some common intervention themes are noted. First the task of ambulation must be practiced for much longer periods in the clinical setting if one wishes to improve this function. Results of this longer practice yield improved ambulation endurance (distance) and speed (velocity). Ambulation practice should occur at faster speeds to meet community ambulation activities. Both LE strength and balance (see Chapter 8) play a role in ambulation enhancement, and the literature supports the notion that performing task specific practice in upright dynamic postures along with ambulation practice, not in place of it, contributes to enhanced locomotion.

OTHER ABNORMAL GAIT PATTERNS

The list of abnormal gait patterns that can appear after stroke is too extensive to be covered completely in a single chapter. Therefore, what follows are examples of abnormal gaits that are particularly challenging to the physical therapist. Each deficit results from damage in the particular part of the brain described.

Table 15-2

Evidence-Based Gait Interventions Poststroke

DESIGN	POPULATION	INTERVENTION GROUPS	TREATMENT DURATION	ASSESSMENT TIMES	OUTCOME MEASURES	RESULTS
RCT-3 groups[75]	Chronic CVA pts on inpt rehab n=45	BWSGT + ES BWSGT Overground walking	20 min/day × 3 wks 55 min/day of trad. PT	Baseline, post completion 6 month retention	10 MWT, 6MWT, dynamic balance time, MMAS	All 3 groups improved significantly across time No difference between the groups
RCT-2 groups pilot study[25]	Chronic CVA pts outpatient setting n=12	LE circuit training UE training	1 hr/ session 3 sessions/wk × 4 wks	Baseline, post completion 2 month retention	10 MWT, 6MWT, step test, TUG Sit-to-stand with force plates	LE circuit group improved significantly more than the other group on 10 MWT, 6 MWT and step test at completion and retention LE circuit group improved peak vertical GRF through affected leg
RCT-3 groups[91]	Chronic CVA pts outpatient setting n=24	BWSTT-slow BWSTT-fast BWSTT-variable	20 min/session 3 sessions/wk × 4 wks	Baseline, middle, post completion 1 month and 3 month retention	10 MWT	All 3 groups improved significantly baseline to completion and continued to improve at 1-month retention Fast group made most improvement
RCT-2 groups[31]	Subacute CVA pts home care n=92	Therex group Usual care	90 min/session 3 sessions/wk × 12 wks	Baseline, post completion	Isometric peak torque (ankle, knee, grip) Fugl Meyer (lower ext. motor score) Berg Balance Scale, Functional Reach test Wolf motor function test, 10 MWT, 6 MWT, peak VO_2	Both groups improved significantly across time Therex group improved significantly more than usual care for Berg, peak VO_2 10 MWT, 6 MWT
RCT-2 groups[2]	Chronic CVA pts n=29	Walking (treadmill/ overground) Home exercise placebo	3×/wk × 4 wks 30 min walking/ session	Baseline, post completion	10 MWT, 6 MWT, Sickness Impact Profile	Significantly improved 10 MWT and 6 MWT compared to placebo group
RCT-2 groups[85]	Chronic CVA pts outpatient setting n=91	LE tasks UE tasks	3×/wk × 6 wks	Baseline, post completion	6 MWT, 5 MWT, TUG, Berg Balance Scale	LE task group improved significantly for all measures at completion
RCT-2 groups[96]	Subacute CVA pts inpt rehab n=100	BWSTT No BWSTT	4 sessions/wk × 6 wks ≤3 trials/ session or ≤ 20 min	Baseline, post completion 3 month retention	Berg Balance Scale, STREAM, 10 MWT, walk endurance (≤320 m)	BWSTT group improved significantly for all measures at completion Both groups improved at 3 month retention compared to completion, but BWSTT group improved more than no BWSTT
Experimental group[9]	Chronic CVA pts n=56	Obstacle ambulation plus overground ambulation	2 sessions/wk × 4 wks	Baseline, post completion 1 month retention	6 MWT, 10 MWT, MMAS (walking section), SF36-PFt, SF36-RPt	Significant improvement noted in all measures except SF36-RPt at completion SF36-PFt and 10 MWT maintained at 1 month

BWSGT, body weight support gait training; *BWSTT*, body weight support treadmill training; *CVA*, cerebrovascular accident; *LE*, lower extremity; *MMAS*, Modified Motor Assessment Scale; *MWT*, minute walk test; *MWT*, meter walk test; *PT*, physical therapy; *RCT*, randomized controlled trial; *SF-36-PFt*, Short Form Health Survey: Physical Function; *SF36-RP*: Short Form Health Survey: Role Physical; *STREAM*, Stroke Rehabilitation Assessment of Movement; *TUG*, timed up and go; *UE*, upper extremity; *VO₂*, maximal oxygen consumption;

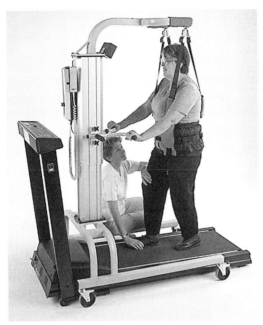

Figure 15-8 LiteGait System. (From Mobility Research, LiteGait, PO Box, 3141, Tempe, AZ 85280; 1-800-332-WALK; www.litegait.com.)

Cerebellar Strokes

A person who has an infarct in the cerebellum caused by occlusion or hemorrhage of a vertebral or a cerebellar artery may exhibit completely different gait deviations than a hemiparetic patient. The cerebellum is composed of three parts or lobes: the flocculonodular lobe, the anterior lobe, and the posterior lobe. The *flocculonodular* lobe also is called the *vestibulocerebellum* because most of its input is from the vestibular nuclei in the pons. The *anterior* lobe also is known as the *spinocerebellum* because most of its input is from the spinocerebellar tracts via the inferior cerebellar peduncle and the superior cerebellar peduncle. The *posterior* lobe also is known as the *neocerebellum* and contains most of the cerebellar hemispheres. The hemispheres receive their major input from the cortex via the middle cerebellar peduncle.

In addition, the cerebellum can be divided longitudinally into functional zones perpendicular to the horizontal fissures dividing the lobes. The medial structure is the vermis. Adjacent to the vermis, on either side, is the pars intermedia (intermediate section) of the cerebellar hemisphere. Lateral to this is the bulk of the cerebellar hemisphere.

Gait is influenced most by the flocculonodular and anterior lobes. Consequently, infarcts in these areas lead to difficulty maintaining a proper stance and walking.[65] Damage to the flocculonodular lobe (vestibulocerebellum) causes head and neck ataxia. Truncal tremor is often severe. The patient often uses a wide-based stance with the feet apart to increase stability. Any attempt to bring the feet together or walk with one foot directly in front of the other causes loss of balance. Ataxia or dysmetria of the limbs is not common.

Damage to the anterior lobe, especially the medial aspect, causes a disruption in the sensory input (via the spinocerebellar tracts) that is related to agonist-antagonist muscle activity. Lower limb ataxia or dysmetria is also present, but upper limb ataxia is usually absent. Lesions in a cerebellar hemisphere result in ipsilateral limb dysmetria or hypotonia, in addition to other deficits. Although the damage does not affect postural stability, the gait appears ataxic and staggering because of the limb dysmetria.[60]

The cerebellum is supplied by three main arteries: the posterior inferior cerebellar artery, the anterior inferior cerebellar artery, and the superior cerebellar artery. These arteries are part of the posterior circulation—the vertebrobasilar system. The posterior inferior cerebellar artery is a branch of the vertebral artery, whereas the anterior inferior cerebellar artery and superior cerebellar artery are branches of the basilar artery. Chapter 1 describes in detail the territories supplied by these arteries and their associated areas.[4,5] In general, these arteries supply the areas of the cerebellum that their names imply, in addition to parts of the brainstem. Some areas of vascularization in the cerebellum overlap because of the many free cortical anastomoses[5] (Fig. 15-9). Although one artery may supply one particular lobe predominantly, this overlapping may result in additional blood coming from the distal branches of another artery. However, as a rule, the superior cerebellar artery supplies the superior cerebellar peduncle, the anterior inferior cerebellar artery supplies the middle

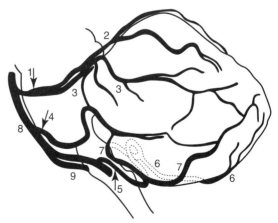

Figure 15-9 Lateral view of cerebellar arteries. *1,* Superior cerebellar artery; *2,* medial branch of superior cerebellar artery; *3,* lateral branch of superior cerebellar artery; *4,* anterior inferior cerebellar artery; *5,* posterior inferior cerebellar artery; *6,* medial branch of posterior inferior cerebellar artery; *7,* lateral branch of posterior inferior cerebellar artery; *8,* basilar artery; *9,* vertebral artery. (From Bogousslavsky J, Caplan L, editors: *Stroke syndromes,* Cambridge, UK, 1995, Cambridge University Press.)

cerebellar peduncle, and the posterior inferior cerebellar artery supplies the inferior cerebellar peduncle.[5]

A cerebellar stroke resulting from occlusion of the posterior inferior cerebellar artery usually is referred to in the literature as a *lateral medullary syndrome* (Wallenberg syndrome)[12,38,95] because it was believed that the posterior inferior cerebellar artery supplied the lateral medulla and parts of the cerebellum. Recently this term has been disputed, based on evidence that the lateral medulla is supplied less frequently by the posterior inferior cerebellar artery than previously thought.[4] If the lateral medulla is spared, an infarct of the posterior inferior cerebellar artery territory is apparent as a headache on the ipsilateral side, vertigo, nausea and vomiting, nystagmus, and limb and gait ataxia. If the lateral medulla is involved, the foregoing signs and symptoms are present. In addition, interruption of the sympathetic nerve fibers can cause Horner syndrome. Cranial nerves V, IX, and X also are affected.[4,94]

Involvement of cranial nerves V, IX, and X results in ipsilateral loss of pain and temperature in the face (V), dysphagia (IX), and dysphonia (X). Pain and temperature may be decreased on the opposite side of the body because of the interruption of the ascending spinothalamic tracts. This combination of cerebellar and medullary signs constitutes Wallenberg lateral medullary syndrome. In either type of posterior inferior cerebellar artery infarct, the inferior cerebellar peduncle and the inferior aspect of the cerebellum are affected. The result is ipsilateral limb ataxia and gait ataxia.[4,94] In addition, the patient tends to fall to the side of the lesion (ipsilateral axial lateropulsion) and has difficulty shifting weight toward the contralateral leg.[4]

Earlier texts reported that posterior inferior cerebellar artery infarcts are the most common,[12] but recent findings have shown that superior cerebellar artery infarcts occur as frequently.[4,5] Superior cerebellar artery infarcts have several different clinical manifestations. Dysarthria is one of the most frequent. Limb dysmetria, gait ataxia, and ipsilateral axial lateropulsion are also common symptoms.[4] Anterior inferior cerebellar artery infarcts are the least common. In addition to vertigo and ataxia, tinnitus and deafness are present. Auditory involvement and peripheral facial palsy are classic signs of anterior inferior cerebellar artery infarcts, which differentiate them from superior cerebellar artery or posterior inferior cerebellar artery infarcts.[4,94]

Gait retraining after a cerebellar stroke is focused on relearning the way to correct balance losses. Patients first must learn the point in space where their center of gravity is positioned optimally over their base of support for stability. Then they must relearn the way to realign their center of gravity constantly with their base of support. This task is most difficult during ambulation when the center of gravity is shifted anterior to the base of support as the body moves forward.[93]

Balance retraining should encourage active problem-solving by the patient (see Chapter 8). Being held upright by the therapist while walking does not promote functional independence. Likewise, assistive devices that require upper extremity weight-bearing (e.g., walkers) may prevent loss of balance but do not promote functional improvement because they do not challenge the patient to relearn balance control.[7,13] The patient is merely stabilized externally and is not required to use or integrate postural reflexes.

Activities that require active weight shifting and goal-oriented reaching are encouraged and practiced while the patient is standing (see Chapter 14). The therapist can introduce progressively more challenging exercises and activities as the patient becomes more adept.[7] Initially, some patients benefit from walking with their nonaffected side next to a high mat. The hand of the nonaffected side is placed on the surface of the mat for support. The patient can advance the dysmetric limb more easily if the opposite (sound side) hip maintains contact with the high mat during stance. Later, the patient uses a cane only to prevent loss of balance or as a cue to shift weight to the less affected side, not as a maximal assistive device.

Contraversive Pushing/Pusher Syndrome

An unusual motor behavior that hemiplegic patients sometimes display in the clinic is ipsilateral pushing. The patients tend to push away from the unaffected side in any position. Davies[24] described the syndrome in 1985 and called it the *pusher syndrome*. The original description of the pusher syndrome was based solely on a practitioner's observation and was most often thought to be associated with left hemiplegia and perceptual deficits (especially left neglect), left visual field neglect with or without homonymous hemianopsia, impaired body scheme and body image, and visuospatial deficits.[24] Recent research activity has attempted to identify the neural correlates and mechanisms for this clinical disorder. Unilateral lesions of the posterior lateral thalamus have been implicated in recent imaging studies.[49,51] Also, diminished perfusion for the intact areas of inferior frontal, middle temporal, and inferior parietal lobes have resulted in pusher syndrome.[92]

The original description of the pusher syndrome was based solely on a practitioner's observation. The behavior was seen in as many as 10% of the 327 stroke patients in the study by Pedersen, Wandell, and Jorgensen.[74] The syndrome appears in both right and left hemisphere damage.[50,74] Neglect and aphasia are also highly associated with pushing behavior.[50]

Karnath and colleagues have suggested through their research that the task of the brain areas damaged or receiving low perfusion in patients with pusher syndrome appears to be control of upright body posture.[49,50,92] They demonstrated that patients with pusher syndrome show normal perception of visual vertical but a severe tilt of perceived body posture in relation to gravity. While seated in a tilting chair, patients with pusher syndrome oriented their bodies upright when they were actually 18 degrees tilted towards the side of the brain lesion. However, they were able to orient the visual world vertically appropriate. In addition, they were able to align their bodies to earth's vertical when they used visual cues from the laboratory surroundings. In the dark, they were also able to orient to visual vertical, suggesting that both visual and vestibular inputs were unaffected.[24]

Karnath and Broetz[48] have identified three characteristic behaviors associated with pusher syndrome (see Chapter 7 for the Clinical Assessment Scale for Contraversive Pushing). First, the patient's longitudinal body axis is tilted toward the paretic side when sitting or standing. Second, the patient actively pushes (abduction and extension of arm or leg) with the nonaffected extremities, which results in a lean toward the hemiplegic side and loss of balance. Third, the patient resists any attempt by the examiner to correct the tilted body axis.

The rehabilitation literature is scant on outcomes and intervention.[72,74,76] Karnath[51] found patients with pusher syndrome have a good prognosis. The behavior was rarely observed after six months of stroke. However, rehabilitation did take 3.6 weeks longer for the patients with contraversive pushing as compared to other stroke patients to achieve similar functional outcomes.

Gait training for patients with contraversive pushing is a definite challenge, as is transfer training. During sit-to-stand activities, some patients project themselves quickly out of a chair toward their hemiparetic side. If left unguarded, they fall. Transferring toward the stronger side is difficult because they always push away from that side. Although easier, transfers toward the hemiparetic side are dangerous because of the lack of motor control on that side. Standing requires assistance to prevent falling to the weak side.

Walking with an assistive device, such as a cane in the stronger hand, is initially unproductive, because these patients tend to use the cane to push themselves toward the hemiparetic leg. They appear unable actively to shift weight onto the strong leg. The more these patients are supported (to prevent falling to the paretic side), the more they push into the helper.

Gait retraining is based on the same principles discussed in the ataxic gaits section. Patients must relearn the way to adjust their center of gravity over their base of support while standing. The patients must regain proper positioning of their trunk in relation to gravitational forces so their center of mass stays within the limits of their strength and base of support (cone of stability). This implies a need for conscious awareness of their loss of balance. Trial and error is encouraged to promote active problem-solving. Two interventions are suggested for

specific use with patients who demonstrate contraversive pushing. Karnath[48] proposed that, since patients' perception of visual vertical are intact but their perception of body vertical is inaccurate, the patients must use the visual vertical to align their bodies. They must be taught that the visual alignment information is correct and the body's perception (feeling) of alignment is incorrect. This can be done through visual feedback of their bodies aligned to an external vertical axis. For example, patients can align their trunks to the vertical axis in a mirror with tape along the vertical line bisecting their body halves. Patients can also use door and window frames to align their trunks. However, they may require external feedback from the therapist simultaneously with a "conscious awareness" that balance is achieved in this position. Using the visual vertical axis for postural alignment takes care of a behavior seen with pusher syndrome.

During dynamic activities such as transferring sit to stand and ambulation, the unaffected upper and lower extremities are called into play to assist with the activity. Active pushing by the nonaffected extremities in a lateral direction toward the hemiplegic side occurs, and often the patient falls to this side when transferring, standing, or walking if not prevented from doing so by the therapist.

The second intervention has been used by clinicians but has not been evaluated systematically in the clinic. Therapists should remove all firm pushing surfaces from patient contact during activities. Thus, when performing sitting activities, the feet may be unsupported initially. In sitting and standing, the patient is not allowed to hold a firm external support with the nonaffected hand, so assistive devices and parallel bars are counterproductive. For example, the patient may be asked to hold a cup of water while transferring from sit-to-stand. When standing or transferring, the patient might be asked to simultaneously perform reach, grasp, and place activities with the nonaffected upper extremity. The items are retrieved or placed on movable surfaces (e.g., hospital tray table or rolling stools). This intervention eliminates the success of the pushing arm in destabilizing the patient, and the therapist can assist the patient to realign the vertical axis of body more easily. If the patient can perform these activities while preferentially shifting their center of mass toward the nonaffected side while receiving external visual and verbal feedback about vertical alignment then he or she can consciously be aware of what body positions create stability (e.g., objects are placed or retrieved from midline and in the direction of the nonaffected side).

Relearning to maintain balance while walking is a formidable task for patients with ipsilateral pushing. The degree of difficulty in relearning to maintain balance while walking is compounded by changes in somatic sensation, strength, motor control, and feedback circuits following the infarction. Patients must regain some control of trunk in dynamic standing activities before ambulation can proceed safely. Visual and tactile goals can be helpful. Having patients walk around a high mat or table while observing themselves in a mirror vertically bisected with a tape may cue patients where to shift their weight to avoid falling. The use of parallel bars is discouraged; patients must learn to weight shift with the trunk to correct balance losses and not merely to pull on a bar to remain upright. If safe for both patient and therapist, using the mirror and ambulating in free space may be possible with the therapist guarding and stabilizing the affected lower limb and trunk side. Patients can advance to using a cane once they have mastered trunk control. Hands-on techniques used by the therapist to facilitate movement are discouraged. The patients simply will push into the hands of the therapist.

At times, leg weakness interferes with a pusher syndrome patient's ability to relearn postural control and weight shifting. Davies[24] advocated splinting the hemiparetic knee in extension while having the patient work on active weight shifting during functional standing activities. Splinting the knee this way might increase loading in the affected patient's affected leg while standing. One can assume that the added stability somehow reassures patients and gives them time to assess accurately whether they are balanced. Perhaps the degrees of freedom have been limited, allowing patients to concentrate on one task, weight shifting, to achieve a functional goal without having to concern themselves with an unstable knee. At this time, only speculations can be made about what reduces the pushing tendency and why. Although treatment techniques were suggested for gait training patients with contraversive pushing, no controlled studies have been done to verify their efficacy, and they are based solely on this and other practitioners' clinical experiences.

Proprioceptive Deficits

Loss of sensation after a stroke can compound motor deficits. In particular, loss of proprioception can greatly impede motor recovery after stroke.[32] Proprioception is conveyed to the cerebellum and to the cerebral cortex. Information about joint position and muscle activity is sent to both, but the information projected to the cerebellum is not recorded as conscious perception. The information is used to ensure coordinated limb movements. In contrast, the information sent to the cortex can be perceived consciously and provides awareness of limb position and movement.[38]

Proprioceptive input from muscle spindles, joint receptors, and cutaneous touch receptors reaches the cerebellum through the inferior cerebellar peduncle via the ipsilateral dorsal spinocerebellar tracts. The same information reaches the somatosensory area of the cerebral cortex via the ipsilateral posterior columns of the spinal cord, which cross in the medulla and ascend in the medial lemniscus to the thalamus and then to the cortex.

Middle cerebral artery strokes can impair awareness of proprioception at the cortical level. Although all sensations can be affected, proprioception and two-point discrimination are usually more impaired than pain and temperature perception.[12] The deficits are manifested in the contralateral arm and leg. Cerebellar artery strokes cause loss of the unconscious, rapid proprioceptive input required for the smooth, automatic movements of gait. Loss of sensory input regarding agonist-antagonist muscle activity disrupts the continuous modulation of these muscles that is required for coordinated gait movements.

A study by Kusoffsky, Wadell, and Nilsson[54] found that patients with proprioceptive loss after cortical stroke were able to regain a greater amount of function in the leg than in the arm. One explanation they gave for this was that gait greatly depends on centrally generated activation patterns, and these patterns in turn do not depend on peripheral sensory mechanisms. These central pattern generators originate in the spinal cord and are controlled by locomotor centers in the brainstem. These centers are influenced by the cerebellum, the basal ganglia, and the cerebral cortex.[40] The physical therapist can take advantage of this phenomenon by emphasizing functional gait as much as possible, as with BWSTT.

Along with vestibular and visual input, proprioceptive information contributes to a patient's ability to maintain a stable upright position. Input from muscle spindles and joint receptors provides valuable information not only about the position of a limb in space but also about the environment.[45,93] The ability to react to uneven surfaces or changes in ground texture depends on this input, and its impairment puts a patient at higher risk of falling. Coordinated limb movements may be decreased, and the person may be unable to judge the step length or limb joint excursions needed for maneuvering in the environment.

Vision can help to compensate for the proprioceptive loss.[38,45,69,93] As with other deficits, the physical therapist should encourage a problem-solving approach. The patient must learn consciously to use visual input, which was not necessary before. Occasionally mirrors are useful, although the therapist should evaluate these aids individually for each patient. Mirrors can hinder as often as they help patients, especially those with visuospatial deficits.

The therapist's role is to provide a variety of settings in which the person can practice using visual cues. In addition, biofeedback can be used to provide auditory cues. One type of biofeedback unit is a limb load monitor that can signal a person when the foot contacts the ground. Standard biofeedback units provide information about the force of muscle contraction during strengthening exercises (see Chapter 10).

Visual Deficits

Visual impairments from strokes also can affect gait. The most common visual deficit in hemiplegic patients is homonymous hemianopsia,[95] which occurs when an infarction involves the optic tract, the lateral geniculate body, or the optic radiation to one occipital cortex. A branch of the internal carotid artery, the anterior choroidal artery, supplies most of the optic tract and the optic radiation, with some coverage by branches of the middle cerebral artery and the posterior cerebral artery.[95] The visual cortex is supplied mainly by the posterior cerebral artery but also is supplied by some middle cerebral artery collaterals.[18] Homonymous hemianopsia also can result from an isolated occlusion of the calcarine branch of the posterior cerebral artery, but in this case, no concurrent hemiplegia or hemisensory loss occurs.[36]

When homonymous hemianopsia is present, visual information about one half of a person's environment is missing. The temporal half of the visual field of one eye and the nasal half of the visual field of the other eye are absent. Loss of the left half of the visual field accompanies left hemiplegia, and loss of right visual field accompanies right hemiplegia. As mentioned previously, balance is maintained by an intricate communication network between the visual, vestibular, and proprioceptive systems. If vision is impaired, one aspect of this network is functioning abnormally. The ability to maintain balance is at risk if the patient does not learn to use other systems for feedback about the environment.[22]

Self-awareness of the visual deficit is crucial for patients. They must test this new awareness in a variety of situations and environments to ensure safety on discharge from the hospital and maximize functional independence (see Chapter 16).

Perceptual Deficits

Perceptual deficits such as left neglect or visual neglect are neurobehavioral deficits that can affect gait. These phenomena and their manifestations, causes, and clinical implications are discussed elsewhere (see Chapters 18 and 19).[10,36] Ipsilateral pushing also may be classified as a neurobehavioral deficit.

Hemineglect and hemianopsia are separate entities that can often coexist.[8] Likewise, neglect and sensory loss can develop together or independently. Communication between the occupational and physical therapists concerning a patient's perceptual status is a necessity and helps determine the best treatment approach to maximize function and ensure consistency of treatment interventions. Information obtained from formal testing by the occupational therapist can provide valuable insights for the physical therapist formulating the gait retraining program.

Orthotic Interventions

An orthosis (from the Greek adjective *orthos*, meaning "straight") is an external device that improves a person's function when applied to a body part.[57] The more commonly used term for an orthosis is a *brace*. Orthoses now are named according to the joints they encompass. Short leg braces are known as *ankle-foot orthoses* (AFOs). A long leg brace is known as a *knee-ankle-foot orthosis* (KAFO) or a *hip-knee-ankle-foot orthosis* if it contains a hip joint and a knee joint. The newer terminology is more descriptive and specific and avoids confusion.

Orthotic devices are prescribed by a physician and fabricated by an orthotist. The physical therapist provides input to the physician and orthotist about which temporary devices have been assessed in the clinic before a permanent orthosis is prescribed. The physical therapist is also responsible for gait training the individual with the orthotic device. Training includes donning and doffing instructions, skin inspections, and patient education as well as the actual gait training.

Orthotic devices are classified in four categories: stabilizing (supportive), functional (assistive), corrective, and protective. All orthoses are used to increase function.

Stabilizing and functional orthoses are the two types most often used with stroke survivors. Stabilizing orthoses are used to prevent unwanted motion such as plantar flexion at the ankle or knee buckling. Functional orthoses have an element that compensates for lost muscle strength by assisting with movement. Stabilizing orthoses are not intended as a way to correct a fixed deformity in an adult; they only can stabilize and accommodate a deformity. Corrective orthoses are used to correct or realign parts of a limb. They are used for infants and young children to help correct flexible skeletal deformities. These orthoses should not be used to correct a fixed deformity in an adult. A stabilization orthosis can be used, but only to support the fixed deformity. Protective orthoses protect a portion of a limb from weight-bearing forces (e.g., a limb with a fracture).[35]

The orthotist adheres to basic physical principles when fabricating an orthosis to control a weak joint. An orthosis that provides three points of pressure is the most common type.[90] One of the three forces is directed toward the joint itself, and the other two end forces are directed opposite to the main force (Fig. 15-10). This principle is important for the occupational therapist to learn because of its relevance to adaptive shoe equipment. Fig. 15-10, *B* illustrates the three points of pressure used with an AFO that is providing a dorsiflexion assist. The main point of pressure is on the dorsum of the foot. The two counter pressures are at the posterior calf and the distal plantar surface of the foot. Elastic laces, often used to facilitate donning a shoe with stroke survivors, eliminate the main point of pressure and result in

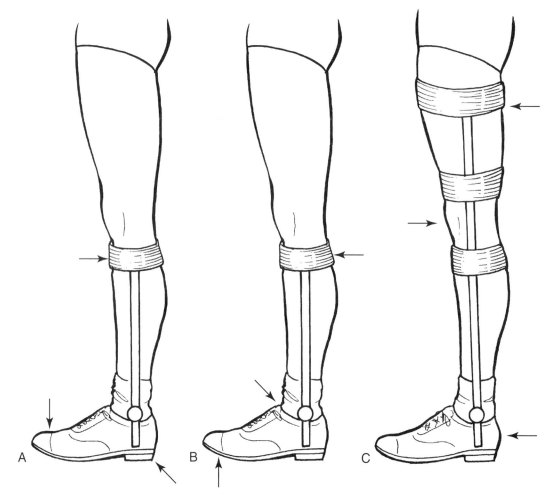

Figure 15-10   **A,** Three points of pressure of an ankle-foot orthosis with dorsiflexion stop. **B,** Three points of pressure of a dorsiflexion assist ankle-foot orthosis. **C,** Three points of pressure of a locked knee-ankle-foot orthosis. (These illustrations are diagrammatic only.)

loss of orthotic effectiveness. Therefore, elastic laces should not be used with dorsiflexion-assist braces. Elastic laces should be used cautiously with solid ankle AFOs that prevent dorsiflexion (see Fig. 15-10, *A*) because the foot needs to be held snugly in the AFO and shoe. This is especially true if plantar flexion spasticity is present.

Another orthotic principle states that the longer the lever arms, the less force needs to be applied at the three points of pressure. Therapists need to consider bony landmarks and superficial nerves when implementing these principles.[90] The orthotic joint axis of motion should be aligned with the skeletal joint; otherwise, abnormal pressures can be applied in the wrong areas, such as under calf bands, with movement or positioning.[35,90]

Orthotic devices can be made of a variety of materials, the most common of which are metal and plastic. Plastic orthoses are in total contact with a limb and are worn inside the shoe. Metal orthoses are attached to a shoe and held in place on the limb with straps or bands.

An AFO is the most commonly used orthosis for patients with a hemiplegic gait and is the most appropriate.[60,77,98] An AFO can affect knee motion and ankle motion. Knee buckling can be reduced, in stance, by adjusting the amount of dorsiflexion at the ankle joint. Similarly, knee hyperextension (genu recurvatum) can be avoided by controlling the amount of plantar flexion. Therefore, the therapist can avoid using a heavier KAFO to control the knee.

Plastic orthoses usually are made from high-temperature thermoplastic materials such as polypropylene. They require high temperatures for molding and therefore are shaped over a model, such as a plaster cast impression of the patient's leg. They are more resistant to continued stress than the low-temperature thermoplastics used for UL orthoses.

The simplest and most commonly used plastic AFO is the posterior leaf splint or spring[35] (Fig. 15-11, *A*). The leaf spring is used when the main gait deviation is "foot

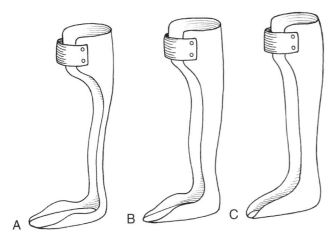

Figure 15-11 **A**, Posterior leaf splint or posterior leaf orthosis. **B**, Modified ankle-foot orthosis. **C**, Solid ankle-foot orthosis.

drop" during the swing phase. The orthosis functions as a dorsiflexion assist device because of its flexibility. The plastic of the calf portion is displaced in stance and then springs back to a 90-degree angle during swing. The ankle joint is held at this 90-degree angle during swing. Foot drop and toe drag are avoided. This orthosis, however, does not afford any mediolateral stability at the ankle joint. If this is of concern, then the therapist can try a more substantial orthosis.

A modified AFO has a wide calf upright with lateral trimline borders that are just posterior to the malleoli (Fig. 15-11, *B*). Usually the foot plate encompasses more of the lateral and medial borders of the foot. This results in more control of calcaneal and forefoot inversion and eversion. The increased width of the calf portion offers somewhat more resistance to plantar flexion in swing and stance.

The most supportive AFO is the solid ankle AFO (Fig. 15-11, *C*). The lateral trim lines extend even farther forward, anterior to the malleoli. Because of its construction, the solid ankle AFO is designed to prevent ankle motion and foot motion in any plane. The device controls dorsiflexion, plantar flexion, inversion, and eversion.

A variety of hinged plastic AFOs are now available to allow certain motions and to block others. The ankle joint components are too numerous to mention, and newer components are being designed continuously. The orthotist can use different combinations of joints and stops to allow, limit, or prevent movement. For example, the therapist may wish to allow dorsiflexion past neutral (90 degrees) in stance to allow normal tibial advancement over the foot but block plantar flexion at neutral to prevent foot drop in swing and knee hyperextension in stance.

Another group of plastic AFOs is referred to as *tone-inhibiting AFOs*. Most of these AFOs initially were designed for use with children with cerebral palsy.[28] Several

types have been designed more specifically for use with adult hemiplegics.[61] The common denominator is the flexibility allowed by these orthoses, in the foot and in the ankle. In theory, this flexibility allows more normal weight-bearing contacts on the plantar surface of the foot throughout stance, which promotes normal mobility in the foot during stance rather than having the foot held in one position. Mueller and colleagues[61] documented the foot-loading patterns obtained when using two different tone-inhibiting AFOs. They assessed biomechanical alignment and foot stability, and one orthosis—the dynamic ankle-foot orthosis—was found to have had significant effects at the lateral forefoot with respect to force. The authors concluded that this effect might support the medial longitudinal arch of the foot and increase the stability of the forefoot as it is loaded. They theorized that this in turn might allow the forefoot to be loaded at a faster velocity. They did not investigate the effects of correct biomechanical alignment on muscle electromyographic activity.

The use of this type of AFO is based on the same principles that underlie the use of serial casting.[19,28] Both were believed, by some practitioners, to reduce abnormal muscle activity. However, the scientific literature so far does not confirm that the prolonged stretch afforded by serial casting has a central inhibitory effect.[1,14,19,27,97] Changes in sarcomere number and connective tissue caused by immobilization, positioning, and stretch can influence muscle contraction force.[1,14,21,41] In addition, muscle length also can influence the manifestation of hyperreflexia.[1,20,21] Perhaps these mechanical properties of muscle are influenced by tone-inhibiting orthoses. By promoting better biomechanical alignment and normal muscle length, these AFOs may exert an effect on peripheral rather than central factors that, over time, could otherwise augment stretch reflexes. Further research is needed—especially long-term, controlled studies—to investigate the many variables that influence motor control and muscle function. The term *tone inhibiting* may have to be reconsidered until a more complete and universally accepted definition of tone exists along with what contributes to normal and abnormal tone.

Metal orthoses were the main type of orthotic devices used before the 1970s.[35] Metal AFOs still are used for certain stroke survivors who cannot tolerate the total contact of a plastic AFO for whatever reason. The components usually consist of two metal uprights attached to an ankle joint. The metal is usually aluminum, but sometimes heavier steel is needed for control. The ankle joint is attached to a stirrup that is fastened beneath the heel of the shoe. The proximal ends of the upright are attached to a calf band.

The metal ankle joint is usually a single- or double-channel (chamber) type (Fig. 15-12). Other types of ankle joints are described in detail elsewhere.[21,35,56]

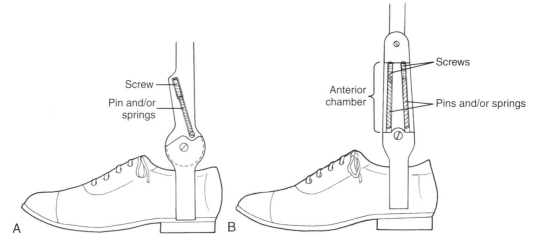

Figure 15-12 **A,** Single-channel (chamber) metal ankle joint. **B,** Double-channel (chamber) metal ankle joint.

A single-channel ankle joint can assist dorsiflexion with a spring placed in the channel. Plantar flexion also can be limited to prevent genu recurvatum by placing a pin in the channel. A double-channel ankle joint can prevent dorsiflexion and plantar flexion by using pins in both channels. Small screws hold the pins in the chambers. The degree of dorsiflexion or plantar flexion (i.e., the ankle joint angle) can be determined by the degree to which the pins are driven into the channels by tightening the screws. Springs and pins can be used in combination to stop one movement and assist another.

The metal uprights attached to the ankle joint and stirrup offer a certain amount of foot and ankle mediolateral control. However, if additional support is needed (e.g., to prevent severe foot inversion), a strap can be added that applies pressure to the lateral malleolus in a medial direction and is secured around the medial upright. Because it prevents varus positioning of the ankle, the strap is called a *varus correction strap*. Force can be applied in the opposite direction with a strap to prevent foot eversion and a valgus foot position. This strap then is called a *valgus correction strap*. A varus correction strap is more common.

The simplest type of metal AFO is the Veterans Administration Prosthetic Center shoe clasp orthosis, which consists of a single narrow metal upright that attaches to the heel counter of a shoe with a metal clasp and a calf strap (Fig. 15-13). The orthosis offers dorsiflexion assist only, with no mediolateral or plantar flexion control.

Occasionally a KAFO with knee locks may be prescribed for a patient who requires additional knee control. However, the additional weight, the prevention of normal knee joint excursions during swing, and increased energy cost caused by these factors greatly limit the potential for functional ambulation.[60,77,98] In addition, donning and doffing a KAFO are difficult for hemiplegic patients (see Fig. 15-10, *C*).[98]

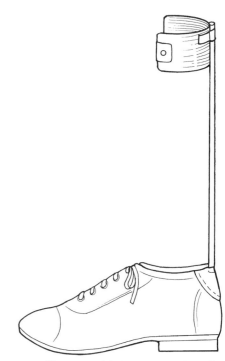

Figure 15-13 Veterans Administration Prosthetic Center orthosis for dorsiflexion assist.

A KAFO combines the features of an AFO with a knee joint and (in the case of a metal orthosis) metal uprights that extend proximally up the thigh. Thigh bands secure the KAFO on the upper leg. The simplest knee joint is a hinge, and the most common locks to maintain knee extension are drop ring locks.[35] The thigh component of plastic KAFOs usually is made of the same thermoplastic material as the AFO component. Metal and plastic combinations also can be used.[33,35,56]

As previously mentioned, KAFOs are seldom used for hemiparetic patients. Occasionally, a preexisting knee joint deformity or ligamentous laxity is exacerbated by walking because of the now weak muscular support. In such instances, no alternative may be available to using a KAFO to allow minimal household ambulation. A KAFO or a knee extension splint sometimes is used as an initial training device to enhance stability. These are used only as temporary measures and not as long-term orthotic devices.[20,60,98]

The physical therapist has the responsibility of reevaluating the orthotic device on an ongoing basis, especially in the outpatient or home therapy setting. In this era of decreased length of hospital stays, patients sometimes are prescribed an orthotic device while still in the early stages of recovery. As motor control improves, the orthotic device may need to be modified or discontinued to allow more active movement by the patient.

ASSISTIVE DEVICES

The assistive devices most commonly used with stroke patients are canes, walkers, and occasionally two crutches. Hemiparetic patients whose balance is impaired minimally and who have functional strength in the opposite upper extremity may use a cane. Two crutches or a walker require at least some functional use of both upper extremities. Both devices provide more external stability, with the walker providing more stability than the crutches. The main function of a cane is to increase the base of support and thereby improve balance.[86] The base of support is increased by providing another contact with the floor. Canes also decrease the need for abductor muscle tension to stabilize the pelvis in stance on the paretic side.[68,86] This in turn helps to prevent dropping of the contralateral pelvis (a positive Trendelenburg sign) in stance when the cane is used in the hand opposite the hemiparetic leg. Using the opposite hand also helps simulate the reciprocal arm and leg movements of a normal gait.

A variety of canes are on the market, ranging from a simple wooden straight cane to a tripod "walk cane" (also called a *hemiwalker*). At a level in between these two canes are the narrow- and wide-based quadruped canes (quad canes) (Figs. 15-14 to 15-17). Widening the base of support provides more stability. Physical therapists may begin training with a wide-based cane because of hemiparesis and impaired balance. They should advance patients as quickly as possible to the least amount of assistance required to ensure a safe, stable gait. Patients often are kept inadvertently on a maximally wide base of support cane when it is no longer needed. This prevents the patient from maximizing functional ambulation for two reasons: (1) normal weight shifting to the hemiparetic leg is limited, and (2) cadence is slower than it is with a smaller device[86] or no device. The key word is *safety*. Maximum use of the involved leg should be encouraged along with normal trunk and pelvic movement, if patient safety is not compromised.

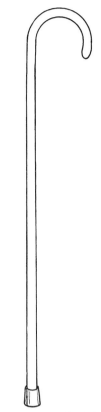

Figure 15-14 Straight cane.

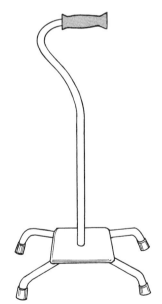

Figure 15-15 Wide-based quad cane.

Two crutches occasionally are used: axillary or (more often) forearm (Lofstrand) crutches (Fig. 15-18). Certain cerebellar stroke patients or others who have impaired balance but functional use of both arms and hands may be trained with these devices. These patients require the

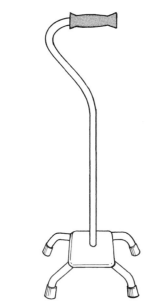

Figure 15-16   Narrow-based quad cane.

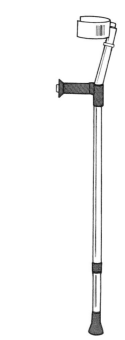

Figure 15-18   Lofstrand crutch.

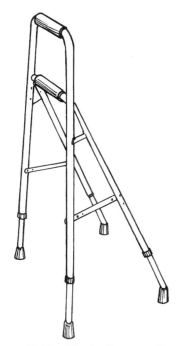

Figure 15-17   Hemiwalker or walk cane.

extra postural support afforded by the second crutch but have enough motor control to be able to advance the crutches reciprocally.

Therapists may use walkers for training stroke patients who have functional use of both arms and hands but need greater outside support than that afforded by two crutches. Occasionally a walker may allow functional use of a hemiparetic arm even though balance is sufficient with a cane. In this case, the patient also should practice gait training with a cane to promote optimum postural control. If patients have sufficient control of the paretic arms, they also

may use walkers when it is necessary for them to transport objects around the house (e.g., in the kitchen).

Standard walkers are the most stable assistive devices because they provide four points of contact with the ground. The base of support is greatly increased. A variety of walkers are available as well. In addition to standard walkers with four legs, rolling walkers with front wheels only, with four wheels, and platform attachments are also available. Rolling walkers allow a more normal reciprocal gait, but the therapist must take care to prevent the walker from "running away" with the patient. A stroke survivor with insufficient arm and hand strength to lift a walker may have the ability to maintain a grip on the rolling walker and push it forward. Some walkers have pressure-sensitive brakes that prevent forward movement when the patient pushes down on the walker.

As mentioned in the cerebellar stroke section, postural control sometimes is sacrificed for stability when a walker is used. The patient has no need to relearn balance and control if the walker provides needed support. As mentioned, safety is the ultimate concern. If safe, functional ambulation is not possible without a walker, then safe, independent ambulation with a walker is the preferred choice.

The type of gait pattern taught to the stroke survivor depends on a number of factors, including balance, strength, and coordination.[68,86] The therapist also should consider cognitive and perceptual deficits, including apraxias.

Smidt and Mommens[89] suggested terminology for describing walking patterns. *Point* refers to the number of contacts made with the floor, including with feet and assistive devices, during the forward progression of the gait cycle (Figs. 15-19 and 15-20). For example, a four-point contralateral gait indicates that two feet and two assistive devices (such as canes being advanced one at a time) are being used (see Fig. 15-20, *A*). The more contacts on the floor at any given moment, the more stable the person is while walking. In addition, the pattern can be called a *delayed pattern* if the assistive device is advanced before the limbs. Delayed patterns provide more stability than moving a limb concurrently with an assistive device. Following are the most common gait patterns taught to stroke patients.

GAIT PATTERNS

Two-Point Contralateral Gait Pattern Using One Device

Hemiparetic patients with a nonfunctional arm often are taught a two-point contralateral gait pattern using one assistive device. A device, such as a cane, is held in the unaffected hand. The cane and the paretic leg are advanced together (one point), and then the unaffected leg is advanced alone (second point) (see Fig. 15-19, *B*). The cane may be advanced first and then the paretic limb followed by the unaffected limb for a more stable pattern.

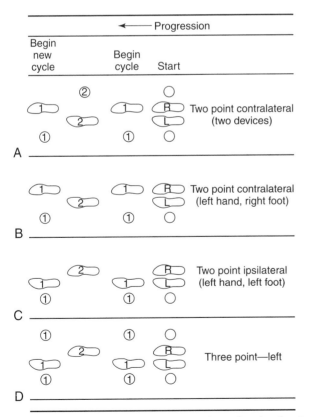

Figure 15-19 **A** to **D**, Diagrammatic view of assisted gaits. (From Smidt G, Mommens MA: Gait patterns. *Phys Ther* 60(5):553, 1980.)

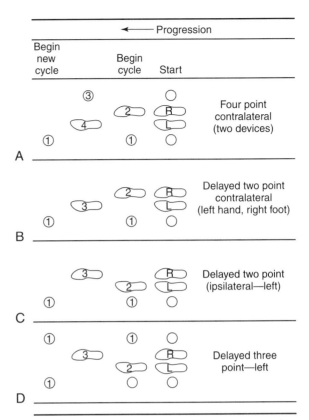

Figure 15-20 **A** to **D**, Diagrammatic view of assisted gaits. (From Smidt G, Mommens MA: Gait patterns. *Phys Ther* 60(5):553, 1980.)

This pattern is a delayed contralateral two-point gait pattern (see Fig. 15-20, *B*). In Figs. 15-19, *B* and 15-20, *B* the right leg is the hemiparetic leg.

Four-Point Contralateral Gait Pattern Using Two Devices

The devices used in a four-point contralateral gait pattern could be canes or crutches. The therapist might choose this type of gait for stroke patients who have functional use of all four limbs but have impaired balance. They require bilateral support but are able to advance each device (two points) and each leg (two points) individually and reciprocally. Although this is a stable gait pattern, it is not used often with hemiparetic patients. Sometimes a patient recovering from a cerebellar stroke will be taught this pattern to encourage coordinated reciprocal arm and leg movements and postural control.

Two-Point Contralateral Gait Pattern Using Two Devices

If the previously mentioned patients regain sufficient postural control, they might be advanced to using a two-point contralateral pattern (see Fig. 15-19, *A*). They still would be using two crutches or canes but would be moving one device and the opposite leg simultaneously (one point) followed by the other device and opposite leg (second point).

Five-Point Gait Pattern Using One Device

Therapists may train patients with a walker if they have functional control of all four extremities but require greater trunk control than that afforded by a cane. For example, certain patients who have had cerebellar strokes may never recover adequate postural stability to be able to use two canes. A walker allows the patient to use five points of contact: the four legs of the walker and one of the patient's legs. The patient advances the walker simultaneously with one leg and then places all four of the walker legs firmly on the floor at the same time as the patient's foot. This pattern is called a *five-point gait pattern* (Fig. 15-21, *B*). If the patient moves the walker first, followed by the patient's leg, the pattern is called a *five-point delayed gait pattern* (Fig. 15-21, *A*). Other authors refer to this gait pattern as a "3-1-point" or "modified 3-point" pattern.[79] The basic sequence is the same, however.

Therapists may train previously mentioned patients with a rolling walker. They may choose this device for two reasons: (1) the walker is in constant contact with the floor while being advanced, therefore affording maximal postural control; and (2) the walker is in constant motion, and the patient is able to take equal step lengths and to increase speed. With the standard walker, the patient is forced to use a "step-to" type of gait pattern (the walker is advanced, then the foot, then the other foot) that prevents a normal stride and limits velocity.[89] In making the decision to use a rolling walker, the physical therapist also must consider the patient's ability to control the continuous forward motion of the walker, as mentioned previously.

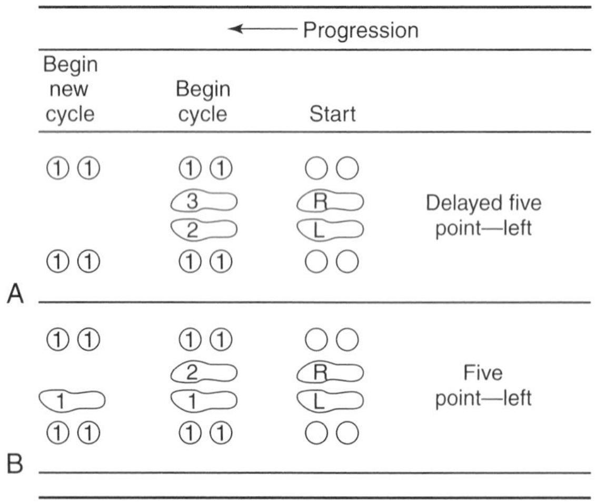

Figure 15-21 **A** and **B**, Diagrammatic view of assisted gaits. (From Smidt G, Mommens MA: Gait patterns. *Phys Ther* 60(5):554, 1980.)

Three-Point Gait Pattern Using Two Devices

Three-point gait patterns seldom are used with stroke patients and are used more often with patients who have orthopedic conditions requiring weight relief on one leg (see Figs. 15-19, *D*, and 15-20, *D*).

GUARDING TECHNIQUES

The goal of gait training after stroke is to have the patient walk as efficiently, safely, and independently as possible. To promote optimum functional ambulation, it is important for the patient to experience postural instability and to relearn the way to correct these imbalances.

With this in mind, the therapist must be as close to patients as necessary to prevent them from falling or injuring themselves and yet not inhibit them from learning the way to right themselves. Therapists must allow patients to take some risks without jeopardizing the patients' safety or their own safety. This is not an easy task, especially for new therapists. The ultimate horror for any therapist is having a patient fall. Obviously, until therapists are comfortable with patients and know how much, if any, outside support they need, guarding too much is better than guarding too little. Regardless, the goal always should be safe, optimal function, and the therapist needs to reevaluate on an ongoing basis how much guarding is needed and in what type of setting and on what type of surface activities should be performed.

Hemiparetic patients walking with a cane most often are guarded on the weaker side. The therapist stands slightly posterior and lateral to the affected side.[79,86] The therapist is then in the best position to assist the patient. Should patients lose their balance or stumble, they may have difficulty preventing a fall to the weaker side because of decreased sensation and decreased strength and control of the paretic leg. The therapist can control patients with the hand closest to them at the hip or pelvis and can control patients' shoulder and trunk with the other hand if necessary.

The use of gait belts or guarding belts varies from therapist to therapist and from institution to institution, but most facilities advocate their use in the initial stages of gait training and on stairs. The patient's safety is of the utmost concern. At times, a patient is uncontrollable without a gait belt. Other times, the belt can be a hindrance to patients relearning postural control if the therapist is inadvertently tugging on the belt with every step. Therapists must evaluate each patient individually. The size of the patient in comparison to the therapist also may need to be considered. The therapist should decide which anticipatory actions need to be taken to protect the patient from harm based on clinical assessment and sound judgment.

When guarding a patient who is ascending stairs, the therapist is positioned posterior and to the weaker side. The patient should be trained using a railing at the stronger side. Initially, the therapist may teach the patient to ascend one step at a time, leading with the stronger leg. When the patient is descending, the therapist stands in front of and lateral to the affected side so as to provide assistance if the patient's knee buckles. Using the railing, the patient steps down one step at a time, leading with the paretic leg. A patient who regains functional strength of the paretic leg may advance to the step-over-step method of stair climbing, with close guarding by the therapist. Ascending and descending stairs with only a cane or two canes is difficult and requires excellent balance. Some home environments may necessitate such training, but it should be undertaken with sufficient guarding, and the therapist carefully should weigh the safety risks.

Guarding techniques need to be taught to family members as soon as possible during inpatient rehabilitation. Family participation in gait training provides the opportunity for practice and repetition of newly learned techniques.

CASE STUDY

Gait Training after Stroke

This case study in no way reflects the patient's whole treatment program because emphasis also is placed on increasing strength and function in the trunk and left arm and in the leg. In addition, frequent sessions of cotreating by the occupational and physical therapists occurred to enhance communication about specific treatment concerns (e.g., the subluxed shoulder) and functional goals.

H.C. is a 54-year-old male who was admitted to the emergency room of a university medical center with sudden onset of left-sided weakness. Two weeks earlier, he had undergone a mitral valve repair and a single coronary artery bypass with a left saphenous vein graft. He had had an uneventful postoperative recovery course and was discharged to his home and prescribed a β-blocker.

On admission, the neurological workup and results included: (1) a computerized tomography scan of the head showing early lucency in the right subcortical area; (2) noninvasive flow studies (on the second day) showing accelerated flow velocities in the right middle cerebral artery suggestive of stenosis and normal flows in the anterior cerebral arteries, posterior cerebral arteries, and basal artery; and (3) a transesophageal echocardiogram revealing trace mitral regurgitation, normal left ventricular function, and no intracardiac or aortic mass or thrombus.

The attending neurologist concluded that H.C. had suffered an infarct in the right corona radiata and putamen in the territory supplied by the lenticulostriate branches of the right middle cerebral artery. The cause of the infarct was probably an embolus of cardiac origin that developed after the mitral valve repair. H.C. was prescribed anticoagulant medication and was stabilized medically. Twelve days later, he was transferred to the rehabilitation unit of the same medical center.

On admission to the rehabilitation unit, H.C. had symptoms of a pure motor syndrome with left upper extremity weakness that was greater than the left leg weakness, minimal left lower facial droop, and no sensory loss. He was alert and oriented and most cooperative although somewhat deconditioned because of the previous cardiac surgery.

Physical assessment revealed normal passive range of motion of the left arm and leg, although both legs manifested tight hamstrings and could perform only a straight leg raise to barely 60 degrees. A finger-width subluxation was present in the left shoulder. Strength testing revealed that the left arm was grossly 2 to 3 out of 5 throughout. He was able to extend the left knee completely while sitting (3 out of 5), but the hip flexors were weaker (2 out of 5). He exhibited no isolated voluntary ankle movement, although dorsiflexion was 2 out of 5 with simultaneous flexion of the hip and knee, and plantar flexion was 2 out of 5 during simultaneous extension of these proximal joints. He did not at that time (or ever) exhibit any spasticity in the limbs during passive testing by the therapist, with the exception of mild, unsustained ankle clonus. He exhibited no ankle edema despite the leg weakness and previous vein graft for the coronary artery bypass graft surgery.

His gait was evaluated initially while he was walking around a high mat with his right side next to the mat, using his right arm and the mat to "unload" the left leg. During static standing, he required contact guarding and verbal cues to extend the left hip and knee actively. He had a tendency to bear most of his weight on the stronger right leg. When cued to stand with equal weight on both legs, he was unable to maintain an upright posture and would fall to the left because the knee would buckle. He required minimal assistance to maintain the hip and knee in extension when bearing weight symmetrically.

Initially he was able to take 10 steps around the mat with minimal assistance. His gait analysis was as follows: Uneven step lengths were observed; the left was greater although less controlled than the right. The shorter step with the right leg resulted in a "step-to" type of gait pattern—the right leg stepping to meet, instead of pass, the left leg. He exhibited a decrease in single-limb stance time on the left leg. His cadence was slow—approximately 40 steps per minute.

Continued

CASE STUDY

Gait Training after Stroke—cont'd

During the left leg stance, the heel did not strike at initial contact; the foot was flat. The loading response resulted in excessive knee flexion that was greater than the normal 10 to 15 degrees. To prevent buckling in midstance, the knee snapped back into hyperextension (genu recurvatum). Instead of bringing his body forward by allowing the tibia to advance over the foot (dorsiflexion), he kept the ankle angle fixed and flexed the hip and trunk over the foot. He did not push off at the end of stance. Instead, he quickly took a short step with the right leg to unload the left one as soon as possible.

Because the resulting right leg position was next to the left leg instead of beyond it, the left leg was unable to assume the normal preswing position of hip extension and 40-degree knee flexion (see Fig. 15-4). Instead, the left hip and knee were in full extension, and he was forced to initiate swing on the left from this position.

During the swing phase of the left leg, H.C. exhibited decreased hip and knee flexion and a foot drop because of the weak dorsiflexors. This resulted in his toes scraping the floor. He displayed mild lateral trunk flexion to the right in an attempt first to initiate swing from the previously mentioned abnormal preswing position and then to clear the toes throughout the swing phase.

H.C. was put on a program of active assistive range of motion and strengthening exercises for the left arm and leg. Treatment of the leg emphasized functional strengthening in weight-bearing positions (e.g., sit-to-stand exercises for hip and knee strengthening).

During the initial stage of gait training, a posterior leaf splint orthosis was used to assist with dorsiflexion during the swing phase on the left side. This splint was chosen to encourage a more efficient swing phase and to discourage the patient from leaning to the right to clear the left leg during swing. Because of its flexibility, the posterior leaf splint did not restrict activity at the left ankle or knee during stance. Although the knee was unstable, H.C. was still in the early stages of recovery. Sacrificing mobility for stability (i.e., blocking any ankle dorsiflexion and knee flexion in stance) was not beneficial. Doing so would have forced him to move compensatorily because it is normal to dorsiflex up to 10 degrees at the ankle during midstance and terminal stance. The therapist offered close supervision to contact guarding at the knee because of possible knee buckling resulting from excessive dorsiflexion. H.C. was taught to be aware of the difference between excessive knee flexion and recurvatum. He was soon able to identify correctly when he was in either of these abnormal positions even if he could not always prevent them.

H.C. quickly advanced from ambulation around the high mat to ambulation with a narrow-based quad cane and then a straight cane. He had the advantage of recovering much of his hip extension and abduction strength, which meant he did not require a large degree of outside support from an assistive device for these muscles.

Functional training included standing balance retraining in single-limb and double-limb weight-bearing positions. Modified versions of activities that the patient previously had enjoyed (soccer) and a few new ones (golf putting and baseball) were introduced. H.C. practiced ambulation in a variety of environments and on both even and uneven terrains in preparation for discharge. H.C. even practiced getting through busy revolving doors.

After 6 weeks of inpatient rehabilitation, H.C. was evaluated for a permanent AFO. His left leg strength had improved enough to allow him to isolate dorsiflexion and plantar flexion in any position grossly in the 2 out of 5 range, ankle inversion and eversion in the 2 out of 5 range, and toe flexion and extension in the 1+ out of 5 range. His hip flexors improved minimally to 2+ out of 5, and knee extension also improved minimally to 3+ out of 5.

During ambulation, H.C. continued to manifest knee recurvatum in stance and did not push off at the end of stance because of weak plantar flexors. During swing, he continued to exhibit a foot drop and toe drag. The physiatrist, physical therapist, and orthotist performed a joint observational gait analysis. Because of the continued plantar flexor and dorsiflexor weakness during the swing and stance phases and less than normal knee extension strength, they decided that H.C. required minimal knee control and ankle control from an AFO. In addition, the weak ankle invertors and evertors necessitated mediolateral control by an orthosis. Therefore a posterior leaf splint was deemed insufficient. However, because H.C. was continuing to progress and did not require maximum support at the knee, a solid ankle AFO was also inappropriate. The general consensus was that H.C. should be allowed to have as much movement at the ankle as possible without jeopardizing his safety to promote development of a normal gait pattern.

For this reason the team decided to order a hinged polypropylene AFO with free dorsiflexion at the ankle and a plantar flexion stop at 90 degrees. The hinged ankle with free dorsiflexion allowed him to move the tibia normally over the foot (dorsiflexion) in midstance and terminal stance. The plantar flexion stop at 90 degrees prevented foot drop in swing and recurvatum in stance. The orthosis improved his gait by allowing the normal joint excursions at the knee and ankle in stance while preventing abnormal movements in stance and swing. The promotion of normal joint excursions at the ankle in stance allowed him to take equal step lengths with both legs.

On discharge to his home, H.C. was able to ambulate independently indoors with a straight cane and the hinged AFO, but he required supervision outdoors. He was able to ascend and descend stairs step-over-step using a railing and ascend and descend curbs and ramps with the straight cane, all with distant supervision. He could perform simple home exercises independently for left leg and arm strengthening. He returned to work as a full-time university professor and continued with outpatient physical therapy three times a week for six months after discharge. He regained full functional use of the left upper extremity including finger function (albeit with decreased coordination), fine motor control, and strength. He also continued to receive occupational therapy for several months as an outpatient.

SUMMARY

The aim of this chapter is to familiarize the occupational therapist with processes used by physical therapists during gait evaluation and training of patients who have had a stroke. The most common type of gait disorders are those resulting from a middle cerebral artery infarction.

The application of orthotic devices is not an exact science. To assume that a particular abnormal gait always requires one specific type of orthotic device is not accurate. Therapists must evaluate devices on an individual trial basis. Use of a specific device or pattern requires individualized attention.

Those well-versed and experienced in motor control research[20,39,42,44,99] believe that the trend in physical therapy is moving away from earlier theoretical models of treatment techniques and toward a motor control model. The emphasis is no longer on specific treatment techniques to "facilitate" movement but on active problem-solving by the patient to promote skilled movement and motor relearning. The practice of specific tasks is to be emphasized during intervention. Treatment programs need to be based on specific motor control deficits, which may require modification or emphasis in the practice of a task which is meaningful to the patient and which takes place in numerous environments. All of the gait intervention research presented in this chapter support this model.

One can no longer assume that certain treatment techniques are effective. Effectiveness needs to be validated by research. As presented earlier, Weinstein and colleagues[99] examined the effect that balance-training and weight shifting activities during standing had on the hemiplegic gait. Although patients who received training improved their standing symmetry significantly, training did not translate into improved weight shifting during ambulation. This study clearly demonstrates the hazards of assuming that transfer of training occurs from a part of one functional task to another. For example, it would be convenient to assume that the techniques used to improve the standing balance of a patient with contraversive pushing will improve the ability to walk. However, no evidence as yet supports this theory. Further research such as that of Weinstein and colleagues[99] is imperative for therapists to validate the rationales for their treatment procedures for stroke patients. To do otherwise denies the patient the most beneficial treatment approach.

The case study was unusual because the patient exhibited no spasticity and had voluntary, isolated control of all muscles but had decreased strength. However, several authors questioned the role of spasticity in preventing normal movement[1,20,21,44] and pointed to weakness as the more limiting factor. Spasticity is well-known to increase the incidence of muscle contracture and thereby alter the biomechanical efficiency of a muscle.[1,20,21,29,41,44] In this respect, only the ankle joint was at risk and minimally so. The patient was a model patient for other reasons. He was not cognitively impaired, and he was motivated to return to work. He was aware (although grudgingly at times) of the need for faithful adherence to a regular exercise program of repeated practice of newly learned motor skills.

Therapists always should be aware of the need for careful physical assessment, individualized treatment programs that are based on research findings, and ongoing reevaluation of the effectiveness of the treatment program in promoting optimum function.

REVIEW QUESTIONS

1. What constitutes a gait cycle?
2. What are the phases and subphases of the gait cycle?
3. What are step, stride, and cadence?
4. What tests would you perform to assess gait speed and gait endurance?
5. What type of cerebral infarct is associated with the typical "hemiplegic gait"?
6. What are some of the variables that can cause a deviation from the normal joint excursions during a gait cycle?
7. In what way does the motor control model differ from the more traditional theoretical models underlying the different therapeutic techniques?
8. How might ambulation recovery be related to hip osteoporosis?
9. What are some of the manifestations of a posterior inferior cerebellar stroke?
10. What makes treatment of patients demonstrating contraversive pushing so challenging?

11. What helps compensate for proprioceptive loss after stroke?
12. What are the main differences between metal and plastic orthotic devices?
13. What orthotic device is used most commonly with stroke patients?
14. What assistive devices are used most commonly with stroke patients?
15. What determines the type of gait pattern that will be taught to a stroke patient?

REFERENCES

1. Ada L, Canning C: Anticipating and avoiding muscle shortening. In Ada L, Canning C, editors: *Key issues in neurological physiotherapy* Boston, 1990, Butterworth-Heinemann.
2. Ada L, Dean CM, Hall JM, et al: A treadmill and overground walking program improves walking in persons residing in the community after stroke: A placebo-controlled, randomized trial. *Arch Phys Med Rehabil* 84(10):1486–1491, 2003.
3. Adams JM, Perry J: Gait analysis: clinical application. In Rose J, Gamble JG, editors: *Human walking*, Baltimore, 1994, Williams & Wilkins.
4. Amarenco P: Cerebellar stroke syndromes. In Bogousslavsky J, Caplan L, editors: *Stroke syndromes*, Cambridge, UK, 2001, Cambridge University Press.
5. Amarenco P: The spectrum of cerebellar infarcts. *Neurology* 41(7):973, 1991.
6. American Thoracic Society Board of Directors. ATS statement: Guidelines for the six-minute walk test. *Am J Respir Crit Care Med* 166(1):111–117, 2002.
7. Balliet R, Harbst KB, Kim D, et al: Retraining of functional gait through the reduction of upper extremity weight bearing in chronic cerebellar ataxia. *Int Rehabil Med* 8(4):148–153, 1987.
8. Barton JJS, Caplan LR: Cerebral visual dysfunction. In Bogousslavsky J, Caplan L, editors: *Stroke syndromes*, Cambridge, UK, 2001, Cambridge University Press.
9. Bassile CC, Dean C, Boden-Albala B, et al: Obstacle training programme for individuals post stroke: feasibility study. *Clin Rehabil* 17(2):130–136,2003.
10. Bingman VP, Zucchi M: Spatial orientation. In Cohen H, editor: *Neuroscience for rehabilitation*, Philadelphia, 1993, JB Lippincott.
11. Bontrager E: Instrumented gait analysis. In DeLisa JA, editor: *Gait analysis in the science of rehabilitation monograph 002*, Baltimore, 1998, Department of Veterans Affairs, Veterans Health Administration, Rehabilitation Research and Development Service, Scientific and Technical Section.
12. Branch EF: The neuropathology of stroke. In Duncan P, Badke MB, editors: *Stroke rehabilitation*, Chicago, 1987, Mosby.
13. Brandt T, Krafczyk S, Malsbenden I: Postural imbalance with head extension: improvement by training as a model for ataxia therapy. *Ann N Y Acad Sci* 374:636, 1981.
14. Brower B, Davidson LK, Olney SJ: Serial casting in idiopathic toe walkers. *J Pediatr Orthop* 20(2):221–225, 2000.
15. Brown DL, Morgenstern LB, Majersik JJ, et al: Risk of Fractures after stroke. *Cerebrovasc Dis* 25(1-2):95–99, 2008.
16. Brust JB: Circulation of the brain. In Kandel ER, Schwartz JH, editors: *Principles of neural science*, ed 4, New York, 2000, McGraw-Hill.
17. Burdett RG, Borello-France D, Blatchly C, et al: Gait comparison of subjects with hemiplegia walking unbraced, with ankle-foot orthosis, and Air-Stirrup brace. *Phys Ther* 68(8):1197, 1998.
18. Caplan LR: Visual perceptual abnormalities. In Bogousslavsky J, Caplan L, editors: *Stroke syndromes*, Cambridge, UK, 2001, Cambridge University Press.
19. Carlson: A neurophysiological analysis of inhibitive casting. *Phys Occup Ther Pediatr* 4(4):31–42, 1984.
20. Carr JH, Shepherd RB: A motor learning model for rehabilitation. In Carr JH, Shepherd RB, editors: *Movement science foundations for physical therapy in rehabilitation*, Gaithersburg, MD, 2000, Aspen.
21. Carr JH, Shepherd RB, Ada L: Spasticity: research findings and implications for intervention. *Physiotherapy* 81(8):421, 1995.
22. Cohen H: Special senses 2: the vestibular system. In Cohen H, editor: *Neuroscience for rehabilitation*, Philadelphia, 1999, JB Lippincott.
23. Craik RL, Dutterer L: Spatial and temporal characteristics of foot fall patterns. In Craik RL, Oatis CA, editors: *Gait analysis, theory and application*, St. Louis, 1995, Mosby.
24. Davies PM: *Steps to follow*, Berlin, 1985, Springer-Verlag.
25. Dean CM, Richards CL, Malouin F: Task-related circuit training improves performance of locomotor tasks in chronic stroke: A randomized, controlled pilot trial. *Arch Phys Med Rehabil* 81(4):409–417, 2000.
26. Dean CM, Richards CL, Malouin F: Walking speed over 10 metres overestimates locomotor capacity after stroke. *Clin Rehabil* 15(4):415–421, 2001.
27. De Deyne PG: Application of passive stretch and its implications for muscle fibers. *Phys Ther* 81(2):819–827, 2001.
28. Diamond M, Ottenbacher K: Effect of tone-inhibiting DAFO on stride characteristics of an adult with hemiparesis. *Phys Ther* 70(7):423, 1981.
29. Dietz V, Quintern J, Berger W: Electrophysiological studies of gait in spasticity and rigidity: evidence that altered mechanical properties of muscle contribute to hypertonia. *Brain* 104(3):431–449, 1981.
30. Dimitrijevic MR, Faganel J, Sherwood AM, et al: Activation of paralysed leg flexors and extensors during gait in patients after stroke. *Scand J Rehabil Med* 13(4):109, 1981.
31. Duncan P, Studenski S, Richards L, et al: Randomized clinical trial of therapeutic exercise in subacute stroke. *Stroke* 34(9):2173–2180, 2003.
32. Duncan PW, Badke MB: Determinants of abnormal motor control. In Duncan PW, Badke MB, editors: *Stroke rehabilitation*, Chicago, 1987, Mosby.
33. Edelstein J: Orthotic management and assessment. In O'Sullivan S, Schmitz TJ, editors: *Physical rehabilitation: assessment and treatment*, ed 4, Philadelphia, 2001, FA Davis.
34. Engardt M, Knutsson E, Jonsson M, et al: Dynamic muscle strength training in stroke patients: effect on knee extension torque, EMG activity, and motor function. *Arch Phys Med Rehabil* 76(5):419–425, 1995.
35. Faculty of Prosthetics and Orthotics, New York University School of Medicine and Post Graduate Medical School: *Lower limb orthotics*, 1986, New York, New York University School of Medicine and Post Graduate Medical School.
36. Ferro JM: Neurobehavioral aspects of deep hemispheric stroke. In Bogousslavsky J, Caplan L, editors: *Stroke syndromes*, Cambridge, UK, 2001, Cambridge University Press.
37. Garland DE, Stewart CA, Adkins RH, et al: Osteoporosis after spinal cord injury. *J Orthop Res* 10(3):371–378, 1992.
38. Gilman S, Newman SW: *Clinical neuroanatomy*, ed 8, Philadelphia, 1992, FA Davis.
39. Giuliani CA: Adult hemiplegic gait. In Smidt GL, editor: *Gait in rehabilitation*, New York, 1990, Churchill Livingstone.
40. Glatt SL, Koller WS: Gait apraxia. In Spivack BS, editor: *Evaluation and management of gait disorders*, New York, 1995, Marcel Dekker.
41. Goldspink G, Williams P: Muscle fiber and connective tissue changes associated with use and disuse. In Ada L, Canning C, editors: *Key issues in neurological physiotherapy*, Boston, 1990, Butterworth-Heinemann.
42. Gordon J: Assumptions underlying physical therapy intervention. In Carr JH, Shepherd RB, editors: *Movement science foundations for physical therapy in rehabilitation*, Gaithersburg, MD, 2000, Aspen.

43. Harro CC, Giuliani CA: Kinematic and EMG analysis of hemiplegic gait patterns during free and fast walking speeds. *Neurol Rep* 11:57, 1987.

44. Held JM: Recovery of function after brain damage: theoretical implications for therapeutic intervention. In Carr JH, Shepherd RB, editors: *Movement science foundations for physical therapy in rehabilitation*, Gaithersburg, MD, 2000, Aspen.

45. Jones LA: Somatic senses 3: proprioception. In Cohen H, editor: *Neuroscience for rehabilitation*, Philadelphia, 1999, JB Lippincott.

46. Jorgensen L, Crabtree NJ, Reeve J, et al: Ambulatory level and asymmetrical weight bearing after stroke affects bone loss in the upper and lower part of the femoral neck differently: Bone Adaptation after decreased mechanical loading. *Bone* 27(5)701–707, 2000.

47. Jorgensen L, Jacobsen BK, Wilsgarrd T, et al: Walking after stroke: Does it matter? Changes in bone mineral density within the first 12 months after stroke. A longitudinal study. *Osteoporos Int* 11(5): 381–387, 2000.

48. Karnath HO, Broetz D. Understanding and treating "Pusher Syndrome." *Phys Ther* 83(12):1119–1125, 2003.

49. Karnath HO, Ferber S, Dichgans J. The origin of contraversive pushing: evidence for a second graviceptive system in humans. Neurology 55(9):1298–1304, 2000.

50. Karnath HO, Ferber S, Dichgans J. The neural representation of postural control in humans. *Proc Natl Acad Sci U S A* 97(25):13931–13936, 2000.

51. Karnath HO, Johannsen L Broetz D, et al: Prognosis of contraversive pushing. *J Neurol* 249(9):1250–1253, 2002.

52. Knutsson E: Gait control in hemiparesis. *Scand J Rehabil Med* 13(2–3):101–108, 1981.

53. Knutsson E, Martensson A: Dynamic motor capacity in spastic paresis and its relation to prime mover dysfunction, spastic reflexes, and antagonist co-activation. *Scand J Rehabil Med* 12(3):93, 1980.

54. Kusoffsky A, Wadell I, Nilsson BY: The relationship between sensory impairment and motor recovery in patients with hemiplegia. *Scand J Rehabil Med* 14(1):27–32, 1982.

55. Lehmann JF: Lower limb orthotics. In Redford JB, editor: *Orthotics etc*, ed 3, Baltimore, 1986, Williams & Wilkins.

56. Lehmann JF, Condon SM, Price R, et al: Gait abnormalities in hemiplegia. *Arch Phys Med* 68(11):763–771, 1987.

57. Licht S: Preface to the first edition. In Redford JB, editor: *Orthotics etc*, ed 3, Baltimore, 1986, Williams & Wilkins.

58. Macko RF, Ivey FM, Forrester LW, et al: Treadmill exercise rehabilitation improves ambulatory function and cardiovascular fitness in patients with chronic stroke: A randomized controlled trial. *Stroke* 36(10):2206–2211, 2005.

59. McComas AJ, Sica RE, Upton AR, et al: Functional changes in motor neurons of hemiparetic patients. *J Neurol Neurosurg Psychiatry* 36(2):183–193, 1973.

60. Montgomery J: Assessment and treatment of locomotor deficits in stroke. In Duncan PW, Badke MB, editors: *Stroke rehabilitation: recovery of motor control*, Chicago, 1987, Mosby.

61. Mueller K, Cornwall MW, McPoil TG, et al: Effect of two contemporary tone-inhibiting AFOs on foot-loading patterns in adult hemiplegics: a small group study. *Top Stroke Rehabil* 1(4):1–16, 1995.

62. Nilsson L, Carlsson J, Danielsson A, et al: Walking training of patients with hemiparesis at an early stage after stroke: A comparison of walking raining on a treadmill with body weight support and walking training on the ground. *Clin Rehabil* 15:515–527, 2001.

63. Norkin C: Gait analysis. In O'Sullivan S, Schmitz TJ, editors: *Physical rehabilitation: assessment and treatment*, ed 4, Philadelphia, 2001, FA Davis.

64. Nyberg L, Gustafon Y. Patient falls in stroke rehabilitation. A challenge to rehabilitation strategies. *Stroke* 26(5):838–842, 1995.

65. Oestreich L, Troost BT: Cerebellar dysfunction and disorders of posture and gait. In Spivack BS, editor: *Evaluation and management of gait disorders*, New York, 1995, Marcel Dekker.

66. Olney SJ, Griffin MP, Monga TN, et al: Work and power in gait of stroke patients. *Arch Phys Med Rehabil* 72(5):309–314, 1991.

67. Olney SJ, Richards CL: Hemiplegic gait following stroke. *Gait Posture* 4(2):36, 1996.

68. Olsson EC, Smidt GL: Assistive devices. In Smidt GL, editor: *Gait in rehabilitation*, New York, 1990, Churchill Livingstone.

69. O'Sullivan SB: Motor control assessment. In O'Sullivan SB, Schmitz TJ, editors: *Physical rehabilitation: assessment and treatment*, ed 4, Philadelphia, 2001, FA Davis.

70. O'Sullivan SB: Stroke. In O'Sullivan SB, Schmitz TJ, editors: *Physical rehabilitation: assessment and treatment*, ed 4, Philadelphia, 2001, FA Davis.

71. Ounpuu S: Clinical gait analysis. In Spivack BS, editor: *Evaluation and management of gait disorders*, New York, 1995, Marcel Dekker.

72. Paci M, Nannetti L: Physiotherapy for pusher behavior in a patient with post-stroke hemiplegia. *J Rehabil Med* 36(4):183–185, 2004.

73. Pathokinesiology Service and Physical Therapy Department: *Observational gait analysis handbook*, Downey, CA, 1991, Professional Staff Association of Rancho Los Amigos Medical Center.

74. Pedersen PM, Wandell A, Jorgensen HS: Ipsilateral pushing in stroke: incidence, relation to neuropsychological symptoms, and impact on rehabilitation—the Copenhagen stroke study. *Arch Phys Med* 77(1):25–28, 1996.

75. Peraula SH, Tarkka IM, Pitkanen K, et al: The effectiveness of body weight-supported gait training and floor walking in patients with chronic stroke. *Arch Phys Med Rehabil* 86(8):1557–1564, 2005.

76. Perennou DA, Amblard B, Laassel EM, et al: Understanding the pusher behavior of some stroke patients with spatial deficits: a pilot study. *Arch Phys Med Rehabil* 83(4):570–575, 2002.

77. Perry J: The mechanics of walking. In Perry J, Hislop H, editors: *Principles of lower extremity bracing*, Washington, DC, 1977, American Physical Therapy Association.

78. Perry J, Garrett M, Gronley JK, et al: Classification of walking handicap in the stroke population. *Stroke* 26(6):982–989, 1995.

79. Pierson FM: Ambulation aids, patterns and activities. In Pierson FM: *Principles and techniques of patients care*, ed 2, Philadelphia, 1999, Saunders.

80. Ramnemark A, Nilsson M, Borssen B, et al: Stroke, a major and increasing risk factor for femoral neck fracture. *Stroke* 31(7):1572–1577, 2000.

81. Ramnemark A, Nyberg L, Borssen B, et al: Fractures after stroke. *Osteoporos Int* 8(1):92–5, 1998.

82. Ramnemark A, Nyberg L, Lorentzon R, et al: Progressive hemiosteoporosis on the paretic side and increased bone mineral density in the nonparetic arm the first year after severe stroke. *Osteoporos Int* 9(3):269–275, 1999.

83. Richards CL, Malouin F, Dumas F, et al: Gait velocity as an outcome measure of locomotor recovery after stroke. In Craik RL, Oatis C, editors: *Gait analysis: theory and application*, St Louis, 1995, Mosby.

84. Richards CL, Olney SJ: Hemiparetic gait following stroke. II. Recovery and physical therapy. *Gait Posture* 4(2):49, 1996.

85. Salbach NM, Mayo NE, Wood-Dauphinee S. A task orientated intervention enhances walking distance and speed in the first year post stroke: a randomized controlled trial. *Clin Rehabil* 18(5):509–519, 2004.

86. Schmitz TJ: Preambulation and gait training. In O'Sullivan S, Schmitz TJ, editors: *Physical rehabilitation: assessment and treatment*, ed 4, Philadelphia, 2001, FA Davis.

87. Shaughnessy M, Michael KM, Sorkin JD, et al: Steps after stroke: Capturing ambulatory recovery. *Stroke* 36(6):1305–1307, 2005.

88. Sisto SA: An overview of the value of information resulting from instrumented gait analysis for the physical therapist. In DeLisa JA, editor: *Gait analysis in the science of rehabilitation monograph 002*, Baltimore, 1998, Department of Veterans Affairs, Veterans Health Administration, Rehabilitation Research and Development Service, Scientific and Technical Section.

89. Smidt GL, Mommens MA: System of reporting and comparing influence of ambulatory aids on gait. *Phys Ther* 60(5):551–558, 1980.

90. Smith E, Juvinall RC: Mechanics of orthotics. In Redford JB, editor: *Orthotics etc*, ed 3, Baltimore, 1986, Williams & Wilkins.

91. Sullivan KJ, Knowlton BJ, Dobkin BH. Step training with body weight support: Effect of treadmill speed and practice paradigms on poststroke locomotor recovery. *Arch Phys Med Rehabil* 83(5):683–691, 2002.

92. Ticini L, Klose U, Nagele T, Karnath HO. Perfusion imaging in Pusher Syndrome to investigate the neural substrates involved in controlling upright body position. *PLoS One* 4(5):e5737, 2009.

93. Tiderksaar R: Falls in older persons. In Spivack BS, editor: *Evaluation and management of gait disorders*, New York, 1995, Marcel Dekker.

94. Timmann D, Diener HC: Cerebellar ataxia. In Bogousslavsky J, Caplan L, editors: *Stroke syndromes*, Cambridge, UK, 2001, Cambridge University Press.

95. Toole JF: *Cerebrovascular disorders*, ed 5, Philadelphia, 1999, Lippincott Williams & Wilkins.

96. Visitin M, Barbeau H, Korner-Bitensky N, et al: A new approach to retrain gait in stroke patients through body weight support and treadmill stimulation. *Stroke* 1998; 29(6):1122–1128.

97. Walsh EG, Wright GW, Brown K, et al: Biodynamics of the ankle in spastic children: effect of chronic stretching on the calf musculature. *Exp Physiol* 75(3):423–425, 1990.

98. Walters RL, Garland DE, Montgomery J: Orthotic prescription for stroke and head injury. In *American Academy of Orthopedic Surgeons. Atlas of orthotics*, ed 2, St Louis, 1985, Mosby.

99. Weinstein CJ, Gardner ER, McNeal DR, et al: Standing balance training: effects on balance and locomotion in hemiparetic adults. *Arch Phys Med* 70(10):755–762, 1989.

100. Whitson HE, Pieper CF, Sanders L, et al: Adding injury to insult: Fracture risk after stroke in veterans. *J Am Geriatr Soc* 54(7):1082–1088, 2006.

101. Wilmet E, Ismail AA, Heilporn A, et al: Longitudinal study of the one mineral content and of soft tissue composition after spinal cord section. *Paraplegia* 33(11):674–677, 1995.

102. Winstein CJ, Gardner ER, McNeal DR, et al: Standing balance training: Effect on balance and locomotion in hemiparetic adults. *Arch Phys Med Rehabil* 70(10):755–762, 1989.

glen gillen

chapter 16

Managing Visual and Visuospatial Impairments to Optimize Function*

key terms

accommodation	hemianopsia	stereopsis
diplopia	orthoptics	strabismus
field cut	pursuits	vergence
fixation	saccades	
figure ground impairment	spatial relations	

chapter objectives

After completing this chapter, the reader will be able to accomplish the following:

1. Understand how visual information is processed by the central nervous system.
2. Understand how everyday living is affected if visual and spatial impairments are present.
3. Be aware of procedures to perform a visual screening after a brain injury.
4. Implement at least five intervention strategies focused on decreasing activity limitations and participation restrictions for those living with visual and spatial impairments.

"Vision is our dominant sense: More than just sight is measured in terms of visual acuity; vision is the process of deriving meaning from what is seen. It is a complex, learned, and developed set of functions that involve a multitude of skills. Research estimates that eighty to eighty five percent of our perception, learning, cognition and activities are mediated through vision."[41]

*This chapter is predominantly excerpted from Gillen G: *Cognitive and perceptual rehabilitation: optimizing function.* Elsevier, 2009, St. Louis.

VISUAL PROCESSING DURING FUNCTIONAL ACTIVITIES

The visual system is commonly impaired after brain damage. Typical visual impairments include visual field deficits, loss of ocular alignment or control, diplopia, and changes in visual acuity.[2,47] Further complex impairments include spatial relations impairments as is discussed later, visual agnosia (see Chapter 19), neglect of visual information contralateral to the brain injury (see Chapter 19), and so on. In order for one to use vision to support participation in daily activities, visual information must be correctly received and recognized (Table 16-1).

The ultimate function of visual processing is to support participation in daily activities via appropriate motor and/ or cognitive response. A relationship exists between visual impairments after acquired brain damage and difficulties with activities of daily living (ADL), increased risk of falls, and poor rehabilitation outcome.[17] Visual processing involves a complex system of peripheral and central structures. Compromised integrity of any of the structures impedes functional performance. To illustrate this complexity, the following examination of processing visual information is based on the example of searching for a gallon of milk that is stored in the left side of the refrigerator. Fig. 16-1 outlines the visual pathways within the central nervous system.

Once the refrigerator is opened, a variety of eye movements occur to locate the milk. This usually systematic visual search is supported by rapid intermittent eye movements (saccades) that occur when the eyes fix on one point after another in the visual field. Each eye is controlled by six muscles (Fig. 16-2). These muscles in turn are controlled by three cranial nerves (cranial nerve III or oculomotor, IV or trochlear, VI or abducens).

The frontal eye fields within the premotor cortex support visual search and guide gaze shifts. The image "lands" on the nasal hemiretina of the left eye and the temporal hemiretina in the right eye once the milk is located in the left visual field. The information is mobilized posteriorly via the optic nerve. At the point of the optic chiasm, information from the right eye's temporal hemiretina remains ipsilateral in the right hemisphere, and the information from the left eye's nasal hemiretina crosses into the right hemisphere.[2,58] Therefore, visual information from the left visual field is processed in the right hemisphere. The optic tract projects to the lateral

Table 16-1

Visual Skills and Their Associated Functions and Resulting Dysfunctions after Stroke[2]

VISUAL SKILL	VISUAL FUNCTION	VISUAL AND PERCEPTUAL DYSFUNCTIONS
Visual acuity	Clarity of vision at near point and distance; 20/20 refraction	Vision blurred in one or both eyes consistently or inconsistently; visual fatigue; task incompletion
Accommodation	Process of focusing whereby the lens changes curvature so that various viewing distances remain clear	Blurred vision; inattention; poor concentration; eyestrain; visual fatigue
Visual fields	The peripheral area of vision up, down, in, and out when both eyes are positioned straight forward	Inability to read or starting to read in the middle of the page; ignoring of food on one half of the plate; difficulty orienting to stimuli in specific areas of space
Oculomotor range of motion; fixation; saccades and pursuits	Ability of both eyes to move within the six cardinal positions of gaze (right, left, inferior, superior, inferior oblique, superior oblique); maintenance of gaze for 10 seconds; small precise eye jumps; following a moving stimulus	Excessive head movement; frequent loss of place; skipping of lines; poor attention span; slow copying; difficulty when driving, reading, writing; difficulty tracking in all planes
Vergence	The ability to bring the eyes together smoothly and automatically along the midline to observe objects singly at near distance (convergence) or to move the eyes outward for single vision of distant objects (divergence)	Difficulty focusing; decreased depth perception; difficulty and confusion in interpreting space; decreased eye-hand coordination in self-care and hygiene; difficulty in driving, sports, communication, and ambulation
Strabismus	Deviation of one eye or one eye at a time from the object of regard, where the eye not in use is turned	Esotropia (inward turn); exotropia (outward turn); hyperopia (upward turn); hypopia (downward turn); double vision or suppression; decreased eye-hand coordination during mobility tasks; overreaching or underreaching; difficulty with reading and near tasks
Functional scanning	Ability to read or write from left to right precisely and smoothly without errors	Omitting letters, words, numbers; losing place when returning to next line; exaggerated head movement; using finger as pointer; abnormal working distance
Color perception	Ability to perceive colors	Muddy or impure color; color may fade out; difficulty finding items by color
Stereopsis	Depth perception and its relationship to spatial judgment	Problematic binocular system; deficits in three-dimensional perception; decreased spatial judgment, especially in fine motor areas

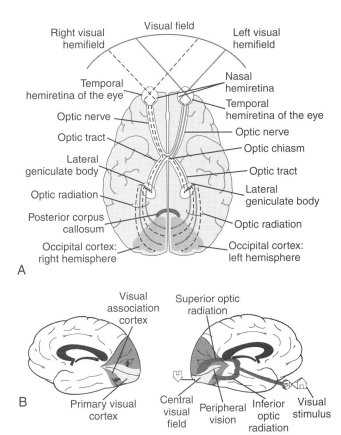

Figure 16-1 The visual pathways. **A,** Inferior view depicting flow of information from the visual fields to the visual cortex (visual fields = 180 degrees). **B,** Medial view of components of the visual cortex and visual processing. (**A,** From Aloisio L: Visual dysfunction. In Gillen G, Burkhardt A, editors: *Stroke rehabilitation: a function-based approach*, ed 2, St Louis, 2004, Mosby. **B,** From Árnadóttir G: *The brain and behavior: assessing cortical dysfunction through activities of daily living*, St Louis, 1990, Mosby).

geniculate nucleus of the thalamus because the lateral geniculate nucleus is the principal subcortical structure that carries visual information to the cortex.[58] The optic radiation "fans out" and carries the visual information to the primary visual cortex around the calcarine fissure in the occipital lobe.

During the radiation, fibers carrying information from the inferior visual field run posteriorly through the parietal lobe, whereas fibers carrying information from the superior visual field loop around the temporal lobe on their way to the visual cortex in the occipital lobe.[2,58] Any lesion in this retino-geniculate-cortical pathway will result in a loss of visual fields (Fig. 16-3). The distribution (e.g., nasal, temporal, inferior, superior, homonymous) of the visual field loss is usually determined by the point of injury. The function of the pathway discussed thus far is to move the visual information from the retina to the cortex, and the direction of flow is primarily anterior to posterior.

At this point the visual information has reached the primary visual cortex in the occipital lobe around the calcarine fissure involved in reception of the visual information. If damage occurs bilaterally around the calcarine fissure, the presentation is usually that of cortical blindness.[3,5] Those living with cortical blindness can usually detect lights and movement but otherwise the visual impairment is severe. Following the processing that occurs in the primary visual cortex, the visual information is mobilized to the visual association cortex. Two pathways allow for sophisticated examination of incoming visual information:[2,3,5,58]

1. The ventral stream or inferior occipitotemporal pathway functions include object recognition via vision, perception of color (e.g., the milk is in a red container), recognition of shapes and forms (the milk is in a rectangular carton), and size discrimination (a quart of milk is smaller than a half gallon). Information from this pathway helps to answer the question, "What am I looking at?"
2. The dorsal stream or the superior occipitoparietal pathway functions include visuospatial perception (the milk is on the top shelf toward the left and behind the butter) and detection of movement. Information from this pathway helps to answer the question: "Where is the object located?"

VISUAL SCREENING

Several authors have described the components of a vision screening.[2,55,56] Prior to developing an intervention plan, a clinician must determine whether difficulties engaging in functional activities are due to a visual deficit, a cognitive or perceptual deficit, or a combination of both. Many dysfunctional behaviors observed or mistakes made during attempts at performing a functional activity can be attributed to one or several underlying impairments that must be differentiated. A person who is having difficulty searching for paperclips in a cluttered drawer may be presenting with poor visual acuity (a decrease in the clarity of vision) versus living with figure-ground impairment (the inability to differentiate foreground from background), necessitating visual acuity testing prior to developing an intervention plan. Similarly, a person who misses the glass when pouring juice from a container may be presenting with a spatial relations impairment related to judging depth or distance versus living with diplopia (double-vision) versus living with monocular vision (information is only obtained via one eye). Finally, not being able to identify an object on a bathroom sink by vision alone may be an issue related to decreased visual acuity versus living with a figure-ground impairment (e.g., not able to identify a white bar of soap on a white sink) versus living with poor contrast sensitivity versus not recognizing the visual information received by the cortex (visual agnosia).

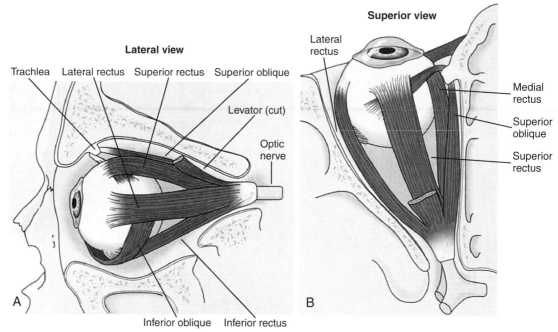

Figure 16-2   The origins and insertions of the extraocular muscles. **A,** Lateral view of the left eye with the orbital wall cut away. **B,** Superior view of the left eye with the roof of the orbit cut away. (From Goldberg ME: The control of gaze. In Kandel ER, Schwartz JH, Jessell TM, editors: *Principles of neural science,* ed 4, New York, 2000, McGraw-Hill.)

A correlation study of adults who sustained a stroke and received occupational therapy examined the relationship between basic visual functions (defined as acuity, visual field deficits, oculomotor skills, and visual attention or scanning) and higher level visual-perceptual processing skills such as visual closure and figure-ground discrimination. The study suggested that a positive relation exists (r=0.75) between basic visual functions and visual-perceptual processing skills. The authors further concluded that the results suggest that evaluation of visual-perceptual processing skills must begin with assessment of basic visual functions so that the influence of these basic visual functions on performance in more complex tests can be taken into consideration.[47] Therefore, it is recommended that a visual screening occur prior to or in conjunction with a full cognitive and perceptual evaluation (Box 16-1). Examples of components of a visual screening include near and far acuity, visual field testing, ocular range of motion or control, ocular alignment, contrast sensitivity, and the like. These skills are often considered the foundation skills for visual processing.[2,53,54]

Specific visuomotor abilities that should be assessed include the following:

- Fixation: The ability to steadily and accurately gaze at an object of regard (e.g., examining the detail of a painting in a museum).

- Pursuits: The ability to smoothly and accurately track or follow a moving object (e.g., watching your dog run through the yard).
- Saccades: The ability to quickly and accurately look or scan from one object to another (e.g., reading or watching a soccer game and trying to locate a certain player).
- Accommodation: The ability to accurately focus on an object of regard, sustain focusing of the eyes, and change focusing when looking at different distances (e.g., maintaining focus when you look from up from a textbook to a clock and back to the textbook).
- Vergence: The ability to accurately aim the eyes at an object of regard and to track an object as it moves toward and away from the person (e.g., watching people walking toward you [convergence] and away from you [divergence] in the mall).

The Brain Injury Visual Assessment Battery for Adults (biVABA)[55] is an example of a battery that includes standardized assessments for evaluation of the visual functions important in ensuring that visual perceptual processing is accurately completed:

- Visual acuity (distant and reading)
- Contrast sensitivity function
- Visual field
- Oculomotor function
- Visual attention and scanning

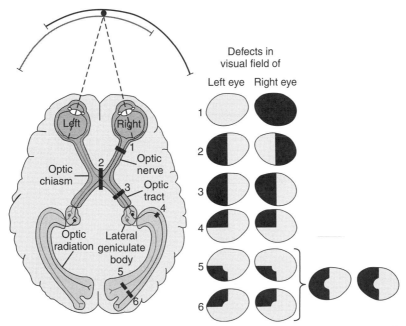

Figure 16-3   Deficits in the visual field produced by lesions at various points in the visual pathway. The level of a lesion can be determined by the specific deficit in the visual field. In the diagram of the cortex, the numbers and the visual pathway indicate the sites of lesions. The deficits that result from lesions at each site are shown in the visual field maps on the right as black areas. Deficits in the visual field of the left eye represent what an individual would not see with the right eye closed rather than deficits of the left visual hemifield. *(1)* A lesion of the right optic nerve causes a total loss of vision in the right eye. *(2)* A lesion of the optic chiasm causes a loss of vision in the temporal halves of both visual fields (bitemporal hemianopsia). Because the chiasm carries crossing fibers from both eyes, this is the only lesion in the visual system that causes a nonhomonymous deficit in vision (i.e., a deficit in two different parts of the visual field resulting from a single lesion). *(3)* A lesion of the optic tract causes a complete loss of vision in the opposite half of the visual field (contralateral hemianopsia). In this case, because the lesion is on the right side, vision loss occurs on the left side. *(4)* After leaving the lateral geniculate nucleus the fibers representing both retinas mix in the optic radiation. A lesion of the optic radiation fibers that curve into the temporal lobe (Meyer loop) causes a loss of vision in the upper quadrant of the opposite half of the visual field of both eyes (upper contralateral quadrantic anopsia). *(5)* and *(6)* Partial lesions of the visual cortex lead to partial field deficits on the opposite side. A lesion in the upper bank of the calcarine sulcus *(5)* causes a partial deficit in the inferior quadrant of the visual field on the opposite side. A lesion in the lower bank of the calcarine sulcus *(6)* causes a partial deficit in the superior quadrant of the visual field on the opposite side. A more extensive lesion of the visual cortex, including parts of both banks of the calcarine cortex, would cause a more extensive loss of vision in the contralateral hemifield. The central area of the visual field is unaffected by cortical lesions *(5)* and *(6)*, probably because the representation of the foveal region of the retina is so extensive that a single lesion is unlikely to destroy the entire representation. The representation of the periphery of the visual field is smaller and hence more easily destroyed by a single lesion. (From Wurtz RH, Kandel ER: Central visual pathways. In Kandel ER, Schwartz JH, Jessell TM, editors: *Principles of neural science*, ed 4, New York, 2000, McGraw-Hill.)

Box 16-1

Components of a Vision Screening

The following is a description of vision screening processes, which should be administered in a well-illuminated room free of glare and reflection.

1. Distance Visual Acuity

   Equipment: Distance acuity chart (Snellen chart), occluder or eyepatch, 20-foot measure

   Setup: Fixate distance acuity chart on a well-lighted wall at client's eye level 20 feet away.

   Procedure: Cover the client's left eye with occluder or patch. Ask the client to identify letters on the 20/40 line. If the client appears confused by the lines and letters, cover all other lines on the chart and expose only the line being used. If necessary, expose only one letter at a time. If the client continues to have problems, attempt to test visual acuity using the Lea Symbols Test. Continue until the individual misses more than 50% of the letters on a line. Cover the client's right eye with occluder or patch and repeat the steps. Record acuity as last line in which the individual can successfully identify more than 50% of the letters.

   Functional implications: If visual acuity is poorer than 20/40 or if a two-line difference or more is evident between the two eyes, a referral is necessary and corrective lenses may need to be prescribed.

2. Near/Reading Visual Acuity

   Equipment: Near acuity chart, occluder or eyepatch, 16-inch measure

   Setup: Hold a near acuity chart in a well-lit room 16 inches away.

   Procedure: The test card is held 16 inches from the person being tested. The test is performed with the client wearing his or her corrective lenses if they are normally used. Binocular vision is tested. The smallest size able to be read correctly is recorded.

   Functional implications: The results of the test will give an idea of the detail that can be discriminated. Near tasks include craft and leisure activities, personal care and hygiene, some work tasks, and reading.

3. Ocular Mobility

   Equipment: Penlight

   Setup: Have client sit facing therapist. Penlight should be approximately 12 inches from the eyes. Do not shine the light directly into the eyes; instead direct the light so that it is pointing slightly above eye level at the brow.

   Procedure: Ask the client to follow the penlight and move it in a large H pattern to the extremes of gaze. Then move the penlight in a large O pattern. Allow the client to fixate on the light for 10 seconds before moving it.

   Functional implications: Observation of pursuits should be smooth and precise without anticipating responses. Note visual fatigue or stress and whether the client reports diplopia (double vision). Observe whether the client looks away, loses the target, or squints or blinks excessively. Inability to attend to visual tasks, difficulty reading or completing writing tasks, and problems with spatial orientation during walking may be displayed.

4. Near Point of Convergence

   Equipment: Penlight and ruler

   Setup: Practice this procedure on a partner to determine when the penlight is positioned at 2, 4, and 6 inches from an individual's eyes.

   Procedure: Slowly move the penlight toward the client at eye level and between the eyes, making sure not to shine the light in the eyes. Ask the client to keep the eyes on the light and state when two lights are seen. After this occurs, move the light another inch or two closer and then begin to move it away. Ask the client to state when only one light is seen. Watch the eyes carefully and observe whether they stop working together as a team—one eye may drift outward. Record the distance at which the client reports double vision and the recovery to single vision.

   Functional implications: Double vision should occur within 2 to 4 inches of the eyes. A recovery to single vision should occur within 4 to 6 inches. A client with a binocular vision problem may not report double vision because the eye that turns out is suppressed. Thus all eye movements should be observed before screening.

5. Stereopsis

   Equipment: Viewer-free random dot test

   Setup: Individual's head position should be vertical. If any head tilt occurs, it negates this screening.

   Procedure: Hold the viewer-free random dot test 16 inches from the client's eyes and ask the client to describe what he or she sees. A person with stereopsis should report seeing a square box in the upper left, an E on the upper right, a circle on the lower left, and a blank box on the lower right. Give the client about 20 to 30 seconds to observe targets. If the client has difficulty, try tilting the target slightly to the left or right.

   Functional implications: The client should be able to identify all three symbols correctly. A client with constant strabismus is unable to identify any of the shapes. Clients with less severe strabismus or phoria may have normal responses. Some people may report double vision on this task, which suggests strabismus.

Box 16-1

Components of a Vision Screening—cont'd

6. Accommodation

   Equipment: Isolated letters and occluder or eyepatch

   Setup: Make a target by photocopying the near visual acuity chart, cutting out the 20/30 targets, and taping them to a tongue depressor. Place one target on each side of the tongue depressor so that you have two screening targets.

   Procedure: Patch the left eye. Hold the tongue depressor with the 20/30 target about 1 inch in front of the right eye. The client should be unable to identify the stimulus on the tongue depressor at this distance. Slowly move the target away and ask the client to report as soon as the target is identifiable. Using a ruler, measure and record the distance at which the person is able to identify the stimulus. Divide 40 by the measurement to determine the amplitude of accommodation. If the client is able to identify the target at 8 inches, divide 40 by 8, which equals 5 diopters. To compare the amplitude of accommodation to the expected amplitude for the client's age, use the following formula: expected amplitude = 18 − one third the client's age. The following are examples of the way to use this equation:

   A 9-year-old child:

   Expected amplitude=18−($\frac{1}{3}$[9]) Expected amplitude=18−3=15 diopters

   A 45-year-old adult:

   Expected amplitude=18−($\frac{1}{3}$[45]) Expected amplitude=18−15=3 diopters

   Functional implications: The amplitude of accommodation should be 2 diopters of the expected finding for the client to pass the screening test. Observe all eye movements. Problems include blurred vision, poor concentration, inattention, visual fatigue, and eyestrain.

7. Saccades

   Equipment: Two fixators with red and green targets and scanning chart

   Setup: Have the client keep the head erect and vertical.

   Procedure: Hold two tongue depressors (one with a red target and one with a green target) 16 inches from the client's face and about 4 inches from the midline. Give the following instructions: "When I say red, look at the red target. When I say green, look at the green target. Do not look until I tell you." Have the client look from one target to the other five round-trips or for 10 fixations.

   Functional implications: Adults without visual impairment should perform perfectly. Any mistake denotes problems with saccadic function, and the client will require further evaluation. Poor saccades result in poor concentration and attention and difficulty reading and writing.

8. Visual Fields: The Confrontation Test

   Equipment: Occluder or eyepatch, black dowels with white targets (are other contrasting colors) on the ends or a wiggling finger

   Setup: Make sure the client is seated facing the examiner.

   Procedure:

   1. One-examiner presentation—the client holds the occluder over the left eye. Wiggle a finger out to the side and ask the client to say "now" when the movement of the wiggling finger is first detected. The client should look at the therapist's nose the entire time and ignore any arm movement. Begin with the hand slightly behind the client about 16 inches away from the head. Slowly bring the hand forward while wiggling a finger. Continue randomly testing different sections of the visual field in 45-degree intervals around the visual field. Proceed to the left eye, asking the client to occlude the right eye. If using the dowel technique, slowly bring it in from the side until the client reports seeing the small pin at the end of the dowel.

   2. Two-examiner presentation—examiner one stands behind the seated client and examiner two sits facing the client about 30 inches in front so that the face of the examiner and client are at the same level.

   Test each eye individually, being careful to patch the other eye. Examiner two closes one eye and instructs the client to "fixate and keep looking at my open eye. Examiner one will show you one or more fingers very quickly. Don't try to look at the fingers. Keep looking at my open eye and when you see a finger or fingers, tell me how many you see."

   Examiner one presents one or two fingers randomly for a one-second duration to each quadrant of the visual field of the client's unpatched eye. The fingers in the upper quadrant point down, and those in the lower quadrant point up. The fingers are presented 18 inches from the client and at approximately 20 degrees from the line of fixation.

Data from Aloisio L: Visual dysfunction. In Gillen G, Burkhardt A, editors: *Stroke rehabilitation: a function-based approach*, ed 2, St Louis, 2004, Mosby; Gianutsos R, Suchoff IB: Visual fields after brain injury: management issues for the occupational therapist. In Scheiman M, editor: *Understanding and managing vision deficits: a guide for occupational therapists*, Thorofare, NJ, 1997, Slack; Gutman SA, Schonfeld AB: *Screening adult neurologic populations*, ed 2, Bethesda, Md, 2009, AOTA Press; and Warren M: Evaluation and treatment of visual deficits following brain injury. In Pendleton H, Schultz-Krohn W, editors: *Pedretti's occupational therapy: practice skills for physical dysfunction*, ed 6, St Louis, 2006, Elsevier Science/Mosby.

MANAGING VISUAL ACUITY IMPAIRMENTS

Assessment of visual acuity has been described in Box 16-1. Visual acuity refers to clarity and sharpness of sight. It is commonly measured using the Snellen chart (or text cards for near acuity) and noted, for example, as 20/20, 20/60, 20/200, and so on. Modifications such as using picture charts or a "tumbling E" chart are available for those with aphasia. A visual acuity of 20/20 means that a person can see detail from 20 feet away the same as a person with normal eyesight would see from the same distance. If a person has a visual acuity of 20/60, that person is said to see detail from 20 feet away the same as a person with normal eyesight would see it from 60 feet away. Visual acuity becomes impaired in various refractive conditions (i.e., impaired focusing of the image on the retina), the most typical being myopia (nearsighted), hyperopia (farsighted), astigmatism (mixed), and presbyopia (age-related decrease in acuity).[2] Chia and associates[9] found that noncorrectable visual acuity impairment (defined as acuity less than 20/40) was associated with reduced functional status and well-being, as measured by the Medical Outcomes Study Short Form-36 (SF-36) (a measure of quality of life, see Chapter 3). Tsai and colleagues[51] documented a relationship between poor visual acuity and depression using the Geriatric Depression Scale. Visual impairment was specifically associated with feelings of worthlessness and hopelessness.

A decrease in visual acuity can result in multiple difficulties in all functional domains. Examples include difficulty reading labels on pill bottles, doing crosswords, unsafe driving, increased fall risk, and so on. A focus on this impairment is warranted to improve participation in daily activities. In general, if visual acuity is worse than 20/40, a referral to an eye care specialist is warranted for evaluation of prescriptive lenses.[2] Other interventions are in line with low-vision rehabilitation techniques. They are pragmatic yet effective and have been outlined by Warren:[56]

- Increase illumination: In general, increasing the amount of light can improve function. Particular attention should be placed on areas of high risk, where activities requiring precision are performed such as cooking, sorting pills into a pill box, and needlework. Task-specific lighting is recommended. Warren warns about maintaining the balance between increasing the amount and intensity of illumination while not increasing glare and recommends halogen, fluorescent, and full-spectrum lights to eliminate casting shadows.
- Increase contrast: Specifically background colors that contrast with objects used for function. Examples are purchasing colored soap to place on a white sink, using dark placemats and white dishes, and placing strips of colored tape on the edge of steps.
- Decrease background pattern: Increased patterns on household objects can further increase the difficulty of finding necessary objects. For example, finding a white sock on a patchwork quilt is much more difficult than finding the same sock on a solid colored bedspread.
- Decrease clutter and organize the environment: A focus should be placed on a having necessary objects placed out neatly and not overlapping.
- Increase size: Commercially available magnification devices, labeling with bold markers, reprinting instructions or daily planners in larger fonts, changing personal computer settings to a larger font are just a few example of this intervention.

MANAGING VISUAL FIELD DEFICITS WITH AN EMPHASIS ON HEMIANOPSIA

The visual fields extend approximately 65 degrees upward, 75 degrees downward, 60 degrees inward, and 95 degrees outward when the eye is in the forward position.[15] Aloisio[2] summarized that:

- The visual fields are essential areas of the visual system that allow the individual to orient effectively to stimuli in specific areas of space.
- In terms of function, they are used when driving, walking, reading, eating, and in all daily living skills.
- In terms of impairment, inferior field loss causes difficulty with mobility, including poor balance, tendency to trail behind others when walking, walking next to walls and touching them for balance, trouble seeing steps or curbs, shortened and uncertain stride while walking, and trouble identifying visual landmarks. In addition, superior field deficit causes difficulty in seeing signs, reading, and writing; misreading of words, poor accuracy, slow reading rate, inability to follow lines of text, and inaccurate check writing are additional difficulties.

Hemianopsia, or hemianopia or hemiopia, means "half-blindness" or a loss of half the fields of vision in both eyes.[38] Homonymous visual field impairments are seen frequently in the clinic after an acquired brain injury. Thirty percent of all clients with stroke and 70% of those with a stroke involving the posterior cerebral artery present with hemianopsia. In addition, those with subarachnoid hemorrhages, intracerebral bleeds, and head trauma also commonly present with this impairment.[34]

Zhang and coworkers[60] examined the medical records of more than 900 people presenting with visual field loss. The authors found that 37.6% were complete homonymous hemianopsias, whereas 62.4% were incomplete. Homonymous quadrantanopsia (29%) was the most common type of incomplete hemianopsia, followed by homonymous scotomatous defects (13.5%), partial homonymous hemianopsia (13%), and homonymous hemianopsia with macular sparing (7%). The causes of homonymous hemianopsias included stroke (69.6%), head trauma (13.6%), tumor (11.3%), after brain surgery (2.4%), demyelination (1.4%), other rare causes (1.4%), and unknown etiology (0.2%). The authors found that the lesions were most commonly located in the occipital lobes (45%) and the optic radiations (32.2%). Almost every type of hemianopsia was found in all lesion locations along the retrochiasmal visual pathways.

The amount and distribution of visual field loss (i.e., nasal, temporal, inferior, superior, homonymous) depends on the location of the lesion. If the optic nerve itself is damaged (i.e., the area between the retina and the optic chiasm), the presentation will be that of monocular visual loss. Damage to the optic tract will result in contralateral hemianopsia. If damage occurs posterior to the lateral geniculate body, the typical presentation is that of either quadrantanopsia or hemianopsia depending on the lesion site (see Fig. 16-3). Although the characteristics of visual field defects can be helpful in lesion location, specific visual field defects do not always indicate specific brain locations.[60]

Zihl[62] summarized that those living with hemianopsia cannot process visual information as compared with those with intact visual fields. Specifically, they demonstrate numerous visual refixations, have inaccurate saccades and disorganized scanning, require longer visual search times, and omit relevant objects in the environment. In addition, they focus on their intact hemifield; their saccades are less regular, less accurate, and too small to allow rapid, organized scanning or reading.[35] The majority of basic and instrumental ADL have the potential to be adversely affected without proper intervention. Reading may be particularly problematic. For example, in those living with a complete right homonymous hemianopsia, rightward saccades during text reading are disrupted ("hemianopsic alexia"), which interrupts the motor preparation of reading saccades during text reading.[25]

In terms of recovery, Zhang and coworkers[59] longitudinally followed 254 clients with homonymous hemianopsia secondary to a variety of brain lesions. The authors documented spontaneous visual field deficit recovery in less than 40% of the cases. They also noted that the likelihood of spontaneous recovery decreased with increasing time from injury to initial visual field testing (p = 0.0003). The probability of improvement was related to the time since injury (p = 0.0003) with a 50% to 60% chance of improvement for cases tested within one month after injury. This chance for improvement decreased to about 20% for cases tested at six months after surgery. In most cases, the improvements occurred within the first three months after injury. The authors warned that spontaneous improvement after six months should be interpreted with caution because it may be secondary to improvement of the disease or to improvement in the client's ability to perform visual field testing reliably. They

recommended that visual field rehabilitation strategies should most likely be initiated early after injury.

The most objective test for mapping the available field is perimetry. This automated test is usually conducted while the person being tested is seated and looking straight ahead at a central target. The person is instructed to press a buzzer when he or she becomes aware of a small light within the visual field. The accuracy of the test depends on the person's being alert and able to concentrate on the central target. The results from this test are printed out by the computer, objectively mapping blind spots in the visual field. A screening technique that grossly measures the visual fields is a confrontation test, which is described in Box 16-1. Although it is common for hemianopsia to occur in conjunction with neglect, there exists a double dissociation between the two impairments—each can occur separately or can coexist. As compared with those living with neglect, awareness of visual filed deficits tends to be better. Nonetheless, clients may benefit from awareness training to make connections between how this impairment will affect a variety of functional activities and to understand the importance of compensating for it (see Chapter 19).

Several interventions are available to those living with visual field loss. The methods are compensatory in nature. These methods include learning oculomotor compensation strategies, strengthening the person's attention to the blind hemifield, improving the ability to direct gaze movements toward the involved side, exploring the involved side more efficiently, improving saccadic exploration toward the blind hemifield, using prisms, and so on.*

Some of the most useful approaches to the treatment of hemianopsia are based on compensating for visual field loss by oculomotor compensation. This training involves psychophysical techniques aimed at strengthening the client's attention to the blind hemifield and improving his or her ability to explore the visual field with saccadic movement.[6] Kerkhoff[18] suggests three types of saccadic training: train people to make broader searches ("visual search field") in the blind hemifield, train people to make large-scale eye movements toward the blind hemifield, and train people to make small-scale eye movements with the goal of improving reading.

In terms of specifically training reading, the minimum visual field required for reading is 2 degrees to the left and right of fixation. This is the area where the text is seen clearly and covers 10 to 12 letters of print at a distance of 25 cm. For fluent reading, the visual span must be extended in the reading direction up to 5 degrees or 15 letters. People with hemianopsia need a minimum of 5 degrees to both sides of fixation to read normally. Less than

---

*References 18, 34, 35, 56, 61, 62.

that amount affects people differently based on whether they are living with a right or a left hemianopsia. Less than 5 degrees preempts proper reading of a given line of text by those with right hemianopia and decreases the ability to locate the beginning of the next line of text by those with left hemianopsia.[48-50] Those with right hemianopsia tend to perform worse on reading tasks and take longer to respond to treatment. Pambakian and Kennard[35] suggest teaching to perceive each word as a whole before reading it. They specifically suggest that those with left hemianopsia should shift their gaze first to the beginning of the line and the first letter of every word in that line. In contrast, those with right-sided hemianopsia are discouraged to read a word before they have shifted their gaze to the end of it. Wang[57] reported the case of a 65-year-old woman who presented with a right homonymous hemianopsia secondary to a left occipital lobe tumor. She was most concerned about her inability to read sheet music and developed an effective compensatory strategy to improve her reading ability. By turning her sheet at right angles (i.e., left-to-right became above-to-below), she could read a line almost as well as prior to the loss of vision. Another possible intervention to assist those with hemianopsia to participate fully in reading tasks is to teach the use of a ruler to assist in keeping track of each line of reading and using the ruler to increase the accuracy of the saccadic eye movements.

Specifically training visual search strategies is also recommended. Pambakian and associates[36] examined 29 subjects with homonymous visual field deficits. Using a videotape, visual search images were projected on a television in subjects' homes for 20 sessions over a one-month period. Prior to beginning the search, subjects fixated on a target in the middle of the screen. Random targets were projected among distracters, and subjects indicated when they appeared. During the training they were encouraged to not move their heads. The researchers found that the subjects had significantly shorter mean reaction times related to visual search after training (p < 0.001). The improvements were confined to the training period and maintained at follow-up. In addition, subjects performed ADL tasks significantly faster after training and reported significant subjective improvements. The researchers found no enlargement of the visual field, but there was a small but significant enlargement of the visual search fields. Findings led the authors to conclude that people with homonymous field deficits can improve visual search with practice and that the underlying mechanism may involve the adoption of compensatory eye movement strategies.

Compensatory visual field training has been tested by Nelles and colleagues.[31] The authors examined 21 subjects with hemianopsia. Compensatory visual field training was accomplished using a 1.25 by 3.05 m training board with right- and left side-wings. Forty red lights

were distributed across the board in four horizontal lines with 10 lights in each line. Clients sat 1.5 m away from the board so that visual fields of subjects were filled out by the board. The subject's heads were kept midline. When the stimulus of the light was presented, the subjects reacted by pressing a button. Training was carried out under two conditions: (1) subjects were required to fixate on a central point on the board and to react to single visual stimuli, and (2) multiple stimuli were randomly presented on the board. Clients were asked to identify a target stimulus (e.g., square of four lights) in each hemifield with use of exploratory eye movements, but without head movements. Detection of and reaction time to visual stimuli were measured during the two conditions. The subjects showed an improvement of detection and reaction time during condition two, but minimum or no change during condition one. Improvements were maintained eight months after training. ADL skills also improved in all clients. Of note was that the size of scotoma (blind area) on computerized perimetry remained stable. Training improved detection of and reaction to visual stimuli without a change of the visual field impairment.

Pambakian and coworkers[34] suggested three steps to improving visual exploration. People with hemianopsia should first practice making large, quick saccades (of amplitude 30 to 40 degrees) into their blind field, to enhance the overshoot of the target. They are then taught to scan for targets among distracters in a systematic way. Finally, these strategies are practiced during real-world activities. These strategies have been tested by Zihl,[61] whose subjects increased their visual field searches from 10 to 30 degrees after four to eight sessions. More recently, Kerkhoff and colleagues[19] had similar findings after examining 92 people with hemianopsia and 30 with additional neglect. Treatment focused on the practice of large saccades to targets in their blind hemifield. Additional focus was on adopting a systematic scanning strategy, either horizontal or vertical scanning. The subjects also practiced searching for targets on projected slides. Training was carried for 30 sessions, and the mean search field size increased from 15 to 35 degrees in those living with hemianopsia. Those with neglect required 25% more training over two to three months to achieve a similar result. At follow-up, almost two years later, there were no further significant changes. The effect of the treatment was independent of variables such as time since lesion, type of field defect, field sparing, and client age. Two noteworthy findings were that those with more severe impairments benefited most from training and that the mean number of required treatment sessions increased dramatically with the frequency and extent of head movements during training. Pambakian and Kennard[35] noted that this finding contradicts the assumption that head movements are helpful to the compensatory mechanisms for those with hemianopsia as is sometimes claimed. The concept of using excessive head movements to compensate for a visual field deficit warrants further investigation.

Optical devices such as prisms also have been used for those with visual field loss. When a prism is applied to glasses, it shifts the peripheral image toward the central area of the retina. Rossi and associates[43] examined the effects of using 15-diopter press on Fresnel prisms on subjects with homonymous hemianopsia and neglect. They found significant improvements on impairment tests of visual perception such as the Motor Free Visual Perception Test, Line Bisection, and Letter Cancellation tests. They found no difference in ADL and mobility scores as measured by the Barthel Index. These findings make sense because the improvements were found only in tabletop measures (i.e., measures that by definition do not encompass large visual fields). The visual image is only subtly shifted when wearing a prism, perhaps not enough to make a positive change in activities such as gait or wheelchair mobility, which require broader visual scans. Tabletop ADL have not been objectively tested, but based on these findings perhaps activities such as balancing a checkbook, doing a crossword puzzle, or leisure reading may be positively affected. On the other hand, several problems are related to wearing prisms, including double vision, a potential blocking of the central field, discomfort, disturbances in spatial orientation, and confusion from the distorted visual image. Prisms may consist of a straight-edged segment of press-on prism applied to the side of the field loss on both lenses or round prisms applied to the lens over one eye. Consultation with an optometrist, ophthalmologist, or neuro-opthamologist mandatory.

MANAGING DIPLOPIA

Diplopia, or double vision, is an all too common visual impairment after a neurological event. During intact processing of visual information, when people look at an object with both eyes, the visual image falls on the fovea (a spot located in the center of the macula, which is responsible for sharp central vision) in each eye, and a single image is perceived. When the eyes are not in alignment, the object we are looking at falls on the fovea in one eye and on an extrafoveal location in the other eye. When this occurs, two images are perceived (i.e., binocular diplopia).[37,44] Diplopia typically resolves completely with monocular vision (i.e., covering one eye). If diplopia is present with monocular viewing, it is unlikely to be neurological in origin.[44] Diplopia may present as the following:[11,44]

- Horizontal (secondary to impaired abduction or adduction of an eye involving the lateral or medial rectus or both)
- Vertical (secondary to impaired elevation or depression of the eye)
- Worse in a particular directional gaze (suggestive of ocular motility being impaired in that direction)

- Worse while viewing objects far away (usually found in conjunction with impaired abduction or divergence of the eyes)
- Worse while viewing near objects (usually found in conjunction with impaired adduction or convergence)

Binocular diplopia is most likely caused by "ocular misalignment" that can be gross or subtle and warrants investigation as to the cause by an optometrist or neuroophthalmologist. The most common causes of misalignment of the visual axes are extraocular muscle dysfunction (see Fig. 16-2).[11]

Ocular alignment should be evaluated in those living with diplopia. Strabismus, or tropia, is a visible turn of one and may result in double vision. The person is unable to keep the eye straight with the power of fusion. In strabismus one eye may turn outward (exotropia), inward (esotropia), upward (hypertropia), or downward (hypotropia).[2] Strabismus may be noncomitant strabismus (the amount of misalignment depends on which direction the eyes are pointed) or comitant (the amount of turn is always the same regardless of whether the person is looking up, down, right, left, or straight ahead). Newly acquired strabismus from a neurological insult is usually noncomitant (i.e., the eye turn changes depend on the direction in which the eyes are looking). Aloiso[2] states that "strabismic disorder may result in an inability to judge distance, underreaching or overreaching for objects, covering or closure of one eye, double vision, head tilt or turn, 'spaced-out' appearance, difficulty reading, and avoidance of near tasks." The term *phoria* is used when there is tendency for the eye to deviate but is controlled with muscular effort. It is not noticeable when a person is focusing on an object.[56] The eyes remain straight as long as fusion is present.

In terms of assessing diplopia, scanning assessments such as convergence and ocular range of motion or ocular mobility should be examined to help determine the weak ocular muscle(s).[2,15] Ocular mobility and convergence assessments as described in Box 16-1 should be evaluated to determine the available ocular range of motion and the observed range of motion lags. During the assessment, the clinician should be aware of the corresponding muscles responsible for the patterns of movements:

- The medial rectus adducts and rotates the eyes inward.
- The lateral rectus abducts and rotates the eyes outward.
- The superior rectus uses elevation and intorsion to move the eyes upward.
- The inferior rectus uses depression and extorsion to move the eyes downward.
- The superior oblique uses depression and intorsion to rotate the eye downward and outward.
- The inferior oblique uses elevation and extorsion to rotate the eye upward and outward (see Fig. 16-2).[2,14]

In addition, the cranial nerves that innervate the various muscles should be considered. The lateral rectus is innervated by the abducens nerve (cranial nerve VI). The medial, inferior, and superior recti and the inferior oblique muscles are innervated by the ocular motor nerve (cranial nerve III). The superior oblique muscle is innervated by the trochlear nerve (cranial nerve IV).[2,14]

Involvement of cranial nerve III results in exotropia, exophoria, convergence insufficiency, accommodative insufficiency, ptosis, and a fixed and dilated pupil. The affected eye is in a down and out position. Damage to the cranial nerve IV results in hypertropia, vertical diplopia, and limited downward gaze. Finally damage to cranial nerve VI manifests as esotropia, esophoria, divergence insufficiency, horizontal diplopia, and limited abduction of the affected eye.[2,11]

In terms of assessment, the Cover-Uncover Test is based on evoking a fixational eye movement and is appropriate for those living with diplopia. If a person is living with an ocular misalignment, only one of the eyes fixates on the particular object while the other eye deviates. If the fixating eye is covered, the deviating eye must refixate in order to align with the particular object. In the cover-uncover test, the person fixates on a distant object, then covers one eye. The examiner observes whether the uncovered eye makes a fixational movement and notes the direction of the movement. Then the occluder is removed and placed in front of the other eye. Again the examiner observes for fixational movements of the uncovered eye. If both eyes are aligned, no movement will be seen during the cover-uncover test (i.e., the test is negative). A positive test is documented if the uncovered eye moves to take up fixation. If refixation is observed, it can be assumed that under binocular viewing conditions the eye is not aligned with fixation, and a deviation is present. Based on the direction of the affected eyes, movement when the nonaffected eye is covered can indicate the type of misalignment. Inward movement of the uncovered eye indicates an exotropia, whereas an outward movement is an esotropia. A vertical deviation may be either a hypotropia or a hypertropia, depending on whether the eye moves up or down.[2,11,56] The Alternate Cover Test is more dissociating than the Cover-Uncover Test, and it may demonstrate phoria more readily.[11] In the Alternate Cover Test, the eyes are rapidly and alternately occluded—from one eye to the other and then back again. This procedure causes breakdown of the binocular fusion mechanism and will reveal refixation movements of each eye now of uncovering. If no tropia is present and the uncovered eye shows refixation during the alternate cover test, the client presents with phoria.

Holmes and coworkers[16] developed a valid, reliable, and responsive questionnaire to quantify diplopia. This self-report measure asks, "Do you always, sometimes, or never see double?" for seven gaze positions (straight ahead, up, downstairs, right, left, reading, any position). The diplopia questionnaire score then ranges from 0 (no diplopia) to 25 (constant diplopia everywhere) and can easily be rescaled to 0 to 100 by multiplying the score by 4 (Fig. 16-4).

In terms of interventions, the overall goal of managing diplopia is to establish clear and comfortable binocular single vision to support engagement in meaningful activities. A typical way to manage diplopia is to apply a patch (i.e., full occlusion or "pirate patching") over one eye. This technique does in fact result in single vision but causes several other problems: issues related to cosmesis and self-image, imposed loss of peripheral vision, eye fatigue, rendering the person monocular, mobility impairments, and safety concerns. Therefore, this technique is not recommended for long-term use.

More recently partial visual occlusion has been used. Proper use of partial occlusion can result in comfortable single vision without the negative side effects of full occlusion, particularly preserving peripheral vision. The "spot patch" is a type of partial visual occlusion. It is a round patch made of translucent tape that is placed on the inside of the client's glasses (corrective or nonprescriptive lens) and directly in the line of sight. The size of the spot patch is approximately 1 cm in diameter, but this varies based on clinical presentation. In general, use the smallest size possible that decreases double vision. The spot patch is effective in eliminating double vision because it blurs central vision in the partially occluded eye.[40]

Another suggested method for partial visual occlusion is to apply a strip of opaque material such as surgical tape to the nasal field of one eye (i.e., the peripheral field is left unoccluded) over prescriptive or nonprescriptive glasses.[56] Similar to the spot patch, this technique results in single vision while sparing the peripheral field. The clinician applies strips of tape systematically to a pair of glasses starting at the nasal field and progressively toward the

Gaze position	Score if Always	Score if Sometimes	Score if Never	Score
Straight ahead in distance	6	3	0	
Up	2	1	0	
Downstairs	4	2	0	
Right	4	2	0	
Left	4	2	0	
Reading	4	2	0	
Any position	1	1	0	
If "always," to all above, can you get rid of it?	−1			
			Total	

Figure 16-4   Diplopia questionnaire. (From Holmes JM, Leske DA, Kupersmith MJ: New methods for quantifying diplopia. *Ophthalmology* 112[11]: 2035-2039, 2005.)

center until a single image is obtained. In general, when using occlusion as an intervention strategy, the nondominant eye is occluded.[56] To determine the nondominant eye, have the person focus on a far target through a 1-inch-diameter hole cut in the center of a piece of white paper. Ask the person to close one eye at a time. Depending on which eye is closed, the target will be visible through the hole. For example, if the person closes the right eye and the left can still see the target through the hole, the left eye is dominant. When the same person closes the left eye while looking through the paper, the target will not be seen with the right eye. Both versions of partial visual occlusion warrant further empirical investigation (Fig. 16-5).

Optical aids such as prisms have been suggested for those with diplopia. Fresnel press-on plastic prisms may be helpful for clients with binocular diplopia up to 40 prism diopters in magnitude. The prisms are available in 1-diopter increments from 1 to 10 and then in 12, 15, 20, 25, 30, 35, and 40 diopters.[44] Rucker and Tomsak recommended placing the Fresnel prism in front of the paretic eye and on only one lens of a person's glasses to minimize blurring of vision. Prisms can be temporary (press-on plastic versions) or permanent (ground into the lens) depending on the trajectory of recovery. Further empirical testing of this intervention related to diplopia that occurs secondary to brain injury is necessary.

The support for eye exercises (orthoptics) in the literature is limited to improving convergence insufficiency.[20,45]

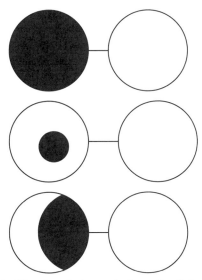

Figure 16-5 Visual occlusion techniques for diplopia. *Top:* Full visual occlusion (e.g., "pirate patch") will result in the person seeing one image, but secondary complications include loss of peripheral vision, body image issues, and so on. Middle and lower figures represent partial visual occlusion such as spot patching with translucent tape *(middle)* and occluding the nasal field of the nondominant eye.

Scheiman and associates[45] compared vision therapy/orthoptics, pencil pushups, and placebo vision therapy/orthoptics as treatments for symptomatic convergence insufficiency in adults ranging from ages 19- to 30-years-old by way of a randomized multicenter trial. The intervention lasted 12 weeks. There were three arms of the trial. The first arm was pencil pushups, in which the subject was instructed to hold a pencil at arm's length directly between his or her eyes, and an index card was placed on the wall 6 to 8 feet away. Each subject was instructed to look at the tip of the sharpened pencil and to try to keep the pencil point single while moving it toward the nose. If one of the cards in the background disappeared, the person was instructed to stop moving the pencil and blink his or her eyes until both cards were present. The client was told to continue moving the pencil slowly toward the nose until it could no longer be kept single and then to try to regain single vision. If the person was able to regain single vision, he or she was asked to continue moving the pencil closer to the nose. If single vision could not be regained, the client was instructed to start the procedure again. The exercises were performed 20 times, three times per day (approximately 15 minutes per day) for 12 weeks.

In the second arm, the vision therapy/orthoptics group received therapy administered by a trained therapist during a weekly, 60-minute office visit, with additional procedures to be performed at home for 15 minutes a day, five times per week for 12 weeks. The exercise protocol[46] included accommodative facility, Brock string exercises, vectograms, computer-assisted orthoptics, and so on.

In the third arm—the placebo office-based vision therapy/orthoptics—clients received therapy administered by a trained therapist during a 60-minute office visit and were prescribed procedures to be performed at home, 15 minutes, five times per week for 12 weeks. The procedures were designed to simulate real vision therapy/orthoptics procedures without the expectation of affecting vergence, accommodation, or saccadic function. Examples included using stereograms monocularly to simulate vergence therapy, computer vergence therapy with no vergence changes, and monocular prism (instead of plus and minus lenses) to simulate accommodative treatment.

The authors found that only clients in the vision therapy/orthoptics group demonstrated statistically and clinically significant changes in the near point of convergence (p = 0.002) and positive fusional vergence (p = 0.001). In addition, clients in all three treatment groups demonstrated statistically significant improvement in symptoms with 42% in office-based vision therapy/orthoptics, 31% in office-based placebo vision therapy/orthoptics, and 20% in home-based pencil push-ups. Although the vision therapy/orthoptics group was the only treatment that produced clinically, more than half of the clients in this group were still symptomatic at the end of treatment; however, their symptoms were significantly reduced.

Rawstron and colleagues[42] systematically reviewed the current evidence regarding the efficacy of eye exercises. The authors reviewed 43 refereed studies (14 were clinical trials [10 controlled studies], 18 review articles, two historical articles, one case report, six editorials or letters, and two position statements from professional colleges). Based on their review, the authors summarized that "eye exercises have been purported to improve a wide range of conditions including vergence problems, ocular motility disorders, accommodative dysfunction, amblyopia, learning disabilities, dyslexia, asthenopia, myopia, motion sickness, sports performance, stereopsis, visual field defects, visual acuity, and general well-being. Small controlled trials and a large number of cases support the treatment of convergence insufficiency. Less robust, but believable, evidence indicates visual training may be useful in developing fine stereoscopic skills and improving visual field remnants after brain damage. As yet there is no clear scientific evidence published in the mainstream literature supporting the use of eye exercises in the remainder of the areas reviewed, and their use therefore remains controversial."

VISUOSPATIAL AND SPATIAL RELATIONS IMPAIRMENTS

Participating in daily living tasks in a meaningful and safe manner relies on higher-order visual processing such as perceiving depth, interpreting spatial relations, and differentiating foreground from background, for example. (Table 16-2). Visuospatial impairments are reportedly one of the most common impairments observed after stroke with a prevalence reported as high as 38%.[32] These deficits have also been reported in those living with Huntington disease,[26] Parkinson disease,[28] traumatic brain injury,[30] and multiple sclerosis.[39]

The presence of visuospatial impairments has been associated with a significant increase in falls,[33] decreased performance of basic ADL and mobility after stroke as measured by the Barthel Index,[32] impairments in both ADL and motor function in those living with Parkinson disease,[27] and difficulties with dressing such as putting one's arm in the correct sleeve[52] (Fig. 16-6).

A qualitative study[22] of those living with visuospatial impairments documented "three main themes comprising six characteristics of how the physical world was experienced in a new, unfamiliar, and confusing way that interfered with the participants' occupational performance and with their experiences of being an individual 'self-person.'" Specific everyday problems that the participants reported included confusion related to space and objects, difficulty reaching for objects, feelings that one's arms were too short, not being able to figure out how to get one's body into a car, feeling unsafe, familiar objects now being unfamiliar, difficulty finding everyday objects, and difficulties with wheelchair maneuvering, for example.

The majority of common instruments to measure the presence of spatial dysfunction use two-dimensional contrived tasks such as overlapping figures, design copying, and so on. The Motor Free Visual Perception Test (MVPT)[10] is only one example of this level of impairment testing. The ability of these types of test to predict performance of everyday tasks performed in context is not clear, and results should be interpreted with caution.[8,29] Specifically validity data have not been collected comparing MVPT scores with real-world tasks requiring visual perception.[29] For example, a retrospective study examined[21] individuals living with a stroke who completed the MVPT and an on-road driving evaluation. The MVPT scores ranged from 0 to 36, with a higher score indicating better visual perception. A structured on-road driving evaluation was performed to determine fitness to drive. A pass or fail outcome was determined by the examiner based on driving behaviors. The author's results indicated that, using a score on the MVPT of less than or equal to 30 to indicate poor visual-perception and more than 30 to indicate good visual perception, the positive predictive value of the MVPT in identifying those who would fail the on-road test was 60.9%. The corresponding negative predictive value was 64.2%. The authors concluded that the predictive validity of the MVPT is not sufficiently high to warrant its use as the sole screening tool in identifying those who are unfit to undergo an on-road evaluation.[21]

An error analysis approach has been suggested to document the effects of impairments on daily living skills.[3,5,52] The Árnadóttir OT-ADL Neurobehavioral Evaluation (A-ONE)[3-5] is one of a select group of standardized assessments that document the effects of spatial impairments on daily living tasks such as mobility, feeding, grooming, and dressing. Specific impairment test items that are scored based on functional observations include spatial relations, visuospatial agnosia, impaired right and left discrimination, and topographic orientation (see Chapter 18). The Assessment of Motor and Process Skills (AMPS)[12,13] may be used to document functional limitations of those living with a variety of impairments, including visual and spatial impairments (see Chapter 21). The Structured Observational Test of Function (SOTOF)[23,24] is a valid and reliable tool that assesses the following:

- Occupational performance (deficits in simple ADL)
- Performance components (perceptual, cognitive, motor, and sensory impairment)
- Behavioral skill components (reaching, scanning, grasp, sequence)
- Neuropsychological deficits (spatial relations apraxia, agnosia, aphasia, spasticity, memory loss)
- Specific visual and spatial impairments (in addition to the above impairments), including figure-ground discrimination, position in space, form constancy, spatial relations, depth and distance perception,

Table 16-2

Visual-Spatial Skills and Their Relationship to Function

SKILL	DEFINITION	FUNCTIONAL ACTIVITIES REQUIRING THE SKILL	COMMENTS
Depth perception (stereopsis)	The processes of the visual system that interprets depth information from a viewed scene and builds a three-dimensional understanding of that scene	Pouring water into a glass, catching a ball, stepping up or down a curb, reaching for cooking equipment with accuracy during meal preparation, parking a car, etc.	Relies primarily on binocular vision but also relies on monocular cues (light and shading, color, relative size). Those living with monocular vision and strabismus will have difficulty perceiving depth.
Spatial relations	Ability to process and interpret visual information about where objects are in space; the process of relating objects to each other and the self	Orienting clothing to your body, applying paste to a toothbrush, orienting/aligning your body in space during a transfer, orienting dentures and glasses to your body Indoor and outdoor mobility during wayfinding, performing math tasks and calculations	Rule out ideational and motor apraxia (see Chapter 18)
Right/left discrimination	Ability to use/apply the concepts of left and right	Following directions related to personal space (e.g., "Dress your right arm first"), applying concepts during mobility ("Make a left turn after the occupational therapy clinic")	Differentiate between personal and extrapersonal confusion related to right/left
Topographic orientation	The ability to use visuospatial (and memory) skills to support wayfinding or route finding	Finding your way via ambulation, wheeled mobility, or driving in familiar environments; learning new routes	
Figure-ground discrimination (foreground from background discrimination)	Inability to distinguish objects in the foreground from objects in the background	Locating a white napkin on a white table, finding a scissors in a cluttered drawer, locating a shirtsleeve on a monochromatic shirt, finding a person in a crowded room, stair climbing (e.g., differentiating when one step ends)	Rule out decreased visual acuity and related basic visual skills

Data from Árnadóttir G: *The brain and behavior: assessing cortical dysfunction through activities of daily living,* St Louis, 1990, Mosby; Árnadóttir G: Impact of neurobehavioral deficits on activities of daily living. In Gillen G, Burkhardt A, editors: *Stroke rehabilitation: a function-based approach,* ed 2, St Louis, 2004, Mosby; Greene JD: Apraxia, agnosias, and higher visual function abnormalities. *J Neurol Neurosurg Psychiatry* 76(Suppl 5):25-34, 2005; Gutman SA, Schonfeld AB: *Screening adult neurologic populations,* ed 2, Bethesda, Md, 2009, AOTA Press; Mazzocco MM, Singh BN, Lesniak-Karpiak K: Visuospatial skills and their association with math performance in girls with fragile X or Turner syndrome. *Child Neuropsychol* 12(2):87-110, 2006; Nori R, Grandicelli S, Giusberti, F: Visuo-spatial ability and wayfinding performance in real-world. *Cogn Processing* 7(5):135-137, 2006.

visual acuity, visual attention, visual scanning, visual filed loss, and neglect. These impairments are detected by the structured observation of simple ADL (eating from a bowl, pouring a drink and drinking, upper body dressing, washing and drying hands).

This relatively quick tool aims to answer the following questions:

- How does the subject perform ADL tasks?
- What behavioral skill components are intact? Which have been affected by neurological damage?
- Which perceptual, cognitive, motor, and sensory impairments are present?
- Why is function impaired?

Although presented here, the SOTOF is appropriate for a variety of the problem areas.

Despite the prevalence of these impairments and the substantial effect on function, little empirical evidence is available to guide interventions focused on decreasing activity limitations and participation restrictions. It has been suggested that a functional approach is the most appropriate intervention for this population.[4,52] This may

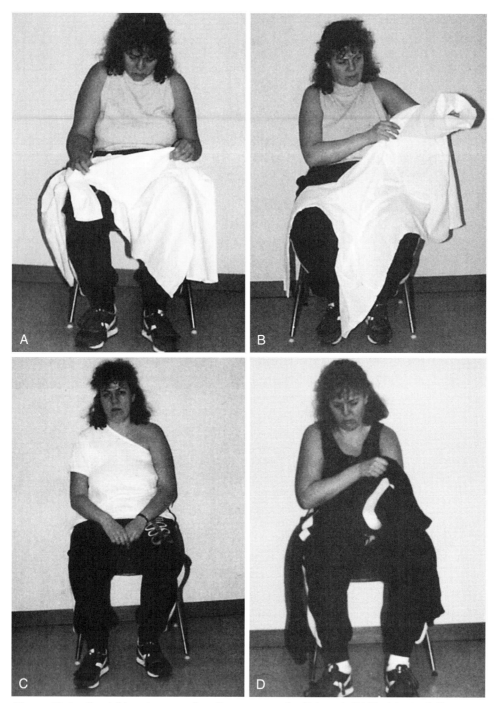

Figure 16-6   Spatial impairments: the effect on everyday living. **A,** Difficulties in differentiating foreground from background. The client has trouble finding the sleeve of a unicolor shirt. **B,** The client is unable to find the right armhole. **C,** The client may start at the wrong hole, placing her arm through the neckhole instead of the left sleeve. **D,** The client is unable to guide the paralyzed arm into the right hole. Pulling more on the shirt at the top of the arm than under it will result in the arm going past the right hole. This deficit can also be related to perseveration.

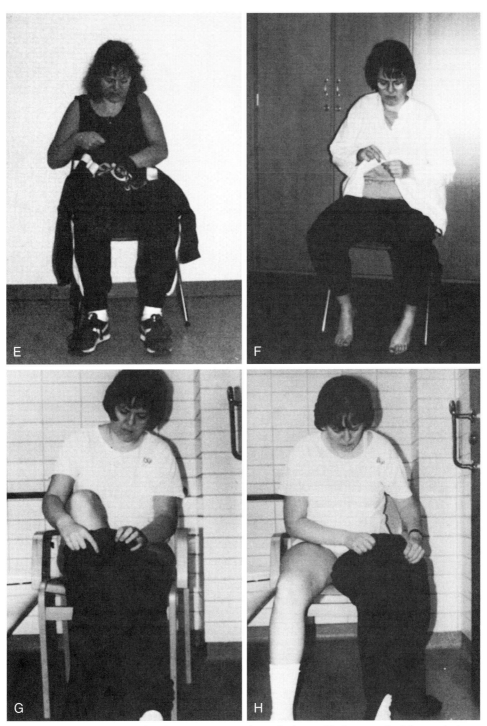

Figure 16-6, cont'd   **E,** The client's arm goes through the neckhole instead of the armhole. **F,** The client matches buttons incorrectly with buttonholes. **G,** The client puts both legs through the same leghole. **H,** The client notices that the pants are turned wrong front to back, with the label at the front, and attempts to correct the mistake by turning the pants with the leg in the leg hole. Ideation also interferes with the client's performance in attempting to correct for the error. See Chapter 18.   *Continued*

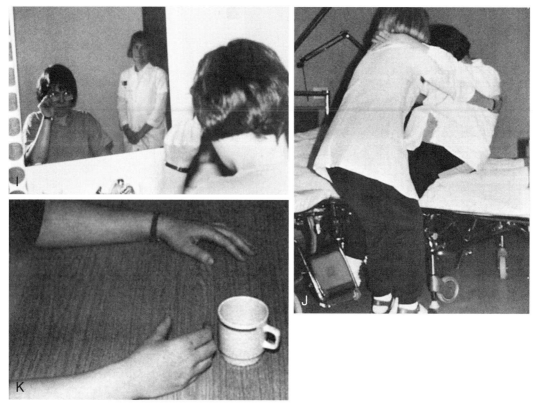

Figure 16-6, cont'd   **I,** The client puts the glasses on upside down. **J,** The client leans backward instead of forward while the therapist attempts to transfer her to a wheelchair. Such a client can be dangerous for the therapist if she is unaware of the problem because the client's actions are unpredictable and often the opposite of what is expected. **K,** Spatial-relation difficulties manifested in underestimation of distances when reaching for the cup. (From Árnadóttir G: *The brain and behavior: assessing cortical dysfunction through activities of daily living,* St Louis, 1990, Mosby.)

consist of task-specific training, strategy training, and environmental modifications (Table 16-3). It also has been suggested that interventions that consist of engaging clients in everyday occupations that are presented to challenge the underlying impairment should be incorporated into treatment.[1,4,7] Abreu and colleagues[1] have proposed an integrated functional approach. In this approach, areas of occupation and context are used to challenge processing skills. With this integrated functional approach, treatment may be focused on a subcomponent skill such as spatial, but daily occupations are used as the modality. Box 16-2 lists potential activity choices.

Table 16-3

Potential Strategies to Improve Function in Those Living with Visuospatial Impairments

DOMAIN OF FUNCTION	POTENTIAL INTERVENTIONS*
Dressing	Deemphasize visual demonstrations during dressing training. Focus on verbal descriptions to retrain the task.
	Decrease the use of spatial-based language (i.e., "under," "over," "right," "left," "behind") when teaching dressing skills. For example, instead of saying "Your left arm is in the right sleeve," say "Wrong sleeve" or "Other sleeve."
	Use cues that facilitate insight into the spatial impairment and that assist in strategy development. For example, if a person puts on the shirt backward, start with a general cue such as, "Are you sure you are finished?" then progress to more specific cues.
	Use clothing that provides cues that can be used to orient the article of clothing to the body. A monochromatic blue T-shirt may be more difficult to orient correctly compared with a baseball jersey in which the sleeves are a different color than the body of the shirt.
	Teach spatial orientation strategies before the client starts to dress, for example, using the label to differentiate front from back or finding a decal on the front shirt.
	Use an audiotape (i.e., does not rely on visual skills) to cue the sequence of dressing.
	The therapist should sit next to and parallel to the person relearning how to dress so that they are working in the same spatial plane.
Meal preparation	Use tactile feedback to increase accuracy when reaching for needed objects (e.g., slide hand across the counter to reach for a pot).
	Decrease clutter. Keep drawers organized to improve foreground from background discrimination.
	Use contrasting colors such as dark dishes on a white counter and vice versa.
	Label or color code needed items or ingredients that are difficult to recognize.
	Organize the kitchen so that cooking equipment is always in the same place. This decreases the amount of time spent search and locating objects.
	Place a piece of colored tape at the edge of the countertop.
	Place colored tape on the handle of the refrigerator and stove controls to ease in spatial localization.
	Use tactile cues before pouring. For example, find the lip of the measuring cup by touch before pouring oil into it.
	Encourage the person to work slowly to ensure safety.
	Label cabinets based on contents.

*May be applied to other functional domains as well; all require further empirical testing.

Box 16-2

Examples of Functional Activities Presumed to Challenge Visuospatial Skills* Based on Activity Analysis

Wrapping a gift
Dressing
Reaching for groceries on shelves of varying distances
Wayfinding/route finding in familiar and new environments
Setting a table
Watering plants
Making a bed
Sorting laundry
Folding clothing

Board games such as checkers
Stair climbing
Sports activities such as playing catch, basketball, or golf
Sorting silverware or coins
Using a mouse on a computer
Playing videogames
Crossword puzzles
Organizing a workspace such as desk or kitchen counter

*Note: This relationship requires further empirical testing.

REVIEW QUESTIONS

1. Name three compensatory interventions that may be used for a person with decreased performance in grooming secondary to spatial impairment.
2. What are the components of a visual screening?
3. Describe the clinical reasoning process to determine why a person cannot locate a spoon in a utensil drawer.
4. Describe three different methods of visual occlusion that may be used with a person presenting with diplopia.
5. What are the potential impairments and the effect on function if a person develops a pathology that adversely affects the dorsal stream (occipitoparietal pathway)?

REFERENCES

1. Abreu, Duval M, Gerber D, et al: Occupational performance and the functional approach. In Royeen CB, editor: *AOTA self-study series: cognitive rehabilitation*, Rockville, MD, 1994, American Occupational Therapy Association.
2. Aloisio L: Visual dysfunction. In Gillen G, Burkhardt A, editors: *Stroke rehabilitation: a function-based approach*, ed 2, St Louis, 2004, Mosby.
3. Árnadóttir G: *The brain and behavior: assessing cortical dysfunction through activities of daily living*, St Louis, 1990, Mosby.
4. Árnadóttir G: Clinical reasoning with complex perceptual impairment. In Unsworth C, editor: *Cognitive and perceptual dysfunction: a clinical reasoning approach to evaluation and intervention*, Philadelphia, 1999, FA Davis.
5. Árnadóttir G: Impact of neurobehavioral deficits on activities of daily living. In Gillen G, Burkhardt A, editors: *Stroke rehabilitation: a function-based approach*, ed 2, St Louis, 2004, Mosby.
6. Bolognini N, Rasi F, Coccia M, et al: Visual search improvement in hemianopic clients after audio-visual stimulation. *Brain* 128 (Pt 12):2830–2842, 2005.
7. Brockmann-Rubio K, Gillen G: Treatment of cognitive-perceptual impairments: a function-based approach. In Gillen G, Burkhardt A, editors: *Stroke rehabilitation: a function-based approach*, ed 2, St Louis, 2004, Elsevier Science/Mosby.
8. Brown GT, Rodger S, Davis A: Motor-Free Visual Perception Test-Revised: an overview and critique. *Br J Occup Ther* 66(4):159–167, 2003.
9. Chia EM, Wang JJ, Rochtchina E, et al: Impact of bilateral visual impairment on health-related quality of life: the Blue Mountains Eye Study. *Invest Ophthalmol Vis Sci* 45(1):71–76, 2004.
10. Colarusso RP, Hammill DD: *Motor-free visual perception test*. ed 3, Novato, CA, 2003, Academic Therapy Publications.
11. Danchaivijitr C, Kennard C: Diplopia and eye movement disorders. *J Neurol Neurosurg Psychiatry* 75(Suppl 4):24–31, 2004.
12. Fisher AG: *Assessment of motor and process skills. vol. 1: development, standardization, and administration manual*, ed 5, Fort Collins, CO, 2003, Three Star Press.
13. Fisher AG: *Assessment of motor and process skills. vol. 2: user manual*, ed 5, Fort Collins, CO, 2003, Three Star Press.
14. Goldberg ME: The control of gaze. In Kandel ER, Schwartz JH, Jessell TM, editors: *Principles of neural science*. ed 4, 2000, McGraw-Hill, New York.
15. Gutman SA, Schonfeld AB: *Screening adult neurologic populations*, 2nd ed, Bethesda, MD, 2009, AOTA Press.
16. Holmes JM, Leske DA, Kupersmith MJ: New methods for quantifying diplopia. *Ophthalmology* 112(11):2035–2039, 2005.
17. Jones SA, Shinton RA: Improving outcome in stroke patients with visual problems. *Age Ageing* 35(6):560–565, 2006.
18. G Kerkhoff: Neurovisual rehabilitation: recent developments and future directions. *J Neurol Neurosurg Psychiatry* 68(6):691–706, 2000.
19. Kerkhoff G, Münssinger U, Haaf E, et al: Rehabilitation of homonymous scotomas in clients with postgeniculate damage of the visual system: saccadic compensation training. *Restor Neurol Neurosci* 4:245–254, 1992.
20. Kerkhoff G, Stogerer E: Recovery of fusional convergence after systematic practice. *Brain Inj* 8(1):15, 1994.
21. Korner-Bitensky NA, Mazer BL, Sofer S, et al: Visual testing for readiness to drive after stroke: a multicenter study. *Am J Phys Med Rehabil* 79(3):253–259, 2000.
22. Lampinen J, Tham K: Interaction with the physical environment in everyday occupation after stroke: a phenomenological study of persons with visuospatial agnosia. *Scand J Occup Ther* 10(4):147–156, 2003.
23. Laver AJ: Clinical reasoning with simple perceptual impairment. In Unsworth C, editor: *Cognitive and Perceptual Dysfunction: A Clinical Reasoning Approach to Evaluation and Intervention*, Philadelphia, 1999, FA Davis.
24. Laver AJ: The structured observational test of function. *Gerontol Special Interest Sec Newslet* 17(1): 1994.
25. Leff AP, Scott SK, Crewes H, et al: Impaired reading in clients with right hemianopia. *Ann Neurol* 47(2):171–178, 2000.
26. Lemiere J, Decruyenaere M, Evers-Kiebooms G, et al: Cognitive changes in clients with Huntington's disease (HD) and asymptomatic carriers of the HD mutation: a longitudinal follow-up study. *J Neurol* 251(8):935–942, 2004.
27. Maeshima S, Itakura T, Nakagawa M, et al: Visuospatial impairment and activities of daily living in clients with Parkinson's disease: a quantitative assessment of the cube-copying task. *Am J Phys Med Rehabil* 76(5):383–388, 1997.
28. Marinus J, Visser M, Verwey NA, et al: Assessment of cognition in Parkinson's disease. *Neurology* 61(9):1222–1228, 2003.
29. McCane SJ: Test review: motor-free visual perception test. *J Psychoeduc Assess* 24(3):265–272, 2006.
30. McKenna K, Cooke DM, Fleming J, et al: The incidence of visual perceptual impairment in clients with severe traumatic brain injury. *Brain Inj* 20(5):507–518, 2006.
31. Nelles G, Esser J, Eckstein A, et al: Compensatory visual field training for clients with hemianopia after stroke. *Neurosci Lett* 306(3):189–192, 2001.
32. Nys GM, van Zandvoort MJ, de Kort PL, et al: Cognitive disorders in acute stroke: prevalence and clinical determinants. *Cerebrovascular Dis* 23(5–6):408–416, 2007.
33. Olsson RH Jr., Wambold S, Brock B, et al: Visual spatial abilities and fall risk: an assessment tool for individuals with dementia. *J Gerontol Nurs* 31(9):45–53, 2005.
34. Pambakian A, Currie J, Kennard C: Rehabilitation strategies for clients with homonymous visual field defects. *J Neuroophthalmol* 25(2):136–142, 2005.
35. Pambakian AL, Kennard C: Can visual function be restored in clients with homonymous hemianopia? *Br J Ophthalmol* 81(4):324–328, 1997.
36. Pambakian AL, Mannan SK, Hodgson TL, et al: Saccadic visual search training: a treatment for clients with homonymous hemianopia. *J Neurol Neurosurg Psychiatry* 75(10):1443–1448, 2004.
37. Pearce JM: Diplopia. *Eur Neurol* 53(1):54, 2005.
38. Pearce JM: Hemianopia. *Eur Neurol* 53(2):111, 2005.
39. Piras MR, Magnano I, Canu ED, et al: Longitudinal study of cognitive dysfunction in multiple sclerosis: neuropsychological, neuroradiological, and neurophysiological findings. *J Neurol Neurosurg Psychiatry* 74(7):878–885, 2003.

40. Politzer T: Visual function, examination, and rehabilitation in clients suffering from traumatic brain injury. In Jay GW, editor: *Minor traumatic brain injury handbook*, Boca Raton, FL, 2000, CRC Press.

41. Politzer T: *Introduction to vision and brain injury* (website). www.nora.cc/client_area/vision_and_brain_injury.html. Accessed May 1, 2007.

42. Rawstron JA, Burley CD, Elder MJ: A systematic review of the applicability and efficacy of eye exercises. *J Pediatr Ophthalmol Strabismus* 42(2):82–88, 2005.

43. Rossi PW, Kheyfets S, Reding MJ: Fresnel prisms improve visual perception in stroke clients with homonymous hemianopia or unilateral visual neglect. *Neurology* 40(10):1597–1599, 1990.

44. Rucker JC, Tomsak RL: Binocular diplopia. A practical approach. *Neurologist* 11(2):98–110, 2005.

45. Scheiman M, Mitchell GL, Cotter S, et al: A randomized clinical trial of vision therapy/orthoptics versus pencil pushups for the treatment of convergence insufficiency in young adults. *Optom Vis Sci* 82(7):583–595, 2005.

46. Scheiman M, Wick B: *Clinical management of binocular vision: Heterophoric, accommodative and eye movement disorders*, ed 2, Philadelphia, 2002, Lippincott Williams & Wilkins.

47. Suchoff IB, Kapoor N, Waxman R, et al: The occurrence of ocular and visual dysfunctions in an acquired brain-injured client sample. *J Am Optom Assoc* 70(5):301–308, 1999.

48. Trauzettel-Klosinski S: Reading disorders due to visual field defects-a neuro-ophthalmological view. *Neuroophthalmology* 27(1):79–90, 2002.

49. Trauzettel-Klosinski S, Brendler K: Eye movements in reading with hemianopic field defects: the significance of clinical parameters. *Graefes Arch Clin Exp Ophthalmol* 236(2):91–102, 1998.

50. Trauzettel-Klosinski S, Reinhard J: The vertical field border in hemianopia and its significance for fixation and reading. *Invest Ophthalmol Vis Sci* 39(11):2177–2186, 1998.

51. Tsai SY, Cheng CY, Hsu WM, et al: Association between visual impairment and depression in the elderly. *J Formos Med Assoc* 102(2):86–90, 2003.

52. Walker CM, Sunderland A, Sharma J, et al: The impact of cognitive impairment on upper body dressing difficulties after stroke: a video analysis of patterns of recovery. *J Neurol Neurosurg Psychiatry* 75(1):43–48, 2004.

53. Warren M: A hierarchical model for evaluation and treatment of visual perceptual dysfunction in adult acquired brain injury, part 1. *Am J Occup Ther* 47(1):42–54, 1993.

54. Warren M: A hierarchical model for evaluation and treatment of visual perceptual dysfunction in adult acquired brain injury, part 2. *Am J Occup Ther* 47(1):55–66, 1993.

55. Warren M: Brain injury visual assessment battery for adults, Birmingham, UK, 1999, visABILITIES Rehab Services.

56. Warren M: Evaluation and treatment of visual deficits following brain injury. In Pendleton H, Schultz-Krohn W, editors: *Pedretti's occupational therapy: practice skills for physical dysfunction.* ed 6, St Louis, 2006, Elsevier/Mosby.

57. Wang MK: Reading with a right homonymous haemianopia. *Lancet* 361(9363):1138, 2003.

58. Wurtz RH, Kandel ER: Central visual pathways. In Kandel ER, Schwartz JH, Jessell TM, editors: *Principles of neural science.* ed 4, New York, 2000, McGraw-Hill.

59. Zhang X, Kedar S, Lynn MJ, et al: Homonymous hemianopias: clinical-anatomic correlations in 904 cases. *Neurol* 66(6):906–910, 2006.

60. Zhang X, Kedar S, Lynn MJ, et al: Natural history of homonymous hemianopia. *Neurology* 66(6):901–905, 2006.

61. Zihl J: Neuropsychologische rehabilitation. In Von Cramon D, Zihl J, editors: *Neuropsychologische rehabilitation: grudlagen, diagnostic, behandlungsverfahren*, Berlin, 1988, Springer-Verlag.

62. Zihl J: Visual scanning behavior in clients with homonymous hemianopia. *Neuropsychologia* 33(3):287–303, 1995.

carolyn a. unsworth

chapter 17

How Therapists Think: Exploring Therapists' Reasoning When Working with Patients Who Have Cognitive and Perceptual Problems Following Stroke

key terms

clinical reasoning	narrative reasoning	procedural reasoning
conditional reasoning	novice therapist	tacit knowledge
expert therapist	phenomenological	generalization reasoning
interactive reasoning	pragmatic reasoning	worldview

chapter objectives

After completing this chapter, the reader will be able to accomplish the following:

- Define clinical reasoning, and identify and define the main forms of clinical reasoning.
- Describe the differences between a more phenomenological approach versus a more biomedical approach to patient care.
- Describe how an understanding of clinical reasoning can enhance practice in the area of cognitive and perceptual dysfunction with patients following stroke.
- Provide examples of situations in which a therapist might use procedural, interactive, conditional, and pragmatic reasoning.
- List the five stages in the development of expertise and the key features of each phase.
- Successfully work through the Review Questions at the conclusion of this chapter.

This chapter reviews how a therapist uses clinical reasoning in the context of practice with patients who have cognitive and perceptual problems following stroke. Because this chapter provides an overview of research literature in the field of clinical reasoning, the content relates to therapists working with all patient groups. However, the case example that illustrates the text is specific to patients with cognitive and perceptual problems following stroke. The chapter examines the different forms of clinical thinking such as scientific versus the phenomenological approaches to patient care and then explores in detail the kinds of reasoning popularly identified in occupational therapy literature, including narrative, procedural, interactive, conditional, and pragmatic reasoning. Influences on clinical reasoning also are explored, such as the therapist's worldview. Because many academics and therapists agree that the use of case studies that demonstrate expert reasoning provides excellent opportunities for students to develop their own reasoning skills, the reasoning processes of an expert therapist obtained during the author's research in this field are used to illustrate the text. The final section of the chapter examines how clinical reasoning skills develop as students or new graduates progress over time from novice to expert. Occupational therapists can use this information to make expert clinical reasoning more explicit and therefore easier for students and novice therapists to learn and incorporate in their practice. Throughout the chapter, the term clinical reasoning is used. However, more recently, occupational therapists are adopting the term professional reasoning since clinical reasoning may be associated with a more medically based approach.[57]

WHAT IS CLINICAL REASONING?

Definition of Clinical Reasoning

Clinical reasoning may be defined as the thinking processes of therapists when undertaking a therapeutic practice. Although occupational therapists have written extensively about clinical reasoning over the past 20 years, they are still just beginning to understand what clinical reasoning is and its importance to practice. Mattingly and Fleming[44] described clinical reasoning as a practical know-how that puts theoretical knowledge into practice and a complex (yet often commonsense) way of thinking to find what is best for each patient.

Unsworth[66] stated, "To me, clinical reasoning is how I think and make decisions when I'm planning to be with a client, when I'm with a client, and afterwards when I reflect on therapy. It involves intuition, judgment, empathy, and common sense.

Clinical reasoning is . . .

   . . . how I think about what the client is telling me and what I observe.
   . . . what I pay attention to and ignore.

   . . . what I respond to immediately or note for future reference.
   . . . the way I try to understand my client as a human being.
   . . . how I draw on my knowledge of previous clients, their difficulties and successful and unsuccessful solutions.
   . . . the way I draw on my theoretical knowledge and apply this in practice.
   . . . the stories I share with other therapists about our clients, the therapy we provide and how we feel about it.
   . . . the way I consider the total picture including how much therapy time I can spend with the client, financial reimbursement issues, and the support available from the client's family.
   . . . the process of deciding what course of action to take with the client, and how I modify or change this over time.

The way I reason has changed over time, due to greater experience and mentoring from expert occupational therapists and other health professionals. The way I reason in my OT [occupational therapy] practice makes me different from other health professionals."*

Development of Clinical Reasoning in Occupational Therapy

Rogers and Masagatani[55] conducted the first empirical study of clinical reasoning in occupational therapy in 1982. The following year, Rogers[53] delivered an Eleanor Clarke Slagle lecture that focused on clinical reasoning. This lecture, coupled with a presentation by Donald Schön (an expert in the analysis of professional practice) to the American Occupational Therapy Association Commission on Education, stimulated the American Occupational Therapy Research Foundation to set up the Clinical Reasoning Study. The study was designed by an anthropologist (Mattingly) and several occupational therapists including Fleming, Gillette, and Cohen and was influenced greatly by Schön as the consultant on the project.[45] The study ran between 1986 and 1990 and was reported extensively in the special issue on clinical reasoning of the *American Journal of Occupational Therapy* in November 1991. In 1994, Mattingly and Fleming[44] published this work in a book. The content of this chapter draws on the foundation laid by Mattingly and Fleming in the Clinical Reasoning Study and extends these ideas using research and theoretical literature from the past 10 years from Sweden, the United Kingdom, Australia, and North America.

---

*Reprinted with permission from Unsworth CA: *Cognitive and perceptual disorders: a clinical reasoning approach to evaluation and intervention,* Philadelphia, 1999, FA Davis.

Clinical Reasoning and Theory

The first consideration is the use of clinical reasoning to explore the practical theories of the profession. One of the aims of the Clinical Reasoning Study was to make explicit the tacit knowledge contained in the practical theories used by the therapists studied. The study argued that this tacit knowledge could be shared if a language to describe therapists' reasoning could be developed. Hence the study aimed to examine the types of reasoning processes used by therapists to use their many practical theories.

Mattingly and Fleming[44] made the distinction between espoused theories and theories-in-use. Espoused theories are those held true by the discipline. These theories are intelligent speculations about the workings of a particular phenomenon, which then usually are tested out and refined through research. Theories-in-use, or practical theories, are those generated by practice. Although many scientists do not support the notion that theory can arise from practice, researchers such as Mattingly and Fleming[44] and Schön[61] believe this is possible. Many of these practical theories pass verbally among therapists when working together, and they often guide therapists in their day-to-day practice. Theories-in-use generally are accompanied by a large fund of tacit knowledge. Often therapists cannot describe what they are doing or why; their expert knowledge is tacit. While this knowledge remains undocumented, it cannot be used to contribute to the fund of knowledge for the profession. Hence a language to describe how and why therapists use certain techniques or communicate in particular ways is needed.

In addition to the way clinical reasoning can be used to explore the practical theories of the profession, one also must consider that the construct of clinical reasoning is itself developing into a theory. Knowledge of clinical reasoning has been growing steadily over the past 20 years and is evolving slowly into a theory derived from practice. If clinical reasoning surfaces into a theory, what is the relationship between this and other theories or frameworks that guide occupational therapy practice? Kielhofner[35] described conceptual practice models as bodies of knowledge developed in occupational therapy for its practice. However, whereas some models can be applied to many patient groups, some are more targeted for patients with particular problems. Hence, Stanton, Thompson-Franson, and Kramer[63] described some conceptual practice models as generic and others as specific to the patients' problem areas. To think about these generic models as umbrella models, such as the Canadian Model of Occupational Performance[11,38] or the Model of Human Occupation,[34] is useful. In the field of cognitive and perceptual dysfunction, an umbrella conceptual practice model is used with a specific practice model such as the Cognitive Disabilities Model,[2] the dynamic interaction approach,[32] the quadraphonic approach,[1] the retraining approach,[32] the neurofunctional approach,[26] or the compensatory or rehabilitation approach.[21,74] The evolving theory of clinical reasoning seems to interface smoothly with all of these conceptual practice models. A clinical reasoning approach cannot replace any model, and yet such an approach can be used to complement these models and add a different perspective to clinical work. Using a clinical reasoning approach with an umbrella and specific practice model ensures that the therapist acknowledges and can describe scientific and phenomenological approaches to patient care (as are described next) and has a language to describe the kinds of thinking that guides practice, including why one chooses a particular practice model. Fig. 17-1 depicts this relationship between a generic occupational therapy (umbrella) conceptual practice model, specific conceptual practice models, and clinical reasoning.

CLINICAL REASONING WITH PATIENTS WHO HAVE COGNITIVE AND PERCEPTUAL PROBLEMS FOLLOWING STROKE

At some point in their careers most occupational therapists work with patients who have cognitive and perceptual problems. One of the largest groups of patients with such problems is the group of stroke survivors. The American Heart Association[4] estimates that each year approximately 795,000 Americans will have a stroke. Documented evidence indicates that at any one time over three million persons in the United States have a stroke-related disability that requires ongoing management and care.[4] Global estimates of incidence of cognitive and perceptual problems following stroke vary enormously because of differences in assessments used, populations studied, and time since stroke onset. However, Kong, Chua, and Tow[36]

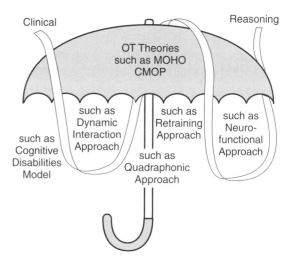

Figure 17-1 Relationship between the evolving theory of clinical reasoning and other conceptual practice models. *CMOP,* Canadian Model of Occupational Performance; *OT,* Occupational therapy; *MOHO,* Model of Human Occupation.

estimate that approximately 41.5% of persons who experience stroke and are more than 75-years-old experience some deficit in this area. Closer examination of specific impairments shows that up to two thirds of individuals with acute right-hemisphere stroke demonstrate signs of unilateral neglect[50] and that 23% of patients have more lasting experience of this problem.[51] The incidence of apraxia is reported to be lower, with estimates of approximately 30% of patients with left hemisphere damage experiencing problems.[17] When occupational therapists work with patients after stroke, the language of clinical reasoning can aid them in describing their practical and espoused theories (and how these translate into day-to-day therapy) to colleagues, students, and the patient and patient's family. Descriptions of the key types of reasoning that form this language are described in the next section.

The conceptual practice model that the therapist adopts guides the kinds of evaluations and interventions that the therapist will undertake,[66,71] and the section on Procedural Reasoning describes this in more detail. For example, a therapist who uses a remedial or bottom-up approach such as the retraining approach[32] assumes that remediation of function is possible, and this fundamental belief helps shape all the reasoning that follows. Such therapists believe that reorganization of brain activity is possible following stroke. Reorganization refers to the ability of the central nervous system to reconfigure and adapt itself in various biological and functional ways to perform an activity. In contrast, a therapist who uses an adaptive, or top-down, framework such as the compensatory or rehabilitation approach[21,74] to patient care believes that the therapist needs to work with patients in the everyday occupations the patients want and need to do and that the environment can be modified or that compensatory strategies can be used to assist patients to complete tasks. The therapist starts at the top, which is the desired occupation rather than working with the patient on the underlying performance components. When using a top-down approach, the therapist does not assume generalization of compensation strategies taught from one activity to another.[66]

Theoretical information provides only the starting point for therapy. Many writers suggest that only through clinical practice can clinical practice develop and creative solutions be found for problems that are not mentioned in texts.[12,60] When problems or obstacles arise in therapy, occupational therapists need to be able to reason to reach a solution. For example, theoretically, therapists know to assess the patient's sensation to exclude these problems before the assessment of complex perceptual problems. But what if the patient has insufficient or unreliable language, making sensory testing impossible? What if the patient is depressed and refuses to undergo sensory testing? Only through learning about clinical reasoning and developing a language to help therapists reason through

these problems and seek answers with colleagues can practice develop.

CASE STUDY: SALLY AND SAM

The next section deals specifically with the different types of clinical reasoning therapists use. To illustrate these different types of thinking, clinical reasoning examples from Sally are provided. Sally is an expert occupational therapist working with a 28-year-old male patient, Sam, who experienced cognitive and perceptual problems along with motor weakness on his right side following a left-sided anterior communicating artery stroke. Sally is the senior therapist in a team of eight therapists at a rehabilitation facility with 60 beds. She manages a caseload of patients with neurological problems following stroke, head injury, or disease processes such as Parkinson. The examples of Sally's reasoning are based on research transcripts in which Sally retrospectively described her therapy sessions with Sam.[68] Three transcripts were recorded, one following an initial outpatient evaluation session with Sam, another following a typical treatment session, and a third when Sam was being discharged from regular outpatient services. Hence transcript excerpts are headed with Evaluation, Intervention, or Discharge Session. These transcripts have been modified (and pseudonyms used) to protect the identity of the patient and therapist or more clearly to illustrate a particular form of reasoning. Sally's description of Sam together with details of his impairments, therapy goals, and the occupational issues he faces are outlined in the following section, which examines the difference between chart talk and narrative reasoning.

A LANGUAGE TO DESCRIBE THE TYPES OF CLINICAL REASONING

This section explores the different types or modes of clinical reasoning. Although several different types of reasoning are described, these types fit into a more biomedical or a more phenomenological approach to patient care. As described by Mattingly,[41] the profession of occupational therapy deals in two practice spheres, the biomedical sphere that focuses on the mechanical body and the social, cultural, and psychological sphere that concerns the meaning of the illness to the person. Hence, Mattingly referred to occupational therapy as the two-body practice. Usually, these more scientific versus more phenomenological approaches to patient care coexist uneasily. However, Mattingly noted that many occupational therapists seem to be able to shift rapidly and easily between thinking about the patient's disease processes (body as a machine or the physical body) and the patient's illness experience (the lived body). Mattingly described how some therapists can integrate these two approaches so seamlessly that "biomechanical means may be used to achieve phenomenological ends or the reverse." The synthesis of these two perspectives into what is called best practice in occupational therapy also reflects the paradigm shifts the professions has undergone over the past 40 years.

Therapists require different types of reasoning when working in these two different spheres and need different ways of communicating this reasoning. When occupational therapists are talking about the patient's medical problem, they are more likely to use a kind of language that Mattingly and Fleming[44] described as chart talk. In contrast, when the therapist thinks about the patient as a person who also has a medical problem, the therapist is more likely to reason in what Mattingly and Fleming described as the narrative form. Mattingly[42] described occupational therapy clinical reasoning as being "largely tacit, highly imagistic, and deeply phenomenological mode of thinking." Mattingly therefore suggested that narrative reasoning is the best basis for most clinical reasoning in occupational therapy. Narrative reasoning means that stories are told or created to assist the therapist to make sense of what is happening with the patient. When thinking about the patient as a person, his or her illness experience, and what therapy will mean for the patient's present life and future, therapists commonly think and talk in the narrative form. These two ways of communicating clinical reasoning are described next.

Narrative Reasoning and Chart Talk

Therapists use narratives or stories to convey their thinking to other professionals, students and novice therapists, and patients. Viewed in this light, narrative reasoning is a way of reporting or giving words to the other forms of clinical reasoning, which are discussed later in this section.[64] Narrative reasoning is also a form of phenomenological understanding. Narratives can take the form of storytelling or story creation. Storytelling can reveal how the therapist treats and interacts with the patient and can be used to explain how the therapist perceives the patient to be managing the disability. Storytelling is most predominant when therapists are carrying out the day-to-day procedures of evaluating and treating patients, trying to understand the patient as a person, and what is happening in therapy.[3] Story creation, however, involves creating a picture of the future with the patient that includes setting goals to work toward in therapy. Story creation is more common when therapists envision a future for the patient, or engage in conditional reasoning (described in detail later). However, the story created for therapy usually does not proceed without the need for revision, and experienced therapists are adept in changing the therapeutic story midstream.[40] In the following example, Sally tells the story of Sam to the researcher. The emphasis of this narrative is on Sam as a person rather than the medical aspects of Sam's stroke.

Evaluation Session, Part 1. "Basically the idea behind this initial outpatient session is just looking at basic home independence for Sam. He was discharged home a couple of days ago, so he is back here every day at the moment as an outpatient. It was actually a self-discharge. We were heading toward that anyway, and the plan was for Sam to live in a bungalow or trailer on his family's property. He used to live in a trailer at the back of their property, but this has rotted out and they've pulled it down. They [his family] actually have a very small house, and it's just not really appropriate for him to be living there since he has teenage stepsiblings, and he is a very independent young man; he wants to have his own space, which you can really understand for a young man, so the idea for him is either to get a bungalow at the back of his family property again or go to a community-based group home. However, that hasn't worked out yet, and so Sam is in the family home for the moment. Sam had his stroke six weeks ago. He was in intensive care for three days, indicating the severity of the infarct, which was in the left anterior communicating artery. The CT [computerized tomography] scan revealed a reasonably large lesion area, and, consistent with his lesion, Sam experiences difficulties with walking, and he is using a 3-point stick. He also has reduced movement in his right arm, and particularly, he has difficulty using his hand since the movements are slowed and his grasp is reduced. He's also got some moderately severe cognitive problems.

"Sam, prior to his stroke, was unemployed, was a drug user, and didn't have a lot that interested him in his life other than playing the guitar, so in terms of finding activities that are meaningful for him, it's been quite hard, and we spent some really worthwhile time in therapy using the Interest Checklist and found that cooking is one activity he loves. He is really motivated; he is a terrific guy; he's really cooperative and tries really hard and seems to always understand the rationale, even though I always explain to him why we are doing what we are doing. So I suppose the two reasons why we chose this cooking activity for today are one, looking toward him in the long-term developing a repertoire of basic meals he can prepare in his own place, and also because it specifically works on improving his planning and problem-solving skills, attention, and his standing tolerance."

In contrast to narrative, reasoning is the kind of language therapists use when speaking with colleagues about a patient's biomedical problems. Although the foregoing example is largely in the narrative form, Sally does slip into another kind or more factual description when she talks about Sam's medical problems. Mattingly and Fleming[44] reported that when therapists discussed procedural aspects of the patient's physical condition, shared treatment goals, and planned evaluations and interventions, they were more likely to use chart talk and scientific forms of reasoning. During these discussions, therapists tended to use a biomechanical way of understanding the patient's problems. For example, in the following excerpt, Sally discusses aspects of Sam's splinting regimen using chart talk.

Intervention Session, Part 1. "A lot of the focus with Sam in the past few weeks has been on him getting functional use of his right hand, which is his dominant hand. He's actually got quite increased muscle tone as you can see there. He has a night splinting regimen, and going back a few weeks ago, he basically forgot he had a right hand; he just wasn't initiating using it, and he quickly taught himself to be left dominant. So we're really pleased with the progress he's making in extending his wrist and MCP [metacarpophalangeal] and PIP [proximal interphalangeal] finger joints. We are talking about his splint at the moment because I did quite a radical change to the splint last Friday, and I was asking him if it was giving him any pain because it does give him a little bit of pain as we have been gradually increasing the extension of his wrist and of his fingers. He told me he took it off midway through the first night, but that he has been able to wear it through the last couple of nights."

Although therapists usually write case notes in the brief and factual language of chart talk, chart talk and narrative reasoning possibly may be interwoven when therapists describe the patient. This idea was suggested previously when noting that occupational therapists seem to be able to weave between a biomedical and phenomenological understanding of the patient. In the first transcripts from Sally, one can see how she slips between discussing Sam as a person and describing the facts of his stroke. Research evidence also supports that therapists interweave these forms of reasoning when discussing and describing their patients.[67,69-70]

The Therapist with the Three-Track Mind

Mattingly and Fleming[44] suggested that when describing the patient's biomedical problems, therapists tended to use chart talk. The kind of reasoning that supports this sphere of patient care draws on scientific reasoning. More specifically, Fleming[23] referred to this kind of thinking in occupational therapy as *procedural reasoning*. When reasoning in the narrative form and considering the meaning of the illness for the patient (when using a phenomenological perspective to patient care), occupational therapists use two other types of reasoning, which Fleming labeled *interactive* and *conditional reasoning*.

Fleming[23] also suggested that therapists seem to be able to think in these reasoning tracks simultaneously. Hence the phrase, "the therapist with the three-track mind" was coined. Therapists seem to monitor the procedural aspects of the treatment, such as the evaluations and interventions to be used with the patient and how the patient is performing, while being able to elicit the patient's cooperation and understand the person's response to the treatment using interactive reasoning.[22] Therapists also seem to engage in considering the patient's condition and how it could alter over time and to imagine how the patient's past, present, and future could be facilitated by occupational therapy intervention. Fleming and Mattingly[25] argued that experienced therapists were able to use these forms of reasoning in rapid succession or use different forms almost simultaneously. Fleming[22] suggested that "Reasoning styles changed as the therapist's attention was drawn from the clinical condition to another feature of the problem, and to how the person feels about the problem, almost simultaneously, using different thinking styles; and they did not 'lose track of' their thoughts about aspects of a problem as those components were temporarily shifted to be the background while another aspect was brought into the foreground."

Although Mattingly and Fleming[44] identified these three modes of reasoning together with narrative reasoning, subsequent theoretical and empirical publications have suggested that these might not be the only forms of reasoning used. In fact, occupational therapists and other allied health scientists have now documented multiple types of clinical reasoning including scientific, diagnostic, pragmatic, management, collaborative, predictive, ethical, intuitive, propositional, and patient-centered.[30,39,54,56] In this chapter, only the most commonly described forms of reasoning are presented, together with comments on their interrelationship. Hence, this chapter explores narrative, scientific, procedural, interactive, conditional, pragmatic reasoning, and a newly identified form of reasoning termed *generalization reasoning*.

Procedural Reasoning. Therapists use procedural reasoning when thinking about the patient's problems and the kinds of evaluation, intervention, and outcome measurement procedures to use. Whereas interactive and conditional reasoning are based more in the phenomenological sphere and therefore are narrative forms of reasoning, procedural reasoning is based more in the biomedical sphere and therefore draws on scientific reasoning. Scientific reasoning almost exclusively forms the basis for medical reasoning and decision-making. Scientific reasoning is the process of hypothesis generation and testing that generally is referred to as hypothetico-deductive reasoning. This form of reasoning most often is used to make a diagnosis of the patient's medical condition. Although occupational therapists are more concerned with identifying the patient's occupational problems rather than the medical diagnosis, therapists do draw on the ideas of scientific reasoning when reasoning procedurally.

In the medical decision-making literature, terms such as *diagnosis, prognosis and prescription, cue identification, hypothesis generation, cue interpretation,* and *hypothesis evaluation* are used commonly.[20] However, in the occupational therapy literature, terms such as *problem identification* and *goal setting* are more common. When determining what the patient's problems might be and selecting appropriate interventions, Fleming[22] identified that therapists were involved in a variety of procedural reasoning strategies and methods of thinking. These methods of thinking include the four-stage model of problem-solving, which is based on the hypothetico-deductive reasoning, goal-oriented problem-solving, task environment, and pattern recognition of the medical model. Each of these methods of thinking is described briefly.

Procedural reasoning generally begins with problem identification, and Elstein, Shulman, and Sprafka[20] developed a four-stage model of problem-solving that focuses on problem identification. Fleming suggests that therapists may use this model when determining the patient's occupational problems.

The four stages in this model are as follows:

1. Cue acquisition: The therapist gathers cues or pieces of information about the patient and the patient's difficulties.
2. Hypothesis generation: The therapist generates several plausible explanations for the observed cues.
3. Cue interpretation: The therapist compares each hypothesis with the cue set and selects the most logical or best hypotheses to explain the cues.
4. Hypothesis evaluation: Finally, the therapist asks what the best hypothesis is by evaluating which cues generally are thought to be necessary for selecting each hypothesis and for the presence of critical cues for selecting each hypothesis. In this way, one hypothesis should be identified as the best.

All problem-solving in occupational therapy is goal directed so that therapists and patients work together to ensure the patient can participate in desired and needed occupations. Although therapy is conducted mostly in clinical environments, therapists think constantly about translating what is being accomplished into the patient's home environments. Hence procedural reasoning also is concerned with considering the environment in which the task is conducted. Pattern recognition refers to a therapist's ability to identify the kinds of patient cues and features that occur together. For example, a therapist who observes a patient go several times to get the necessary toiletries for the morning bathroom routine may question whether the patient has a planning and organization problem or difficulties with memory. However, adding this information to many other observations of difficulties with planning, judgment, and problem-solving prompts the therapist to consider difficulties with executive functions. The ability to recognize patterns of cues and behaviors becomes part of the therapist's tacit knowledge.[22] The therapist recognizes these patterns without needing actually to think through or articulate the emerging trend. Finally, current practice culture is driven by providing evidence to support the evaluations and interventions therapists select to use with patients. Therefore, an occupational therapist reasons procedurally when asking, "What evidence is there to support the treatments I offer?"

In the following example that illustrates procedural reasoning, Sally describes setting up a cooking task with Sam.

Intervention Session, Part 2

Interviewer: I notice you just set up the fry pan, so tell me about that.

Sally: Yes. I basically set it up due to the timeframe for this session and the demands on Sam. We've been gradually upgrading the task demands on Sam, but today I said to Sam that I would set the fry pan up and also because reaching that would be extremely hard for him. He would have to lean right over the table, and also I was planning to put the rice on to cook, just to let him focus on the one task today.

Interviewer: So, you would do the rice, and he would do the stir-fry vegetables in the pan?

Sally: Yes and that's sort of been from past experience because when he has to attend to two things, he will forget one of them, like the rice. So once we sort of feel that he's managing cooking one dish well, then we'll upgrade it and include the second dish, the rice, and we would probably have something like a prompt sign on the table for him to remind him to check the rice and also the timer, which we always use.

In the example of procedural reasoning, Sally talks about some of the difficulties that Sam has with the cooking task because of his memory and planning difficulties. However, more that just looking at Sam's problems, in this transcript excerpt, Sally goes on to incorporate into the activity her understanding of how Sam learns. This kind of reasoning is referred to as interactive reasoning and is described in the next section.

Intervention Session, Part 3

Sally: I think with Sam, he's the sort of guy that learns from repetition. So, by letting him go in and make mistakes—you will see later, he comes back to the table and I've actually let him come back without the can opener and all those things—so that's a way for him to stop and think what he needs.

Interactive Reasoning

Therapists use interactive reasoning to consider the best approach to communicate with the patient and to understand the patient as a person. In the Clinical Reasoning Study, Mattingly and Fleming[44] found that although therapists reported their procedural practices, they did not report their interactions with the patient. Hence, the authors referred to interactive reasoning as the underground practice. Therapists often see patients at difficult times in their lives; their health or well-being is challenged, and they may be experiencing their body in a new way. This can be frightening for the patient, who may respond with confusion or anger. The skilled therapist needs the ability to communicate effectively with the patient so as to share information about the patient's progress and prognosis, and the therapist can gain an understanding of how the patient perceives the disability and views the future.[44] However, because many patients who experience stroke also have a clinical lack of insight to their problems, the therapist faces the additional difficulty of collaborating with patients who may not have any understanding of their problems. Therapists need to take extra care with these patients to establish meaningful and realistic goals.

In its most simple form, interactive reasoning is concerned with how the therapist communicates with the patient. In the following example, Sally reasons about the way she interacts with Sam to make sure he can follow through with what she wants him to do.

Evaluation Session, Part 2

"I'm just sort of basically explaining to Sam the actual movement I want him to do. Often, if I can, I try to decrease the verbal cues and actually look at giving some physical cues as well. That carries right over to all of his program. So, for example, when we do personal care, I really have to use a combination of both physical cues and verbal prompting. I'm certainly trying to decrease that. I think with Sam and a lot of patients with stroke or brain injuries, it just takes much longer for them to respond. It just doesn't go in as quickly as it does with us. My strategy with Sam at the moment is give him the instruction or prompt him and then give him some time to respond, and then go on to give him some physical guidance as well."

More than just basic communication, interactive reasoning is also about understanding the patient as a person who has interests, needs, values, and problems, so that the therapist can understand the disability from the patient's perspective. Interactive reasoning stems from the way therapists value the patient as an individual and the therapist's deeply held humanistic beliefs. In the following example, Sally indicates that she understands Sam as an easygoing person who might want to take the easy way, even though he often can achieve more than he thinks.

Intervention Session, Part 4

Sally: That's another one of the jokes we have. He's been asking me for months about having elastic shoelaces, and I just said, "No way, you're not having elastic shoelaces. You don't need them."

Interviewer: How does he know about them?

Sally: I don't know. He just came out of the blue one day, and I said, "Who told you about those?" And he is the kind of guy that will say to you, "Anything to make my life easier, I will do." He will say, "I'm a bit slack," and that's his personality. I was having a joke with him before saying, "At least I believed in you," because now he's doing his shoelaces independently. I just said to him, "Imagine if we got you elastic shoelaces. You would look a bit silly out there with these big elastic shoelaces." So joking around with him has worked really well.

In this example, Sally talks about joking around with Sam as a way of building a shared language between them and gaining his cooperation in therapy. In the following example, Sally elaborates further on this use of humor in therapy.

Intervention Session, Part 5.
"Yes, and I use humor as well. That's the approach I often take with people but especially with people like Sam, who are really laid back and low key; that really works well. Sam responds much better to a friendship sort of approach, just encouragement, rather than the dictator sort of approach. That's not something Sam goes for. In fact, he bumps up against that approach, and I think that's been a pattern throughout his life. . . . With Sam in particular, like I said, sort of having our own private joke, like I say, "I'm the hand police," and so if I see him not using his hand, I only have to say "hand police," and we can have a bit of a laugh. And we can also laugh a bit at some of the failures he's had, and you obviously have to pick the people you do that with. You wouldn't do that with someone who has got poor insight, but Sam has excellent insight. But, like I said, that's my approach with a lot of people, but with other people you just don't use it because it's not appropriate, and they get very upset if you sort of stir them up a little bit, but with Sam, no, he's not problem at all."

Using a variety of authors' works, Mattingly and Fleming[44] put together a list of purposes for which interactive reasoning is used:

1. Engage the patient in therapy.[43]
2. Know the patient as a person.[13]
3. Understand the patient's disability from the patient's point of view.[43]
4. Individualize the therapy for the patient to match the treatment goals with the person, disability, and experience of the disability.[24]
5. Convey a sense of acceptance/trust/hope to the patient.[37]
6. Break tension through humor.[62]
7. Build a shared language of actions and meanings.[15]
8. Monitor how the treatment session goes[24] and demonstrate interest in the patient and the patient's concerns without indicating disapproval or distaste of the condition.[10]

Hence, interactive reasoning is concerned with collaborating with the patient as a partner in the therapy process. Together the therapist and patient must devise goals that are meaningful to the patient and that also serve to promote the patient's occupational functioning. Humor seems to be one way to facilitate patients to collaborate in the therapy process, and Mattingly and Fleming[44] discussed several other strategies that therapists use to engage patients in this collaboration. These strategies include the following:

"1. Creating choices. Therapists try to engage clients in therapy by providing choices in relation to problem areas the client wants to work on, and the specific occupations or activities they might use in therapy.

"2. Individualizing treatment. A therapy program that is uniquely tailored for the client, through both the ingenuity of the therapist and the involvement of the client, generally keeps the client engaged in therapy. While the goals of therapy for a client with a memory problem may be quite similar, the way the therapy program is structured, and the activities that the client and therapist choose are usually different for each client.

"3. Structuring success. Therapists often structure, or manipulate therapy to provide the client with opportunities for success, and thus promote their alliance. Therapists are often in the business of revealing problems, and then working with the client to reduce their impact. Unless the client has some successes along the way, it is very hard to keep the client motivated, or to maintain a positive relationship with the client. Therapists often talk about keeping the client optimally challenged. This includes pushing the client to achieve, but not so far that he fails. This has been described as the 'just right challenge.'[9,16]

"4. Joint problem solving. Another approach therapists use to facilitate client engagement in therapy is to ask the client to help them in the problem solving process. For example, if the therapist has difficulty in using a piece of equipment, or in devising a strategy for a transfer, calling on the client for his input enables him to take a strong and active role in therapy if only for a short time.

"5. Gift exchange. The final two strategies that Mattingly and Fleming[44] found [that] therapists use to build an alliance with their clients were more personal in nature. The researchers found that therapists would go out of their way, or their formal roles to do something nice for the client such as bake a cake for a client's birthday. In this way the therapist shows a willingness to care for the client in a more personal way. In exchange, clients often feel more committed to co-operate in therapy. Clients may also give gifts to the therapist. These may be as simple as a flower, a few words of thanks or a hug, all of which demonstrate their personal thanks for the therapists' involvement in their treatment.

"6. Exchanging personal stories. Exchanging personal experiences is another powerful way to develop a bond with a client. Mattingly and Fleming[44] found this was commonly used by clinicians to engage the clients in therapy, and that clinicians were usually aware of the value of this strategy."*

Sally talks about the importance of patients choosing their own therapy activity. This illustrates the point made before about creating choices for the patient and supports the idea of a patient-centered practice.

Intervention Session, Part 6. "Now we're upgrading his program, and we have a hand function group that Sam will start coming to. In this group we are looking at a lot of active wrist and finger extension because that's what he really needs to work on, and a lot of gross grasp because he really has trouble extending his third, fourth, and fifth fingers at this stage. Even in the hand function group, although I don't actually run it, two of the other OTs [occupational therapists] do; it's actually fantastic, and the therapists find out what it is the person who wants to do. We have had people in the group eating using chopsticks in their other hand or practicing putting CDs in and out of their player. We really try and keep people motivated by choosing their own therapy activities, and it's a really great fun group that people get a lot out of, I think, more than doing therapy on a one-to-one basis. A lot of my patients, from my experience working here, if they can't see or understand why they are doing a stupid exercise, you just lose them. As I said, we really try to emphasize here that patients choose meaningful activities."

Finally, the following transcript excerpt shows an example of how Sally structures the therapy session to ensure that Sam has some success. The motivating effect of this success pushes patients forward in their therapy programs.

Evaluation Session, Part 3. "We've just finished making toasted cheese sandwiches with Sam, and he did so well. And I made sure that Sam could do nearly all of this activity, since I'm challenging him with the stir-fried vegetables, so its good to balance this a bit with a cooking task that he can complete successfully. I was telling him how well his right hand is working now, and he was like so many other patients who say. 'Gosh, couldn't I use my hand at the start?' and we'll say, 'No,' and they'll just be amazed, so yes, having this success in an activity just keeps them going, I think."

Conditional Reasoning. Conditional reasoning was the last mode identified in the Clinical Reasoning Study. In describing the emergence of this mode, Fleming[22] wrote,

---

*Reprinted with permission from Unsworth CA: *Cognitive and perceptual disorders: a clinical reasoning approach to evaluation and intervention*, Philadelphia, 1999, FA Davis.

"Later we realized that there was a third type of reasoning that therapists employed when they thought of the whole problem within the context of the person's past, present, and future; and within personal, social and cultural contexts. This was an especially useful form of reasoning, which therapists used when they wanted to, as they say, 'individualize' the treatment for the particular person. We called this 'conditional reasoning' because it took the whole condition into account."

Conditional reasoning takes the whole of the patient's condition into account as the therapist considers the patient's temporal contexts (past, present, and future), and his personal, cultural, and social contexts. Fleming[22] proposed that this form of reasoning is based in the cultural and social processes of understanding one's self and others and is used when the therapist wishes to understand the patient from a phenomenological perspective. A therapist uses this form of reasoning in trying to understand what is meaningful to patients in their world by imagining what their life was like before the illness or disability, what it is like now, and what it could be like in the future. In the following transcript excerpt, Sally thinks through the issues surrounding Sam's life at home and what the future holds. This example not only illustrates conditional reasoning (e.g., discussing how Sam's condition has changed and on what his residential care situation is conditioned) but also shows aspects of what some authors describe as ethical reasoning,[5] where Sally imagines how Sam might behave in different residential settings and how his drug use may affect other residents.

Discharge Session, Part 1. "Now, we're talking about a big issue for Sam at the moment; it's the breakdown of his residential situation at home. He's still in his parents' house, but he can't stay there much longer, and they want him out. It's really hard because a lot of the residential settings [supervised housing such as nursing homes] are too low level for him, or the ones that he could live in and have day-to-day contact with someone in attending care support, there's no vacancies or he doesn't like them, and the other issue with him is if he goes into a group home, other people are at risk. He actually, unfortunately, shares his drugs around, and most of these houses have young men with brain injuries, and so we have a responsibility to ensure, you know—they can't obviously make an informed decision about whether to take the drugs Sam offers them. With Sam it's a premorbid thing, and essentially we have come to the realization he is not going to change. He's tried drug counseling, then we had a consultant, then social workers have tried, his mum has tried, and she is tearing her hair out, but he just—it's something he likes to do no matter what we say. He acknowledges there is a high risk of psychotic incidences and all these things, but he just doesn't really

budge from that. You know, when it comes down to the crunch, he just can't resist the temptation.

"So, essentially the two things we are trying to do at the moment is one, structure all of his time, since its when he's bored that he starts smoking drugs and things. Secondly, looking into attendant care so that he has someone helping him to live in a shared house, because if we look at him coming to our transitional living house, which is just across the road here, and I was also, at the end of the session, discussing with him the increased responsibilities that would be on him, and he is a very capable young man. He can make basic meals for himself now. Like, you didn't see him walk in, but he is now mobile with a stick, which he is hardly using. He has really well exceeded all of our expectations for someone with such a serious stroke. He still has ongoing cognitive impairments with things like memory and problem-solving and planning, but with repetition and things, he can really learn to do things himself. It's really hard at the moment until we find out whether there's a bed available in one of the nearby group share houses. He is quite keen about that idea, but still his favored option is for himself to get a trailer or a bungalow on his family block."

Fleming[22] described the third form of reasoning as the most elusive. Conditional reasoning is not always conscious and therefore is more difficult to get at, understand, and describe. Conditional reasoning requires more than a simple knowledge of the patient's condition; it also calls for an understanding of how the condition has affected the individual's work, social situation and leisure, and view of self. Fleming[22] reported that therapists who were more interested in patients' medical conditions or occupational therapy treatment procedures than the patients themselves did not seem to use conditional reasoning. This is often the case with less experienced therapists who are still grappling with the patients' medical conditions and are still learning about putting an occupational therapy treatment program together. Hence conditional reasoning seems to be more pervasive in the thinking of experts rather than novice therapists.[28,67]

To convey a sense of the patient's past, present, and future and to map out how therapy is progressing, the therapist may remind the patient (and self) of a time when the patient could not do a task or activity. This may be particularly useful when therapy is progressing slowly or some of the routine aspects have become boring. Importantly, these reminders show the patient and therapist how the condition is progressing and that together they may yet reach their shared vision of the future.[22] For example, to encourage Sam, Sally talks about how much improvement he has made and how this helps him toward his goal of independent living.

Intervention Session, Part 7. "I'm just saying to him, 'Sam, you've made such great progress.' I remind him of when he first started in the kitchen and his endurance really limited how long he could work, and we used to make really simple meals like toasted sandwiches. And now he can make a stir-fry, and he can use his right hand to stabilize very effectively when he chops vegetables, and how he can concentrate for much longer on the job. I find Sam responds really well to reminders of how far he's come and how far this will get him in the future in terms of living in a more independent home environment, and that's a real motivator to keep going in therapy."

To summarize, Mattingly and Fleming[44] use the term *conditional* in three different ways. In its most simple form, the therapist thinks about the patient's whole condition and the meaning attached to this. The therapist also thinks about how the patient's condition could change and what this would mean for the patient, and finally the therapist thinks about whether the imagined life will be achieved and realizes that this is conditioned on the patient's participation in the therapy program and the shared image of the future.

Pragmatic Reasoning

Schell and Cervero[56] reviewed Fleming's[23] conceptualization of the three tracks of clinical reasoning and postulated theoretically that this account of reasoning neglected the reasoning surrounding the environmental influences that affect thinking and the therapist's personal context. They referred to these kinds of reasoning as pragmatic reasoning. They suggested that organizational, political, and economical constraints and opportunities affect a therapist's ability to provide an occupational therapy service, as do personal motivation, values, and beliefs. In the following example, Sally describes how at the facility in which she works, she must use the Functional Independence Measure (Adult FIM, 1995) as an outcome measure.[27]

Evaluation Session, Part 4. "Last week just before Sam's discharge from inpatient care, I rescored his FIM and discussed that with the team as well. We use FIM as one of our outcome measures here. I don't really mind doing it, but like I have no choice anyway since that's what management has said we'll do."

Therapy often is constrained or promoted by issues over which the therapist may have little control, such as reimbursement for service, the kinds of services and equipment that can be provided given the patient's length of stay, whether the patient can afford to purchase equipment, and the kinds of services available in the community for the patient on discharge.[69] Another important note is that pragmatic reasoning as influenced by the environmental/practice context appears to interface directly with therapists' procedural, interactive, and conditional reasoning. In the earlier example, when reasoning conditionally, Sally

also reasoned pragmatically about how Sam's residential options were constrained by the number of available supported community housing places.

Time pressures are another common source of pragmatic reasoning. Therapists must consider what can be achieved in one session or across the patient's admission. Therapists feel the pressure of patients waiting for them and having to treat more than one patient at a time. Sally also talks about having to share therapy time when the patient is at his or her best.

Evaluation Session, Part 5. "We are trying to gradually increase his endurance, but you get to the stage where his face is going to fall into his cereal, [and] there's no point. You just have to sort of respect that fatigue and also respect the role of the other therapists, because if I see him first, it's not fair if I exhaust the guy, and everyone else gets nothing out of him, either in physical therapy or neuropsych. assessment or whatever it may be."

The author's empirical research has shown that although many instances of pragmatic reasoning were found in the transcripts relating to the therapist's practice context, few related to the therapist's personal context.[69] Hence one really must question whether pragmatic reasoning is in fact only concerned with the practice context and whether the therapist's personal context is not related to clinical reasoning but to something else.

Worldview

Worldview is a useful term to describe the influence of the therapists' personal views about life on their thinking and reasoning. Although Schell and Cervero[56] proposed that these personal belief and values form the personal context component of pragmatic reasoning, one has difficulty imagining that therapists could reason actively with their deeply held sociocultural beliefs.[69] Rather, personal context seems to be something that influences clinical reasoning. The term *worldview* seems to be the best way to describe the factors that make up one's personal context.[72,76] Worldview commonly is understood as an individual's underlying assumptions about life and reality.[31] Hence it encompasses the therapist's ethics, values, beliefs, faith and spirituality, and motivation. If the therapist's worldview influences reasoning, then the therapist also must acknowledge that this may be a positive or negative influence. Therapists also must recognize that they have varying degrees of insight to the influence of their worldviews on reasoning and therefore varying ability to modulate this influence if desired. The most popular method of researching clinical reasoning is for the researcher to ask the therapist to tell what he or she is thinking about after a therapy session has ended.[68] As mentioned previously, in the author's research, it was discovered that therapists rarely if ever revealed any information about their worldviews or how this influenced their reasoning. This is not surprising given that worldview beliefs are deeply held and that individuals find that they cannot, or may not want to, articulate these beliefs. Hence, it is difficult to research and gain an understanding of the influence of worldview on clinical reasoning.[69] However, in some brief glimpses to her worldview, Sally's transcripts did reveal the personal satisfaction she gains from working with patients who have neurological problems.

Evaluation Session, Part 6. "I think OTs [occupational therapists] are really great at empowering people and help them to feel they are in control and they have some say. I think OTs do that better than a lot of other professions. . . . I love to work with people with disabilities, so I think if you actually enjoy the contact and seeing people achieve things, it's such a rewarding job. That comes across in your approach."

The transcripts also revealed Sally's disappointment that Sam cannot achieve what she considers his potential because of drug use.

Discharge Session, Part 2. "Even though he's motivated and you can say, 'Sam, you've just made such amazing gains,' when he does use drugs, he just loses all his cognition basically. He sits there, and his mother reports he spaces out for 24 hours at a time, and it's a real shame. I have seen this fellow going from being full assistance in absolutely every activity of daily living to being fully independent in personal care, basic domestic activities, and basic community activities, so he really has done remarkably well, so it's a bit disappointing. You try not to dwell on it too much, but it is disappointing from a therapist's point of view because you think he could just keep on improving, but the drug use is holding him back, but at the same time that's his life."

Although Mattingly and Fleming[44] did not describe worldview specifically or its relationship to clinical reasoning, their text is rich with descriptions of how the therapist's personal qualities, abilities, or style influences therapy. Further research is required, perhaps using interview techniques, to explore the relationship of therapists' worldview to clinical reasoning.[69]

Generalizing Form of Reasoning

Finally, in each of the forms of reasoning discussed before (procedural, interactive, conditional, and pragmatic), research has shown that therapists seem to draw on their experiences to enrich the kind of reasoning in which they are engaged.[70] Rather than being described as a separate form of reasoning, this form of reasoning seems to be an extension of the other forms. The author calls this *generalization reasoning*. Although generalization reasoning has similarities to simple pattern recognition (as described in relation to pragmatic reasoning), it appears to go beyond simple pattern recognition of a set of cues. Therapists seem to reason initially about a particular issue or scenario with a patient, then reflect on their general experiences related to the situation (i.e., making generalizations), and then refocus the reasoning on the patient. This seems to occur in rapid succession, as in the following excerpt in which Sally reasons interactively about how she is communicating with the patient.

Intervention Session, Part 8. "Often, if I can, I try to decrease the verbal cues and actually look at giving some physical cues as well. That carries right over to all of his program. Physically, even though he has significant problems in all areas in terms of transfers and bed mobility and everything. So, for example, when we do personal care, I really have to use a combination of both physical cues and verbal prompting. I'm trying to certainly decrease that. I think with Sam and a lot of patients with stroke or brain injuries, it just takes much longer for them to respond. It just doesn't go in a quickly as it does with us. My strategy with Sam at the moment is give him the instruction or prompt him and then give him some time to respond, and then go on to give him some physical guidance as well."

In summary, this generalization form of reasoning seems to enrich the other reasoning modes and also seems to be used more frequently by expert rather than novice therapists.[70]

Embodied Knowledge

This chapter has explored the clinical reasoning and thinking that underpins occupational therapy practice. However, this reasoning is a product of cognitive or mental processes and body experiences. Therapists' bodies obtain a great deal of information as they work with clients. For example, their bodies tell them about the client's smell, and the feel of their muscles and how their body moves in ways that the therapists' own bodies recognize or "know" but that they might not be able to put into words. This is referred to as embodied knowledge.[58] In the case study illustrating this chapter, Sally described how she would automatically smell Sam as soon as he arrived at therapy to help determine if he had been smoking drugs. Although occupational therapists have long recognized the importance of information from their bodies about their clients, the embodied nature of clinical reasoning is a relatively new area for research in occupational therapy.

Putting It All Together: A Summary of the Different Modes of Reasoning

Before summarizing the different kinds of clinical reasoning and influences on reasoning such as worldview, exploration of the interaction of the three tracks of clinical reasoning is important. Although some researchers examine procedural, interactive, and conditional reasoning in isolation from each other,[28] it seems that these forms of reasoning can occur in rapid succession or even simultaneously. As described earlier, Fleming[22] described how therapists can think in "many tracks simultaneously." For example, Fleming[23] writes "in using conditional reasoning, the therapist appears to reflect on the success or failure of the clinical encounter from both the procedural and interactive standpoints and attempts to integrate the two." Although the notion of the simultaneous use of the three tracks should not be taken too literally, therapists certainly can see evidence in their clinical reasoning transcripts of the rapid blending of different modes of reasoning. For example, Sally uses all three forms of reasoning in the following brief explanation of one aspect of her therapy session. Procedural reasoning is underlined, conditional reasoning is in bold, and interactive reasoning is italicized.

Intervention Session, Part 9. <u>"Another thing I'm working on with Sam is his speed. He's very slow to process information and therefore slow in executing tasks,</u> *and I find that he also tends to self-distract a fair bit by chatting.* <u>But at the same time that's hard because I'm Sam's case manager, which means that I monitor his whole program,</u> and since he's just gone home, ***we have been having long chats about how he was coping at home since*** <u>***I want to find out how he's doing and what he's having difficulty with, whether he's following through by making his own breakfast and using his dressing aids***</u> ***and things like that,*** *so in a way I'm distracting him a little bit,* <u>*but he has to learn to cope with distractions in his environment.*</u>"

The relationship between the three main modes of reasoning can be illustrated by the use of a Venn diagram in which the three circles each represent a different mode of reasoning and yet show that each mode does not occur in isolation from the others.[70] These three forms of reasoning are related to the other modes described in this chapter, as illustrated in Fig. 17-2.[69] Fig. 17-2 presents the relationships between the different forms of reasoning, or influences on clinical reasoning, using the analogy of the basic structures of the brain. Starting at the top of this figure is worldview. This was described previously in the chapter as an influence on reasoning rather than a form of reasoning. Worldview is at the top of the diagram because it influences all the modes of reasoning, and like the idea of higher cortical function, worldview represents fairly sophisticated thinking that includes one's morals, ethics, and sociocultural perspective. The next level of the brain can be described crudely as the engine or working areas. Hence, this is where the main forms of reasoning (procedural, interactive, and conditional) occur, as illustrated using a Venn diagram. These forms of reasoning are more scientific (such as procedural reasoning) or draw more on

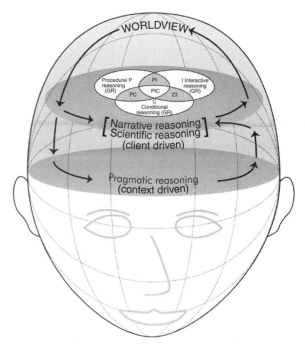

Figure 17-2 The relationship between the different forms of clinical reasoning within the patient-centered practice of occupational therapy. *GR,* Generalized reasoning. (From Unsworth CA: Clinical reasoning: how do pragmatic reasoning, worldview and client-centredness fit? *Br J Occup Ther* 67[1], 10-19, 2004.)

phenomenological forms of thinking and therefore can be described as narrative forms of reasoning (such as interactive and conditional reasoning). At this level, the therapist's reasoning is basically driven by the patient (such as the patient's strengths and weaknesses, goals, and desires). Finally, at the most basic level of operation, which is similar to the brainstem, is pragmatic reasoning. Similar to fundamental brain functions such as breathing, pragmatic reasoning involves thinking related to things over which therapists often do not have much control. For example, the therapist reasons pragmatically about what might be achieved with a particular patient given the patient's maximum length of stay, which often is dictated by the payment or reimbursement system. In contrast to the patient-driven forms of reasoning described previously, pragmatic reasoning is context driven. Generalized reasoning can occur in connection with procedural, interactive, conditional, and pragmatic reasoning. The arrows that flow around Fig. 17-2 indicate that each influence on reasoning or form of reasoning influences the others to a greater or lesser extent. Finally, one must acknowledge that this representation of clinical reasoning operates within the patient-centered practice of occupational therapy. In other words, this diagram assumes that therapists practice within a patient-centered framework. Hence, the client's goals, values, beliefs, and life experience are at the forefront of the therapist's reasoning and drive the therapy process.

CLINICAL REASONING AND EXPERTISE

Differences between the Clinical Reasoning of Novice and Expert Therapists

Over the past 15 years, research in health sciences has shown consistently that experts have better general problem-solving and clinical reasoning skills than novice therapists.[65] The occupational therapy literature contains a wealth of information about the differences in the clinical reasoning of novice and expert therapists[14,28,52,64] and how students can improve their reasoning skills.[12,33,46-49] The purpose of this section is to review what is known about the clinical reasoning of expert therapists and strategies to enhance clinical reasoning so that students and novice therapist can hasten their own journey to expert status.

Like most skills, clinical reasoning can be graded along a continuum. Different points along the continuum are marked by certain characteristics that indicate an individual's skill level. Dreyfus and Dreyfus[18,19] presented a five-stage model of skill acquisition based on their study of chess players and airline pilots. They suggested that as students develop a skill, they pass through five stages of proficiency: novice, advanced beginner, competent, proficient, and expert. Benner[6] and Benner and Tanner[8] incorporated this model in their studies of the acquisition of skill in nursing, and since that time, most health science research regarding clinical reasoning incorporates the Dreyfus and Dreyfus model. Benner[6] suggested that as a therapist passes through the five stages of proficiency, changes in three aspects of skilled performance occur. A shift in reliance from abstract principles to past experiences occurs, a change in perception of the situation occurs (i.e., a shift from perceiving all parts of the picture equally to viewing the whole situation in which only parts are relevant), and a change from detached observer to involved performer occurs. Based on the work of Dreyfus and Dreyfus,[18] Benner,[6] and Benner and Tanner,[8] Table 17-1 outlines the stages in the development of expertise and some of the characteristics of therapists at each stage.

Research with occupational therapists and other allied health professions has revealed a variety of aspects of clinical reasoning processes that differ between novices and experts. For example, Collins and Affeldt[14] suggested that whereas novices tend to focus on one aspect of a situation and one observation triggers one association, experts can focus on many aspects of a situation and a single observation can trigger multiple associations. Although a more experienced therapist may reason holistically and react quickly to a problem with a total solution, a novice may reason step by step and react more slowly to a problem with only a partial solution. Robertson[52] supported this empirically through research that found that more experienced therapists had more integrated problem representations (that is, a well-organized body of knowledge).

In addition, because occupational therapists reason in narratives, therapy is like telling or creating a story.[44] Mattingly and Fleming[44] suggested that expert therapists have a greater capacity than novices to make revisions to the story as therapy progresses.

Other differences between novices and experts include the way experts reason intuitively and have more tacit knowledge. This contrasts to the reasoning of a new practitioner, which seems to require conscious effort. Strong and colleagues[64] reported that experts viewed gaining an understanding of their patients in terms of their illness and disability and of patients' perceptions of the effect of these on their lives as more important than did student therapists. Students placed a higher value on knowledge and understanding of the patient's problems, whereas expert therapists placed more emphasis on good communication skills. Hallin and Sviden[28] also found that expert therapists seemed to have an excellent understanding of the patient.

Finally, my research on the differences between the clinical reasoning of novices and experts[67] found that experts make complex skills look simple. The experts in this study were articulate and able to present the clinical reasoning that supported their therapy with confidence. Similar to the findings of Mattingly and Fleming,[44] Hallin and Sviden,[28] and Benner, Hooper-Kyriakidis, and Stanard,[7] experts seem to draw on their past experiences when planning and executing therapy and use this knowledge to anticipate patient performance and modify or change the therapy plan as needed. In addition, although the students in this study had had recent exposure to literature on patient-centered practice, the expert therapists appeared to have embraced this concept and were incorporating this approach in their work. Robertson[52] also noted this trend. Finally, expert therapists seemed to have a greater capacity to undertake an activity that met several patient goals or were more likely to be doing several things with the patient at once. Rather than suggesting that they were impatient or pressured by time, this finding indicated an efficiency of time use that novices had not yet developed.

Enhancing the Student's Clinical Reasoning Skills

The progression of a therapist from novice to expertise is not assured. Although some therapists reach competent or proficient practice levels of expertise, they may never attain expert status. In addition, as can be understood from the foregoing examples, expertise is not necessarily reflected in the depth or breadth of experience nor years of practice. Therefore, a relatively young therapist might possibly possess an intuitive grasp of the situation, generate therapy from patient-generated cues, recognize patient strengths and weaknesses based on past experience, and thus be considered an expert. This section presents a summary of ideas from occupational therapy literature

Table 17-1

Stages and Characteristics in the Development of Expertise

STAGE	THERAPIST CHARACTERISTICS
1. Novice	Novices do not have experience of the situations in which they will be involved. To enter the clinic and gain experience in these areas, students are taught about theories, principles, and specific patient attributes.
	A novice is usually rigid in the application of these rules, principles, and theories. However, rules cannot guide the therapist to do all the things that need to be done in the multitude of situations and contexts in which the therapist works.[6] A clinician can acquire only "context-dependent judgment" through participation in real situations.[49]
2. Advanced beginner	Advanced beginners have been involved in enough clinical situations to realize, or to have had pointed out to them, the recurring themes and information on which reasoning is based. An advanced beginner may begin to modify rules, principles, and theories to adapt them to the specific situation.
	Advanced beginners do what they are told or what the text dictates as the correct procedure but may have difficulty prioritizing in more unusual circumstances those parts of the procedure that are least important or those aspects that are vital.
	Advanced beginners have to concentrate on remembering the rules and therefore have less ability to apply them flexibly.
	Dreyfus and Dreyfus[18] suggest that an awareness of the client as a person beyond the technical concerns does not usually develop until the student has advanced to this stage.
3. Competent	Competent therapists are able to adjust the therapy to the specific needs of the patient and the situation but may have difficulty altering initial treatment plans. Benner[6] suggests that therapists are competent once they are consciously aware of the outcome of their actions. This is typical of a therapist who has been in the job for 2 to 3 years. However, a competent therapist is said to lack the speed and flexibility of the proficient therapist. Efficiency and organization are achieved at this stage through conscious or deliberate planning.
4. Proficient	Proficient therapists are flexible and are able to alter treatment plans as needed. Proficient therapists have a clear understanding of the patient's whole situation rather than an understanding of the components alone. Proficient practitioners have a perception of the situation based on experience rather than deliberation. Given that the proficient therapist has a perspective of the overall situation, components that are more and less important stand out, and the therapist can focus on the problem areas.
5. Expert	Expert therapists approach therapy from patient-generated cues rather than preconceived therapeutic plans. Experts anticipate and quickly recognize patient strengths and weaknesses based on their experience with other patients. The expert therapist does not need to rely on rules and guidelines to take appropriate action but rather has an intuitive grasp of the situation. Experts often find it difficult to explain this intuition.[49]

From Unsworth CA: *Cognitive and perceptual disorders: a clinical reasoning approach to evaluation and intervention*, Philadelphia, 1999, FA Davis.

that examines how students and novice therapists can improve their clinical reasoning and thus hasten their journey from novice to expert. More specific details of teaching strategies to enhance student's development of clinical reasoning skills may be found in Higgs[29] and Neistadt.[46]

The following list provides example strategies for novice and student therapists to try that will assist them better in honing clinical reasoning skills.

- Learn about clinical reasoning and the different modes of reasoning. When undertaking cognitive and perceptual dysfunction coursework, try to integrate this with knowledge of clinical reasoning techniques.[46,66] In these courses, scientific and procedural forms of reasoning can dominate to the extent that insufficient attention is paid to the patient's experience of the disability, priorities, and life story.[49]

- Spend time reflecting on the patient's experience of the illness and disability and the patient's perceptions of how these affect his or her life. One might achieve this after a patient interview in which the student/therapist asks the patient about what the disability means to him or her and its effect on life.[59,64]

- Use case scenarios from experts to make expert therapist reasoning and hypothesis generation more explicit. In this way, students can learn to model their practice on an expert's.[52] Students can generate their own case studies and work in pairs to describe evaluation and treatment processes and thus facilitate self-evaluation and critical reflection.[46] As Mattingly and Fleming's study[44] revealed, mentoring from an expert therapist is just as influential as formal education is on a novice's practice.
- Note significant similarities and differences between patients and reflect on how these differences can influence treatment.[14]
- Develop relationships among data so that treatment planning is guided by a thorough understanding of the problem situation.[52]
- Explore probable consequences of treatments before enactment.[14]

Finally, an important way to enhance student development of clinical reasoning skills is to provide them with structured ways to reflect on their clinical encounters. A key aspect of clinical reasoning is the ability to reflect on what has been experienced in therapy and to go forward in response to this reflection. Having told stories, novice therapists need time to reflect on their meaning and significance. Expert reasoning relies on the ability to reflect on, and learn from, therapeutic encounters as an individual and from sharing experiences with other therapists. Much has been written in the medical[61] and education literature[73,75] regarding the training of doctors and teachers to be reflective. Also important is teaching occupational therapy students and novice therapists to become more reflective by writing diary entries following therapy sessions and providing opportunities to reflect on their therapy encounters with more experienced occupational therapists.

SUMMARY

Occupational therapists who work with patients who have cognitive and perceptual problems following stroke often find themselves working in environments dominated by the medical model. This means that in subtle or more obvious ways, occupational therapist do not always fit in with the approach taken by the rest of the team. Although most occupational therapists seem to marry scientific and phenomenological approaches to patient care successfully in practice, explaining this practice to others may prove more difficult. These explanations are hindered by the tacit nature of much of this knowledge. This chapter has explored the ways that therapists think and reason. Using Mattingly and Fleming's foundation work[44] in this field, the chapter has presented a language to describe the clinical reasoning that supports the more scientific and phenomenological approaches to patient

care. Using this language helps novice and expert therapists to explain practice to colleagues and patients and helps therapists to articulate more clearly their goals and the methods used to reach them. In the challenging area of treating patients with cognitive and perceptual problems following stroke, the ability to communicate the clinical reasoning that supports practice is particularly important. The chapter concluded by presenting an overview of what we know about the differences between novice and expert practice and the role of clinical reasoning in expert practice and highlighted techniques that novice therapists can use to hasten their journey from novice to expert therapist status.

ACKNOWLEDGMENT

I would like to thank Sheridan Vines (BAppSc.[Occ. Ther], AccOT) for sharing her rich knowledge and intuitions during a clinical reasoning research program conducted through the School of Occupational Therapy, La Trobe University. Thanks also to Geoffrey Campbell (graphic designer at Amanda Roach Designs, Windsor, Melbourne), who patiently translated my drawings of the relationship between the different modes of clinical reasoning into Fig. 17-2.

REVIEW QUESTIONS

1. What is clinical reasoning in occupational therapy?
2. Describe the difference between narrative and scientific forms of reasoning. How do Fleming's three tracks of reasoning relate to narrative and scientific forms?
3. Using first-person writing style, write a short narrative about one of your clinical encounters with a patient. Reflect on this encounter and identify in the margins what kinds of reasoning you were using at different times during the session.
4. The case study used to illustrate the chapter described Sally and Sam. Sam recently had discharged himself to home. Imagine that Sam was married with a child rather than single and that he had returned home to this environment. Also consider that Sam was working as a printer before his stroke and that he is keen to get back to this and does not use drugs. Write a chart report of your outpatient goals for Sam (i.e., a one paragraph summary that could be placed in Sam's medical record). Then write a short narrative indicating your therapy aspirations for what you and Sam hope to achieve over the next two months. Indicate the kind of future you predict for Sam and what kind of treatment activities you might use.
5. What are some of the hallmarks of clinical expertise?
6. What are three approaches novice therapists can use to hasten their journey from novice to expert therapist status?

REFERENCES

1. Abreu BC: *The quadraphonic approach: Management of cognitive and postural dysfunction*, New York, 1990, Therapeutic Service Systems.
2. Allen CK, Earhart CA, Blue T: *Occupational therapy treatment goals for physically and cognitively disabled*, Rockville MD, 1992, American Occupational Therapy Association.
3. Alnervik A, Sviden G: On clinical reasoning: patterns of reflection on practice. *Occup Ther J Res* 16(2):98–110, 1996.
4. American Heart Association: *Heart disease and stroke statistics 2009. Update at a glance (website)*. www.american heart.org. Accessed June 1, 2009.
5. Barnitt R, Partridge C: Ethical reasoning in physical therapy and occupational therapy. *Physiother Res Int* 2(3):178–94, 1997.
6. Benner P: *From novice to expert: excellence and power in clinical nursing practice*, Menlo Park, CA, 1984, Addison-Wesley.
7. Benner P, Hooper-Kyriakidis P, Stanard D: *Clinical wisdom and interventions in critical care: a thinking-in-action approach*, Philadelphia, 1999, Saunders.
8. Benner P, Tanner C: Clinical judgment: how expert nurses use intuition. *Am J Nurs* 87(1):23–31, 1987.
9. Berlyne DE: Laughter, humor, and play. In Lindzert G, Aronson E, editors: *The handbook of social psychology*, Reading, Mass, 1969, Addison-Wesley.
10. Bradburn SL: *Psychiatric occupational therapists' strategies for engaging patients in treatment during the initial interview*, Unpublished master's thesis, Medford, MA, 1992, Tufts University.
11. Canadian Association of Occupational Therapists: *Enabling occupation II: Advancing an occupational therapy vision for health, well-being and justice through occupation*, Ottawa, 2007, The Association.
12. Cohn ES: Clinical reasoning: explicating complexity. *Am J Occup Ther* 45(11):969–971, 1991.
13. Cohn ES: Fieldwork education: shaping a foundation for clinical reasoning. *Am J Occup Ther* 43(4):240–244, 1989.
14. Collins LF, Affeldt J: Bridging the clinical reasoning gap. *Occup Ther Pract* 1:33–35. 1996.
15. Crepeau EB: Achieving intersubjective understanding: examples from an occupational therapy treatment session. *Am J Occup Ther* 45(11):1016–1025, 1991.
16. Csikszentmihalyi M: Play and intrinsic rewards. *Humanistic Psychol* 15(3):41–63, 1975.
17. Donkervoort M, Dekker J, Van den Ende E, et al: Prevalence of apraxia among patients with a first left hemisphere stroke in rehabilitation centres and nursing homes. *Clin Rehabil* 14(2):130–136, 2000.
18. Dreyfus HL, Dreyfus SE: *Mind over machine: the power of human intuition and expertise in the era of the computer*, New York, 1986, Free Press.
19. Dreyfus SE, Dreyfus HL: *A five-stage model of the mental activities involved in directed skill acquisition*, Unpublished report supported by the Air Force Office of Scientific Research, USAF (Contract F49620–79–C–0063), Berkley, 1980, University of California.
20. Elstein AS, Shulman LS, Sprafka SA: *Medical problem solving: An analysis of clinical reasoning*, Cambridge, MA, 1978, Harvard University Press.
21. Fisher AG: An expanded rehabilitative model of practice. In Fisher AG, editor: *Assessment of motor and process skills*, ed 2, Fort Collins, CO, 1997, Three Star Press.
22. Fleming MH: The therapist with the three track mind. In Mattingly C, Fleming MH, editors: *Clinical reasoning: forms of inquiry in a therapeutic practice*, Philadelphia, 1994, FA Davis.
23. Fleming MH: The therapist with the three-track mind. *Am J Occup Ther* 45(11):1007–1014, 1991.
24. Fleming MH: *Proceedings of the institute on clinical reasoning for occupational therapy educators*, Medford, MA, 1990, Clinical Reasoning Institute, Tufts University.
25. Fleming MH, Mattingly C: Giving language to practice. In Mattingly C, Fleming MH, editors: *Clinical reasoning: Forms of inquiry in a therapeutic practice*, Philadelphia, 1994, FA Davis.
26. Giles GM, Wilson JC: *Rehabilitation for the severely brain-injured adult*, ed 2, London, 1999, Nelson Thornes.
27. *Guide for the Uniform Data Set for Medical Rehabilitation* (Adult FIM), (1995). Version 5.0 Buffalo, NY: State University of New York at Buffalo.
28. Hallin M, Sviden G: On expert occupational therapists' reflection-on practice. *Scand J Occup Ther* 2(2):69–75, 1995.
29. Higgs J: Developing clinical reasoning competencies. *Physiotherapy* 78(8):575–581, 1992.
30. Higgs J, Jones M, Loftus S, Christiansen N: *Clinical reasoning in the health professions*, ed 3, Melbourne, Australia, 2008, Butterworth-Heinemann.
31. Hooper B: The relationship between pretheoretical assumptions and clinical reasoning. *Am J Occup Ther* 51(5):328–338, 1997.
32. Katz N: *Cognition and occupation across the life span: models for intervention in occupational therapy*, ed 2, Bethesda, MD, 2005, AOTA Press.
33. Keponen R, Launiainen H: Using the model of human occupation to nurture an occupational focus in the clinical reasoning of experienced therapists. *Occ Ther Health Care* 22(2-3):95–104, 2008.
34. Kielhofner G: *A model of human occupation: theory and application*, ed 4, Baltimore, 2008, Lippincott Williams & Wilkins.
35. Kielhofner G: *Conceptual foundations of occupational therapy*, ed 3, Philadelphia, 2004, FA Davis.
36. Kong KH, Chua KS, Tow AP: Clinical characteristics and functional outcome of stroke patients 75 years and older. *Arch Phys Med Rehabil* 79(12):1535–1539, 1998.
37. Langthaler M: *The components of a therapeutic relationship in occupational therapy*, Unpublished master's thesis, Medford, MA, 1990, Tufts University.
38. Law M, Baptiste S, Carswell A, et al: *Canadian Occupational Performance Measure*, ed 4, Toronto, 2005, CAOT Publications Ace.
39. Lyons KD, Crepeau EB: The clinical reasoning of an occupational therapy assistant. *Am J Occup Ther* 55(5):577–581, 2001.
40. Mattingly C: The narrative nature of clinical reasoning. In Mattingly C, Fleming MH, editors: *Clinical reasoning: forms of inquiry in a therapeutic practice*, Philadelphia, 1994, FA Davis.
41. Mattingly C: Occupational therapy as a two-body practice: the body as machine. In Mattingly C, Fleming MH, editors: *Clinical reasoning: forms of inquiry in a therapeutic practice*, Philadelphia, 1994, FA Davis.
42. Mattingly C: What is clinical reasoning? *Am J Occup Ther* 45(11):979–986, 1991.
43. Mattingly C: *Thinking with stories: stories and experience in a clinical practice*, Unpublished doctoral dissertation, Cambridge, MA, 1989, Massachusetts Institute of Technology.
44. Mattingly C, Fleming MH: *Clinical reasoning: forms of inquiry in a therapeutic practice*, Philadelphia, 1994, FA Davis.
45. Mattingly C, Gillette N: Anthropology, occupational therapy, and action research. *Am J Occup Ther* 45(11):972–978, 1991.
46. Neistadt ME: Teaching strategies for the development of clinical reasoning. *Am J Occup Ther* 50(8):676–684, 1996.
47. Neistadt ME: The classroom as clinic: applications for a method of teaching clinical reasoning. *Am J Occup Ther* 46(9):814–819, 1992.
48. Neistadt ME: Classroom as clinic: a model of teaching clinical reasoning in occupational therapy education. *Am J Occup Ther* 41(10):631–637, 1987.
49. Neistadt ME, Atkins A: Analysis of the orthopedic content in an occupational therapy curriculum from a clinical reasoning perspective. *Am J Occup Ther* 50(8):669–675, 1996.
50. Parton A, Husain M: Spatial neglect. *ACNR* 4(4):17–18, 2004.

51. Pedersen PM, Jorgensen HS, Nakayama H, et al: Hemineglect in acute stroke-incidence and prognostic implications: the Copenhagen stroke study. *Am J Phys Med Rehabil* 76(2):122–127, 1997.

52. Robertson LJ: Clinical reasoning, part 2: novice/expert differences. *Br J Occup Ther* 59(4):212–216, 1996.

53. Rogers JC: Eleanor Clarke Slagle Lectureship—1983; Clinical reasoning: the ethics, science, and art. *Am J Occup Ther* 37(9):601–616, 1983.

54. Rogers JC, Holm MB: Occupational therapy diagnostic reasoning: a component of clinical reasoning. *Am J Occup Ther* 45(11):1045–1053, 1991.

55. Rogers JC, Masagatani G: Clinical reasoning of occupational therapists during the initial assessment of physically disabled adults. *Occup Ther J Res* 2:195–219, 1982.

56. Schell BA, Cervero RM: Clinical reasoning in occupational therapy: an integrative review. *Am J Occup Ther* 47(7):605–610, 1993.

57. Schell BA, Schell J: *Clinical and professional reasoning in occupational therapy*, Philadelphia, 2008, Lippincott Williams & Wilkins.

58. Schell BA, Harris D: Embodiment: reasoning with the whole body. In Schell BA, Schell J, editors: *Clinical and professional reasoning in occupational therapy*, Philadelphia, 2008, Lippincott Williams & Wilkins.

59. Schell JW, Schell BA: Teaching for expert practice. In Schell BA, Schell J, editors: *Clinical and professional reasoning in occupational therapy*, Philadelphia, 2008, Lippincott Williams & Wilkins.

60. Schön DA: *Educating the reflective practitioner*, San Francisco, 1988, Jossey-Bass.

61. Schön DA: *The reflective practitioner: how professionals think in action*, New York, 1983, Basic Books.

62. Siegler CC: *Functions of humor in occupational therapy*, Unpublished master's thesis, Medford, MA, 1987, Tufts University.

63. Stanton S, Thompson-Franson T, Kramer C: Linking concepts to a process for working with clients. In Townsend E, editor: *Enabling occupation: an occupational therapy perspective*, Ottawa, 1997, Canadian Association of Occupational Therapists.

64. Strong J, Gilbert J, Cassidy S, et al: Expert clinicians' and students' views on clinical reasoning in occupational therapy. *Br J Occup Ther* 58(3):119–123, 1995.

65. Thomas SA, Wearing AJ, Bennett M: *Clinical decision making for nurses and health care professionals*, Sydney, Australia, 1991, Harcourt Brace Jovanovich.

66. Unsworth CA: *Cognitive and perceptual disorders: a clinical reasoning approach to evaluation and intervention*, Philadelphia, 1999, FA Davis.

67. Unsworth CA: Clinical reasoning of novice and expert occupational therapists. *Scand J Occup Ther* 8(4):163–173, 2001.

68. Unsworth CA: Using a head-mounted video camera to study clinical reasoning. *Am J Occup Ther* 55(5):582–588, 2001.

69. Unsworth CA: Clinical reasoning: How do worldview, pragmatic reasoning and client-centredness fit? *Br J Occup Ther* 67(1):10–19, 2004.

70. Unsworth CA: Using a head-mounted video camera to explore current conceptualizations of clinical reasoning in occupational therapy. *Am J Occup Ther* 59(1):31–40, 2005.

71. Unsworth CA, Warburg CL: Assessment and treatment planning strategies for cognitive and perceptual dysfunction. In O'Sullivan SB, Schmitz TJ, editors: *Physical rehabilitation: assessment and treatment*, ed 5, Philadelphia, 2006, FA Davis.

72. Van Belle HA: *Basic intent and therapeutic approach of Carl Rogers*, Burnaby, British Columbia, 1980, Academy Press, Wedge Publishing Foundation.

73. Valli L: *Reflective teacher education: cases and critiques*, Albany, NY, 1992, State University of New York Press.

74. Vining Radomsky M, Trombly Latham CA: *Occupational therapy for physical dysfunction*, ed 6, Baltimore, MD, 2007, Lippincott Williams & Wilkins.

75. Witherell C, Noddings N: *Stories lives tell: narratives and dialogue in education*, New York. 1991, Teachers College Press.

76. Wolters AM: On the idea of worldview and its relationship to philosophy. In Marshall PA, Griffioen S, Mouw R, editors: *Stained glass: worldviews and social science*, New York, 1989, University Press of America.

guðrún árnadóttir

chapter 18

Impact of Neurobehavioral Deficits on Activities of Daily Living

key terms

A-ONE
activities of daily living
activity analysis
agnosia
aphasia
areas of occupation
assessment methods
body functions

body neglect
client factors
clinical reasoning
context
deficit-specific approach
executive control functions
ideational apraxia
motor apraxia

neurobehavior
occupational performance
perseveration
praxis
spatial neglect
spatial relations
task analysis
top-down approach

chapter objectives

After completing this chapter, the reader will be able to accomplish the following:

1. Establish a relationship between neurobehavioral concepts and task performance.
2. Apply the theory on which the Árnadóttir OT-ADL Neurobehavioral Evaluation (A-ONE) is based as a structure for clinical observations of stroke patients.
3. Provide conceptual and operational definitions for neurobehavioral impairments and disability.
4. Apply clinical reasoning skills based on the A-ONE theory for hypothesis testing.
5. Relate the *International Classification of Functioning, Disability and Health and the Occupational Therapy Practice Framework*, 2nd Edition, to the concepts used in the A-ONE.
6. Provide examples of how strokes can cause different patterns of impairments affecting task performance.

Referrals to occupational therapy for patients who have had a stroke are usually made when the resulting impairments are suspected to affect activity performance. When neurobehavioral impairments result from a stroke, they can affect the performance of daily activities. This chapter contains discussions on the effect of neurobehavioral impairments on activity performance. Topics such as occupational performance, neurobehavior, function of the cerebral cortex, activity limitation, patterns of impairment resulting from different types of strokes, and application of clinical reasoning during assessment are discussed. However, before considering these issues, the following questions might be useful to consider: What are activities of daily living (ADL)? What is neurobehavior? What is neurobehavioral impairment? How is neurobehavior related to activity performance? How is the effect of neurobehavioral impairments on activity performance detected?

ACTIVITIES OF DAILY LIVING

ADL are defined by the U.S. Department of Health and Human Services[72] as basic daily activities such as eating, grooming, toileting, and dressing. The Center for Disease Control and Prevention refers to ADL as "bathing or showering, dressing, eating, getting in or out of bed or chairs, using the toilet, including getting to the toilet, and getting around inside the home."[25] The *Occupational Therapy Practice Framework: Domain and Process*, 2nd Edition (Framework-II),[4] defines ADL as activities "that are oriented toward taking care of one's own body." These activities include, similarly to the definitions mentioned previously, bathing or showering, bowel and bladder management, dressing, eating, feeding, functional mobility, personal hygiene and grooming, and toilet hygiene. Thus all three definitions agree on characterizing ADL as self-care tasks and functional mobility. Additionally personal device care and sexual activity are included in the Framework's definition of ADL. To locate ADL within the whole domain of occupational therapy, ADL are classified as one of eight areas of occupation, according to the Framework-II. The other seven areas of occupation are instrumental activities of daily living (IADL): rest and sleep, education, work, play, leisure, and social participation. In addition to areas of occupation, five other aspects of the domain of occupational therapy to which occupational therapists attend during the process of providing services are defined in the Framework-II. These are client factors, performance skills, performance patterns, contexts, environments, and activity demands.

Client factors, including body functions and structures, values, beliefs and spirituality, are the foundation of human performance, according to the Framework-II. These fundamental factors residing from within the individual are required for successful performance of different tasks. The eight main groups of body functions in the Framework-II based on the *International Classification of Functioning, Disability and Health (ICF)*,[77] a document developed by the World Health Organization, include a group of mental functions (affect, cognition, perception) divided into global functions and specific functions; a group of sensory functions and pain; neuromusculoskeletal and movement-related functions; cardiovascular, hematological, immunological, and respiratory functions; voice and speech functions; digestive, metabolic, and endocrine functions; genitourinary and reproductive functions; and functions of skin and related structures. Each of these groups can be subdivided into smaller units or factors. Table 18-1 shows important aspects of the domain of occupation as presented in the Framework-II, in view of the main themes of this chapter—neurobehavior and ADL—and relates the Framework's terminology to the classification systems of the ICF and items used in the Árnadóttir OT-ADL Neurobehavioral Evaluation (A-ONE).[6] The A-ONE has more recently been referred to as the ADL-focused Occupation-based Neurobehavioral Evaluation.[12,14]

The ICF describes two parts: functioning and disability, and contextual factors. Each of these parts has two components. Functioning and disability includes the components of body structures and body functions referring to anatomical parts of the body and functioning of body structures that can become impaired; activities (referring to execution of task or activity by an individual) and participation (involvement in a live situation), thus referring to capacity and performance that can become limited or restricted; and environmental factors that can act as facilitators and barriers of performance.[77] As can be seen in Table 18-1, the ICF does not differentiate between activity and participation, nor does it use the terms ADL and IADL tasks. Rather, what has been referred to as ADL earlier in this section spans several terms classified under activities and participation, i.e., self-care tasks, mobility, and communication.

NEUROBEHAVIOR: THE PROCESS OF LINKING OCCUPATION TO NEURONAL ACTIVITY

According to Árnadóttir,[10,17] neurobehavior is defined as behavior based on neurological function. Neurobehavior can be linked to occupation (defined as a series of actions in which one is engaged)[35] and occupational performance (defined as accomplishment of selected activity resulting from the dynamical transaction among the person, context, and activity in the Framework-II),[4] as elements of neurobehavior include different types of sensory stimuli evoked by different tasks. These stimuli are processed by different mechanisms of the central nervous system (CNS) and result in different types of behavioral responses. Feedback

Text continued on p.462

Table 18-1

Comparison of Terms Used in Different Classifications Systems

FRAMEWORK-II	ICF	A-ONE

Areas of occupation
■ Activities of daily living*
  ■ Dressing*
  ■ Personal hygiene and grooming*
  ■ Personal device care
  ■ Toilet hygiene*
  ■ Bathing, showering*
  ■ Bowel and bladder management
  ■ Functional mobility*
  ■ Eating*
  ■ Feeding*
  ■ Sexual activity
■ Instrumental activities of daily living
■ Rest and sleep
■ Education
■ Work
■ Play
■ Leisure
■ Social participation
	Activities and participation
	■ Self-care*
	  ■ Dressing*
	  ■ Washing*
	  ■ Caring for body parts*
	  ■ Toileting*
	  ■ Eating*
	  ■ Drinking*
	  ■ Looking after one's health
	■ Communication*
	■ Mobility*
	  ■ Changing and maintaining body position*
	  ■ Changing, moving, and handling objects
	  ■ Walking and moving*
	  ■ Moving around using transportation
	■ Domestic life areas
	■ Interpersonal interactions and relationships
	■ Major life areas
	  ■ Education
	  ■ Work and employment
	  ■ Economic life
	■ Community, social, and civic life
	■ General tasks and demands
	■ Learning and applying knowledge purposeful sensory experiences
	■ Activity limitation
	■ Participation restriction
		Activity performance; activities of daily living (ADL)*
		■ Dressing
		  ■ Put on shirt/upper body garments
		  ■ Put on pants
		  ■ Put on socks
		  ■ Put on shoes
		  ■ Manipulate fastenings
		■ Grooming and hygiene
		  ■ Wash face and upper body
		  ■ Comb hair
		  ■ Shave beard/apply cosmetics
		  ■ Brush teeth
		  ■ Perform toilet hygiene
		  ■ Bathe or shower
		■ Transfers and mobility
		  ■ Sit up in bed
		  ■ Transfers from sitting
		  ■ Maneuver around
		  ■ Transfer to toilet
		  ■ Transfer to tub
		■ Feeding
		  ■ Drink from glass/cup
		  ■ Use fingers to bring food to mouth
		  ■ Bring food to mouth by fork or spoon
		  ■ Use knife to cut and spread
		■ Communication
		  ■ Comprehension
		  ■ Expression
		
		Activity limitation: errors in task performance and possible limitation/restriction of independence resulting in required assistance
		■ Supervision needed during task performance
		■ Verbal assistance needed during task performance
		■ Physical assistance needed during task performance

Performance skills
■ Motor and praxis skills
■ Sensory-perceptual skills
■ Emotional regulation skills
■ Cognitive skills
	Activities and participation
	■ Learning and applying knowledge
	  ■ Basic learning
	  ■ Applying knowledge
		Observed and used in reasoning about body functions and their effect on activity performance, but not specifically addressed as items
		
		Addressed in comments but not labeled in a standardized way

Performance patterns
- Routines
- Roles
- Habits
- Rituals

Context and environment
- Environment
  - Physical
  - Social
- Context
  - Cultural
  - Personal
  - Temporal
  - Virtual

Client factors (based on ICF; see next column)
- Body functions*
- Body structures

Activities, participation, and personal contextual factors
- General tasks and demands (routines)
- Habits included under personal factors and not classified in ICF
- Limited participation

Contextual factors
- Environmental factors
  - Physical environment
  - Social environment
  - Attitudinal environment
- Personal factors

Body functions*
- Neuromusculoskeletal and movement-related functions:
- Functions of joints and bones
- Muscle functions*
  - Power (strength)
  - Tone (flaccid/spastic)
  - Endurance
- Movement functions*
  - Motor reflex
  - Involuntary movement reaction (righting and supporting reactions)
  - Control of voluntary movement (eye-hand coordination, bilateral integration, eye-foot coordination)
  - Involuntary movement functions (tremors, ticks, motor perseveration)
  - Gait pattern functions

Habits and routines are noted and used in reasoning about body functions, but not specifically addressed as items

Contextual factors
- Environmental factors: their influence on activity performance is considered and helping aids used are listed.
- Personal factors considered for ADL:
  - Age
  - Gender
  - Social Background
  - Profession

Central nervous system function
- Motor function

Addressed in comments but not labeled specifically

Contextual restrictions
- Environmental factors and possible restrictions are considered and listed.
- Personal factors considered and listed during ADL performance:
  - Age
  - Gender
  - Profession
  - Social background

Neurobehavioral dysfunction/impairments
- Motor dysfunction
  - Diminished strength
  - Altered tone: spasticity/rigidity/flaccidity
  - Athetosis, tremor, or
  - Involuntary movements
  - Motor perseverations
  - Motor impersistence
  - Dysarthria

Continued

Table 18-1

Comparison of Terms Used in Different Classifications Systems—cont'd

FRAMEWORK-II	ICF	A-ONE
	Sensory functions* and pain • Proprioception • Touch/temperature • Seeing (visual acuity, visual fields) • Hearing • Vestibular • Taste • Smell • Pain	Sensory reception and simple gnosis • Tactile • Proprioceptive/kinesthetic • Visual • Auditory **Agnosia** • Astereognosis • Visual agnosia • Auditory agnosia related to comprehension
	Mental functions (affective, cognitive, perceptual) Global mental function: • Consciousness* • Orientation (to person, place, time, self, and others)* • Sleep • Temperament and personality* • Energy and drive (motivation,* impulse control,* interests,* values)	General performance • Alertness • Orientation is considered under memory and topographical disorientation • Initiative • Motivation • Temperament and personality are considered in relation to emotional functions **Impaired general performance** • Impaired alertness • Impaired initiative • Impaired motivation
	Specific mental function: • Attention*	• Attention **Attention and arousal dysfunctions** • Impaired alertness • Altered attention • Distractibility • Performance latency
	• Memory*	• Memory **Memory dysfunction** • Working and short-term memory • Long-term memory • Orientation • Confabulation
	Mental functions of sequencing complex movement (praxis)*	• Praxis • Ideation • Sequencing and timing of activity steps • Programming of motor movement **Apraxia** • Ideational apraxia • Motor apraxia • Impaired organization and sequencing of activity steps

- Perception*
  - Spatial relations
    - Foreground/background
    - Depth/distances
    - Body scheme
      - Spatial relations dysfunction
      - Spatial relations impairment
      - Topographic disorientation
      - Body scheme dysfunction
      - Anosognosia
      - Somatoagnosia
      - Unilateral body neglect
  - Auditory agnosia
- Thought* (recognition, categorization, generalization, awareness of reality, logical/coherent thought, appropriate thought content)
- Higher-level cognition* (judgment, insight, abstraction, organization and planning, concept formation, time management, problem solving)
  - Higher cognitive and executive functions
    - Judgment
    - Insight
    - Abstract thinking
      - Comprehension
      - Cognitive disturbances
      - Lack of judgment
      - Decreased insight
      - Concrete thinking
      - Confusion
- Calculation
- Psychomotor functions
- Experience of self and time functions
- Emotional functions
  - Emotional functions
    - Emotional disturbances
      - Apathy
      - Depression
      - Lability
      - Euphoria
      - Irritability
      - Aggression
      - Frustrations
      - Restlessness
- Mental functions of language* (reception and expression)
  - Language functions
    - Comprehension
    - Expression
      - Language dysfunction
      - Sensory (Wernicke's)
        - Aphasia
        - Jargon aphasia
        - Anomia
        - Paraphasia
      - Expressive (Broca's)
        - Aphasia
        - Dysarthria
- Voice and speech functions
  - Articulation functions
  - Fluency and rhythm of language functions
  - Alternative vocalization functions
- Impairments
- Body structures
- Nervous system*

*Item relates to A-ONE terminology.

From Árnadóttir G: A-ONE training course: lecture notes, Reykjavík, Iceland, 2009, Guðrún Árnadóttir. Material drawn from Occupational therapy practice framework: domain and process (2nd ed.), *Am J Occup Ther* 62(6):625–683, 2008; World Health Organization: The international classification of functioning, disability and health—ICF, Geneva, 2001, WHO; and *The brain and behavior: assessing cortical dysfunction through activities of daily living*, St Louis, 1990, Mosby. Selected samples related to occupational performance with a specific focus on activities of daily living and neurology.

A-ONE, Árnadóttir OT-ADL Neurobehavioral Evaluation; *FRAME WORK-II, Occupational Therapy Practice Framework; Domain and Process* 2nd Edition; *ICF*, International Classification of Functioning, Disability and Health.

from the responses affects new sensory stimuli."[6,9] Neurobehavior therefore includes the different types of pertinent neurological *body functions* necessary for performing different aspects of occupation. "All tasks provide sensory stimuli. Some functions relate to the reception of sensory stimuli, others to CNS processing of that information including for example different functions associated with perception, cognition, emotion, and praxis. Additional functions relate to different behavioral responses, such as affect and movement. The mechanism of nervous-system processing and neurobehavior leading to occupational performance is a complex interaction where different combinations of factors are involved depending on the task."[6,9,17] Fig. 18-1 illustrates the elements of neurobehavior. A *neurobehavioral deficit* has been defined by Árnadóttir[6,17] as a functional impairment of an individual manifested as defective task performance resulting from a neurological processing dysfunction that influences body functions such as affect, body scheme, cognition, emotion, gnosis, language, memory, motor movement, perception, personality, praxis, sensory awareness, spatial relations, and visuospatial skills. Árnadóttir[10,17] further defined occupational error as any deviations from flawless responses when performing occupation. Indications of neurobehavioral impairments that limit ADL task performance are based on detection of occupational errors through task analysis of the observed ADL performance. The observed errors are subsequently classified and scored by use of operational definitions of neurobehavioral impairments included in the A-ONE test manual.

DETECTING THE EFFECT OF NEUROBEHAVIORAL DEFICITS ON ACTIVITY PERFORMANCE

The therapist can detect occupational errors through observation of occupational performance, with these errors indicating the effect of neurobehavioral deficits on task performance. Subsequently, the therapist can hypothesize about the impaired body functions that caused the error. As neurobehavioral deficits often interfere with independence, therapists can benefit from detecting errors in occupational performance while observing ADL and thereby gain an understanding of the impairments affecting the patient's activity limitation.

Therapists can use the information based on observed task performance in a systematic way as a structure for clinical reasoning to help them assess functional independence related to the performance and to subsequently detect impaired neurological body functions. Such information can be important when intervention methods are aimed at addressing occupational errors[6] during any of the following types of intervention programs classified by Fisher[36] as adaptive, acquisitional, and restorative occupation, or occupation-based education programs, i.e., programs for families or caregivers of persons with neurological impairments. This method therefore allows the therapist to analyze the nature or cause of a functional problem that requires occupational therapy intervention, as recommended by Holm and Rogers,[42,60] and so make the analysis from the view of occupations.

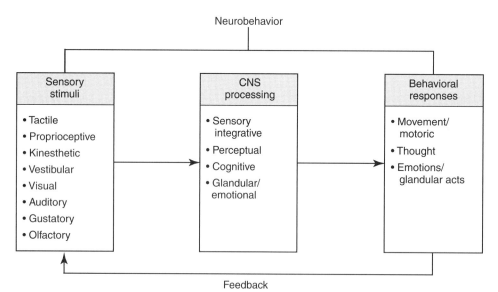

Figure 18-1   Elements of neurobehavior include different types of sensory stimuli. These stimuli are processed by different mechanisms in the central nervous system (CNS) and result in different types of behavioral responses. Feedback from the responses affects new sensory stimuli. (Adapted from Llorens LA: Activity analysis: agreement among factors in a sensory processing model. *Am J Occup Ther* 40(2):103, 1986.)

The use of different terms and definitions related to "analysis" in the field of occupational therapy is rather inconsistent and can lead to confusion. The following definitions were in mind when writing this chapter. Activity analysis has commonly been referred to as the process of examining activities in detail by breaking them into their components in order to understand and evaluate the activity. Therapists study body functions that are needed to perform specific tasks and the effects impaired body functions have on task performance.[6,46] Activity analysis can be based on particular theories and conceptual frameworks or focused on specific body functions.[27,70] Performance analysis is defined by Fisher[36] as the "observational evaluation of the quality of a person's occupational performance" taking into account how effectively the goal directed actions are performed. Task analysis, on the other hand, refers to interpretation of cause be it related to body functions, context, or environmental factors. Latham[70] discussed performance focused activity analysis. The therapist in this analysis observes the person perform role related occupations. The role includes tasks that are divided into several activities that are subsequently separated into actions that are based on capacities. Performance focused activity analysis examines these from the top-down by observing the person perform.

When applying the A-ONE principles to evaluate occupational performance and subsequently dysfunctional body functions that limit the performance, the therapist applies different types of clinical reasoning, according to Árnadóttir.[7,17] These are interactive reasoning, as interaction between the client and therapist takes place; and procedural reasoning,[51] which is also termed *diagnostic*[42,60] or *scientific reasoning*[23] and refers to hypothesis formation following interpretation of cues about the nature of problems that interfere with occupational performance. When using the A-ONE, the therapist observes performance of an ADL task and while classifying level of assistance needed identifies observed errors in performance. The errors can subsequently be used in the clinical reasoning process required for analyzing the task, as they can contribute to hypotheses about different impairments and possible manifestations of CNS dysfunction. They are used to help identify the cause of the dysfunction. During the instrument development of the A-ONE, information based on neurologically focused activity analysis, used to determine which body functions are necessary for performance of the ADL tasks and task analysis based on behavioral observations of persons with neurological dysfunctions, were used to operationalize impairments. The analyses were performed to determine how dysfunction of specific neurological body functions is revealed by neurobehavioral responses and occupational errors during performance of activities. For clinical reasoning during the A-ONE focused task analysis, the therapist keeps in mind different possible neurological body functions and

impairments and the theoretical definitions of functional and dysfunctional behavior. An example might explain this process better. A meaningful task, such as eating, calls for a goal directed, purposeful response. Various context and environmental factors are involved, such as food and cutlery, and body functions such as visuospatial relationships, muscle tone, and emotional state. Carrying out the behavior required to eat requires different body functions. When analyzed with the required factors in mind, the quality of the response reveals information not only about independence in ADL but also regarding neurobehavioral impairments—the problems that interfere with independence, such as misjudging distances when reaching out for a cup or not knowing how to use cutlery[6] (Fig. 18-2).

Function of the Cerebral Cortex: The Foundation of Task Performance

Occupational therapists observe performance of daily activities regularly as they work with stroke survivors. With the use of clinical reasoning combined with task analysis, detection of impaired neurological body functions is possible. These functions are necessary for optimal task performance. Subsequently, therapists can detect the type and degree of severity of neurobehavioral impairments that interfere with activity performance. For forming hypotheses from ADL observation and errors affecting performance, the therapist commonly draws on his or her neurological knowledge and relates the body functions to functional areas of the brain responsible for different neuronal processing functions. Many body functions are based on neurological function, which takes place at different levels of the CNS. According to Árnadóttir,[6] several CNS areas may contribute to a particular type of neuronal processing, resulting in simultaneous or parallel processing at different locations, which contributes to the development of the same body functions. During activity performance, different types of processing may take place simultaneously. Neuronal processing in the brain varies in complexity. It is common to view three levels of functional complexity in the cortex based on Luria's theories,[47,48] which are usually called *primary, secondary,* and *tertiary cortical zones* or *projection areas.*

Functional Localization for Neurological Processing of Body Functions

During task analysis, the therapist draws on information about neurological functions in the clinical reasoning process when forming and testing hypotheses about impaired functions; a short summary of functional localization follows. Fig. 18-3 illustrates location of different cortical areas, the shades indicating primary, secondary, and tertiary projection areas. The frontal lobes are responsible for motor functions, including motor speech; motor praxis; emotions; intelligence; cognition including attention and working memory; and executive control functions such as

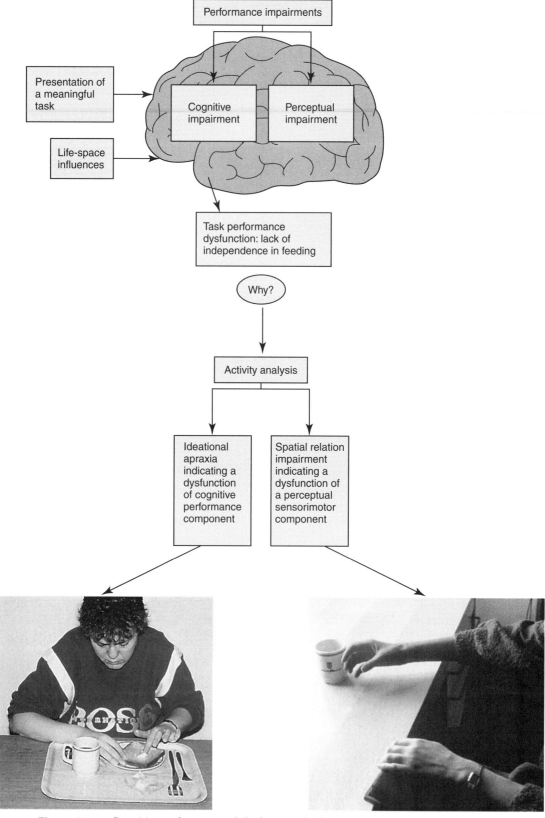

Figure 18-2   Cognitive and perceptual dysfunction leading to ideational apraxia and spatial relations impairment revealed by performance errors observed during feeding and detected by task analysis. (Adapted from Árnadóttir G: *The brain and behavior: assessing cortical dysfunction through activities of daily living,* St Louis, 1990, Mosby.)

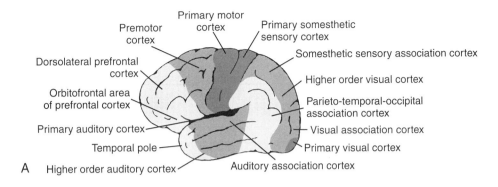

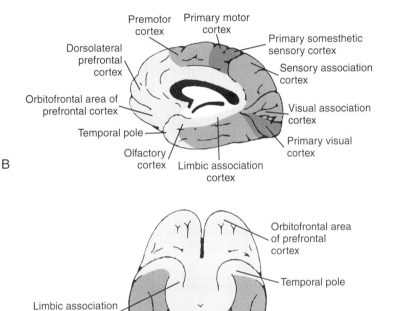

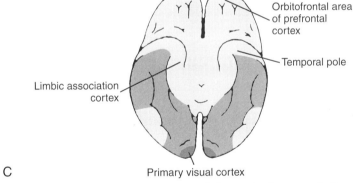

Figure 18-3 Functional organization of the cerebral cortex. **A,** Lateral surface. **B,** Medial surface. **C,** Inferior surface. The different shades refer to primary, secondary, and tertiary functional areas of the cortex. The darkest shades are primary areas, the medium shades are secondary areas, and the lightest shades are tertiary areas. (From Árnadóttir G: *The brain and behavior: assessing cortical dysfunction through activities of daily living*, St Louis, 1990, Mosby.)

ideation, intention, judgment, and motivation. This refers to neuromusculoskeletal and movement-related functions, including muscle and movement functions, according to the ICF terminology; voice and speech functions; and global and specific mental functions. The parietal lobes are concerned with the processing of somesthetic information—and more complex sensory input from different sources, which includes sensory reception of somesthetic information—and specific mental functions related to memory and sequencing of complex movement and to perception and emotional functions, according to the ICF. The occipital lobes process visual information (i.e., visual sensory functions and specific mental functions related to visual perception), and the temporal lobes process auditory information and long-term memory, emotion, and motivation. These functions are classified by the ICF as sensory functions of hearing, voice, and speech functions; global mental functions of temperament and personality; and specific mental functions of memory, perception of hearing, and emotional functions. Table 18-2 summarizes the functions of the different cortical lobes of the brain and relates them to primary, secondary, and tertiary functional areas in these lobes. As indicated in the table, several functional areas in different lobes may contribute to a

Table 18-2

Functions of the Cerebral Cortex

FUNCTIONAL AREA	ANATOMICAL AREA	NEUROLOGICAL BODY FUNCTIONS
Frontal lobes		
Primary motor area	■ Precentral gyrus	■ Execution of movement
Secondary association area	■ Premotor cortex ■ Frontal eye field ■ Broca's area in the left inferior frontal gyrus ■ Supplementary motor area	■ Planning and programming of movement ■ Sequencing, timing, and organization of movement ■ Voluntary eye movements ■ Programming of motor speech ■ Intention of movement
Tertiary association area	■ Orbitofrontal and dorso-lateral prefrontal cortex	■ Ideation ■ Concept formation ■ Abstract thought ■ Intellectual functions ■ Sequencing, timing, and organization of action and behavior ■ Initiation and planning of action ■ Judgment ■ Insight ■ Intention ■ Attention ■ Alertness ■ Personality ■ Working memory ■ Emotion
Parietal lobes		
Primary somesthetic sensory area	■ Postcentral gyrus	■ Fine touch sensation, proprioception, kinesthesia
Secondary somesthetic sensory association area	■ Superior parietal lobule	■ Coordination, integration, and refinement of sensory input ■ Tactile localization and discrimination ■ Stereognosis
Tertiary association area	■ Inferior parietal lobule	■ *Gnosis*: recognition of received tactile, visual, and auditory input ■ *Praxis*: storage of programs or visuokinesthetic motor engrams or praxicons necessary for motor sequences ■ *Body scheme*: postural model of body, body parts, and their relation to the environment ■ *Spatial relations*: processing related to depth, distance, spatial concepts, position in space, and differentiation of foreground from background
Occipital lobes		
Primary visual sensory area	■ Calcarine fissure	■ Visual reception (from the opposite visual field)
Visual association area	■ Brodmann areas 18 and 19	■ Synthesis and integration of visual information ■ Perception of visuospatial relationships ■ Formation of visual memory traces ■ Prepositional construction of language comprehension and speech

Table 18-2

Functions of the Cerebral Cortex—cont'd

FUNCTIONAL AREA	ANATOMICAL AREA	NEUROLOGICAL BODY FUNCTIONS
Temporal lobes		
Primary auditory sensory area	■ Superior temporal gyrus	■ Auditory reception
Secondary association area	■ Superior and middle temporal gyri (Wernicke's area)	■ Language comprehension ■ Sound modulation ■ Perception of music ■ Auditory memory
Tertiary association area	■ Temporal pole, parahippocampus	■ Long-term memory ■ Learning of higher-order visual tasks and auditory patterns ■ Emotion ■ Motivation ■ Personality
Limbic lobes		
Tertiary association area	■ Orbitofrontal cortex in frontal lobe, temporal pole, and parahippocampus in the temporal lobe ■ Cingulate gyrus in frontal and parietal lobes	■ Attention ■ Motivation ■ Emotions ■ Long-term memory

Adapted from Árnadóttir G: *The brain and behavior: assessing cortical dysfunction through activities of daily living,* St Louis, 1990, Mosby.

particular neurological function. Therefore, different cortical areas may be responsible for processing particular neurological body functions. Although function can be related to different anatomical areas, one must remember that plasticity permits deviations from the usual localization sites under certain conditions such as injury or developmental abnormality.

When considering CNS localization of body functions necessary for task performance, the therapist must keep in mind that the cortex does not function in isolation. The cortex communicates by various pathways with other CNS areas such as the thalamus, the basal ganglia, cerebellum, and brainstem that also contribute to neuronal processing.

Processing of Praxis

Although certain neurological functions can be assigned to specific cortical or subcortical locations within lobes, several CNS areas help process particular neurological body functions. Árnadóttir[6] summarized neurological information resulting in several processing models indicating processing sites of different functions in the cortex. One example is the processing model for praxis. Praxis takes place in two steps:[18] ideation, referring to concept formation related to an activity and classified by the ICF as specific mental function related to thought and higher level cognition including sequencing of complex movement; and planning and programming of

movement, which can be related to the neuromusculoskeletal and movement-related functions of the ICF. The result of praxis is motor execution. The ideation involved in praxis requires function of the frontal lobes (prefrontal and premotor areas) and of areas around the lateral fissure. The formulas for movement (praxicons) are stored in the left inferior part of the parietal lobe,[40] the left hemisphere in general being superior in storing routinely used codes.[39] Access to the left inferior parietal lobe is needed for either side of the body to move. Information flows from this area to the premotor area, which programs movement before the information is conveyed to the primary motor cortex in the left hemisphere (which controls execution of movements of the right side of the body). The premotor cortex on the left side connects with the premotor cortex of the right side by way of the anterior fibers of the corpus callosum and in turn relays the visuokinesthetic motor information to the right hemisphere. The right premotor cortex programs movements and instructs the adjacent primary motor cortex on the execution of movement of the left side of the body (Fig. 18-4).

PROCESSING DURING TASK PERFORMANCE

Motor praxis (as described previously) is only one type of neurological body function related to neurobehavior. The type of body function and the degree of involvement

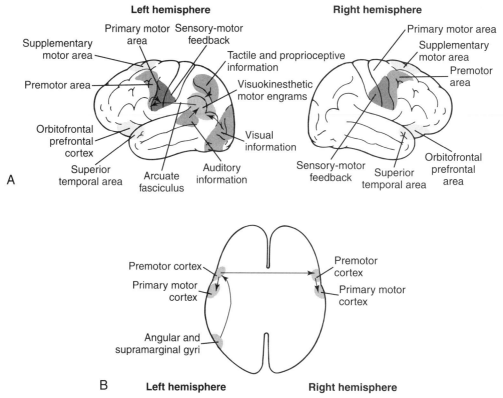

Figure 18-4   Processing of motor praxis. **A,** Active functional areas of the left and right hemispheres during praxis. **B,** Transverse view of the most commonly accepted sequential processing model of motor praxis.[40] (From Árnadóttir G: *The brain and behavior: assessing cortical dysfunction through activities of daily living,* St Louis, 1990, Mosby.)

depend on the task performed. As mentioned, several processing mechanisms may be involved simultaneously in the performance of a particular activity. Árnadóttir has demonstrated this through analysis of task such as brushing hair.[6] A person sitting in front of a mirror by a sink where the brush is located has at least three routes by which sensory information related to this particular task will reach the cortex. The person notes the brush visually, and this information travels through the visual pathway to the primary visual cortex where it is synthesized and further analyzed by the association areas. Memories and ideational processes are brought into play; as a result, the person gets the idea to want to brush the hair. Similarly, when the person is instructed verbally to brush the hair, this auditory input travels over the auditory pathway to the primary auditory area of the cortex in the temporal lobe where it is processed by the association areas. Subsequently, the input is compared with information in memory stores, yielding an idea based on the auditory information. The third pathway is somesthetic. A person who grasps or is handed a brush receives tactile and proprioceptive information, which (after it reaches the primary sensory cortex in the parietal lobe) is analyzed by the association areas and integrated with prior experiences.

Information from all three pathways travels from the pertinent primary receptive areas to secondary and tertiary areas where further processing takes place. Attention processes, memory processes, emotions, and higher-order thought are brought into play. The sensory information is integrated with previous experiences, and responses are planned. A response may be emotional or motoric, resulting in different processing mechanisms depending on the nature of the response. Simultaneous processing of information takes place as information from the different secondary association areas is fed into the limbic system, the tertiary association areas in the prefrontal lobe, and the temporal pole, where higher cognitive functions including emotion and memory take place. Different fiber connections in a hemisphere, between hemispheres, and between the cortex and other CNS structures play important roles in this processing.

During processing, ideation, intent to perform an action, and preparation of a sequenced plan of action occur; all result in flow of information to the primary motor cortex and ultimately in the functional response of picking up the brush. This process requires praxis. The intention to perform an action is relayed to the frontal lobes and supplementary motor areas. From the lower left parietal lobe (which houses movement formulas also called visuo-kinesthetic motor engrams or, more recently, praxicons), information travels to the left premotor cortex (which is responsible for planning and sequencing of movement) on its way to the middle part of the primary motor cortex of the frontal lobe in the left hemisphere (which is responsible for movement performed by the right hand). A series of feedback movement interactions and readjustments follow. This series is based on continuous sensory information from the activity. During the complex process of performing "simple" activity, other responses (e.g., emotional and verbal) may be elicited. Such responses require function of processing areas different from the ones mentioned previously. Fig. 18-5 illustrates some of the processing components that take place during the activity of brushing hair. Observation of task performance that results from this kind of neuronal processing and analysis of the errors detected by observation during the performance may reveal substantial information about function and subsequent dysfunction of the cerebral cortex. Therapists' neurological knowledge is important and needs to be incorporated into their clinical reasoning when forming hypotheses about impairments and differentiating between hypotheses.

DYSFUNCTION OF THE ACTIVITIES OF DAILY LIVING AREA OF OCCUPATION DUE TO STROKE

A stroke may affect neurological body functions. Dysfunction of these factors may interfere subsequently with primary ADL. Neurobehavioral impairments may be related to dysfunction of neurological body functions, which have been classified into four groups according to the ICF.[77] These groups are (1) neuromuscular functions, (2) sensory functions and pain, (3) mental functions, and (4) voice and speech functions. These functions have been related previously to concepts used in the A-ONE theory in Table 18-2. Concepts may be defined in two ways. Conceptual definition is general and abstract, but an operational definition refers to how particular concepts are measured and observed (e.g., test items with which particular concepts can be measured). The content of the following sections are based on concepts from the A-ONE.

Conceptual Definitions of Terms

The frontal lobes process functions related to neuromusculoskeletal and movement-related body functions including muscle and movement functions, according to the ICF terminology; voice and speech functions; and global and specific mental functions.[17] Dysfunction of the frontal lobes, for example, may affect neuromusculoskeletal body functions processed in the primary motor and premotor areas. Subsequently, the therapist may observe impairments

including paralysis of the contralateral body side, muscle weakness, and spasticity. The distribution of impairments is related to lesion localization in the primary motor cortex. Table 18-3 includes definitions of impairments or dysfunction of neurological body functions and relates these to different cerebral lobes.[6,17]

The parietal lobes process somatosensory and complex sensory information from multimodal stimuli. When a dysfunction of the parietal lobes occurs, impairments related to different functional areas may develop, and these can be related to dysfunctions of body functions, in particular somesthetic sensory functions and specific mental functions.[6] Dysfunction of the inferior parietal lobe, which processes information from the secondary association areas of all three posterior lobes, for example, may lead to impairments related to perceptual and motor processing of body functions, in particular specific mental functions related to sequencing of complex movement, memory, and perception. These impairments include bilateral motor- and ideational apraxia, if the left inferior parietal lobe is involved, because the movement formula or praxicons are stored in this area. Spatial relations disorders also may be present when the right hemisphere is involved. These disorders have been defined conceptually as difficulties in relating objects to each other or to the self. Such difficulties may include difficulties with foreground and background perception, depth and distance perception, perception of form constancy and perception of position in space. Further dysfunction of the right inferior parietal lobe may lead to body scheme disturbances including unilateral body neglect. Unilateral spatial neglect may also be present.[6] See Table 18-3 for definitions of terms and different lesion sites.

The occipital lobe houses primary and secondary processing areas for visual information. The tertiary area for visual processing is located mainly in the inferior parietal lobe. If a dysfunction of the occipital lobe occurs, impairments are related to visual sensory functions and specific mental functions related to perception of visual information referring to the ICF.[17] Lesions of the association area, for example, cause visual agnosia. Different types of visual agnosias exist, including visual object agnosia; visuospatial agnosia, which is a spatial relations disorder of visual origin; prosopagnosia; color agnosia; and associative visual agnosia.[6] Visual object agnosia is defined conceptually as the inability of a patient to recognize, name, or demonstrate use of objects seen and results from distorted visual perception, regardless of visual acuity.[65] The affected person can see and describe the components of the object but cannot recognize the object itself (see Table 18-3 for additional definitions of terms and lesion sites).[6]

The temporal lobes are involved with two types of processing—auditory and limbic—that can be related to sensory functions of hearing, voice and speech functions, global mental functions of temperament and personality,

Text continued on p.476

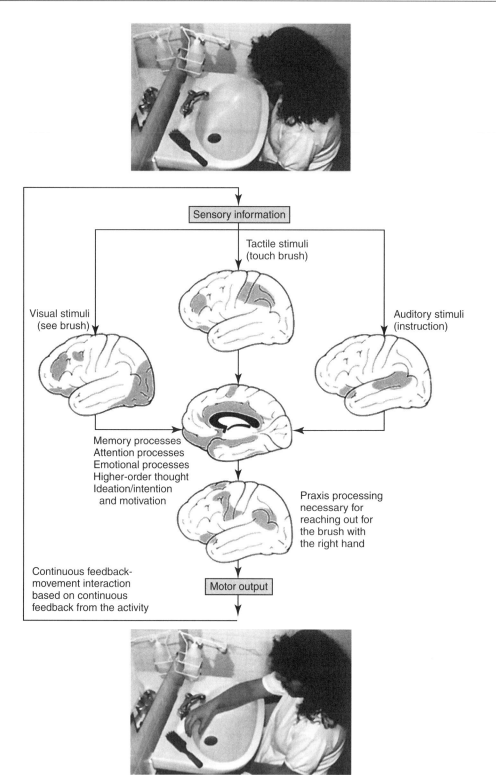

Figure 18-5 Different cortical areas involved in processing of various client factors during an activities of daily living task. A person sitting by a sink preparing for grooming is asked to brush her hair. Note that three types of sensory stimulation can lead to performance. (From Árnadóttir G: *The brain and behavior: assessing cortical dysfunction through activities of daily living*, St Louis, 1990, Mosby.)

Table 18-3

Cortical Impairments as Related to Anatomical Location and Definitions of Terms*

IMPAIRMENT AND CORTICAL LOCATION	CONCEPTUAL DEFINITION	OPERATIONAL DEFINITION
Anosognosia ■ Right inferior parietal lobule ■ Specific sensory thalamic nuclei, reticular formation, basal ganglia ■ Prefrontal and premotor frontal lobe[62]	■ Denial or lack of awareness of a paretic extremity accompanied by lack of insight regarding the paralysis ■ Paralyzed extremities may be referred to as objects or perceived out of proportion to other body parts.	■ Does not identify a paralyzed body part as own ■ May deny it completely as a separate object or recognize it and reject it (e.g., patient may complain about "somebody's" arm and not recognize it as own)
Apathy ■ Prefrontal cortex ■ Posterior internal capsule, basal ganglia[62] ■ Medial forebrain bundle and reticular formation	■ Shallow affect, psychomotor slowing, blunted emotional responses, lack of interest in the environment and inaction	■ Has a lack of emotion or feeling during activity performance and communication, lack of interest in things that generally are found exciting, and indifference during performance
Impaired attention ■ Prefrontal cortex, thalamus, reticular formation	■ Inability to attend to or focus on a specific stimulus ■ Possible distraction from presence of other irrelevant environmental stimuli ■ Inability to screen out irrelevant stimuli	■ Does not continue an activity ■ Does not attend to instruction or activity ■ Does not attend to mistakes ■ May focus attention on irrelevant details and not on global environment
Confabulations ■ Prefrontal cortex	■ Unconscious fabrication of stories or excuses to fill in memory gaps ■ May be within limits of reality or patient may not consider rules of reality and then will be identified easily ■ Associated with lack of inhibitions and lack of judgment, as well as memory problems	■ Does not remember what happened during weekend and comes up with an explanation not grounded in reality
Confusion ■ Prefrontal and diffuse dysfunction—bilateral ■ Thalamus and reticular formation	■ Lack of ability to think clearly, resulting in disturbed awareness and orientation regarding time, place, and person ■ Impaired interpretation of external environment and slowed responses to verbal stimuli[29] ■ Cognitive disturbance	■ Talks about past as present ■ Talks out of context ■ Not oriented to time and place
Depression ■ Left frontal lobe and left basal ganglia, right frontal and right parietal lobes[62]	■ Affective disorder manifested as sadness, hopelessness, or loss of general interest in usual performance ■ May be accompanied by loss of appetite, loss of energy, sleeping disorders, and feelings of worthlessness	■ Has sad affect or expression during activity performance

*Conceptual definitions of some common impairments seen in individuals with cerebrovascular accidents and examples of operational definitions from the A-ONE instrument. Relation of impairments to dysfunctional central nervous system areas is simplified. Adapted from Árnadóttir G: A-ONE training course: lecture notes, Reykjavík, Iceland, 2009-2010.

Continued

Table 18-3

Cortical Impairments as Related to Anatomical Location and Definitions of Terms—cont'd

IMPAIRMENT AND CORTICAL LOCATION	CONCEPTUAL DEFINITION	OPERATIONAL DEFINITION
Distractibility ■ Prefrontal cortex, reticular formation	■ Diversion of attention	■ Becomes distracted by environmental stimuli such as conversation in next room or somebody entering the room
Field dependency ■ Prefrontal cortex	■ Uninhibited, inadequate, and irrelevant stereotypical actions that replace selective goal directed actions corresponding to specific tasks ■ Impulsiveness related to elementary orienting reflex[49] ■ Field dependency thus has a dysfunction of an attention component and perseverative component.	■ Becomes distracted from particular task performance by specific stimuli (e.g., is washing hands, suddenly sees denture brush, and incorporates it into the hand-washing activity by scrubbing the hands with the denture brush) ■ Note two components of field dependency: distraction and perseveration.
Frustration ■ Prefrontal cortex, hypothalamus	■ An appearance of agitation and intolerance in behavior that may be manifested emotionally, verbally, or physically	■ Becomes excited or intolerant when trying hard to perform or unable to perform (may be manifested emotionally, verbally, or physically)
Homonymous hemianopsia ■ Primary visual cortex around calcarine fissure in either hemisphere	■ Loss of a visual hemifield contralateral to a cerebral lesion	■ Has visual field defect to visual field that is contralateral to a cerebral lesion ■ Is usually aware of deficit and tries to compensate for it by using head movements to scan both visual fields
Ideational apraxia ■ Prefrontal and premotor cortex in either hemisphere, left inferior parietal lobule, and corpus callosum	■ A breakdown of knowledge of knowing what is to be done to perform that results from loss of a neuronal model or a mental representation about the concept required for performance ■ Lack of knowledge regarding object use ■ Also refers to sequencing of activity steps or use of objects in relation to each other (NOTE: Therapist should rule out comprehension difficulties)	■ Does not know what to do with toothbrush, toothpaste, or shaving cream ■ Uses tools inappropriately (e.g., smears the toothpaste on face) ■ Sequences activity steps incorrectly so that there are errors in end result of tasks (e.g., puts socks on top of shoes)
Impaired initiative ■ Prefrontal cortex and supplementary motor cortex[28]—predominantly right hemisphere	■ Inability to initiate performance of an activity when need to perform is present	■ Sits without initiating an activity ■ Can describe activity performance but displays inertia in initiating it
Decreased insight ■ Prefrontal cortex	■ Insight—a discovery stage, with increasing awareness of the whole self ■ Decreased insight—lack of insight into personal condition and disability	■ Does not have insight into disease or disability ■ Does not make realistic statement regarding future plans ■ Makes unrealistic comments regarding disability

Deficit	Location	Definition	Impact on ADL
Irritability	Prefrontal cortex—particularly orbitofrontal cortex and hypothalamus	Excessive sensitivity to stimulation; Includes quick excitability manifested as annoyance, impatience, or anger	Appears annoyed; May verbally indicate dislike or be physically agitated out of proportion to stimulus that evoked behavior
Impaired judgment	Prefrontal cortex	Inability to make realistic decisions based on environmental information; Unable to make use of feedback from own errors	Does not turn off water taps after washing; Does not put brakes on wheelchair and makes unsafe transfers; Goes to dining room without dressing or combing hair; Does not care whether clothes are turned inside out or back to front, even when those facts have been pointed out
Lability	Prefrontal cortex	Pathological emotional instability; Alternating states of gladness and sadness, including inappropriate crying	Has mood swings; Cries or laughs inappropriately
Impaired motivation	Prefrontal cortex, particularly orbitofrontal cortex, medial forebrain bundle, and hypothalamus	Lack of willingness to perform, with or without a perceived need	Does not initiate or continue an activity unless really accepting the need, although physical ability to perform is present (e.g., does not attempt to eat at mealtimes and may refuse to participate in activity); Refuses to get up in morning or perform activities, although physically able to perform and has been motivated previously to perform by same activities
Motor apraxia	Premotor frontal cortex of either hemisphere, left inferior parietal lobe, corpus callosum, basal ganglia, and thalamus	Loss of access to kinesthetic memory patterns so that purposeful movement cannot be achieved because of defective planning and sequencing of movements, even though idea and the purpose of task are understood; Used as a synonym for ideomotor apraxia	Has difficulties related to motor planning (e.g., cannot sequence and plan movements necessary to adjust grasp on a hairbrush when moving it from one side of head to other to turn the bristles toward hair)
Impaired motor function	Primary motor cortex, anterior internal capsule, basal ganglia, thalamus, and cerebellum	Flaccidity, decreased strength, rigidity, spasticity, ataxia, athetosis, tremor	Has difficulty stabilizing objects such as containers that must be opened; Has difficulty reaching unaffected axilla when washing; Has difficulty dressing because of a paralyzed arm or inability to button because of tremor

Continued

Table 18-3

Cortical Impairments as Related to Anatomical Location and Definitions of Terms—cont'd

IMPAIRMENT AND CORTICAL LOCATION	CONCEPTUAL DEFINITION	OPERATIONAL DEFINITION
Impaired organization and sequencing ■ Prefrontal cortex	■ Inability to organize thoughts with activity steps properly sequenced (component of ideational apraxia but can occur separately as the first indication of impairment in a progressive disease process or last step of regressing ideational problems)	■ Has difficulties sequencing and timing steps of an activity ■ Does not complete one activity step before starting another (e.g., does not take off glasses before taking off a T-shirt with a tight neck hole; puts on shoes before putting on the trousers; washes too quickly, resulting in poor performance)
Paraphasia ■ Prefrontal cortex or left lateral temporal lobe	■ Expressive speech defect characterized by misuse or replacement of words or phonemes during active speech	■ Replaces words with incorrect similar or dissimilar words (e.g., may identify an apple as an orange because both are fruits)
Perseveration ■ Premotor and/or prefrontal cortex	■ Repeated movements or acts during functional performance as a result of difficulty in shifting from one response pattern to another ■ Refers inertia on initiation or termination of performance[47,48] ■ Prefrontal perseveration—repetition of whole actions or action components ■ Premotor perseveration—compulsive repetition of the same movement	■ Repeats movements or acts and cannot stop them once initiated (e.g., attempts to put on shirt without any progress—may pull a long sleeve up arm past wrist [premotor perseveration]; moves comb toward mouth instead of hair after having brushed teeth [prefrontal perseveration])
Restlessness ■ Prefrontal cortex	■ Uneasiness, impatience, inability to relax	■ May be impatient (e.g., cannot wait for therapist to start an activity) ■ May have trouble staying in one place during activity
Short-term memory loss ■ Limbic system and limbic association cortex in orbitofrontal areas or temporal lobes	■ Lack of registration and temporary storing of information received by different sensory memory modalities, be it somatosensory, auditory, or visual ■ Refers to working memory in that a person must keep different aspects in mind while working on different memory tasks such as reasoning, comprehension, and learning ■ Length of working or short-term memory depends on nature of assignments	■ Does not remember instructions throughout evaluation ■ May have to be reminded to comb hair several times

Term	Location	Definition	Impact on Activities of Daily Living
Somatoagnosia	Right inferior parietal lobule	■ Disorder of body scheme ■ Diminished awareness of body structure and failure to recognize own body parts and their relationship to each other[80] ■ Difficulty relating own body to objects in external environment	■ Puts legs into armholes or arms into legholes ■ Brushes mirror image of teeth instead of own teeth or washes mirror image of face instead of own face ■ Attempts to dress the therapists arm
Somesthetic sensory loss	Postcentral gyrus in either parietal lobe, posterior internal capsule, specific thalamic sensory nuclei	■ Loss of tactile sensation, proprioception, or kinesthesia	■ Has difficulty manipulating objects because of lack of sensation ■ Is aware of sensory loss and tries to compensate (e.g., using visual clues)
Spatial relations impairment	Usually right inferior parietal lobule	■ Difficulty relating objects to each other or to self ■ Synonymous with visuospatial agnosia when such difficulties are due to visuospatial impairment	■ Is unable to find armholes, legholes, or bottom of shirt ■ Pulls sleeve in wrong direction ■ Overestimates or underestimates distances when reaching for objects
Topographic disorientation	Inferior parietal lobule or occipital association cortex	■ Difficulty finding way in space due to amnestic or agnostic problems ■ Manifested as problems finding way in familiar surroundings or learning new routes	■ Does not know way to bedroom or bathroom
Unilateral body neglect	Inferior parietal lobule, right cingulate gyrus, prefrontal cortex, reticular formation, specific sensory thalamic nuclei; posterior internal capsule	■ Failure to report, respond, or orient to a unilateral stimulus presented to body side contralateral to a cerebral lesion ■ Can result from defective sensory processing or attention deficit, which causes ignorance or impaired use of extremities (used as a synonym for unilateral body inattention) ■ Usually affects left side of body	■ Does not dress affected body side ■ Does not pull shirt all the way down on affected side ■ Gets shirt stuck on affected shoulder and does not try to correct it or does not realize what is wrong
Unilateral spatial neglect	Inferior parietal lobule, right cingulate gyrus, prefrontal cortex, reticular formation, specific sensory thalamic nuclei; posterior internal capsule	■ Inattention to or neglect of visual stimuli presented in extrapersonal space of side contralateral to a cerebral lesion because of visual perceptual deficits or impaired attention[41] ■ It may occur independently of visual deficits or with hemianopsia[80] (synonymous with unilateral visual neglect)	■ Does not account for objects in visual field on affected side—usually left side ■ When moving, runs into furniture, doorways, or walls located in affected visual field

Courtesy G. Árnadóttir, Reykjavik, Iceland.

and specific mental functions of memory, perception of hearing, and emotional functions. The lateral sides of the hemispheres house primary and secondary processing sites for auditory stimuli and perceptual processing of such information. The tertiary processing area for these functions is located in the inferior part of the parietal lobe.[17] A lesion of the auditory association cortex in the left hemisphere, for example, can cause anomia because the memory stores for nouns are located in this area. Anomia is loss of the ability to name objects or retrieve names of persons; the person does have fluent speech. As previously mentioned, Table 18-3 relates defined impairments to dysfunction of different cortical and subcortical areas.

Manifestation of Neurobehavioral Impairments during Task Performance: Operational Definitions of Concepts

Operational definitions are how concepts are measured and observed. Following is a review based on Árnadóttir's operational definitions of terms[6] from the A-ONE regarding how one can detect neurobehavioral impairments during task performance in the areas of grooming and hygiene, dressing, functional mobility, and eating. Each of these performance areas comprises several tasks. For successful completion of each of the tasks, involvement of several neurological body functions is necessary. Dysfunction of body functions resulting in the previously defined impairments is manifested differently during performance. The following examples indicate the effect of different impairments on task performance manifested by occupational errors in the various performance areas. This review refers to the terms used in the classification systems of the *Framework* and the ICF (see Table 18-3 for conceptual and operational definitions of terms). Some impairments affect specific ADL areas. Other impairments are more pervasive and may appear in any ADL performance area or may need to be addressed specifically. One must keep in mind that behavior is flexible and neurobehavioral impairments are complex. The following behavioral examples are guidelines for detecting impairments. However, they cannot be taken for granted without knowledge of neurobehavior, cortical function, activity and task analysis, and clinical reasoning because similar behaviors may result from different impairments at times. Thus the behavior of not washing one arm during the task of washing the upper part of the body may be caused by unilateral body neglect when it occurs in an individual with right hemisphere dysfunction. However, an individual with left hemisphere dysfunction may need assistance to wash the affected arm, partly because of motor paralysis, and also may need guidance to wash the other arm and body parts because of ideation problems and difficulty in organizing and sequencing the activity steps of the task. The patient also may have comprehension difficulties, which complicates the situation. The behavior of not washing an arm

therefore may result from unilateral body neglect or ideational apraxia, depending on the situation. Therefore the following examples are to be used only as guidelines. Clinical reasoning and knowledge of neurobehavioral impairments and how the impairments group together in different diagnostic categories are crucial for effective differentiation and classification of impairments.

Personal Hygiene and Grooming Performance Area. Three activities listed in the Framework-II are included in the grooming and hygiene domain of the A-ONE: personal hygiene and grooming, toilet hygiene, and bathing or showering. The performance of grooming and hygiene activities comprises several tasks; for example, washing the face and body and bathing or showering; performing oral hygiene (including brushing teeth); combing hair; shaving; applying cosmetics, deodorants, or perfumes; and performing toilet hygiene. These tasks may be affected by dysfunction of different body functions, resulting in various behavioral outcomes. Dysfunction of neuromusculoskeletal and movement-related functions can result in paralysis, muscle weakness, and spasticity. Paralysis or muscle weakness may be manifested as difficulty in washing the affected arm or axilla (Fig. 18-6, *A*). The individual may need to learn to use one-handed techniques to overcome the impairment. Adapted equipment also may be needed for the individual to reach body parts such as the back or, if balance is poor, the feet. Stabilizing objects may be a problem; the individual may need a nonslip pad under the soap. While brushing teeth, the person may have problems opening the tube of toothpaste and may need to learn to compensate by stabilizing it between the knees or teeth. The same applies to other containers and the opening of lids. If the individual uses dentures, an adapted toothbrush or a suction brush for stabilization may be necessary (see Chapter 28).

Dysfunction of sensory functions can result in impaired tactile and proprioceptive sensation, astereognosis, or hemianopsia with a loss of a visual field, or a loss of part of a visual field may be present. Problems with tactile sensation, proprioception, or stereognosis affect object manipulation. An individual with such problems who does not suffer from inattention or neglect will be aware of the impairment and attempt to compensate for it (e.g., by using vision for sensory feedback). If a part of a visual field is defective or hemianopsia is present, an individual may have to compensate by turning the head. If an individual only has this impairment and not neglect, the individual will be aware of the problem and will be able to describe it, with insight into the dysfunction, and compensate for it.

Dysfunction of sequencing complex movement, classified as specific mental functions, can lead to motor apraxia and motor perseveration. Individuals with motor apraxia have difficulty with motor planning; they may have difficulty adjusting the grasp of a razor when moving from

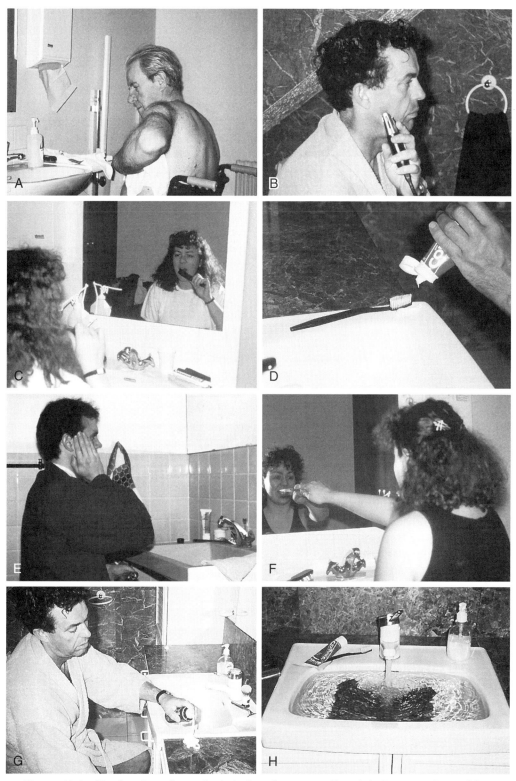

Figure 18-6 Dysfunction of neurological client factors manifested during grooming and hygiene tasks. **A,** Paralysis results in difficulty washing the affected axilla. **B,** Motor apraxia makes manipulation of razor difficult. **C,** Prefrontal perseveration, a part from the previous task of brushing the teeth, is perseverated during combing so that the comb is moved toward the mouth instead of the hair. **D,** Spatial relations impairment results in underestimation of distances when the individual attempts to place toothpaste on a toothbrush. **E,** Unilateral body inattention during shaving. Aftershave lotion spills from a bottle held in left hand while individual is reaching with right hand to face and looking into mirror. **F,** Somatoagnosia. Woman cannot differentiate between a mirror image and her own body when brushing her teeth. **G,** Ideational apraxia. Man does not know what to do with shaving cream. **H,** Lack of judgment. Water has been left running with the washcloth in the sink, producing a safety hazard.

one side of the face to another or when moving the razor to the chin. This requires sequencing and planning of fine finger and wrist movements so that the razor is turned toward the face for effective use (see Fig. 18-6, *B*). Similarly, motor apraxia may influence the ability to comb or brush hair. The performance may be adequate on the side where the individual starts brushing but when moving the brush to the other side of the head or to the back, the individual has difficulty adjusting the hand movements required to turn the brush toward the hair. Manipulating a toothbrush and other items may be similarly difficult and manifested as "clumsiness."

Premotor perseveration may be manifested as repetition of the movements of washing the face; the individual cannot stop the movements and take the washcloth to other body parts. Prefrontal perseveration is perseveration of whole acts. The affected individual, having completed one task such as brushing the teeth, begins another activity such as combing but perseverates a part of the previous action program. As a result, the individual approaches the mouth with the comb (see Fig. 18-6, *C*).

If a dysfunction of the perceptual processing aspect of the specific mental functions is present, a spatial relation disorder, difficulty with left-right discrimination, unilateral body inattention or neglect, unilateral visual inattention or neglect, anosognosia, or somatoagnosia may be expected. Spatial relation disorder may be manifested during hygiene and grooming tasks as difficulty in determining distances. An individual reaching for a toothbrush may overestimate or underestimate its distance. When the individual squeezes toothpaste onto the toothbrush, the paste may end up beside the brush (see Fig. 18-6, *D*). When trying to stabilize objects, the individual may reach next to the object, resulting in ineffective performance. For example, an individual may reach with the washcloth into the space next to the water faucet instead of under the faucet. When manipulating objects such as dentures, the individual may have problems determining the top from the bottom part of the dentures and the front from the back and left from right.

Impairments related to neglect or inattention can result from dysfunction of the specific mental function of perception or attention. In unilateral body neglect, or inattention, the individual does not use the affected limb according to available control. For example, the individual may not use the arm for stability while attempting to open a bottle. An individual with unilateral body neglect may not wash the affected side but washes other body parts systematically. The same may apply to other tasks as well, such as shaving and combing, in that the individual only attends to one side of the face or hair. A man holding an aftershave bottle in the left hand while looking at his own face in the mirror and reaching with the right hand to the face may tilt the bottle without noticing it and spill the liquid (see Fig. 18-6, *E*).

In unilateral spatial inattention or neglect, the individual randomly may locate all items in the affected visual field only when accidentally seeing them or may not notice an object at all in the affected visual field and does not systematically compensate for the impairment by rotating the head as required. An individual with somatoagnosia cannot differentiate between the mirror image and self. An individual thus affected may attempt to wash the mirror image of the face instead of the actual face (see Fig. 18-6, *F*). These individuals may not be able to differentiate between their own body parts and those of others. For example, an individual may grab another person's arm and attempt to use it to hold onto objects. *Somatoagnosia* is defined in the A-ONE as a severe dysfunction that usually is accompanied by ideational apraxia and often by spatial relation disorders.

Dysfunctions of global and specific mental functions with an effect on grooming and hygiene tasks include ideational apraxia, organization and sequencing problems related to activity steps, impaired judgment, decreased level of arousal, lack of attention, distraction, field dependency, impaired memory, and impaired intention. Ideational apraxia may appear during grooming and hygiene activities; an individual may not know what to do with the toothbrush, toothpaste, or shaving cream or may use these items inappropriately (e.g., smear toothpaste over the face or spray the shaving cream over the sink; (see Figure 18-6, *G*). An individual with organization and sequencing difficulties only may have the general idea of how to perform but may have problems timing and sequencing activity steps. Such a patient may not complete one activity step before starting another or may perform activities too quickly due to problems in timing activity steps, resulting in a poor performance.

Lack of judgment may appear as an inability to make realistic decisions based on environmental information, providing that perception of those impulses is adequate. An individual so affected may leave the sink area without turning off the water taps or may leave the wash cloth in the sink, not noticing that the water level is increasing and threatening to overflow (see Fig. 18-6, *H*).

Field dependency has an attention component and a perseveration component. Individuals with this dysfunction may be distracted from performing a particular task by specific stimuli that they are compelled to act on or incorporate into the previous activity. For example, if an individual with field dependency sees a denture brush while washing the hands, then that person may incorporate the brush into the activity and scrub the hands with the denture brush.

An individual with short-term memory problems may not remember the sequence of activity steps or instructions throughout activity performance. The therapist may have to remind an individual several times to comb the hair, even though the individual does not have comprehension problems.

Lack of initiation may occur during performance of grooming and hygiene tasks; the individual may sit by the sink without performing, even after being asked to wash. With repeated instructions to begin, the individual may indicate that the activity is about to start, yet nothing happens. After several such incidents and if the therapist asks for a plan, the individual may state a detailed plan of action in which the water will be turned on, the washcloth will be picked up and put under the running water, soap will be put on the cloth, and washing will begin. The individual has a plan of action but cannot start the plan. This impairment may be associated with ideational problems as well.

Dressing Performance Area. The dressing performance includes the tasks of dressing the upper part of the body, including putting on items such as underwear, T-shirts, pullovers, sweaters, shirts, bras, cardigans, or dresses; dressing the lower part, such as putting on pants, socks, pantyhose, and shoes; and manipulating fasteners, such as zippers, buckles, laces, or Velcro. Following are some examples of the effect of neurobehavioral impairments on task performance in this area. Dysfunction of neuromusculoskeletal and movement-related body function affecting this performance area can result in paralysis of a body side. Individuals with one-sided paralysis must learn one-handed dressing techniques (Fig. 18-7, *A*).

Dysfunction of the mental factor of sequencing complex movement can manifest as perseveration. Premotor perseveration may appear during dressing; the individual is unable to stop movements that have been initiated. For example, when the individual is placing an arm in a sleeve, the individual may keep pulling the arm into the sleeve until the end of the sleeve is up to the elbow or shoulder. Similarly the person may repeatedly pull up on a sock, even though it has already covered the foot (see Fig. 18-7, *B*).

Defective specific mental function factor of perception may result in spatial relation disorders such as difficulty figuring out the front and back, the inside and outside, and the top and bottom of an article of clothing. Although the individual knows that the shirt goes on the upper part of the body and tries to get the arm through the sleeve, the arm may go through the neckhole instead of the sleeve or in the right sleeve instead of the left. An individual may place both legs in the same leghole (see Fig. 18-7, *C*) or may not perceive that one of the legholes is turned inside out. Right-left disorientation can be related to visuospatial problems; for example, an individual may put the right

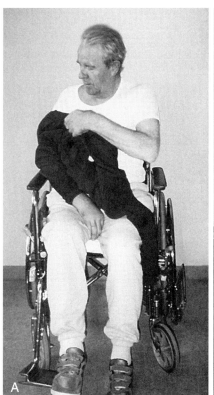
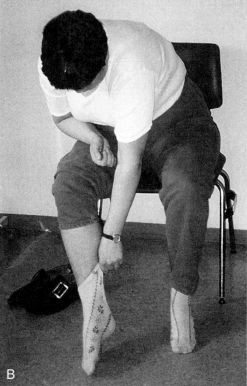

Figure 18-7 Dysfunction of neurological client factors manifested during dressing tasks. **A,** Paralysis requires use of one-handed dressing techniques. **B,** Premotor perseveration results in repetitions of movements so that the leghole may be pulled up to the knee; the patient pulls the sock repeatedly, although it is already in place.   *Continued*

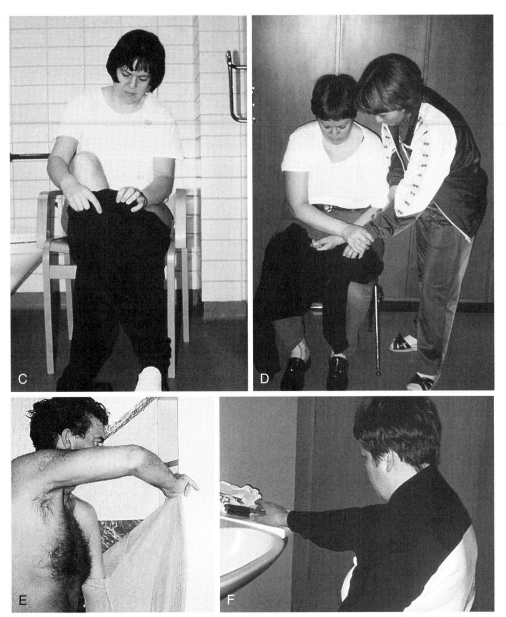

Figure 18-7, cont'd **C,** Spatial relations impairment, in which the patient places both legs in the same leghole. **D,** Somatoagnosia. Woman attempts to dress the therapist's arm instead of her own. **E,** Unilateral body neglect. Man attempts to hang up his gown without having undressed his left arm. **F,** Field dependency. The sight of a comb distracts a woman in the middle of a dressing task. Woman discontinues dressing and begins combing.

shoe on the left foot. An individual with spatial relation disorder may pull the sleeve in the wrong direction when attempting to put on a shirt. The individual may be unable to tie shoelaces because of difficulty handling the spatial relations aspects of manipulating shoestrings. Velcro fastenings on shoes may be folded back on themselves instead of being passed through the D-loop before being folded backward. Somatoagnosia may manifest as a patient attempting to dress a therapist's arm instead of his or her own (see Fig. 18-7, *D*) or when he or she attempts to

place his or her legs into the armholes of a shirt. Thus, the individual has problems with differentiating his or her own body from the therapist's body and relating objects to corresponding body parts. This is not only a spatial relation problem but also a defect in body image. An individual with only a visuospatial problem cannot find the correct armhole but realizes that a shirt is related to the upper body. This realization is not evident in individuals with somatoagnosia because of his or her body scheme dysfunction.

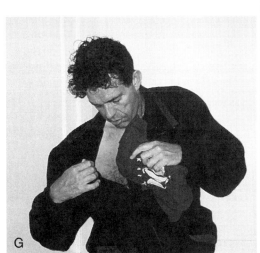
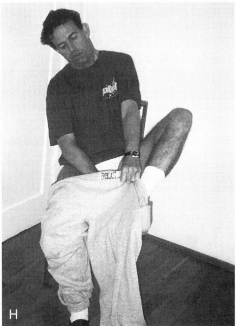

Figure 18-7, cont'd **G,** Ideational apraxia. Man knows that the T-shirt should go under the sweater but does not know how to accomplish the goal. **H,** Organization and sequencing impairment. Man puts on socks and shoes before trousers, resulting in difficulties donning trousers.

Unilateral body neglect may be severe, or less severe unilateral body inattention may be present. In severe cases an individual may not dress or undress the affected arm. The individual may even leave the arm in the armhole when undressing and attempt to hang the shirt on a clothes peg on the wall, not cognizant that the arm is still in the armhole (see Fig. 18-7, *E*). However, the problem is not always this severe or apparent. At times the shirt may get stuck on an affected shoulder without the individual noticing it, or the shirt may not be pulled properly down on the affected side. An individual with unilateral visual neglect or inattention may not put on clothes that are placed in the left visual field because they remain unnoticed.

Dysfunction of global and specific mental functions may be seen as field dependency, ideational problems, or impaired judgment. Field dependency is illustrated by an individual in the middle of the activity of putting on a sweater. Having placed both arms through the correct armholes and the neck through the neckhole, the patient is distracted by the sight of a comb. The activity of dressing subsequently is discontinued immediately as the individual grabs the comb and starts combing his or her hair. After combing, the individual may or may not go back to the task of putting on the shirt (see Fig. 18-7, *F*). A person might not know what to do with the clothes or how to put them on. A person with ideational apraxia may be able to perform certain activities automatically, such as putting on a sweater. Difficulty arises when the person realizes the T-shirt or undershirt has not been put on under the sweater. The individual may not be able to plan the necessary activity steps to correct the mistake. The T-shirt may be tucked down the neckhole instead of the sweater being removed and the activity started over (see Fig. 18-7, *G*). An individual with ideational apraxia also may attempt to put a sock on over a shoe. An individual who only has organization and sequencing problems might put shoes on before putting on trousers (see Fig. 18-7, *H*). However, the general ideas of how to put the clothes on and where they fit are intact. Organization and sequencing problems may appear when an individual dresses the unaffected arm before the affected one and then runs into difficulty dressing the affected arm. The therapist also may detect impaired judgment during dressing performance. An individual may be improperly dressed in the hallways or the dining area, indicating a lack of social judgment. Spatial relation disorder also may affect dressing performance. An affected individual may not be able to differentiate the front and the back of the clothes. Trousers may be put on with the front pockets and fastenings turned backward. Because these spatial relations deficits are of visual origin, the affected individual may not be able to identify the mistakes. However, when a therapist points out that the trousers are backwards, an individual with a lack of judgment might comment that it does not matter how the trousers are worn. A subject with intact judgment would attempt to make corrections, ask for assistance, or otherwise indicate a desire to have the performance corrected.

Functional Mobility Performance Area. The performance area of functional mobility includes the tasks of rolling over and sitting up in a bed, transferring to and from a bed, transferring to and from a chair, transferring to and from a toilet, transferring to and from a bathtub or a shower, and moving from one room to another. The previously defined impairments may interfere with the tasks of this performance area (see Chapter 14). Following are some examples of how these dysfunctions may be manifested.

If a dysfunction of the neuromusculoskeletal and movement-related functions, such as paralysis is present, it affects strength and control of one body side and thus affects mobility and balance. An individual therefore may need assistance with transfers, require a wheelchair or walking aids, or require supervision or personal assistance for mobility (Fig. 18-8, *A*).

Dysfunction of the specific mental functions of sequencing complex movement may lead to perseveration and motor apraxia as previously mentioned. Individuals with premotor perseveration may not be able to stop the movements of wheeling a wheelchair; as a result, they continue wheeling and moving after reaching the desired destination.

Dysfunctions of the specific mental functions perceptual factor may result in spatial relation disorders in which the affected individual may misjudge distances. The individual may park a wheelchair too far from a bed or chair for a transfer. An individual with unilateral body neglect or inattention may not account for the affected body side when moving. Such an individual may hit furniture with the affected arm or walk into obstacles such as doorways. When transferring from the bed to a chair, an individual may only move the unaffected side to the chair, leaving the affected side in bed or off the chair (see Fig. 18-8, *B*). An individual with severe neglect also may have the impairment of anosognosia. These individuals may deny that they are paralyzed or that their affected arm or side is a part of themselves. The affected limb may be referred to as an object, or these individuals may claim that someone else's arm is lying in bed with them. One man with anosognosia was heard to comment that he was going to occupational therapy and that he would "need to bring the arm along," because the occupational therapist "always works on the arm." Unilateral spatial neglect or inattention refers to the phenomenon in which the individual does not account for visual stimuli from the

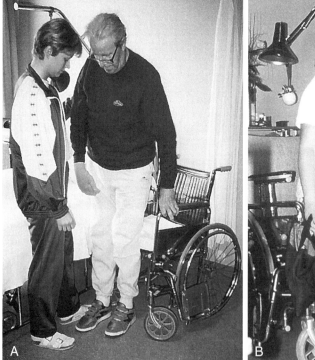 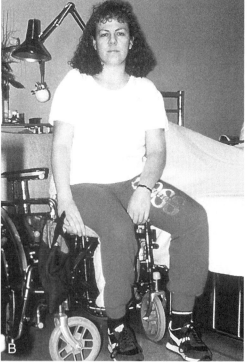

Figure 18-8 Dysfunction of neurological client factors manifested during functional mobility tasks. **A,** Paralysis affects strength and balance. Individuals require assistance when transferring from bed. A wheelchair is needed for mobility. **B,** Unilateral body neglect. Woman only moves intact body side over to wheelchair and leaves affected side in bed.

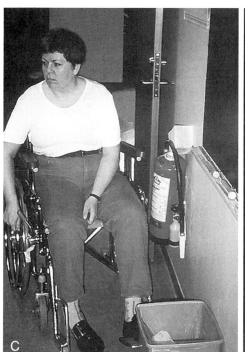
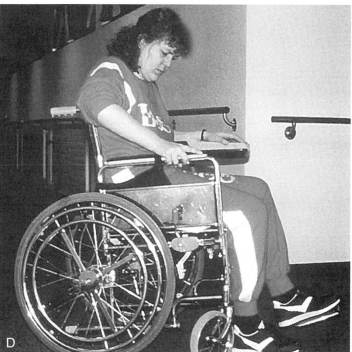
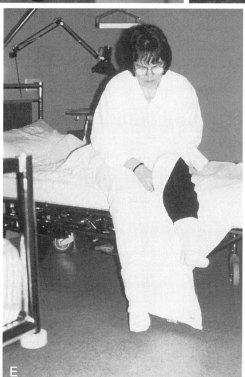
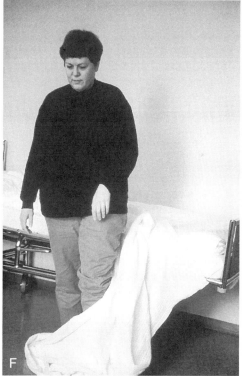

Figure 18-8, cont'd **C,** Unilateral spatial neglect. Woman wheels into a garbage can in a neglected left visual field. **D,** Ideational apraxia. Woman does not know how to propel the wheelchair and pushes down on the armrest instead of the wheel. **E,** Organization and sequencing impairment. Woman does not lift off the blanket before sitting up in bed. **F,** Organization and sequencing impairment and ideational apraxia. Woman attempts to walk away from bed without having moved the blanket.

affected visual field. The individual may walk or wheel into obstacles such as garbage cans, furniture, doorways, or other individuals (see Fig. 18-8, *C*). Topographic disorientation, in which the person has visuospatial problems or memory problems regarding spatial locations also may be present. The individual does not know the way to different, familiar locations such as the bathroom, dining room, bedroom, or therapy department.

If a dysfunction of the global and specific mental factors is present, ideational apraxia or organization and sequencing problems may occur during transfers and mobility tasks. Individuals with ideational apraxia may not know how to get into bed. They literally may throw themselves into the bed. An individual may not know how to wheel a wheelchair and may push down repeatedly on the armrest (see Fig. 18-8, *D*). (However, the therapist should rule out attention problems.) An individual with organization and sequencing problems may sit up in bed without taking off the blanket but will remove the blanket before standing up (see Fig. 18-8, *E*). However, an individual with additional ideational apraxia may sit up without lifting the blanket off and then attempt to stand up and walk away without moving the blanket, thus producing a safety hazard (see Fig. 18-8, *F*). An individual with organization and sequencing problems only may not put on wheelchair brakes before transferring or take them off before moving. This particular performance difficulty might occur when memory problems are present as well. If memory problems without impaired judgment are present, the results of the unsafe transfers (e.g., instability) may remind these individuals to lock the brakes.

Eating Performance Area. Neurobehavioral impairments or dysfunction of the previously mentioned body functions may affect dysfunction of eating performance, such as chewing and swallowing, drinking from a glass or a cup, eating without utensils (only using the fingers), eating with a fork or a spoon, and using a knife to cut or spread. Many of these tasks are accomplished earlier in the developmental sequence than some of the tasks mentioned previously.

A dysfunction of the neuromusculoskeletal and movement-related factors may result in paralysis of one side of the body, resulting in poor sitting balance and use of only one arm. Tactile and proprioceptive sensation in the affected hand and arm may be impaired because of defective sensory functions. All these impairments may affect eating tasks that require sitting balance and bilateral integration of the arms (e.g., stabilizing a slice of bread while buttering it or a slice of meat while cutting it, eating an egg, or peeling an orange). Because of the impairments, these eating tasks may require different performance techniques, helping aids, or personal assistance.

An individual with motor apraxia classified as dysfunction of the specific mental factor of sequencing complex movement according to the ICF classification system may spill soup when moving the spoon from the bowl to the mouth, a task that requires much significant adjustment of fine finger and wrist movements to keep the spoon level. Motor apraxia may result in "clumsy movements" when spreading butter, resulting in problems manipulating the knife (Fig. 18-9, *A*). Premotor perseveration is demonstrated when an individual cannot stop the movements of bringing the spoon to the mouth from the bowl after having finished the soup. Another example is the continuation of chewing movements after the food has dissolved in the mouth. Prefrontal perseveration, or perseveration of actions rather than movements (a cognitive factor), may manifest when an individual who has finished eating yogurt with a spoon reaches out for the spoon again to use it to get a sip of milk from a glass rather than drink directly from the glass (see Fig. 18-9, *B*).

Dysfunction of specific mental perceptual factors affecting eating behavior may result in spatial relation disorders; an individual trying to stabilize a slice of bread to butter it may misjudge distance and grab the plate instead of the bread (see Fig. 18-9, *C*). The individual may also overestimate or underestimate distances and reach beside the cup instead of grabbing the cup. Unilateral body neglect may occur during eating when the individual does not use the hand in a natural relation to its available function. Individuals may start eating bread using the left hand, "forget" that the bread is in the hand, and proceed to eat other items as the hand holding the bread slides off the table (see Fig. 18-9, *D*). Unilateral spatial neglect may manifest in that the individual may not attend to objects or food in the affected visual field. For example, an individual may not notice a fork in the left visual field and attempts to solve the problem by grabbing the next person's fork located by a plate in the right visual field (see Fig. 18-9, *E*). Individuals may not eat food located in the affected visual field, although they enjoy that particular type of food.

Dysfunction of global and specific mental function factors may result in ideational apraxia in which the affected individual does not know which utensils to use or how to use them. The individual may simplify the activity by using the fingers to eat meat instead of a fork. The person also may misuse objects. An individual may attempt to eat the soup with a knife. Activity steps may be left out of the sequence, resulting in defective performance. An affected individual may not take the shell off an egg before attempting to eat it or may not peel an orange before biting it. An individual may have the proper object in hand but may not know how to use it for the situation at hand: the individual may open a teabag, remove the tea leaves, and place them in the cup instead of placing the bag in the cup. Individuals may misuse objects; for example, they may sprinkle salt on the butter container (see Fig. 18-9, *F*). Field dependency may be manifested during feeding activities. Individuals may start grabbing food items before

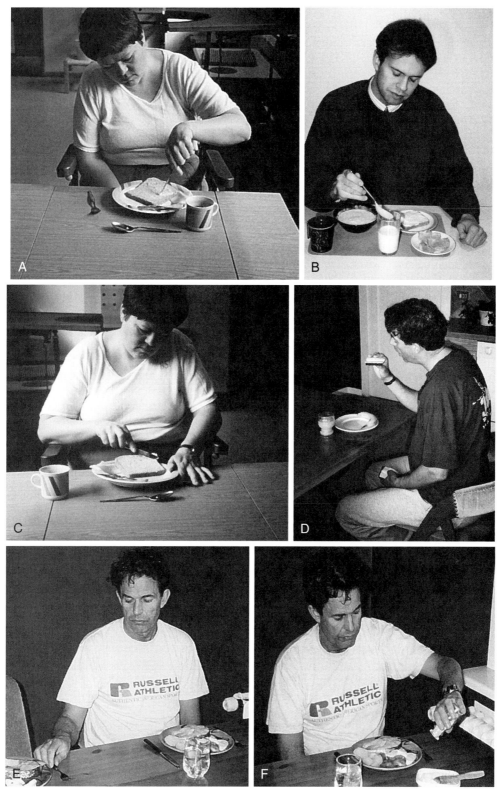

Figure 18-9 Dysfunction of neurological client factors manifested during feeding and eating tasks. **A,** Motor apraxia makes manipulation of a knife difficult when buttering bread. **B,** Prefrontal perseveration. Man continues to move the spoon toward the glass instead of drinking from it, after having used the spoon to eat yogurt. **C,** Spatial relations impairment. Woman attempts to stabilize a piece of bread but misjudges distances and grabs the side of the plate instead. **D,** Unilateral body neglect. Man does not attend to a piece of bread in left hand; hand slides unnoticed off the table, and man grabs another slice with right hand. **E,** Unilateral spatial neglect. Man does not notice fork in his left visual field but solves problem by borrowing a fork from the next plate in the right visual field. **F,** Ideational apraxia. Man does not know what salt is used for and shakes it over butter container.

having positioned themselves properly at the table. Individuals also may grab items as they are seen, although the items are inappropriate for the activity at hand.

Pervasive Impairments. According to the A-ONE classification,[6,8,17] impairments can be classified as specific or pervasive in relation to activity performance. The impairments described in the previous sections and affecting specific tasks of an ADL domain are classified as specific because they are observed in relation to the particular task, whereas other impairments are not task-specific. Thus some impairments are not necessarily tied to a particular performance area but can occur in relation to any performance area. Emotional and affective disturbance classified by ICF as global mental functions, such as apathy, depression, frustration, irritability, aggression, and lack of motivation, are examples of this because they may affect task performance in different areas of occupation.

As stated earlier, different impairments have different effects on task performance. The behavioral examples described in this chapter are intended as guidelines to assist therapists in detecting impairments revealed by errors observed during task performance for assessment purposes. This information, used with the appropriate theoretical background and clinical reasoning, is important in determining intervention strategies. Occasionally, differentiation between impairments with similar behavioral manifestations may be difficult, particularly for less experienced therapists. Knowledge of neurological function and of how impairments are grouped in different diagnostic categories may be valuable for clinical reasoning in such instances.

PATTERNS OF IMPAIRMENTS RESULTING FROM STROKES

In a preceding section, neurobehavioral impairments were defined and related to different cortical areas. Involvement of dysfunction affecting neurological body functions depends on various pathological conditions resulting in stroke and the different anatomical areas involved. The cerebral blood supply depends mainly on three arteries in each hemisphere: the middle and anterior cerebral arteries, which are branches of the internal carotid artery, and the posterior cerebral artery, which is a branch of the basilar artery, formed by the union of the vertebral arteries.[45] Two major types of cerebrovascular dysfunction cause neurological lesions: (1) ischemia, or insufficient blood supply to the brain, which is responsible for 70% to 80% of all strokes, and (2) hemorrhage, or bleeding, caused by a ruptured blood vessel, which accounts for the remaining 15% to 20% of strokes.[2,6,24,72] Hemorrhage results in swelling and compression of brain tissue. Different subtypes of strokes occur. Ischemia is subdivided into thrombosis, or blood flow obstruction caused by a local process in one or more blood vessels; embolism, in which blood flow obstruction is caused by materials from distant parts of the vascular system; and decreased systemic perfusion, or hypoperfusion, in which low systemic perfusion pressure results in reduced blood flow.[6,24,72]

Hemorrhage is subdivided into subarachnoid hemorrhage, which occurs at the surface of the brain and intracerebrally, and intraparenchymal hemorrhage, or bleeding in the cerebral tissue.[2,6,24] Each type of stroke results in different patterns of impairment. The type of impairment and severity depend mainly on the anatomical location of the lesion.[3,24] These further depend on the rate of arterial occlusion, adequacy of the collateral circulation, resistance of brain structures to ischemia,[24] duration and severity of ischemia, hematoma size, and underlying mechanism of hypoperfusion[79] and on edema.

Dysfunction of different arteries leads to different patterns of impairments. If the middle cerebral artery, for example, is occluded, affecting blood supply to the lateral aspect of the hemisphere, the impairments vary depending on which branches of the artery and which hemisphere is affected. If the insult affects the upper trunk of the middle cerebral artery, which supplies the lateral aspects of the frontal and parietal lobes, hemiplegia is expected on the contralateral body side, especially of the face and arm, along with hemisensory loss, including tactile and proprioceptive information. This type of insult also may cause impairment of a visual field to the opposite site of the lesion. If the right hemisphere is impaired, unilateral neglect of space and body may result, as well as attention deficits, including unilateral body inattention and unilateral spatial inattention, anosognosia, spatial relation dysfunction, unilateral motor apraxia of the left side (if not paralyzed), lack of judgment, lack of insight, field dependency, and organization of behavior and activity steps. Emotional disturbances such as apathy, lability, and depression also may be present. If the left hemisphere is involved, speech and language functions may be impaired, and bilateral motor apraxia may be observed. Ideational apraxia and perseverations and emotional disturbances such as depression and frustration may be a consequence. If the lower trunk of the middle cerebral artery is affected, visual field defect of the contralateral visual field, Wernicke's aphasia caused by involvement of the left hemisphere, and emotional disturbances may be present.[6,24] Table 18-4 indicates patterns of impairments as they relate to dysfunction of different cerebral arteries and systemic hypoperfusion, a diffuse cerebral dysfunction affecting the watershed regions or the border zones in the periphery of the major cerebral arteries, and different CNS areas, because of various vascular pathological conditions (see Chapter 1).

Table 18-4

Cerebral Artery Dysfunction: Cortical Involvement and Patterns of Impairment

ARTERY	LOCATION	POSSIBLE IMPAIRMENTS

Middle cerebral artery: upper trunk	Lateral aspect of frontal and parietal lobe	■ Dysfunction of either hemisphere
		  ■ Contralateral hemiplegia, especially of the face and the upper extremity
		  ■ Contralateral hemisensory loss
		  ■ Visual field impairment
		  ■ Poor contralateral conjugate gaze
		  ■ Ideational apraxia
		  ■ Lack of judgment
		  ■ Perseveration
		  ■ Field dependency
		  ■ Impaired organization of behavior
		  ■ Depression
		  ■ Lability
		  ■ Apathy
		■ Right hemisphere dysfunction
		  ■ Left unilateral body neglect
		  ■ Left unilateral visual neglect
		  ■ Anosognosia
		  ■ Visuospatial impairment
		  ■ Left unilateral motor apraxia
		■ Left hemisphere dysfunction
		  ■ Bilateral motor apraxia
		  ■ Broca's aphasia
		  ■ Frustration

Middle cerebral artery: lower trunk	Lateral aspect of right temporal and occipital lobes	■ Dysfunction of either hemisphere
		  ■ Contralateral visual field defect
		  ■ Behavioral abnormalities
		■ Right hemisphere dysfunction
		  ■ Visuospatial dysfunction
		■ Left hemisphere dysfunction
		  ■ Wernicke's aphasia

Middle cerebral artery: both upper and lower trunks	Lateral aspect of the involved hemisphere	■ Impairments related to both upper and lower trunk dysfunction as listed in previous two sections

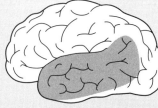

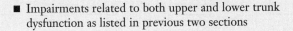

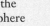

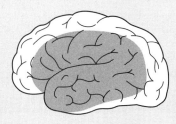

Continued

Table 18-4

Cerebral Artery Dysfunction: Cortical Involvement and Patterns of Impairment—cont'd

ARTERY	LOCATION	POSSIBLE IMPAIRMENTS
Anterior cerebral artery	Medial and superior aspects of frontal and parietal lobes	■ Contralateral hemiparesis, greatest in foot ■ Contralateral hemisensory loss, greatest in foot ■ Left unilateral apraxia ■ Inertia of speech or mutism ■ Behavioral disturbances

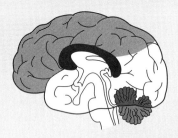

ARTERY	LOCATION	POSSIBLE IMPAIRMENTS
Internal carotid artery	Combination of middle cerebral artery distribution and anterior cerebral artery	■ Impairments related to dysfunction of middle and anterior cerebral arteries as listed previously
Anterior choroidal artery, a branch of the internal carotid artery	Globus pallidus, lateral geniculate body, posterior limb of the internal capsule, medial temporal lobe	■ Hemiparesis of face, arm, and leg ■ Hemisensory loss ■ Hemianopsia[24]
Posterior cerebral artery	Medial and inferior aspects of right temporal and occipital lobes, posterior corpus callosum and penetrating arteries to midbrain and thalamus	■ Dysfunction of either side 　■ Homonymous hemianopsia 　■ Visual agnosia (visual object agnosia, prosopagnosia, color agnosia) 　■ Memory impairment 　■ Occasional contralateral numbness ■ Right side dysfunction 　■ Cortical blindness 　■ Visuospatial impairment 　■ Impaired left-right discrimination ■ Left side dysfunction 　■ Finger agnosia 　■ Anomia 　■ Agraphia 　■ Acalculia 　■ Alexia

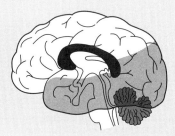

ARTERY	LOCATION	POSSIBLE IMPAIRMENTS
Basilar artery proximal	Pons	■ Quadriparesis ■ Bilateral asymmetrical weakness ■ Bulbar or pseudobulbar paralysis (bilateral paralysis of face, palate, pharynx, neck, or tongue) ■ Paralysis of eye abductors ■ Nystagmus ■ Ptosis ■ Cranial nerve abnormalities ■ Diplopia ■ Dizziness ■ Occipital headache ■ Coma[24]

Table 18-4

Cerebral Artery Dysfunction: Cortical Involvement and Patterns of Impairment—cont'd

ARTERY	LOCATION	POSSIBLE IMPAIRMENTS
Basilar artery distal	Midbrain, thalamus, and caudate nucleus	■ Papillary abnormalities ■ Abnormal eye movements ■ Altered level of alertness ■ Coma ■ Memory loss ■ Agitation ■ Hallucination[24]
Vertebral artery	Lateral medulla and cerebellum	■ Dizziness ■ Vomiting ■ Nystagmus ■ Pain in ipsilateral eye and face ■ Numbness in face ■ Clumsiness of ipsilateral limbs ■ Hypotonia of ipsilateral limbs ■ Tachycardia ■ Gait ataxia[24]
Systemic hypoperfusion	Watershed region on lateral side of hemisphere, hippo-campus and surrounding structures in medial temporal lobe	■ Coma ■ Dizziness ■ Confusion ■ Decreased concentration ■ Agitation ■ Memory impairment ■ Visual abnormalities caused by disconnection from frontal eye fields ■ Impaired eye movements ■ Weakness of shoulder and arm ■ Gait ataxia[24]

CLINICAL REASONING INVOLVED IN USING THE A-ONE

As mentioned in an earlier section of this chapter, the therapist applies different types of clinical reasoning when applying the A-ONE principles to evaluate task performance and dysfunctional body functions that limit the performance. Further exploration is necessary in relation to the reasoning that goes into the A-ONE. When observing dressing performance, the therapist may detect a critical cue such as not dressing one arm. The therapist interprets this cue, and other cues, by using previously described conceptual and operational definitions from the theory behind the A-ONE instrument and forms hypotheses. Possible hypotheses might be (1) lack of somesthetic sensory input from the arm, (2) unilateral body neglect—in which the person does not attend, usually to the left arm—that may or may not be paralyzed, (3) organization and sequencing problems in which the person is leaving an activity step out of the performance, or (4) ideational apraxia, in which the person does not have an idea of what to do with the shirt or how to put it on. In addition to considering definitions of terms when choosing the appropriate hypotheses, or determining which impairment is most likely to cause the particular activity limitation, the therapist keeps in mind indications of impairments during other activities because these might support a particular hypothesis. The neurological information on functional localization and patterns of impairments as related to different diagnoses or different cerebral arteries described in the previous section also would be included in the reasoning and hypothesis formation. Thus, if the patient (1) knows in general how to use objects, not to mention if the patient can state a plan of action for the activity performance, but does not use the left hand according to muscle strength, or (2) has other impairments that fit with the picture of right hemisphere dysfunction such as spatial relations impairment, one would probably suspect unilateral body neglect or inattention to body side as a result of right hemisphere dysfunction. The therapist would consider sensation in the arm because this may or may not be defective if neglect or inattention exists and could affect arm use. The therapist also would check insight into activity limitations and occupational errors by using operational definitions from the pervasive scale. If sensory loss exists, the patient is aware of the problem and how it affects performance. If neglect or inattention exists, the patient will not be aware consistently of the impairment and its effect on activity performance. If, however, cues indicate the patient is having difficulties with object use in other activities as well, cannot state a plan of action, or has language problems that might indicate a defect in inner language and problems forming a plan of action, one might conclude that the impairment of ideational apraxia limits the dressing performance. Thus, the therapist might hypothesize that ideational apraxia caused by left hemisphere dysfunction might be the nature of the problem that interferes with task performance.[17] This information may be useful combined with other types of reasoning such as conditional reasoning[51] (see Chapter 17) when making decisions regarding intervention methods, as discussed later.[17]

ASSESSMENT METHODS

Occupational therapists use basically two evaluation and intervention approaches when working with patients with neurological conditions: deficit-specific approach, also termed *bottom-up, restorative,* or *remedial approach;* and functional adaptation or compensation approach, also referred to as *top-down,* or *adaptive approach.* Evaluation tools used when applying the deficit-specific approach are aimed at the impaired body structures and functions, using the ICF terminology. The evaluation tools of the functional approach target the activity level or occupational performance. Today, different authors within occupational therapy emphasize the importance of focusing on task performance or occupational functioning in a top-down fashion when assessing patients rather than focusing on impairments.[13,36,38,54] They also stress the importance of using standardized evaluation methods that relate occupational performance to body functions,[13,36,38,42,50] or performance skills.[21]

The previous sections have described how the therapist can detect neurobehavioral impairments during observation of task performance by the use of task analysis based on the A-ONE theoretical framework. Functional assessments may include nonstandardized and standardized observations. According to Unsworth,[71] a nonstandardized hypothesis testing approach for evaluation could be useful for therapists who have not had the chance to complete the required training for standardized assessments such as the A-ONE and the Assessment of Motor and Process Skills[34] (see Chapter 21). Most authors agree that standardized assessments have established, during their developmental process, uniform standards regarding assessment conditions, materials, and instructions for collecting and analyzing information that must be followed precisely. Furthermore, particular assessments may require specific training programs.[5,19,20,58,61] The development of conceptual and operational definitions can further be considered an important aspect of providing uniform standards.

Determining for which purpose information is needed is a crucial prerequisite for choosing an evaluation method. For gathering information for goal setting and choice of intervention, either standardized or nonstandardized evaluations may serve the desired purpose. However, if the purpose is to measure change in performance, standardized methods are not enough. Most instruments used in rehabilitation have ordinal scales. Such scales can be used as a base for descriptions of performance, but in order to measure performance interval scales are mandatory.[22,52,78] Thus, in rehabilitation, increased emphasis is being placed on use of scales that have measurement properties[67] both for clinical and research use. Such scales allow for measuring change over time and comparisons of different groups.

In contrast to the nonstandardized method reviewed earlier in this chapter and based on the A-ONE, the A-ONE instrument, a criterion based method, is standardized; that is, it includes detailed administration and scoring instructions. Several studies of validity and reliability have been conducted to ensure the A-ONE does what its developer claims it does and that it measures the traits consistently (Table 18-5). The instrument requires a training seminar for therapists to ensure reliability.[17,63] The original development of the instrument was based on traditional psychometric methods and use of ordinal scales, as the purpose was to gather useful information for goal setting and intervention ideas, not to evaluate change. Increased demand for evidence-based practice and efficacy in rehabilitation services call for instruments with measurement potential. For this reason, the new test theory was used to revalidate the A-ONE and explore if the original ordinal scales could be converted to interval scales. The ADL scale of the A-ONE has successively been Rasch analyzed, and development of conversion tables to convert the ordinal scores recorded after observation of ADL performance to interval scores is taking place.[12] Interval scales have also recently been constructed based on the ordinal neurobehavioral impairment scales of the A-ONE, by application of Rasch analysis.[14] Thus, the revalidated A-ONE instrument permits comparison between patients in addition to monitoring of progress, regardless of which trained therapist administers and interprets the evaluation. The results provide useful information to guide the choice of intervention method based

Table 18-5

Instrument Development and Samples of A-ONE Reliability and Validity Studies

STUDY	PURPOSE	DESIGN AND SUBJECTS	RESULTS	CONTRIBUTION TO INSTRUMENT DEVELOPMENT
		Traditional Psychometric Studies		
Interrater reliability[6]	Provide interrater reliability for the scales of the A-ONE.	Four occupational therapists rated 20 patients (2 therapists at the time). Sample of convenience.	Average kappa coefficient $(\kappa) = 0.84$	Establishment of interrater reliability
Interrater reliability[11]	Provide interrater reliability for the scales of the A-ONE.	Five therapists evaluated 20 videotapes of 4 children and 16 disabled adults.	Functional Independence (FI) scale: $ICC = 0.98$ Kendall $\tau = 0.92$ $\kappa w = 0.9$ Neurobehavioral Specific Impairment Subscale (NBI specific scale): $ICC = 0.93$ $\kappa w = 0.74$	Establishment of interrater reliability
Item correlations[6]	Examine interitem correlations	Scores from 89 subjects with cortical neurological diagnoses on the FI scale were correlated within and across domains. Subsequently scores obtained from the FI scale were correlated with scores of the NBI specific subscale	Item correlations within domains ranged from $r = 0.3$ to 0.9. Item correlations across domains ranged from $r = 0.1$ to 0.8 Item correlations across scales (independence/neurobehavior) were significant for 75% of comparisons.	Support for the theoretical statement of neurobehavioral dysfunction affecting performance in self-care activities, resulting in diminished independence.
Exploratory factor[6] analysis.	Explore factors. Contribute to construct validity	Factor analysis: varimax rotation. 89 subjects with CNS diagnoses	Three factors emerged from the FI scale. Two factors emerged from the Neurobehavioral Specific Impairment Subscale.	Contribution to construct validity.

Continued

Table 18-5

Instrument Development and Samples of A-ONE Reliability and Validity Studies—cont'd

STUDY	PURPOSE	DESIGN AND SUBJECTS	RESULTS	CONTRIBUTION TO INSTRUMENT DEVELOPMENT
		Traditional Psychometric Studies		
Item correlations[63]	Explore construct validity	60 subjects with and without neurological diagnoses	Items from the 4 domains of dressing, grooming and hygiene, transfers and mobility, and eating had high item correlations ranging from 0.82 to 0.93. Correlations for items in the communication domain to items in other domains were unacceptable.	Contribution to construct validity.
Concurrent validation[63]	Explore concurrent validity	Scores from 60 subjects on the FI scale of the A-ONE and Barthel Index were compared. Scores from 42 subjects on the NBI scale of the A-ONE and Mini Mental State Examination (MMSE) were compared.	Correlations of A-ONE FI scale and Barthel Index, $r = 0.85$. Correlations of A-ONE NBI scores and Mini Mental State Examination (MMSE), $r = 0.7$	Contribution to concurrent validation
Concurrent validation[37]	Explore if persons diagnosed with right and left cerebral vascular accidents perform differently on the scales of the A-ONE. Explore which NBI items interfere most frequently with ADL	Prospective study of performance of 42 subjects diagnosed with right and left stroke (R stroke, L stroke)	Only one ADL item out of 20 showed difference between subjects with R stroke and L stroke. Significant difference was obtained between groups for the impairments of unilateral body and spatial neglect, motor and ideational apraxia and organization and sequencing. Most frequently detected items were: "organization and sequencing," "spatial relations impairment," unilateral body neglect, Wernicke's aphasia, and Broca's aphasia.	Contribution to concurrent validity and construct validity

Concurrent validation[55]	To explore association of therapists hypothesis about lesion location based on clinical observations and results of technological evaluation methods	Results from the A-ONE hypothesis for 21 stroke and transient ischemic attack subjects were compared to results of computerized tomography (CT scans) and computerized mapping of electroencephalography (CMEEG)	Kappa coefficients revealed: A-ONE to CT scans $\kappa = 0.75$, A-ONE to CMEEG $\kappa = 0.63$, CT to CMEEG $\kappa = 0.53$	Contribution to concurrent validity and construct validity

New test theory, Rasch analysis

Rasch analysis of the ADL scale[12]	Explore the internal scale validity and structure of the ADL scale of the A-ONE with need for revision in mind. Examine possibility of converting the ordinal A-ONE ADL scale to an interval scale and revising the instrument.	Retrospective design including 209 persons with stroke or dementia	Unidimentionality of items on the ADL scale of the A-ONE can be achieved with minor revision of the instrument. Revision would increase power of the instrument as a tool to measure change. Information for conversion tables.	Contribution to internal validation of the ADL scale (construct validity).
Rasch analysis of the NBI scale[14]	Explore the internal scale validity and structure of the NBI scale of the A-ONE with need for revision in mind. Examine possibility of converting the ordinal A-ONE NBI scale to an interval scale and revising the instrument.	Retrospective design including 206 persons with stroke or dementia. Items were dichotomized.	Unidimentionality of items on the NBI scale of the A-ONE can be achieved with specific scales for different diagnostic groups. Revision would increase power of the instrument as a tool to measure change. Information for conversion tables.	Contribution to internal validation of the NBI scale (construct validity).
Further Rasch analysis of the NBI scale for different diagnostic groups[15,16]	Explore the internal scale validity and structure of different versions of the NBI scale for combination of different diagnostic groups. Examining the research use of scales for combined diagnostic groups	Retrospective design including 422 persons diagnosed with stroke and 216 persons with R stroke and L stroke.	Unidimentionality of items on the ADL scale of the A-ONE can be achieved for combined diagnostic groups. Revision would increase power of the instrument as a tool to measure change and compare individuals from different groups. Information for conversion tables	Contribution to internal validation of the NBI scale

Courtesy G. Árnadóttir, Reykjavik, Iceland.
From Árnadóttir G: A-ONE training course: lecture notes, Reykjavik, Iceland, 2009-2010.
CNS, Central nervous system; *FI,* Functional Independence; *NBI,* Neurobehavioral Impairment.

on strengths and weaknesses of the patient, from the perspective of task performance and body functions.

The way in which the A-ONE provides information on task performance dysfunction in different ADL domains and the neurobehavioral impairments that might affect ADL performance, becomes evident by exploring the case study that follows this review. The therapist first fills in scores for the level of assistance needed for task performance. Observations are written in the comments and reasoning sections about ineffective actions observed as errors in task performance. Subsequently the therapist reasons, based on the content of the observed errors, about the type of impairment responsible for the error. The neurobehavioral impairment is then scored based on whether the impairment is present or not and how much assistance is needed to complete the task.

The case study illustrated in Fig. 18-10 describes a patient who sustained a right hemispheric stroke. The A-ONE assessment was used to evaluate ADL performance and the type and severity of neurobehavioral impairments that interfered with task performance. The study demonstrates how neurobehavioral impairment interferes with ADL performance and how the two types of dysfunction—impaired neurological body functions and their effect on task performance—may be evaluated by different scales of the same assessment.

The case study presents an individual who needs physical assistance with all items in the dressing domain of the Functional Independence Scale of the A-ONE (Fig. 18-10, *A*). The limitations in ADL task performance resulting in diminished independence are related to several neurobehavioral impairments including unilateral body neglect, spatial relations impairment, unilateral spatial neglect, organization and sequencing problems, and left hemiplegia (as indicated by scores on the Neurobehavioral Specific Impairment Subscale of the A-ONE). The dressing domain is one of five domains on the Functional Independence Scale of the A-ONE. Summary sheets from the A-ONE indicating scores in the other functional domains and different neurobehavioral impairments are also shown (see Fig. 18-10, *B* and *C*). A subsequent evaluation performed three months later indicated observed improvement in ADL performance. Measures of person ability were obtained by comparing the raw scores to conversion tables. Comparison of the ability measures from the initial evaluation (0.58 logits) to the follow-up evaluation (2.39 logits) revealed significant improvement (1.81 logits) in the magnitude of the measures.

Some authors have suggested use of deficit-specific tests as a follow-up of the functional evaluation under specific conditions. These conditions include circumstances in which the therapist has difficulties defining deficits, when a new therapist needs to refine observation skills,[56,57] when therapists require an aid in quantification of the severity of the deficit,[57] and/or when the therapist needs to report

efficacy of treatment in research studies.[50] A therapist interested in applying a deficit-specific approach to evaluate dysfunction of body functions (e.g., muscle strength and tone, motor apraxia, spatial relations, neglect, and memory) has a choice of applying test batteries or evaluations aimed at specific impairments. Examples of test batteries used by occupational therapists to evaluate a range of impairments in patients with stroke are the Lowenstein Occupational Therapy Cognitive Assessment (LOTCA)[43] and the Rivermead Perceptual Assessment Battery (RPAB).[73] Examples of standardized deficit-specific tests available for evaluating some of the impairments mentioned in the case presented in Fig. 18-10 are the Behavioral Inattention Test (BIT)[76] for unilateral neglect or inattention; the Motor-Free Visual Perception Test—Vertical (MVPT—V),[53] a deficit-specific evaluation that could be used to examine presence of spatial relations impairments; the Test of Every Day Attention (TEA)[59] for attention deficits; the Behavioral Assessment of the Dysexecutive Syndrome (BADS)[74] for evaluating prefrontal dysfunction; Rivermead Behavioral Memory Test (RBMT)[75] for everyday memory functions; the Self-Reporting Awareness Test[1] and the Assessment of Awareness of Disability[68] for evaluating insight; a test for imitating gestures[30] used to evaluate ideomotor apraxia; and a test for ideational apraxia.[31] See Chapter 19.

Several studies have explored the relationship of scores from ADL instruments to scores from different cognitive, perceptual, and motor instruments for different reasons. These include examination of the associations between disability and impairment, search for prognostic factors useful for rehabilitation, and establishment of ecological validity for different scales. Sample size, type and number of items, scales, and psychometric methods used vary considerably in these studies. However, most of the obtained results support the notion that impairments and lowered ADL function are associated, although the reported strength of the association varies between studies. Correlations of scores from cognitive and perceptual scales to ADL scales most frequently range from small to moderate ($r = 0.2$ to 0.6).[26,32,33,38,66] Correlations of motor functions to ADL scores sometimes reach higher values than cognitive and perceptual comparisons.[45,66] Gillen[38] pointed out in his consideration for evaluation of those with functional limitations secondary to neurological impairments that separate evaluations of cognitive and motor tasks reveal different results from using tasks that combine different body functions. Further, the performance of more than one task at the time, as is often the case in natural context as opposed to deficit-specific testing situations, may lead to worse performance. Thus, it is emphasized here that information from deficit-specific tests cannot replace information from observation in a natural context. Further, no other evaluation format can replace observation of task performance in natural settings.[6,13,36]

**Functional Independence Scale and
Neurobehavioral Specific Impairment Subscale**

Name Ms. Wilson   **Date** 6/13/03

Independence Score (IP):

4 = Independent and able to transfer activity to
other environmental situations.
3 = Independent with supervision.
2 = Needs verbal assistance.
1 = Needs demonstration or physical assistance.
0 = Unable to perform. Totally dependent on assistance.

Neurobehavioral Score (NB):

0 = No neurobehavioral impairments observed.
1 = Able to perform without additional information, but some
neurobehavioral impairment is observed.
2 = Able to perform with additional verbal assistance, but
neurobehavioral impairment can be observed during
performance.
3 = Able to perform with demonstration or minimal to considerable
physical assistance.
4 = Unable to perform due to neurobehavioral impairment. Needs
maximum physical assistance.

List helping aids used:

• Wheelchair
• Nonslip for soap and plate
• Adapted toothbrush
• Velcro fastening on shoes

Primary ADL activity   Scoring   Comments and reasoning

Dressing	IP Score					Comments and reasoning
Shirt (or dress)	4	3	2	(1)	0	Include one armhole, fix shoulder
Pants	4	3	2	(1)	0	Find correct leghole
Socks	4	3	2	(1)	0	One-handed technique, balance
Shoes	4	3	2	(1)	0	Balance
Fastenings	4	3	2	(1)	0	Match buttonholes, Velcro through loop
Other						

NB Impairment	NB Score					
Motor apraxia	(0)	1	2	3	4	
Ideational apraxia	(0)	1	2	3	4	
Unilateral body neglect	0	1	2	(3)	4	Leaves out left body side
Somatoagnosia	(0)	1	2	3	4	
Spatial relations	0	1	2	(3)	4	Finding correct holes, front/back
Unilateral spatial neglect	0	1	(2)	3	4	Leaves out items in left visual field
Abnormal tone: right	(0)	1	2	3	4	
Abnormal tone: left	0	1	2	(3)	4	Sitting balance/bilateral manipulation
Perseveration	(0)	1	2	3	4	
Organization/sequencing	0	1	(2)	3	4	For activity steps
Other						

Note: All definitions and scoring criteria for each deficit are in the evaluation manual.

A

Figure 18-10   **A,** Árnadóttir OT-ADL Neurobehavioral Evaluation (A-ONE): sample from
the dressing domain of the Functional Independence Scale and the Neurobehavioral Specific
Impairment Subscale for Ms. Wilson.   *Continued*

Árnadóttir OT-ADL
Neurobehavioral Evaluation
(A-ONE)

Name ___Ms. Wilson___   **Date** ___6–13–03___

Birthdate ___4–15–1943___   **Age** ___60___

Gender ___Female___   **Ethnicity** ___Caucasian___

Dominance ___Right___   **Profession** ___Dressmaker___

Medical Diagnosis:
Right CVA 6/20/03. Ischemia.

Medications:

Social Situation:
Lives alone in an apartment building on third floor
Has two adult daughters

Summary of Independence:
Needs physical assistance with dressing, grooming, hygiene, transfer, and mobility tasks because of left-sided paralysis and perceptual and cognitive impairments. Is more or less able to feed herself if meals have been prepared. No problems with personal communication, although perceptual impairments will affect reading and writing skills. Also has lack of judgment and memory impairment, which affect task performance. Is not able to live alone at this stage. If personal home support becomes available, will need a home evaluation because of physical limitation and wheelchair use. Needs recommendations regarding removal of architectural barriers or suggestions for alternative housing. Unable to return to previous job as a dressmaker.

Functional Independence Score (optional)

Function	Total Score	% Score
Dressing	1,1,1,1,1 = 5/20	
Grooming and hygiene	1,2,1,1,3,0 = 8/24	
Transfer and mobility	1,1,1,1,1 = 5/20	
Feeding	4,4,4,3 = 15/16	
Communication	4,4 = 8/8	

B

Figure 18-10, cont'd   B, A-ONE ADL summary sheet.

List of Neurobehavioral Impairments Observed:

Specific impairment	D	G	T	F	C
Motor Apraxia					
Ideational Apraxia					
Unilateral Body Neglect	3	3	3	1	
Somatoagnosia					
Spatial Relations	3	3	3	1	
Unilateral Spatial Neglect	2	2	3	1	
Abnormal Tone: Right					
Abnormal Tone: Left	3	3	3	1	
Perseveration					
Organization	2	2	2	1	
Topographic Disorientation			3		
Other					
Sensory Aphasia					
Jargon Aphasia					
Anomia					
Paraphasia					
Expressive Aphasia					

Pervasive Impairment	ADL
Astereognosis	✓
Visual Object Agnosia	
Visual Spatial Agnosia	✓
Associative Visual Agnosia	
Anosognosia	
R/L Discrimination	✓
Short-Term Memory	✓
Long-Term Memory	
Disorientation	✓
Confabulation	
Lability	✓
Euphoria	
Apathy	
Depression	✓
Aggressiveness	
Irritability	
Frustration	

Pervasive Impairment	ADL
Restlessness	
Concrete Thinking	✓
Decreased Insight	✓
Impaired Judgment	✓
Confusion	
Impaired Alertness	
Impaired Attention	✓
Distractibility	✓
Impaired Initiative	
Impaired Motivation	
Performance Latency	
Absentmindedness	
Other	
Field Dependency	✓

Use (✓) for presence of specific impairments in different ADL domains (D = dressing, G = grooming, T = transfers, F = feeding, C = communication) and for presence of pervasive impairments detected during the ADL evaluation.

Summary of Neurobehavioral Impairments:
Needs physical assistance for most dressing, grooming, hygiene, transfer, and mobility tasks because of left-sided paralysis, spatial relations impairments (e.g., problems differentiating back from front of clothes and finding armholes and legholes), and unilateral body neglect (i.e., does not wash or dress affected side) finding. Does not attend to objects in the left visual field and needs verbal cues for performance. Also needs verbal cues for organizing activity steps. Does not know her way around the hospital. Does not have insight into how the CVA affects her ADL and is thus unrealistic in day-to-day planning. Has impaired judgment resulting in unsafe transfer attempts. Leaves the water running after hygiene and grooming activities if not reminded to turn it off. Is emotionally labile and appears depressed at times. Is not oriented regarding time and date. Presents with impaired attention, distraction, and defective short-term memory requiring repeated verbal instructions.

Treatment Considerations:

Occupational Therapist:

A-ONE Certification Number:

C

Figure 18-10, cont'd **C,** A-ONE neurobehavioral summary sheet. (Courtesy G. Árnadóttir, Reykjavík, Iceland.)

SUMMARY

The information in this chapter has provided guidelines for the observation of stroke patients during task performance with the purpose of detecting impairments that interfere with independent performance. The conceptual and operational definitions provided in this text, based on the A-ONE, are important to ensure consistency of the method. The review allows therapists to interpret cues and to form hypotheses regarding impairments and activity limitation. However, this information has limitations and as presented in this text is not standardized. The standardized A-ONE instrument has recently been revalidated, adding measurement properties to previously established reliability and validity. The instrument aids therapists in understanding the reasons for the activity limitations. The instrument aids the therapist in analyzing the nature or cause of a functional problem requiring occupational therapy intervention. Subsequently, therapists can speculate about the best intervention for activity limitation and impaired body functions (see Chapter 19). Therapists can base the decision on information from the evaluation and the therapist's knowledge of different intervention methods. Whether they are focused on the level of activity performance only or choosing to consider the CNS level of body functions as well either in influencing choice of tasks and environments or informing the patient's support system about what to expect in terms of impairments and activity limitations in the persons performance. However, one must keep in mind that at present no functional assessment prescribes treatment, and therefore clinical reasoning is necessary to combine evaluation results with available treatment choices, and patient's specific conditions such as conceptual factors. Furthermore, research studies are needed to test the efficacy of intervention and theories.[49,64,69] For such testing, valid and reliable instruments are mandatory.

REVIEW QUESTIONS

1. Which kind of lesions may produce unilateral motor apraxia of the left side of the body and how might that impairment affect task performance of brushing teeth?
2. You observe a person placing both legs in the same leghole of a pair of pants. Which impairment(s) might cause such an error in performance and what is your reasoning for the decision(s) you made?
3. If an individual does not wash both sides of the body spontaneously, impairments such as unilateral body neglect, organizational and sequencing problems, or ideational apraxia might be suspected. How could you use clinical reasoning to differentiate among the different possible impairments?
4. What is the difference between expected impairments in the presence of a right middle cerebral artery dysfunction compared with expected impairments of a left middle cerebral artery dysfunction?
5. How might impairments of the left middle cerebral artery limit task performance in dressing?

REFERENCES

1. Abreu BC: Evaluation and intervention with memory and learning impairments. In Unsworth C, editor: *Cognitive and perceptual dysfunction: a clinical reasoning approach to evaluation and intervention*, Philadelphia, 1999, FA Davis.
2. American Heart Association: *American Stroke Association: types of stroke* (website). www.strokeassociation.org/presenter.jhtml?identifier=1014. Accessed August 20, 2009.
3. American Heart Association: *American Stroke Association: effects of stroke* (website). www.strokeassociation.org/presenter.jhtml?identifier=1052. Accessed August 20, 2009.
4. American Occupational Therapy Association: Occupational therapy practice framework: domain and process, ed. 2. *Am J Occup Ther* 62(6):625–683, 2008.
5. Anastasi A, Urbina S: *Psychological testing*, ed. 7, Upper Saddle River, NJ, 1997, Prentice Hall.
6. Árnadóttir G: *The brain and behavior: assessing cortical dysfunction through activities of daily living*, St Louis, 1990, Mosby.
7. Árnadóttir G: *Impact of neurobehavioral deficits on ADL: Theoretical principles behind the Árnadóttir OT-ADL Neurobehavioral Evaluation (A-ONE)*. Poster presentation at the twelfth World Congress of Occupational Therapists. Montréal, Canada, 1998, World Federation of Occupational Therapists.
8. Árnadóttir G: Evaluation and intervention with complex perceptual impairment. In Unsworth C, editor: *Cognitive and perceptual dysfunction: a clinical reasoning approach to evaluation and intervention*, Philadelphia, 1999, FA Davis.
9. Árnadóttir G: *Neurobehavior: the key to occupation*. Poster presentation at the thirteenth World Congress of Occupational Therapists, Stockholm, Sweden, 2002, World Federation of Occupational Therapists.
10. Árnadóttir G: *Development versus dysfunction: Neurobehavioral perspective related to errors in occupational performance*. Poster presentation at the seventh European Congress of Occupational Therapy, Athens, Greece, 2004, European Congress of Occupational Therapy.
11. Árnadóttir G: *Árnadóttir OT-ADL Neurobehavioral Evaluation (A-ONE): interrater reliability*. Poster presentation at the At Forum, Stockholm, Sweden, 2005, Förbundet Sveriges Arbetsterapeuter.
12. Árnadóttir G, Fisher AG: Rasch analysis of the ADL scale of the A-ONE. *Am J Occup Ther* 62(1):51–60, 2008.
13. Árnadóttir G: Árangur af iðjuþjálfun einstaklinga með taugaeinkenni: Hentug ADL matstæki. *Iðjuþjálfinn* 30(1):28–39, 2008.
14. Árnadóttir G, Fisher AG, Löfgren B: Dimensionality of nonmotor neurobehavioral impairments when observed in the natural contexts of ADL task performance. *Neurorehabil Neural Repair* 23(6):579–586, 2009.
15. Árnadóttir G, Löfgren B, Fisher AG: Neurobehavioral functions evaluated in naturalistic contexts: Rasch analysis of the A-ONE Neurobehavioral scale. Manuscript submitted for publication, 2009.
16. Árnadóttir G, Löfgren B, Fisher AG: The impact of neurobehavioral dysfunction on ADL performance in clients with right versus left hemispheric stroke. Unpublished manuscript, 2009.
17. Árnadóttir G: *A-ONE training course: lecture notes*, Reykjavík, Iceland, 2009–2010, Guðrún Árnadóttir.
18. Ayres AJ: *Developmental dyspraxia and adult onset apraxia*, Torrance, CA, 1985, Sensory Integration International.

19. Bailay DM: *Research for the health professional: a practical guide*, ed. 2, Philadelphia, 1997, FA Davis.
20. Benson J, Schell BA: Measurement theory: application to occupational and physical therapy. In Deusen JV, Brundt D, editors: *Assessment in occupational therapy and physical therapy*, Philadelphia, 1997, Saunders.
21. Bernspång B, Fisher AG: Differences between persons with right or left cerebral vascular accident on the assessment of motor and process skills. *Arch Phys Med Rehabil* 76(12):1144–1151, 1995.
22. Bond TG, Fox CM: *Applying the Rasch model: fundamental measurement in the human sciences*, ed. 2, Mahwah, NJ, 2007, Erlbaum.
23. Boyt Schell BA: Clinical reasoning: the basis of practice. In Crepeau EB, Cohn ES, Boyt Schell BA, editors: *Willard and Spackman's occupational therapy*, ed. 10, Philadelphia, 2003, Lippincott-Williams & Wilkins.
24. Caplan LR: *Stroke: a clinical approach*, ed. 2, Boston, 1993, Butterworth-Heinemann.
25. Center for Disease Control and Prevention: *Health policy data requests—Limitations in ADL and IADL* (website). www.cdc.gov/nchs/health_policy/ADL_tables.htm. Accessed July 2, 2009.
26. Cooke DM, McKenna K, Fleming J, Darnell R: Construct and ecological validity of the Occupational Therapy Adult Perceptual Screening Test (OT-APST). *Scand J Occup Ther* 13(1):49–61, 2006.
27. Crepeau EB, Boyt Schell BA: Analyzing occupations and activity. In Crepeau EB, Boyt Schell BA, Cohn ES, editors: *Willard and Spackman's occupational therapy*, ed. 11, Philadelphia, 2008, Lippincott-Williams & Wilkins.
28. Damasio AR, Anderson SW: The frontal lobes. In Heilman KM, Valenstein E, editors: *Clinical neuropsychology*, ed. 3, New York, 1993, Oxford University Press.
29. Daube JR, Sandok BA: *Medical neurosciences: an approach to anatomy, pathology and physiology by systems and levels*, Boston, 1978, Little, Brown.
30. De Renzi E, Fabrizia M, Nichelli P: Imitating gestures: a quantitative approach to motor apraxia. *Arch Neurol* 37(1):6–10, 1980.
31. De Renzi E, Lucchelli F: Ideational apraxia. *Brain* 111(5):1173–1185, 1988.
32. Donkervoort M, Dekker J, Deelman BG: Sensitivity of different ADL measures to apraxia and motor impairments. *Clin Rehabil* 16(3):299–305, 2002.
33. Edmans, JA, Lincoln, NB: The relation between perceptual deficits after stroke and independence in activities of daily living. *Br J Occup Ther* 53(4):139–142, 1990.
34. Fisher AG: Assessment of motor and process skills. In *Development, standardization, and administration manual*, vol 1, ed. 6, Fort Collins, CO, 2006, Three Star Press.
35. Fisher, AG: Overview of performance skills and client factors. In McHugh Pendleton H, Schultz-Krohn W, editors: *Pedretti's occupational therapy practice skills for physical dysfunction*, ed. 6, St. Louis, 2006, Mosby.
36. Fisher AG: *Occupational therapy intervention process model: A model for planning and implementing top-down, client-centered, and occupation-based interventions*, Fort Collins, CO, 2009, Three Star Press.
37. Gardarsdóttir S, Kaplan S: Validity of the Árnadóttir OT-ADL neurobehavioral evaluation (A-ONE): performance in activities of daily living in persons with left and right hemisphere damage. *Am J Occup Ther* 56(5):499–508, 2002.
38. Gillen G: *Cognitive and perceptual rehabilitation: Optimizing function*. St Louis, 2009, Elsevier.
39. Goldberg E, Costa LD: Hemisphere differences in the acquisition and use of descriptive system. *Brain Lang* 14(1):144, 1981.
40. Heilman KM, Gonzalez Rothi LJ: Apraxia. In Heilman KM, Valenstein E, editors: *Clinical neuropsychology*, ed. 3, New York, 1993, Oxford University Press.
41. Heilman KM, Watson RT, Valenstein E: Neglect and related disorders. In Heilman KM, Valenstein E, editors: *Clinical neuropsychology*, ed. 3, New York, 1993, Oxford University Press.
42. Holm MB, Rogers JC: The therapists thinking behind functional assessment II. In Royeen CB, editor: *AOTA self study series: assessing function*, Rockville, MD, 1989, American Occupational Therapy Association.
43. Itzkovich M, Elazar B, Averbuch S, et al: *Lowenstein occupational therapy cognitive assessment: LOTCA™ Manual*, Pequannock, NJ, 1990, Maddack.
44. Kiernan JA: *Barr's the human nervous system: an anatomical viewpoint*, ed. 8, Philadelphia, 2005, Lippincott-Williams & Wilkins.
45. Korpelainen JT, Niileksela, E, Myllylä VV: The Sunnaas Index of Activities of Daily Living: Responsiveness and concurrent validity in stroke. *Scand J Occup Ther* 4(1):1–36, 1997.
46. Llorens LA: Activity analysis: agreement among factors in a sensory processing model. *Am J Occup Ther* 40(2):103–110, 1986.
47. Luria AR: *The working brain: an introduction to neuropsychology*. New York, 1973, Basic Books.
48. Luria AR: *Higher cortical functions in man*, ed. 2, New York, 1980, Basic Books.
49. Ma HI, Trombly CA: A synthesis of effects of occupational therapy for persons with stroke II. Remediation of impairments. *Am J Occup Ther* 56(3):260–274, 2002.
50. Mathiowetz V: Role of physical performance component evaluations in occupational therapy functional assessment. *Am J Occup Ther* 47(3):225–230, 1993.
51. Mattingly C, Fleming MH: *Clinical reasoning: forms of enquiry in a therapeutic practice*, Philadelphia, 1994, FA Davis.
52. Merbitz C, Morris J, Grip JC: Ordinal scales and foundations of misinference. *Arch Phys Med Rehabil* 70(4):308–312, 1989.
53. Mercier L, Hebert J, Colarusso RP, et al: *MVPT-V Motor free visual perception test—vertical format—manual*, Novato, CA, 1997, Academic Therapy Publications.
54. Neistadt ME: *Occupational therapy evaluation for adults: a pocket guide*, Baltimore, 2000, Lippincott Williams & Wilkins.
55. Nuwer MR, Árnadóttir G, Martin AA, et al: A comparison of quantitative electroencephalography, computed tomography, and behavioral evaluations to localize impairment in patients with stroke and transient ischemic attacks. *J Neuroimaging* 4(2):82–84, 1994.
56. Okkema K: *Cognition and perception in the stroke patient: a guide to functional outcomes in occupational therapy*, Gaithersburg, MD, 1993, Aspen.
57. Phillips ME, Wolters S: Assessment in practice: common tools and methods. In Royeen CB, editor: *AOTA self study series: stroke—strategies, treatment, rehabilitation, outcomes, knowledge and evaluation*, Bethesda, MD, 1996, American Occupational Therapy Association.
58. Polgar JM: Critiquing assessments. In Crepeau EB, Cohn ES, Boyt Schell BA, editors: *Willard & Spackman's occupational therapy*, ed. 9, Philadelphia, 1998, Lippincott-Raven.
59. Robertson I, Ward T, Ridgeway Y, et al: *The test of everyday attention (TEA)*. Bury St Edmunds, England, 1994, Thames Valley Test Company.
60. Rogers JC, Holm MB: The therapists thinking behind functional assessment I. In Royeen CB, editor: *AOTA self study series: assessing function*, Rockville, MD, 1989, American Occupational Therapy Association.
61. Royeen CB: *A research primer in occupational and physical therapy*, Bethesda, MD, 1997, American Occupational Therapy Association.
62. Starkstein SE, Robinson RG: Neuropsychiatric aspects of stroke. In Coffey CE, Cummings JL, editors: *Textbook of geriatric neuropsychiatry*, Washington, DC, 1994, American Psychiatric Press.
63. Steultjens EM: A-ONE: De Nederlandse Versie. *Ned Tidskrift Ergoterapie* 26:100–104, 1998.
64. Steultjens EM, Dekker J, Bouter LM, et al: Occupational therapy for stroke patients: a systematic review. *Stroke* 34(3):676–687, 2003.
65. RL Strub, FW Black: *The mental status examination in neurology*, ed 2, Philadelphia, 1985, FA Davis.

66. Sveen U, Bautz-Holter E, Sødring KM et al: Association between impairments, self-care ability and social activities 1 year after stroke. *Disabil Rehabil* 21(8):372–377, 1999.

67. Tesio L: Measuring behaviours and perceptions: Rasch analysis as a tool for rehabilitation research. *J Rehab Med* 35(3):105–115, 2003.

68. Tham K, Bernspång B, Fisher AG: Development of the assessment of awareness of disability. *Scand J Occup Ther* 6(4):184–190, 1999.

69. Trombly CA, MA HI: A synthesis of effects of occupational therapy for persons with stroke. I. Restoration of roles, tasks and activities. *Am J Occup Ther* 56(3):250–259, 2002.

70. Trombly Latham CA: Occupation as therapy: Selection, gradation, analysis and adaptation. In Radomski MV, Trombly Latham CA, editors: *Occupational therapy for physical dysfunction*, ed. 6, Philadelphia, 2008, Lippincott Williams & Wilkins.

71. Unsworth C: Reflections on the process of therapy in cognitive and perceptual dysfunction. In Unsworth C, editor: *Cognitive and perceptual dysfunction: a clinical reasoning approach to evaluation and intervention*, Philadelphia, 1999, FA Davis.

72. US Department of Health and Human Services: *Clinical practice guideline number 16: post-stroke rehabilitation*, Rockville, MD, 1995, US Department of Health and Human Services.

73. Whiting S, Lincoln N, Bhavnani G, et al: *The Rivermead Perceptual Assessment Battery*, Windsor, 1985, NFER-NELSON.

74. Wilson BA, Alderman P, Burgess H, et al: *Behavioral assessment of the dysexecutive syndrome (BADS)*, Bury St Edmunds, England, 1996, Thames Valley Test Company.

75. Wilson BA, Cockburn J, Baddely A: *The Rivermead behavioural memory test*, Suffolk, England, 1989, Thames Valley Test Company.

76. Wilson BA, Cockburn J, Halligan P: *Behavioral inattention test: manual*, Suffolk, England, 1987, Thames Valley Test Company.

77. World Health Organization: *The international classification of functioning, disability and health—ICF*, Geneva, Switzerland, 2001, WHO.

78. Wright BD, Linacre JM: Observations are always ordinal; Measurements, however, must be interval. *Arch Phys Med Rehabil* 70(12):857–860, 1989.

79. Yatsu FM, Grotta JC, Pettigrew LC, et al: *Stroke: 100 maxims*, St Louis, 1995, Mosby.

80. Zoltan B: *Vision, perception, and cognition: a manual for the evaluation and treatment of the neurologically impaired adult*, ed. 3, Thorofare, NJ, 1996, Slack.

glen gillen
kerry brockmann rubio

chapter 19

Treatment of Cognitive-Perceptual Deficits: A Function-Based Approach

key terms

apraxia	integrated functional approach	problem-solving
attention	memory	spatial relations
cognition	neurobehavior	unilateral neglect
concrete thinking	organization/sequencing	
executive dysfunction	perception	
poor insight/awareness	perseveration	

chapter objectives

After completing this chapter, the reader will be able to accomplish the following:

1. Understand the different approaches to treatment of cognitive and perceptual impairments and be aware of research conducted on each approach.
2. Integrate performance-based assessments to guide intervention planning.
3. Discuss different treatment approaches to individual neurobehavioral impairments.
4. Realize the relevance and importance of occupation-based activities in the treatment of cognitive and perceptual impairments.

Few things are more interesting or frustrating to a therapist than observing a stroke survivor with severe neglect or apraxia attempting unsuccessfully to perform an activity. Cognitive and perceptual (processing) impairments can severely impair a person's ability to participate in everyday activities. Frequently, the priority for occupational therapists is to determine what can be done to improve the performance in activities for stroke patients with processing impairments.

This chapter focuses on assessment and interventions for those living with functional deficits secondary to cognitive/perceptual impairments. It reviews studies and other literature on treatment approaches and discusses suggestions for treating processing impairments that frequently are found in persons who have sustained a stroke. The reader should review Chapters 17 and 18 for a full overview of this topic.

NEUROBEHAVIOR

Neurobehavior has been defined as any behavioral response resulting from central nervous system processing. Neurobehavior is considered the basis of performance in activities of daily living (ADL).[6] In this chapter, neurobehavior refers to cognitive and perceptual components of behavior, including praxis, attention, memory, spatial relations, sequencing, and problem-solving.

TREATMENT APPROACHES

Approaches to stroke rehabilitation can be directed at the level of impairment, activity limitations, or participation restrictions. *Impairment* refers to body dysfunction; *activity limitation*, to task performance dysfunction; and *participation restriction*, to problems in life situations. Approaches aimed at the level of participation restrictions have the greatest

impact on the stroke survivor's quality of life.[62] Unfortunately, many times in current practice, participation restrictions are deemphasized, whereas impairment or activity limitation is stressed. Therapists must strive to provide service in all three areas of need while promoting issues relevant to the patient's quality of life. See Chapter 3.

Treatment approaches to perceptual or cognitive impairments generally are classified in one of two categories: (1) the functional or adaptive approach or (2) the remediation or restoration approach.[34] The functional or adaptive approach underscores techniques to assist the patient in adapting to deficits, changing the environmental parameters of a task to facilitate function, and using a person's strengths to compensate for loss of function. Remediation, or restoration, highlights the use of techniques to facilitate recovery of the actual cognitive or perceptual skills affected by the stroke. Each approach has strengths and limitations, and therapists often use both approaches during stroke rehabilitation (Table 19-1).

Functional/Adaptation Approach

The functional approach uses repetitive practice in particular activities, usually daily living tasks, to help the patient become more independent. This approach is

Table 19-1

Traditional Classifications of Interventions

REMEDIATION	ADAPTATION
Also known as a restorative or transfer of training approach	Also known as a functional approach
Focused on the decreasing impairment(s)	Focused on decreasing activity limitations and participation restrictions
Focused on the cause of the functional limitation. Assumes cortical reorganization takes place	Focused on the symptoms of the problem
Typically uses deficit-specific cognitive and perceptual retraining activities chosen based on the pattern of impairment	Typically uses practice of functional activities chosen based on what the person receiving services wants to do, needs to do, or has to do in his or her own environment
Examples of interventions: cognitive and perceptual table-top "exercises," parquetry blocks, specialized computer software programs, cancellation tasks, block designs, pegboard design copying, puzzles, sequencing cards, gesture imitation, picture matching, design copying	Examples of interventions: meal preparation, dressing, generating a shopping list, balancing a checkbook, finding a number in the phonebook, environmental adaptations (i.e., placing all necessary grooming items on the right side of the sink for a person with neglect), compensatory strategy training approaches (i.e., using a scanning strategy such as the "Lighthouse Strategy" to improve attention to the left side of the environment for those living with; an alarm watch to remember to take a medication for those with memory impairment)
Requires the ability to learn and generalize the intervention strategies to a real world situation	Using a compensatory strategy requires insight to the functional deficits and accepting that the impairment is relatively permanent. Environmental modifications do not require insight or learning on the part of the person receiving services.
Assumes that improvement in a particular cognitive-perceptual activity will "carryover" to functional activities	Does not assume that the underlying impairment is even affected by the intervention

From Gillen, G. *Cognitive and perceptual rehabilitation: optimizing function*, St. Louis, 2009, Mosby/Elsevier.

designed to treat symptoms rather than the cause of the dysfunction.[33] Some occupational therapists believe their role in cognitive and perceptual rehabilitation lies solely in the realm of a functional approach, involving training in compensatory techniques and only with tasks directly related to functional performance.[76] This approach appears most compatible with research indicating that family members and financial providers rank independence in ADL as the highest priority for rehabilitation.[29,72]

Therapists use the functional approach to train patients to function by compensating. An example of compensation is the use of an alarm watch to remind someone with poor memory to take medication. Compensation circumvents the problem. Some therapists believe the use of compensation should be limited to patients who have accepted the permanence of the perceptual or cognitive deficit.[77] Only persons who can benefit from compensation should be taught these strategies; they must have a basic understanding of their skills and the permanence of their limitations because the use of compensation for disability requires that the individual recognize the need to compensate. The patient must be a self-starter, must be goal directed, have insight/awareness of the functional consequences of his or her impairments, and must want to learn new strategies. Successful compensation requires practice, repetition, and overlearning of the strategies.[116]

Environmental adaptation is more appropriate for those who cannot use compensatory strategies because of poor insight of disability. Adaptation involves changing the characteristics of the task or environment. This technique is used in patients with poor learning potential. An example of adaptation is the use of contrasting colors for a plate and placemat for someone with figure-ground difficulties. Establishing a routine and constant environment with repeated participation in familiar activities is often the most successful strategy for these individuals. The adaptive approach relies on caregivers to implement treatment strategies.[116]

A significant limitation of the functional approach is the task specificity of the strategies and lack of generalizability to other tasks.[25] For example, the use of an alarm timer to take medications on time does not help the patient remember a repertoire of other activities, such as to take a shower, start meal preparation, or get to a doctor's appointment, unless the patient specifically has been trained to do so.

Remedial Approach

Remediation (or restoration or transfer of training) emphasizes restoration of the function or skill lost due to the stroke. Remedial treatment relies on several assumptions: the cerebral cortex is malleable and can adapt, and the brain can repair and reorganize itself after injury. Practice and repetition are assumed to result in learning. In turn, learning results in a more organized, functional system. Another assumption is that table-top activities, such as pegboard tasks or computer activities, directly affect the underlying processing skills

required for the patient to perform those activities. The most important assumption is that improved task performance of table-top activities will be carried over to improved performance in functional activities.[25,33,67]

Although this approach has been successful when used in the initial stages of treatment,[33] most studies show only short-term results, generalization only to similar tasks,[104] or little effectiveness from remedial training for neurobehavioral impairments.[33,44] For this approach to be successful, treatment sessions must be frequent and lengthy.

Neistadt[67] believes that only those patients who show transfer of learning to tasks that are different in multiple characteristics are appropriate candidates for the remedial approach to processing impairments. Therapists widely agree that practice of a subcomponent skill, such as problem-solving or attention to task, must occur in multiple contexts for successful transfer of learning.[116] According to Neistadt,[68] therapists always should train for transfer of skills because the patient's home environment is always different from the clinical setting. Those who can transfer learning only to similar tasks should be restricted to a functional/adaptive approach to maximize their training potential.[66]

Recommended Approach

Determination of the appropriate treatment approach for the stroke patient with processing impairments relies on the results of the assessment. Important questions include the following:

- Does the patient have the potential to learn?
- Is the patient aware of errors during task performance; and if so, does the patient have the potential to seek solutions to those errors?

If the patient has poor learning potential or poor awareness and is unlikely to benefit from the use of cues or task modification, a strictly functional approach involving domain-specific training would be recommended.[101] Domain-specific training requires little or no transfer of learning (generalizability) and involves repetitive performance of a specific functional task using a system of vanishing cues. (*Vanishing cues* are cues that are provided at every step of task performance but then gradually are removed. The goal is to establish a program in which the patient can successfully perform the task with a minimum number of cues.) This type of training is hyperspecific, and the learning associated with it persists only if the task and environmental characteristics remain unchanged.

Traditionally the therapist has used a restorative or functional approach; however, Abreu and colleagues[1] have proposed an integrated functional approach to treatment using principles from both approaches simultaneously. In this approach, areas of occupation and context are used to challenge processing skills. Because individuals engage in occupations as integrated wholes—not as separate attention machines, categorizers, or memory coders—

treatments that are not aimed at real life contexts are irrelevant to real life. With this integrated functional approach, treatment may be focused on a subcomponent skill such as sustained attention, but daily occupations are used as the modality. For example, a self-feeding task can be used to improve sustained attention to task. Mealtime is often distracting. Eating can be a difficult task if attention deficits are present. A system of vanishing cues and a gradual increase in the amount of environmental distraction can be used to address inattention to task and activity participation.

The use of a functional approach is supported by today's health care industry, which seeks documentation of patient's functional competence in ADL. Only cost-effective interventions that directly affect functional status are embraced in today's health care environment.

Any functional task can be used to address a myriad of neurobehavioral impairments. For occupational therapists to use their skills in activity analysis to evaluate an activity for its effectiveness in addressing particular cognitive or perceptual deficits is imperative. Box 19-1 contains an example of using everyday function to address neurobehavioral performance skills.

ASSESSMENT DECISIONS

The assessment of the impact of cognitive and perceptual deficits on daily function is a complex process (see Chapter 18). To increase the efficiency and use of this process, the following recommendations are made:
- As opposed to pen and paper/table-top measures, performance-based assessments are recommended. See Table 19-2 and other samples within this chapter for examples. Pen and paper or "table-top" assessments typically include items that attempt to detect the presence of a particular impairment (i.e., deficit-specific). Test items are usually contrived and are usually nonfunctional tasks such as copying geometrical forms, pegboard constructions, constructing block designs, matching picture halves, drawing tasks, sequencing pictures, remembering number strings, cancellation tasks, identifying overlapping figures, completing body puzzles, etc. It may be argued that this type of test has low ecological validity. Does the ability to sequence a series of picture cards predict the ability to plan, cook, and clean up a family meal? Does failure to accurately create a three-dimensional block

---

Box 19-1

Tooth-Brushing Task: Treatment of Neurobehavioral Impairments

SPATIAL RELATIONS/SPATIAL POSITIONING
- Positioning of toothbrush and toothpaste while applying paste to toothbrush
- Placement of toothbrush in mouth
- Positioning of bristles in mouth
- Placement of toothbrush under faucet

SPATIAL NEGLECT
- Visual search for and use of toothbrush, toothpaste, and cup
- Visual search and use of faucet handle

BODY NEGLECT
- Brushing of affected side of mouth

MOTOR APRAXIA
- Manipulation of toothbrush during task performance
- Manipulation of cap from toothpaste
- Squeezing of toothpaste onto toothbrush

IDEATIONAL APRAXIA
- Appropriate use of objects (toothbrush, toothpaste, cup) during task

ORGANIZATION/SEQUENCING
- Sequencing of task (removal of cap, application of toothpaste to toothbrush, turning on water, and putting toothbrush in mouth)
- Continuation of task to completion

ATTENTION
- Attention to task (for greater difficulty, distractions such as conversation, flushing toilet, or running water may be added)
- Refocus on task after distraction

FIGURE-GROUND
- Distinguishing white toothbrush and toothpaste from sink

INITIATION/PERSEVERANCE
- Initiation of task on command
- Cleaning parts of mouth for appropriate period of time and then moving bristles to another part of mouth
- Discontinuation of task when complete

VISUAL AGNOSIA
- Use of touch to identify objects

PROBLEM-SOLVING
- Search for alternatives if toothpaste or toothbrush is missing

Table 19-2

Selected Performance-Based and Self-Report Assessments for Use with Those Experiencing Limitations in Daily Function Secondary to Cognitive and Perceptual Impairments

INSTRUMENT	INSTRUMENT DESCRIPTION
Comprehensive assessments	
Árnadóttir Occupational Therapy-ADL Neurobehavioral Evaluation (A-ONE)[6,7] See Chapter 18.	Structured observation of basic ADL including feeding, grooming and hygiene, dressing, transfers, and mobility to detect the impact of multiple underlying impairments Provides information related to how neurobehavioral deficits affect everyday living Includes items related to ideational apraxia, motor apraxia, unilateral body neglect, somatoagnosia, spatial relations dysfunction, unilateral spatial neglect, perseveration, organization and sequencing dysfunction, topographical disorientation, motor control impairments, agnosias (visual object, associative visual object, visual spatial), anosognosia, body scheme disturbances, emotional/affective disturbances, impaired attention and alertness, memory loss, etc. Requires training
Assessment of Motor and Process Skills (AMPS)[36,37] See Chapter 21.	An observational assessment used to measure the quality of a person's ADL assessed by rating the effort, efficiency, safety, and independence of 16 motor and 20 process skill items Includes choices from 85 tasks Provides information related to everyday function Requires training
Brief measure of cognitive functional performance	
Kettle Test[46]	Provides a brief performance-based assessment of an instrumental ADL task designed to tap into a broad range of cognitive skills. The task consists of making two hot beverages that differ in two ingredients (one for the client and one for the therapist). The electric kettle is emptied and disassembled to challenge problem-solving skills and safety judgment, and additional kitchen utensils and ingredients are placed as distracters to increase attention demands.
Assessing apraxia	
ADL Observations to measure disabilities in those with apraxia[106,107]	Structured observation of four activities: washing face and upper body, putting on a shirt or blouse, preparing food, an individualized task chosen by the occupational therapist Scored based on initiation, execution, and control
The ADL Test for those with apraxia[41]	Observation of spreading margarine on bread, putting on a T-shirt, brushing teeth, or putting cream on hands Scores based on reparable or fatal errors relate to selection of objects, movements, or sequencing
Assessing unilateral neglect	
Catherine Bergego Scale (CBS)[9,18]	Examines the presence of neglect related to direct observation of functional activities such as grooming, dressing, feeding, walking, wheelchair navigation, finding belongings, positioning self in a chair. Has been used as a self-assessment with results compared with therapist's ratings to objectify anosognosia (awareness) Measures personal and extrapersonal neglect
Behavioral Inattention Test (BIT)[45,113]	Assessment for unilateral neglect using 6 pen-and-paper tests and 9 behavioral tests. Behavioral tests consist of *simulated* tasks.
Comb and razor/compact test[19,64]	Analyzes attention to both sides of the body during hair combing followed by *simulating* shaving or applying makeup Each task is 30 seconds.
Wheelchair collision test[75]	The person is asked to propel a wheelchair to pass four chairs arranged in two rows. Screening tool only
Baking Tray Task[5,99]	Clients are asked to spread out 16 cubes on a 75 × 50 cm board or A4 paper (8.27 × 11.69 inches) "as if they were buns on a baking tray." *Simulated* task
Fluff test[28]	24 white cardboard circles are adhered to various areas on a person's clothing (15 on the left side of the body and 9 on the right). The person must find and remove the targets from the clothing.

Continued

Table 19-2

Selected Performance-Based and Self-Report Assessments for Use with Those Experiencing Limitations in Daily Function Secondary to Cognitive and Perceptual Impairments—cont'd

INSTRUMENT	INSTRUMENT DESCRIPTION
Assessing impairments of attention	
Test of Everyday Attention[80]	Considered an ecologically valid test of various types of everyday attention such as sustained attention, selective attention, attentional switching, and divided attention Includes several subtests. It is one of the few tests of attention that *simulates* everyday life tasks. The test is based on the imagined scenario of a vacation trip to the Philadelphia area of the United States.
Cognitive Failures Questionnaire[21]	*Self-report* measure of the frequency of lapses of attention and cognition in daily life. Includes items related to memory, attention, and executive dysfunction.
Assessing executive function impairments	
Executive Function Performance Test (EFPT)[12]	Assesses executive function deficits during the performance of real world tasks (cooking oatmeal, making a phone call, managing medications, and paying a bill). The test uses a structured cueing and scoring system to assess initiation, organization, safety, and task completion and to develop cuing strategies.
Multiple Errands Test[2,30,58,85]	Tasks include purchasing 3 items, picking up an envelope from reception, using telephone, posting the envelope, writing down four items (i.e., price of a candy bar), meeting assessor, and informing assessor that the test was completed.
Behavioural Assessment of Dysexecutive Syndrome (BADS)[111,114]	Includes items that are sensitive to those skills involved in problem solving, planning, and organizing behavior over an extended preiod of time. The battery is designed to access capacities that are typically required in everyday living using simulated tasks. It includes the six subtests that represent different executive abilties such as cognitive flexibility, novel problem solving, planning, judgment and estimation, and behavioral regulation.
Assessing memory loss	
Rivermead Behavioral Memory Test[112]	Ecologically valid test of everyday memory. Uses simulations of everyday memory tasks. The original version is used for those with moderate to severe impairments while an extended version is available for those with subtle memory loss. Modifications are available for those with perceptual, language, and mobility impairments.
Everyday Memory Questionnaire[81,93,95]	Subjective report of everyday memory. A metamemory questionnaire. Self-report or via proxy.
Prospective and Retrospective Memory Questionnaire[55,88]	Measure of prospective and retrospective failures in everyday life. Self-rated or proxy-rated. Norms are published.

design from a two-dimensional cue card mean that an individual will not be able to dress or bathe independently? The use of this type of assessment procedure as the basis for clinical assessment needs to be questioned if the goal of the cognitive and perceptual assessment is to determine if/how impairment(s) will affect functioning in the real world. In contrast, a performance-based test uses functional activities commonly engaged in during daily life as the method of assessment. The use of structured observations to detect underlying impairments is a not only clinically valid [6,84,93,107] but provides the clinician with detailed information regarding how the underlying impairments directly *impacts* task performance.

- The environment chosen to conduct the assessment must be carefully considered. Typically these assessments are conducted in a quiet room, free of distractions. This may

be an appropriate starting point, but the findings might underestimate the impairment. Sbordone[82] emphasized that the typical assessment environment (a quiet room without environmental distracters) is not the real world. Specific concerns with a typical testing environment include:

- Conditions of testing are set up in such a way as to optimize performance.
- Distraction-free
- Overstructured
- Clear and immediate feedback is provided.
- Time demands are minimized.
- Repeated and clarified instructions to optimize performance.
- Problems with task initiation, organization, and follow-through are minimized as the clinician provides multiple cues for task progression, and the tests tend to

include discrete items that are performed one at a time as opposed to a sequence of events.[17]

TREATMENT CONSIDERATIONS

Therapists must consider many factors while preparing a treatment plan. A stroke survivor may not have the same needs as a person with a closed-head injury, encephalitis, or a gunshot wound to the head. All have brain injury, but they have different patterns of behavior and recovery. Likewise, one must remember that no two stroke survivors are alike. Each person with a stroke is a unique individual with special needs, goals, and problems.

Environment

The importance of the environment or setting in which treatment takes place cannot be underestimated. Patients plan and perform ADL differently[73] at home than in the clinical setting.[69] Exposure to different environments and contexts requires patients to adapt strategies and solve problems,[51] leading to greater independence in a variety of situations.

The adaptation of purposeful activities to ensure success is important in occupational therapy (OT). Success depends on the therapist's ability to analyze the activities and the patients' strengths, weaknesses, and needs to present the most relevant and challenging activity.

Generalization

One of the biggest challenges to providing interventions to this population is the issue of generalizing or transfer of what is learned in therapy sessions to other real world situations. Examples include generalizing the use of the skills learned on an inpatient rehabilitation related to meal preparation to making a meal at home on discharge, use of a scanning strategy used to read a newspaper article or to locate an item of clothing in a closet, or use of tactile feedback to identify objects on a meal tray or when shopping for grooming items. The consistent perspective on the idea of generalization is that it will not occur spontaneously but will instead need to be addressed explicitly in an intervention plan.[66,90,101,102,103]

Suggestions have been made in the literature to enhance generalization of cognitive and perceptual rehabilitation techniques:

- Avoid repetitively teaching the same activity in the same environment.[101,102,103] Consistently practicing bed mobility and wheelchair transfers in a person's hospital room does not guarantee that the skill will generalize to the ability to transfer to a toilet in a shopping mall.
- Practice the same strategy across multiple tasks (see Chapter 5). For example, if the "lighthouse strategy" (see later in this chapter) is successfully used during the treatment of an individual with spatial neglect to

accurately read an 8½ by 11 inch menu, the same strategy should be consistently and progressively practiced to read a newspaper, followed by reading the labels on spices in a spice rack, followed by a street sign, etc.
- Practice the same task and strategies in multiple natural environments.[101,102,103] Practice of organized visual scanning for an inpatient should be done in the therapy clinic, in the person's hospital room, in the facility's lobby and gift shop, in the therapist's office, etc.
- Include metacognitive training in the intervention plan to improve awareness.

Toglia[101,102,103] identified a continuum related to the transfer of learning and emphasized that generalization is not an all or none phenomenon. She discussed grading tasks to promote generalization of learning from those that are very similar to those that are very different. Toglia's[101,103] criteria for transfer included:

- Near transfer. Only one to two of the characteristics are changed from the originally practiced task. The tasks are similar, such as making coffee as compared to making hot chocolate or lemonade.[103]
- Intermediate transfer. Three to six characteristics are changed from the original task. The tasks are somewhat similar, such as making coffee as compared to making oatmeal.
- Far transfer. The tasks are conceptually similar but share only one similarity. The tasks are different, such as making coffee as compared to making a sandwich.
- Very far transfer. The tasks are very different, such as making coffee as compared to setting a table.

Based on her research and review of the literature, Neistadt[67] suggested that only those individuals who have the ability to perform far and very far transfers of learning are candidates for the remedial approach to cognitive and perceptual rehabilitation. She suggested that, on the other hand, those who are only capable of near and intermediate transfers of learning are candidates for the adaptive approach, as described earlier. Similarly, near transfers seem to be possible for all individuals regardless of severity of brain damage, while intermediate, far, and very far transfers may be possible only for those with localized brain lesions and preserved abstract thinking, and with those who have been explicitly taught to generalize.[67] While these statements should continue to be tested empirically, they give clinicians guidelines related to intervention planning.

NEUROBEHAVIORAL IMPAIRMENTS IN THE STROKE POPULATION

Processing impairments in the stroke population are part of an interactive process involving the patient, the activity at hand, and the context in which the task is being performed.[103] Cognition and perception are a dynamical process, constantly changing and reacting to internal and external stimuli. Therapists must address neurobehavioral impairments in the context of the situation and according to the person's needs and goals. This is why a generic, general approach does not work for the patients included in this population.

Neurobehavioral impairments often are noted in stroke survivors. Lesions from a stroke may cause localized loss of function such as language comprehension. More often, strokes cause a variety of neurobehavioral impairments associated with the severity of the infarct. General treatment strategies for persons with cognitive and perceptual impairments after stroke are addressed next. Commonly noted neurobehavioral impairments are discussed individually later in the chapter.

INTERVENTION STRATEGIES

Activity Processing

Activity processing is especially helpful in cognitive rehabilitation because the therapist discusses the purpose and results of the activity with the patient. The therapists can discern awareness by the patient from feedback provided during and after activity participation. Activity processing enhances the patient's metacognition (knowledge of one's own cognitive ability and ability to monitor one's own performance) and general knowledge. Activity processing emphasizes the purpose of the activity in the rehabilitation process.[23] For example, when practicing spatial positioning during a dressing task, the therapists should instruct the patient on the spatial requirements for each step of the activity and the purpose of using the dressing task to improve spatial skills. As the patient performs the task, the patient and the therapist should discuss performance and strategies to perform the activity.

Behavior Modification

Use of behavior modification techniques such as prompting, shaping (reinforcing responses that increasingly resemble the sought-after behavior), and contingent reinforcement (reward contingent on an appropriate response) are common in the stroke and/or brain injury population. Behavior modification techniques with intermittent praise and reinforcement to improve independence in daily activity have been successful.[43,53]

Group Treatment

Group treatment in the stroke population is often effective. It can yield situations more like real life, because they are less structured and can generate unpredictable events and provide distractions. In a group, patients can get feedback from their peers (which is often more meaningful), share similar experiences, and exchange problem-solving and coping strategies. Group treatment allows patients to learn from others' mistakes, practice monitoring their own behavior, and see that their problems are not unique.

TREATMENT APPROACHES FOR SPECIFIC NEUROBEHAVIORAL IMPAIRMENTS

Therapists rarely observe perceptual or cognitive deficits in isolation. Usually these deficits overlap and are difficult to interpret because of their complexity. Little research has been conducted or published on outcomes of specific treatment approaches for isolated perceptual and cognitive deficits, with the possible exceptions of memory impairments and unilateral neglect. However, therapists continue to assess these impairments individually, and using a combination of general and specific treatment approaches to neurobehavioral impairments does help sometimes. With this thought in mind, information on distinct treatment approaches related to specific impairments follows.

Decreased Awareness

Most authors recommend that self-awareness should be evaluated before initiating an intervention program focused on retraining living skills. Findings from standardized evaluations of self-awareness will clearly guide intervention choices. For example, a person who exhibits insight into an everyday memory deficit may be a candidate for teaching compensatory strategies such as using a diary or notebook However, a person who does not realize he or she is presenting with a severe unilateral neglect may not be able to learn compensatory strategies but may require environmental modifications (e.g., all clothing hung on the right side of the closet) to improve everyday function. In addition, ascertaining the level of insight to a disability is one factor that may determine how motivated one is to participate in the rehabilitation process. In the most simplistic interpretation, one must be aware and concerned about a deficit in everyday function to be motivated to participate in what may be a long and difficult rehabilitation process.

A variety of assessment measures are typically recommended to ascertain a person's level of self-awareness, including questionnaires (self or clinician rated); interviews; rating scales; functional observations; comparisons of self-ratings and ratings made by others such as significant others, caretakers, or rehabilitation staff; and comparisons of self-ratings and ratings based on objective measures of function or cognitive constructs. In addition, naturalistic observations can provide further information related to how decreased awareness interferes with performance of everyday tasks.

Simmond and Fleming[86,87] summarized that a comprehensive and clinically relevant assessment should:

- Be preceded by an assessment of intellectual awareness (e.g., the Self-Awareness of Deficits Interview) as intellectual awareness seems to be a prerequisite to online awareness.

- Allow a client to rate his or her own performance before, during, and after the assessment.
- Use meaningful activities.
- Use activities that allow enough flexibility to challenge clients.
- Be goal focused. The assessment findings should be used to work toward acceptance of a disability followed by interventions to improve function.

Sohlberg[89] further suggested that five assessment questions should be answered to comprehensively manage a lack of awareness. Sohlberg's suggestions for resources to answer each question follow as well:

1. *What is an individual's knowledge or understanding of strengths and deficits?* Sohlberg suggested gleaning information from standardized questionnaires and rating scales, and interviews with the client and significant others.

2. *How much of the problem is denial versus organically-based unawareness?* This complicated question may be answered via a review of medical history, cognitive assessment, standardized questionnaires and rating scales, interviews with the client and significant others, observations (strategy use, use of prediction, self-evaluation, and error response), and response to feedback.

3. *Is unawareness generalized or modality specific and does it accompany other cognitive impairments?* Similar to the previous question, Sohlberg recommended collecting data from multiple sources including a review of medical history, cognitive assessment, standardized

questionnaires and rating scales, interviews with the client and significant others, and observations (strategy use, use of prediction, self-evaluation, error response, and response to feedback).

4. *Does the individual consciously or unconsciously accommodate changes in functioning?* This question may be answered via interviews with the client and significant others, and through observations (strategy use, use of prediction, self-evaluation, error response, and response to feedback).

5. *What are the consequences of awareness?* Similar to question 4, this may be answered via interviews with the client and significant others, and through observations (strategy use, use of prediction, self-evaluation, error response, and response to feedback).

See Table 19-3 for a summary of assessments used to ascertain level of awareness.

Use of prompts and cues is key to successful cognitive and perceptual rehabilitation. Cues can be faded by reducing the number, frequency, or specificity of the prompts.[117] For example, a therapist initially may provide detailed cues at every step of task performance, such as "Look to the left to find the soap." Cues should be tapered and should become less detailed as the patient progresses (e.g., "Have you remembered all the steps?"). Therapists should provide prompts and cues in a calculated and graded fashion. The use of cues and prompts is part of cognitive and perceptual rehabilitation and is an essential way of facilitating patient insight, error detection, and strategy development (Table 19-4). See Box 19-2 for awareness training interventions.

Table 19-3

Recommended Measures of Awareness

INSTRUMENT AND AUTHOR	VALIDITY	COMMENTS
Self-Awareness of Deficits Interview[38]	Correlated with the Self-Regulation Skills Interview and the Awareness Questionnaire Correlated with work status Discriminates between those with brain injury and spinal injury	Measures intellectual awareness via a rating scale Rated by clinicians
Self-Regulation Skills Interview[71]	Discriminates between brain injured and non-brain injured subjects for awareness Correlated with the Self-Awareness of Deficits Interview and Health and Safety Scale Correlated with work status	Rated by clinicians As area of difficulty is determined by the client, it requires a level of intellectual awareness and includes items related to emergent and anticipatory awareness.
Awareness Interview[4]	Correlated in the expected direction with the Wechsler Adult Intelligence Scale and measures of temporal disorientation	Measures intellectual awareness via a discrepancy score compared with performance on standardized neurological tests
Assessment of Awareness of Disability[97,98]	A Rasch analysis suggested acceptable scale validity, construct validity, and person response validity	Used in conjunction with the Assessment of Motor and Process Skills (AMPS)

Table 19-4

Prompting Procedures

PROMPTS	RATIONALE
"How do you know this is the right answer/ procedure?" or "Tell me why you chose this answer/procedure."	Refocuses patient's attention to task performance and error detection.
"That is not correct. Can you see why?"	Can patient self-correct with a general cue?
	Provides general feedback about error but is not specific
	Can patient find error and initiate correction?
"It is not correct because . . ."	Provides specific feedback about error
	Can patient correct error when it is pointed out?
"Try this [strategy]" (e.g., going slower, saying each step out loud, verbalizing a plan before starting, or using a checklist)	Provides patient with a specific, alternate approach
	Can patient use strategy given?
Task is altered. "Try it another way."	Modifies task by one parameter. Can patient perform task? Begin again with grading of prompting described previously.

Adapted from Toglia JP: Attention and memory. In Royen CB, editor: *AOTA self-study series: cognitive rehabilitation*, Rockville, Md, 1993, American Occupational Therapy Association; and Toglia JP: Generalization of treatment: a multicontext approach to cognitive perceptual impairment in adults with brain injury. *Am J Occup Ther* 45(6):505, 1991.

Apraxia

According to Ayres,[8] praxis is one of the most important connections between brain and behavior; it is what allows persons to interact with the physical world. Apraxia is a dysfunction of purposeful movement that does not result primarily from motor, sensory, or comprehension impairments.[6] Although many different types of apraxia have been named and defined, the labels used to classify them are not universally accepted.[11] For relevance in this chapter, however, they fit into two general categories: motor and ideational apraxia. See Chapter 18 for examples of how the various types of apraxia affect daily living skills.

Patients with apraxia are often unaware of their deficits,[96] creating a dilemma for planning therapeutic interventions. However, one study concluded that patients with more severe cognitive (and motor) impairments showed the most significant improvement in ADL.[108] The study demonstrated the obvious potential for improvement

with severely apraxic patients using compensatory strategy training for ADL skills and therefore negates the idea that severely apraxic patients have poor potential for improvement. Box 19-3 lists general treatment guidelines for patients with apraxia. See Box 19-4 for a specific example of a performance-based assessment.

If physical guiding of the limbs is used during a task, incorporate the suggested principles of guiding,[22] including:

- Place their hands over the patient's whole hand, down to the fingertips.
- Keep talking to a minimum.
- Guide both sides of the body when possible.
- Move along a supported surface to give the patient maximal tactile feedback.
- Involve the whole body in the task to challenge posture.
- Provide changes in resistance during the activity.
- Allow the patient to make mistakes to give opportunities to solve problems (Figs. 19-1 and 19-2).

Encourage tactile exploration of functional objects and tools to enhance performance as somatosensory feedback from the tool may play a role in organizing movements.[42] Related to the above, object affordances (the functional use of particular objects within a context) positively affects motor performance.[42] Using meaningful objects and tasks will yield better results than movements performed in isolation.[61] As those with apraxia have compromised learning of old and new tasks, increased repetitions and practice will be necessary. Goals should be scaled accordingly. Encourage practice of learned skills outside of therapy and throughout the day. For those with ideomotor apraxia, experiment with decreasing the degrees of freedom (i.e., number of joints) used to perform the task (i.e., encourage a woman who is attempting to apply makeup to keep her elbow on the table). Grade the number of tools and distracters used in a task (i.e., finger feeding [no tools], followed by eating applesauce with only a spoon available, followed by eating applesauce with the choice of one to three utensils, followed by eating a meal requiring the choice of various tools for different aspects of the task [spoon to stir coffee, knife to cut and spread butter, etc.], followed by a meal with the necessary and usual utensils and distracter tools such as comb and toothbrush).[40]

- Grade the number of steps of an activity via chaining procedures. The whole task should be completed for each trial.
- Grade the number of tasks that will be performed in succession such as during a morning routine.
- Use clear and short directions.
- Use multiple cues to elicit functions: visual demonstration, verbal explanation, tactile guiding.
- Demonstrate the task while sitting parallel to the person with apraxia to help develop a visual model of the task.
- Encourage verbalization of what to do.

Box 19-2

Suggestions for Improving Awareness

Have clients perform tasks of interest and then provide them with feedback about their performance. The goal is to have clients monitor and observe their behavior more accurately so that they can make more realistic predictions about future performance and gain insight into their strengths and weaknesses.

Encourage self-questioning during a task and self-evaluation after a task (e.g., "Have I completed all of the steps needed?").

Provide methods of comparing functioning pre- and postinjury to improve awareness.

Use prediction methods. Have the client estimate various task parameters such as difficulty, time needed for completion, number of errors, and/or amount assistance needed before, during, or after a task and compare with actual results.

Help clients develop and appropriately set their personal goals.

Allow clients to observe their own performance during specific tasks (i.e., via videotape) and compare actual performance to what they state they can do.

Group treatments and peer feedback may be used because one person can receive feedback on performance from multiple individuals.

Use role reversals. Have the therapist perform the task, make errors, and have the client detect the errors.

The development of a strong therapeutic alliance is critical in managing both denial and lack of self-awareness. This alliance should be open and based on trust. Coaching clients to make better choices and understand how defensive strategies affect daily function.

Use familiar tasks that are graded to match the person's cognitive level ("just the right challenge") to develop self-monitoring skills and error recognition.

Provide education related to deficit areas for clients and families.

Integrate experiential feedback experiences. This method has been called "supported risk taking" and "planned failures" and is used during daily activities to gently demonstrate impairments. High levels of therapist supported are mandatory during this intervention.

Monitor for increased signs of depression and anxiety as awareness increases.

Increase mastery and control during performance of daily tasks to increase awareness.

Use emotionally neutral tasks to increase error recognition.

Use tasks that offer "just the right challenge" to increase error recognition/correction.

Provide feedback in a sandwich format (negative comments are preceded and followed by positive feedback).

Data from Fleming JM, Strong J, Ashton R: Cluster analysis of self-awareness levels in adults with traumatic brain injury and relationship to outcome. *J Head Trauma Rehabil* 13(5):39-51, 1998; Klonoff PS, O'Brien KP, Prigatano GP, et al: Cognitive retraining after traumatic brain injury and its role in facilitating awareness. *J Head Trauma Rehabil* 4(3):37-45, 1989; Lucas SE, Fleming JM: Interventions for improving self-awareness following acquired brain injury. *Austr Occup Ther J* 52(2):160-170, 2005; Prigatano GP: Disturbances of self-awareness and rehabilitation of patients with traumatic brain injury: a 20-year perspective. *J Head Trauma Rehabil* 20(1):19-29, 2005; Sherer M, Oden K, Bergloff P, et al: Assessment and treatment of impaired awareness after brain injury: implications for community re-integration. *NeuroRehabilitation* 10:25-37, 1998; Tham K, Tegner R: Video feedback in the rehabilitation of patients with unilateral neglect. *Arch Phys Med Rehabil* 78(4):410-413, 1997; Toglia J: A dynamic interactional approach to cognitive rehabilitation. In Katz N, editor: *Cognition and occupation across the life span*, Bethesda, Md, 2005, AOTA Press; Toglia JP: Generalization of treatment: a multicontext approach to cognitive perceptual impairment in adults with brain injury. *Am J Occup Ther* 45(6):505-516, 1991; and Toglia J, Kirk U: Understanding awareness deficits following brain injury. *NeuroRehabilitation* 15(1):57-70, 2000.

Further Interventions for Apraxia

The following paragraphs summarize evidenced-based interventions for those living with functional limitations secondary to apraxia.

Strategy Training. van Heugten and colleagues[105] described an intervention study designed for use by occupational therapists and based on teaching patients strategies to compensate for the presence of apraxia. In addition to interest checklists, the decision as to which activities to focus on was a joint decision between the therapist and patient. The focus of the intervention was determined by the specific problems observed during standardized ADL

observations (see Box 19-4). Specifically, interventions focused on errors related to:

- Initiation: inclusive of developing a plan of action and selection of necessary and correct objects
- Execution: performance of the plan
- Control: inclusive of controlling and correcting the activity to ensure an adequate result

Difficulties related to *initiation* were treated via specific instructions. Instructions were hierarchical in nature and could include verbal instructions, alerting the patient with tactile or auditory cues, gesturing, pointing, handing objects starting the activity together, etc. Assistance was the intervention provided when problems related to

Box 19-3

Potential Interventions for Those Living with Functional Limitations Secondary to Apraxia

Use functional tasks (previously learned and new tasks that are necessary to perform secondary to neurological impairments) for the interventions, i.e., an individualized task-specific approach.

"Tap into" an individual's routines and habits.

Collaborate with the client and his or her significant others/caregivers in order to choose the tasks to focus on and become the goals of therapy, i.e., a client-centered approach.

Practice these activities in the appropriate environments and at the appropriate time of day, i.e., context-specific with full contextual cues.

Use strategy training interventions to develop internal or external compensations during the performance of functional activities.

Focus interventions based on the errors made during the task: initiation, execution, and or control, i.e., error-specific interventions.

Practice functional activities with vanishing cues.

Provide graded assistance via providing graded instructions, assistance, or feedback during task performance.

Practice functional activities using errorless learning (preempting the error via assistance) approaches.

execution of the activity occurred. Also hierarchical, assistance could range from various types of verbal assist, stimulating verbalization of steps, naming the steps of the activity, to physical assistance such as guiding movements (see Figs. 19-1 and 19-2). Feedback is provided when patients have difficulty with *control* (i.e., patients do not detect or correct the errors they make during the activity) and can be verbal feedback related to the results of performance, verbal feedback focused on having the patient use a variety of senses to evaluate the results, or physical feedback focused on knowledge of results. The specific strategy training intervention protocol is included in Box 19-5. The strategy training approach for apraxia has been tested with promising results.[32]

A pretest/posttest study design[105] demonstrated significant improvements and large effects for three different ADL measures (Barthel Index; a standardized evaluation of personal hygiene, dressing, preparing food, and a patient chosen activity; and an ADL questionnaire that was filled out by both therapists and patients). In addition, significant improvements were documented on tests of apraxia (small to medium effects) and motor function (small effects). Improved ADL function was still significant after correcting for the improvement on the apraxia measures, motor measure, and time post-stroke. Of the patients in this study, 84% perceived complete recovery or substantial improvement because

of the intervention. While the intervention did not explicitly focus on decreasing the apraxic impairment, the strategy training approach during participation in functional activities decreased *both* activity limitations and severity of impairment.

Donkervoort and colleagues[32] also tested this intervention via a large randomized clinical trial comparing usual OT to strategy training integrated into usual OT. After intervention, those receiving strategy training improved significantly on ADL observations (small to medium effect size) and the Barthel Index (medium effect size) as compared to those who received usual care.

A posthoc analysis of Donkervoort and colleagues data performed by Geusgens and colleagues[39] focused on whether or not the strategy training approach resulted in transfer of training to untrained tasks. The analyses revealed that both intervention groups (traditional OT and traditional OT combined with strategy training) demonstrated significantly improved scores on nontrained tasks. Change scores of the nontrained activities were significantly larger in the strategy training group as compared to usual OT.

Errorless Completion and Training of Details. Goldenberg and Hagman[42] tested a method of specifically training ADL for those living with apraxia. They specifically examined spreading margarine on a slice of bread, putting on a T-shirt, and brushing teeth or applying hand cream. When an activity was being trained, the focus was on errorless completion of the whole activity. As opposed to trial and error learning, errorless learning or completion is a technique in which the person learns the activity by doing it. The therapist intervenes to prevent errors from occurring during the learning process. Specific interventions included:

- Guiding the hand through a difficult aspect of the activity (see Figs. 19-1 and 19-2)
- Sitting beside the patient (parallel position) and doing the same action simultaneously with the patient
- Demonstrating the required action and asking the patient to copy it afterwards

In addition, the intervention focused on training of details. This was aimed at directing the patient's attention to "the functional significance of single perceptual details and to critical features of the actions associated with them" (p.133).[42] Specific difficult steps of the activity were trained using this approach. To promote knowledge of object use, key details of ADL objects, such as the bristles on a toothbrush and the teeth on a comb, were explored and examined. Actions connected to the details were then practiced (i.e., searching for and positioning a shirt sleeve for a person with dressing difficulties) outside of therapy. Specific necessary motor actions were also practiced in other activities and contexts (i.e., squeezing paint from tubes as a similar action as squeezing toothpaste).

Box 19-4

Assessment of Disabilities in Stroke Patients with Apraxia

OBSERVATION AND SCORING OF ACTIVITIES OF DAILY LIVING

Purpose:

- To assess the presence of disabilities resulting from apraxia
- To gain an insight in the style of action of the patient and the sort of errors made
- To prepare treatment goals for specific training

Method:

The therapist observes the following activities and scores the findings for each activity and each aspect.
1. Personal hygiene: washing the face and upper body
2. Dressing: putting on a shirt or blouse
3. Feeding: preparing and eating a sandwich
4. The therapist chooses an activity that is relevant for the patient or standard at the department

I. Score of independence

    0—The patient is totally independent, can function without any help in any situation.
    1—The patient is able to perform the activity but needs some supervision.
    —The patient needs minimal verbal assistance to perform adequately.
    —The patient needs maximal verbal assistance to perform adequately.
    2—The patient needs minimal physical assistance to perform adequately.
    —The patient needs maximal physical assistance to perform adequately.
    3—The patient cannot perform the task despite full assistance.

II. The course of an activity

In every aspect, the patient can encounter problems; however, for each aspect only one score can be entered.
    A. Initiation
    0—There are no observable problems: the patient understands the instruction and initiates the activity.
    1—The verbal instruction has to be adapted or extended.
    —The therapist has to demonstrate the activity.
    —It is necessary to show pictures or write down the instructions.
    —The objects needed to perform the task have to be given to the patient.
    2—The therapist has to initiate the activity together with the patient.
    —The activity has to be modified in order to be performed adequately.
    3—The therapist has to take over.
    B. Execution
    0—There are no observable problems; the activity is performed correctly.
    1—The patient needs verbal guidance.
    —Verbal guidance has to be combined with gestures, pantomime, and intonation.
    —Pictures of the proper sequence of action have to be shown.
    2—The patient needs physical guidance.
    3—The therapist has to take over.
    C. Control
    0—There are no observable problems; the patient does not need feedback.
    1—The patient needs verbal feedback about the result of the performance.
    —The patient needs physical feedback about the result of the performance.
    2—The patient needs verbal feedback about the execution.
    —The patient needs physical feedback about the execution.
    —It is necessary to use mirrors or video recordings.
    3—The therapist has to take over.

From van Heugten C, Dekker J, Deelman B et al: Assessment of disabilities in stroke patients with apraxia: internal consistency and inter-observer reliability. *Occup Ther J Res* 19(1):55-73, 1999.

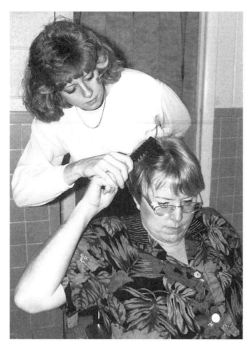

Figure 19-1   Patient is guided through a hair-brushing task.

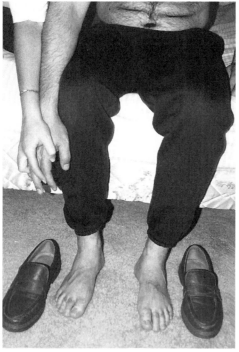

Figure 19-2   Guiding of the patient's hand along a supported surface (leg) as he reaches for a shoe.

Goldenberg and Hagman[42] tested this intervention by examining 15 patients with apraxia with repeated measures of ADL function. Success of therapy was based on the reduction of errors of specific tasks. The authors differentiated between reparable errors (the patients succeeds in continuing the task) or fatal errors (the patient is unable to proceed without help, or the task is completed but did not fulfill its purpose). Across the whole group, the number of fatal errors decreased significantly while the number of reparable errors did not significantly change.

Direct Training of the Whole Activity versus Exploration Training. Goldenberg and colleagues[41] developed and compared two therapy interventions aimed at restoring the ability to engage in complex ADL for those living with apraxia. Exploration training focused on having patients infer function from structure and solve mechanical problems embedded in tasks. During treatment, the therapist directed the patient's attention to functionally significant details of the object (i.e., prongs on a fork, serrations on a butter knife, bristles on a toothbrush). The therapist explained the functional significance via verbal, gestural, and pointing cues. The patients *did not* practice use of the tools. Specific interventions related to exploration training included explanation, touching, and comparing objects with photographs.

The direct training focused on the patient carrying out the whole activity with a minimum of errors. The technique is similar to errorless completion as reviewed previously and includes guided movements, with the therapist sitting beside the patient to perform the task simultaneously. During the training, particularly difficult components of the activity were practiced, but the whole activity was always completed. Specific interventions for direct training included guided performance of the whole activity, passive guidance, guidance by example, and rehearsal of steps.

Goldenberg and colleagues[41] tested these interventions related to the training of four complex ADL. The authors found that exploration training had no effect on performance, while direct training resulted in a significant reduction of errors and the amount of assist required to complete the task. Follow-up three months later revealed that gains were maintained.

Task-Specific Training. Poole[74] examined the ability of those living with apraxia to master the technique of one-handed shoe tying (commonly a necessary skill to be mastered after brain injury). She compared those living with a stroke without apraxia, those living with stroke with apraxia, and healthy adults. The task was taught using published standardized procedures via demonstration and simultaneously verbalizing instructions. Repetition was used until the task was achieved. The mean number of trials to learn the task was higher for those with apraxia ($M = 6.4$) as compared to those stroke survivors without apraxia ($M = 3.2$) versus healthy controls ($M = 1.2$). While the number of trial required to learn the task was greater, the majority of those with apraxia were able to retain the task.

Box 19-5

Protocol for Strategy Training for Those Living with Functional Deficits Secondary to Apraxia

The specific interventions are built up in a hierarchical order, depending on the patient's level of functioning. The therapist can use instructions, assistance, and feedback.

INSTRUCTIONS

The occupational therapist can give the following instructions:
- Start with a verbal instruction.
- Shift to a relevant environment for the task at hand.
- Alert the patient by:
  - Touching
  - Using the patient's name
  - Asking questions about the instruction
- Use gestures, point to the objects.
- Demonstrate (part of) the task.
- Show pictures of the activity.
- Write down the instruction.
- Place the objects near the patient, point to the objects, put the objects in the proper sequence.
- Hand the objects one at a time to the patient.
- Start the activity together with the patient one or more times.
- Adjust the task to make it easier for the patient.
- Finally, take over the task because all efforts did not lead to the desired result.

ASSISTANCE

The following forms of assistance can be given by the therapist:
- There is no need to assist the patient during the execution of the activity.
- Verbal assistance is needed:
  - By offering rhythm and not interrupting performance.
  - To stimulate verbalization of the steps in the activity.
  - To name the steps in the activity or name the objects.
  - To direct the attention to the task at hand.
- Use gestures, mimics, and vary intonation in your speech.
- Show pictures of the proper sequence of steps in the activity.
- Physical assistance is needed:
  - By guiding the limbs.
  - In positioning the limbs.
  - To use the neurodevelopmental treatment method.
  - To use aids to support the activity.
  - To take over until the patient starts performing.
  - To provoke movements.
- Finally, take over the task.

FEEDBACK

Feedback can be offered in the following ways:
- No feedback is necessary because the result is adequate.
- Verbal feedback is needed in terms of the result (knowledge of results).
- Verbal feedback by telling the patient to consciously use the senses to evaluate the result (tell the patient see, hear, feel, smell, or taste).
- Physical feedback is needed in terms of the result (knowledge of results):
  - To evaluate the posture of the patient.
  - To evaluate the position of the limbs.
  - To support the limbs.
- Physical feedback is given by pointing or handing the objects to the patient.
- Verbal feedback is needed in terms of performance (knowledge of performance).
- Physical feedback is needed in terms of performance (knowledge of performance).
- Place the patient in front of a mirror.
- Make video recordings of the patient's performance and show the recordings.
- Take over the control of the task and correct possible errors.

From van Heugten C, Dekker J, Deelman B, et al: Outcome of strategy training in stroke patients with apraxia: a phase II study. *Clin Rehabil* 12(4):294-303, 1998.

Wilson[110] documented a task-specific training program for a young woman status post an anoxic brain injury. The program focused on two tasks: drinking from a cup and sitting on a chair followed by positioning it correctly at the table. Functional performance was improved for this woman via the techniques of breaking down the steps of the tasks followed by practice of the steps, chaining procedures, and verbal mediation. The author noted that generalization to untrained tasks was not evident.

Perseveration

Perseveration is demonstrated by the inability to shift from one concept to another or to change or cease a behavior pattern once having started it. Perseveration also refers to the inability to translate knowledge into action (initiation of a task). The person is "stuck in set"—unable to discard the previous set of behaviors—or is unable to "activate" for a new situation. The person stuck in set attempts to solve another problem with information relevant to a previous problem.

Bringing perseveration to a conscious level and training the patient to inhibit the perseverative behavior has been successful.[48] Other strategies include redirecting attention, assisting the patient in initiating a new movement or task, and engaging the patient in tasks that involve repetitive action (e.g., washing the face or body, stirring food, or sanding wood) to promote successful task participation.

Unilateral Neglect

Unilateral neglect has been defined as "the failure to report, respond, or orient to novel or meaningful stimuli presented to the side opposite a brain lesion, when this failure cannot be attributed to either sensory or motor defects."[47] Unilateral neglect is most often seen when right-side brain damage occurs; therefore, the most frequent clinical presentation is that of left unilateral neglect. Although the mechanisms underlying neglect are still debated, a common hypothesis is that neglect is related to attention-based impairments and has been described as a lateralized attention deficit. Behaviors observed during everyday activities lend support to the attentional hypothesis, including the following:

- Not being aware of incoming stimuli on the side opposite the brain lesion (e.g., *hypo*attentive to the left side)
- A bias in attention to information presented on same side of the lesion (e.g., *hyper*attentive to the right side)
- Not being able to disengage from right-side stimuli.

The fact that those living with neglect *most often* present with left neglect also supports the attentional hypothesis because the right hemisphere is thought to be dominant for attention. That being said, right unilateral neglect is possible.[92] Beis and associates[15] documented right

neglect in 10% to 13.2% of those they examined. They concluded that right neglect caused by left hemispheric involvement is an elusive phenomenon and is less consistent than right hemispheric neglect. In addition, the frequency of occurrence of right neglect was, as expected, much lower than that reported in a study using the same assessment battery in right brain damage stroke clients.

Unilateral neglect can present with or without a concurrent visual field cut (see Chapter 16 and Table 19-5). In addition, neglect can interfere with attending to personal space (body neglect), near space, and/or far space (Table 19-6). Therefore, the recommended assessment method is a performance-based approach to give the therapist multiple opportunities to evaluate the impact of neglect on tasks that occur in the various aspects of space. Examples include the A-ONE (see Chapter 18) and the Catherine Bergego Scale (Fig. 19-3). Evidenced interventions to decrease the functional impact of neglect include the following.

Awareness Training

Tham and coworkers[98] developed an intervention to improve awareness related to the effect of neglect on functional performance. Purposeful and meaningful (for the participant) daily occupations were used as therapeutic change agents to improve awareness of disabilities. Specific interventions include the following:

- Encourage the participants to choose motivating tasks as the modality of intervention.
- Discuss task performance. Examples include encouraging the participants to describe their anticipated difficulties, to link their earlier experiences of disability to new tasks, and to plan how they would handle new situations; and asking the participants to evaluate and describe their performance and to think about whether they could improve performance by doing the task in another way.
- Provide feedback about the observed difficulties including verbal feedback (describe to the participant difficulties with reading and understanding the text in the left half of the page of the newspaper), visual feedback (give visual guidance to show the "neglected" text in the left half of the page), and physical guidance.
- When participants could describe their difficulties, the therapists and participants discussed compensatory techniques that could improve task performance.
- The participant performed the task again, using the newly learned compensatory techniques.
- The home environment was used to confront difficulties in familiar settings.
- Video feedback was used (see later).
- Interviews were used to reflect on and heighten awareness.

Table 19-5

Suggestions to Differentiate between Neglect and Visual Field Loss Based on Analysis of Behaviors

VISUAL FIELD LOSS	NEGLECT
Objectively tested via confrontation testing (screening) or via formalized perimetry testing (see Chapter 16)	Objectively tested using a battery of assessments to identify body/personal, extrapersonal (near and far), and motor neglect
Awareness of deficits emerge early in the recovery process.	Lack of awareness is more severe and persistent.
Compensatory strategies such as head turning are observed early and relatively easily taught.	Compensatory interventions are difficult, may require multiple sessions, or may not be effective.
Postural alignment is usually not affected.	Postural alignment of the head, neck, and trunk may bias toward the right side.
Sensory-based deficit	Attention-based deficit
Visual deficit only	Multiple sensory systems may be involved (visual, auditory, tactile).
Effective compensatory strategies result in positive functional outcomes.	Functional outcomes tend to be poor as compared to those without neglect.
Cortical representation of the "whole real world" is intact.	Decreased representation of the left side of space while describing a room from memory
Movement into both hemifields is not affected.	Resistance to moving actively (akinesia) or passively into the left field
	Long delays related to moving into the affected field (hypokinesia)
Extinction is not present.	Extinction may be present.
Early leftward eye movements noted	Rightward-biased eye movements
Not fully effective but consistent scanning patterns	Haphazard scanning patterns biased to the right
Comparatively, not as severe a deficit	A severe deficit related to functional outcome, rehabilitation needs, and caregiver burden

Scanning Training

Scanning training has long been considered a critical aspect of intervention programs for those with neglect. Scanning training has been documented to include the following:

- Rotation activities (trunk, head/neck)
- Scanning while static
- Scanning while mobile (ambulation or wheelchair navigation)
- Using perceptual anchors (the left arm on the table or a brightly colored strip of tape on the left side of an activity)
- Specific reading, writing, and mathematical calculations training

Lighthouse Strategy (LHS)

The specific intervention is outlined as follows:[65]

- A cancellation test is administered during the initial evaluation.
- The test is scored, and the person is shown the letters missed on the test.
- The therapist makes introductory statements such as, "I teach a strategy to help people pay better attention to their left [or right]. See how you missed these on this side? I can help you fix this problem."

- The LHS is introduced as a strategy for helping people pay better attention to their left and right and is explained fully. The person is shown a simple line drawing of the Cape Hatteras lighthouse, with the light beams and top lights highlighted with a yellow marker. The person is told to imagine that his or her eyes and head were like the light inside the top of the lighthouse, sweeping to the left and to the right of the horizon to guide ships to safety. The person is then asked to think about what would happen if the lighthouse only provided light to the right (or left) side of the ocean and horizon. The therapist probes for consequences of the lighthouse illuminating only one side.
- The picture of the lighthouse is placed on the table to the right and in front of the person.
- The therapist then introduces a task requiring full scanning of the left and right fields. The person is asked to close the eyes while the therapist sets up objects across the table in front of the person. The person is asked to find these objects.
- Each time an object is missed, the person is asked to turn the head "like a lighthouse, left and right, like this" while the therapist demonstrates the proper degree and pace of head turning. The person is shown how to line the tip of the chin first with the top of the right and then the top of the left shoulder.

Table 19-6

Spatial Aspects of Neglect during Functional Activities*

TYPE OF NEGLECT	FUNCTIONAL ACTIVITY DIFFICULTIES
Personal or body neglect	Does not shave left side of face
	Does not comb left side of head
	Does not apply makeup to left side of face
	Does not wash or dry left side of body
	Does not integrate left side of body during bed mobility and transfers
	Does not use left side of body
Near extrapersonal (peripersonal [within arms' reach]) neglect	Cannot find objects on left side of sink
	Cannot find objects on left side of desk
	Inability to read
	Inability to locate numbers on the left side of the phone
	Does not eat food on left side of the plate
	Cannot find wheelchair brakes on left side of the chair
Far extrapersonal neglect	Cannot locate clock on left side of wall
	Gets lost easily during ambulation or wheelchair mobility
	Cannot navigate doorways
	Difficulty watching TV
	Cannot locate source of voices

*Spatial neglect includes both near and far extrapersonal space.

From Gillen G: *Cognitive and perceptual rehabilitation: optimizing function*, St. Louis, 2009, Mosby/Elsevier.

- The person is then asked to find the objects again, this time using the LHS.
- A tactile cue such as a light tap on the left shoulder may be given in addition to the verbal cue.
- The person is asked to notice how many more objects can be seen when the LHS is used.
- A copy of the lighthouse poster is placed on the wall of the person's room, to the right of the bed.
- All therapists are given copies of the poster and asked to use it to cue the person when task performance requires attention to both the right and left fields (i.e., grooming, feeding, mobility.).

Limb Activation

Limb activation is based on the idea that any movement of the contralesional side may function as a motor stimulus, activating the right hemisphere and improving neglect. It has been shown across a series of studies that unilateral neglect can be improved by encouraging clients to make even small movements with some part of the left side of their body if these movements are performed in the left hemispace. In general, the principle behind this approach is to "find" the affected limb and encourage movements of the affected limb in the neglected hemispace (i.e., spatiomotor cueing). It is hypothesized that these movements lead to summation of activation of affected receptive fields of two distinct but linked spatial systems for personal and extrapersonal space, resulting in improvements in attentional skills and appreciation of spatial relationships on the affected side.[52,79] A counter hypothesis is that the movements in the left hemispace serve as perceptual cues such as an anchor. Studies have demonstrated a reduction in the severity of neglect when subjects actively engage their left hand in a task.

Partial Visual Occlusion

In a randomized study, Beis and colleagues[14] examined 22 subjects with left unilateral neglect. Interventions included the use of right half-field patches (*n* = 7), a right monocular patch (*n* = 7), and a control group (*n* = 8). Patches were worn throughout the day during inpatient rehabilitation. Results of paired comparison tests showed significant differences between the control group and the group with the half-eye patches for the total Functional Independence Measure score and objective measures of displacements of the right eye in the left field. No significant differences were found between the control group and the group with the right monocular patch.

Videotaped Feedback of Task Performance

Using videotaped feedback of task performance has been suggested as a strategy to decrease the effects of unilateral neglect. When viewing one's own performance on a TV screen during video playback, one can see and attend to the neglected left side on the right side of the TV monitor (i.e., neglect behaviors can be observed in the non-neglected space). This may be a key therapeutic factor. In usual care, the therapist describes the neglect behavior, but the person with neglect may not be able to "see" his or her mistakes. Visualizing the mistakes, followed by processing them with the therapist, may help insight building and subsequent strategy formation.

Environmental Adaptation

Some people will not recover spontaneously or respond to "active" interventions such as teaching a new strategy to perform a task. Similarly, those who have poor awareness and insight and who don't respond to awareness training may not respond to interventions that require self-generated compensatory strategies. In these cases, a person's functional performance may be enhanced by implementing and teaching caregivers or family members environmental strategies (Table 19-7).

	0	1	2	3
1. Forgets to groom or shave the left part of his/her face	☐	☐	☐	☐
2. Experiences difficulty in adjusting his/her left sleeve or slipper	☐	☐	☐	☐
3. Forgets to eat food on the left side of his/her plate	☐	☐	☐	☐
4. Forgets to clean the left side of his/her mouth after eating	☐	☐	☐	☐
5. Experiences difficulty in looking towards the left	☐	☐	☐	☐
6. Forgets about a left part of his/her body (e.g., forgets to put his/her upper limb on the armrest, or his/her left foot on the wheelchair rest, or forgets to use his/her left arm when he/she needs to)	☐	☐	☐	☐
7. Has difficulty in paying attention to noise or people addressing him/her from the left	☐	☐	☐	☐
8. Collides with people or objects on the left side, such as doors or furniture (either while walking or driving a wheelchair)	☐	☐	☐	☐
9. Experiences difficulty in finding his/her way towards the left when traveling in familiar places or in the rehabilitation unit	☐	☐	☐	☐
10. Experiences difficulty finding his/her personal belongings in the room or bathroom when they are on the left side	☐	☐	☐	☐

Total score (/30)

0=no neglect; 1=mild neglect; 2=moderate neglect; 3=severe neglect

Figure 19-3   Catherine Bergego Scale. A test of functional neglect including personal, peripersonal, and extrapersonal aspects of neglect. Score of 0 is given if no spatial bias is noted. Score of 1 is given when the patient always first explores the right hemispace before going slowly and hesitatingly toward the left space and shows occasional left sided omissions. Score of 2 is given if the patient shows clear and constant left-sided omissions and collisions. Score of 3 is given when the patient is totally unable to explore the left hemispace. (From Bergego C, Azouvi P, Samuel C, et al: Validation d'une échelle d'évaluation fonctionnelle de l'héminégligence dans la vie quotidienne: l'échelle CB. *Ann Readapt Med Phys* 38:183-189, 1995.)

Organization/Sequencing Deficits

The ability to organize thoughts requires the integration of multiple skills, including praxis, sequencing, and problem-solving. *Sequencing* refers to the ability to plan and carry out events in proper order, progression, and time.[6] Sequencing and organization deficits represent the breakdown of a complex integration of skills, including use of sensory feedback and organization. Patients with sequencing and organization deficits can be trained to use a daily planner, tape recordings, or cue cards (depending on whether they perform better with auditory or visual cues) to help sequence the steps of daily tasks. Gradually increasing the number of steps in a task can increase a patient's tolerance and ability to perform more complex tasks (Box 19-6). Note those living with ideational apraxia will also present with organization and sequencing deficits.

Spatial Relations Syndrome

Spatial relations syndrome is the label given to disorders with impairment in the perception of spatial relationship of objects. These disorders include impairments with figure-ground, position in space, spatial relations, and form and space constancy skills. Topographical disorientation also is classified sometimes as part of spatial relations syndrome. Recommendations for spatial impairments include training patients to move slowly through their environments, encouraging patients to touch objects in the environment frequently, teaching patients to handle objects by the base, and using verbal cues or feedback instead of gestures.[70] Perceptual impairments are often difficult for families to understand. Educating the caregivers about these disorders and instructing them on how they can help their loved ones (Box 19-7) is especially important. See Chapter 16.

Spatial Relation Dysfunction

Spatial relation dysfunction is an impairment in relating objects to one another or to the self. Some examples of functional activities for patients with spatial deficits include identification and orientation of clothing during a dressing activity. This includes matching buttons and buttonholes together on a shirt or working on the ability to

Table 19-7

Sample Environmental Strategies to Improve Function in Those with Neglect

FUNCTION	STRATEGIES
Feeding	Place food, utensils, napkin, etc., on the right side of plate and placemat. Note: This intervention may be *combined* with the use of cue on the left side of the placemat such as a colored anchor (strip of tape or nonslip material) and/or the person's left arm on the table to be used as a spatiomotor cue. Situate person at the table so that other diners are biased to the right to enhance socialization.
Table games	Rotate the person's chair 45 degrees to the left to place key game items in the intact field. Situate person at the table so that other players are biased to the right.
Home management	Organize closets, drawers, refrigerator, etc. so that the person's necessary items are on the right.
Bed side care	Call bell *always* placed on right. Orient bed so that incoming stimuli (doorway, television, seating) are in the right field.*
Mobility	Colored markers on furniture that be an obstacle; signs posted on right side of hall, i.e., "Turn left here"

*In the acute stages, this may be controversial because the therapist may want to "force" the person to respond to the left side of the environment.
From Gillen G: *Cognitive and perceptual rehabilitation: optimizing function*, St. Louis, 2009, Mosby/Elsevier.

orient shoelaces during a one-handed tie. Wheelchair transfers require the ability to position the body in relation to a bed or other object and spatial orientation to maneuver wheelchair brakes and armrests in the correct direction. Simple meal preparation is another activity that requires spatial orientation and positioning because of tasks as locating and selecting needed items, stirring food, and setting the table.[50]

The use of the computer for visuospatial retraining has little or no effect on visuospatial skills and no carryover to functional activities.[44] Thus the use of computer programs aimed solely at addressing visuospatial skill retraining appears to be an ineffective remediation technique. A computer screen provides information as a two-dimensional image. Spatial relation impairment is a three-dimensional problem. For persons who use the computer for work or leisure, however, the use of the keyboard or mouse while

Box 19-6

SEQUENCING DEFICITS: TIPS FOR FAMILY MEMBERS

- Frustration and error can be lessened by step-by-step directions written in a simple format (e.g., a checklist).
- Maps and diagrams may be useful.
- Visual aids often prove helpful, especially when combined with verbal instructions or physical guiding.
- Frequent, routine practice should help reinforce the sequencing of daily activities.

Box 19-7

PERCEPTUAL PROBLEMS: TIPS FOR FAMILY MEMBERS

- Overstimulation from visual information may increase the problem.
- Getting rid of unnecessary objects and equipment lessens the demands on the patient and simplifies the task. For example, the table-top should be cleared of objects that look alike so that the patient does not confuse them.
- Slowing down while reaching for an object or walking into a new area is usually helpful.

working on the computer can be an effective, challenging, and meaningful modality.

Spatial Positioning Impairment
The concept of spatial positioning involves accurate placement or positioning of objects, including body parts. That impairment may be associated with impaired proprioception, however. This disorder is linked with language comprehension. Concepts such as *above*, *in*, and *under* are interpreted according to position in space and language skills.

Treatment for spatial positioning impairment should include increasing the patient's awareness of the impairment and teaching compensatory strategies. Matching colored markers for correct placement of objects can be helpful. Treatment ideas include having the patient practice placing a glass on top, in front, to the right, and to the left of a plate on command, placing certain objects (cups or utensils) in a row and having the patient identify which object is in a position different from those of the others. If language skills are impaired, the patient can be asked to create a place setting from a model. Repetition of specific spatial concepts, with emphasis on attention to detail and compensatory strategies (e.g., Velcro shoe strap goes toward the colored marker), may be helpful.

Treatment techniques for right-left discrimination problems include providing activities that stress right and left differences, such as dressing and grooming. In addition, therapists may use color or other markers to distinguish the right from the left side of items such as clothing and shoes.

Figure-Ground Impairment

Figure-ground deficits involve the inability to distinguish the foreground from the background. Treatment strategies for figure-ground deficits should include teaching the patient to be cognitively aware of the deficit and to slow down enough during task performance to identify all the relevant objects or stimuli before handling or manipulating them. The environment can be adapted to make it simple and uncluttered (e.g., organizing drawers or shelves). The use of stark contrast between objects (e.g., the plate and table during mealtime) is helpful for patients with this disorder. Sorting objects such as utensils from a kitchen drawer or nuts and bolts from a toolkit can be a good therapeutic activity; the sorting can be made more difficult with the addition of smaller and larger objects, thereby adding the element of size discrimination. The sorting should have a purpose, such as using the utensils for a cooking task.

Topographical Disorientation

Topographical disorientation is difficulty finding direction in space.[6] The use of compensatory techniques and environmental adaptation, progressively reduced as the patient demonstrates learning, is often successful in the treatment of this disorder. Therapists can use markers such as colored dots to identify a route the patient must travel every day. The therapist gradually removes cues as the patient memorizes the route. One successful treatment program described by Borst and Peterson[20] used the patient's intact skills of right-left discrimination and language to assist with functional mobility. In this treatment program, the patient practiced following directional instructions (e.g., "Go left at the next door."). The patient then was asked to draw the path from room to room on a map of the clinical area. Such an exercise would be especially helpful in the home setting. At first the therapist may need to assist the patient with correctly orienting the map with each turn. The therapist should withdraw verbal cues slowly. Next, the patient should attempt to go from room to room with only brief glances at the map. The last step is to withdraw the use of the map altogether. Generalization of this type of treatment is unlikely; therefore, treatment should take place only in the most meaningful environment.

Agnosia

Agnosia typically is defined as the inability to recognize sensory stimuli. Agnosia presents as a defect of one particular sensory channel, such as visual, auditory, or tactile. Examples include finger agnosia, visual agnosia, somatoagnosia, simultanagnosia, and tactile agnosia. These disorders are rarely seen in isolation, and little data have been published regarding treatment techniques for agnosia. However, because the defining principle of agnosia is impairment of one

specific sensory modality, treatment usually focuses on teaching the patient to use the intact sensory modalities. For example, in tactile agnosia—the inability to recognize objects by handling them—the patient is taught to use visual, olfactory, and auditory senses to recognize objects (Box 19-8 and Box 19-9).

Memory Impairments

Although memory impairments are not as common in persons who have sustained strokes as they are in those with closed-head injuries, dementia, or encephalitis, difficulty retaining information is nonetheless common in the stroke population.

Human memory is composed of multiple and distinct systems[10,90] that are required to support daily activities and participate in the community. Examples include remembering your significant other's birthday, remembering to take your medications, remembering to feed the dog, remembering how to type, remembering events that occurred during a vacation, and so on. Even this "simple" list of memory tasks requires intact functioning of multiple memory systems and includes knowledge of facts and events, procedures, and remembering future intentions. Clearly, memory serves as a key cognitive support to facilitate independent living.

The steps or stages of memory have been well-documented.[10,90] The flow of these stages follows (Table 19-8):

Attention $\rightarrow$ Encoding $\rightarrow$ Storage $\rightarrow$ Retrieval

Box 19-8

Difficulties during Everyday Function and Agnosia

VISUAL (OBJECT) AGNOSIA

Inability to find the razor on the sink despite adequate scanning abilities. The razor can only be located by touch.

VISUOSPATIAL AGNOSIA

Misjudging the distance while reaching for a cup resulting in an inappropriate endpoint (i.e., the hand end up several inches from the cup)

Difficulties orienting a shirt to one's body. See Chapter 16.

TACTILE AGNOSIA

Difficulty with clothing fasteners despite intact motor function

Inability to recognize objects that are in one's pockets unless vision is also used

Data from Árnadóttir G: *The brain and behavior: assessing cortical dysfunction through activities of daily living,* St Louis, 1990, Mosby.

Box 19-9

More Interventions for Agnosia, Based on the Literature

VISUAL AGNOSIA

Teach compensation via the use of other senses such as tactile information.

Teach awareness of deficits focusing on consequences of the impairments because those with visual agnosia may underestimate the consequences of the deficit.[83]

Teach recognition of figures and shapes by kinesthetic sense combined with visual information.[96]

Teach tracing with eyes and fingers such as tracing letters to improve recognition.[96]

Moving an object or moving the head relative to an unrecognizable object and tracing the outline may facilitate recognition.[54] Encourage head movements when examining objects and encourage observing items related to depth cues.[27,100]

Teach the use of spatial and location cues to recognize objects, people, etc. Examples include organizing a bedroom or classroom so that needed objects are assigned to specific spatial locations such as school clothes on the right side of the dresser and casual clothes on the left.[83] Teach the use of unique identifying features and idiosyncratic cues to assist recognition (e.g., color or shape).[83] Use knowledge of relevant and critical features to identify objects. For example, when looking for Swiss cheese in the refrigerator, focus on color (white) and shape (cube shaped) to narrow down the number of objects that must be examined.

Teach a piecemeal reconstruction approach using feature-by-feature analysis.[83]

Teach reliance on verbal memory skills and verbal reasoning to interpret the piecemeal visual information into a whole (e.g., "it's a person, no it's a dress, it's short, it must be a shirt").[83]

Use color cues, labels, or textures on objects or environments (e.g., Velcro on the phone receiver or red tape on doorknobs).[24,60]

Encourage overt verbalization of the visual characteristics of objects before producing a name.[26]

Practice identification of real objects vs. line drawings. Real objects are more easily recognized than drawings or pictures. Focus attention to depth cues, surface texture, and colors.[100] Real objects provide cues based on surface detail (different luminance and textures), color shades, and provide depth information.[27]

Use landmarks such as a sofa to route find.[60]

Use cues from other people to help generate a strategy. For example, if during a meal one cannot find utensils, watching others during the meal may help locate these items.[60]

ALEXIA

Read via letter tracing.[24]

Trace letters on the palm of the hand.

Use books on tape.

Text to speech software programs such as Kurzweil 1000 or RealSpeak.

PURE WORD DEAFNESS

Teach use of contextual cues, intonation, gestures, and facial expressions.[24]

Use written directions and information.

PROSOPAGNOSIA

Use gait clues to identify people (e.g., speed, sound of shoes).[83]

Teach voice recognition.[13,83]

Using clothing sounds or clues to recognize.[13] Use localization clues (e.g., Ann sits behind me in the classroom, and John is to my right).[83]

Highlight distinguishing features such as eye color, a scar, or mustache.[24]

TOPOGRAPHICAL DISORIENTATION SECONDARY TO AGNOSIA AND RELATED DISORDERS

Teach navigation in home environments by always starting at the same point such as the front door.[24]

Focus on past memories of the home to assist in navigation or relearning directions using kinesthetic and vestibular cues.

Use color markers on key rooms (e.g., a blue circle is my room).

Teach the use of kinesthetic memory for route finding such as the number of turns or steps.[83]

TACTILE AGNOSIA AND/OR ASTEREOGNOSIS

Begin practicing with identifying simple shapes via tactile information. Practice recognition of two-dimensional and three-dimensional objects because recognition may not be consistent.[78]

Use combined tactile and visual recognition.

From Gillen G: *Cognitive and perceptual rehabilitation: optimizing function*, St. Louis, 2009, Mosby/Elsevier.

Table 19-8

Stages of Memory

STAGE OF MEMORY	DESCRIPTION	NEUROANATOMICAL AREA OF FUNCTION
Attention	The processes that allow a person to gain access to and use incoming information. Inclusive of alertness, arousal, and various attention processes such as selective attention.	Brainstem Thalamic structures Frontal lobes
Encoding	How memories are formed. An initial stage of memory that analyzes the material to be remembered (visual vs. verbal characteristics of information). Correct analysis of information is required for proper storage of the information.	Dorsomedial thalamus Frontal lobes Language system (e.g., Wernicke area) Visual system (e.g., visual association areas)
Storage	How memories are retained Transfer of a transient memory to a form or location in the brain for permanent retention/access	Hippocampus Bilateral medial temporal lobes
Retrieval	How memories are recalled Searching for or activating existing memory traces	Frontal lobe

Data from Sohlberg MM, Mateer CA: Memory theory applied to intervention. In Sohlberg MM, Mateer CA, editors: *Cognitive rehabilitation: an integrative neuropsychological approach*, New York, 2001, Guilford Press.

A variety of memory impairments have been documented and each impact daily function differently (Table 19-9).

Interventions focused on those with memory deficits can be categorized as restorative approaches to improve underlying memory deficits, strategy training, use of non-electronic memory aids, and electronic memory aids or assistive technology. Techniques aimed at improving the underlying memory impairment such as memory drills have been unsuccessful in terms of generalizing to meaningful activities. An improvement may be detected on a laboratory-based measure of memory without a corresponding change in daily function or subjective memory reports.

As will be discussed later, the most promising interventions to improve function in those living with memory deficits rely at least partially on compensatory techniques. When using a compensatory approach, choosing the correct system of compensation is critical. Kime[57] suggested a comprehensive evaluation that includes the following:

- Severity of injury
- Severity of memory impairment
- Presence of comorbidities including physical impairments, language deficits, and other cognitive deficits
- Social supports
- Client needs (e.g., will the system be used for work, home management)

Memory Notebooks and Diaries

Sohlberg and Mateer[90] published a systematic, structured training sequence for teaching individuals with severe memory impairments to independently use a compensatory memory book. The training sequence they proposed incorporates principles of learning theory and procedural memory skills, which may be preserved in many clients with even severe memory impairments. Their paper described the components of a functional memory book. In addition, they explained a three-stage approach to using the notebook.

- Acquisition or how to use it
- Application or where and when to use it
- Adaptation or how to update it and use it in novel situations

Sohlberg and Mateer[90] highlighted that successful memory book training takes time, requires that all staff and family need to be trained in its use, that the person carry the book at all times, and that its use is individualized and function-based. They documented the effectiveness of this approach to memory book training via a case study in which the intervention was successfully used to support daily living and employment, despite persistent memory deficits.

Donaghy and Williams[31] suggested that the diary or notebook include a pair of pages for each day of the week. The notebook is set up to aid scheduling things to do in the future and record activities done in the past. Within each pair of pages, the left-hand page contains two columns: one with a timetable for the day, and the other with the to-do items. The right-hand page contains the memory log. A "Last Week" section at the back stores previous memory log entries. A full year calendar allows for appointments to be recorded. Donaghy and Williams[31] published their training protocol and two case studies to support use of the notebook.

Table 19-9

Terminology Related to Memory Impairments

TERM	DEFINITION	EXAMPLES OF EVERYDAY BEHAVIORS
Anterograde amnesia	A deficit in new learning. An inability to recall information learned *after* acquired brain damage. An inability to form new memories after brain damage occurs	Not able to recall staff names, easily gets lost secondary to topographical disorientation, not able to recall what occurred in therapy this morning, difficulty learning adaptive strategies to compensate for memory loss
Retrograde amnesia	Difficulty recalling memories formed and stored *prior to* the disease onset. May be worse for recent events as opposed to substantially older memories	Inability to remember autobiographical information (address, social security number, birth order), not able to remember historical events (war, presidential elections, scientific breakthroughs), and/or personally experienced events (weddings, vacations)
Short-term memory	Storage of limited information for a limited amount of time	Difficulty remembering instructions related to the use of adaptive equipment, not able to remember the names of someone just introduced at a dinner party, not able to remember "today's specials" in a restaurant
Working memory	Related to short-term memory and refers to actively manipulating information in short-term storage via rehearsals	Unable to remember and use the rules of the game while playing a board game, not able to perform calculations mentally while balancing the checkbook, difficulty remembering and adapting a recipe.
Long-term memory (LTM)	Relatively permanent storing of information with unlimited capacity	May affect declarative memory of knowledge, episodes, and facts or nondeclarative memories such as those related to skills and habits
Nondeclarative/ implicit or procedural memory	Knowing *how* to perform a skill, retaining previously learned skills and learning new skills. Form of LTM	Driving, playing sports, hand crafts, learning to use adaptive ADL equipment or a wheelchair.
Declarative/ explicit memory	Knowing that something was learned, verbal retrieval of a knowledge base such as facts, and remembering everyday events. Includes episodic and semantic information. Form of LTM (see following)	See episodic and semantic memory.
Episodic memory	Autobiographical memory for contextually specific events. Personally experienced events. Form of declarative LTM	Remembering the day's events, what one had for breakfast, occurrences on the job, the content of therapy sessions
Semantic memory	Knowledge of the general world, facts, linguistic skill, and vocabulary. (Note: may be spared after injury.) Form of declarative LTM	Remembering the dates of holidays, the name of the president, dates of world events
Explicit memory	Explicit memories consist of memories from events that have occurred in the external world. Information stored in explicit memory is about a specific event that happened at a specific time and place.	Remembering places and names, and various words. See declarative memory.
Implicit memory	Does not require conscious retrieval of the past. Knowledge is expressed in performance without the person being aware of possessing this knowledge. Consists of memories necessary to perform events and tasks, or to produce a specific type of response.	Memory of skills, habits, and subconscious processes. See nondeclarative memory.
Prospective memory	Remembering to carry out future intentions	Remembering to take medications, return phone calls, buy food, pick up children from school, mail the bills. A critical aspect of memory to support everyday living

Table 19-9

Terminology Related to Memory Impairments—cont'd

TERM	DEFINITION	EXAMPLES OF EVERYDAY BEHAVIORS
Metamemory	Awareness of your own memory abilities	Knowing when you need to compensate for memory capacity (making a list of errands, shopping list, writing down a new phone number or driving directions), recognizing errors in memory

Data from Baddeley AD: The psychology of memory. In Baddeley AD, Kopelman MD, Wilson BA, editors: *The essential handbook of memory disorders for clinicians*, Hoboken, NJ, 2004, John Wiley; Bauer RM, Grande L, Valenstein E: Amnesic disorders. In Heilman KM, Valenstein E, editors: *Clinical neuropsychology*, ed 4, New York, 2003, Oxford University Press; Markowitsch HJ: Cognitive neuroscience of memory. *Neurocase* 4(6):429-435, 1998; and Sohlberg MM, Mateer CA: Memory theory applied to intervention. In Sohlberg MM, Mateer CA, editors: *Cognitive rehabilitation: an integrative neuropsychological approach*, New York, 2001, Guilford Press.

Errorless Learning

Errorless learning is a learning strategy that is in contrast to trial and error learning or errorful learning. Interventions using an errorless learning approach are based on differences in learning abilities. People with memory impairments typically remember their own mistakes as results of their own action more successfully than they remember the corrections to their mistakes occurring via explicit means (e.g., a therapist's cue). People may remember their mistakes but not the correction. With errorless learning, a person learns something by saying or doing it, rather than being told or shown by someone. In addition, the person is not given the opportunity to make a mistake (i.e., there are no mistakes to be remembered). The hypothesis is that reduction or prevention of incorrect or inappropriate responses facilitates memory performance. The technique is straightforward and involves preventing clients from making any errors during learning via physical and verbal support or cues from the therapist, reducing the use of trial and error and avoiding mistakes.

Evans and colleagues[35] presented nine experiments, in three study phases, which tested the hypothesis that learning methods that prevent the making of errors (*errorless learning*) will lead to greater learning than *trial and error* learning methods among those who are memory impaired because of acquired brain injury. Errorless learning techniques include the following:

- *Providing the correct answer immediately:* For example, when showing a picture of unfamiliar face, the therapist would ask, "What is this person's name? His name begins with M; his name is Michael." The authors found that this technique was beneficial for remembering names by first letter–cued recall as compared to learning names by trial and error.
- *Backward chaining:* Used to teach multistep tasks. In this approach the therapist shows or prompts all of the steps of the task. On the next trial, all of the steps except for the last one are demonstrated or prompted

and the person being taught the skill must demonstrate it. After each trial, prompts are withdrawn and the technique progresses until all of the steps are learned. The authors found that this technique was beneficial for learning names by first letter–cued recall as compared to trail and error.

- *Forward chaining:* Also used to teach multiple step tasks. The therapist prompts or demonstrates the first step on the first trial, the first two steps on the second trial, and continues until the whole sequence is remembered.
- *Combined imagery with errorless learning:* Associations between faces and names were taught by having the subject create a mental image based on facial features; for example, the wave in the person's hair looks like a W; his name is Walter. The authors documented improved free recall of names using this technique.

The authors' results suggest that tasks and situations that facilitate retrieval of implicit memory for the learned material (e.g., learning names with a first letter cue) will benefit from errorless learning methods, whereas those that require the explicit recall of novel associations (such as learning routes or programming an electronic organizer) will not benefit from errorless learning. The more severely memory-impaired clients benefited to a greater extent from errorless learning methods than those who were less severely memory impaired, but the authors cautioned that this may apply only when the interval between learning and recall is relatively short.

Assistive Technology

Several studies have documented the success of using simple assistive technology to compensate for memory loss and improve daily function (Box 19-10). Interventions for those with memory impairments must consider social networks as well. Including significant others in all interventions may be the key factor to ensure success (Box 19-11).

Box 19-10

Assistive Technology for Those with Memory Loss

Handheld computers
Paging systems
Voice recorders
Personal data assistants
Alarm watches
Smartphones
Electronic pill box
Microwave with preset times
Adaptive stove controls to turn off an electric stove after a certain period of time or when heat becomes excessive
A phone with programmable memory buttons (affix pictures to the buttons)
A phone with buttons programmed to speak the name of the person being called
A key locator attachment
Tape recorders used to cue a behavioral sequence such as morning care

From Gillen G: *Cognitive and perceptual rehabilitation: optimizing function*, St. Louis, 2009, Mosby/Elsevier.

Attention Deficits

Attention is an essential element in successful task performance. Poor ability to attend to a task often is misinterpreted as a lack of motivation or neglect. Accurate assessment of an attention impairment is important to implementing appropriate treatment techniques. One method that may be helpful in managing attention problems is changing the way occupational therapists speak to patients. The goal is to couple the patient's attention with the intended action; instructions should be in the logical sequence of the action. Instead of instructing a patient to "Scoot forward," the therapist would say, "Your bottom [*pause*]. Move it forward to the edge of the chair." The wording should correspond with the order in which the steps are to be executed and should allow the patient to attend to each step. The pause is important to allow the patient enough time to shift focus and process the information.[25]

Use of systematic training incorporating a series of tasks with progressively increasing attentional demands has resulted in improvements in memory and attention to task,[16] although other studies have failed to demonstrate support for remedial training in attention.[102]

Family members often are frustrated when their loved ones are distracted easily or are unable to focus on a task. Family members must be informed that stroke survivors do not behave erratically on purpose. Teaching the family the way to create a supportive environment is important (Box 19-12).

Box 19-11

Strategies for Significant Others Living with Those Living with Memory Impairment after Stroke

Understand that in many cases this impairment may not be reversible.

Become very familiar with the specific type of compensatory memory strategies that have been prescribed.

Keep daily schedules as consistent as able. Stick with habits and routines.

Simplify the environment by decreasing clutter and keeping the living areas organized.

Decrease excessive environmental stimuli.

Help by organizing calendars, clocks, and reminders posted around the house.

Be proactive in identifying potential safety issues.

Use short and direct sentences.

Make sure that the most important information comes at the beginning the sentence.

Highlight, cue, and emphasize key aspects of communication (i.e., repeat, point.)

Avoid conversations that rely on memory (i.e., keep conversations in the present).

Repetition of sentences may be inevitable.

Summarize conversations.

Remember that in many cases, intelligence may remain intact.

Keep "a place for everything and everything in its place."

Use photographs, souvenirs, and other appropriate items to help access memories.

Understand that fatigue, stress, sleep disorders, and depression can exacerbate memory loss.

Keep back-up items (glasses, spare keys, etc.).

Help create to-do lists. Remind loved ones to check it off or highlight the item when the task is completed.

Label items, drawers, and shelves.

Attention has been described as having four distinct domains: alertness, selective attention, sustained attention, and divided or alternating attention. Therapists must train patients in each domain skill individually, and generalization from one domain to another should not be expected after training.[63]

Selective Attention Impairment

The ability to focus on relevant stimuli while screening out irrelevant stimuli is referred to as *selective attention*. Training patients to react to certain environmental cues and ignore distractions may improve selective attention. For example, the therapist can ask a patient to follow audio-recorded instructions for a hygiene task (or meal preparation, if a more complex task is desired). After the patient is able to complete the task successfully, the therapist can add elements of distraction, such as a radio or television, one by one.

Box 19-12

Attention Deficits: Strategies for Clinicians and Caretakers

Avoid overstimulating/distracting environments.

Face away from visual distracters during tasks.

Wear earplugs.

Shop or go to restaurants at off-peak times.

Use filing systems to enhance organization.

Label cupboards and drawers.

Reduce clutter and visual distracters.

Use self-instruction strategies.

Use time pressure management strategies.

Teach self-pacing strategies.

Control the rate of incoming information.

Self-manage effort and emotional responses during tasks.

Teach monitoring or shared attentional resources when multitasking.

Manage the home environment to decrease auditory and visual stimuli. Keep radios and phones turned off. Close doors and curtains. Keep surfaces, cabinets, closets, and refrigerators organized and uncluttered.

Use daily checklists for work, self-care, and instrumental activities of daily living.

Data from Cicerone KD: Remediation of "working attention" in mild traumatic brain injury. *Brain Inj* 16(3):185-195, 2002; Fasotti L, Kovacs F, Eling Paul ATM et al: Time pressure management as a compensatory strategy training after closed head injury. *Neuropsychol Rehabil* 10(1)47:-65, 2000; Michel JA, Mateer CA: Attention rehabilitation following stroke and traumatic brain injury, a review. *Eura Medicophys* 42(1):59-67, 2006; and Webster JS, Scott RR: The effects of self-instructional training on attentional deficits following head injury. *Clin Neuropsychol* 5(2):69-74, 1983.

Sustained Attention Impairment

Sustained attention is the ability to maintain attention over a period. Focusing and sustaining attention is improved by gradually increasing the attentional demands of activities, through choosing activities with longer duration and additional distractions. For example, a task such as combing hair in a quiet bathroom without a mirror initially may require less than 30 seconds of focused attention to complete (and have few inherent distractions). As the patient successfully completes these types of tasks, the therapist should choose activities that require focused attention to detail and have more distractions (e.g., straight razor shaving task with the radio playing in the background). Some support exists for providing specific training for attention to improve alertness and sustained attention, but no evidence exists that attention training affects functional abilities.[63]

Alternating Attention Impairment

Alternating attention is shifting focus from one stimulus to another. For the brain-injured population, the therapist should plan graded activities from simple to complex that initially require the patient to shift attention from one stimulus to another. For example, a simple activity may consist of participating in a ceramics painting project (in which the patient alternates attention from the paint to ceramic vase); a more complex task would be to have the patient perform a dressing task while watching the news on television and having the patient repeat important daily events after completing the task. Initially, tasks should require only attention shifts between two focal points. As the patient successfully completes these tasks, the therapist should use activities incorporating more focal points (e.g., a meal preparation task in which focus must alternate among planning, following directions, searching for supplies, monitoring other foods, timing, and place setting).

Concrete Thinking

Inflexible thought processes characterize persons who use concrete thinking. They have difficulty generalizing information from one situation to another and rely heavily on available sensory information.

Persons with impaired abstraction skills usually have poor ability to recognize and learn the cognitive and perceptual skills needed for a specific task. Therefore, they may benefit only from learning splinter (nongeneralizable) skills in treatment and may demonstrate training only in those tasks that are similar to those learned.[67] Box 19-13 reviews suggestions for family members to facilitate communication and task performance with this population.

Executive Function Impairments

Executive functions is an umbrella term that refers to complex cognitive processing requiring the coordination of several subprocesses to achieve a particular goal.[34a] This term has been defined as "a product of the coordinated operation of various processes to accomplish a particular goal in a flexible manner"[38a] or "those functions that enable a person to engage successfully in independent, purposive, self-serving behavior."[60a] These higher-order mental capacities allow one to adapt to new situations and

Box 19-13

COGNITIVE INFLEXIBILITY: TIPS FOR FAMILY MEMBERS

- Make statements and questions as simple and uncomplicated as possible.
- Explain the reasons for certain procedures. The person may have difficulty understanding the long-term effects of therapy or medical procedures. Explain these with smaller goals that are easier to accomplish.
- If possible, structure tasks so they consist of a series of related tasks rather than many unrelated tasks.

achieve goals. They include multiple specific functions such as decision-making, problem-solving, planning, task switching, modifying behavior in the light of new information, self-correction, generating strategies, formulating goals, and sequencing complex actions.[12,60a] Clearly these executive functions support engagement in daily life activities and participation in the community, most important during new, nonroutine, complex, and unstructured situations.[60a] (Table 19-10). Intervention approaches for these problems are somewhat lacking in the stroke survivor population. Available information is summarized in Boxes 19-14 and 19-15.

GOALS

The ability to document OT evaluation and treatment information appropriately is more important than ever. The insurance industry reimburses for OT services according to information provided to them through documentation; the goals set for a patient are critical to the support of the plan of care by the insurance company. Functional outcomes have gained increasing support and, in many cases, are required by insurance companies for reimbursement. Therefore, goals should be meaningful and sustainable; they must be valued and carried out by the patient outside the clinical environment. Examples include:

- Patient will properly sequence dressing tasks involving the legs with fewer than two verbal cues in three out of three trials.
- Patient will use grab bars or other objects for stability and safety during dressing task with close supervision in three out of three trials.

Table 19-10

Examples of Executive Functions Related to Everyday Living: Preparing a Salad

EXECUTIVE FUNCTION	ASSOCIATED TASKS
Initiation	Starting the task at the appropriate time without overreliance on prompts
Organization	Organizing the work space and performing the task efficiently (e.g., gathering necessary vegetables at the same time from the refrigerator)
Sequencing	Sequencing the steps of the task appropriately (e.g., gather tools and vegetables, wash vegetables, chop and slice vegetables, mix in bowl, add dressing)
Problem-solving	Solving the problem of using a knife that is too dull to slice

Box 19-14

Categories of Interventions for Those Living with Impairments of the Executive Functions

Environmental modifications: Examples include using antecedent control, manipulating the amount of distractions and structure in the environment, organizing work and living spaces, and ensuring balance of work, play, and rest.

Compensatory strategies: Examples include the use of external cueing devices such as checklists, electronic pagers, use of reminder systems, organizers.

Task-specific training: Training of specific functional skills and routines including task modifications.

Training in metacognitive strategies to promote a functional change by increasing self-awareness and control over regulatory processes: These include self-instruction strategies, teaching problem-solving, and goal management training.

Data from Cicerone KD, Giacino JT: Remediation of executive function deficits after traumatic brain injury. *NeuroRehabilitation* 2(3):12-22, 1992; Sohlberg MM, Mateer CA: Management of dysexecutive symptoms. In Sohlberg MM, Mateer CA, editors: *Cognitive rehabilitation: an integrative neuropsychological approach*, New York, 2001, Guilford Press; and Worthington A: Rehabilitation of executive deficits: the effect on disability. In Halligan PW, Wade, DT, editors: *Effectiveness of rehabilitation for cognitive deficits*, Oxford, 2005, Oxford University Press.

- Patient will demonstrate appropriate and independent use of pillbox for medication schedule in three out of three trials.
- Patient will prepare a shopping list from a recipe with all needed ingredients with minimal assist in two out of three trials.
- Patient will independently use 75% of objects and eat 75% of food placed on left side of midline, without verbal cues, in three out of three trials.
- Patient will prepare a simple, familiar meal with 80% recognition of errors in three out of five trials with close supervision.
- Patient will use objects appropriately in hygiene tasks without assistance in two out of three trials.
- Patient will attend to and perform all steps of audio-cued grooming task in three out of three trials with distant supervision.
- Patient will plan and participate in community activities once a week in three out of five trials with supervision.

Box 19-15

Further Strategies to Manage Functional Deficits Secondary to Dysexecutive Symptoms*

1. Organize living and work spaces such as:
   - Labeling and organizing drawers, cabinets.
   - Organizing shelves in kitchen cabinets and the refrigerator based on categories (e.g., by meal, food category, products used together).
   - Use paper-based organization systems such as organizers, calendars, and appointment books.
   - Color code or use in/out tray systems for work and home tasks (e.g., blue dots indicate priority work such as bills to be paid, or files in the bottom tray can be reviewed next week).
   - Use organizing technology such as personal data assistants, alarm watches, handheld organizers, and personal information manager software (these may include e-mail applications, a calendar, task and contact management, note taking, and a journal).
   - Post lists of usual and typical sequenced tasks in appropriate locations (e.g., a morning ADL routine posted on the bathroom mirror, night tasks such as lock the door and make lunch posted on the nightstand, arrive-at-work tasks such as check e-mail and phone messages posted on the computer screen).
   - Use timer functions while cooking.
2. Decrease environmental distractions.
   - Keep office door closed.
   - Use "do not disturb" signs when appropriate.
   - Turn off background radio and television.
   - Shut window blinds.
   - Keep workspaces (desks, kitchen counters, coffee tables) clear of clutter.
   - Use phone-answering systems.
   - Post office hours.
3. Plan and organize the day
   - Avoid multitasking
   - Families should establish structured routines (e.g., dinner at 7 PM each day, laundry is done on Saturday mornings).
   - Avoid situations in which multiple people are speaking at once.
   - Use clear and concise instructions.
   - Integrate relaxation breaks throughout the day.
   - Establish several "check your work and progress" points throughout the day (time to tick off checklists for completed tasks, check organizer for tasks that still need to be completed).

Data from Cicerone KD, Giacino JT: Remediation of executive function deficits after traumatic brain injury. *NeuroRehabilitation* 2(3):12-22, 1992; Sohlberg MM, Mateer CA: Management of dysexecutive symptoms. In Sohlberg MM, Mateer CA, editors: *Cognitive rehabilitation: an integrative neuropsychological approach*, New York, 2001, Guilford Press; and Worthington A: Rehabilitation of executive deficits: the effect on disability. In Halligan PW, Wade, DT, editors: *Effectiveness of rehabilitation for cognitive deficits*, Oxford, 2005, Oxford University Press.

CASE STUDY 1

Neurobehavioral Deficits after Stroke

G.W., a 49-year-old man, was working as a security guard at a prison when he sustained a massive right middle cerebral artery stroke. He was hospitalized for seven days and subsequently received OT on an outpatient basis. G.W.'s neurobehavioral deficits initially included severe left-side spatial and body neglect, anosognosia, and difficulty with spatial relationships, along with hemiparesis, resulting in total dependence in mobility and all ADL except eating (for which he needed moderate assistance).

Initial treatment plans focused on setting up functional activities such as eating, grooming, hygiene, and dressing. G.W. was required visually to scan the left side of space to find needed objects or use both arms to practice use of the left side of the body. (This was achieved through use of guiding techniques because no independent movement of left arm was present.) Diminishing verbal cues were used for G.W. to learn to attend to the left side of his body and left side of space during functional task performance. G.W.'s greatest initial impediment was his steadfast denial that his left arm and leg belonged to him (known as *anosognosia*). Fortunately, this denial diminished and was no longer present four weeks after the stroke.

Techniques such as matching color markers were minimally successful in treating spatial deficits. However, adaptive devices, such as elastic shoelaces (to prevent the need spatially to execute one-handed shoelace

Continued

CASE STUDY 1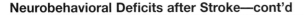

Neurobehavioral Deficits after Stroke—cont'd

tying), and compensatory strategies, such as slowing down movements and keeping hands on supported surfaces while reaching, were highly successful in increasing G.W.'s independence in daily task performance.

As G.W.'s awareness of his disability improved, use of awareness questioning was emphasized. G.W. initially was questioned after (and then before) each task; he later learned to ask himself questions such as, "What do I do before I start?" "Do I see everything I need?" "Is there anything I forgot?" and "Did I pay attention to my left side?" Awareness questioning was the most successful technique for improving G.W.'s ability to achieve independent performance of basic self-care and eventually perform instrumental ADL without assistance. Initially he lived with his mother and brother after the stroke, but he returned to independent living in his apartment and at the time of discharge was working with vocational rehabilitation services to explore employment options.

CASE STUDY 2

Role of Family in Overcoming Neurobehavioral Deficits after Stroke

M.A., an 82-year-old man, sustained a stroke in the left hemisphere at the age of 80 and subsequently underwent above-the-knee amputation of his right leg due to peripheral vascular disease. M.A. was placed in a skilled nursing facility, and soon thereafter OT services were initiated. Neurobehavioral impairments noted at the time of evaluation included global aphasia, motor and ideational apraxia, and severe attention deficits. M.A. depended on others for all mobility and ADL skills, including eating. M.A.'s family was supportive and visited him daily at lunch and dinnertime. Much of the OT was focused on patient, family, and staff education. The family was taught to use guiding techniques, which they implemented at mealtime and for grooming and hygiene tasks. The family and staff were taught ways to facilitate communication through tactile and visual cues and guiding techniques, ways to decrease environmental stimulation and distractions, and ways to approach M.A. to help him attend to tasks. M.A. responded well to guiding techniques, requiring only occasional tactile cues after initiating the task (through guiding) to eat, comb his hair, and wash his face in a low-stimulus environment. OT continued for seven weeks (because M.A. also was seen for contracture management), and eventually M.A. was discharged from the skilled nursing facility to his family's care.

REVIEW QUESTIONS

1. How is the integrated functional approach different from traditional functional approaches, and why is it the recommended approach for cognitive and perceptual impairments?
2. What neurobehavioral components are required to perform a hair grooming task? How can this task be used in the treatment of motor apraxia?
3. How can caregivers adapt environments to assist loved ones with cognitive or perceptual impairments?
4. What are two interventions that can be used to increase function in those living with unilateral neglect? Apraxia? Memory loss?

REFERENCES

1. Abreu B, Duval M, Gerber D, et al: Occupational performance and the functional approach. In Royeen CB, editor: *AOTA self-study series: cognitive rehabilitation*, Rockville, MD, 1994, American Occupational Therapy Association.
2. Alderman N, Burgess PW, Knight C, et al: Ecological validity of a simplified version of the Multiple Errands Shopping Test. *J Clin Exp Neuropsychol* 9(1):31–44, 2003.
3. Deleted.
4. Anderson SW, Tranel D: Awareness of disease states following cerebral infarction, dementia, and head trauma: standardized assessment. *Clin Neuropsychol* 3:327–339, 1989.
5. Appelros P, Karlsson GM, Thorwalls A, et al: Unilateral neglect: further validation of the baking tray task. *J Rehabil Med* 36(6): 258–261, 2004.
6. Árnadóttir G: *The brain and behavior: assessing cortical dysfunction through activities of daily living*, St Louis, 1990, Mosby.
7. Árnadóttir G: Evaluation and intervention with complex perceptual impairment. In Unsworth C, editor: *Cognitive and perceptual dysfunction: a clinical-reasoning approach to evaluation and intervention*, Philadelphia, 1999, FA Davis.
8. Ayres AJ: *Development dyspraxia and adult onset apraxia*, Torrance, CA, 1985, Sensory Integration International.
9. Azouvi P, Olivier S, de Montety G, et al: Behavioral assessment of unilateral neglect: study of the psychometric properties of the Catherine Bergego Scale. *Arch Phys Med Rehabil* 84(1):51–57, 2003.
10. Baddeley AD: The psychology of memory. In Baddeley AD, Kopelman MD, Wilson BA, editors: *The essential handbook of memory disorders for clinicians*, Hoboken, NJ, 2004, John Wiley.
11. Baggerly J: Sensory perceptual problems following stroke. *Nurs Clin North Am* 26(4):997–1005, 1991.
12. Baum CM, Edwards DF, Morrison T, et al: The reliability, validity, and clinical utility of the Executive Function Performance Test: a measure of executive function in a sample of persons with stroke. *Am J Occup Ther* 62(4):446–455, 2008.
13. Behrmann M, Marotta J, Gauthier I, et al: Behavioral change and its neural correlates in visual agnosia after expertise training. *J Cogn Neurosci* 17(4):554–568, 2005.
14. Beis JM, Andre JM, Baumgarten A, et al: Eye patching in unilateral spatial neglect: efficacy of two methods. *Arch Phys Med Rehabil* 80(1):71–76, 1999.
15. Beis JM, Keller C, Morin N, et al: French collaborative study group on assessment of unilateral neglect (GEREN/GRECO). Right spatial neglect after left hemisphere stroke: qualitative and quantitative study. *Neurology* 63(9):1600–1605, 2004.
16. Ben-Yishay Y, Piasetsky EB, Rattok J: *A systematic method for ameliorating disorders in basic attention*, New York, 1987, Guilford Pres.

17. Bennett TL: Neuropsychological evaluation in rehabilitation planning and evaluation of functional skills. *Arch Clin Neuropsychol* 16(3):237–253, 2001.

18. Bergego C, Azouvi P, Samuel C, et al: Validation d'une échelle d'évaluation fonctionnelle de l'héminégligence dans la vie quotidienne: l'échelle CB. *Ann Readapt Med Phys* 38:183–189, 1995.

19. Beschin N, Robertson IH: Personal versus extrapersonal neglect: a group study of their dissociation using a reliable clinical test. *Cortex* 33(2):379–384, 1997.

20. Borst MJ, Peterson CQ: Overcoming topographical orientation deficits in an elderly women with a right cerebrovascular accident. *Am J Occup Ther* 47(6):551, 1993.

21. Broadbent DE, Cooper PF, FitzGerald P, et al: The Cognitive Failures Questionnaire (CFQ) and its correlates. *Bri J Clin Psychol* 21 (Pt 1):1–16, 1982.

22. Brockmann-Rubio K, Gillen G: Treatment of cognitive-perceptual impairments: A function-based approach. In Gillen G, Burkhardt A, editors: *Stroke rehabilitation: a function-based approach*, ed 2, St Louis, 2004, Elsevier Science/Mosby.

23. Bruce MA: Cognitive rehabilitation: intelligence, insight, and knowledge. In Royeen CB, editor: *AOTA self-study series: cognitive rehabilitation*, Rockville, MD, 1994, American Occupational Therapy Association.

24. Burns MS: Clinical management of agnosia. *Top Stroke Rehabil* 11(1):1–9, 2004.

25. Calvanio R, Levine D, Petrone P: Elements of cognitive rehabilitation after right hemisphere stroke. *Behav Neurol* 11(1):25–57, 1993.

26. Carlesimo GA, Casadio P, Sabbadini M, et al: Associated visual agnosia resulting from a disconnection between intact visual memory and semantic systems. *Cortex* 34(4):563–576, 1998.

27. Chainay H, Humphreys GW: The real-object advantage in agnosia: evidence for a role of surface and depth information in object recognition. *Cogn Neuropsychol* 18(2):175–191, 2001.

28. Cocchini G, Beschin N, Jehkonen M: The fluff test: a simple task to assess body representation neglect. *Neuropsychol Rehabil* 11(1):17–31, 2001.

29. Condeluci A, Ferris LL, Bogdan A: Outcome and value: the survivor perspective. *J Head Trauma Rehabil* 7(4):37, 1992.

30. Dawson DR, Anderson ND, Burgess P, et al: Further development of the Multiple Errands Test: standardized scoring, reliability, and ecological validity for the Baycrest version. *Arch Phys Med Rehabil* 90(11 Suppl):S41–51, 2009.

31. Donaghy S, Williams W: A new protocol for training severely impaired patients in the usage of memory journals. *Brain Inj* 12(12):1061–1076, 1998.

32. Donkervoort M, Dekker J, Stehmann-Saris FC et al: Efficacy of strategy training in left hemisphere stroke patients with apraxia: A randomized clinical trial. *Neuropsychol Rehabil* 11(5):549–566, 2001.

33. Edmans JA, Lincoln NB: Treatment of visual perceptual deficits after stroke. *Int Disabil Stud* 11(1):25–33, 1989.

34. Edmans JA, Webster J, Lincoln NB: A comparison of two approaches in the treatment of perceptual problems after stroke. *Clin Rehabil* 14(3):230–243, 2000.

34a. Elliott R: Executive functions and their disorders. *Br Med Bull* 65(1):49–59, 2003.

35. Evans JJ, Wilson BA, Schuri U, et al: A comparison of "errorless" and "trial-and-error" learning methods for teaching individuals with acquired memory deficits. *Neuropsychol Rehabil* 10(1):67–101, 2000.

36. Fisher AG: *Assessment of motor and process skills. vol. 1: development, standardization, and administration manual*, ed 5, Fort Collins, CO, 2003, Three Star Press.

37. Fisher AG: *Assessment of motor and process skills. vol. 2: user manual*, ed 5, Fort Collins, CO, 2003, Three Star Press.

38. Fleming JM, Strong J, Ashton R: Self-awareness of deficits in adults with traumatic brain injury: how best to measure? *Brain Inj* 10(1):1–15, 1996.

38a. Funahashi S: Neuronal mechanisms of executive control by the perfrontal cortex. *Neurosci Res* 39(2):147–165, 2001.

39. Geusgens C, van Heugten C, Donkervoort M, et al: Transfer of training effects in stroke patients with apraxia: An exploratory study. *Neuropsychol Rehabil* 16(2):213–29, 2006.

40. Gillen, G: *Cognitive and perceptual rehabilitation: optimizing function*, St. Louis, 2009, Mosby/Elsevier.

41. Goldenberg G, Daumuller, Hagmann S: Assessment and therapy of complex activities of daily living in apraxia. *Neuropsychol Rehabil* 11(2):147–169, 2001.

42. Goldenberg G, Hagmann S: Therapy of activities of daily living in patients with apraxia. *Neuropsychol Rehabil* 8(2):123–141, 1998.

43. Guiles, GM, Clark-Wilson J: use of behavioral techniques in functional skills training after severe brain injury. *Am J Occup Ther* 42 (10):658–665, 1988.

44. Hajek VE: The effect of visuo-spatial training in patients with right hemisphere stroke. *Can J Rehabil* 6(3):175, 1993.

45. Halligan PW, Cockburn J, Wilson BA: The behavioural assessment of visual neglect. *Neuropsychol Rehabil* 1(1):5–32, 1991.

46. Hartman-Maeir A, Harel H, Katz N: The Kettle Test—a brief measure of cognitive functional performance: reliability and validity in stroke rehabilitation. *Am J Occup Ther* 63(5):592–599, 2009.

47. Heilman KM, Watson RT, Valenstein E: Neglect and related disorders. In Hilman KM, Valenstein E, editors: *Clinical neuropsychology*, ed 4, New York, 2003, Oxford.

48. Helm-Estabrooks N, Emory P, Albert ML: Treatment of aphasic perseveration. *Arch Neurol* 44(12):1253–1255, 1987.

49. Deleted.

50. Jabri J: Providing visuoperceptual remediation treatment for stroke patients in the home setting. *J Home Health Care Pract* 4(4):36. 1992.

51. Jarus T: Motor learning and occupational therapy: the organization of practice. *Am J Occup Ther* 48(9):810–816, 1994.

52. Kalra L, Perez I, Gupta S, et al: The influence of visual neglect on stroke rehabilitation. *Stroke* 28(7):1386–1391, 1997.

53. Katzmann S, Mix C: improving functional independence in a patient with encephalitis through behavior modification shaping techniques. *Am J Occup Ther* 48 (3):259–262, 1994.

54. Kertesz A: Visual agnosia: the dual deficit of perception and recognition. *Cortex* 15(3):403–419, 1979.

55. Kim HJ. Craik FI. Luo L. Ween JE. Impairments in prospective and retrospective memory following stroke. *Neurocase* 15(2):145–56, 2009.

56. Deleted.

57. Kime SK: *Compensating for memory deficits using a systematic approach*, Bethesda, MD, 2006, AOTA Press.

58. Knight C, Alderman N, Burgess PW: Development of a simplified version of the multiple errands test for use in hospital settings. *Neuropsychol Rehabil* 12(3):231–256, 2002.

59. Kottorp A, Tham, K: *Assessment of Awareness of Disability (AAD), manual for administration, scoring, and interpretation*, Stockholm, Sweden, 2005, Karolinska Institutet, NEUROTEC Department, Division of Occupational Therapy.

60. Lampinen J, Tham K: Interaction with the physical environment in everyday occupation after stroke: a phenomenological study of persons with visuospatial agnosia. *Scand J Occup Ther* 10(4):147–56, 2003.

60a. Lezak MD: Executive function and motor performance. In Lezak MD, Howieson DB, Loring DW, editors: *Neurological assessment*, New York, 2004, Oxford University Press.

61. Lin K, Wu C, Tickle-Degnen L, Coster W: Enhancing occupational performance through occupational embedded exercise: A meta-analytic review. *Occup Ther J Res* 17(1) 25–47, 1997.

62. Lincoln N: Stroke rehabilitation. *Curr Opin Neurol Neurosurg* 5(5):677–681, 1992.

63. Lincoln NB, Majid MJ, Weyman N: Cognitive rehabilitation for attention deficits following stroke. *Cochrane Database Syst Rev* (4):CD002842, 2000.

64. McIntosh RD, Brodie EE, Beschin N, et al: Improving the clinical diagnosis of personal neglect: a reformulated comb and razor test. *Cortex* 36(2):289–292, 2000.

65. Niemeier JP: Visual imagery training for patients with visual perceptual deficits following right hemisphere cerebrovascular accidents: a case study presenting the Lighthouse Strategy. *Rehabil Psychol* 47(4):426–437, 2002

66. Neistadt ME: A meal preparation treatment protocol for adults with brain injury. *Am J Occup Ther* 48(5):431–438, 1994.

67. Neistadt ME: The neurobiology of learning: implications for treatment of adults with brain injury. *Am J Occup Ther* 48(5):421–430, 1994.

68. Neistadt ME: Perceptual retraining for adults with diffuse brain injury. *Am J Occup Ther* 48(3):225–233, 1994.

69. Nygard L, Bernspang B, Fisher AG, et al: Comparing motor and process ability of persons with suspected dementia in home and clinic settings. *Am J Occup Ther* 48(8):689–696, 1994.

70. Olson E: Perceptual deficits affecting the stroke patient. *Rehabil Nurs* 16(4):212–213, 1991.

71. Ownsworth TL, McFarland KM, Young RM: Development and standardization of the Self-regulation Skills Interview (SRSI): a new clinical assessment tool for acquired brain injury. *Clin Neuropsychol* 14(1):76–92, 2000.

72. Papstrat LA: Outcome and value following brain injury: a financial provider's perspective. *J Head Trauma Rehabil* 7(4):11, 1992.

73. Park S, Fisher AG, Velonzo C: Using the assessment of motor and process skills to compare occupational performance between home and clinic settings. *Am J Occup Ther* 48(8):697–709, 1994.

74. Poole JL: Effect of apraxia on the ability to learn one-handed shoe tying. *Occup Ther J Res* 18(3) 99–104, 1998.

75. Qiang W, Sonoda S, Suzuki M, et al: Reliability and validity of a wheelchair collision test for screening behavioral assessment of unilateral neglect after stroke. *Am J Phys Med Rehabil* 84(3):161–166, 2005.

76. Radomski MV: Cognitive rehabilitation: advancing the stature of occupational therapy. *Am J Occup Ther* 48(3):271–273, 1994.

77. Radomski MV, Dougherty PM, Fine S, et al: Case studies in cognitive rehabilitation. In Royeen CB, editor: *AOTA self-study series: cognitive rehabilitation*, Rockville, MD, 1994, American Occupational Therapy Association.

78. Reed CL, Caselli RJ, Farah MJ: Tactile agnosia: underlying impairment and implications for normal tactile object recognition. *Brain* 119(Pt 3):875–888, 1996.

79. Robertson IH, North N: Spatio-motor cueing in unilateral left neglect: the role of hemispace, hand and motor activation. *Neuropsychologia* 30(6):553–563, 1992.

80. Robertson IH, Ward T, Ridgeway V, Nimmo-Smith I: The structure of normal human attention: the Test of Everyday Attention. *J Clin Exp Neuropsychol* 2(6):525–534, 1996.

81. Royle J. Lincoln NB. The Everyday Memory Questionnaire-revised: development of a 13-item scale. *Disabil Rehabil* 30(2): 114–21, 2008.

82. Sbordone RJ: Limitations of neuropsychological testing to predict the cognitive and behavioral functioning of persons with brain injury in real world settings. *Neurorehabilitation* 16(4):199–201, 2002.

83. Schiaveto A, Decaile J, Flessas J, et al: Childhood visual agnosia: a seven-year follow-up. *Neurocase* 3(1):1–17, 1997.

84. Schwartz MF, Segal M, Veramonti T, et al: The Naturalistic Action Test: A standardised assessment for everyday action impairment. *Neuropsychol Rehabil* 12(4):311–339, 2002.

85. Shallice T, Burgess PW: Deficits in strategy application following frontal lobe damage in man. *Brain* 114(Pt 2):727–741, 1991.

86. Simmond M, Fleming JM: Occupational therapy assessment of self-awareness following traumatic brain injury. *Br J Occup Ther* 66(10):447–453, 2003.

87. Simmond M, Fleming J: Reliability of the self-awareness of deficits interview for adults with traumatic brain injury. *Brain Inj* 17(4):325–337, 2003.

88. Smith G, Della Sala S, Logie RH, Maylor EA: Prospective and retrospective memory in normal ageing and dementia: a questionnaire study. *Memory* 8(5):311–321, 2000.

89. Sohlberg MM: Assessing and managing unawareness of self. *Semin Speech Lang* 21(2):135–151, 2000.

90. Sohlberg MM, Mateer CA: Training use of compensatory memory books: a three stage behavioral approach. *J Clin Exper Neuropsychol* 11(6):871–891, 1989

91. Sohlberg MM, Mateer CA: Memory theory applied to intervention. In Sohlberg MM, Mateer CA, editors: *Cognitive rehabilitation: an integrative neuropsychological approach*, New York, 2001, Guilford Press.

92. Stone SP, Patel P, Greenwood RJ, et al: Measuring visual neglect in acute stroke and predicting its recovery: the visual neglect recovery index. *J neurol Neurosurg Psych* 55(6):431–436, 1992.

93. Sunderland A, Harris JE, Baddeley AD: Do laboratory tests predict everyday memory? a neuropsychological study. *J Verbal Learn Verbal Behav* 22(3):341–357, 1983.

94. Sunderland A, Harris JE, Baddeley AD: Assessing everyday memory after severe head injury. In Harris JE, Morris PE, editors: *Everyday memory, actions, and absent-mindedness*, London, 1984, Academic Press.

95. Sunderland A, Walker CM, Walker MF: Action errors and dressing disability after stroke: an ecological approach to neuropsychological assessment and intervention. *Neuropsychol Rehabil* 16(6):666–83, 2006.

96. Tanemura R: Awareness in apraxia and agnosia. *Top Stroke Rehabil* 6(1):33–42, 1999.

97. Tham K, Bernsprang B, Fisher AG: Development of the assessment of awareness of disability. *Scand J Occup Ther* 6:184–190, 1999.

98. Tham K, Ginsburg E, Fisher A, et al: Training to improve awareness of disabilities in clients with unilateral neglect. *Am J Occup Ther* 55(1):46–54, 2001.

99. Tham K, Tegner R: The baking tray task: a test of spatial neglect. *Neuropsychol Rehabil* 6(1):19–25, 1996.

100. Thomas RM, Forde EM, Humphreys GW, et al: A longitudinal study of category-specific agnosia. *Neurocase* 8(6):466–479, 2002.

101. Toglia JP: Generalization of treatment: a multicontext approach to cognitive perceptual impairment in adults with brain injury. *Am J Occup Ther* 45(6):505–516, 1991.

102. Toglia JP: Attention and memory. In Royeen CB, editor: *AOTA self-studies series: cognitive rehabilitation*, Rockville, MD, 1993, American Occupational Therapy Association.

103. Toglia JP: A dynamic interactional approach to cognitive rehabilitation. In Katz N, editor: *Cognitive and occupation throughout the lifespan*. Bethesda, MD, 2005, AOTA.

104. Trombly C: Clinical practice guidelines for post-stroke rehabilitation and occupational therapy practice. *Am J Occup Ther* 49(7): 711–714, 1995.

105. van Heugten C, Dekker J, Deelman B, et al: Outcome of strategy training in stroke patients with apraxia: A phase II study. *Clin Rehabil* 12(4):294–303, 1998.

106. van Heugten C, Dekker J, Deelman B, et al: Assessment of disabilities in stroke patients with apraxia: internal consistency and inter-observer reliability. *Occup Ther J Res* 19(1):55–73, 1999.

107. van Heugten C, Dekker J, Deelman B, et al: Measuring disabilities in stroke patients with apraxia: a validity study of an observational method. *Neuropsychol Rehabil* 10(4):401–414, 2000.

108. van Heugten CM, Dekker J, Deelman BG, et al: Rehabilitation of stroke patients with apraxia: the role of additional cognitive and motor impairments. *Disabil Rehabil* 22(12):547–554, 2000.

109. Deleted.
110. Wilson BA: Remediation of apraxia following an anaesthetic accident. In West J, Spinks P, editors: *Case Studies in Clinical Psychology*, Bristol UK, 1988, John Wright.
111. Wilson BA, Alderman N, Burgess PW, et al: *Behavioural assessment of the dysexecutive syndrome*, Edmunds, UK, 1996, Thames Valley Test Company.
112. Wilson B, Cockburn J, Baddeley AD, Hiorns R: The development and validation of a test battery for detecting and monitoring everyday memory problems. *J Clin Exp Neuropsychol* 11(6):855–870, 1989.
113. Wilson B, Cockburn J, Halligan P: Development of a behavioral test of visuospatial neglect. *Arch Phys Med Rehabil* 68(2):98–102, 1987.
114. Wilson BA, Evans JJ, Emslie H, et al: The development of an ecologically valid test for assessing patients with dysexecutive syndrome. *Neuropsychol Rehabil* 8(3):213–228, 1998.
115. Wu C, Trombly C, Tickle-Degnen L: Effects of object affordances on movement performances: A meta-analysis. *Scand J Occup Ther* 5(2) 83–92, 1998.
116. Yuen HK: Increasing medication compliance in a woman with anoxic brain damage and partial epilepsy. *Am J Occup Ther*

SUGGESTED READINGS

Gillen, G. Cognitive and Perceptual Rehabilitation: Optimizing Function. St. Louis, Mosby/Elsevier, 2009.
Katz, N. (Ed.): Cognitive and Occupation Throughout the Lifespan. Bethesda, AOTA, 2005.

celia stewart
karen riedel

chapter 20

Managing Speech and Language Deficits after Stroke

key terms

anarthria	conduction aphasia	spastic dysarthria
anomic aphasia	dysarthria	transcortical motor aphasia
aphasia	fluent aphasia	transcortical sensory aphasia
Broca's aphasia	locked-in syndrome	unilateral upper motor neuron dysarthria
Cognitive communication disorder	mutism	Wernicke's aphasia
	nonfluent aphasia	

learning objectives

After completing this chapter, the reader will be able to accomplish the following:

1. Understand the impact of communication impairment following stroke.
2. Be aware of the incidence and prevalence of communication disorders.
3. Understand the various types of communication problems following stroke.
4. Understand the presentation and management of various communication disorders.

Communication disorders have a devastating effect not only on the rehabilitative process, but on the overall quality of life of the stroke survivor.[35,50] The objectives of this chapter are, first, to inform the occupational therapist and others regarding communication disorders found in stroke to increase the effectiveness of their intervention and, second, to discuss the ways in which the speech-language pathologist and occupational therapist can work collaboratively to foster better outcomes in the survivor's life participation. The chapter begins with a discussion about communication in general, and is followed by a description of the nature and the range of communication problems associated with stroke and the incidence and prevalence of communication disorders. Some guidelines provided may be helpful for the occupational therapist in enhancing communication with patients following stroke.

SCOPE OF COMMUNICATION

Communication is simply the transfer of information from one individual to another.[12,22,35] Human communication in all of its many forms fits within this definition, but for members of a human community, communication in all of its forms has much more meaning.[17,64] Humans' individual personality is displayed in their style of communication. They use gestures, facial expression, and vocal emphasis to convey more than facts. Their various modes of communication signify engagement and intention in their interaction with others. In addition, they communicate differently at home than they do in negotiating the tasks of daily life in the community. Furthermore,* their social interactions with their friends require different communicative skills than those required in most work settings.

The intricacy of human communication is compounded by the range and variety of skills with which they communicate.[64] Society's emphasis on communication has expanded with advances in communication technology. To be a successful communicator, one must not only be able to speak and comprehend spoken messages, but also understand and produce written and electronically transmitted information.[8] One cannot view communication in a vacuum of merely sender and receiver.[31] Cultural values, not only those associated with different languages and ethnic groups but with each life setting, have their own rules of interaction, which are internalized by the communication partners.[21,44,67,76]

IMPACT OF COMMUNICATION IMPAIRMENT FOLLOWING STROKE

The reaction of the stroke survivor to communication impairment is unique to the individual. The very suddenness of a stroke may overwhelm one's sense of well-being.[94] The alteration of communication in the first few days and weeks following the "brain attack" results in a range of emotions, from sheer terror in some individuals to indifference in those with little awareness of their deficits.[63,66] These responses depend on a variety of factors, including the locus and extent of the lesion, the nature of the deficits, the accompanying medical and physical problems, and the individual's personality characteristics.[68] In addition, the premorbid abilities of persons with communication disorders vary across the continuum, from those whose livelihood and identity are defined by speaking several languages, writing books, and/or giving speeches to those whose identity is based on activities other than spoken language.[27,68] Many stroke survivors describe issues of loneliness, social isolation, loss of independence/privacy, restricted activities, loss of work/income, and social stigmatization.[94,95] Sarno[95] has stated that the loss of communication in aphasia, for example, is a loss of personhood or

of personal identity. For some, these changes in communication alter one's roles in life and influence one's sense of personal identity.[27,68,94] These reactions and the reactions of friends and family are crucial considerations in the overall management plan.

Families of persons with communication impairment following stroke are more prone to difficulties in psychosocial adaptation than those with similar physical changes but intact communication.[27,35] Although family members' responses are individual and wide-ranging, their coping patterns are established prior to the onset of stroke and are found to be rather stable.[27,35,104] A greater than normal burden is placed on the caregiver when individuals require significant assistance in expressing themselves.[27,35,52]

Living successfully with communication impairments requires adaptations in life and consciously making choices.[27,35,104] These qualities are embedded in the person's personality and also in the coping strategies of the patient's significant others. Qualities of resilience in the face of challenges include the ability to maintain a distinct sense of self throughout the recovery process and not allowing for the development of overdependency.[53,70] Having a caregiver that can be flexible in changing roles, both in assuming the role of caregiver and relinquishing the role when appropriate, facilitates successful adaptation. Staying engaged in life helps one avoid boredom and depression.[70,104] Understanding that one can be valued and participate in life even with significant communication impairment is essential.[35,71,104] Openness to venturing out and having fun or pursuing something new is also a characteristic of those who live successfully following stroke.[70,104]

Cultural responses are relevant to the patient's willingness to participate in rehabilitation. The stroke survivor has internalized the values of his or her society for speech and communication function.[94] When communication disorders are identified, the survivor may fear that he or she is mentally challenged.[68] Family and friends hold similar cultural values and, as the closest group to the patient, may reinforce the sense of incompetence by making rehabilitation decisions without the survivor's input and unwittingly adding to the shame and embarrassment.[35,68] The fact that it is difficult to overcome and address these cultural biases argues for education of various types in multiple languages.[15,108] The need for current information in many languages about stroke is increasing with the steady expansion of the multilingual population.[15] Furthermore, access to medical care, to social settings, and to vocational options is constrained by the interaction of social, cultural, and linguistic factors.[15] Grassroots organizations, such as the National Stroke Association, American Stroke Association,[4] and Aphasia Association, are attempting to modify these misconceptions about stroke and communication disorders. In addition, the National Aphasia Association[86] is confronting the stigmatization that society gives to individuals who exhibit an obvious speech problem through raising awareness and by providing education in many languages.[86]

INCIDENCE AND PREVALENCE OF COMMUNICATION DISORDERS

Valid statistical information about the incidence of speech and language disorders following stroke is not available. However, according to the American Heart Association,[3] in 2006 there were around 6.5 million stroke survivors alive, and "on average, every 40 seconds someone in the United States has a stroke."[3] The percentage of strokes that have the initial symptom of speech and/or language issues is unknown. Around 25% to 40% of acute strokes result in aphasia, according to the National Aphasia Association.[86] However, the presence of aphasia may not be the most common communication symptom following stroke. The incidence and prevalence of dysarthria and cognitive communicative impairment following stroke are unavailable and may be more common and debilitating than aphasia.[33]

It is almost impossible to quantify the percentage of persons with communication problems. Included in the well-publicized "stroke warning signs" is the presence of changes in speech.[4] Medical records of hospital admissions for stroke often include patient complaints of "slurred speech." Many of these initial speech symptoms disappear shortly after, but other subtle changes in communication may be undetected by both the patient and health care professionals.[77] This lack of concern is understandable in the initial stages, since the focus is on acute medical treatment, preserving life, and intervening to preserve brain function, thus mitigating possible long-term disability.[79] Consequently, the less obvious changes in cognitive communicative function are not of paramount concern. The reduced hospital stay for patients with stroke, and the shortened admission to acute and subacute rehabilitation results in limited access to treatment, and under the best of current practices, this leaves many patients either unidentified or undertreated.[56]

THE TYPES OF COMMUNICATION PROBLEMS FOUND IN STROKE

Stroke results in three general categories of communication disorders: dysarthria, aphasia, and cognitive communicative impairment.[28,33] Each type of disorder is associated with a particular site of the damage in the peripheral and central nervous system. Although these three types can and do occur together, they will be discussed as separate categories.

1. Dysarthria is "a collective name for a group of neurologic speech disorders resulting from abnormalities in the strength, speed, range steadiness, tone, or accuracy of movements required for control of the respiratory, resonatory, articulatory, and prosodic aspects of speech production. The reasonable pathophysiologic disturbances are due to central or peripheral nervous system abnormalities and most often reflect weakness; spasticity; incoordination; involuntary movements; or excessive, reduced, or variable muscle tone."[33]

2. *Aphasia* is an acquired communication disorder caused by brain damage, characterized by an impairment of language modalities: speaking, listening, reading, and writing; it is not the result of a sensory or motor deficit, a general intellectual deficit, confusion, or a psychiatric disorder.[47]

3. Cognitive-communication disorders encompass difficulty with any aspect of communication affected by disruption of cognition. Communication may be verbal or nonverbal and includes listening, speaking, gesturing, reading, and writing in all domains of language (phonological, morphological, syntactic, semantic, and pragmatic). Cognition includes cognitive processes and systems (e.g., attention, perception, memory, organization, executive function). Areas of function affected by cognitive impairments include behavioral self-regulation, social interaction, activities of daily living, learning and academic performance, and vocational performance.[110]

THE ROLE OF THE SPEECH-LANGUAGE PATHOLOGIST ACROSS THE CONTINUUM OF CARE

The field of speech-language pathology has a relatively long history of investigating, defining, and treating communication disorders. However, the treatment of stroke-related communication disorders by speech-language pathology is relatively recent and grew out of a medical specialty in physical rehabilitation (physiatry).[95] Physical rehabilitation as a specialty had its beginning after World War II.[10,39,97] Prior to World War II, little attempt had been made to ameliorate debilitating conditions such as those following stroke. The experience of treating the war injured revealed the positive effects of physical treatment and pointed to the need for rehabilitation of similarly disabled individuals in the civilian population.[10,39] The field of speech-language pathology, along with occupational therapy, physical therapy, psychology, and social work were seen as integral to the team approach, which characterized the new field of physiatry (Physical Medicine and Rehabilitation).[20,42,97,111]

The inclusion of speech-language pathology into the rehabilitation model greatly expanded its scope of practice. Most people now take for granted that the rehabilitation team is the optimal model for stroke management.[20,111] The focus of rehabilitation medicine goes beyond other medical specialties in three ways: (1) its concern for the "whole" person rather than the illness or condition for which service was required, (2) the notion of "living with a condition" and "maximizing function" as opposed to curing chronic conditions, and (3) the inclusion of a psychosocial perspective that recognizes that the stroke happens not only to the survivor, but also to the family and friends.[96] The hallmark of rehabilitation has been its focus on function, and the contribution of that model to speech-language pathology is to focus on functional communication.[104,112]

Currently, stroke management is spoken of in terms of a continuum of care and a multiple phase process. Stroke management begins in the emergency department with a focus on rapid medical treatment and extends to years poststroke as the survivor learns to live with chronic impairments.[48,111] The speech-language pathologist may intervene at various points in this continuum. The settings include the emergency department, acute medical hospital stay, acute rehabilitation, home care, outpatient and long-term care, and community integration.[56] In each of these settings, the role of the speech-language pathologist changes. Although in all settings they begin with an evaluation of motor control of the speech mechanism, an assessment of language function, and an analysis of cognitive factors affecting communication, the comprehensiveness of the evaluation and the focus of treatment or management varies.[48,57] Rehabilitation services that facilitate the process of integration into the community and assumption of vocational/avocational endeavors are limited. While speech-language pathologists are focusing on "life participation" activities for individuals with aphasia,[16] almost no attention is given to the process of integration for those with other communication disorders.

THE MANAGEMENT OF COMMUNICATION DISORDERS

Major Dysarthrias Associated with Stroke

Normal speech production requires the exquisite coordination of a large number of muscle groups, which control respiration, phonation (voice production), resonation, and articulation.[28,31] The complexity of the control is due to established movement patterns that are unique to each language and are automatic. For example, the respiratory cycle is modified to have an increased duration during speech, and the vocal folds vibrate more quickly at the end of questions to raise the pitch.[11] Conversational articulation involves approximately 500 different oral shapes per minute, and even a minor deviation in control patterns can influence the precision of speech production.[31] Remarkably, the average speaker performs these actions automatically with no awareness or conscious planning.[28] Any disturbance in the control of movements

of respiration, phonation, resonation, and articulation may be reflected in speech, which is the primary modality of human communication.[28] The resulting speech disorders that may emerge following stroke include unilateral upper motor neuron dysarthria, spastic dysarthria, anarthria, and ataxic dysarthria.[33]

Unilateral Upper Motor Neuron Dysarthria

One of the easiest speech pathologies to identify, and probably the most common speech disorder following stroke, is known as "unilateral upper motor neuron dysarthria," which is relatively mild and often resolves in the weeks following stroke.[33,35,38] This impairment in the precision of consonant articulation is due to unilateral changes in muscle tone and accompanying weakness of the muscles of the speech mechanism.[33,38,82]

The speech-language pathologist evaluates the impact of this disorder on intelligibility of speech and effectiveness of communication.[82,114] Although unilateral upper motor neuron dysarthria may occur after either left or right hemisphere strokes, the specific abilities probed and assessment tools selected depend on the location of the stroke.[33,38] When the dysarthria persists as part of the sequelae of right brain stroke, it involves not only the accuracy of articulation but also changes in voicing and delivery that include rate and inflection of speech.[34,38,49,82] There is often an accompanying lack of facial affect. Sometimes these patients are somewhat hypoaroused and lethargic.[32] These characteristics may influence the quality of communication almost as much as the motor speech disorder.[33,38]

There are many opportunities for collaboration between occupational therapy and speech-language pathology with patients who have right brain injured unilateral upper motor neuron dysarthria.[42] Individuals with this dysarthria, though fairly intelligible, are often unaware of when they are not being understood.[33,38] In partnership with the speech-language pathologist, the occupational therapist may provide feedback to patients and increase their awareness of the deviations in their speech output.[42] Because many right brain injured patients are concrete in their interpretation of what is said to them, it is helpful for the feedback to be specific and concrete. For example, say, "I had difficulty understanding you because your voice was not loud enough" rather than simply requesting that the patient repeat what was said. For the individual with a right gaze preference and left neglect, reinforcement by all members of the team to look at the speaker when communicating may increase communication effectiveness. Given the change in awareness and reasoning, collaborative treatment and reinforcement of goals increases the transfer of learning.[33,38] See Chapter 19.

Following a left stroke of the unilateral upper motor neuron pathways, aphasia (language disorder) may accompany the dysarthria.[24,33] Without aphasia, the stroke survivor with left unilateral upper motor neuron dysarthria may function fully in life participation, even with persisting motor speech deficits, as long as speech is intelligible to the listener. Diagnosis of a concurrent language difficulty is sometimes obscured by the dysarthria and requires a comprehensive examination to identify subtle language changes.[33,38] These language disorders are discussed later in this chapter. On the other hand, individuals with left hemisphere unilateral upper motor neuron dysarthria may appear to have a language disorder when none is present.[33] They may speak less frequently, use shorter phrases, simplify sentences, but in fact not show any language dysfunction when formally assessed. These reductions in speech may simply reflect a motor speech disability rather than an underlying language problem.

Spastic Dysarthria (Bilateral Upper Motor Neuron Dysarthria)

The impact of bilateral upper motor lesion strokes on communication is substantial and is not simply the addition of the two upper motor neuron dysarthrias, but is a different speech disorder. Historically, this dysarthria is associated with the term "*pseudobulbar palsy*."[28,38] According to Darley and associates,[28] there are four muscular abnormalities that affect function in pseudobulbar palsy: spasticity,* weakness, limited range of movement, and slowness of movement.

The patient with spastic dysarthria has a strained-strangulated hoarse (rough) low-pitched voice.[28,33,38,82] He speaks slowly, with effort and extreme hypernasality and is monotonal in his delivery. Due to the absence of the sensitive coordination of timing of the onset of voicing, often his articulation of /p/ is said as a /b/, and similar confusions exist with /t - d/ and /k - g/.[28] These deviations in speech affect intelligibility and efficiency of communication. Individuals with spastic dysarthria tend to speak rarely, not because they are necessarily aphasic, but because of the effort that is required to speak. In addition, these patients manifest a flat affect but also display emotional outbursts in the form of emotional lability.[33,38] Speaking of even mildly emotional topics may trigger laughing or crying in inappropriate contexts. This lability is known as "*pseudobulbar affect*."[28,38] The location of the brain damage determines whether language function is spared or affected. Because of bilateral damage, these patients may have considerable upper extremity limitations affecting their ability to gesture, write, and use a computer.[28]

There are some general guidelines to follow when working with individuals with spastic dysarthria:[28,33,72] (1) acknowledge the effort needed to speak by providing extra time for the speech process; (2) validate (confirm) that the message was understood by repeating back what was said and thus give the patients a sense of control by confirming that they have been understood; (3) recognize that increasing spasticity in one part of the body (e.g., the upper extremity) may result in increased stiffness in the speech mechanism, and therefore do not expect speech during activities that increase spasticity; and (4) remind patients that the emotional lability is not within their control. Sometimes therapists have provided a notice to listeners that the patient's crying does not necessarily mean that he or she is sad, but that crying "just happens." Occupational therapists can assist the patient's recovery of Communication effectiveness by addressing team goals that target the previous behaviors.[42]

Anarthria and Locked-In Syndrome (Brainstem and Bilateral Midbrain Lesions)

In order to provide appropriate care to individuals without speech, differential diagnosis must distinguish among anarthria, locked-in syndrome, and mutism.[26,28,33,85] Anarthria is the absence of speech due to severe motor speech impairment.[33] Duffy reported that this condition is different from mutism, which is due to a cognitive dysfunction limiting the production of speech.[33] When the profound impairment of speech is accompanied by immobility of the body except for vertical eye movements, the disorder is called locked-in syndrome. Duffy described locked-in syndrome as a "special and dramatic manifestation of anarthria."[33] Intact language generation is often demonstrated once a communicative system is established. In his personal account, *The Diving Bell and the Butterfly*, Jean-Dominique Bauby[7] described blinking to indicate letters of the alphabet as the communication partner spoke the letters. When working with individuals without speech, the speech-language pathologist must determine the presence or absence of cognitive/linguistic function.

Medical treatment for locked-in syndrome has changed significantly over time.[85] Individuals with this rare condition have a better long-term survival rate than in the past.[33] Those who survive over many months require intensive rehabilitation to maximize their function. Establishing a basic communication system of "yes" and "no" is the first step and may be based on an eye blink system.[65] Once this is established, one can move on to more elaborate communication systems including letter boards and electronic systems. The painstaking effort described by Bauby is greatly reduced when more sophisticated augmentative and alternative communicative assistive devices are used. This technology is continuing to be developed and a brain computer interface may be available that allows individuals without movement to communicate by using electroencephalography activity to control a cursor on a computer screen.[109] Augmentative communication is an area where occupational therapists and speech-language pathologists work closely together. The most

---

*Note: Medical treatments such as baclofen or surgical treatments such as dorsal rhizotomy that reduce general body spasticity are known to improve motor speech production.[75]

important message for treatment of individuals with locked-in syndrome is that they may be intact cognitively and linguistically. Therefore, it is important that staff use natural adult speech and language because patients react to style and tone of communication.[35] In addition, to ensure that the patient is included in all decisions about care, staff should address the patient and the caregivers about the particulars of the rehabilitation plans.[42]

Some patients who are initially without speech progress to the point where they have some vocalization and some mobility of the upper or lower extremities.[65] Small movements can be used to activate a switch for alternative communication. The emerging voice production is effortful, strained, and similar to the voice heard in individuals with spastic dysarthria.[28,33] Even when the vocalization is limited to one sound, the individual can use the sound to call out to the caregiver. More articulate speech may not be possible, but some develop a small repertoire of words that are intelligible to familiar listeners. Communication can be enhanced by using the same strategies as identified for spastic dysarthria. The key points to remember are (1) give the patient lots of time to respond, (2) collaborate with the speech-language pathologist in designing low-tech tools that are visually and spatially accessible to the patient who has limitations in upper extremity functions, (3) indicate that you have understood the message by repeating it, and (4) validate the patient's cognitive competence by treating the individual in an appropriately mature manner.[92]

Ataxic Dysarthria (Cerebellar Lesions)

Most cases of ataxic dysarthria are not the result of stroke. Nevertheless, vascular lesions primarily in the posterior inferior cerebellar artery and anterior inferior cerebellar artery may result in ataxic dysarthria.[28,33] Furthermore, ataxic dysarthria in stroke is rare. The primary speech symptoms are slow rate, abnormal prosody, and intermittently imprecise articulation.[14,28,33] Typically the patient's cognition is intact, but speech, though intelligible, may sound quite bizarre and unnatural.[14,28,33,38]

Rehabilitation of these communicative disorders is dependent on the patient's age and vocational and avocational needs. The person may be more concerned with physical dysfunction than the speech changes, as the limb ataxia affects the ability to write, type, or use a computer mouse. These graphomotor disorders may affect more of the individual's ability to communicate and require more intervention than the motor speech disorders. See Chapter 10. Team treatment with this type of dysarthria should recognize that these individuals probably have intact cognitive and language skills.

Mixed (Any Combination of the Previous Conditions)

Multiple strokes can affect various components of the motor speech system and result in mixed dysarthria. Certain combinations of dysarthria are more likely to occur than

others are.[28,33] The most common mixed motor speech disorder is a combination of an upper motor neuron dysarthria affecting the right side of the oral musculature and apraxia of speech.[33] This combination occurs frequently in left middle cerebral artery strokes, and its symptoms are addressed in the discussion of aphasia. Moreover, single brainstem strokes might produce a mixed flaccid, spastic, and cerebellar dysarthria. This combination occurs because of the closeness of the upper and lower motor neuron brain structures and the proximity to cerebellar control circuits.[33]

LANGUAGE DISORDERS ASSOCIATED WITH STROKE

Occupational therapists often question the speech-language pathologist about the complex and fascinating syndromes of acquired language disorders known as aphasia. Patients with aphasia say unusual and, at times, bizarre things. For example, a patient may make up a meaningless word (neologism) and use it as if it is a real word or take a real word and use it inappropriately (paraphasia).[43] Symptoms such as a verbal stereotypy (saying a recurrent utterance such as "keep the key" or "ho doe ho doe ho doe" with appropriate melody and intonation) are remarkable phenomena.[35,43] A patient with aphasia reports that he "knows exactly what I want to say, but the words don't come out." The person with aphasia searches for the number word to indicate the number of children he has and is forced to start with "one...two" and say the whole series until he arrives at the number word that he is trying to say.[35,43]

The unevenness of communication issues among the various language modalities is confusing to the professional unfamiliar with aphasia.[35,43] For example, a patient may write normally but be unable to read what he or she has written, or a patient may not understand a word or sentence when spoken, but immediately "gets it" when it is written down.[35,43] These unexpected combinations of language strengths and weaknesses pose challenges to the rehabilitation professional. Another issue surrounds the term "*expressive*" aphasia, which leads one to believe that there is no "*receptive*" component when in fact for most patients, the difficulty understanding language is the most functionally limiting component of the syndrome.[43] Reduced auditory comprehension keeps persons with aphasia from returning to their work environment, participating comfortably in some social events, and enjoying language-based activities such as television, movies, and reading.[55] The communication partner is prone to overestimate the patient's comprehension of spoken language because the patient often appears to understand.[37] This misconception is a reflection of the aphasic person's socially appropriate affect and response to the environment and can lead to misunderstandings and miscommunication.[37]

Historically, aphasiologists have categorized aphasias differently depending on their particular bias.[35,43] In the last half of the twentieth century, the most common categorization system was based on a classical typology which used the fluency of speech production and spoken language comprehension attributes to group the types of language issues.[43] These classical groups are Broca's, Transcortical Motor, Wernicke's, Conduction, Transcortical Sensory, and Anomic aphasias. The most severe form is global aphasia and results from large or multiple lesions of the left hemisphere. Most modern aphasiologists simplify this classification into two general forms: nonfluent and fluent aphasia.[43] It is understood that pure forms of any of these types are relatively rare (Table 20-1).

Broca's Aphasia

Broca's aphasia, which many refer to as "expressive" aphasia, is regularly associated with a middle cerebral artery stroke affecting the third frontal convolution of the frontal lobe (classical Broca's area, Brodmann's areas 44 and 47)[1,25,26,40] and extending into the white matter, the internal capsule. This lesion is anterior to the inferior portion of the precentral gyrus, clarifying the connection of this syndrome with the reductions in motor control in the right upper extremity.[43,61,62,80,105] In the acute stage, these patients may be mute.[43] Their speech production may evolve over the next few weeks to a few automatic expressions and perhaps a spoken "Yes."[43] These patients are typically alert, aware of their surroundings, and frustrated by the absence of speech.[13,61] Their preserved affect can mislead the untrained observer to overestimate the language competency of the patient.[100] The five main features of the evolving pattern are awkward labored articulation, difficulty initiating speech, reduced utterance length, telegraphic speech, and reduction in melodic contours.[13,43] The following is an example of a patient with Broca's aphasia describing the "Cookie Theft Picture."[43] See Fig 20-1.

"Boy . . . Cuh . . . Cuh . . . Cookie . . . girl . . . mama . . . kay . . . water . . . sinking . . . ice . . . ay . . . ch . . . ch . . . no . . . water . . . sinking . . . ee . . . why?" Given the limited flow of speech, one would think that little is being communicated. However, the words are substantive and appropriate, so that giving the patient with Broca's aphasia time and using context to anticipate content allows the individual to

Table 20-1

General Suggestions for Improving Post stroke Communication

	GUIDELINES FOR ENHANCEMENT OF COMMUNICATION
To enhance expression	■ Use phrase "I know you know___" to show that you understand that the problem is one of expression, not knowledge. ■ Give person to time to talk. ■ Tolerate patient's silence, but encourage person to take part in the conversation. ■ Talk about personally relevant topics and shared experiences. ■ Engage patient's family/friends in providing topics. ■ Talk about items in the immediate environment. ■ Accept and encourage nonverbal expression (gestures, facial expression). ■ Keep paper and pencil handy. ■ Provide choices when necessary. ■ Acknowledge breakdowns in communication and encourage patient to repair.
To enhance comprehension	■ Identify hearing loss. ■ Slow the rate of your speech, but maintain normal intonation. ■ Reduce distractions (noise free, visually simple environment). ■ Use face-to-face communication. ■ Use short phrases interspersed with appropriate pauses. ■ Use simple direct sentences. ■ Signal topic shifts and provide a context for the next topic, e.g., "On another topic . . . ." ■ Use visual props when needed.[100] ■ Write down important words or instructions. ■ Identify communication breakdowns and use repair strategies (rephrase, use simpler word, slow rate of speech, etc.). ■ Emphasize important words. ■ Simplify written instructions for homework. ■ Have only one person (or few persons) talk at a time .

Adapted from Hedge,[51] and Simmons-Mackie,[103]

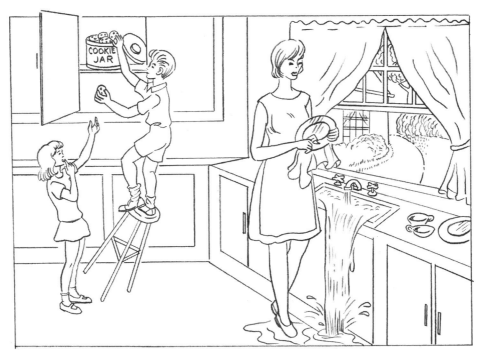

Figure 20-1 The Cookie Theft picture. (From Goodglass H, Kaplan E, Barresi B: *The assessment of aphasia and related disorders*, ed 3, Philadelphia, 2001, Lea & Febiger.)

be successful in communicating substance.[35,42,61,95] In addition, using visual stimuli, key words, or simple pictures to supplement context and accepting gestures and drawing makes it possible for the patient with severe Broca's aphasia to communicate not only thoughts and feelings but also specific information.[18,71,99,101]

The comprehension of spoken language in Broca's or nonfluent aphasia is better than the production of speech, but it is far from perfect, at least in the early stages of the condition.[43,61] Comprehension tends to improve faster in these types of aphasia than in other forms.[61,62] Probably the major error made in working with patients with Broca's aphasia is to overestimate the patient's adequacy of comprehending spoken language.[51] Some of the signs of overestimation are "the patient fails to carry out the activities that I have told him, and he understands everything I say" or "the patient comes at the wrong time . . . too early or too late . . ." Many patients with Broca's aphasia do not process spoken number words. Providing a written appointment slip helps ensure that the patient with aphasia understands the scheduled appointment time. Communication can be further enhanced by using simple, clear direct adult sentences.[51] Breakdowns of comprehension occur with complex grammar (tense, number, negation, comparison, words relating to space) that may be difficult for the patient.[30] One needs to provide processing time for comprehension of more complex language,[51,61,101] which can be done by inserting pauses between phrases or thought groups. It is a good idea to

verify that the patient with Broca's aphasia comprehends communication to him, no matter how intact the social behavior appears.

Reading and writing are also impaired in patients with Broca's aphasia.[61] Patients with severe Broca's aphasia read the content words (nouns and verbs) and guess at the overall meaning of the sentences.[43] Their ability to read improves over time, but the elements of asyntactic comprehension limit reading of most adult level reading material. Writing is impaired not only by the motor component, since the patient may have limited use of the dominant right hand, but also because of the language component.[61] Spelling and letter formation may be extremely difficult. The use of computer-assisted programs may be helpful but are sometimes difficult. Some patients improve sufficiently to use computer-based typing, text messaging and e-mailing to communicate with friends.[60]

Recovery with Broca's aphasia has a longer course than with other types of aphasia.[6] In the authors' clinical experience, persons with Broca's aphasia can continue to improve their communication skills long after the acute stages. This improvement corresponds with an amelioration of the motor component associated with Broca's aphasia (i.e., apraxia of speech) and a gradual improvement in speech comprehension.[93] If in the early stages, the aphasia is mild, and it may improve to a relatively mild anomic aphasia or resolve almost completely.[62,95]

In the authors' experience, occupational therapists often address functional language-based daily tasks. For example, following written instructions on medication, reading written instructions for upper extremity exercises, or following written recipes in the kitchen all have elements that can be most impaired in nonfluent aphasia. Any activity involving numbers (e.g., check writing and reconciliation of a bank account) may be impossible for the person with Broca's aphasia to complete. It is important to set realistic therapy goals with respect to these tasks. Whenever possible, collaboration with the speech-language pathologist may be helpful when planning compensatory and supportive techniques to facilitate these language-based activities.

Apraxia of Speech

Apraxia, a common speech disorder resulting from a middle cerebral artery stroke, is controversial,[2] because aphasiologists have described it differently according to different theoretical biases. Duffy[33] listed 25 different terms for apraxia of speech that researchers have used to define it. Many speech-language pathologists, including Duffy, view it as a separate specific type of motor speech disorder independent of aphasia.[33] However, in the authors' experience, this motor disorder that is not dysarthria usually occurs with a nonfluent Broca's aphasia or mixed dysarthria. Speech production is effortful, slow, and dysrhythmic, resulting in impaired prosodic variation (i.e., melody of speech).[28,33,38] The cardinal feature articulatory effort is visible and is apparent groping for the articulatory positioning and sequencing.[33,38] These patients are generally aware and frustrated by their speech disorder and say things such as "I know what I want to say but it will not come out."[13,28,33] In addition, these individuals have great difficulty imitating words and phrases.[28,33,38]

In general, these individuals are highly motivated to improve their speech and are unusually focused on their speech production.[28,33,38] In the authors' experience, their concentration on the speech component can be so strong that it supersedes their interest in other therapies and overrides efforts to ameliorate other linguistic disturbances. Although it would seem reasonable to introduce supplementary or communicative alternatives (i.e., a communication book or a computerized communication device), the authors find that these patients initially reject these devices. Interestingly, younger patients who are familiar with text messages and e-mail are more receptive to facilitating their communication through these avenues.

It is helpful for the occupational therapist to remember that these patients may have a subtle language comprehension disorder despite their appearing to be completely cognitively intact.[28,33,38] Their struggle may be alleviated by providing additional time to communicate, giving verbal choices, using supplementary written material, and having an attitude of calmness around their communication.[33,38] Typically, the listener is counseled not to provide a word when it is known what the individual is attempting to say, but in this case, for efficiency,

the occupational therapist might choose to do so with the patient's permission.

Prognosis for individuals with apraxia of speech ranges depending on the severity of the apraxia and the underlying linguistic disorders.[38] However, patients with good comprehension tend to improve over a longer period and clear to a milder version of apraxia of speech.[38,107] Slow speech, intermittent articulation errors, and reduced prosodic variation may persist in the chronic state.[38,107] Nevertheless, their communication is effective. The authors find that these individuals can become the advocates for public awareness of aphasia, because they are intensely focused on the alteration of their speech and its impact on their lives. See Table 20-2.

Transcortical Motor Aphasia

Transcortical motor aphasia is a rare type of aphasia is due to a small subcortical lesion superior to Broca's area, or to a lesion outside of the anterior language areas of the left hemisphere.[26,40] Because of the location of the lesion in the frontal lobe, transcortical motor aphasia includes both language and cognitive components. The person with transcortical motor aphasia has difficulty spontaneously initiating speech but repeats even long sentences effortlessly and accurately.[43,62] Consequently, the listener is required to initiate the topic and to structure the question in order to facilitate a verbal response.[2,69,92] For example, when asked an open-ended question such as "what did you do yesterday?" the patient is known to say, "I . . . I . . . I can't . . . I can't . . . yesterday . . . I did many things." However, when asked to describe a picture, the output is in the form of a simple declarative sentence that is usually grammatically correct, appropriate, but lacking in elaboration.

The main communication problem in transcortical motor aphasia is maintaining the flow of fluent speech, which is due to an underlying difficulty organizing the content of communication.[89] This form of aphasia displays cognitive failures that result in limited and disorganized output both in speech and writing.[92] However, comprehension of spoken language or even syntactically complex sentences are often well-preserved.[43] Frequently, reading comprehension and oral reading are also excellent.[59]

The patient with transcortical motor aphasia may be indifferent to the reduction in his communication.[13] In the authors' experience, the patient's apathy elicits frustration in the staff working with him or her because they may overestimate his or her ability to perform. The staff may expect the patient to initiate the use of a memory book, to structure a meaningful activity, or to set priorities for daily activities, none of which this patient can do without prompting. The authors have found that the patient requires structure and repetition to perform and constant prompting to initiate and follow through with tasks. The patient's lack of appreciation of the goals of therapy and

Table 20-2

Suggestions for Improving Communication: Broca's Aphasia and Apraxia

BROCA'S APHASIA: SPEECH AND LANGUAGE SYMPTOMS*	GUIDELINES FOR COMMUNICATION ENHANCEMENT†
May be mute at onset	Give patient plenty of time to speak
Impaired "flow" of speech	Encourage participation in conversation
Halting and hesitant speech	Encourage patient to use alternate means of
Impaired prosody and intonation	communication (gesture, drawing)
Awkward effortful articulation	Use visual supports (key words, word books)
Short simple utterances	Ask the person to tell you if he or she wants you to fill in
Telegraphic style	the missing words
Intact content with poor sentence structure	If you do not understand what the person is saying, let
and grammar	him or her know
Self-correction of errors	Pay close attention to body language and facial expression
Aware of errors and frustrated	Try not to over estimate comprehension
Impaired speech repetition	Write down numbers (time, date, address, etc.)
Impaired comprehension	Avoid using semantically reversible sentences like "the
Dyslexia (reading problems)	girl was hit by the boy"
Dysgraphia (writing problems)	Simplify grammatical structures when you do ADL tasks,
Dyscalculia (calculation problems)	(e.g., before/after, negatives, comparatives)
	Ask SLP regarding level of reading comprehension
	before giving written instructions
	Highlight key words
	Pair written words with auditory stimuli (electronic
	books)
	Enlarge print as necessary
	Provide model for written material

APRAXIA OF SPEECH: SPEECH AND LANGUAGE SYMPTOMS‡	GUIDELINES FOR COMMUNICATION ENHANCEMENT ‡
May be mute at onset	Strategies for enhanced expression are the same as the
Speech symptoms are often similar to the previous	ones previously listed
symptoms listed with the addition of:	For the patient with severe apraxia of speech augmenta-
Sequential speech movements are difficult	tive and alternative devices may be considered
(diadochokinesis)	May not require the modifications for comprehension
Sound clusters simplified ("splash" becomes	indicated previously
" . . . plash")	
Errors increase as a function of increased word length	
Heightened awareness of speech errors	
High level of frustrations	
Fairly preserved speech comprehension	

* Adapted from Goodglass and associates[43] and Hedge.[51]
† Adapted from Hedge[51] and Simmons-Mackie.[103]
‡ Adapted from Duffy.[33]
SLP, Speech-language therapist.

inability to connect the procedures to the goals impedes his ability to respond to treatment.[2,42,69]

If the transcortical motor aphasia is mild in the early stages, it may resolve to an anomic variety.[43,92] Nevertheless, the authors have found that persistence in the reduction of speech initiation and organization of discourse may prevent the patient from resuming normal social and vocational activities. These deficits most likely reflect dysexecutive function that may be more debilitating than the language disorder.[9]

The occupational therapist can facilitate communication with the patient who has transcortical motor aphasia by structuring the communication environment and providing many cues for communication. Despite the preservation of some communication modalities, the individual is dependent on the listener to initiate, maintain, and repair conversation breakdowns.[69] In addition, the patient will need prompting to use his or her calendar, notebook, and other augmentative systems. See Table 20-3.

Fluent Aphasias (Wernicke's, Conduction, Transcortical Sensory, and Anomic)

Fluent syndromes are relatively common among elderly poststroke patients. These individuals may not be referred for occupational therapy if they do not present with concurrent difficulties in daily living. However, some of these patients have a right visual field cut, and they may eventually find their way to occupational therapy for evaluation and treatment. The major language characteristics of fluent aphasia are the ease of speech production and the normal utterance length.[43] Various types and severities of speech characteristics are found among the fluent syndromes. In addition, a variety of speech comprehension, reading, and writing deficits may occur.[43]

Wernicke's Aphasia

The diagnosis of Wernicke's aphasia rests on a triad of characteristics, including fluent paraphasic speech, reduced speech comprehension, and anosognosia (lack of

awareness of the erroneousness of output).[43] Although speech is produced with normal fluency and prosody, the content is severely limited.[43] Speech contains a mixture of real words and neologisms (made up new words) and usually is empty of meaning.[13,45] The severe reduction in nouns and verbs and vagueness of content is reflected in the following example. When shown the Cookie Theft picture[43] (Fig. 20-1), a patient said "had that before . . . chories . . . this guy is a messo . . . she is okay. He has a mess on . . . all over here. She is just stupid. Oh, what is that? That's just . . . those are nice, pretty . . . and that's a mess and then goots (cups). He's pretty stupid. She is okay. She's cute. This is inside . . . outside." These patients have been incorrectly labeled confused or demented, or diagnosed with having psychiatric disorders when in fact the syndrome of aphasia causes the bizarre output.[74]

In the early stages, a patient with Wernicke's aphasia may be unaware of his or her language disorder, deny that he or she has had a stroke, and confabulate the reason for the hospitalization.[13,43,45] Since a patient is unable to understand what is being asked of him or her and is unaware of his or her deficits, initial language testing may make little or no sense to him or her.[13,29,45] The patient's willingness to participate in therapy increases as spontaneous recovery of language occurs and he or her develops more insight into the nature of his or her communication problem.[29,45] He or she begins to have a nagging awareness of something amiss in the process of communication, but he or she may not recognize that the communicative breakdown is due to aphasia.

People with Wernicke's aphasia are said to have "*receptive aphasia.*" This term suggests that their communication difficulty is simply a failure to understand spoken language.[45] However, from the previous description, aphasia obviously has both receptive and expressive components. Furthermore, comprehension of spoken language is uneven and at times unexpected.[43,45,99] For example, the authors have found the simple instruction "pick up the spoon and put it in the bowl" is usually more difficult than the whole body command "stand up and turn around." If the person catches the right word or interprets the context sufficiently, responses may be surprisingly appropriate and may obscure the severity of the language comprehension problem.[43,45,74]

Comprehension can be facilitated by discussing topics of personal relevance, giving the patient time to process the information, signaling changes in topic, stating the same idea in different words, and providing visual cues.[74] The staff also needs to remember the patient's difficulty in detecting a communication breakdown, so it is up to the communicative partner to fill in and assist in any way possible with the needed repair.[45] Comprehension of written language is impaired so that use of written cues, written homework, and schedules may not be helpful for these patients, particularly in the early stages.[74] Most of these patients will

---

Table 20-3

Suggestions for Improving Communication: Transcortical Motor Aphasia

TRANSCORTICAL MOTOR APHASIA: SPEECH AND LANGUAGE SYMPTOMS*	GUIDELINES FOR COMMUNICATION ENHANCEMENT†
May be mute at onset	Prompting required for speech engagement and initiation:
Difficulty initiating speech	
Flat affect	
Sentence repetition is fluent and effortless	Prompt the patient to use a notebook for daily activities
Sentence length is reduced	
Comprehension of spoken and written language is generally spared	Use written cues to prompt communication (i.e., when asking patients if they did their exercises, write down the anticipated response)
Impaired executive function (i.e., organization of speech output, narrative skills, all varieties of discourse, engagement evident both in spoken and written output)	

*Adapted from Goodglass and associates[43] and Hedge.[51]
†Adapted from Hedge[51] and Simmons Mackie.[103]

have no right upper extremity weakness and that writing may be fluently executed. However, the content of writing samples usually mirrors speech production and contains neologisms, meaningless content, and inappropriately spelled words.[43,74]

Depending on their social behavior and their communication partners, these individuals can live a rich life after stroke.[74] In time, many patients with Wernicke's aphasia successfully use a "communication book" that contains nouns of personal relevance.[106] Some of these patients are remarkably independent despite the global severity of their aphasia.[74] See Table 20-4.

Conduction Aphasia

The neuroanatomical correlate for conduction aphasia is somewhat controversial, but most agree that it is usually due to a small lesion in the supramarginal gyrus.[26]

The outstanding feature of conduction aphasia is relatively fluent spontaneous speech with disproportionately poor sentence repetition.[13,43] Spontaneous speech is characterized by "abundant literal paraphasias"[13] (sound substitutions), especially in the early stages. The progressive approximation or targeting of sound sequences is common. For example, to say the word "bench," the individual may make the following attempts to arrive at the required word "chench . . . nech . . . pench . . . spench . . . bench."

These word finding problems and anomia can range from mild to severe.[13,102,103] Persons with conduction aphasia also have difficulty reading aloud and make frequent sound errors.[13] This function improves over time but limits the use of written scripts as a treatment procedure. Writing varies in effectiveness, but graphic production typically contains some errors in grammar, spelling, and word retrieval.[13] Patients with conduction aphasia are aware of their errors and may be highly frustrated by their inability to properly string together the sequence of sounds required to say polysyllabic words such as "statistical analysis."[43] This syndrome is fairly rare and has a relatively good prognosis, evolving in time to a mild anomic aphasia.[13,102,103]

It is the authors' experience that when working with this group, professionals need to support the patient's attempts to communicate by being an active communication partner and accepting imprecise productions. The production of complex scientific terms, medical terminology, and the names of pharmaceuticals will always be difficult for the patient with conduction aphasia. Inaccurate production of words, if the words resemble the target sufficiently, may not limit the transfer of ideas. The therapist should avoid requesting verbatim repetition of instructions including repetition of numbers (telephone numbers, dates, etc.) and recall of specific complicated words.

Table 20-4

Suggestions for Improving Communication: Wernicke's Aphasia

WERNICKE'S APHASIA: SPEECH AND LANGUAGE SYMPTOMS*	GUIDELINES FOR COMMUNICATION ENHANCEMENT†
Speech initiation is easy (hyperfluent)	Stop strategy: Use gestures to cue a patient to stop the flow of speech
Fluent uninterrupted strings of words	Refocus patient to change topics
Well-articulated	Provide written nouns (key words or pictures to convey information)
Neologisms and verbal paraphasia	
Jargon	Allow circumlocution
Grammatically coherent: small words fall into place automatically	Simplify written and spoken material
Inability to repeat words	Provide meaningful contexts for tasks—personal relevance is helpful
Intact prosody and intonation	Speak slowly clearly and at normal loudness levels
Little awareness of errors	Face the person when you talk to them
Poor speech comprehension	Give the person time to understand
Unaware of comprehension limitation	Write down key words to change topics and support comprehension
Dyslexia and dysgraphia	Use common words and simple direct sentence structures
	Say the same thing differently
	Rely on the speech-language pathology evaluation to guide choice of reading material level
	Anticipate writing difficulty

*Adapted from Goodglass and associates[43] and Hedge.[51]

†Adapted from Marshall.[74]

Communication can also be improved by realizing that the person probably understands even complex language, reads sophisticated material silently, and responds well to cues. In addition, the person can learn new material and develop new skills.[102,103] See Table 20-5.

Anomic Aphasia

Since all syndromes of fluent aphasia are characterized by a reduction in the retrieval of nouns, the use of the term *"anomic aphasia"* becomes arbitrary, as it is both a symptom and diagnostic category.[13,41] It is also well-accepted that anomic aphasia is regularly the end point of other aphasias, and because of this feature, there is no one neuroanatomical site associated with the classification of anomic aphasia.[13]

According to Goodglass, Kaplan, and Barresi,[43] the "major feature of anomic aphasia is the prominence of word-finding difficulty in the context of fluent, grammatically well-formed speech."[43] There are few paraphasias, and comprehension is "relatively intact."[43] Patients with anomic aphasia may be underidentified because their speech is fluent and their content is substantive. In contrast, on confrontation naming tasks, their speech is "empty" and they use frequent circumlocutions. Their naming difficulty poses a significant functional limitation in situations where clear, concise verbal function is required.[13]

In anomic aphasia, comprehension of spoken and written material is marred by subtle deficits.[13] For example, the patient may have no difficulty following conversation when talking about pictures in a photograph album or listening to a paragraph about current events where context supports comprehension.[43] On the other hand, the authors have found that they may do rather poorly on specific nonredundant content (e.g., the Revised Token Test instructions, "Point to the green square and the white circle.")[78]

The occupational therapist needs to be aware that it is easy to miss the language deficits in individuals with anomic aphasia and needs to look for difficulty with confrontation naming. For example, these patients have difficulty both saying and understanding unfamiliar names (staff members, pharmaceuticals, locations, and names of medical conditions), putting them at risk for making errors.[42] The listener might be tempted to overestimate the communicative skills of the person with anomic aphasia and to expect the individual to return to work. Therefore, recognizing the disorder and developing strategies that enhance the person's ability to perform on the job are essential.[42] The authors find that collaboration with the vocational rehabilitation counselor facilitates reintegration into the individual's work life (Table 20-6).

Global Aphasia

Global aphasia is common, especially in the acute phase after a large left middle cerebral artery stroke.[26,40] Sometimes this aphasia is also found when a patient has two or more smaller left hemisphere strokes.[26] The main feature is that all language modalities are severely impaired.[18] It is important to remember that "global" when describing aphasia does not mean "total."[18,19] Speech may be limited to automaticisms ("yes," social greetings, and curse words) and recurrent utterances (e.g., "ah-dig-ah-dig-ah-dig" or "television . . . television . . . television"). Speech repetition can be limited to serial speech (counting, days of the week, and overlearned material such as prayers and lyrics of familiar songs).[43] In the early stages, patients with global aphasia have only rudimentary comprehension of spoken language. The patient appears to rely almost entirely on facial expression, vocal intonation, and contextual cues to understand others. Speech comprehension almost always improves to some extent; some patients can be reclassified as a milder aphasia, such as Broca's or conduction aphasia.[18] However, speech comprehension remains impaired in many cases, and small gains in language comprehension do not always change the aphasia diagnosis.[18] In the beginning, reading may be restricted to familiar nouns and

Table 20-5

Suggestions for Improving Communication: Conduction Aphasia

CONDUCTION APHASIA: SPEECH AND LANGUAGE SYMPTOMS*	GUIDELINES FOR COMMUNICATION ENHANCEMENT
Fluent conversational speech, but unusually poor speech repetition	Refrain from expecting verbatim repetition of numbers, words, sentences
Abundant literal paraphasia (sound substitutions)	Allow circumlocution
Some word substitutions	Encourage alternate methods of supplying target words
Polysyllabic words are more difficult than shorter words	Give plenty of time to express self
Naming is variable (from poor to good)	Encourage patient to use shorter simpler words or to use pantomime
Preserved speech comprehension	
Oral reading is poor; characterized by words containing phonemic paraphasia (literal)	Encourage patient to use own cueing strategies
Silent reading comprehension is good	Refrain from activities requiring reading aloud, e.g., scripts
Writing can be comparable to speech	Rely on the speech-language pathology evaluation to guide writing activities

*Adapted from Goodglass and associates[43] and Hedge.[51]

Table 20-6

Suggestions for Improving Communication: Anomic Aphasia

ANOMIC APHASIA: SPEECH AND LANGUAGE SYMPTOMS*	GUIDELINES FOR COMMUNICATION ENHANCEMENT
Object naming is disproportionally impaired relative to preserved speech fluency	Allow patient to refer to word lists to locate target word
Word substitutions and circumlocution are common	Encourage patient to describe target noun
Repetition is sometimes quite preserved	Allow circumlocution
Comprehension of spoken and written material relatively preserved but variable	Refrain from confrontation naming tasks
Writing parallels speaking	Ask patient if he or she wants the listener to supply the word
	Consider use of word prediction software for writing tasks
	Refrain from overestimating adequacy of comprehension

*Adapted from Goodglass and associates[43] and Hedge.[51]

verbs, and writing is usually limited to random lines on a page or single letters. Writing of one's own name and some numbers may improve in time. In the chronic phase, gestures and nonoral means of communication are often effective compensations for the severe reduction in language abilities.[18]

Patients with global aphasia may be withdrawn and unaware or they may be alert, oriented, and extremely aware.[18] The alert patient is usually described as having better comprehension than is actually the case.[101] Frustration tolerance is variable and may be related to the patient's self-awareness.[18]

To facilitate rehabilitation, the occupational therapist should speak to the patient in direct, short instructions that pair simple and explicit language structures with modeling and manual cues[18] (i.e., "right arm first" followed by a gentle touch on the right arm, rather than "don't use your left arm for this") The mere use of too many words may overwhelm the individual with global aphasia.[18] Communication partners need to be aware that gestures and facial expressions are cues that the patient with global aphasia uses to understand his or her world.[18] Therefore, clinicians need to pay attention to facial expression and use a natural and appropriate vocal tone.[18] The simple social language used to begin conversations is necessary in establishing rapport and trust.[18]

Topic shifting is enhanced if the communicative partner uses visual prompting such as providing key word choices from which a patient can choose the word(s). The writing of key words to support communication is essential in enabling the patient to participate actively in conversation.[18,58] In a therapeutic session, it is helpful to limit the goals and procedures to one or two, provide breaks, extra time, and a set routine to facilitate successful communication in individuals who have global aphasia.[18] See Table 20-7.

COGNITIVE COMMUNICATION IMPAIRMENT

Common etiologies of cognitive communicative impairment are right hemisphere stroke and vascular dementia (formerly known as "multi-infarct dementia").[84] The unifying factors for this disorder are reductions in attention, concentration, memory, and problem-solving. The impact of these factors ranges widely, and the resulting communication disorder is complex.[84]

Right Brain

Although most patients with a right brain stroke "do well in straightforward conversation,"[84] their communication abilities are not "normal." Some individuals with right brain damage have speech and/or language problems and an upper motor neuron dysarthria.[84] This dysarthria is characterized by slight imprecision of articulation, harsh voice quality, and monotonal delivery.[33] Rarely is overall speech intelligibility affected.[33] These patients often lack appropriate and meaningful vocal inflection, and emotional display is blunted.[84] In addition, speech rate, rhythm, and melody are sometimes abnormal.[33] Some right brain damaged (RBD) patients also have mild language deficits and display difficulty on clinical tasks such as confrontational naming, divergent naming (category naming), and word recall.[84] These language problems seem more related to cognitive deficits of attention and memory than language dysfunction.[84] Frequently, there is a reduction in comprehension of word meanings and difficulty processing metaphors that result in unusual and concrete decoding of language.[83] On rare instances, RBD patients present aphasia; however, the aphasia is atypical (also known as "crossed aphasia").[26,83]

Another component of right brain injury cognitive communicative impairment is an alteration in pragmatic communication and discourse.[84] When describing an event, the patient with right brain communicative deficits will become tangential and overly detailed and show a tendency toward hyperverbosity.[87,88] Although relatively infrequent, some patients use confabulation to make up stories to help them explain events that they do not understand.[83] The patient's discourse is sometimes redundant and irrelevant.[84] These issues can be seen in this description of the "Cookie Theft" picture[43] (see Fig. 20-1): "The

Table 20-7

Suggestions for Improving Communication: Global Aphasia

GLOBAL APHASIA: SPEECH AND LANGUAGE CHARACTERISTICS*	GUIDELINES FOR COMMUNICATION ENHANCEMENT†
All aspects of language are severely impaired	For both expression and comprehension:
Speech limited to automaticisms (e.g., "yes" "OK" numbers in series)	Rely on visual (nonlanguage) cues
Unable to repeat	Pictures
Unable to produce speech sounds voluntarily	Gestures
Jargon may be present	Facial expression, body language
Auditory comprehension limited to simple material of high personal relevance	Signs and signal
Appears to understand when patient does not	Emphasize important words in a sentence
Silent reading limited to recognition of own name	Provide simple verbal or written word choices when appropriate
Unable to read aloud	Keep all stimuli personally relevant
Unable to write words	Accept any and all modes of communication
Awareness of/reliance on social cues may be good	Encourage inclusion in social conversation and singing activities
	Encourage speech activities (e.g., counting, prayers)
	Focus on doing things together rather than talking about things

*Adapted from Goodglass and associates[43] and Hedge.[51]
†Adapted from Simmons-Mackie.[103]

woman just got home from work and she is thinking about dinner. She might go to the restaurant so doesn't have to cook and clean up. The kitchen is pretty clean for someone who works. The curtains are clean." This description highlights the communication issues frequently observed in RBD patients: the absence of the relationship of the individuals in the picture (woman rather than mother), irrelevant and tangential content that misses the activity of the picture (washing the dishes and ignoring her children), misses the emotion (the woman's distraction while the water overflows the sink), neglect of the left side of the page (the description misses the children on the left side of the picture), and the focus on inconsequential details ("the curtains are clean").

Furthermore, a lack of insight and concreteness may reduce the patient's ability to participate in the setting of rehabilitation goals. Goals, such as reducing impulsivity or increasing safety awareness, have little meaning to the RBD patient. For example, when the authors ask the patients if they have noticed that they tend to neglect the left side of space, they probably will deny the problem.[84] However, they may readily acknowledge that people repeatedly tell them "look to the left." In the authors' experience, the patient will not appreciate the goal or meaningfulness of the activity unless the therapist makes the consequence of the neglect evident to the patient (i.e., not seeing dangers on the left). In the authors' experience, clinicians sometimes ascribe the failure to work

productively in treatment to a lack of motivation or decreased initiation. However, the failure seems, to the authors, most likely a consequence of the alterations in cognition, particularly the reduction of insight.[84] This failure to derive implied meaning from what is said affects decisions at every stage of the rehabilitation process.[84] The patient may not understand that his or her impairments affect the ability to live independently or return to work because of his or her inability to connect the impairment with the failure to negotiate the tasks of daily life.

The cognitive communication deficits described previously are exacerbated by nonlinguistic communicative impairments that include left neglect, reduced and disturbed attention, anosognosia (failure to recognize deficits) prosopagnosia; and visual and spatial perception deficits.[73,83] The factors that most affect communication are neglect, inattention, reduced awareness, and impulsivity. The failure to respond to speakers in the left visual field affects the pragmatic interaction with communication partners.[5,73,84] In addition, left neglect can be paired with cognitive issues that affect reading and writing.[73,84] Difficulty reading prescriptions and inadequacies in filling out medical forms affect the patient's compliance in medical care. While these skills are not central to communication, they seriously influence the rehabilitation team's decisions about prognosis, discharge, and burden of care.[84]

Little is known about the recovery of communication deficits in the RBD patient.[73,84] Speech-language pathology intervention is frequently focused on specific tasks that show concrete changes.[84] Direct unambiguous cues can sometimes be successful in inhibiting the hyperverbosity.[84] When working on a task that requires listening to directions, following written instructions, writing checks, or filling out forms, the attention and concentration impairments are being addressed in concrete everyday communicative tasks. There is literature on improvement of left neglect[5] in reading and writing, an area of possible collaboration between speech-language pathology and occupational therapy. See Chapter 19.

Vascular Dementia

This underappreciated dementia[32,81] was formerly known as "multi-infarct dementia" or "hardening of the arteries," and it may resemble Alzheimer disease in the severity of the functional cognitive impairments. But vascular dementia differs from Alzheimer in important characteristics.[54] While the disease is progressive, it is stepwise rather than sloping in progression.[46] There are periods of slight but sometimes meaningful improvements in communication.[90] In general, the disease is most often described as "microvascular" or "small vessel disease."[81] The symptoms are heterogeneous and based on the lesion site.[54]

Prognosis is dependent upon effectiveness of medical treatment for hypertension and on anticoagulation.[90] Early on, the progression may be slow and subtle with little specific functional difficulty, so that many of these individuals are never hospitalized or evaluated by rehabilitation professionals.[54] Patients are usually identified after a major stroke or other medical event.[90] Their rehabilitation course must take into account the severity of cognitive impairment.[54] Strategies used with other forms of dementia (e.g., low-tech memory and communication systems such as memory notebooks or wallets) are sometimes helpful in assisting patients become better oriented and foster improved communication.[54] Occupational therapists and speech-language pathologists regularly work together to establish the goals and determine content and use of these augmentative systems. Many of the techniques and suggestions made for people with aphasia or right hemisphere damage are appropriate (i.e., giving time to process information, speaking in direct simple sentences). Prognosis for this common progressive vascular disease is unstable and variable.[54]

SUMMARY

In acknowledging the complexity and centrality of human communication, this chapter has emphasized the importance of the changes in communication that often follow stroke.

The stroke-related communication difficulties encompass a broad range of disorders, each with its own unique characteristics. Having an understanding of the relative strengths and difficulties of the various communicative disorders allows the occupational therapist to detect and understand the communicative issues their stroke patients present. Better understanding of speech, language, and cognitive disorders can only increase communicative competence and minimize the impact of the patient's communication disorder on rehabilitation.

REVIEW QUESTIONS

1. What is the difference between Broca's aphasia and apraxia of speech?
2. Name three strategies that would be helpful when working with a client presenting with Wernicke's aphasia.
3. Name three strategies that would be helpful when working with a client presenting with Broca's aphasia.
4. Name three strategies that would be helpful when working with a client presenting with global aphasia.
5. What is the clinical presentation of conduction aphasia?

REFERENCES

1. Alexander MP, Naeser MA, Palumbo C: Broca's area aphasia. *Neurology* 40:353–362, 1990.
2. Alexander MP, Schmitt MA: The aphasia syndrome of stroke in the left anterior cerebral artery territory. *Arch Neurol* 37(2):97–100, 1980.
3. American Heart Association: *Heart disease and stroke statistics: our guide to current statistics and the supplement to our heart and stroke facts: 2009. update at-a-glance* (website). www.americanheart.org/downloadable/heart/1240250946756LS-1982 Heart and Stroke Update.042009.pdf. Accessed July 19, 2009.
4. American Stroke Association: *Stroke warning signs* (website). www.americanheart.org/presenter.jhtml?identifier=4742. Accessed July 19, 2009.
5. Appelros P, Nydevik I, Karlsson GM, et al: Recovery from unilateral neglect after right-hemisphere stroke. *Disabil Rehabil* 26(8):471–477, 2004.
6. Basso A Capitani E Zanobio ME: Pattern of recovery of oral and written expression and comprehension in aphasic patients. *Behav Brain Res* 6(2):115–128, 1982.
7. Bauby JD: *The diving bell and the butterfly*, New York, 1997, Knopf.
8. Beeson PM and Henry ML: Comprehension and production of written words. In Chapey R, editor: *Language intervention strategies in aphasia and related neurogenic communication disorders*, ed. 5, Philadelphia. 2008, Lippincott Williams & Wilkins.
9. Binder JR, Desai RH, Graves WW, et al: Where is the semantic system? a critical review and meta-analysis of 120 functional neuroimaging studies, Cerebral cortex advance access. *Cereb Cortex* 19(12):2767–2796, 2009.
10. Blum N, Fee E: Voices from the past: Howard A. Rusk (1901–1989) from military medicine to comprehensive rehabilitation. *Am J Public Health* 98(2):256–257, 2008.
11. Boden GJ, Harris KS, Raphael LJ: *Speech science primer: physiology acoustics and perception of speech*, Philadelphia, 2003, Lippincott Williams & Wilkins.

12. Borden GA, Gregg RB, Grove TG: *Speech behavior and human interaction*, Englewood Cliffs, NJ, 1969, Prentice Hall.

13. Brown JW: *Aphasia, apraxia, and agnosia*, Springfield, IL, 1972, Charles C Thomas.

14. Cannito MP, Marquardt TP: Ataxic dysarthria. In McNeil MR, editor: *Clinical management of sensorimotor speech disorders*, New York, 2009, Thieme.

15. Centeno JG: Issues and principles in service delivery to communicatively-impaired minority bilingual adults in neurorehabilitation. *Semin Speech Lang* 30(3):139-153, 2009.

16. Chapey R. Cognitive stimulation: stimulation of recognition/comprehension, memory, and convergent, divergent and evaluative thinking. In Chapey R, editor: *Language intervention strategies in aphasia and related neurogenic communication disorders*, ed. 5, Philadelphia, 2008, Lippincott Williams & Wilkins.

17. Cherry C: *On human communication*, ed. 2, Cambridge, MA, 1968, MIT Press.

18. Coelho CA, Sinotte MP, Duffy JR: Schuell's stimulation approach to rehabilitation. In Chapey R, editor: *Language intervention strategies in aphasia and related neurogenic communication disorders*, ed. 5, Philadelphia, 2008, Lippincott Williams & Wilkins.

19. Collins: Global aphasia. In LaPointe LL, editor: *Aphasia and related neurogenic language disorders*, ed. 2, New York, 546 1997, Thieme.

20. Commission on Accreditation of Rehabilitation Facilities: *Medical Rehabilitation Accreditation Manual*, Tucson AZ, 2005, CARF.

21. Connor LT, Obler LK, Tocco M, et al: Effect of socioeconomic status on aphasia severity and recovery. *Brain Lang* 7(2):254–257, 2001.

22. Critchley M: *Aphasiology*, London, 535 1970, Edward Arnold.

23. Croot K: Diagnosis of AOS: Definition and criteria. *Semin Speech Lang* 23(4):267–279, 2002.

24. Damasio AR: Aphasia with nonhemorrhagic lesions in the basal ganglia and internal capsule. *Arch Neurol* 39(1):15, 1982.

25. Damasio H: Neuroanatomical correlates of the aphasias. In Sarno MT, editor: *Acquired aphasia*, San Diego, 1991, Academic Press.

26. Damasio H: Neural basis of language disorders. In Chapey R, editor: *Language intervention strategies in aphasia and related neurogenic communication disorders*, ed. 5, Philadelphia, 2008, Lippincott Williams & Wilkins.

27. Darley FL: *Aphasia*, Philadelphia, 1982, Saunders.

28. Darley FL, Aronson AE, Brown JR: *Motor speech disorders*, Philadelphia, 1975, Saunders.

29. Davis GA: *A survey of adult aphasia and related language disorders*, Englewood Cliffs, NJ, 1993, Prentice Hall.

30. Davis GA: Investigating symptoms and syndromes. In Davis GA, editor: *Aphasiology: disorders and clinical practice*, Boston, 2000, Allyn & Bacon.

31. Denes PB, Pinson EN: *The speech chain*, Berkeley Heights, NJ, 1963, Bell Telephone Laboratories.

32. Dubois MF, Hebert R: The incidence of vascular dementia in Canada: A comparison with Europe and East Asia. *Neuroepidemiology* 20(3):179–187, 2001.

33. Duffy JR: *Motor speech disorders: Substrates differential diagnosis and management*, ed 2, St Louis, 2005, Mosby.

34. Duffy JR, Folger NW: Dysarthria associated with unilateral central nervous system lesions: a retrospective study. *J Med Speech Lang Pathol* 4(2):57, 1996.

35. Eisenson J: *Adult aphasia*, Englewood Cliffs, NJ, 1984, Prentice Hall.

36. Enderby P, Emerson J: *Does speech and language therapy work? A review of the literature*, London, 1995, Whurr.

37. Flowers CR, Beukelman DR, Bottorf LE, et al: Family members' predictions of aphasic test performance. *Aphasia, apraxia, agnosia* 1:18–26, 1979.

38. Freed D: *Motor speech disorders: diagnosis and treatment*, San Diego, CA, 2000, Singular.

39. Gelfman R, Peters D, Opitz J, et al: The history of physical medicine and rehabilitation as recorded in the diary of Dr. Frank Krusen: Part 3. Consolidating the position (1948–1953). *Arch Phys Med Rehabil* 78(5):556–561, 1997.

40. George KP, Viklingstad E, Silbergleit R, et al: Brain imaging in acquired language disorders. In Johnson AF, Jacobson BH, editors: *Medical speech-language pathology: a practitioner's guide*, ed 2, New York, 2007, Thieme.

41. Goldstein K: *Language and language disturbances*, New York, 1948, Grune and Stratton.

42. Golper LA: Teams and partnerships in aphasia intervention. In Chapey R, editor: *Language intervention strategies in aphasia and related neurogenic communication disorders*, ed. 5, Philadelphia, 2008, Lippincott Williams & Wilkins.

43. Goodglass H, Kaplan E, Barresi B: *The assessment of aphasia and related disorders*, ed 3, Philadelphia, 2001, Lea & Febiger.

44. Gordon C, Ellis-Hill C, Ashburn A: The use of conversational analysis: nurse-patient interaction in communication ability. *J Adv Nurs* 65(3):544–553, 2009.

45. Graham-Keegan L, Caspari I: Wernicke's aphasia. In LaPointe LL, editor: *Aphasia and related neurogenic language disorders*, ed 2, New York, 1997, Thieme.

46. Hachinski VD, Iliff LD, Zilhka E, et al: Cerebral blood flow in dementia. *Arch Neurol* 32(9):632–637, 1975.

47. Hallowell B, Chapey R: Delivering language intervention services to adults with neurogenic communication disorders. In Chapey R, editor: *Language intervention strategies in aphasia and related neurogenic communication disorders*, ed. 5, Philadelphia, 2008, Lippincott Williams & Wilkins.

48. Hallowell B, Chapey R: Introduction to language intervention strategies in adult aphasia. In Chapey R, editor: *Language intervention strategies in aphasia and related neurogenic communication disorders*, ed. 5, Philadelphia, 2008, Lippincott Williams & Wilkins.

49. Hartman DE, Abbs JH: Dysarthria associated with focal unilateral upper motor neuron lesion. *Eur J Disord Commun* 27(3):187–196, 1992.

50. Hasan R: The uses of talk. In Sarangi S, Courlthard M, editors: *Discourse and social life*, Essex, UK, 2000, Pearson Education.

51. Hedge MN: *A course book on aphasia and other neurogenic language disorders*, ed 3, Clifton Park, NY, 2006, Thomson Delmar Learning.

52. Herrmann M, Britz A, Bartels C, et al: The impact of aphasia on the patient and family in the first year post-stroke. *Top Stroke Rehabil* 2(1): 5–19, 1995.

53. Holland A: *Counseling for communication disorders: A wellness perspective*, San Diego, 2007, Plural.

54. Hopper T, Bayles KA: Management of neurogenic communication disorders associated with dementia. In Chapey R, editor: *Language intervention strategies in aphasia and related neurogenic communication disorders*, ed. 5, Philadelphia, 2008, Lippincott Williams & Wilkins.

55. Horenstein S: Effects of cerebrovascular disease on personality and emotionality. In Benton AL, editor: *Behavioral change in cerebrovascular disease*, New York, 1970, Harper.

56. Johnson AF, Jacobson BH: The scope of medical speech-language pathology. In Johnson AF, Jacobson BH, editors: *Medical speech-language pathology: a practitioner's guide*, ed. 2, New York, 2006, Thieme.

57. Johnson AF, Valachovic AM, George KP: Speech-language pathology practice in the acute care setting: a consultative approach. In Johnson AF, Jacobson BH, editors: *Medical speech-language pathology: a practitioner's guide*, ed. 2, New York, 2006, Thieme.

58. Kagan A: Supported conversation for adults with aphasia, methods and resources for training conversations partners. *Aphasiology* 12(9): 816–830, 1998.

59. Kaplan E: Aphasia-related disorders. In Sarno MT, editor: *Acquired aphasia*, ed. 2, San Diego, 1991, Academic Press.

60. Katz RC: Computer applications in aphasia treatment. In Chapey R, editor: *Language intervention strategies in aphasia and related neurogenic communication disorders*, ed. 5, Philadelphia, 2008, Lippincott Williams & Wilkins.

61. Kearns LL: Broca's aphasia. In LaPointe LL, editor: *Aphasia and related neurogenic language disorders*, ed 2, Stuttgart, 1997, Thieme.

62. Kertez A, Harlock W, Coates R: Computer tomographic localization lesion size and prognosis in aphasia and nonverbal impairment. *Brain Lang* 8(1):34–50, 1979.

63. Lafond YJ, Lecours AR: The person and aphasia. In Lafond D, DeGiovani R, Joanette Y, et al, editors: *Living with aphasia: psychological issues*, San Diego, 1993, Singular.

64. LaPointe LL: *Adaptation, accommodation, aristos. Aphasia and related neurogenic language disorders*, New York, 1997, Thieme.

65. Laureys S, Pellas F, Van Eckhout P, et al: The locked-in syndrome: what is it like to be conscious but paralyzed and voiceless? *Prog Brain Res* 150:495–511, 2005.

66. Lebrun Y: Awareness of the problem. In Lafond D, DeGiovani R, Joanette Y, et al, editors: *Living with aphasia: psychological issues*, San Diego, 1993, Singular.

67. Lemay MA: The person with aphasia and society. In Lafond D, DeGiovani R, Joanette Y, et al, editors: *Living with aphasia: psychological issues*, San Diego, 1993, Singular.

68. Letourneau PY: The psychological effects of aphasia. In Lafond D, DeGiovani R, Joanette Y, et al, editors: *Living with aphasia: psychological issues*, San Diego, 1993, Singular.

69. Luria AR, Tsvetkova LS: The mechanism of 'dynamic aphasia.' *Foundations of Language* 4, 1968.

70. Lyon JG: Resuming daily life with expressive forms of severe aphasia: observations of adults who have successfully made life transitions and clinical implications. *Perspect Neurophysiol and Neurogenic Speech Lang Disord* 19:23-29, 2009.

71. Lyon JG, Helms-Estabrooks N: Drawing: its communicative significance for expressively restricted aphasic adults. *Top Lang Disord* 8:61–71, 1987.

72. Mackenzie C, Lowit A: Behavioral intervention effects in dysarthria following stroke: communication effectiveness intelligibility and dysarthria impact. *Int J Lang Commun Disord* 42(2):131–153, 2007.

73. Manly T: Cognitive rehabilitation for unilateral neglect: review. *Neuropsychol Rehabil* 12(4):289–310, 2002.

74. Marshall RC: Early management of Wernicke's aphasia: a context-based approach. In Chapey R, editor: *Language intervention strategies in aphasia and related neurogenic communication disorders*, ed. 5, Philadelphia, 2008, Lippincott Williams & Wilkins.

75. Mason C, Gilpin P, McGowan S, et al: The effect of intrathecal baclofen on functional intelligibility of speech. *Int J Lang Commun Disord* 33(Suppl):24–5, 1998.

76. Mavis I: Perspectives on public awareness of stroke and aphasia among Turkish patients in a neurology unit. *Clin Linguist Phon* 21(1):55–70, 2007.

77. McClenahan R, Johnson M, Densham Y: Misperceptions of communication difficulties of stroke patients in doctors nurses and relatives. *J Neurol Neurosurg Psychol* 53(8):700–701, 1990.

78. McNeil MR, Prescott TE: *Revised token test*, Baltimore, 1978, University Park Press.

79. Mlcoch AG, Metter EG: Medical aspects of stroke rehabilitation. In Chapey R, editor: *Language intervention strategies in aphasia and related neurogenic communication disorders*, ed. 5, Philadelphia, 2008, Lippincott Williams & Wilkins.

80. Mohr JP, Pessin MS, Finkelstein S, et al: Broca's aphasia: Pathologic and clinical aspects. *Neurology* 28(4):311–324, 1978.

81. Mungas D: Contributions of subcortical lacunar infarcts to cognitive impairment in older persons. In Paul RH, Ott BR, Cohen R, editors: *Vascular dementia: Cerebrovascular mechanisms and clinical management*, Totowa NJ, 2005, Humana Press.

82. Murdock BE, Ward EC, Theodoros DG: Spastic dysarthria. In McNeil MR, editor: *Clinical management of sensorimotor speech disorders*, New York, 2008, Thieme.

83. Myers PS: Right hemisphere syndrome. In LaPointe LL editor: *Aphasia and related neurogenic language disorders*, ed. 2, New York, 1997, Thieme.

84. Myers PS, Blake ML: Communication disorders associated with right hemisphere damage. In Chapey R, editor: *Language intervention strategies in aphasia and related neurogenic communication disorders*, ed. 5, Philadelphia, 2008, Lippincott Williams & Wilkins.

85. Nagaratnam N, Nagaratnam K, Ng K, et al: Akinetic mutism following stroke. *J Clin Neurosci* 11(1):25–30, 2004.

86. National Aphasia Association, Aphasia Frequently Asked Questions (website). www.aphasia.org/Aphasia%20Facts/aphasia_faq.html. Accessed July 19, 2009.

87. Rehak A, Kaplan JA, Gardner H: Sensitivity to conversational deviance in right-hemisphere damaged patients. *Brain Lang* 42(2):203–217, 1992.

88. Rehak A, Kaplan JA, Weylman ST, et al: Story processing in right-hemisphere damaged patients. *Brain Lang* 42(3):320–336, 1992.

89. Roland PE, Larsen B, Lassen NA, et al: Supplementary motor area and other cortical areas for organization of voluntary movements in man. *J Neurophysiol* 43(1):118–136, 1980.

90. Roman GC: Clinical forms of vascular dementia. In Paul RH, Ott BR, Cohen R, editors: *Vascular dementia: Cerebrovascular mechanisms and clinical management*, Totowa, NJ, 2005, Humana Press.

91. Rosenbeck JC, Jones HN: Principles of treatment for sensorimotor speech disorders. In McNeil MR, editor: *Clinical management of sensorimotor speech disorders*, New York, 2009, Thieme.

92. Rothi LJG: Transcortical motor sensory and mixed aphasias. In LaPointe LL, editor: *Aphasia and related neurogenic language disorders* ed. 2, New York, 1997 Thieme.

93. Sands ES, Freeman FJ, Harris KS: Progressive changes in articulatory patterns in verbal apraxia: a longitudinal case study. *Brain Lang* 6(1):97–105, 1978.

94. Sarno JE: The psychological and social sequelae of aphasia. In Sarno MT, editor: *Acquired aphasia*, San Diego, 1991, Academic Press.

95. Sarno MT: Recovery and rehabilitation in aphasia. In Sarno MT, editor: *Acquired aphasia*, San Diego, 1991, Academic Press.

96. Sarno MT: Ethical-moral dilemmas in aphasia rehabilitation. In Lafond D, DeGiovani R, Joanette Y, et al, editors: *Living with aphasia: psychological issues*, San Diego, 1993, Singular.

97. Sarno JE, Rusk HA, Diller L, Sarno MT: The effect of hyperbaric oxygen on the mental and verbal ability of stroke patients. *Stroke* 3(1):10–15, 1972.

98. Schnakers C, Majerus S, Goldman S: Cognitive function in the locked-in syndrome. *J Neurol* 255(3):323–30, 2008.

99. Schuell H: Auditory impairment in aphasia: Significance and retraining techniques. *J Speech Hear Disord* 18(1):14–21, 1953.

100. Schuell H: *Aphasia theory and therapy*, Baltimore, MD, 1974, University Park Press.

101. Schuell H, Carroll V, Street R: Clinical treatment of aphasia. *J Speech Hear Disord* 21:43–53, 1955.

102. Simmons-Mackie N: Conduction aphasia. In LaPointe LL, editor: *Aphasia and related neurogenic language disorders*, ed. 2, New York, 1997, Thieme.

103. Simmons-Mackie N: Social approaches to aphasia intervention. In Chapey R, editor: *Language intervention strategies in aphasia and related neurogenic communication disorders*, ed. 5, Philadelphia, 2008, Lippincott Williams & Wilkins.

104. Tanner DC: *The family guide to surviving stroke and communication disorders*, Boston, 1999, Allyn & Bacon.

105. Deleted

106. Tonkonogoy J, Goodglass H: Language function foot of the third frontal gyrus and rolandic operculum. *Ann Neurol* 38(8):486–490, 1981.

107. Wallace GJ, Canter G: Effects of personality relevant language materials on the performance of severely aphasic individuals. *J Speech Hear Disord* 50(4):385–390, 1985.

108. Wertz RT: Response to treatment in patients with apraxia of speech. In Rosenbek R, McNeil, M, Aronson A, editors: *Apraxia of speech: phonology acoustics linguistic management*, San Diego, 1984, College-Hill Press.

109. Whitworth A, Sjardin H: The bilingual person with aphasia—the Australian context. In Lafond D, DeGiovani R, Joanette Y, et al, editors: *Living with aphasia: psychological issues*, San Diego, 1993, Singular.

110. Wolpaw JR, McFarland DJ, Vaughan TM: Brain-computer interface research at the Wadsworth Center, Rehabilitation Engineering. *IEEE Transactions* 8(2):222–226, 2000.

111. Working Group on Cognitive-Communication Disorders of ASHA's Special Interest Division I Language Learning and Education and Division 2 Neurophysiology and Neurogenic Speech and Language Disorders: *ASHA roles of speech-language pathologists in the identification diagnosis and treatment of individuals with cognitive-communication disorders: position statement* (website). www.asha.org/docs/html/PS2005–00110.html. Accessed August 5, 2009.

112. World Health Organization: *International classification of functioning disability and health ICF*, Geneva, Switzerland, 2006, WHO.

113. Yorkston KM, Bukelman DR: an analysis of connected speech samples of aphasic and normal speakers. *J Speech Hear Disord* 45(1): 27–36, 1980.

114. Yorkston KM, Strand EA, Kennedy RT: Comprehensibility of dysarthric speech: implications for assessment and treatment planning. *Am J Speech Lang Pathol* 5:55, 1996.

birgitta bernspång
josefine lampinen

chapter 21

Enhancing Performance
of Activities of Daily Living

key terms

occupational therapy intervention
process model

assessment of motor and process
skills

chapter objectives

After completing this chapter, the reader will be able to accomplish the following:

1. Understand the occupational therapy process using a client-centered top-down approach.
2. Recognize the effect of a stroke on a person's engagement in activities of daily living.
3. Discuss the occupational therapy reasoning process for enhancing engagement in activities of daily living.
4. Understand the basics for documentation and goal writing during the whole intervention process.
5. Understand the different models of interventions used for instrumental activities of daily living.

In this chapter, two cases will be presented where the occupational therapist has used an intervention process to enhance the performance of activities of daily living (ADL) after stroke. The process model used is occupation-based, top-down, and client-centered. The Occupational Therapy Intervention Process Model (OTIPM)[3] has been used at the hospital where the two cases are being treated for over ten years and is the base for a general program used for all patients at the occupational therapy (OT) department. The complete process model is shown in Fig. 21-1, and all steps will be described in the two cases, Astrid and August. This chapter focuses on leading the reader through the

client-centered intervention process and on showing how the Assessment of Motor and Process Skills (AMPS) can be used as a guide in planning OT interventions.

Within stroke rehabilitation, there is a growing body of knowledge that patients will benefit from a team approach to rehabilitation, from the acute to the later stages of the rehabilitation.[9] At the rehabilitation department where the cases in this chapter participated, the team works with an interdisciplinary view where the client is included in the team as a member. Together with the client, all team members participate and formulate the goals at the initial planning meeting. The occupational therapist's contribution to this team approach has a clear

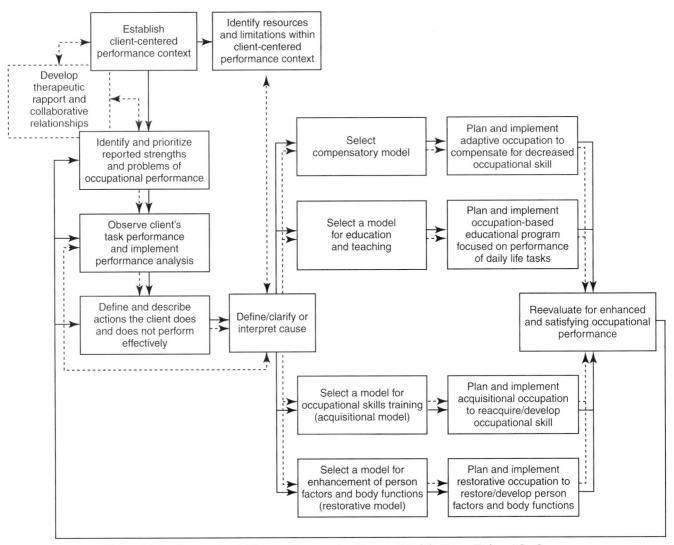

Figure 21-1   Occupational Therapy Intervention Process Model. (From Fisher AG: *Occupational therapy intervention process model,* Fort Collins, Colo, 2009, Three Star Press.)

focus on the client's ability to perform those daily tasks that he or she wants the ability to do and that hold meaning given the circumstances in which the client lives.[15] It is, therefore, important that the occupational therapist start the intervention process by finding out the areas of interest and meaning for each individual client. To do so means that the occupational therapist uses so called *top-down* reasoning, which immediately gives the occupational therapist knowledge about the areas in the client's everyday life that he or she views as most important, given the current situation. Top-down reasoning is separated from *bottom-up* reasoning, where the occupational therapist initially focuses on evaluating the client's body functions and/or environmental factors. The identified decreased functions are then viewed as the cause of the client's problems in the everyday doings.

In Sweden, where these cases take place, it is common practice to develop an OT program that describes the

services that OT may provide to a specific client group in a particular setting. In Västerbotten County, a group of occupational therapists developed a general program from which more specific programs can be developed. These programs are based on Fisher's OTIPM;[3] the general OT program developed in Sweden is also included in Fisher's text.[3] The OTIPM describes the process from the first meeting with the client and the different OT interventions and through the whole rehabilitation process until the final meeting with the client. The description of the two cases will use this model to clarify the process and to suggest interventions for the specific cases. The OTIPM will be used to demonstrate how OT services can be provided in a manner that is top-down, client-centered, and occupation-based.

The cases will be described according to the OTIPM model and, according to the OT program used at this particular rehabilitation unit (see Fig. 21-1).

As the intervention process progresses, evaluations will be used to help each step of the process. One of the main sources of information gathering on the actual ability to perform daily tasks is the AMPS.[2] Other standardized assessments can also be used to document the status of performance of ADL after stroke and are summarized in Table 21-1.

The AMPS is a standardized evaluation of personal and instrumental ADL, which can be performed with persons with any diagnosis and at any age from 2-years-old to over 100-years-old, as long as the person is interested in and has experience doing daily tasks. To become a trained and calibrated AMPS rater, the occupational therapist must attend a five-day training course and test 10 people after the course. When the potential rater demonstrates the ability to score AMPS in a valid and reliable manner, he or she becomes a calibrated AMPS rater and has full access to reports generated by the AMPS computer scoring program. The use of these reports in practice will be demonstrated in this chapter.

The AMPS is an observational method of evaluating a person's skills in daily tasks. In all, 36 skills are evaluated: 16 ADL motor skills and 20 ADL process skills (Box 21-1). There are 86 different standardized tasks that are standardized in the AMPS. Both personal and instrumental ADL tasks are included. The tasks represent several different cultures and levels of difficulties. Each person is observed doing two or more tasks and is scored on each of the 36 items for each task. Examples of standardized tasks are listed in Box 21-2. To implement an AMPS observation, the process includes finding out relevant and challenging tasks for the client to perform in order to get the most complete and comprehensive evaluation of the client's performance. Several steps are required in order to conduct an AMPS evaluation according to the standardized procedures.[2] After the observation, the scores are then entered into the AMPS software, and several reports can be generated that will assist the occupational therapist in the intervention planning process.

When the AMPS is used in its full potential as a standardized tool, it will generate two ability measures that will inform the therapist and the client about ADL ability in relation to effort, efficiency, safety, and independence. Occasionally, the occupational therapist calibrated as an AMPS user meets a client where none of the 85 tasks are relevant to the client. In those occasions, the occupational therapist can perform a nonstandardized AMPS evaluation by observing the client doing a task of relevance that is an appropriate challenge and chosen by the client. During this instance, the therapist cannot use the AMPS software, but can get detailed information on which of the skill items the client has problems performing and can use that information in the documentation and the continuing process of planning and implementing interventions.

There is also another ADL assessment available to use as a structure during a first meeting with a client."[14,16] This *ADL-taxonomy* is conceptualized as a divided large circle where each area of daily tasks has its own slice (Fig. 21-2, *A* and *B*). All slices are then divided into the actions included in each task domain according to a hierarchy of difficulty. The areas include eating and drinking, mobility, going to the toilet, dressing, personal hygiene, grooming, communication, transportation, cooking, shopping, cleaning, and washing. Located at the top of the circle is a blank slice where the occupational therapist can add areas of importance to the client that are not included in the listed areas (i.e., leisure tasks).

In rehabilitation departments in Sweden and elsewhere, it is common to work with interdisciplinary teams.[5] This means that several professions are involved in the whole rehabilitation process, and members contribute their specific expertise to the team through their profession specific assessments, which allows them to get the full picture of the patient needs. The team members collaborate closely and assist each other in solving problems that arise during the rehabilitation process. The patient is a member of the team. The patient's rehabilitation goals are the basis for the goals of the team, and they guide the decision about which team members to involve in the rehabilitation process, a decision that can also change over time as the goals change.[5,11] The following two cases show when and how this interdisciplinary teamwork is implemented in the rehabilitation process.

GERIATRIC DAY REHABILITATION: CLIENT LIVING IN COMFORT (ASSISTED) LIVING

Astrid is a 72-year-old woman who had a stroke eight months ago. The computerized tomography (CT) scan showed a cerebral hemorrhage in the basal ganglia through to the ventricles on the left side of the brain. She had a right-sided hemiparesis, aphasia, and she was substantially depressed. Initially, she had low arousal due to the cerebral edema and received rehabilitation for two weeks on the stroke unit in the hospital.

During this period:

- She required substantial assistance to transfer into her recliner wheelchair. The staff used a sling attached to the ceiling to move her from bed to chair.
- She required a two person assist for her hygiene and dressing, which was done bedside, although she did try to participate when she was able.
- She had aphasia, but she could answer yes and no to questions, and she did understand simple encouragements.
- She fatigued easily.

Two weeks after her stroke, she was moved to the geriatric rehabilitation unit and met an occupational therapist the first day. Since Astrid had difficulty speaking and was easily

Table 21-1

Standardized Assessments

RIVERMEAD ADL ASSESSMENT	ADELAIDE ACTIVITIES PROFILE	FRENCHAY ACTIVITIES INDEX	NOTTINGHAM EXTENDED ADL SCALE	INSTRUMENTAL ACTIVITY MEASURE	LAWTON INSTRUMENTAL ADL SCALE
Authors					
Whiting and Lincoln, 1980[17]	Bond and Clark, 1998[1]	Holbrook and Skilbeck, 1983[6]	Nouri and Lincoln, 1987[12]	Grimby and colleagues, 1996[4]	Lawton and Brody, 1969[8]
Meal preparation					
Prepare a meal	Prepare main meal	Prepare main meals	Make a hot drink	Cook a main meal	Prepare a meal
Prepare a hot drink	Wash dishes	Wash dishes	Make a hot snack	Prepare simple meal	
Prepare a snack			Wash dishes		
			Take hot drinks between rooms		
Domestic activities					
Heavy cleaning	Heavy housework	Heavy housework	Housework	Cleaning house	Laundry
Light cleaning	Light housework	Light housework	Wash small clothing items	Washing clothes	Housekeeping
Handwash clothes	Wash clothes	Wash clothes	Full clothes wash		Manage medications
Iron clothes	Household or car maintenance	Household or car maintenance			Manage finances
Hang out washing					
Bed making					
Gardening					
	Light gardening	Gardening	Manage own garden		
	Heavy gardening				
Productive activities					
	Voluntary or paid employment	Gainful work			
	Care for other family members				

Shopping/community activities						
Carry shopping Cope with money	Household shopping Personal shopping	Local shopping	Shopping Manage own money	Large scale shopping Small scale shopping	Shopping	
Transportation						
Use public transportation: bus Transport self to shop	Drive a car or organize transport	Drive car or go on bus Travel outings or car rides	Use public transportation Drive a car	Use public transportation	Use public transportation Car/taxi	
Leisure/social activities						
Community social activities Outdoor social activities Invite people to home Hobby Telephone calls to family/friends Attend religious events Outdoor recreation or sporting activity	Social occasions Hobby Reading books		Go out socially Use the telephone Read newspapers or books Write letters		Use telephone	
Mobility: outdoors						
Outdoor mobility Crossing roads Get in and out of car	Walk outdoors	Walk outside	Walk outside Cross roads In/out of car Walk on uneven ground	Locomotion outdoors		

Continued

Table 21-1

Standardized Assessments—cont'd

RIVERMEAD ADL ASSESSMENT	ADELAIDE ACTIVITIES PROFILE	FRENCHAY ACTIVITIES INDEX	NOTTINGHAM EXTENDED ADL SCALE	INSTRUMENTAL ACTIVITY MEASURE	LAWTON INSTRUMENTAL ADL SCALE
Mobility: indoors					
Indoor mobility			Climb stairs		
Mobility to lavatory					
Move bed to chair					
Move floor to chair					
Basic self-care					
Drinking			Feed yourself		
Clean teeth					
Comb hair					
Wash face and hands					
Apply makeup or shave					
Eating					
Undress					
Dressing					
Wash in bath					
In and out of bath					
Overall wash					

Modified from Park S: Enhancing engagement in instrumental activities of daily living: an occupational therapy perspective. In Gillen G, Burkhardt A, editors: *Stroke rehabilitation: a function based approach*, ed 2, St. Louis, 2004, Elsevier.

Box 21-1

The Items Observed and Evaluated in the Assessment of Motor and Process Skills (AMPS)

List of the motor and process skills observed during task performance:

MOTOR SKILLS	PROCESS SKILLS
Body position	**Sustaining performance**
Stabilizes	Paces*
Aligns	Attends
Positions	Heeds
Obtaining and holding objects	**Applying knowledge**
Reaches	Chooses
Bends	Uses
Grips	Handles
Manipulates	Inquires
Coordinates	
	Temporal organization
Moving self and objects	Initiates
	Continues
Moves	Sequences
Lifts	Terminates
Walks	
Transports	**Organizing space and objects**
Calibrates	
Flows	Searches/locates
	Gathers
Sustaining performance	Organizes
	Restores
Endures	Navigates
Paces*	
	Adapting performance
	Notices/responds
	Adjusts
	Accommodates
	Benefits

*Paces is considered both a motor and a process skill
From Fisher AG: *Assessment of motor and process skills*, ed 6, Fort Collins, Colo, 2006, Three Star Press.

Box 21-2

Examples of Standardized AMPS Tasks

PADL	IADL
Putting on shoes and socks	Making breakfast
Brushing teeth	Repotting a small houseplant
Upper body grooming/bathing	Fresh fruit salad
	Sweeping the floor
	Raking grass cuttings or leaves
	Shopping

fatigued, the main information was gathered via medical records and through telephone contact with one of Astrid's daughters.

The rehabilitation goals at this subacute stage included:

1. To be able to propel independently in the wheelchair on a flat surface
2. To transfer from wheelchair to bed or toilet with verbal instructions and support handles
3. To know the day of the week, time of day, and the date
4. To adjust the temperature of the water from the faucet
5. To manage upper body grooming and dressing independently
6. To make own breakfast (i.e., make cooked oatmeal independently)

At the time for discharge from the geriatric rehabilitation unit three months later, the first four goals were met. Tasks included in goal numbers five and six still required physical assistance. A referral was sent to the geriatric day rehabilitation unit for continuing rehabilitation. Astrid moved to a "comfort living" complex for elderly and had access to home care 24 hours a day. Comfort living is the client's own apartment in a complex for older persons with access to jointly owned areas and dining room.

Establish Client-Centered Performance Context

About two months later and now five months after the stroke, Astrid was admitted to the geriatric day rehabilitation unit. She arrived with her ex-husband Emil at the first visit with the occupational therapist. The occupational therapist, Maria, carried out an initial interview to establish the client-centered performance context, and she asked Astrid to describe for her how a usual day was laid out. For guidance in the first step, Maria used the OTIPM and ADL-taxonomy, which helped her visualize

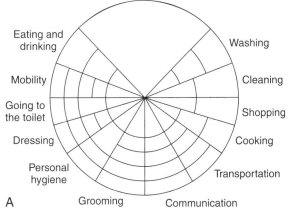

Figure 21-2 A, The ADL Taxonomy.

Continued

ACTIVITIES	ACTIONS
Eating and drinking Defined as getting food from the table, to eat and drink. The activity comprises the following actions:	1. Eating, that is, getting food from a plate or equivalent into one's mouth and eating 2. Drinking, that is, getting the liquid from a glass or cup or equivalent into one's mouth and drinking 3. Getting food and liquid and cutting up/preparing food
Mobility Defined as goal directed mobility of the body from one place to another. The activity comprises the following actions:	1. Transfer in bed, that is, changing positions, turning over and sitting up 2. Transferring the body from bed to chair or between two chairs 3. Walking or moving from one room to another (the same floor) 4. Walking or moving from one floor to another 5. Walking or moving in and out of the house 6. Walking or moving in the neighborhood
Going to the toilet Defined as getting to the toilet room in time and performing the necessary elimination. The activity comprises the following actions:	1. Bowel and urine elimination, volitional 2. Getting on and off the toilet and cleaning oneself after elimination 3. Arranging clothes and equipment such as pads and sanitary towels, washing hands 4. Getting to and from the toilet room in time
Dressing Defined as getting the necessary clothes and shoes, dressing and undressing. The activity comprises the following actions:	1. Undressing 2. Dressing upper trunk 3. Dressing lower trunk 4. Pulling on stockings/pantyhose/shoes 5. Getting necessary clothes from closets and drawers
Personal hygiene Defined as getting to and from the hygiene room, washing hair and body, and getting dry. The activity comprises the following actions:	1. Washing hands and face 2. Washing body/bathing/showering 3. Washing one's hair 4. Getting to and from the hygiene room
Grooming Defined as other hygiene activities concerning one specific part of the body. The activity comprises the following actions:	1. Combing one's hair 2. Brushing teeth 3. Shaving/make-up 4. Manicuring 5. Pedicuring
Communication Defined as transferring information between a transmitter and a receiver and managing actual equipment. The activity comprises the following actions:	1. Calling for attention/communicate 2. Taking part in a conversation 3. Using the telephone 4. Reading 5. Writing by hand and/or using a word-processor
Transportation Defined as getting to, in and out of public or private transportation. The activity comprises the following actions:	1. Going by car 2. Going by bus, tram, tube 3. Going by train, boat, airplane 4. Riding bicycle/moped 5. Driving car/motorcycle
Cooking Defined as planning, and taking out equipment, preparation, cooking, laying the table, and washing the dishes. The activity comprises the following actions:	1. Preparing a cool meal 2. Heating up liquid or prepared food 3. Cooking a hot meal
Shopping Defined as making plans for shopping, getting to the store, taking out groceries, paying for them, and bringing them home. The activity comprises the following actions:	1. Making plans for shopping (shopping list/order) 2. Daily or small quantity shopping in neighborhood shop 3. Weekly or large quantity shopping
Cleaning Defined as light cleaning: making the bed, "clearing away/tidying up," wiping off, dusting. Heavy cleaning; vacuum cleaning/washing floors, washing toilet and bathroom. The activity comprises the following actions:	1. Daily light cleaning 2. Weekly heavy cleaning
Washing Defined as transportation of laundry to and from the washing place, sorting, washing/ironing/mangling the laundry. The activity comprises the following actions:	1. Light washing by hand 2. Light washing in washing machine 3. Heavy washing in washing machine (e.g., sheets)

B

Figure 21-2, cont'd
For legend see opposite page

Figure 21-2, cont'd B, Operational Definitions of Activities and Actions included in the ADL Taxonomy. (A is from Törnqvist K, Sonn U: Towards an ADL taxonomy for occupational therapists, *Scand J Occup Ther* 1[2], 69-76, 1994. B is from Sonn U, Törnqvist K, Svensson E: The ADL taxonomy - from individual categorical data to ordinal categorical data. *Scand J Occup Ther* 6[1]:11-20, 1999.)

the daily tasks for the client. Maria summarized Astrid's occupational performance context according to the ten dimensions in the process model, OTIPM.

Environmental Dimension

Astrid had recently moved to a comfort living complex for elderly persons (55+). Her apartment has two rooms and a kitchen, and it is adapted for functional limitations. The bedroom has a bed with rails, a book shelf, and a bedside table close by with a telephone, a digital day and night calendar. The living room has a sofa, armchairs, a TV, and a dining room table with two chairs close to the kitchen area. In the kitchen, there is a refrigerator and microwave oven located high up. Astrid can reach the lowest shelf in the refrigerator from her wheelchair. The apartment has a large bathroom with a shower, including a shower stool and toilet with a raised seat and armrests. The bathroom also has a washing machine and tumbler. In her current living arrangement, Astrid has access to home care staff 24 hours and can also use the jointly owned areas of the living complex, i.e., dining room, library, TV room, and spa unit. Astrid does not use these areas because of her current problems with mobility, and she cannot propel the distance required for this.

Social Dimension

Astrid has a lot of support from her ex-husband Emil, who is now responsible for her finances. She has some close friends as well. Prior to her stroke, she lived alone in her own apartment and managed all her daily tasks on her own. Astrid is divorced and has two grown daughters, one in the south of the country and one abroad. Earlier she often traveled to her daughters and their families and spent a lot of time with her grandchildren. Now they will have to travel to her instead.

Role Dimension

Astrid is a mother and caretaker. Previously Astrid spent a lot of time in the forest, picking wild berries and mushrooms, and enjoying walks. She also has a great interest in gardening. Being together with friends and participating in the city's culture such as theatre, concerts, and movies have also been important interests of hers.

Cultural Dimension

Astrid is a typical Swedish woman, and her cultural beliefs, values, customs and where and how she performs her daily life tasks are similar to other persons in Sweden of the same age.

Motivational Dimension

Astrid enjoyed keeping her home nice and tidy. She has also read several journals about gardening and home decorating and fictional books. She is motivated to invite her friends to her apartment and wants to be able to do that independently. When she currently has visitors, the guests have to make their own coffee. She also wishes to be able to eat a meal using the usual utensils, since it bothers her that others see her using only her fork while eating (in Sweden it is customary to use both knife and fork during a meal, with knife in right hand and fork in left hand during the whole eating process). Because of this, she does not want to eat in the dining room but instead chooses to have the staff prepare her food for her in her apartment. Due to the same reason, she would like to be able to walk without assistive devices.

Astrid would like to be able to manage her daily tasks herself again, such as inviting her friends for coffee, make her own breakfast, make her own sandwich, and manage going to the toilet by herself and safely.

Institutional Dimension

Astrid has several resources available to her of which she now needs to make use:

- The home help staff to help with her personal hygiene, dressing, and toileting. The staff also helps her to prepare her meals, and they supervise transfers among wheelchair, bed, and toilet. She also receives help with cleaning and shopping.
- Her ex-husband and daughters are responsible for her finances, and her ex-husband supports her in other situations.
- Currently she also has support from the team at geriatric day rehabilitation.

Body Function Dimension

Astrid presents with right-sided hemiparesis and aphasia. She initially presented with low arousal secondary to cerebral edema. Right after the stroke, she sat in a recliner wheelchair and was lifted with a mechanical lift. She also presented with fatigue and depression (which was treated medically). Currently, Astrid's memory problems and decreased ability to use her right arm and hand are her biggest problems. She has pain in her right shoulder, causing her to have problems moving her arm effectively, although she has good ability to grip with her right hand. Some of her problems can also be related to her apraxia. Astrid wants to be able to walk independently and safely with her rolling walker. Astrid usually sits in her wheelchair and has problems propelling herself, as the chair is too high for her to strike her heel.

Task Dimension

Astrid expressed that her greatest problem today is to move herself. She would like to be able to safely walk with her rolling walker. She also thinks it is important to manage by herself as much as possible during her daily tasks. She would like to manage to perform simple everyday tasks on her own, and her highest priority is to again be able to make coffee with cookies for her friends, make her breakfast (oatmeal), make an open-faced sandwich, and eat with knife and fork. She also wishes to be able to write with her right hand again.

Temporal Dimension

One ordinary day in Astrid's life starts when the staff at her living complex comes in and wakes her up at 7:30 AM. They help her to her wheelchair, into the bathroom, and onto the toilet. Astrid can do these actions herself with supervision and verbal assistance. She transfers herself to the shower stool and receives help with showering and dressing. She tries to participate as much as possible. After the morning hygiene routine, the staff makes her breakfast. She eats and reads the daily newspaper. She then lies down to rest until lunchtime. The staff then returns, helps her to the bathroom, and makes her lunch. Presently, the staff needs to cut the food into small pieces, so that she can eat with her fork in the left hand. After lunch, Astrid usually has a session of practicing walking with the staff. She will use her rolling walker, and the staff uses a gait belt. In the afternoons, she will often have visitors, who will prepare the afternoon snack for themselves and her. Astrid will rest again before dinner, when the staff comes to her room and helps her to the bathroom and to prepare dinner. In the evening, she watches TV and reads the newspaper. She goes to bed around 9:00 PM. Astrid still fatigues during the day and needs to rest several times. But in between her rests, she would like to manage more daily tasks herself.

Astrid lives at home in the comfort living complex and uses the option to take a taxi (mobility service) to the geriatric day rehabilitation two afternoons every week (between 1:00 and 3:00 PM). She will continue to do so until she meets her rehabilitation goals.

Adaptation Dimension

Astrid has difficulty fully participating in an effective manner due to her lack of initiative. Her fatigue also limits her today. Therefore, she needs support from the staff at her living complex and from relatives, so that the rehabilitation can continue during the whole day. The helping staff need to be familiar with Astrid's problems, so they can best supervise and support Astrid in her daily tasks.

Develop Therapeutic Rapport and Collaborative Relationships

When Maria, the occupational therapist, met Astrid, and Emil, they started to develop rapport and identified persons to include in the collaborative relationship during the intervention process.

During this first meeting, Astrid had Emil as a support. His role was to confirm what she tried to say and to provide moral support for her, and as such, he is involved in the collaborative relationship. Astrid managed the interview to a great extent by herself and only occasionally looked at her ex-husband for support when she was unsure. Maria tried to identify the problems that Astrid described as they discussed her everyday habits. Maria also was keen to listen and to show empathy for the situation that Astrid described.

Identify Resources and Limitations within Client-Centered Performance Context

Due to their first meeting, Maria has gathered the information from Astrid that she herself can identify and consider as current resources and limitations. This information will be important for the occupational therapist as background information that she can use throughout the intervention process. The occupational therapist tries to have a focus on occupations as she documents the information that she has gathered from Astrid.

Documentation of initial OT evaluation:

Background Information and Reason for Referral

Background: Astrid is a 72-year-old retired woman that lives in a small apartment in a comfort living complex for elderly and has around the clock service. A rehabilitation plan is made together with the team and Astrid. She uses a wheelchair and would like to be able to walk independently with a rolling walker and to manage simple daily chores herself (i.e., to make her own breakfast, invite friends for a coffee snack, eat with cutlery). She also wishes to be able to use the toilet independently. She survived a left-sided stroke about 5 months ago. She is weaker in the right hand and leg, still has some aphasia (she can make herself understood and understands most conversations), and has impaired memory, impaired initiative, and fatigue.

Reason for referral: Referred to the geriatric day rehabilitation for rehabilitation by the interdisciplinary team. Will be evaluated and receive interventions in daily tasks by the occupational therapist.

Identify and prioritize reported strengths and problems of occupational performance.

Another outcome from the first meeting between the client and the occupational therapist is the client's self-reported strengths and problems of performance. At this meeting, the occupational therapist can use the Canadian Occupational Performance Measure (COPM),[7] ADL taxonomy[14,16] or other available instruments that guide the interview and give a structure that can support the client in identifying and prioritizing important limitations with daily occupations. Since Astrid has both aphasia and some memory loss, it was difficult to use the COPM. The ADL taxonomy was easier to use with Astrid during this first time, and one of Astrid's daughters was contacted for further information.

Documentation from initial OT evaluation, part II: reported level of performance and prioritized task performance.

Maria documented the identified strengths and problems according to Astrid's information as follows:

Self-Reported Level of Performance

Astrid describes that she feels dependent on other persons around her all the time. As she currently requires substantial assistance for her everyday doings, she would like to be able to perform some everyday tasks herself. She prioritizes highest to be able to make coffee and snacks for her friends, to make her own breakfast, eat with cutlery, make an open-faced sandwich, and write with the right hand again.
Priorities:

- Make coffee snack (brew coffee, serve coffee and cookies at the table)
- Make a portion of hot oatmeal independently
- To cut/separate the food on the plate and eat with cutlery
- Make an open-faced sandwich independently
- To write with right hand again

Observe Client's Task Performance and Implement Performance Analysis

Presently in the rehabilitation process, it was time for Maria to observe Astrid's actual performance before they decide about which intervention to initiate. At the next visit, Maria thus had planned for an observation of Astrid's performance. Astrid chose to make her breakfast. There was no formal AMPS evaluation made at this time, and

Astrid chose to make cooked oatmeal for one person, since she usually ate that for breakfast. Although the AMPS was not used as a standardized tool, the occupational therapist could still use the skills of the AMPS to describe the performance. The AMPS skills observed during the performance are inserted in the next section in parentheses.

Observation in Prioritized Task

To Make Breakfast. Astrid was observed in the clinic kitchen as she cooked oatmeal and served jam, milk, and oats. As they set up the environment before the performance of the task, they decided to move the objects that were located high in the cupboards down to the lower shelf so Astrid could reach them. Before the observation, Maria and Astrid located all the tools and materials needed in the task. Astrid started to perform the task and collected all the materials and tools that she needed to make the oatmeal, but she does not gather the salt (initiates, search/locates, gathers). She had an ineffective ability to move herself in the wheelchair in the kitchen, since the wheelchair was too high for her (moves, reaches, bends). She also took a lot of time and effort to gather the objects and to place them for easy access (paces, endures, organizes). She was ineffective as she scooped the oats from the bag with a measuring cup as she held the measuring cup with her right hand and could not reach the oats in the bag that she held with her left hand (grips, coordinates, navigates, handles). She stopped, hesitated, and then moved the bag of oats to her right hand and the measuring cup to her left hand (continues, notice/responds, accommodates). She was now able to gather the amount of oats that she needed from the bag. Astrid then asked for salt, and the therapist gave her a general cue/clue where to find it (inquires, search/locates). Astrid did not organize the materials in an effective manner on her workspace, and there was a risk that she would knock over the milk carton with her left elbow when she reached over to pick up the jam jar (organizes, navigates). She tried to open the jar, but did not have enough strength to open the lid and asked for needed help (coordinates, calibrates, accommodates). She also needed verbal assistance to keep the pan on counter while she scooped the oats into the bowl; she tried with her right hand and then with her left hand, but needed assistance to scoop the oats in a safe manner (coordinates, handles). She served the oats in the bowl at the kitchen table, and restored all items to their original storage place. This task took 45 minutes to complete.

Initial Evaluation: Observed Current Level of Performance

Global Baseline: Cooking Oatmeal. Astrid was moderately inefficient and showed moderate increase in effort, from being able to firmly touch the floor with her feet to move a wheelchair properly. She also had a minimal need for verbal assistance for finding the salt, and a moderate degree of physical assistance to open the jam jar and scoop the cooked oats into bowl.

Specific Baseline. Astrid moved herself in her wheelchair with moderate effort, which affected her ability to position herself in relation to the task in order to enhance task performance (e.g., she sat with her left side toward the workplace where her right side was too far away to reach effectively with her right hand). Her awkward sitting affected her ability to organize the tools and material on the workplace. All task objects were placed very close together, and she then bumped into the milk carton with the elbow when she reached for jam. She also had limited ability to safely scoop the oatmeal from the pan. Astrid mobilized herself and task objects in an ineffective manner.

When Astrid was made familiar with the environment in the kitchen, Maria completed a standardized AMPS evaluation to evaluate her OT in an effective manner. The standardized ADL assessment will help the occupational therapist get more detailed information on actions problematic for Astrid. The AMPS is well-suited for the evaluation phase since it will define and describe the actions of performance that Astrid performs effectively or not.

AMPS Evaluation

The stroke affects Astrid in many aspects of her everyday life and to a great extent. The occupational therapist uses the information she has about Astrid to decide that Astrid must choose tasks that are calibrated as average or easier than average in the AMPS process task hierarchy. Drawing on the list of prioritized tasks that Astrid made earlier, the occupational therapist presented a list of five possible task choices: sweeping the floor, folding laundry, setting a table for four persons, making an open-faced sandwich with meat and a vegetable, and handwashing dishes. Astrid prioritized some of these tasks and wanted to be able to do them independently again.

Astrid chose to make a sandwich with cheese and sliced vegetable (average task difficulty) and to sweep the floor (easier than average task). She decided to start her performance making the sandwich, since she now felt familiar in the kitchen and had knowledge of the location of things she would need. Before the observation, the occupational therapist and Astrid set up the environment to make sure that Astrid had tried to open all cupboards and drawers, including the refrigerator door, and knew the location of all the things she needed. The setting up of the environment is also done prior to each task, so the client has an environment that is as similar to her own home as possible to perform the task. The objects needed in this task were moved from the upper cupboards down into drawers within reach for Astrid sitting in her wheelchair. The actions marked in parentheses in the following text are actions that

were recorded as ineffective or markedly deficit according to AMPS criteria.

Astrid chose to start with the task of making a sandwich and decided to make a cheese sandwich with sliced cucumber on top. Astrid demonstrated an inefficient ability to reach into the refrigerator for needed objects, as she placed herself far from the refrigerator with her wheelchair and sat leaning back in the wheelchair (stabilize, reach, bend). She was ineffective in transporting herself in the wheelchair as the chair is too high for her. She placed herself diagonally in relation to the work area, which led to an ineffective way to use her right hand. She tried to spread the butter on the sandwich with the knife in the right hand. She lost her grip on the knife, and, after sometime, she switched to the other hand (grips, manipulates, coordinates, calibrates, flows). The objects in the task were organized close together, leading to problems for her to navigate the workspace. She also had a decreased ability to accommodate and adjust to the situations during the task (organize, navigate, accommodate, adjust). She showed a decreased ability to use objects, as she chose a knife to pick up a slice of cheese and then continued to use the knife to pick up slices of cucumber as well. The task took about 20 minutes for her to accomplish, primarily due to her limited ability to transport herself with the wheelchair in the kitchen.

Since Astrid still had energy, she also wanted to do the second task, sweeping the floor of the kitchen. The verbal contract was that she should sweep the whole floor in the kitchen and move lightweight furniture that were in her way. During this task, she had the same inefficient way of transporting herself (moves), and she tried but was not able to move chairs, which meant that she did not reach (reach) visible crumbs, although she tried to bend forward (markedly decreased ability to adjust). She gripped the brush with her right hand but changed to the left hand and swept with the left hand instead (manipulates, coordinates, accommodates). She navigated inefficiently, and her wheelchair became stuck on a chair that she was not able to move in order to sweep the floor (organize). She did not sweep the whole floor and did not restore until a verbal cue (restore, heed) was given. She asked if she should restore the brush to original place and was scored down for the item terminates.

The occupational therapist, Maria, then filled in the AMPS score form and entered the results into the AMPS computer software. See a summary of Astrid's Motor and Process Skills from the Summary report in Figs. 21-3 and 21-4.

The AMPS software also generates a graphic report (Fig. 21-5) of the motor and process skills indicated on linear measures. Each scale also has a cutoff, where a score below the cutoff indicates problems of performance in terms of effort, efficiency, safety, or need for assistance.

ASSESSMENT OF MOTOR AND PROCESS SKILLS (AMPS)
PERFORMANCE SKILL SUMMARY

Caution: Item and total raw scores are not valid representations of client performance, and they cannot be used for documentation or statistical analyses. Raw scores must be analyzed using the AMPS computer-scoring software to create ADL ability measures. Only ADL ability measures are valid for measuring change.

Client: **Evaluation date:**

Id: 37   **Occupational therapist:**

Task 1:   F-7: Open-face meat or cheese sandwich with sliced vegetable (Average)

Task 2:   J-1: Sweeping the floor (Average)

Overall performance in each skill area is summarized below using the following scale:

A = Adequate skill, no apparent disruption was observed

I = Ineffective skill, moderate disruption was observed

MD= Markedly deficient skill, observed problems were severe enough to be unsafe or to require
         therapist intervention

MOTOR SKILLS: Skills observed when client moved self and objects during task performance	A	I	MD
Body Position			
STABILIZES: Does not lose balance when interacting with task objects		X	
ALIGNS: Does not persistently support oneself during task performance		X	
POSITIONS the arm or body effectively in relation to task objects		X	
Obtaining and Holding Objects			
REACHES effectively for task objects		X	
BENDS or twists the body appropriate to the task		X	
GRIPS: Securely grasps task objects		X	
MANIPULATES talk objects as needed for task performance		X	
COORDINATES two body parts to securely stabilize task objects		X	
Moving Self and Objects			
MOVES: Effectively pushes/pulls task objects and opens/closes doors or drawers			X
LIFTS task objects effectively		X	
WALKS effectively within the task environment		X	
TRANSPORTS task objects effectively from one place to another		X	
CALIBRATES the force and speed of task-related actions		X	
FLOWS: Uses smooth arm and hand movements when interacting with task objects		X	
Sustaining Performance			
ENDURES for the duration of the task performance	X		
PACES: Maintains an effective rate of task performance		X	

Figure 21-3   Astrid's AMPS summary report at baseline: Motor Skills.

The graphic report shows that Astrid's motor ability is below the cutoff on the motor scale. Astrid's motor ability indicates that she has increased effort when performing ADL tasks. Approximately 95% of well, elderly persons of her age have ADL motor ability between 1.07 and 3.27 logits, and her ability at 0.01 logits is thus lower than age expectations. Astrid's process ability is also below the cutoff on the process scale. This indicates that she experiences decreased safety, independence, and/or efficiency when she performs familiar ADL tasks. About 95% of healthy persons of Astrid's age have an ADL process ability measure between 0.59 and 2.55 logits, thus her ADL process ability at 0.45 logits is lower than age expectations. An

ADL process ability measure below 1.0 logits indicates that the person needs assistance. Approximately 93% of persons below the ADL process cutoff need assistance to live in the community. Both Astrid's cognitive and motor impairments after her stroke affects her ADL performance. More information about the AMPS scales and cutoff can be found in the AMPS manual.[2]

After the observation using the standardized AMPS, the occupational therapist can also look at the hierarchy of the standardized tasks in the AMPS manual and make assumptions about other tasks in the hierarchy that will be easier or harder for Astrid to perform. For example, since she showed increased effort and decreased efficiency making a sandwich

ASSESSMENT OF MOTOR AND PROCESS SKILLS (AMPS)
PERFORMANCE SKILL SUMMARY

Caution: Item and total raw scores are not valid representations of client performance, and they cannot be used for documentation or statistical analyses. Raw scores must be analyzed using the AMPS computer-scoring software to create ADL ability measures. Only ADL ability measures are valid for measuring change.

Client: Evaluation date:

Id: 37   Occupational therapist:

Task 1:   F-7: Open-face meat or cheese sandwich with sliced vegetable (Average)

Task 2:   J-1: Sweeping the floor (Average)

Overall performance in each skill area is summarized below using the following scale:

A = Adequate skill, no apparent disruption was observed

I = Ineffective skill, moderate disruption was observed

MD= Markedly deficient skill, observed problems were severe enough to be unsafe or to require therapist intervention

PROCESS SKILLS: Skills observed when client (a) selected, interacted with, and used task tools and materials; and (b) modified task actions, when needed, to complete the task performance	A	I	MD
Sustaining Performance			
PACES: Maintains an effective rate of task performance		X	
ATTENDS: Does not look away from task performance	X		
HEEDS the goal of the specified task		X	
Applying Knowledge			
CHOOSES appropriate tools and materials needed for task performance		X	
USES task objects according to their intended purposes		X	
HANDLES task objects with care		X	
INQUIRES: Asks for needed task-related information		X	
Temporal Organization			
INITIATES actions or steps of task without hesitation			X
CONTINUES task actions through to completion	X		
SEQUENCES the steps of the task in a logical manner	X		
TERMINATES task actions or steps appropriately		X	
Organizing Space and Objects			
SEARCHES for and effectively LOCATES task tools and materials	X		
GATHERS tools and materials effectively into the task workspace	X		
ORGANIZES tools and materials in an orderly and spatially appropriate fashion		X	
RESTORES: Puts away tools and materials and cleans the workspace			X
NAVIGATES: Maneuvers the hand and body around obstacles in the task environment		X	
Adapting Performance			
NOTICES and RESPONDS to task-relevant cues from the environment		X	
ADJUSTS: Changes workplaces or adjusts switches and dials to overcome problems			X
ACCOMMODATES: Modifies one's actions to overcome problems		X	
BENEFITS: Prevents task-related problems from persisting		X	

Figure 21-4   Astrid's AMPS summary report at baseline: Process Skills.

and sweeping the floor, she would have fewer problems with tasks such as folding laundry or making the bed.

Define and Describe the Actions of Performance the Client Does and Does Not Perform Effectively. Also available from the AMPS software is the possibility to print a narrative report of the observed performance. This report gives information about the AMPS, the observed tasks, and some information about the strengths of the performance. It also includes information on how well the performance compares to persons in the same age group.

**ASSESSMENT OF MOTOR AND PROCESS SKILLS (AMPS)
GRAPHIC REPORT**

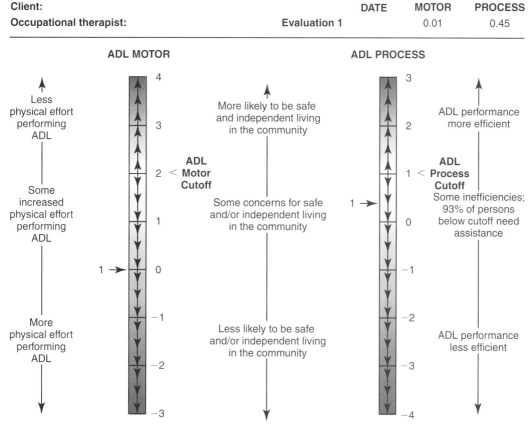

Client:		DATE	MOTOR	PROCESS
Occupational therapist:	Evaluation 1		0.01	0.45

Figure 21-5 AMPS graphic report of Astrid's performance at baseline. The numbers on the Activities of Daily Living (ADL) motor and ADL process scales are units of ADL ability (logits). The results are reported as ADL motor and ADL process measures plotted in relation to the AMPS scale cutoffs. Measures below the cutoffs indicate that there was diminished quality or effectiveness of performance of instrumental and/or personal ADL. See the AMPS Narrative Report for further information regarding the interpretation of a single AMPS evaluation.

Grouping Skills of Most Concern into Meaningful Clusters. The next step was to group the skills found to be of most concern into meaningful clusters. These clusters can help document the problems observed in Astrid's performance. Astrid's limitations could thus be summarized into the following clusters:

Cluster 1: Moves and Positions. Astrid had problems related to moving around in the task environment in an effective manner, which resulted in problems related to positioning herself in an effective way to use the task objects.

Cluster 2: Reaches and Bends. She had problems reaching for and reaching into the refrigerator, despite the fact that she tried to bend forward (also due to cluster 1).

Cluster 3: Grips and Coordinates. Astrid tried to sweep the floor with the broom in her right hand, but could not hold her grip effectively, and had problems getting the dirt onto the dust-pan.

Cluster 4: Paces. Due to problems in moving herself effectively, she had problems maintaining an acceptable tempo throughout the task. Every task took a long time to finish.

Cluster 5: Organizes. Astrid placed the objects too close to each other, which resulted in problems (i.e., in spreading the butter on the bread as the container was too close to the bread).

The strengths of Astrid's performance are also summarized, since her strengths could be used as interventions were planned with Astrid during her rehabilitation period. Astrid's strengths could be summarized into the following cluster.

Cluster 6: Endures, Attends, Continues, Sequences, Searches/Locates, Gathers. Astrid was motivated and endured through both tasks. She stayed focused and continued the performance to the end of the tasks. She completed all of the actions in the correct order and had no problems finding and gathering the tools and materials she needed for the tasks.

Define/Clarify or Interpret Cause

When the occupational therapist has evaluated the quality of the performance of the client, the occupational therapist is ready to clarify or interpret the cause of the problems of occupational performance. When the occupational therapist looked through her notes that summarized the ten dimensions, what she had documented in the patient files, and the information gathered from the other members of the team, it became clear that Astrid's problems were due to both her limited motor skills and the cognitive impairments that she had acquired from her stroke eight months earlier (body function dimension).

Astrid also demonstrated problems related to organizing the tools and materials in the environment, such as moving the furniture, organization in kitchen, and wheelchair use (environmental dimension). Currently she also did not receive the support to be as independent as possible that she needed from the staff at her living complex.

Documentation from Initial Occupational Therapy Evaluation: Interpretation of Cause

This is what Maria documented in Astrid's files:

Interpretation

Limited motor skills and cognitive impairments limit the quality of ADL task performance. Lack of sufficient support from others and limited possibility to try and perform daily tasks after stroke further hinder ADL task performance.

Document Client's Baseline and Goals. From the AMPS results, it might be important to verify and maybe change some of the rehabilitation goals set together with Astrid. Thus, Maria reasoned together with Astrid that a more realistic goal was to manage some of the tasks with supervision instead of a goal of being independent. She wanted, for example, to make coffee for her friends, and after having observed Astrid, the occupational therapist was aware that it might be more realistic for her to aim to perform this task with some supervision. With the support from her daughter, Astrid was very clear in what she wished to accomplish during her rehabilitation. After the initial evaluation phase, it was time for the team to have a joint meeting and to plan the continuous care and rehabilitation for Astrid. This happened as Astrid arrived for her fifth meeting at the geriatric day rehabilitation. The goals that Astrid and the occupational therapist had agreed upon, and were prioritized by Astrid, are written below. These tasks will be the focus during the following OT visits at the geriatric day rehabilitation two times a week for some time. The following goals were also included in the common team goals.

Goal 1. Astrid will, with supervision, safely manage to serve coffee and cookies to her friends. This includes brewing coffee, taking out cookies and placing on a plate, setting the table with coffee cups and saucers, and serving at a table (Fig. 21-6).

Goal 2. Astrid will, with verbal support from the staff at her living complex, initiate and, in an effective and safe way, make herself a portion of warm oatmeal using an adapted work chair (the chair will allow her to reach her cupboards and at the same time allow her to propel her chair in an effective manner).

Goal 3. Astrid will independently and efficiently make her own sandwich with one spread (i.e. easy spread butter), sliced cheese, and pre-sliced vegetable, using a nonslip device and a rolling work chair.

Goal 4. Astrid will independently and effectively manage to eat a meal with both cutlery (i.e. knife and fork, simultaneously).

Goal 5. Astrid will manage to write a sentence from a newspaper or book by herself with the right hand.

Select Intervention Model and Plan and Implement Occupation-Based Interventions

As this step in the OT process is reached, it is now time to select the interventions, as described in the OTIPM. The four models suggested include: the restorative

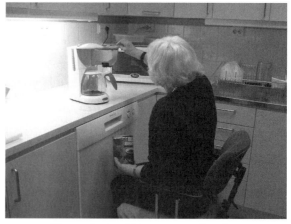

Figure 21-6 Client-centered goal 1.

occupation model, the acquisitional occupation model (Fig. 21-7), the adaptive occupation model (Fig. 21-8), and the occupation-based educational programs (Fig. 21-9).

Together with Astrid, the team discussed how to prioritize the goals and with which goal to start the intervention. Before each intervention session, the occupational therapist observed the client doing each of the prioritized tasks to evaluate the resources and limitations of the performance, according to the process model in OTIPM.

Implementing Occupation-Based Interventions

In the OTIPM, four different models of interventions are described, which all have a focus on occupation. The four models of praxis are: (1) *Adaptive Occupation* to compensate for decreased occupational skill; (2) *Acquisitional Occupation* to reacquire, develop, or maintain occupational skill; (3) *Restorative Occupation* to restore, develop, or maintain

person factors or body functions; and (4) *Occupation-Based Educational Programs* focused on performance of daily life tasks. Astrid's occupational therapist used three of the models, and the plan in each area is described below:

Intervention Plan

Adaptive occupation:
- Trying out technical aides: work chair with wheels, antislip device, new wheelchair cushion
- Adaptation of tasks: presliced cucumber and cheese
- Adaptation of environment: relocating tools and materials in kitchen

Education program:
- Supervision of caring staff: during ADL tasks prioritized by Astrid

Acquisitional occupation:
- Training of tasks: eating with cutlery, handwriting

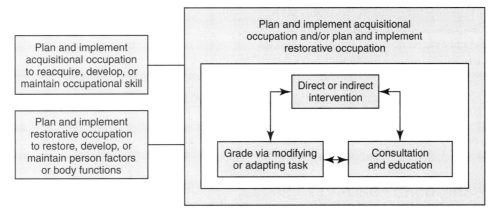

Figure 21-7 Acquisitional and restorative occupation. (From Fisher AG: *Occupational therapy intervention process model*, Fort Collins, CO, 2009, Three Star Press.)

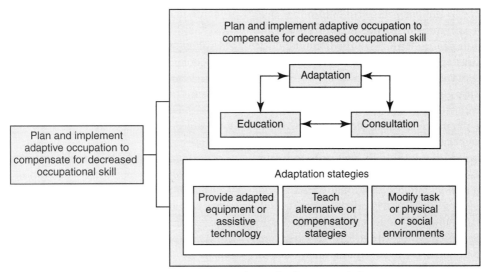

Figure 21-8 Adaptive occupation. (From Fisher AG: *Occupational therapy intervention process model*, Fort Collins, CO, 2009, Three Star Press.)

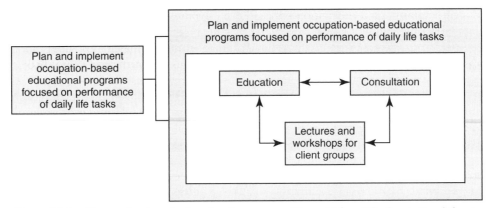

Figure 21-9   Occupation-based educational programs. (From Fisher AG: *Occupational therapy intervention process model*, Fort Collins, CO, 2009, Three Star Press.)

After reading through the notes that she had taken so far, the occupational therapist, together with Astrid, reached the conclusion that they would start by making adjustments to the wheelchair that was far too high for Astrid to propel herself effectively. This had consistently been the biggest struggle for her in all observed tasks and was a prerequisite to reach her goals. Therefore, the occupational therapist chose the model of adaptive compensation at this stage.

Adaptive Occupation

Wheelchair. The occupational therapist arranged for Astrid to change her seat cushion to one that was not so thick, which meant that Astrid was immediately able to propel herself forward both effectively and quickly by using her feet. After trying this cushion for a few days, Astrid still wanted to change back to the higher cushion. The occupational therapist then tried to find a wheelchair that had a lower seat, but was not successful. At the same time, Astrid made progress with the physiotherapist and started to be able to walk with a rolling walker and an assistant. Since the occupational therapist wanted to take this into account, she thought through Astrid's situation once again (through all the steps in OTIPM) and reached the conclusion that Astrid might be able to use a rolling work chair, with a brake and adjustable height seat, for her to use at home instead of a wheelchair (see Fig. 21-6). This chair would make reaching easier for Astrid, since she also had difficulty reaching up to the fridge and upper cupboards. It was still hard to imagine how safely Astrid would learn to walk in the future, so for the time being, Astrid could have this chair on loan. Astrid thought that this was a good idea, and the occupational therapist ordered the chair from the technical aides department. When she received the chair, it needed to be adjusted to fit Astrid, and she needed training in how to maneuver and use it in a safe manner (i.e., locking the brakes before sitting down onto the chair, before standing up, or raising it to the highest level [maximum seat height 75 cm]). After

this initial practice, she also needed supervision in how to use it in the tasks that she had prioritized (i.e., making warm oats, making coffee for her friends, or making a sandwich). Simultaneously the staff at her living complex received supervision from the occupational therapist on how to support Astrid when she used the chair, how to tend to the chair, and how to use it in a safe manner.

Goal: To Make a Sandwich

Assistive Devices/Domestic Technical Aides. During the observation of Astrid when she prepared a sandwich, it became clear that she had problems gripping the sandwich in an effective way; the sandwich was close to falling off the table into her lap, and it slid over the table while she was spreading the butter. Astrid tried a nonslip mat used to hold the bread in the same place as she spread the butter. She was very satisfied after she had tried it. With this mat under her sandwich, she could safely spread butter. After this purchase, Astrid practiced with the occupational therapist a few times, and within two weeks, Astrid could make her own sandwich with presliced cheese and cucumber for her afternoon snack at the day rehab.

After this goal was met, the occupational therapist and Astrid continued working on the next goal (to make coffee and cookies for her friends and make cooked oats). To reach these goals, the occupational therapist reasoned that she would need to use two different models. She decided to use the compensatory model and the model for education and teaching.

Goals: Make Coffee and Cookies for Her Friends and Make Cooked Oats for Breakfast

Environmental Adaptation. Since it is not possible to carry out all of the rehabilitation initiated at the geriatric day rehabilitation in the clients home, the occupational therapist, together with the client, will adapt the kitchen in the clinic to be as similar to the client's home as possible (i.e., the objects needed in the different tasks were placed in a way to imitate the situation in Astrid's home). This was possible to accomplish after the home visit that the occupational therapist had done earlier and became aware of how Astrid had her home organized. While the rehabilitation sessions mostly took place at the clinic, the occupational therapist had a few opportunities during the rehabilitation period to evaluate the progress in Astrid's home. In Astrid's home, it became obvious that Astrid needed to reorganize some of the kitchen cupboards to enhance her ability to reach the objects she wanted to use more frequently (either as she was using the wheelchair or the work chair). In both the clinic and Astrid's home, there was limited ability to adapt all; for example, the coffee maker was not possible to move at both locations, since it must be close to an electric outlet and to the sink.

Occupation-Based Education Program

The occupational therapist continued to reason in relation to the results from the AMPS observation. Since Astrid had process skill ability at 0.45 logits, which indicates a need for assistance, the occupational therapist considered her need for help to safely make coffee (decreased ability to reach, place, use, handle, organize, accommodate, adjust) by educating the staff in how to best support Astrid without doing the task for her. The occupational therapist informed the staff that it is important that Astrid performs as many actions as possible by herself in each task. At the same time, the staff would need watch over and intervene in case of safety risks. The occupational therapist thus used educational principles.

Acquisitional Occupation

After some time in the day rehabilitation program, Astrid had reached her first goals, and they now started to work on goals 4 and 5. To reach these goals, the occupational therapist chose the acquisitional model, which is used for occupational skills training.

Goal: To Eat With Knife and Fork Again. Initially the occupational therapist simulated the task of eating with knife and fork using a slice of bread to imitate a thin slice of beef, and Astrid tried to cut it up using the cutlery and then eat it. They practiced this situation once every time they met for two weeks. When Astrid mastered this simulated task, the occupational therapist went to Astrid's home to observe her during a meal. The staff at her living complex let Astrid cut her own food herself in order for her to practice in a natural (ecologically relevant) condition.

Goal: To Write with Her Right Hand. Astrid had some remaining aphasia and apraxia and had a hard time writing spontaneously, which was revealed already as the occupational therapist observed her. The occupational therapist started with simple writing exercises, like writing a word to describe a picture. Astrid also wanted to have homework that she could do in between the times at

the clinic. Initially during the practice, Astrid had a hard time holding the pen, and the occupational therapist had to place it in her hand for her to be able to use it. Maria gave her simple crosswords to solve at home. As soon as she could hold the pen herself, it was also easier for her to write. First she used block letters, and after about three weeks of training, she was able to write script again with some effort. While she was able to manage to copy text or solve a simple crossword, it was not possible for Astrid to write spontaneously, due to her aphasia.

Reevaluate for Enhanced and Satisfying Occupational Performance

The next section will describe the change in occupational performance for some of the goals that Astrid had set together with the occupational therapist.

Baseline: Make a Portion of Hot Oatmeal Independently. Astrid needed both verbal support in finding the salt and holding the pan to serve the oats and physical assistance to open the jam jar when she made cooked oats. Her performance was moderately ineffective, and she performed the task with moderate effort and needed supervision.

Goal. Astrid will, with verbal support from the staff at her living complex, initiate and, in an effective and safe way, make herself a portion of warm oatmeal using an adapted work chair.

Current Status. When the occupational therapist observed Astrid to evaluate this goal during a home visit, Astrid managed to make her cooked oats with only verbal assistance and support for safety. When Astrid used the rolling chair, she performed the task without effort and effectively.

Result. Goal was met.

Baseline: Make an Open-Faced Sandwich Independently. Astrid managed to make a sandwich with presliced cheese and cucumber if the objects were located within reach for her in the chair. It was with great effort that she could transport herself and place herself appropriately in relation to the actions required for the task. The task took a long time for her to accomplish, and she was moderately ineffective.

Goal. Astrid will independently and efficiently make her own sandwich with one spread (i.e., easy spread butter), sliced cheese, and presliced vegetable, using a nonslip device and a rolling work chair.

Current Status. Astrid managed to make a sandwich readily and effectively when using a nonslip pad and can reach all needed tools and materials.

Result. Goal was met.

During the continuing time at the rehabilitation unit, the occupational therapist and Astrid continued to work toward the set goals in the same manner as described previously.

Reevaluation Using the AMPS

As the goals that Astrid set together with Maria, the occupational therapist, have been reached, it is important to notice the changes that have occurred and to document these changes. To do so, both formal standardized evaluations of performance and of the client's satisfaction with the results can be used. Since Maria used the AMPS initially to observe and evaluate the performance skills initially, it is appropriate to use the AMPS at the end of the treatment period to find out if ability has increased during the rehabilitation period.

Five days before Astrid was discharged, Maria completed a new AMPS evaluation. Astrid chose the same tasks that she performed at the first evaluation: sweeping the floor and making a sandwich with cheese and a vegetable. The AMPS summary report showed the scoring of the motor and process skills for the two observed tasks and documents if the performance was adequate, ineffective, or markedly deficient (Figs. 21-10 and 21-11). The AMPS graphic report showed a significant change in her motor skills, from 0.01 logits to 0.84 logits. No significant

---

ASSESSMENT OF MOTOR AND PROCESS SKILLS (AMPS)
PERFORMANCE SKILL SUMMARY

Caution: Item and total raw scores are not valid representations of client performance, and they cannot be used for documentation or statistical analyses. Raw scores must be analyzed using the AMPS computer-scoring software to create ADL ability measures. Only ADL ability measures are valid for measuring change.

Client: **Evaluation date:**
Id: 37   **Occupational therapist:**

Task 1:   J-1: Sweeping the floor (Average)
Task 2:   F-7: Open-face meat or cheese sandwich with sliced vegetable (Average)
Overall performance in each skill area is summarized below using the following scale:

  A = Adequate skill, no apparent disruption was observed

  I = Ineffective skill, moderate disruption was observed

MD= Markedly deficient skill, observed problems were severe enough to be unsafe or to require
        therapist intervention

MOTOR SKILLS: Skills observed when client moved self and objects during task performance	A	I	MD
Body Position			
STABILIZES: Does not lose balance when interacting with task objects	X		
ALIGNS: Does not persistently support oneself during task performance	X		
POSITIONS the arm or body effectively in relation to task objects			X
Obtaining and Holding Objects			
REACHES effectively for task objects		X	
BENDS or twists the body appropriate to the task		X	
GRIPS: Securely grasps task objects		X	
MANIPULATES task objects as needed for task performance	X		
COORDINATES two body parts to securely stabilize task objects		X	
Moving Self and Objects			
MOVES: Effectively pushes/pulls task objects and opens/closes doors or drawers		X	
LIFTS task objects effectively		X	
WALKS effectively within the task environment		X	
TRANSPORTS task objects effectively from one place to another	X		
CALIBRATES the force and speed of task-related actions		X	
FLOWS: Uses smooth arm and hand movements when interacting with task objects		X	
Sustaining Performance			
ENDURES for the duration of the task performance	X		
PACES: Maintains an effective rate of task performance		X	

Figure 21-10   AMPS summary report for Astrid at discharge: Motor Skills.

ASSESSMENT OF MOTOR AND PROCESS SKILLS (AMPS)
PERFORMANCE SKILL SUMMARY

Caution: Item and total raw scores are not valid representations of client performance, and they cannot be used for documentation or statistical analyses. Raw scores must be analyzed using the AMPS computer-scoring software to create ADL ability measures. Only ADL ability measures are valid for measuring change.

Client: **Evaluation date:**
Id: 37   **Occupational therapist:**

Task 1:   J-1: Sweeping the floor (Average)
Task 2:   F-7: Open-face meat or cheese sandwich with sliced vegetable (Average)

Overall performance in each skill area is summarized below using the following scale:

A = Adequate skill, no apparent disruption was observed

I = Ineffective skill, moderate disruption was observed

MD= Markedly deficient skill, observed problems were severe enough to be unsafe or to require therapist intervention

PROCESS SKILLS: Skills observed when client (a) selected, interacted with, and used task tools and materials; and (b) modified task actions, when needed, to complete the task performance	A	I	MD
Sustaining Performance			
PACES: Maintains an effective rate of task performance		X	
ATTENDS: Does not look away from task performance	X		
HEEDS the goal of the specified task		X	
Applying Knowledge			
CHOOSES appropriate tools and materials needed for task performance		X	
USES task objects according to their intended purposes		X	
HANDLES task objects with care		X	
INQUIRES: Asks for needed task-related information		X	
Temporal Organization			
INITIATES actions or steps of task without hesitation	X		
CONTINUES task actions through to completion	X		
SEQUENCES the steps of the task in a logical manner	X		
TERMINATES task actions or steps appropriately		X	
Organizing Space and Objects			
SEARCHES for and effectively LOCATES task tools and materials	X		
GATHERS tools and materials effectively into the task workspace	X		
ORGANIZES tools and materials in an orderly and spatially appropriate fashion		X	
RESTORES: Puts away tools and materials and cleans the workspace		X	
NAVIGATES: Maneuvers the hand and body around obstacles in the task environment		X	
Adapting Performance			
NOTICES and RESPONDS to task-relevant cues from the environment		X	
ADJUSTS: Changes workplaces or adjusts switches and dials to overcome problems		X	
ACCOMMODATES: Modifies one's actions to overcome problems			X
BENEFITS: Prevents task-related problems from persisting			X

Figure 21-11   AMPS summary report for Astrid at discharge: Process Skills.

change was noted on process skills. See the graphic report in Fig. 21-12.

Astrid reached all her goals according to the plan and was discharged knowing she would be able to manage the tasks she wanted with the support from the staff at her living complex.

GERIATRIC DAY REHABILITATION: CLIENT LIVING AT HOME

In the second case, the focus will be on the day rehabilitation services for the client, August. Initially some background will be given.

**ASSESSMENT OF MOTOR AND PROCESS SKILLS (AMPS)
GRAPHIC REPORT**

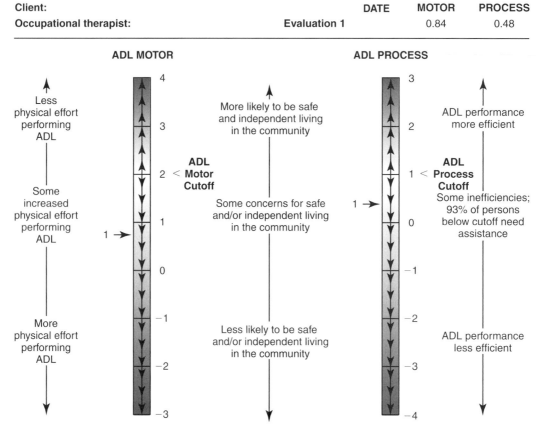

Figure 21-12 AMPS graphic report for Astrid at discharge. The numbers on the activities of daily living (ADL) motor and ADL process scales are units of ADL ability (logits). The results are reported as ADL motor and ADL process measures plotted in relation to the AMPS scale cutoffs. Measures below the cutoffs indicate that there was diminished quality or effectiveness of performance of instrumental and/or personal ADL. See the AMPS Narrative Report for further information regarding the interpretation of a single AMPS evaluation.

Acute

August, 66-years-old, woke up in the morning four months ago with a left-sided hemiparesis. CT showed "demarked ischemic areas on the right side temporal and frontal in the basal ganglia." He was admitted as an inpatient to the hospital's stroke unit. During the stay at the hospital, August suffered from fatigue and memory impairments. After inpatient rehabilitation, he was able to walk with the support of two persons and needed help with personal ADL.

Subacute

After the acute phase of the stroke, he was moved to a geriatric stroke rehabilitation ward two weeks after his stroke and met an occupational therapist the same day. Together the occupational therapist and August set the

goals for the rehabilitation, and those goals were:
1. Managing daily hygiene.
2. Manage dressing independently.
3. Manage visits to the toilet independently.

Six weeks later August was discharged, having met his goals. August was also able to walk independently with a rolling walker. August was discharged to his home, and was placed on a waiting list for continuous training at the geriatric day rehabilitation unit.

In the beginning of the following year, about four months after his stroke, August started at the geriatric day rehabilitation unit. At his first visit, he met the occupational therapist, Maria, who conducted an interview with him. She had prepared herself by reading the referral and earlier patient files from when he was an inpatient. Maria worked with the OTIPM as her frame of reference, which guided her work as an occupational therapist. At this first meeting, August informed her about his illness and described a typical day for him at this stage. The occupational therapist listened for the daily life tasks that he described as problematic, and she asked him several questions to clarify his strengths and problems in ADL. After their meeting, to get a clear picture of August and his circumstances and concerns, she documented the key information she collected from the patient files, according to the ten dimensions described in the OTIPM. As August became a day patient at the geriatric day rehabilitation unit, he met with all the professionals in the team to establish the focus of the rehabilitation at the time. The team worked interdisciplinary, as suggested in the literature, in order to deliver quality geriatric care.[10] To work interdisciplinary means that the patient is a natural member of the team, and the patient's goals are formulated as common team goals for the rehabilitation of the patient. The needs of the patient dictate which members of the team will be involved and participate in the rehabilitation of the patient. The members of the team can shift during the rehabilitation process. The occupational therapist on the team will use the patient's prioritized tasks as her focus during rehabilitation.

BEGINNING OF THE OCCUPATIONAL THERAPY INTERVENTION PROCESS MODEL

Establish Client-Centered Performance Context

When his occupational therapist, Maria, began the intervention process with August, she first met him for an interview to find out August's current situation/status and his goals for the future. During this interview, the client and the therapist also developed a therapeutic rapport and a collaborative relationship. The information that the therapist gathered during this first meeting were used to identify and prioritize strengths and problems with occupational performance, and hindrances and resources in the client-centered performance context that supported and limited his occupational performance. Some information was also "stored" for use later in the process, especially information about resources and limitations within the client-centered performance context. She learned the following information as she established a global picture of the client-centered performance context.

Environmental Dimension

August lives with his wife and dog in a house with three bedrooms, kitchen, and living room, in a farming village outside the main city in northern Sweden. They have three adult children and two grandchildren. Their house is on one level; the toilet has a raised seat with armrests, and the shower has a shower stool. There are no thresholds in the house, but there is a small level change (one step is 45 cm) at the main entrance, where August usually enters the house. He has received supportive railings on both sides of the entrance to manage the different levels.

There is a home office with a computer, office chair (no brakes), and a telephone. He manages most of his company's bookkeeping in this office. He can manage the office chair safely. It is hard for him to manage the telephone with his left hand, but he can manage the computer with his right hand. His house is located nearby the forest, and there are a bicycle and a car parked in front of the house.

Social Dimension

August's wife is supportive, and she and August seem to have a good relationship. The three children are also available in times of need. August also has many friends and relatives that he frequently visits during his leisure time.

Role Dimension

August and his wife have a traditional, Swedish role distribution in the home (i.e., August takes care of the maintenance of the house and the outdoors, and his wife is responsible for the domestic care). August's role is to maintain the outside of their house. During winter, that means snow shoveling, but now he gets help with snow-clearance from a neighbor. August would like to manage this independently. In the summer, maintaining the house means mowing the lawn, which August would like to manage by himself. August will prepare simple ready-made food and also makes "fika" (coffee and cookies), while his wife cooks food from scratch.

Before his stroke, August worked in his own company together with his wife. His main tasks were bookkeeping. He is worried about what will happen to the company in the future, and if he will be able to manage as before.

August identifies himself as a traditional man in the village where he lives (i.e., as a hunter and fisherman, and "knowledgeable in most things"). He also worries about being able to hunt again or taking the dogs for walks in the forest. Currently he cannot perform these tasks.

Cultural Dimension

August lives in a farmer village where "everybody knows everybody else." He shares the customs, habits, values, and beliefs with the other people in the area, a traditional village in the north of Sweden. August had a hard time initially as he was not able to manage his "typical male" tasks in the home: snow clearance, walking the dog, driving the car/motorbike, and mowing the lawn.

Motivational Dimension

In his leisure time, August spends a lot of time in nature, mainly hunting and fishing. He hunts mainly for moose and small game. This is something that he enjoys, and he would like to regain this ability. He was also responsible, together with a friend, for managing the local shooting range. He hopes to be able to continue this during the upcoming hunting season. August used to make daily walks together with his hunting dog, walking in the forest or biking, and he wants to pursue this again. He is also interested in motors and has his own motorbike and has enjoyed ballroom dancing.

Institutional Dimension

August's wife supports him, and he has no demands from society to go back to work since he had planned to retire during this year. He has the whole team at the day rehabilitation unit supporting him for the time during his rehabilitation. There are no medical restrictions related to August's impairments that limit him from doing the tasks that he has done before.

Body Function Dimension

August survived a right-sided stroke about four months ago. He has a weakness in both left hand/arm and leg, but can walk safely and independently with a rolling walker. August feels depressed and has a hard time sleeping at night. He is easily fatigued.

Task Dimension

August describes his biggest problems, which are his highest priorities. He wants to manage to hold a telephone receiver with left hand at the same time as he makes notes with his right hand. He also wants to hold his hunting weapon in a correct way, and hopefully later he would like to continue to hunt. He also mentions wanting to hold a potato on the fork with one hand and peel it with the knife in the other hand. Another task that he wishes to do is walking the dog. For him to do this, he needs to be able to walk safely with a walking stick and manage to lead the dog on a leash without the dog pulling him. Due to his decreased balance and gait, this is currently not possible.

Temporal Dimension

A usual day in August's life right now is that he rises up early in the morning, completes his bathroom routine, gets dressed, eats breakfast, and reads the daily newspaper. He then exercises for one hour, eats another small snack in midmorning, and then takes a rest and watches TV. He has a coffee midday and exercises for another half hour. Afterwards he cooks/warms dinner and watches TV in the evening. He goes to bed around 10:00 PM.

August lives at home during the outpatient rehabilitation and goes by taxi the 30 km into town two mornings a week between 9:00 and 11:30 AM. This will continue until he meets the rehabilitation goals documented together with the team, in about two to four months.

August has progressed well during his rehabilitation mainly because he is motivated and is in otherwise very good physical condition.

Adaptation Dimension

August has the ability to adjust to his current circumstances and takes in instructions for exercise/training and continues the training at home by himself in between the rehabilitation visits.

He uses his wife and friends to increase his activity repertoire in his everyday life and makes sure that he can try to regain activities/tasks that he has done earlier himself (i.e., walking the dog and mending inventories at the shooting range).

Develop Therapeutic Rapport and Collaborative Relationships

August was motivated for the continuous rehabilitation and positive that he would be able to practice more at the rehabilitation unit. He told the occupational therapist, Maria, how he managed during the days at home and reviewed areas of difficulty. Maria listened carefully and asked follow-up questions as needed, so that she would get a complete picture of August's performance context. They both felt they had a nice therapeutic relation after this conversation.

Identify and Prioritize Reported Strengths and Problems of Occupational Performance

After the collection of information on the ten dimensions needed to establish the client-centered performance context, the occupational therapist needs to summarize the information. As the OTIPM is followed, two parts are documented: (1) resources and limitations within the client-centered performance context, and (2) self-reported strengths and problems of occupational performance.

The documentation at this stage is described below.

Background information: August is 66-years-old and lives in a village outside a major city with his wife. They run a company together. August is responsible for the bookkeeping. The rehabilitation starts by the team developing a rehabilitation plan together. August's main interests are hunting, caring for his dog, and being outside in the forest. August expresses problems using his left hand the way he wants to (i.e., holding his hunting rifle), and his weak left leg interferes with performing his other interests.

Reason for initial referral: August was referred to day rehabilitation unit in the geriatric department for interdisciplinary team rehabilitation. August will meet with Maria, the occupational therapist, for evaluation and intervention.

The first part is to identify the resources and limitations within this client's performance context, and how the limitations hinder the client's engagement in his life roles. From the list of tasks discussed, the client prioritizes which he finds to be most important. The performance of tasks that support the clients engagement in life roles are the strengths, while those tasks that the client experience as problems to perform and that hinder the engagement in life roles are limitations. At this stage, it might be appropriate to use another instrument to verbalize the strengths and limitations and to prioritize

them. The Canadian Occupational Performance Measure (COPM)[7] is a tool that can be used, since it will clarify and describe the strengths and limitations of the client. Maria administered the COPM at the beginning of the rehabilitation period. The COPM helped Maria and August priorities for intervention. See August's COPM results in Fig. 21-13.

August also put priority on driving again, but in Sweden there is a common rule that each person who has a stroke is not allowed to drive during the first six months after the stroke.

STEP 1A: Self-Care — Importance

Personal Care (e.g., dressing, bathing, feeding, hygiene): Eat with cutlery — 9

Functional Mobility (e.g., transfers, indoor, outdoor): Walk in the forest — 10; Bike — 8

Community Management (e.g., transportation, shopping, finances): Drive a car — 10

STEP 1B: Productivity

Paid/Unpaid Work (e.g., finding/keeping a job, volunteering): Speak in telephone and simultaneously take notes — 9; Bookkeeping — 7

Household Management (e.g., cleaning, doing laundry, cooking): Shovel snow — 7; Cut grass — 7

Play/School (e.g., play skills, homework)

STEP 1C: Leisure

Quiet Recreation (e.g., hobbies, crafts, reading)

Active Recreation (e.g., sports, outings, travel): Walk the dog — 9; Hunting — 10; Manage local shooting range — 8; Barn dance — 5

Socialization (e.g., visiting, phone calls, parties, correspondence)

Figure 21-13 Results from August's interview using step 1 of the Canadian Occupational Performance Measure. (Modified from Law M, Baptiste S, Carswell A, et al: *Canadian occupational performance measure*, Toronto, Ontario 1994, CAOT Publications ACE.)

Identified Level of Performance:

August manages his morning routines and simple domestic chores independently, although he cannot manage peeling his potatoes at mealtime since he cannot grasp the fork in his left hand.* He has problems talking on the phone and simultaneously taking notes, which he needs to do to run his company. August is unable to walk his dog in the forest, which was his duty earlier. He also reports that he is not able to attend to his house and garden chores in a safe manner, due to his limited balance and limited grip with his left hand. He also wants to be able to hold his rifle in a correct way and, if possible, also hunt during the fall again.

Reported priorities:

■ Being able to eat with both cutlery again (knife and fork)
■ Talk in the telephone and simultaneously take notes
■ Hold a rifle in a safe and "right way" (shooting position)
■ Walk the dog in the forest independently

In Swedish culture, it is common for each person to peel boiled potatoes by holding the potato in the air, supported on a fork held in one hand, while the person simultaneously removes the peel using a knife held in the other hand (Fig. 21-14).

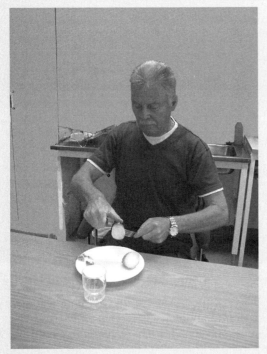

Figure 21-14   Relearning to use cutlery.

Observe Client's Task Performance and Implement Performance Analysis

As the OTIPM is followed, it is time for Maria to observe August doing some of the tasks that he identified as being problematic for him. This first performance analysis will give Maria the opportunity to evaluate the quality of the client's performance when executing a chosen task. Maria planned to use a standardized instrument to evaluate August's performance, and she decided to use the AMPS, for her performance analysis. Since the tasks that August had problems performing were not available as task choices in the AMPS, she did the observation with her "AMPS eyes" and could thus describe his performance using the AMPS vocabulary, but she was not able to enter the information into the AMPS software. The information was still very valuable and helped her in her documentation of August's performance.

Make a Phone Call and Take Notes. In August's case, the occupational therapist wanted to observe the client perform some daily tasks that he experienced difficulties performing and that he had prioritized. August chose to start by showing how he used the telephone. The observation was carried out at the OT department, using the telephone of the occupational therapist. It became obvious that August was not able to hold the receiver in an effective manner, as it slid out of his hand. He was not able to hold it long enough, so that he would be able to make notes at the same time with the pen in his right hand.

After the observation, Maria and August discussed how he had experienced the task, and the occupational therapist told him what she had observed as his strengths and limitations during his performance. Maria also suggested that he could do the task by leaning the elbow on the table, but August expressed a need to do the task without elbow support.

Peel Boiled Potatoes with Knife and Fork. At the third observation, August performed the task of peeling a boiled potato on a plate in front of him at the kitchen table. He sat on a chair by the table and had the plate with potatoes in front of him, with cutlery on the side of the plate (fork to the right and knife to the left of the plate). It was hard for August to turn his left hand in an effective manner to put the fork into the potatoes. As he pierced the potato on the fork, he had difficulty holding it to peel the skin off with the knife in his right hand. His arm was unsteady, and he was not able to hold the position for the amount of time needed to peel the whole potato. He managed slightly better when he leaned his left lower arm on the table, but still did not have an effective performance.

Define and Describe Actions the Client Does and Does Not Perform Effectively

The occupational therapist made a note in the patient file about the observed and measured baseline.

Baseline: August managed to perform the task "making a phone call" with a mild degree of effort (the grip on the receiver), a modest degree of disorganization, and an undesirable use of time (he lost his grip and needed to use his right hand instead), which resulted in the inability to make notes at the same time as he spoke on the phone.

Grouping Skills of Most Concern into Meaningful Clusters. August's limitations can be summarized into the following clusters:

Cluster 1: Positions and Coordinates. August needs to place the arm in a position that facilitates continuation of the task and coordinate both limbs. August has limited ability to hold the arm in the needed position long enough to make notes with his right hand.

Cluster 2: Grips, Manipulates with His Left Hand, and Lifts. August has a limitation in holding the fork in his left hand in a position to facilitate peeling with the knife in the right hand.

Cluster 3: Attends and Organizes. August showed limitations in listening to the conversation on the telephone at the same time as he took notes. The limitation was increased as the pen and paper were placed too far away at the desk

Cluster 4: Paces, Heeds, Chooses, Continues, and Sequences. August also had strengths. August shows a nice pace as he performs the tasks, and he also works toward completion of the task. He chooses the tools and materials, and works continuously without interruption and completes both tasks in an orderly sequence.

Initial Evaluation
Baseline: Observed. When Maria, the occupational therapist, has summarized the strengths and limitations, she continues to document August's baseline, both the global baseline and the specific baseline. Both these baselines will be documented in the patient files and will be used as the base as the team plans the rehabilitation, including setting the goals with August.

Global Baseline: Making Phone Call. The occupational therapist documented in the files the observed and measurable global baseline: August managed the task of making a phone call with mild degree of effort and was moderately effective, which limited him to make the notes at the same time.

Specific Baseline: Making Phone Call. August had the pens far away from his sitting position, which made him have to reach far to pick one up in order to make notes. This provided some limitation since he had trouble holding the receiver with his left hand at the same time. He had limited ability to grip and coordinate. He was also limited in attending to the task of talking in the phone, since he needed to concentrate on holding the receiver in his left hand and simultaneously making notes with his right hand. August was ineffective in accommodating his actions and his work area.

Global Baseline: Peeling Potato. August performed the task of peeling the potatoes using cutlery with moderate effort and a mild degree of disorganization.

Specific Baseline: Peeling Potato. August had problems manipulating the fork in a necessary way with his left hand, which resulted in limitations in the ability to pierce the fork into the potato and position it for ease of peeling with the knife in the right hand. His elbow was angled out from the body as he performed the task. He hesitated before he accommodated by putting the arm onto the table for support.

In the same manner, Maria evaluated the other highly prioritized tasks: to shoot with a hunting rifle and to walk the dog. These observations were made at a shooting range and at home as he walked his dog.

Define/Clarify or Interpret the Cause. When Maria had evaluated the quality of her client's performance, she continued to clarify or interpret the cause of the limitations observed. This can be done by taking into account all information collected during the establishment of the client-centered performance context, by thinking about that the observations made on the client's performance, and by administering other evaluations through interviews and nonstandardized or standardized evaluations. To underscore the unique focus in OT on activity and participation, activity and participation must be documented.

When Maria looked through her notes from the ten dimensions, she saw that August's problem was mainly related to his hemiparetic left arm and leg. Maria also noted that August had a swollen left hand, increased spasticity, and decreased coordination in the elbow and hand. This influenced his occupational performance and primarily the fine motor aspects of the performance. Due to his left-sided weakness, he also had problems with balance; however, Maria did not need to investigate that further, since she had information from the interdisciplinary team members to confirm these observations. During the team conference held once a week, the whole team received a very thorough picture of the client, as all members of the team presented their results of evaluations and tests to the other team members.

Initial Occupational Therapy Evaluation and Interpretation of Cause

Decreased motor function in the left side, increased tone, and decreased balance influenced how August performed his prioritized daily tasks. Decreased fine motor control, a swollen hand, and decreased strength in his left hand had disrupted his ability to grip and manipulate objects. Attending to two things simultaneously was also limited. The decreased balance and muscle weakness in his leg affected his ability to walk in the forest and walk the dog.

Document Client's Baseline and Goals

The interdisciplinary team met with August to plan and set goals to reach during the rehabilitation period. Maria brought her notes of the global and specific baselines, and together they set the following goals:

- To eat a meal using both knife and fork without effort and in an efficient manner
- To talk on the phone and make simultaneous notes effectively and with minimal effort
- To hold a rifle in a safe and effective way
- To walk the dog independently and safely in the forest.

Maria needed to select an intervention model, and plan and implement occupation-based interventions. Each member of the team worked according to his or her specific focus and towards those goals. For example, the physiotherapist worked with training of underlying body functions (i.e., increase balance, muscle strength, endurance, fine motor) to strengthen August's body, so that he could meet his goals. The occupational therapist continued her process in line with OTIPM and now the time had come to choose a model for intervention that would cover the goals and focus on occupations.

Occupation-Based Interventions in Instrumental Activities of Daily Life

Intervention Plan

Acquisitional occupation: making phone calls, eating with cutlery

Adaptive occupation: using the air gun (available in OT department), sitting at a table with support under arm, taking the dog for a walk, and doing "Nordic walking" with poles with supervision from wife

Restorative occupation: introduced to a program to practice training with affected hand using therapeutic putty at home. Received a glove for compression of hand to prevent edema of the hand

August visited the day rehabilitation unit and met the occupational therapist twice a week. In between, he practiced everyday at home with a self-training program and other home tasks. Since the occupational therapist had made a home visit earlier, she was able to give precise and concrete advice on what to do and how to go about performing tasks at home. For example, she encouraged him to answer the phone at home using his left hand, turning on the switch of the lights also using his left hand, practicing peeling potatoes at meals at home, and, with his wife, taking walks with their dog using walking poles.

Acquisitional Occupation to Reacquire, Develop, or Maintain Occupational Skill

At the day rehabilitation clinic, Maria and August decided to start training the task of making a phone call and taking notes, and the task of peeling boiled potatoes using a knife and fork, since both these goals were possible to reach in a short time. August practices these two tasks at every occasion during OT (two times, 45 minutes each week). To use the cutlery, the training was done in the training kitchen at the clinic, and the telephone practice was done in the OT office. The aim of the practice was for August to practice to use efficient grips as much as possible, and to practice multiple repetitions of the task. For example, in the early sessions August peeled one to two potatoes, and it took him up to 10 minutes, and at the end of therapy, he managed five to six potatoes in the same time frame. The occupational therapist also encouraged him to practice in between sessions at home. After about one month, the goals were met.

Adaptive Occupation to Compensate for Ineffective Actions

When those first goals were met, they proceeded with the goal focused on shooting with a hunting rifle. Since the goal was to shoot with his own rifle, it was safer for both August and Maria to start with an air gun inside a shooting range. The occupational therapist thus used a shooting range available at another OT department in the hospital. August started to practice sitting in an office chair with wheels that needed to be locked before starting. The chair was placed in front of a table with a large piece of foam-rubber to be used as a support for the elbow under his left arm (Fig. 21-15). He practiced shooting about 30 to 35 minutes each session.

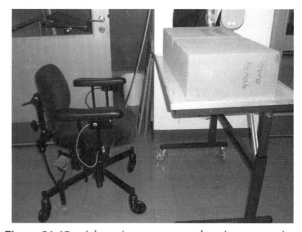

Figure 21-15   Adaptations to support hunting occupation.

Initially he needed frequent breaks, but as he continued to practice, he became stronger and needed fewer breaks. August was skilled and managed to perform the task in an effective and safe manner after some practice. But as time came to discharge August, there was concern that his own heavier hunting rifle would be too difficult for him to use. Since Maria and the rest of the team had the opinion that August did not have any serious cognitive impairments after his stroke, they encouraged August to practice with his own rifle in their shooting range when he felt he was ready. August also thought of acquiring an elbow support, a portable telescope pole with a "u" for the elbow, for use when he hunted in the forest.

Restorative Occupation to Restore Personal Factors and Body Function

Initially in the rehabilitation period, the occupational therapist prepared a program for hand training with therapeutic putty that August could use himself to practice, intensify the home training, and hopefully minimize the edema in his left hand. Maria also tried out a compression glove for treatment of the edema. She informed August to use the glove during day time when the hand was not engaged.

Intervention Summary

- Occupational training to peel boiled potatoes and make phone calls
- Home exercise program with training therapeutic putty and eating with cutlery at home
- Air-rifle shooting at a shooting range
- Reevaluate for enhanced and satisfying occupational performance

Documentation of Client's Current Ability and Result

When August made progress, it was important for the occupational therapist to document this in his files. Since August could evaluate his own ability in an adequate manner, Maria also assessed August by asking him how he managed in the different occupations. In this way, she did not have to observe him in all tasks to appraise his progress.

After one month of training, August managed to safely hold the receiver of the telephone and simultaneously make notes (Fig. 21-16). He could also peel potatoes using a knife and fork and eat with all cutlery again. The more August used his left hand actively in daily tasks, the more the edema diminished. When he was discharged after five and a half months (i.e., 34 treatment sessions), the goal to be able to walk in the forest and to safely walk the dog using a pole for support also were achieved. He was also able to shoot with an air gun with support under his elbow. He had not been able to try hunting yet, since the hunting season had not yet started. See evaluation of results in Table 21-2.

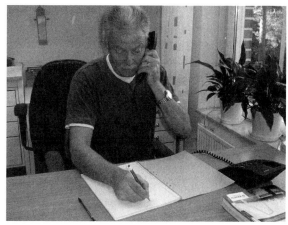

Figure 21-16 Improved occupational performance related to work tasks.

Table 21-2

Evaluation of Results

GOAL	BASELINE STATUS	CURRENT STATUS
To eat a meal using both knife and fork without effort and in an efficient manner	August performed the task of peeling the potatoes using cutlery with moderate effort and a mild degree of disorganization.	August can manage to eat a meal without effort and effectively with both cutlery.
To talk on the phone and take simultaneous notes effectively and with minimal effort	August managed the task of making a phone call with mild degree of effort and was moderately effective, which limited his taking notes at the same time.	August can talk in the telephone and take notes simultaneously in an effective manner and without effort.
To hold a rifle in a safe and effective way	August could hold an air gun in shooting position, with support under left elbow, safely and with mild ineffectiveness.	August can shoot with an air gun, sitting with support under left elbow, in a safe and effective manner
To walk the dog independently and safely in the forest	August needed support from one person and walking sticks to safely walk in the forest.	August can walk the dog in the forest independently and safely if using a walking pole.

Results. August had reached all his goals according to the initial plan from when he started his rehabilitation. After another three months, a follow-up phone call was made, and he then informed the team that he was able to use his hunting rifle at the shooting range when he had the elbow support attached to his left elbow. Less than one year after his stroke, August also was able to return to hunting.

REVIEW QUESTIONS

1. What are the key components of the OTIPM?
2. What are four examples of motor and process skills included on the AMPS?
3. What are examples of interventions that would be considered *adaptive occupation*?
4. What are examples of interventions that would be considered *acquisitional occupation*?
5. What are examples of interventions that would be considered *restorative occupation*?
6. What are examples of interventions that would be considered *occupation-based educational programs*?

REFERENCES

1. Bond MJ, Clark MS: Clinical applications of the Adelaide Activities Profile. *Clin Rehabil* 12(3):228, 1998.
2. Fisher AG: *AMPS Assessment of motor and process skills. Volume 2: User manual* (6th ed.), Fort Collins, CO, 2006, Three Star Press.
3. Fisher AG: *Occupational therapy intervention process model*, Fort Collins, CO, 2009, Three Star Press.
4. Grimby G Andren, E Holmgren E, et al: Structure of a combination of functional independence measure and instrumental activity measure items in community-living persons: A study of individuals with cerebral palsy and spina bifida. *Arch Phys Med Rehabil* 77(11):1109, 1996.
5. Hall P, Weaver L: Interdisciplinary education and teamwork: a long and winding road. *Med Educ* 35(9):867–875, 2001.
6. Holbrook M, Skilbeck CE: An activities index for use with stroke patients. *Age Ageing* 12(2):166, 1983.
7. Law M, Baptiste S, Carswell A, McColl MA, et al: *Canadian occupational performance measure* (Rev. 4th ed.), Ottawa, Ontario, 2005, CAOT Publications ACE.
8. Lawton, MP, Brody, EM: Assessment of older people: Self-maintaining and instrumental activities of daily living. *Gerontologist* 9(3):179–186, 1969.
9. Legg LA: Therapy-based rehabilitation services for stroke patients at home. *Cochrane Database Syst Rev* (1):CD002925, 2003.
10. Leipzig RM, Hyer K, Ek K, et al: Attitudes toward working on interdisciplinary healthcare teams: A comparison by discipline. *J Am Geriatr Soc* 50(6): 1114–1148, 2002.
11. National Board of Health and Welfare: *A grant to stimulate early and coordinated rehabilitation— about the rehabilitation process, content and application*. (in Swedish: "Stimulansbidrag för tidig och samordnad rehabilitering— om rehabiliteringsprocessen, innebörd och tillämpning".) 2000. 04 ISSN 1403–338, 2000.
12. Nouri FM, Lincoln NB: An extended activities of daily living scale for stroke patients. *Clin Rehabil* 1(4):123, 1987.
13. Park S: Enhancing Engagement in Instrumental Activities of Daily Living: An Occupational Therapy Perspective. In Gillen G. & Burkhardt A, editors: *Stroke Rehabilitation: A Function Based Approach*, 2nd edition, St. Louis, 2004, Elsevier.
14. Sonn U, Törnqvist K, Svensson E: The ADL taxonomy— from individual categorical data to ordinal categorical data. *Scand J Occup Ther* 6(1):11–20, 1999.
15. Steultjens EMJ, Dekker J, Bouter LM, et al: Evidence of the efficacy of occupational therapy in different conditions: an overview of systematic reviews. *Clin Rehabil* 19(3):247–254, 2004.
16. Törnqvist K, Sonn U: Towards an ADL taxonomy for occupational therapists. *Scand J Occup Ther* 1(2):69–76, 1994.
17. Whiting S, Lincoln NB: An ADL assessment for stroke patients. *Bri J Occup Ther* 43:44, 1980.

judith rogers
megan kirshbaum

chapter 22

Parenting after Stroke

key terms

adaptive baby care equipment   one-handed baby care   visual history

adaptive baby care techniques   transition tasks

chapter objectives

After completing this chapter, the reader will be able to accomplish the following:

1. Describe visual history.
2. Describe transitional tasks.
3. Have a basic understanding of one-handed baby care task performance.
4. Identify examples of adapted baby care equipment.
5. Apply parent child collaboration to a baby care task.
6. Identify an emotional or cognitive problem that can affect baby care.
7. Appreciate the importance of teamwork between occupational therapists and mental health practitioners in services to parents who have had strokes.

This chapter will discuss caring for an infant or child by those who have had a stroke. The chapter will raise issues that caregivers and prospective caregivers may encounter and will provide options available to them. The focus is mainly on physical caring of infants, but also includes emotional and cognitive issues relevant to parenting children of varied ages. The goal of this chapter is to provide practical advice to occupational therapists, so they can help caregivers find adaptive methods to carry out the tasks of childcare.

Although strokes are most common after the age of 65-years-old, they can occur at any age. For example, women may have a stroke during pregnancy or during the postpartum period. Men or women may have strokes before considering parenthood or when they already have

children. Grandparents who have had strokes may want to participate fully in the lives of their grandchildren or may need to act as primary caregivers.

Some people may feel that the task is insurmountable, but experience has indicated that bringing up a child is an achievable goal for many stroke survivors. In fact, working toward this goal can increase confidence, help reintegrate the family, enhance general functioning, and reduce feelings of depression.

Material in the chapter is based primarily on intervention and research with parents with physical or cognitive disabilities and their children at *Through the Looking Glass* (TLG) in Berkeley, California, since its founding in 1982. TLG is a disability culture and independent living-based organization that has pioneered research, training, resource development, and services for families in which a family member has a disability or medical issue, and is The National Center for Parents with Disabilities and their Families, funded by National Institute on Disability and Rehabilitation Research (NIDRR), U.S. Department of Education. Illustrative examples in this chapter are based on services provided to TLG clients who had strokes and raised babies and children. This research and intervention framework is summarized, as follows, focusing on points that are particularly salient for serving parents who have experienced strokes.

RESEARCH ON PARENT/CHILD COLLABORATION

The groundbreaking study of the interaction of mothers with physical disabilities and their babies (funded by the National Easter Seal Research Foundation, 1985 to 1988) documented the reciprocal and natural process of adaptation to disability obstacles as it developed between 10 mothers and their babies.[6] Basic care (feeding, bathing, lifting, carrying, dressing/diapering) was videotaped from birth through toddlerhood. These families were not receiving intervention or baby care adaptations. Analysis of videotapes mapped the gradual mutual adaptation process during interaction between parent and infant. Results documented the mothers' ingenuity in developing their own adaptations, the infants' early adaptation, and the mothers' facilitation of the infants' adaptation.

Based on the natural adaptation process recorded in this study, subsequent intervention was developed that facilitated collaboration between parent and infant during baby care tasks, such as that described in the Adaptive Techniques and Strategies section of this chapter.

RESEARCH ON BABY CARE ADAPTIVE EQUIPMENT

In the 1990s, TLG conducted three research projects (funded by NIDRR, U.S. Department of Education), specifically focused on developing and evaluating the impact of baby care adaptations for parents with physical disabilities.[6,12,14] The equipment development was informed by adaptations invented by mothers in the previous Easter Seal study. For example, in that study, several mothers lifted their babies with one hand by grasping their babies' clothing. In the subsequent baby care equipment development projects, TLG designed and used lifting harnesses as a more secure version of this natural adaptation. All three equipment studies used analyzed videotapes of care and interaction prior to and subsequent to providing baby care adaptive equipment. Such equipment was found to have a positive effect on parent/baby interaction, in addition to reducing difficulty, pain, and fatigue relating to baby care. The equipment also seemed to prevent secondary disability complications from

overstressing the body during care and to help reduce depression associated with postnatal onset or worsening of disability. By increasing the caregiving role of the parent with a disability, stress was lessened in the couple; there was more balance of functioning in the family system.

VISUAL HISTORY

TLG has emphasized the use of videotaping in both research and intervention because of the lack of images of parenting by individuals with physical disabilities, which affects diverse professionals, including occupational therapists, and parents and their family members. The occupational therapy (OT) team coined the term *visual history* to refer to the mental image most people have of the way a task is accomplished.[12] For example, when people imagine holding a baby, they think of a baby in someone's arms. Such limited visual histories may interfere with the goal of learning to accomplish a task in a new way. Thus, occupational therapists and clients need to be aware of their limited visual history and the need to expand and change it. For instance, holding a baby can be accomplished by attaching an infant car seat to a wheelchair (Fig. 22-1). In order to expand visual history regarding parenting, TLG has developed DVDs showing different techniques of accomplishing baby care tasks, including one-handed techniques often needed in parents who have experienced strokes.

OCCUPATIONAL THERAPY ASSESSMENT TO GUIDE BABY CARE ADAPTATIONS

TLG developed an assessment tool to guide occupational practice with parents with disabilities and their babies and toddlers. The assessment provides a framework for understanding the complexity of OT support of caring for a baby when a parent has a physical disability. This

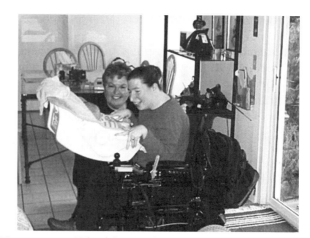

Figure 22-1   Wheelchair and infant car seat adaptations to support parenting occupations.

assessment tool, *The Baby Care Assessment for Parents with Physical Limitations or Disabilities*,[15] guides the OT practitioner in intervention work and analyzing potential obstacles. It brings together the parent's perspective and the occupational therapist's skill in task analysis. This tool provides an extensive review of all baby care functioning within the home and community relative to the parent's needs and/or wishes. The tool identifies the parent's strengths and highlights the obstacles that are interfering with his or her ability to complete the task in the least demanding, most efficient, safe, and ergonomic manner and with a method that supports and enhances the parent-child relationship. This assessment tool also has a parent interview section, which helps the occupational therapist find the activities important to the parent. It incorporates the disability philosophy of independent living, i.e., having opportunities to make decisions that affect one's life and to choose which activities one wants to pursue. It should be noted that the assessment emphasizes visiting in the home and community.

INTERVENTION MODEL

TLG's research has informed its intervention with thousands of parents with disabilities and their children. The intervention model has been described and rigorously evaluated since the 1980s, demonstrating positive outcomes with particularly stressed families in which parent and/or child has a disability.[5,6] The intervention model includes multidisciplinary teamwork emphasizing:

1. Infant/parent and family relationships, integrating infant mental health and family systems expertise
2. Parenting and intervention adaptations to address diverse disability issues
3. Developmental expertise regarding infants and children
4. Integrating and respecting personal/family disability and cultural experience
5. Functioning in the natural environment, through home and community-based assessment, intervention, monitoring, and referrals

A family in which a parent has experienced a stroke is usually served in the home and community by an occupational therapist who assesses and provides baby care adaptations, introduces cognitive adaptations, consults on environmental access, and monitors infant/child development issues and continued safety and appropriateness of the adaptations over time. The occupational therapist works closely with the home visiting mental health practitioner who attends to the emotional issues in parent, child, and family, such as grieving, loss, depression, volatility or impulse control, management of children's behavior, couple conflict, and changes in family roles and functioning. Both providers facilitate interaction between parents and their infants or children and monitor safety and well-being of

the child. Ongoing training and reflective supervision are integral to these services.

Working with Pregnant Women Poststroke

Working with a woman who is trying to decide whether to become pregnant or who is in the first trimester of pregnancy is a challenge for the OT practitioner who has to imagine both how pregnancy may impact the client's mobility and how her limitations may affect her ability to care for the baby. It is helpful for women to understand that physical difficulties from a stroke need not close off the option to have a child. During pregnancy, mobility generally is affected from the latter part of the second trimester, when the center of gravity has changed, to delivery.[10] This change in the center of gravity will most likely affect walking, standing up, and/or transferring in and out of bed, cars, etc. See Chapters 14 and 15. The woman may benefit from a mobility device (walker or wheelchair/scooter). It might be beneficial to consult a physical therapist. If the leg is mildly involved, a rollator (four-wheeled walker) would be a good choice. It could not only make her stable but also could be used for carrying her baby around the house. If the affected leg is very involved, walking can be difficult, and a motorized wheelchair/scooter could be the most appropriate choice. See Chapter 26.

Willingness to accept a motorized vehicle (wheelchair or scooter) can be problematic for the prospective mother. It is important for the future mother to understand that the wheelchair/scooter would make her more comfortable, less likely to fall, and more able to conserve energy and care for the baby after birth. If she tries a motorized piece of equipment for an activity such as shopping, she may realize how easy some activities can be. She may also be concerned about how she will be able to care for the baby. A discussion of the adaptive techniques described in this chapter may ease her mind about solutions to physical limitations. However, a crucial issue in decision-making about parenthood is how the stroke has affected emotional and cognitive functioning.

Facilitating Relationships between Babies and Parents Poststroke

Without appropriate supports, a stroke occurring late in pregnancy or postpartum can be devastating to a mother, family, and infant/parent relationship. Since hospitalization creates a separation between mother and child, it is critical to consider the need to promote attachment during the subacute phase of rehabilitation. The occupational therapist should have attachment activities as part of the treatment plan. Attachment activities will change depending on the age of the baby or child. All baby care activities can support the relationship between parent and child. However, if the baby is under 9-months-old, holding, feeding, and soothing are particularly essential activities.

If the caregiver has sustained a stroke when his or her child is a toddler, or if the caregiver who had sustained an earlier stroke comes in seeking help, the emphasis is more on supporting and scaffolding interaction between parent and child, for instance during play, snack, snuggle time, and outings, in order to promote the parent and child relationship.

Facilitating Physical Care by the Parent

Being able to provide physical care to the baby is one of the essential elements in parenting. For a caregiver who has had a stroke to pursue the dream of caring for a baby, he or she may need baby care equipment, appropriate durable medical equipment (DME), and adaptive techniques. *Transitional tasks* refer to tasks that are necessary before accomplishing or between basic baby care tasks. Therefore, it is important to begin intervention with these tasks: (1) holding, (2) carrying and moving, (3) transfers, and (4) positional change.[12]

- Holding: The task of holding is a prerequisite for carrying, transferring, feeding, changing, burping, or comforting your child.
- Carrying and moving: The task of carrying is a prerequisite for moving around the house and community. If a caregiver cannot carry or move the baby, then he or she will be confined to functioning in one room.
- Transfers: The task of transfer is a prerequisite to being able to do several activities such as diapering and putting the baby into a crib or high chair
- Positional change: The task of positional change is a prerequisite for being able to burp a baby or diaper change a baby. A positional change is defined as changing a position of the baby while the baby remains on the same surface.

Holding

Holding involves contact with the baby, whether it is directly in the mother's arms or with the aid of a holding device. It is essential that the parent feel confident that the baby is secure and for the baby to experience this security. Useful positions and holding devices for a parent with limited sitting balance include:

- Side lying for both baby and parent
- Parent's bed at 45 degree angle, sitting
- Sling, nursing pillows, wedge pillow

CASE STUDY 1

Darla had a cerebellar stroke at 8½ months of pregnancy. Immediately following the stroke, her son David was delivered by caesarean section. He was healthy and weighed 6 pounds 10 ounces. His lungs were fully developed, and he did not need hospitalization, so he was discharged at 3-days-old and went home with John, his dad. Darla's parents moved in to help with David. Darla was in a coma in intensive care unit for several days. As soon as she was transferred to the subacute unit, her family was able to bring David to her. The hospital staff put David in a sling baby carrier. Although David was secured in the sling, Darla feared that he would fall. The hospital staff was unaware that her concern was because of her need for some support when sitting. She had not yet gained sufficient trunk control and increased sitting balance, so holding her baby increased her anxiety. In this situation, the occupational therapist could have checked with Darla and discovered why she felt insecure holding her baby, and then a more appropriate position could have been found. One such position would have been to have her lie on her more affected side with David side lying on her arm, so that they could look at each other and so that Darla could kiss and touch him.

Carrying and Moving

TLG has recommended a four-wheeled walker, also known as a rollator, for safely moving the baby around the house. This walker has been used successfully with caregivers with hemiplegia (where half of the body is paralyzed) and with those with ataxia (problems with coordination), because it keeps both baby and parent physically stable. This piece of equipment consists of a baby carrier securely attached to a walker seat. The baby carrier can be a bouncy seat or a booster seat, although the former is more difficult to attach. TLG prefers a feeding seat that can be positioned in several ways, such as reclining for an infant or more upright for the older baby. Moreover, having a baby seat on the walker positions the baby at an optimal height for transfers (Fig. 22-2).

When the walker is introduced depends on the stability of the parent. It has been successfully used during inpatient physical therapy to help prepare the caregiver for going home. However, it is designed to be used only within a household. Extreme caution needs to be used if the adapted walker is moved over any uneven or raised surface since it is top heavy with a baby on it. In consultation with a rehabilitation engineer, adding weights to the lower part of the walker can be considered to compensate for the added weight of the baby. Otherwise, strategies are used by parents with physical disabilities that may be less feasible with parents that also have cognitive difficulties, i.e., putting the back wheels over the raised surface separately, lifting one of the sides of the walker over the raised surface with an arm, or using a leg to nudge one side of the walker at a time. The occupational therapist should

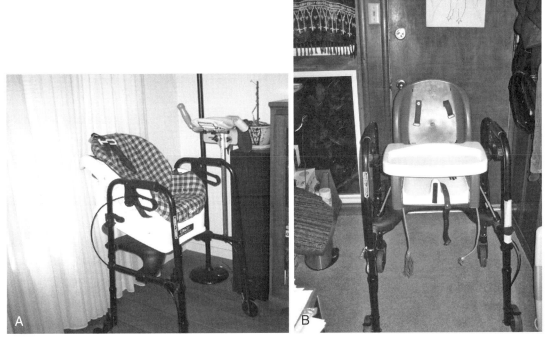

Figure 22-2 **A** and **B,** Walker and baby seat adaptations to support parenting occupations.

carefully assess the safe use of the adapted walker during home visits.

If the parent prefers or needs to use a manual or motorized wheelchair, there are several types of devices for holding the baby.[11] The following adaptations are especially easy to use. Using a wedged piece of form as wide as the parent's lap, 8 inches thick at the parent's knees, and slanted down to 3 inches thick at the parent's waist can provide a surface for moving, feeding, and playing with the baby. The wedge should be covered in washable fabric and have a strap attached to go around the parent's waist, and a strap attached to hold the baby securely on the pillow (Fig. 22-3). Another design that can be used for an older baby with good head control is

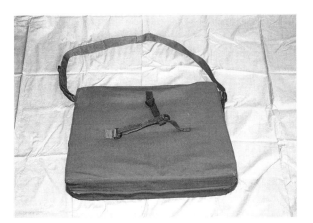

Figure 22-3 Adapted wedge to support parenting occupations.

the double neck pillow, which consists of two neck pillows.

Positional Changes
Positional change examples are described in the discussion of burping and diapering in the Adaptive Techniques and Strategies section of the chapter.

Transfers
Lifting an infant who does not yet have head control can pose a challenge for people with limited upper extremity use. The easiest solution is to use a baby carrier sling (see equipment chart). If the baby does not accept the sling, the following technique can be used while a parent is in a sitting position in order to transfer from lap to surface. (1) Choose or arrange surfaces that are high enough to avoid back strain. (2) Place the functional hand under the baby's head. (3) Bend over and simultaneously pull the baby to caregiver's chest. The chest acts like another arm to support and hold the baby. (4) Straighten up and move the baby. A caregiver can wear a fanny pack stuffed full of soft material that can provide additional support for the baby's bottom (Fig. 22-4). It is crucial to assess whether a parent can move in a balanced and secure way from a sit to a standing position holding the baby in this manner.

Caregivers have been successful using a lifting harness to transfer the baby from one surface to another. Note that the lifting harness cannot be used until the baby has head control, so prior to this period parents should use

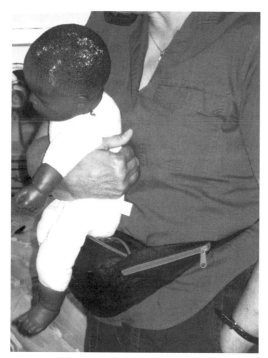

Figure 22-4   Adapted fanny pack to support parenting occupations.

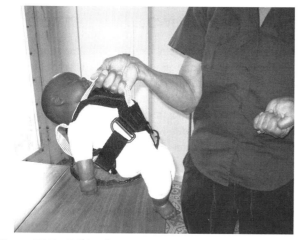

Figure 22-5   Lifting harness to support parenting occupations.

an infant carrier sling. A good template for making a harness is using a baby vest on the market (www. babybair.com) with added straps using one inch webbing (Fig. 22-5). Lifting a toddler with a harness can produce repetitive stress injury, because of the added weight. Therefore, toddlers should be taught to climb onto the desired surface using parent-child collaboration techniques. If the surface is too high, TLG has found steps with short risers, making them easier for toddlers to climb.

Michael, an older father and the primary caregiver of his son, had a stroke affecting his left hemisphere shortly after his son Sam's birth. His wife Karen worked full time. His right arm was more involved than his leg. When Sam was 1-year-old, he was in the 70% percentile in height and weight. Michael was still successful using the lifting harness to transfer Sam. Michael wanted to continue using it even though he was experiencing considerable pain in his left shoulder. An occupational therapist from TLG showed him the adaptive technique of giving Sam a boost up to a higher surface by reaching between his legs from behind Sam's back. This approach provided enough advantage for Sam to climb up and importantly reduced the use of Michael's shoulder muscles and lessened his pain. The occupational therapist's developmental background helped her know when to introduce Sam to climbing that would help with care. She brought steps, so Sam could climb into the high chair.

Providing Adaptive Baby Care Equipment

Appropriate equipment can make caring for a child possible for a person who has had a stroke. Some equipment is essential for use in conjunction with certain techniques, while other items simply make the tasks easier or may be crucial to care.

Bedtime

TLG gets more calls about issues with bedtime than any other topic. For most clients, the greatest difficulty occurs in the course of the transfer activity of putting the baby in bed. The parent can often enjoy the ritual of dressing his or her child in night clothes, reading a book, cuddling, and perhaps singing a song, but since most cribs are inaccessible, the soothing bedtime activities feel incomplete, resulting in frustration for parent and child alike.

Some commercially available infant beds allow the child to sleep with the parent, but these have flaws. The Co-Sleeper, which attaches to the adult bed, poses problems for parents with disabilities, since it can make it difficult to get out of bed. The parent must slide to the foot of the bed to get out. Another make, the Snuggle Nest, lasts only a few months because only the youngest infants fit into them.

Commercially available cribs can be adapted to meet the needs of parents with physical disabilities, but the occupational therapist must be careful to consider safety in choosing an adaptation. TLG does not recommend cribs with gate openings because the baby can roll out when the parent backs away in order to open the side. TLG recommends use of a sliding door design, so that the parent can block the entrance with her body as the door slides to the side. When using a sliding door, one needs to install a lock that is workable for the parent but not for the child. TLG has used a two-step lock, but this could be difficult for a parent who has apraxia or sequencing issues. TLG does not recommend using a top bar to stabilize the sliding door because babies can hit their heads coming out, especially if the baby is already crying and upset. Adaptations of commercially available cribs cause problems to structural integrity; therefore, adapted cribs need to be frequently checked to assure safety (Fig. 22-6).

Childproofing

Home visiting is essential to address childproofing. Some childproofing can be adult proofing, since devices may be too complicated for a parent because of cognitive and physical difficulty. It is necessary to try several types of devices to see which one is successful. The process will be an opportunity to assess visual and visual neglect issues, apraxia, sequencing, and motor planning. See Chapters 16 to 18. It should be noted that access without raised thresholds for walkers and wheelchair access needs to be considered when using safety gates.

Diapering Equipment

Following a stroke, some parents find it more comfortable to sit when diapering, while others still prefer to stand. For those who prefer to sit, there are several options using computer tables. Computer tables come in different sizes, shapes, and costs. For families who may not have space for another table and need to conserve space in their house, a dining room table works well. If a table is used for another activity, it is important to have a diapering surface that can be removed from the table. Whether the parent sits or stands, it is very helpful to use a toy mobile that uses interactive toys to keep the baby occupied during the diapering process. Using a concave diapering pad and a safety strap is essential to prevent the baby from rolling off a desk or table. If the pad is put on a table, it may slip around. If the pad is attached to plywood, the pad will be prevented from slipping around, and a toy mobile can be used.

To make this piece of equipment, use a piece of plywood 1½" wider than the concave diapering pad, and cover the bottom of the wood with nonslip shelving material. A threaded phalange is added to the plywood, so PVC piping for the mobile can be attached to the plywood. Drilling holes into the polyvinyl chloride (PVC) piping and fastening an electrical cord affixes interactive toys, such as squeaky animals or plastic books (Fig. 22-7).

Examples of Equipment on the Market

Prior to customizing or developing new baby care adaptations, the occupational therapist should explore the changing options of commercially available equipment that can support baby care by a parent who has experienced a stroke (Table 22-1).

Durable Medical Equipment

In addition to baby care equipment, the caregiver may need assistive mobility technology, such as a power wheelchair, scooter, or four-wheeled walker. Transporting the baby safely can increase the need for this equipment. DME can be an issue to a caregiver within the household or if he or she cannot keep up with the family out in the community. Unfortunately, the caregiver may face difficulties acquiring appropriate mobility equipment, as there may be no coverage if he or she can walk within the household or inadequate coverage of costs (such as for a motorized wheelchair).

Adaptive Techniques and Strategies

These techniques were devised for the caregiver who has the use, or partial use, of one arm.[16] Many of these techniques also emphasize baby collaboration with the parent.

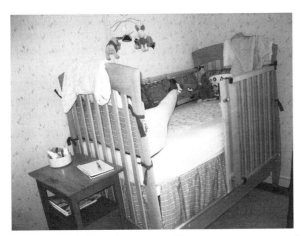

Figure 22-6 Adaptations to crib to support parenting occupations.

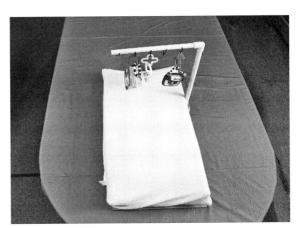

Figure 22-7 Adapted diapering surface to support parenting occupations.

Table 22-1

Commercially Available Baby Care Equipment

ACTIVITY OR TASK	COMMERCIALLY AVAILABLE EQUIPMENT
Bed time Cosleeper (attached to the parent's bed)	Arms Reach cosleeper (can make it difficult for the caregiver to get out of bed)
Cosleep in parent's bed	Snuggle Nest
Diapering	1. A computer table can be used to change the baby while sitting. 2. A concave diapering pad should be used. 3. A toy mobile with interactive toys to entertain the baby during long diapering.
Dressing	1. Long one-piece suits with zippers by Gerber and others with key rings attached to zippers 2. Onesies (T-shirt closure at the crotch) with Velcro closure 3. Fleece bunting with no legs for winter
Holding equipment	1. Infant carrier sling can be used lying down, seated, and standing. 2. Nursing pillows (Hugster, Boppy, Kid Kozy, My Baby Nest) can be used lying down and seated.
Breastfeeding	1. Easy Expression bra supports the breast and can hold a pump in place. 2. Breast shield or breast shell
Bottle feeding	Bottle holders
Burping	Lifting harness adapted from (Babybair) vest
Carrying and moving for a parent who has hemiplegia/paresis and/or ataxia	Four-wheeled walker (Rollator) with seat attached
Wheelchair user (motorized) with use of one hand	Sling (see previously)
Transfers	Lifting harness adapted from (Babybair) vest
Going out into the community	1. Car seats (try fastening the straps at the store) 2. Walking harness: toddler backpack, child safety harness backpack 3. Stroller (look for attributes: lightweight, easy to collapse, easy to open, easy to transfer baby)

During inpatient rehabilitation services, the OT clinician can introduce baby care techniques. It is important to include baby care tasks in the treatment plan. For example, some of the patient's own activities can serve two purposes. As the caregiver learns how to dress herself, he or she can also learn how to dress the baby. This can motivate the parent and help reduce depression.

Feeding: Combining Adaptive Baby Care Equipment and Techniques

Feeding is one of the most important aspects of care in the formation and maintenance of a parent/child relationship.

Breastfeeding. Being able to breastfeed can be important for the relationship between mother and baby and can give the mother self-confidence and hope that she can continue her role as mom. If the mother's stroke was due to high blood pressure, she may need blood pressure medication and/or blood thinners, which could affect breast milk and therefore breastfeeding. Prior to breastfeeding, it is important to consult with physicians

regarding possible harm to the baby from medications being used. An additional source of this information is the Organization of Teratology Information Specialists at (866) 626-6847.

If the mother breastfed prior to hospitalization and she would like to continue breastfeeding during hospitalization, it will require the availability of the family or other support people, so the baby can breastfeed regularly. If she wants to breastfeed but is unable to see the baby often enough, a breast pump can be used to express milk until she reunites with her baby. The breast milk can help her feel connected with her baby and feel that she is the source of the best possible nourishment. A useful bra for pumping is one that contains the pump, so it is hands-free (Easy Expression). In addition, the bra exposes the areola, making it easier for the baby to latch on since the breast tissue is held back and hand use is not needed. A "breast shield" or "breast shell," also used for flat or inverted nipples, can also be used to hold the areola back.

Finding a good position to feed the baby is critical. To hold and feed the baby on the nonaffected side can be emotionally disconcerting, because the mother cannot use her functional arm. Therefore, it is usually best to position the baby on a pillow rather than the nonaffected arm. It is important to try various breastfeeding pillows on the market to see what works best, and it is best to use a pillow with a waist strap, so it will be secured on the mother's lap.

Bottle Feeding. Sometimes the new mother may decide to bottle feed, which can be a good choice and should be respected. Bottle feeding is another task that promotes the parent/child relationship, but holding a bottle can be difficult. A bottle holder can eliminate the frustration a parent may experience when trying to hold both the baby and bottle steady. Bottle holders can be found on the Internet. Important problems relating to formula preparation are dealt with in the Cognitive Issues section.

Burping
Whether breastfeeding or bottle feeding, most people with the use of one functional arm need a technique to help the infant burp. Typically, visual history involves a picture of burping a baby over the shoulder. For many parents with a disability, burping over the shoulder can be difficult or impossible, as it requires both coordination and the use of two arms. However, there are other equally effective techniques, and learning them can increase the caregiver's sense of confidence and independence. One of the successful techniques developed by TLG is called the *sit and lean.* This is an example of a positional change, a transitional task discussed earlier. Using this method, the caregiver holds the baby on his or her lap facing away from the body. Supporting the baby by placing one arm across the baby's chest, the caregiver then leans forward. This puts gentle pressure on the baby's stomach and facilitates a burp.[16]

Another technique is to lay the baby prone (face down) on the caregiver's lap and pat the baby's back.[10] Alternatively, the caregiver can lay the baby on the right side, rolled slightly towards the stomach and rub on the back.

A third technique begins with lifting the baby's legs up before putting the baby into a sit, with the parent then putting his or her hand under the baby's bottom and bouncing upwards.

Diapering
In diapering a child, application of the parent-child collaborative technique is essential. Most babies can be "trained" to do the "bottoms up" technique. Parents can teach their baby to lift his or her bottom by lifting the baby's bottom with the working arm and saying, "Up, up" simultaneously. With time, many babies will then lift their bottoms when cued with the words "up, up or butt up." With infants who are premature or still mostly in the flexed position, the caregiver can rest the baby's bottom on the caregiver's functional palm and lift the child onto the diaper.

Fastening the Diaper. After the caregiver places the diaper under the baby and brings the diaper through the legs, the front of the caregiver's wrist should rest on the baby's pelvis in order to secure the diaper. The thumb and one to two fingers grab the tab or corner, and then the remaining fingers of the same hand walk the tab over to fasten it down. On the other side of the diaper, some of the fingers hold the diaper tab or corner, while the remaining fingers and palm hold the diaper steady to fasten the tab

Nighttime. Many parents find it more difficult to be coordinated in the middle of the night. One mother devised a method to help her overcome this problem. She put two diapers on her baby at bedtime. The only thing she had to do in the middle of the night was to pull the interior diaper out and then refasten the remaining one.

Position. Parents have varied preferences for their positions during diapering. Some caregivers prefer to have their functional arm closer to the baby's feet, while others prefer to have their functional arm closer to the baby's head, and still others prefer to face the baby's feet. Therefore, it is important for the caregiver to try each of those positions to find the most comfortable one.

Undressing and Dressing
Birth to 3-Years-Old. Dressing is one of the most difficult baby care activities to do one-handed. Many times parents with disability think that they should dress the baby as most people do, on the diapering surface. However, having a baby on the diapering table is generally harder for a parent who has the use of just one hand because they don't have enough advantage and control at such a distance from their body. The following techniques can help the caregiver make this task less difficult. In all cases, it is helpful if the clothing is a little too large, since it will come on and off more easily.

Dressing a Younger Baby. It is important to position the infant as close to one's body as possible, since it gives the best advantage. Using a nursing pillow such as the Hugster or Boppy will place the infant in a good position on the caregiver's lap and make maneuvering clothes over the baby's head easier. Easy open fasteners will facilitate dressing and undressing the baby. Snaps can be difficult to undo with one hand. Velcro closures and zippers are good substitutes for snaps.

Undressing a Younger Baby. After the clothing is unfastened, the parent begins with the sleeves, even if the baby is dressed in a one-piece garment. First, the hem of the sleeve needs to be pulled away from the baby with a slight shaking of the clothing, which will encourage the baby to flex a limb to withdraw it from the sleeve. The parent may need to ensure that the garment is not stuck on the elbow by pulling it around the joint. Once the elbow is out, the rest of the arm and hand should follow easily. This process should be repeated with the other arm. To remove a shirt, the front of the garment should be grasped and scrunched together from the neckline to the lower hem. Then it can be pulled away from the baby's face and lifted over the head from the front.

For dressing an infant in a "onesie" (a shirt that is prevented from riding up due to a closure between the legs) or shirt, the garment can be put on the top of the head as the baby lies on the nursing pillow. The front of the garment can be scrunched together from top to bottom and pulled over the back of the infant's head. The baby's head is held between the parent's forearm and chest. The front of the garment is scrunched up in the parent's hand, pulled away from the baby's face, and pulled down. Then the back of the baby's garment can be pulled down and the infant's arms pulled into the sleeves.

If the garment has a zipper, it does not matter if the arms or legs are put in first, though many parents prefer to put the arms in first and then the legs before fastening the zipper.

Dressing an Older Baby. When the baby is too large to fit on the caregiver's lap, it is helpful to place the baby near the parent such as on a bed and to use a nursing pillow for support. As with infants, it is important to find garments that have easy fasteners. To put a baby into a one-piece garment, first the fasteners should be undone and the item laid on the dressing surface near the parent. Next the baby is placed on top of the one-piece, the legs are put in first, and then the arm is directed into the sleeve. By pushing slightly on the elbow, the baby will be encouraged to extend his or her arm fully into the sleeve. These steps need to be repeated with the other sleeve and with the pant leg, encouraging the knees to extend.

Undressing an Older Baby. Removing a one-piece garment can be accomplished by using the following technique: After unzipping, pull the opening of the one-piece garment toward a shoulder. Pull the garment off the baby's shoulder. Then pull down from the hem of the sleeve to encourage the baby to withdraw the arm, and shake the clothing to encourage the baby to remove the arm entirely from the clothing. To remove the legs from the one-piece suit, the parent will pull the foot part of the clothing or pant legs away from the baby. If the baby has been encouraged with "butt up," the baby can help with lifting his or her butt and legs up while the pant legs are pulled off.

Socks. Putting on a baby sock is easier for the caregiver than putting on his or her own socks. The caregiver grabs one side of the sock of the open end and catches the baby's big toe with the other side. After the sock is on the big toe, the caregiver pulls the rest of the sock onto the rest of the toes and continues to pull the sock onto the foot. The caregiver then grabs the sock from the underside and pulls the sock over the heel.

Dressing and Undressing a Toddler. This age is one of the most demanding, because the children try to assert their independence and therefore are less cooperative. Once the baby crawls and walks, the bed may not be a workable surface. Because the bed affords the child with plenty of room to attempt an escape, the couch is a better choice as it is more contained.

Putting on the shirt or one-piece garment is easier if the toddler is on the parent's lap. Having a strong collaboration between toddler and parent will help greatly in this process. As with the infant and baby, it is helpful to use a larger size shirt with a large opening at the neck.

Car Seats

Latching safety straps of car seats is essential, but fastening them can be difficult even for people with two hands. It is important for the caregiver to experiment with a variety of brands in order to find the easiest to use. The chest strap must be narrow enough to be grasped and closed with one hand. Engaging the straps is easier if the crotch strap is short and stable, so that it does not wobble. Caregivers will find it easier to sit with the affected arm next to the car seat and to use the functional arm across his or her own midline to provide more strength and advantage.

Placing Children in Car Seats
Infants
1. Place the infant car seat in the middle of the back seat.
2. Sit with the functional arm next to the car seat.
3. Cradle the baby in the elbow of the functional arm.
4. Lean across the car to position the baby correctly in the car seat. While leaning, the upper arm will support the baby's head.
5. Slide the baby in place and gently remove the hand.

Once the infant can be lifted with a harness, the caregiver should sit in the back seat with the affected side next to the car seat to make it easier to latch the safety straps.

Crawling Babies. The caregiver sits in the back seat, with the affected side next to the car seat and the baby on the lap. With practice, babies can learn to crawl into the car seat. The therapist or another adult can help during the learning process.

Toddlers. It is too hard to lift a toddler into the car and car seat. Instead, the caregiver should have the toddler climb into the car seat. If the seat is too high for the toddler to climb up into, a step-stool can be placed on the floor. To protect the caregiver's back, he or she should sit on the back seat while attaching the straps.

Cognitive Issues

Cognitive impairment is present in the majority of patients with stroke, so it is crucial to identify any impairment and assess the impact on parenting.[3] The caregiver may lose many aspects of cognitive functioning: the ability to speak, read, or follow directions (completely or partially), and other impairments may occur. See Chapters 16 to 20. Cognitive assessment can pinpoint the cognitive difficulties and strengths, so that interventions can be developed to compensate for parenting difficulties. The occupational therapist must determine which specific parenting tasks may be problematic and which impairments lead to these difficulties. TLG currently has a project developing parenting adaptive strategies in relation to cognitive impairments, such as those identified in the cognitive assessment. For example, if the parent has hemianopsia or visual neglect, it can affect keeping track of a moving baby. Attaching bells in the baby's clothing and/or shoes securely, or buying shoes with built-in squeakers (search the Internet for squeaky shoes for children) could help. If the parent has figure-ground problems that affect distinguishing between the diaper and diaper pad, a dark cover for the diapering surface, visually contrasting with a diaper, could help. The parent may have trouble making formula because of difficulty with following directions, sequencing, or motor planning/apraxia. Infants can develop failure to thrive or seizures from improperly diluted formula, so it is crucial to monitor this area of the parent's functioning and the infant's weight gain. An occupational therapist can work closely with the other home visitors, public health nurse, pediatrician, and family to accomplish this. When the parent has problems making formula and qualifies for the Women, Infant, Children (WIC) program, federal regulations of WIC support the provision of premixed formula.

Some cognitive difficulties are much more challenging during parenting, of course, such as difficulties with attention, multitasking, and judgment. When parents have these problems, the use of adaptive equipment and techniques can be more complex. The process needs to be more closely monitored during home visiting by occupational therapists working as a team with mental health, other home visitors, and family members.

minutes. If Jerry did not want a bottle, Bob did not know what to do. Bob became overwhelmed and perseverated on only giving the bottle. TLG offered a mental health clinician, but the offer was declined. The occupational therapist tried varied strategies, such as relaxation techniques, which were not successful. She tried having Bob take Jerry outside more frequently in order to create a new pattern. Since Bob could read, she introduced a picture of a crying baby with captions of "try diaper changing, try putting baby to sleep, try going outside." Because Bob's impairment was significant and the occupational therapist's interventions were only partially successful, an outside caregiver was recommended and brought in to help for part of the day. Additional strategies would have been possible with support from cognitive therapy and mental health specialists. In retrospect, it might have been helpful to use a tape of the baby crying with repeated practice of calming the baby and putting the baby in the crib; if these were unsuccessful, then the practice of options that calmed the father (e.g., music) might have helped. A list of calming strategies for the father might have been tried. However, when progress is slow or uncertain to succeed, the priority is the welfare of the baby, and community supports may be crucial to support the family.

Emotional Issues

When parents have significant difficulties with communication, both cognitively and emotionally, there can be a profound effect on parenting, and teamwork between occupational therapists and mental health practitioners is crucial. However, it is important to keep in mind that all parents need support; all parenting is interdependent. Many people now live away from their immediate family, which can be stressful for both parent and partner. If a partner who has been providing assistance goes back to work, it is important that the parent who has had a stroke has enough support or is safe and confident to care for the baby by himself or herself. A social worker/therapist can help assess the situation, support the family in adjusting to new roles, provide referrals of community resources, and help integrate outside support into the family system. Otherwise the role of a spouse can be so focused on care that the couple relationship suffers, or an older child can be inappropriately used as a caregiver.

CASE STUDY 3

Bob had a stroke during his wife's pregnancy. Bob became the primary caregiver, while his wife Carol became the bread winner. Bob had a great deal of difficulty caring for Jerry when Jerry cried for longer than two

CASE STUDY 4

Janice, a mother with school-age children, had a new baby. A month after the birth, she had a stroke and had left hemiplegia as a result. Janice was discharged from the hospital following basic rehabilitation without any

Continued

CASE STUDY 4

information on how to care for her baby Lois. Her husband had to work full-time at this point. Janice felt her only alternative was to keep her older daughter Sandy home from school to do baby care. When the home visits began, both an occupational therapist and a mental health clinician went in as a team due to the level of the mother's anxiety about her ability to provide care with a disability. As an experienced mother, she had a strong "visual history" of care as a nondisabled mother. The occupational therapist gave Janice baby care equipment (rollator with baby seat) and taught one-handed baby care techniques so she could care for her baby without support. Since her cognitive problems were minimal, she absorbed information readily. Almost immediately, Janice was able to independently care for her child, and her daughter Sandy went back to school. The mental health clinician was able to ease Janice's anxiety and facilitate the relationships between mother, infant, and older child.

Care by Others

Other stroke survivors may receive help from their in-laws or their own parents. Grandparents may be concerned about both their own child and the new baby, and want to decrease the stress on everyone. When grandparents live nearby, they may step in with good intentions but may not give the new parent sufficient opportunity to learn how to take care of the baby. The insufficient contact between parent and baby can impede the attachment and adaptation process, and intensify depression and grieving in the parent. When this happens, the occupational therapist may need to bring in a mental health consultant to help with family dynamics.[4] In addition, grandparents should be included in OT sessions, so the grandparents can observe how well the parent is doing.

When the parent uses a personal assistant or attendant, it is also important that the parent interact with the baby sufficiently to develop and maintain the parent/child relationship. Even during an assistant's care, the parent can participate and hold the baby's attention (e.g., by talking or touching), and can appear more psychologically central to the baby by verbally directing the care.[2]

Mental health professionals' involvement can help identify and address the common psychological difficulties associated with stroke, including anxiety, depression, and grief. Problems of frustration, reduced emotional control, and anger especially call for mental health assessment and intervention regarding their impact on parenting. Experiencing cognitive impairment or aphasia can be associated with or can deepen the depression. The long-term negative impact of maternal depression on infants

and the crucial role of early mental health intervention have been well-established.[7,9]

TLG has found that limit-setting or behavior management is often challenging for parents with cognitive disabilities, partially due to difficulties with consistency. When parents who have had strokes have emotional control or anger management in addition to communication and physical difficulties, it is important that occupational therapists and mental health providers work collaboratively in this difficult yet essential area of parenting.

Discipline from Crawling through Toddling

In order for caregivers who have had a stroke to discipline successfully, it is important to teach parent and child to collaborate. Parent/child collaboration helps facilitate development of the baby and creates a special bond. To restore and maintain the parent/child relationship it is crucial to support enjoyable interaction between them, e.g., identifying roles and play where the parent can be effective, offering adaptations to support positive mutual experiences. Children tend to be more collaborative and act out less when they have fun with the parent and see them in effective roles.

To understand how to discipline with a physical disability, it is important to change the "visual history" people have about discipline. For instance, with a cruising baby, the best practice is for the occupational therapist to help the parent learn to entice the baby to come to him or her. A crawling baby is hard to pick up in the middle of a room when the parent is standing up. This can put the parent at risk for secondary injury (back injury and/or shoulder pain) and falling. Developmentally, toddlers enjoy and learn from the game of chase. Typically, they love to run away from their parents. For a parent with physical disabilities, it is essential to teach the toddler to chase the parent.

CASE STUDY 5

Alicia had a stroke and returned home when her child, Ramon, was one and just learning to walk. The occupational therapist taught Alicia to entice Ramon to come to her. Having an arsenal of enticing items, such as a bottle, toy cell phone, car, etc., is essential to engage the baby and make the baby want to crawl over to the parent. Since Ramon liked to crumple paper and chew on it, he was shown a piece of paper, which was shaken to make noise; he was told, "Look, look at the paper!" Once Ramon came over to get his paper, Alicia was able to lift him onto the couch where she was sitting by using a one-handed technique, bringing her hand down Ramon's back and lifting him up from under his crotch. Alicia said, "The technique helped reduce my anxiety by knowing that my baby will come to me.

The worry that he might get into trouble was making me tense, and this technique gave me the feeling that I was in control." The mental health clinician also addressed Alicia's anxiety, anger, and depression, which could have created more obstacles in the parent/child relationship.

Temper Tantrums

When a toddler throws a temper tantrum, it is usually impossible to have the child go to the parent, but there are other techniques. Most parents with a stroke cannot pick up kicking and screaming children and take them to their room. However, the belief that taking a misbehaving child to his or her room is the only appropriate response is due to visual history preventing caregivers from seeing alternative approaches. It is important to remember that the point of the separation is separation. Having the parent leave the room is equally effective. It is, of course, important to have rooms child-proofed and ensure that the child will be safe when left alone.

TRANSITION NAVIGATING SOCIAL OBSTACLES INTEGRAL TO PARENTING

Getting Out in the Community

Going out in the community is a typical family activity, but can pose problems for a caregiver with a disability.

Transportation

In a national survey and in national and regional task force reports, parents with disabilities have reported that the availability of transportation had more of an impact on being able to parent with a disability than any other issue.[8,13] Since many people who have experienced a stroke can no longer drive, they are often left relying on paratransit services for individuals with disabilities. Unfortunately, there are many problems involved in using this service, especially for parents with disabilities transporting their children. One such difficulty is that paratransit does not provide car seats for children. This becomes especially problematic when the child requires a car seat for children from 20 to 60 pounds, given the bulk of such carriers. Parents using paratransit are therefore forced to lug bulky car seats around with them during the day, which is impossible for many parents with physical disabilities. See Chapter 23.

Recreation

Being able to take child to a playground is a common outing for parents; however, recreation is an area fraught with problems for parents with physical and/or cognitive disabilities. The task force reports and national survey of parents with disabilities have identified access problems during recreation: "Public recreational sites such as playgrounds and parks are either inaccessible altogether or only accessible for young children with disabilities—rarely for a parent/adult with a disability."[8] Parents also reported needing assistance in recreation with their children. Parents with attention problems or difficulties with the authority required to manage behavior in public places may need mental health services to facilitate interaction and possibly an ongoing adult companion during outings. When a parent with a physical and/or cognitive disability goes out in the community with a toddler, it is important to have a walking harness. One good type of harness is a backpack with a tether. The harness can prevent the toddler from running away, but will not stop the screaming of a toddler having a tantrum. One good technique for the parent to try during the tantrum is making a call on a cell phone as a diversion technique, taking advantage of the desire of toddlers and preschoolers to engage with or talk with parents whenever they get on the phone.

Parenting Older Children

Since a stroke can occur at any time, it can happen when a parent has school-age children. If a parent has had a stroke prior to birth, the parent's disability is integral to the child's experience of the parent. For an older child whose parent has a stroke, the changes in the parent are typically experienced as loss of the parent as the child has known him or her, and grieving about this loss can take the form of depression or acting out. Providing continuity in contacts between parent and child, including during hospitalization, can be helpful, so that loss is less complicated by separation. Older children are often acutely aware of social stigma directed toward the parent, and teasing and embarrassment about differences may be issues. Parent and child can strategize together about responses to teasing. One parent taught her child to answer "So what?!" and this was successful in ending the hostile comments. Some parents have found that ongoing participation in the classroom helped. Communication with older children about the social prejudice and barriers can raise their consciousness about social justice issues (e.g., transportation obstacles can make it difficult for the older child to participate in organized sports and other events when there is not another available adult or adequate paratransit services). The role of mental health practitioners is heightened for the child and for the parent, since depression is so problematical during parenting.

Occupational therapists have a crucial role in facilitating functioning, so the child and parent can navigate new obstacles and enjoy interaction and play. If the caregiver has lost the ability to read, being able to use computer software or other devices that can read books is an alternative. There are options of software on all subjects that can help the caregiver be present while the child learns a skill and does homework. When there is no parent or family member who can assist with homework, TLG also recommends tutoring for school-age children, ideally including or coordinated with respectful services to the parent providing assistance (e.g., in structuring time and place to complete homework). Some family recreation choices may have become too difficult (e.g., hiking, beachcombing). However, there are outdoor activities that have been adapted for people who are disabled (e.g., skiing, bicycling, sailing, horseback riding) that the family can join.

CASE STUDY 6

Jim and Mary had two older children in junior high and high school when a surprise pregnancy occurred. Soon after Sharon was born, Jim had a left hemisphere stroke resulting in aphasia and right hemiplegia. Jim was not the only one in the family who had depression; his wife and older children also did. They felt they had lost their father/husband who had had a great sense of humor and enjoyed the outdoors. A TLG family mental health clinician and the occupational therapist helped the family change how they looked at their recreational activities. The mental health clinician and occupational therapist worked together to help the family adjust to new activities that were fun for them, such as playing card games or board games. TLG was able to help them join another disability community program that provided outdoor activities. The family started doing adapted bike trips every month.

Although there can be pitfalls for parents who have had strokes, there are also many beautiful success stories. TLG has funded scholarships for high school seniors or college students whose parents have disabilities. One of the 2009 national winners has a father who experienced a stroke. He wrote:[1]

The Impact of Growing Up with a Parent with a Disability

Some people will look at him and see weakness, but I look at him and see nothing but strength and fortitude. Some people may look at him and see a man who cannot get his words out as well as he wants too, but I look at him and see a man who speaks volumes to me. Some people may look at him and see a man whose hand doesn't work quite right, but I look at him and see a man who gives hugs and handshakes as strong and comforting as they ever were. Some people may look at him and see a man who walks with a limp on his right side, but I see a man who hopped to first base at our father-son baseball game, unashamed of his deficits and the obstacles that lay before him, because he just wants to be there for me, his son.

My father suffered a major stroke in 2004, and many of the effects of that stroke are still with him today . . . Witnessing his strength and tenacity has taught me to be strong just like he is. He has also taught me the value of family, and that it is the best thing you can have in life. Lastly, but probably the greatest thing he ever taught me is to always work hard toward your dreams and never give up hope . . . Not a day goes by where my father doesn't work hard to get back to normal. He is unable to work as a cabinetmaker and can't use his right hand or speak clearly. He may not know it now, but he has helped me so much to become stronger, just by watching how hard he worked. Living with a disabled parent has made me stronger when I am faced with harsh conditions and has taught me to always work hard to get where I need to be . . . . . Since I could walk, the only thing I have wanted to do in life is play baseball, and I hope to play professionally one day . . . I figured out that I had to work hard to achieve my dreams. I remembered my dad and how he struggled with physical therapy every day until he was sweating and crying, and I started lifting weights at school, stayed after practice an hour longer than the other players, [and] got extra help from my coach and other instructors, so I could be a better player. I feel so blessed that my dad taught me this lesson of working hard to "get better" because I have now been recruited by several colleges to play on their baseball teams . . .

Seeing my dad have the stroke has done nothing but add fuel to my fire to get to where I want to be. My dad has not missed a game since he got out of the hospital, and he still does his best to teach me how to play the game . . . I only hope that when I am older that I can be half the man my father is. You see, I consider myself lucky to be living with the man who can't get the words out all the time, whose right hand doesn't work quite right, and who walks with a limp, because the alternative is something that I don't want to think about. I live with the man who suffered a severe stroke in 2004, but since then has taught me enough lessons to last me multiple lifetimes.

TLG has assisted many parents who have had strokes to find ways to navigate and enjoy the caregiving experience. Teamwork between occupational therapists and mental health practitioners can increase the parent's role and effectiveness, address obstacles, support the relationship between parent and child, and assist the functioning of the entire family system.

REVIEW QUESTIONS

1. Describe techniques that would be useful in helping a parent with hemiplegia burp a child independently.
2. Name the four transitional tasks to master as the starting point of intervention.
3. What is an appropriate diapering technique to teach a parent with hemiplegia?
4. What are the steps to teaching dressing and undressing a younger baby? An older baby?
5. What is the correct sequence of placing an infant in a car seat for a parent who has unilateral upper extremity impairment?

REFERENCES

1. Anonymous 2009. Through the Looking Glass Scholarship Recipient. Unpublished essay.
2. Groah SL, editor: *Managing spinal cord injury: A guide to living well with spinal cord injury*, Washington, DC, 2005, NRH Press.
3. Hoffman M, Schmitt F, Bromley E: Comprehensive cognitive neurological assessment in stroke. *Acta Neurol Scand* 119(3):162–171, 2009.
4. Kirshbaum M: *Disabilities in the family: Babycare assistive technology for parents with physical disabilities: Relational, systems, & cultural perspectives*, AFTA Newsletter 20–26, Spring 1997.
5. Kirshbaum M: A disability culture perspective on early intervention with parents with physical or cognitive disabilities and their babies. *Infants Young Child* 13(3):9–20, 2005.
6. Kirshbaum M, Olkin R: Parents with physical, systemic, or visual disabilities. *Sex Disabil* 20(1):65–80, 2002.
7. Lyons-Ruth K, Zoll D, Connell D, Grunebaum HU: The depressed mother and her one-year-old infant: Environment, interaction, attachment, and infant development. *New Dir Child Dev* (34):61–82, 1986.
8. Preston P: *Visible, diverse and united: A report of the Bay Area parents with disabilities and deaf parents task force meeting*, Berkeley, 2006, Through the Looking Glass.
9. Radke-Yarrow M: Attachment patterns in children of depressed mothers. In Parkes CM, Stevenson-Hinde J, editors: *Attachment across the life cycle*, New York, 1991, Tavistock/Routledge.
10. Rogers J: *Disabled woman's guide to pregnancy and birth*, New York, 2006, Demos Medical Publishing.
11. Through the Looking Glass: *Adaptive parenting equipment: Idea book 1* (NIDRR Grant No. H133G10146), Berkeley, 1995, Through the Looking Glass.
12. Through the Looking Glass: *Developing adaptive equipment and techniques for physically disabled parents and their babies within the context of psycho-social services, Final Report* (NIDRR Grant No. H133G10146), Berkeley, 1995, Through the Looking Glass.
13. Toms Barker LT, Maralani V: *Challenges and strategies of disabled parents: Findings from a national survey of parents with disabilities, Final Report* (NIDRR, Rehabilitation Research and Training Grant No. H133B30076), Berkeley, 1997, Through the Looking Glass.
14. Tuleja C, Rogers J, Vensand K, et al: *Continuation of adaptive parenting equipment development*, Berkeley, 1998, Through the Looking Glass.
15. Tuleja C, Rogers J, Kirshbaum M, et al: *Baby care assessment for parents with physical limitations or disabilities: An occupational therapy evaluation*, Berkeley, 2005, Through the Looking Glass.
16. Vensand K, Rogers J, Tuleja C, et al: *Adaptive baby care equipment: Guidelines, prototypes & resources*, Berkeley, 2000, Through the Looking Glass.

susan l. pierce

chapter 23

Driving and Community Mobility as an Instrumental Activity of Daily Living

key terms

driving and community mobility
driver rehabilitation therapist
ecological validity
independent transportation

mobility prescription
occupational therapy generalist in driving
occupational therapy specialist in driving

on-road evaluation
predriving clinical evaluation
transportation choices

chapter objectives

After completing this chapter, the reader will be able to accomplish the following:

1. Define *driving* and *community mobility* as instrumental activities of daily living.
2. Identify the role of occupational therapy in addressing driving and community mobility issues at different stages of rehabilitation and recovery for the stroke survivor.
3. Understand the legal issues associated with involvement of driving issues and how to manage liability risks.
4. Identify performance skill deficits related to a stroke and client factors that can interfere with the occupation of driving.
5. Understand the current accepted practice for a comprehensive driving evaluation for the stroke survivor.
6. Identify resources for information, education, and referral in addressing driving and community mobility as an instrumental activity of daily living.

Following a stroke, the occupational therapist considers the many types of occupations in which the client engages. The Occupational Therapy Practice Framework[1] defines instrumental activities of daily living (IADL) as activities "to support daily life within the home and community that often require more complex interactions than self-care used in ADL." Driving and community mobility are included within the domain of occupational therapy (OT) and in the profession's scope of practice.[1] *Community mobility* is defined in the framework[1] as "moving around in the community and using public or private transportation, such as driving, walking, bicycling, or accessing and riding in buses, taxi cabs or other transportation systems." The OT practitioner during evaluation and intervention considers the client's own perspective of how driving and community mobility meets his or her needs and interests.

Evaluation and intervention for functional and community mobility should center on safe mobility for the patient in the home and in the community for meeting his or her life needs and interests. For some following a stroke, driving may play a major role in getting to and from a job or it may be the means of obtaining nourishment and medications. Driving a motor vehicle is a common form of transportation used by clients recovering from a stroke, and therefore, addressing driving and/or community mobility is a crucial IADL that must be addressed by OT.

In 2005 American Occupational Therapy Association's (AOTA) Representative Assembly adopted an official statement on Driving and Community Mobility.[36] The document stated that "All occupational therapists and occupational therapy assistants possess the education and training necessary to address driving and community mobility as an IADL. Throughout the evaluation and intervention process, all practitioners recognize the impact of clients' aging, disability, or risk factors on driving and community mobility. Through the use of clinical reasoning skills, practitioners use information about client strengths and weaknesses in performance skills, performance patterns, contexts, and client factors to deduce potential difficulties with occupational performance in driving and community mobility." In the continuum of activities of daily living (ADL), the occupational therapist must consider mobility in the rehabilitation process of the patient recovering from a stroke.

As with all other ADL and IADL, the occupational therapist considers the occupation of driving for a client with the holistic approach of examining the client factors, the performance skills, the performance patterns and habits, the contextual and environmental factors, and the activity demands. A determination is made as to any difficulties or issues in these areas that affect occupational performance for driving. Intervention is then structured to improve or enhance the problem areas prior to discharge from OT. If independent driving cannot be a short- or long-term goal for the client who is recovering from a stroke, then the occupational therapist must address the community mobility issues by examining the client's resources in the community and assisting the client and family with good and safe transportation choices.

A century ago, individuals could walk to work, shops, friends' homes, churches, and most other destinations. Today, with the primary mode of transportation being the personal vehicle and with the distance separating homes and businesses in the suburbs, few destinations are now within walking distance. Impairments and activity limitations caused by a stroke or age can further shorten

distances traversable on foot. Reduced mobility in the community by an individual can result in a lower self-esteem, depression, and feelings of uselessness, loneliness, and unhappiness.

The performance skills necessary for safe driving begin to deteriorate around the age of 55-years-old and dramatically decline after age 75-years-old.[27] Approximately 72% of strokes occur in persons older than 65-years-old. In addition to normal aging conditions, the brain damage from a cerebral infarct and its clinical manifestations can affect the person's driving skills. The specific motor, sensory, and cognitive deficits depend on the location and severity of the cerebrovascular damage (see Chapters 1 and 18). This damage can cause one or more temporary or permanent impairments. Of the approximately 80% of persons who survive the initial period, 75% are left with residual perceptual-cognitive dysfunction.[21] These or other impairments or additional client factors not related to the stroke may affect safe driving for this person. The occupational therapist must evaluate each patient recovering from a stroke individually, because the location and nature of the stroke can produce different problems and deficits, and everyone will have a different occupational profile.

Achieving or not achieving independent transportation for a stroke survivor can impede or affect greatly all other IADL. Carp,[5] a California psychologist who has studied older drivers, used the conceptual model in Fig. 23-1 to detail the determinants of emotional and social well-being. Life maintenance needs to include nourishment, clothing, medical care, banking, and pharmaceuticals. Community resources for meeting these needs include grocery and drug stores, department stores, physician's offices, and banks. If a person has no access to these resources, independent living becomes nearly impossible. Other needs, labeled higher order, include needs for social interaction, usefulness, recreation, and religious experience. Carp's research of investigative studies supported the idea that "if life is to have an acceptable quality, higher-order needs such as those expressed in trips for relaxation and enjoyment and religious activities are also essential."

The Occupational Therapy Practice Framework[1] supported Carp's ideas by articulating that OT has a contribution "to promote the health and participation of people, organizations, and populations through engagement in occupation." The Framework[1] continued that "all people need to be able or enabled to engage in the occupations of their need and choice, to grow through what they do, and to experience independence or interdependence, equality, participation, security, health and well-being."

The threat of losing a driver's license may have devastating effects on a stroke survivor's motivation to maintain independence in other areas of daily living. The primary fear of elderly persons is not death but losing

Qualities of Mobility   **Need/Resource**   **Outcomes**

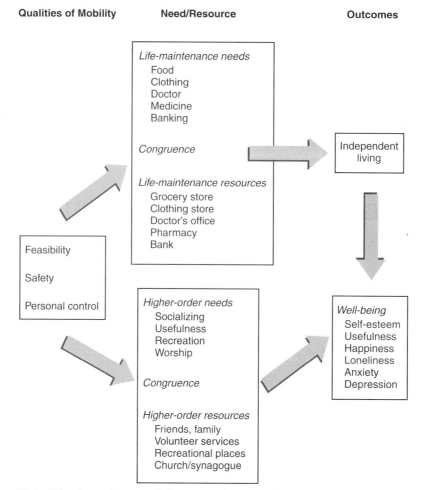

Figure 23-1 The determinants and dynamics of emotional and social well-being. (Modified from Transportation Research Board—National Research Council, Special Report 218, *Transportation in an aging society*, Washington, DC, 1988.)

their independence and becoming burdens to their loved ones.[3] Carp[5] stated the following:

Loss of license is a serious fear among drivers, a threat to their autonomy, usefulness, and self-esteem . . . A century ago people could walk to work, shops, others' homes, religious services, and most destinations. Few destinations [today] lie within walking distance for any person . . . Mobility is a key influence on the congruence term in the model . . . Satisfaction of life-maintenance and higher order needs require going out into the community . . . The loss of a license would mean inability to go where they needed to go and therefore meet their needs independently . . . Just as receipt of the first driver's license is an important rite of passage to adulthood and independence, license loss formally identifies one as "over the hill."

Driving or being independent in community mobility by another means is inseparable with being one's own person and taking care of oneself. The issue is more than just one of losing mobility. Rendering an opinion as to whether the patient recovering from a stroke is capable of driving has lasting implications. Driving is one of the

more complex ADL and therefore must be taken with careful thought and serious consideration by using the best critical thinking methods by the rehabilitation team. Law enforcement officers or driver licensing personnel cannot address this issue effectively, which has potentially dangerous consequences to the stroke survivor or to pedestrians or other road users. Elderly drivers who do not self-regulate effectively are not detected easily with standard licensing procedures.[21] Furthermore, doubt exists as to whether most licensing staffs have the skills necessary to detect these problem drivers.[8]

DRIVING AND COMMUNITY MOBILITY IS A CRUCIAL ACTIVITY OF DAILY LIVING SKILL

Community mobility is paramount to the patient recovering from stroke and attempting to maintain a productive lifestyle in the work, home, or social arenas. The occupation of driving and community mobility is such an important activity that it requires inclusion with other

ADL issues in OT. If the rehabilitation team addresses safety in functional mobility or safety in the kitchen for the stroke survivor, then safety in driving demands addressing. If driving and community mobility is within the domain of OT, then it is the occupational therapist's responsibility to address it as with any other ADL such as dressing, cooking, bathing, and functional ambulation. "Each area of mobility requires a certain skill level in occupational performance. A hierarchy of skills dictates the order in which each area is addressed. Mobility in basic activities of daily living (BADL) is first, followed by mobility in instrumental activities of daily living (IADL). Some occupational therapy (OT) goals for motor, sensory, perceptual, and cognitive functioning must be achieved prior to ADL training and specifically mobility training."[29]

The occupational therapist should begin to discuss driving and community mobility early on in the stroke survivor's rehabilitation and recovery intervention. Such discussion will lead to patient and family education and acceptance early to reinforce their responsibility and requirements in the process of the patient's regaining independent driving or his or her need to investigate alternative transportation choices. The early discussion also will lessen the family's stress and anxiety over the issue of driving for their family member, for they will not have to shoulder the burden of telling the person that he or she cannot drive and then dealing with an angry family member.

"As an activity that contributes to independence and quality of life, driving falls squarely within the province of occupational therapy practice," Johansson stated.[18] The discipline of OT has been given the role of evaluating clients regarding their ability to drive a motor vehicle primarily because of the wide spectrum of physical, cognitive, and perceptual skills that fall under the realm of OT.[19] In addition, occupational therapists have a background in psychosocial dysfunction that can be key in giving the therapist the necessary therapeutic attitude and approach to this sensitive issue to understand how it can affect the psychosocial and emotional well-being of the patient. The AOTA has identified older driver evaluation and retraining as an important specialty area for practitioners to consider because of the broad approach of the profession to evaluation and treatment. Eberhard, a former senior research psychologist at the National Highway and Traffic Safety Administration, said that he "envisions a key role for the OT profession in maintaining elders' automotive proficiency. OT practitioners have clear insights into the need for mobility. They have the skills to assess functional mobility and the skills to enhance it."[26]

In all settings, the occupational therapist is concerned with the performance level of ADL, with mobility being at the top of the pyramid (Fig. 23-2). The daily living task of functional mobility involves bed and wheelchair mobility, transfers, and functional ambulation while performing

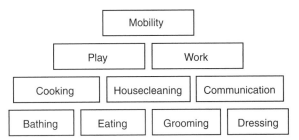

Figure 23-2 Pyramid model for rehabilitation of activities of daily living.

activities. Functional mobility tasks allow an individual to function independently by moving from one place to another. Successful community mobility allows a person to move about his or her community and environment and the person's ability to drive or use other transportation choices may make the difference in the stroke survivor returning to his or her living situation prior to the stroke. Because persons of all ages can suffer a stroke, driving or transportation choices as a community mobility issue must be on the ADL repertoire for the occupational therapist to explore, evaluate, and provide intervention as necessary. The occupational therapist must understand the significance of community mobility for the total well-being of the client. A holistic view presents driving as a vital link between the client and the outside world.

REHABILITATION TEAM'S RESPONSIBILITY

The entire rehabilitation team must address the issue of driving or transportation for the stroke survivor, with members addressing the issue within their own professional expertise (Fig. 23-3). The rehabilitation team must get involved with this issue because they are concerned with the overall functioning of the client and his or her resulting quality of life after a stroke. They are in the best position to identify any existing or potential contributors to driving risk. In addition, families need assistance and guidance with this highly sensitive issue before they take the family member home. The rehabilitation team must define a fair and reasonable course of action. They must weigh client-physician or client-therapist confidentiality versus public safety. The social and ethical dilemma faced by medical professionals and the department of driver licensing is to strike a balance between protecting the person's privilege to drive and the safety of other road users, including pedestrians, other drivers, and vehicle passengers.

Each team member has a role and responsibility and should be ready to address related issues as they arise. For example, the physician, as the head of the rehabilitation team and medical authority, must take a leading role with this issue. The physician should be the first to inform the client and family that because of its complexity

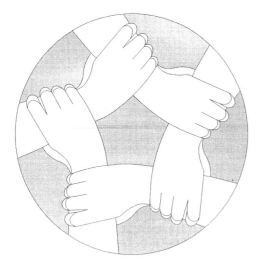

- Physician
- Social worker
- Occupational therapist
- Physical therapist
- Rehabilitation nurse
- Speech therapist
- Neuropsychologist

Figure 23-3 Driving should be addressed as appropriate by each member of the rehabilitation team following the same policies and procedures. The process depends on good communication among the team members.

and demand of high functional levels of skills, driving will be one the last activities addressed in the person's rehabilitation and recovery.

Other team members also play a role in addressing the occupation of driving in relation to their specific area of knowledge and skill. For example, the nurse can provide a list of medications with which the client will be discharged home and note any side effects that could affect safe driving. The speech-language pathologist may address the need for a client with aphasia to begin carrying a personal identification card, so that if he or she is involved in an accident or is stopped by a police officer, the card would explain the speech difficulties. The speech-language pathologist also may inform the occupational therapist of any language deficits that might be contraindicated for safe driving. For example, if the stroke survivor has global aphasia and needs to be evaluated for driving using driving aids, he or she may have difficulty with verbal instructions on a new task, with directions, or with reading road signs. The physical therapist can reinforce the reality that the person with dense right hemiplegia will not be able to use the right foot for driving because of lack of necessary motor and sensory function. The physical therapist can also work on the goal of the client entering and exiting a vehicle with or without an orthotic device. The social worker can counsel the family to reinforce the team's discharge recommendations related to referral for a formal driving evaluation if deemed necessary after discharge and can assist the OT Generalist in Driving and the family members in identifying alternative transportation choices in their specific community environment.

The OT practitioner will play the largest role and the greatest responsibility in addressing the occupation of driving for the stroke survivor. The roles of the OT practitioner have been defined in an AOTA online course entitled Driving and Community Mobility for Older Adults: Occupational Therapy Roles:[16] "Occupational therapists are already educated and trained to address many of the important issues associated with driving and community mobility, and they must be ready to take on the role of the occupational therapy Driving and Community Generalist whatever the practice setting. In addition, an increasing number of occupational therapists must prepare and be available to assume the role of the Occupational Therapy Driver Rehabilitation Specialist." The Occupational Therapy Driving and Community Mobility Generalist (Generalist in Driving) is defined as "all occupational therapists and occupational therapy assistants with all the education, training and credentials necessary to practice occupational therapy but who do not possess specialized training and experience in driver evaluation or driver rehabilitation." The Occupational Therapy Driver Rehabilitation Specialist (Specialist in Driving) is defined as occupational therapists and OT assistants with all the education, training, and credentials of an OT practitioner in addition to the advanced knowledge and skills in the specialty field of driver evaluation and driver rehabilitation (including intervention, vehicle modifications, and adapted driving equipment).

While the OT Generalist in Driving begins addressing issues and skills as they relate to the activity of driving early on for the stroke survivor, it may be necessary to seek the expertise of an OT Specialist in Driving at some point for an on-road evaluation. The physician should inform the stroke survivor and the family that the client should not drive until the team and the OT Generalist in Driving or Specialist in Driving has considered all aspects necessary to evaluate the occupation of driving.

OCCUPATIONAL THERAPISTS' CHANGING ROLE WITH THE STROKE SURVIVOR

"Occupational therapists are responsible for all aspects of OT service delivery and are accountable for the safety and effectiveness of that service delivery process."[1] The occupational therapist's unique background and training in evaluation and intervention in the performance skill areas of motor and praxis skills, sensory-perception skills, emotional regulation skills, cognitive skills, and communication and social skills coupled with the understanding of client factors and environment and contextual factors assist the therapist to understand all issues related to the occupation of driving. In addition, the occupational therapist's background and understanding of psychological and emotional issues assists the therapist greatly in handling the delicate issue of driving when just speaking of driving can cause anxiety, defensiveness, and other psychological stress for not only the stroke survivor but also family members. The occupational therapist's role many times is to educate, listen, and counsel not only the client but also family members. The occupational therapist's keen ability to look at the "whole person" is important to the process in considering all aspects of engagement in community mobility, including driving, and how all the different aspects are interrelated and have transactional relationships.

The occupational therapist's role changes during different phases as the stroke survivor moves through acute care hospitalization, inpatient and outpatient rehabilitation, discharge, and community follow-up. As the person moves through these phases, the occupational therapist addresses issues of driving relevant to each phase. The level of involvement varies during each phase. Driving or community mobility should be an established IADL goal early on with all other ADL goals and have a well-defined intervention plan toward the stroke survivor's stated outcome with this activity. The outcome regarding this IADL is the end-result of the OT process throughout each recovery stage with the stroke survivor. Each occupational therapist that the stroke survivor sees along the continuum of care must understand his or her role and responsibility at the level that he or she treats the client.

Acute Care Phase

During the initial hospital phase following a stroke, the role for the occupational therapist is primarily one of inquiry and fact finding. One of the most common questions initially asked by a person in this phase is "Can I drive again?" or "When will I be able to drive again?" The therapist must be able to answer the question when asked and to speak with confidence about how this activity will be addressed along the continuum of care. The therapist can inquire whether the stroke survivor had been a licensed driver before and what was the frequency and circumstances of driving. For example, did the person drive to work or drive his or her children to school? Does the person live in a rural or suburban area? Was the person the primary driver in the family? Did the person drive intrastate, interstate, or just locally? Is the person at a stage at which he or she already had begun to limit driving to daylight only or within short distances of home? Is independent driving a goal for the person now? If the client has memory, cognitive, or speech deficits, the family may need to be consulted to obtain or verify the information given by the client. If the stroke survivor passes through the hospital phase quickly, then these questions may need to be explored more completely by

the therapist in the next phase. The point is that driving should be addressed early and as commonly as dressing, grooming, and other mobility issues. Whether the appropriate time is in the acute care phase or the rehabilitation phase, the therapist should be equipped to address driving in an appropriate way.

Rehabilitation Phase

As the stroke survivor moves into the rehabilitation phase, the foregoing information would be passed on to the rehabilitation unit therapist. The primary rehabilitation occupational therapist would pick up the issue by addressing driving as an IADL in the initial evaluation for an intervention plan with the stroke survivor as for other ADL such as dressing, bathing, and cooking. To address driving as an IADL and assess factors that may affect safe driving, the occupational therapist requires an understanding of all factors and skills involved in driving and activity demands of driving. With an understanding of the level of skill performance demanded in the driving task, the occupational therapist can include intervention, with driving in mind, much as the therapist would for other ADL tasks.

Driving an automobile is a complex task involving a hierarchy of skills. Adequate motor response and physical control of the vehicle are essential skills but are secondary to accurate perception and understanding of ever-changing traffic environments and unpredictable situations. A driver processes information and makes conscious or unconscious decisions using (1) environmental information such as traffic lights, road markings, road signs, and other road users; (2) attention and perceptual mechanisms using visual search, spatial relations, and time and space management; (3) reasoning, problem-solving, and planning to analyze each situation and understand cause and effect; and (4) response by physical control, adjustment, and compromise. Table 23-1 gives an overview of occupational performance in driving.

Preexisting or Progressive Age-Related Conditions

In addition to conditions or problems associated with the primary diagnosis of a stroke, the therapist should explore other preexisting medical or aging conditions that require attention. Stressel[39] writes the following:

In general, aging results in the normal deterioration of the physical, cognitive, and visual functioning. People age at different rates, and age-related problems that are known to affect driver performance do not occur in all people at the same rate or to the same degree. The rate of decline is very individualized, and chronological age is not a good predictor of an individual's capabilities. As the prevalence of disease increases with age, it becomes more difficult to differentiate between functional losses due to the effects of disease versus functional loss associated with the aging process. The process of aging is inescapable. Age-related changes are characteristically detrimental in nature,

Table 23-1

Occupational Performance in Driving for a Stroke Survivor

BASIC SKILL AREAS	PERFORMANCE FACTORS
Physical demands	
One functional upper extremity and lower extremity	Operation of primary/secondary vehicle controls with or without adaptive equipment
Visual demands	
Visual acuity: 20/40 in at least one eye	Reading/understanding road signs
	Reading odometer and dash gauges
	Can influence depth perception
	Identification of stimuli seen in side vision
Peripheral vision: >130 degrees of total field of vision with both eyes	Awareness of stimuli in side vision
	Visual scanning
	More useful than visual acuity
Good eye function/quality of vision: disease or age-related problems	Cataracts: poor glare recovery, poor night vision
	Diabetic retinopathy: blind spots, see incomplete driving scene
	Glaucoma: blurriness, blindness
Visual-perceptual demands	
Spatial relations	Reading/responding to road signs/markings; perception of space around car
Figure-ground	Maneuvering through parking lot; finding road signs in a visually busy environment
Visual closure	Discrimination of high- and low-priority issues; seeing the whole picture with incomplete cues
Visual memory	Time and space management; delay response time
Form constancy	Visual analysis in busy and/or low-light environments
Visual discrimination	Analysis of road signs by shape and color
Cognitive demands	
Strategic skills	Choice of route
	Time of day to take trip
	Planning a sequence of trips or stops
	Evaluating general risks in traffic (under varying traffic, road, and weather conditions)
Tactical skills	Anticipatory driving behavior
	Adjusting speed to varying traffic conditions
	Quick decisions related to expected or unexpected situations
	Judgment/reasoning to estimate risks
Operational skills (combines physical, visual, and cognitive)	
Attention:	
Focused	Responding to specific stimuli
Sustained	Maintaining focus during continuous driving
Selective	Maintaining focus in face of distractions
Alternating	Mental flexibility to focus between several tasks requiring attention
Divided	Responding simultaneously to multiple tasks or multiple task demands
Complex reaction time (appropriateness and timeliness of response)	
Memory skills	
Recent	Remembering destination, path to take, and event
Procedural	Subconscious operation of vehicle controls as old, learned behavior

cumulative and irreversible over time, but often lack sharply defined points of transition. Changes begin at different chronological ages, progress at varying rates, and do not affect each body system in the same way. Although some diseases and deterioration may present themselves suddenly, generally there is a slow accumulation of deficits.

Several examples to illustrate this point are the stroke survivor who has had insulin-dependent type 2 diabetes for 25 years. He was diagnosed with diabetic retinopathy and had two laser surgeries for treatment. Another stroke survivor has been on kidney dialysis for two years after having an allergic reaction to a medication that damaged the kidneys. Each of these preexisting conditions, separate from any deficits related to the stroke, could increase risk factors associated with safe driving and should be addressed separately in terms of the affect on the driving task. Box 23-1 lists other examples of nonstroke factors to consider. Communication with the family, rehabilitation physician, neurologist, and perhaps the primary care physician is important to synthesize the patient's entire medical history and consider all potential client factors that may affect the stroke survivor returning to independent driving.

After driving and community mobility are addressed in the initial gathering of the occupational profile, the second stage of involvement for the occupational therapist during the rehabilitation period is the crucial area of education of the stroke survivor and the family regarding individual responsibility in the whole process. In this phase, the client must be informed how, when, and by what process driving and community mobility will be addressed. The therapist should be able to speak with authority and confidence of the process of addressing driving, the timing, the referral procedure if referral to an OT driver rehabilitation specialist is necessary, and the available resources. The therapist must speak with first-hand knowledge of the value of the on-road evaluation, if necessary, so that the client and family will equally value the comprehensive driver evaluation services of the OT Specialist in Driving. The stroke survivor and family should know at that point that the client cannot drive until a conclusion has been reached by the collaboration of the OT practitioner and the rehabilitation team. By the OT practitioner giving the client the information at an early stage, the client will be prepared and more cooperative in moving through the process and knowing what to expect along the way. Speaking specifically about the activity of driving will help the client understand that the intervention plan includes treatment along the continuum of care that will improve and enhance his or her performance skills related to driving an automobile.

Driving is one area that scares many family members of stroke survivors. They need to be informed as well, so they can provide the necessary assistance and support for the client throughout the process in regards to the issue of driving. The family can begin dealing with the reality and can plan for alternative transportation choices for the stroke survivor until it has been finally determined that they have the driver competency to begin driving again. This should lessen the family's fears and anxiety and bring them into an active role in the process while allowing them to remain in the background regarding the ultimate decisions about driving. In other words, the family cannot be blamed for the stroke survivor's temporary or permanent loss of driving privileges. By addressing the driving issue in the medical setting, the family is relieved of having to address the issue themselves with the stroke survivor, which many times can cause frustration and emotional stress from the stroke survivor's anger, lack of insight, or poor judgment.

Medical Reporting with Driver Licensing Authorities

Each state has licensing requirements and reporting laws. Many states do not require a driver to report a new medical episode resulting in disability between license renewals. Some states allow only a doctor to report a medical condition that may preclude safe driving. Other states may allow professionals such as a law enforcement officer or allied health professional or even nonprofessionals such as a neighbor or family member to report a driver's medical condition or to raise a concern. Occupational therapists should investigate the requirements for the state in which they work to develop a consistent procedure to use with every client that includes a set policy

---

Box 23-1

Nonstroke Medical Factors That Potentially Can Affect Driving Safety

- Previous history of stroke or transient ischemic attack
- Diabetes
- Visual problems such as cataracts, glaucoma, macular degeneration, or diabetic retinopathy
- Arthritis and osteoarthritis
- Surgeries that caused limitations such as hip/knee replacements or cervical laminectomy
- Respiratory conditions such as emphysema or chronic obstructive pulmonary disease
- Amputations
- Other neuromuscular conditions such as polio, multiple sclerosis, or muscular dystrophy
- Dementia or Alzheimer
- Polypharmacy: multiple medications with interacting effects; prescription and over-the-counter looked at separately and in synergistic combination
- Psychological diagnoses such as bipolar disease, depression, or schizophrenia
- Parkinson's disease

approved by the administration and legal departments of the facility and understood by each team member. Many states have medical advisory boards to their departments of driver licensing that are good resources for licensing requirements and the medical reporting process.

The American Association of Motor Vehicle Administrators (AAMVA) at www.aamva.org is a nonprofit organization that develops model programs in motor vehicle administration, police traffic services, and highway safety. The AAMVA works with the National Highway Traffic Safety Administration to review Medical Advisory Boards and driver licensing renewal procedures throughout the United States. This information can be accessed from their website. The AAMVA also serves as an information and awareness resource regarding older driver issues.

That testing procedures in driver examination offices do not evaluate fully all skills related to driving is common knowledge, particularly when the driver may have a medical condition or deficit that is not physically obvious. Examiners may not have knowledge of an applicant's diagnosis unless the person informs them or a physician provides written notification. These examiners do not have an understanding of possible implications of disability on driving skills. For example, a person with a complete right homonymous hemianopsia, which is a common vision deficit after a stroke, usually does not pass the visual requirements of most states for a minimum of 125 to 140 degrees of continuous field of vision. The typical methods of vision testing by driver licensing offices measure only visual acuity and not visual fields. A person can have 20/40 visual acuity, which is acceptable in most states; however, the driver examiner may never know the person has homonymous hemianopsia.

Predriving Clinic Screening

A comprehensive driving evaluation for a person who has had a stroke may include the steps illustrated in Fig. 23-4. The process for addressing driving and community mobility as an IADL starts during the initial OT in the acute care setting and continues through inpatient rehabilitation therapy, outpatient rehabilitation therapy, and beyond. Along this continuum of care, the occupational therapist should continue including the IADL of driving and/or community mobility until the conclusion is drawn and the outcome decided. A successful completion of this process depends on many factors that can influence the outcome, as noted in Fig. 23-5. A predriving screening by the occupational therapist should be completed prior to the client being discharged from inpatient rehabilitation and outpatient therapy. The purpose of the predriving screen near discharge is multifaceted. The OT Generalist in Driving should:

1. Evaluate for any residual deficits in the performance skill areas of motor and praxis skills, sensory-perceptual skills, emotional regulation skills, cognitive

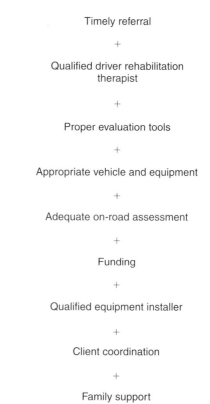

Evaluation of IADL of driving by OT Generalist in Driving to develop intervention plan and to improve or enhance driving performance skills during initial therapy and rehabilitation.

↓

If determination is made that an on-road evaluation is needed, then referral to OT Specialist in Driving for a comprehensive driver evaluation

↓

Vehicle/equipment evaluation

↓

On-road evaluation

↓

Additional driver training if needed

↓

Mobility prescription for equipment needs

↓

Vehicle inspection/fitting

Figure 23-4   The driving evaluation process for a stroke survivor.

Timely referral

+

Qualified driver rehabilitation therapist

+

Proper evaluation tools

+

Appropriate vehicle and equipment

+

Adequate on-road assessment

+

Funding

+

Qualified equipment installer

+

Client coordination

+

Family support

Figure 23-5   Factors that influence the driving evaluation process.

skills, and communication and social skills, and determine whether any of these deficits could or would interfere with driving performance skills.

2. Determine with the full team's input if the client can begin driving or should not drive upon inpatient discharge, and document in the medical records that the client was informed of the conclusion.

3. Determine if a more in-depth driver evaluation by an OT Specialist in Driving is necessary, and begin the referral process.

4. Determine if the client can benefit from further therapy to improve and enhance his or her skills in outpatient therapy, and pass on the intervention goal of driving to the outpatient occupational therapist.

The inpatient and outpatient occupational therapist should have knowledge of the appropriate state licensing laws and understand the necessary level required in each performance skill area needed for safe driving so that the appropriate information can be passed on to the OT Specialist in Driving. For example, if the patient has left neglect or serious visual-perceptual deficits, these conditions are contraindicative for safe driving unless they resolve early. Another example is the field of vision requirement already discussed. If a stroke survivor has a complete homonymous hemianopsia, then the therapist should tell the client and family that a return to driving is not possible because of the requirements of the state unless the condition resolves itself enough to meet the field of vision requirements. Table 23-2 has examples of problem areas to note.

When structuring the predrive clinical screening, the therapist should be guided by common sense and evidence-based practice where applicable to use appropriate clinical tools and tests as they relate to driving. Although typical clinical tools and equipment in an OT department can be used for this screening, the therapist may need additional specialized equipment for more relevance to driving. Clients may be more cooperative with the clinical evaluation for the IADL of driving if they appreciate its relevancy to the driving task. For example, the client may feel frustrated and angry working on a puzzle or paper maze during the therapist's predrive clinical screening but may understand the importance of a test that provides specific data related to driving such as reaction time, driving risk behavior assessed using a clinical tool to measure divided and selective attention, and a measuring of cognitive abilities for safe driving with a clinical tool that

Table 23-2

Examples of Stroke-Related Deficits to Identify during Initial Assessment That May Impact Driving Performance

DEFICIT	POTENTIAL ISSUES FOR FUTURE RETURN TO DRIVING
Left or right neglect	May not see or respond to road signs or markings; may ride to extreme right or left of lane; may miss turning lanes; will not look to affected side at intersections
Loss of field of vision	Will be surprised by unexpected stimuli or events that move into field of vision suddenly from blind area, may collide with something the driver did not even see such as a person stepping off a sidewalk or a car lane changing from the field loss side
Dense hemiplegia	May require adaptive devices to compensate for motor dysfunction in one or both affected extremities
Seizure	Most states have a required period of being seizure-free, with or without medication.
Complex regional pain syndrome type I (reflex sympathetic dystrophy)	Pain or strong medications may affect mood and be a distracting factor; associated motor deficits may require adaptive equipment for driving; posturing of the affected limb while driving is important.
Sensory-perceptual	Body positioning behind the steering wheel is difficult due to visual neglect or body imaging issues, inadequate spatial relations or time/space management, and poor depth perception, leading to short following distance and stopping distance, inadequate determination of speed and distance of approaching vehicle for making a safe unprotected left turn.
Communicate difficulties such as aphasia	Misreads signs or other road user cues; becomes distracted when attempting to talk
Impulsivity, poor inhibition	Responds or reacts without thinking or seeing the consequences; does not see the entire driving picture to make sound judgments and decisions
Denial, poor insight	Does not see or understand overall performance skill deficits or how the deficits interfere with safe driving; improvement difficult because he or she does not feel there is any need for improvement
Memory	May not remember where destination is or how to get there; becomes confused and anxious when cannot find street, misses a street, or is faced with a detour

assesses memory, judgment, decision-making, attention, and motor speed abilities. The therapist should describe the relevance of any test given, so the client will be motivated to perform well on the test. The assessment of motor/praxis skills and sensory-perceptual skills is generally easy for the therapist to set up because the assessment and techniques used in these areas are similar to those used in other settings and with other disabilities. The difference is that the therapist must keep a mind set on the activity demands of driving as they do similarly with cooking, dressing, and other ADL they consider.

The therapist should attempt to use clinical tools and tests during this phase that have the most significance to the driving task. Box 23-2 lists some of the more common clinical tests. Additional tools and devices are available on the market that can be used in the clinic with driver-related tasks and have a degree of face validity and statistical correlation (Box 23-3).

Engum and colleagues[9] noted the following: "Knowing the patient's diagnosis or pathology typically does not yield predictions about the patient's ability to drive.... Even loss of brain mass is not deemed to be an exact predictor of driving skills ... neuropsychological tests, which can detect gross organic impairment or provide useful catalogs of patients' impairments and abilities, do not seem to assess driver potential." The OT Generalist in Driving must collaborate with the OT Specialist in Driving to coordinate the tests and tools used, so duplication is not done.

Their four-year research project with more than 230 brain-damaged patients led to the development of the Cognitive Behavioral Drivers Inventory (CBDI). This inventory is designed to assess aspects of cognitive

Box 23-2

Examples of the Common Clinical Tests Used as Needed

- Trailsmaking Part A and B
- Gardner Test of Visual Perceptual Skills
- Motor-Free Visual Perceptual Test—3
- Cognitive Linquistic Quick Test
- Rey-Osterreith Complex Figure Test
- Digit Symbol
- Gardner Reversal
- Neglect (HVN) Screen
- Short Blessed Test or Mini-Mental Status Exam
- Draw-a-Clock or Draw-a-Person test
- DriveABLE Assessment
- DriveSafe Simulator
- Simple reaction time
- Road smart judgment test
- Gross Impairments Screening Battery of General Physical and Mental Abilities (GRIMPS)
- Porteus Maze Test
- Raven Progressive Matrices

Box 23-3

Clinical Evaluation Tools with Face Validity and/or Correlation to On-Road Driving Performance

Cognitive Behavioral Driver's Inventory
Psychological Software Services
www.neuroscience.cnter.com/pss/

Elemental Driving System
Life Science Associates
1 Fenimore Road
Bayport, NY 11705
(631) 472–2111
lifesciassoc@pipeline.com

Braking Test Computer
Vericom Computers
14320 James Road, Suite 200
Rogers, MN 55374
1–800–533–5547
www.vericomcomputers.com

functioning such as attention, concentration, rapid decision-making, visual-motor speed and coordination, visual scanning and acuity, and shifting attention from one task to another. Their results demonstrated that more than 95% of the patients receiving passing scores on the CBDI were judged independently by an on-road driving test as safe to operate a motor vehicle. Conversely, all patients who failed the CBDI were judged as unsafe drivers in the independently administered road test.[9] A subsequent study by some of the same authors in 1988 completed a double-blind test of the validity of the CBDI. Again, the authors found a high correlation between the results of the CBDI and the independent road test.[8] Although the CBDI is psychometrically strong, it has no face validity. The CBDI is useful, but the Elemental Driver Simulator has face validity and may be better understood by patients as being relative to driving because it involves operating simulated primary car controls (Fig. 23-6).

Gianutsos,[11] the originator of the Elemental Driving Simulator, stated, "road tests lack the basic psychometric requisites of tests—standardization, reliability and empirical validity." She described the Elemental Driving Simulator as a "computer-based quasi-simulator that is based on objective, norm-referenced measures of the cognitive abilities regarded as critical for driving." These cognitive abilities include mental processing efficiency, simultaneous information processing, perceptual-motor skills, and impulse control. The Elemental Driving Simulator also attempts to measure insight and judgment by comparing self-appraisal with performance. Research by Gianutsos[11] and Engum and colleagues[9] indicated a significant correlation in the Elemental Driving Simulator and CBDI. These

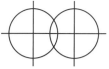
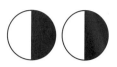
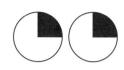
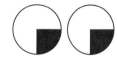

for Vision Testing Equipment

ration
lome St.
N 46545
25

ew
review.com

ng Equipment
Main Ave.
A 18504

ical Company
optical.com

Normal visual field

Right homonymous hemianopsia

Right superior quadranopsia

Right inferior quadranopsia

Figure 23-10   Representation of normal visual field in the eyes and typical visual field defects.

areas arise, the stroke survivor should be an eye care specialist. If the patient does not state requirements, an eye care specialist the patient before an on-road assessment. For the stroke survivor does not meet the state's irement for peripheral vision, then he or she nily should be educated on this fact and never the OT Specialist in Driving. This informald be reported to the state's medical review h the Department of Driver Licensing, so the make a decision to suspend the person's driving (see Box 23-4).

states allow a loss of vision in the upper quadrant the lateral median in the superior quadrant is Fig. 23-10). The exact degree of visual field availch eye should be assessed quantitatively. Gianutsos hoff[13] have suggested that perimetric and funcual fields also are important to assess. A patient plete homonymous hemianopsia may have only rees of total visual field. Whenever an occupaherapist suspects that a patient has any degree of ral vision loss, an objective test using machines the Goldman or Humphrey perimeter test should l. An OT clinic generally cannot afford expensive, bjective perimeter machines that can quantitatively e exact degrees of visual fields in all quadrants. The ist can perform a finger confrontation test or use a ntal perimeter tool, and while this will confirm a ete hemianopsia, the test is not inclusive or objecBefore concluding that the patient cannot drive with npairment, the therapist must make a referral to a eye care specialist that uses one of the machines previously to get an accurate report of the exact of vision.

Aside from visual deficits that may occur because of the stroke, the occupational therapist also must consider the normal change in visual skills occurring due to the person's age. Testing eye range of motion, tracking, pursuits, and saccades can be done quickly with a few handheld sticks or a tracking ball. As does any organ in the body, the eye loses some of its capability with age. The pupil of the eye becomes less elastic and restricts the amount of light let into the retina. Many elderly patients complain of difficulty driving at night or during weather conditions when the illumination is poor, such as in rain, fog, or snow. Cataracts, glaucoma, and macular degeneration are common among elderly persons. Cataracts, a clouding of the lenses, also can affect night driving and can produce hazy vision during the day. Cataract surgery has a 90% success rate in a healthy older person who does not have comorbidities. Glaucoma, an increase in ocular pressure that damages the optic nerve and retinal nerve fibers, begins by affecting side vision first and eventually compromises central vision. It is a treatable condition, and a referral to the appropriate eye care specialist is important before performing the on-road assessment. The therapist should consider diabetic retinopathy for a person with a history of diabetes. When the degree of macular degeneration is so great that it affects the central vision to a point that the person cannot see anything in this visual area, then the patient needs to stop driving. Therapists can assess visual scanning, awareness, and attention in the clinic by using some of the subtests in the visual-perceptual and cognitive tests discussed later in this chapter.

Because speed and movement can influence visual a visual-perceptual skills, the therapist must make the determination of the proficiency and effectivene

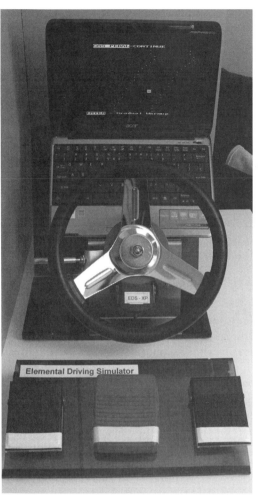

Figure 23-6   The Elemental Driving Simulator. (Courtesy Life Science Associates, Bayport, NY.)

researchers believe that their results confirm the reliability and validity of their clinical driving assessment programs. By using the Elemental Driving Simulator or CBDI, the therapist obtains not only objective data but also recorded information relevant to the driving task. More importantly, data from these tests have demonstrated reliability and validity with published norms and standardized rules. The drawbacks to these tools are that they are expensive, time consuming to give, and require the use of a proper computer, which can be intimidating for an older person.

The predriving clinical evaluation can be organized similar to or along with a typical discharge evaluation of performance skill areas and an ADL and IADL evaluation. The screening would be an obvious emphasis on driving skill requirements in an attempt to determine if the person is ready for referral for the on-road assessment or if the referral should be delayed to a better time. One should remember that if the person is referred too early, the results may produce negative consequences for the person's driving privileges.

The 2008 OT Practice Framework[1] describes performance skills as observable, concrete, goal directed actions that a client uses to engage in daily life occupations. Multiple factors, such as the context in which the occupation is performed, the specific demands of the activity being attempted, and the client's body functions and structures, affect the client's ability to demonstrate performance skills. With this in mind, the OT Generalist in Driving should evaluate the stroke survivor's performance skills for driving with consideration of all of the client factors, contextual/ environmental factors, and the activity demands of the occupation of driving for this particular individual.

Discussion of the components of a predriving clinical evaluation at this stage follows.

Motor and Praxis Skill Assessment

The motor and praxis skill assessment should involve a brief functional look at the patient's active range of motion, muscle strength, sensory modalities, bilateral and unilateral gross and fine motor coordination, and any abnormalities such as muscle tone, spasticity, stereotypical patterns, and associated reactions. A slowing of physical functioning can affect reaction time in responding to stimuli in the environment. Slower reaction time among older drivers may be caused by motor change or delayed visual processing. The loss of strength and range of motion can prevent the person from safely operating the primary or secondary controls of the vehicle. If the person has the necessary isolated control in the affected arm with appropriate sensation and smooth coordination, he or she may be able to continue using this arm for two-handed steering. For liability reasons, the OT Generalist in Driving will not evaluate or recommend adaptive equipment for driving but should be familiar with options available for the stroke survivor, so that the intervention plan may include education of the client and family on the importance of seeing the OT Specialist in Driving. The OT Generalist in Driving should also consider the person's functional mobility in regards to ambulating to and from a vehicle and loading any assistive devices. Preintervention in this area can save time for the OT Specialist in Driving.

In driving, an affected limb cannot be used at all if the necessary functional skills are not available since it could be unsafe and cause the driver to lose control of the vehicle. An example would be an upper extremity that has a stereotypical flexor pattern with little isolated control. If the patient cannot use the affected arm safely, then various kinds of adaptive equipment and driving aids are available that can be used to aid one-handed steering or for reach of secondary control functions that the impaired extremity should operate. For example, the left hand generally operates the turn signals and the right hand generally operates the gear selector. Fig. 23-7 gives examples of adaptive equipment for driving that is recommended by the OT Specialist in Driving to assist with various vehicle controls. Some states require a spinner knob even if the person can

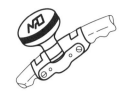

Spinner knob

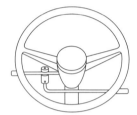

Left foot accelerator

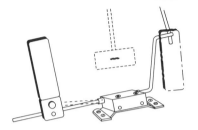

Turn signal crossover

Figure 23-7 Typical driving aids for a person recovering from stroke. (Courtesy Mobility Products and Design, Winamac, Ind.)

palm the wheel and control it well with the remaining good arm. Compensatory techniques with special equipment can assist only with physically controlling a vehicle and do not resolve the person's other potential problem area with cognitive and sensory-perceptual skills.

Regarding lower extremity function, if the patient does not have isolated control in the right lower extremity, then the person will require a left foot gas pedal (see Fig. 23-7). If the person has recovery in muscle strength, sensation, and coordination in the right leg, then the patient may be able to continue using this leg normally on the pedals. If the person wears a lightweight short leg brace and has some minimal movement in the ankle, and all other factors—such as strength, sensation, and coordination—are good, then this person still may be able to use the right leg for gas and brake operation or just gas operation. If movement to the brake pedal is slow with or without a brace, or the hip or knee fatigues quickly, then teaching a two-footed driving method may be possible if this is allowed in the state of residence and the person has plantarflexion and dorsiflexion in the affected ankle. Proprioception is necessary and should be evaluated carefully. The OT Specialist in Driving will determine if the stroke survivor has good foot placement, good pedal regulation, and acceptable reaction time using the affected leg. The in-vehicle and on-road evaluation will determine which method and what

equipment, if any, is viable and necessary. After the moving assessment, the therapist may determine that the person requires equipment when initially it was thought he or she could use the affected upper or lower limb.

For secondary controls that are operated in a stationary position, the stroke survivor may be able to use compensatory methods for these controls; for example, using the left hand for inserting and turning the ignition key or operating the gearshift lever. If this is difficult, adaptive aids such as a gear selector crossover and key extension may be appropriate. Special panoramic mirrors can be beneficial when neck range of motion is limited or to increase visual awareness to the rear, sides, and blind spots (Figs. 23-8 and 23-9). These mirrors do not compensate for loss of peripheral vision, so they are not useful for correction of homonymous hemianopsia.

Sensory-Perceptual Assessment

A visual assessment is crucial because driving depends so much on visual input. A visual assessment in regards to the task of driving is more than mere checking of a patient's visual acuity and depth perception. Scheiman,[32] a rehabilitation optometrist who works with patients with various diagnoses, stated that good vision is more than clear vision: "the individual must have the ability to use his eyes for extended periods of time without discomfort, be able to analyze and interpret the incoming

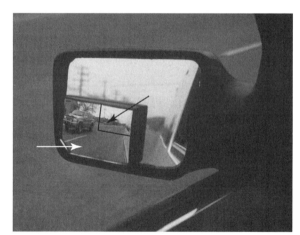

Figure 23-8 SmartView Mirror by Interactive Driving Systems. This mirror eliminates the confusion noted in the typical spot convex mirror and increases rear vision by dividing the mirror into two areas. The outside half of the SmartView mirror (*white arrow*) shows objects in the blind spot of the vehicle, or Danger Zone. If a car is detected in the Danger Zone, the driver must not move in front of it. In this photograph, the car shown is detected by the mirror to be in the driver's Danger Zone. The upper inside quadrant of the mirror (*black arrow*) is boxed and shows the Safe Zone. If a car is seen in the box—and stays in the box—the driver may move in front of it. (Courtesy Interactive Driving Systems, Cheshire, Conn.)

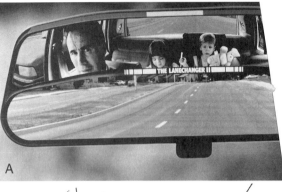

A

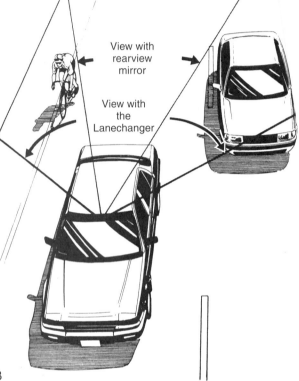

View with rearview mirror

View with the Lanechanger

B

Figure 23-9 **A,** The Lanechanger mirror combines a standard rearview mirro mirror. **B,** This convex mirror provides a wider angle of vision and increased sa The Lanechanger, Quebec, Canada.)

information, and respond to what is being seen." His experience indicates that nearly half of the patients admitted to a rehabilitation center with stroke or traumatic brain injury have visual system deficits, primarily in the area of binocular vision and accommodation. Other commonly reported vision problems include reduced visual acuity, decreased contrast sensitivity, visual field deficits, visual neglect, strabismus, oculomotor dysfunction, and accommodative and stereopsis dysfunction. See Chapter 16.

The stroke survivor should be evaluated visually according to the vision requirements for licensing of the state. This usually includes visual acuity of 20/40 in at least one eye and a total field of vision of at least 130 to

140 degrees. Eye test char visual acuity. A commerciall sion tester that is self-contair licensing agencies may be app In addition to visual acuity, t for depth perception or stere road sign recognition, phoria perimeter vision. These ma that the therapist must take i using them and interpreting tl stereoscopic vision testers rely patient does not possess binocu reason, this machine can be used Box 23-4 lists vision testing reso

of problei
referred to
meet basi
should see
example,
visual req
and the fa
referred
tion sho
board wi
state can
privilege
Some
as long
normal
able in e
and Su
tional v
with co
110 de
tional
periph
such a
be use
large
meas
thera
horiz
com
tive.
this
loca
note
field

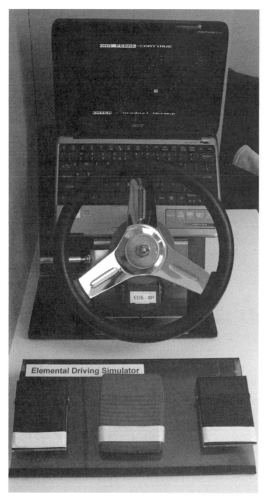

Figure 23-6 The Elemental Driving Simulator. (Courtesy Life Science Associates, Bayport, NY.)

researchers believe that their results confirm the reliability and validity of their clinical driving assessment programs. By using the Elemental Driving Simulator or CBDI, the therapist obtains not only objective data but also recorded information relevant to the driving task. More importantly, data from these tests have demonstrated reliability and validity with published norms and standardized rules. The drawbacks to these tools are that they are expensive, time consuming to give, and require the use of a proper computer, which can be intimidating for an older person.

The predriving clinical evaluation can be organized similar to or along with a typical discharge evaluation of performance skill areas and an ADL and IADL evaluation. The screening would be an obvious emphasis on driving skill requirements in an attempt to determine if the person is ready for referral for the on-road assessment or if the referral should be delayed to a better time. One should remember that if the person is referred too early, the results may produce negative consequences for the person's driving privileges.

The 2008 OT Practice Framework[1] describes performance skills as observable, concrete, goal directed actions that a client uses to engage in daily life occupations. Multiple factors, such as the context in which the occupation is performed, the specific demands of the activity being attempted, and the client's body functions and structures, affect the client's ability to demonstrate performance skills. With this in mind, the OT Generalist in Driving should evaluate the stroke survivor's performance skills for driving with consideration of all of the client factors, contextual/ environmental factors, and the activity demands of the occupation of driving for this particular individual.

Discussion of the components of a predriving clinical evaluation at this stage follows.

Motor and Praxis Skill Assessment

The motor and praxis skill assessment should involve a brief functional look at the patient's active range of motion, muscle strength, sensory modalities, bilateral and unilateral gross and fine motor coordination, and any abnormalities such as muscle tone, spasticity, stereotypical patterns, and associated reactions. A slowing of physical functioning can affect reaction time in responding to stimuli in the environment. Slower reaction time among older drivers may be caused by motor change or delayed visual processing. The loss of strength and range of motion can prevent the person from safely operating the primary or secondary controls of the vehicle. If the person has the necessary isolated control in the affected arm with appropriate sensation and smooth coordination, he or she may be able to continue using this arm for two-handed steering. For liability reasons, the OT Generalist in Driving will not evaluate or recommend adaptive equipment for driving but should be familiar with options available for the stroke survivor, so that the intervention plan may include education of the client and family on the importance of seeing the OT Specialist in Driving. The OT Generalist in Driving should also consider the person's functional mobility in regards to ambulating to and from a vehicle and loading any assistive devices. Preintervention in this area can save time for the OT Specialist in Driving.

In driving, an affected limb cannot be used at all if the necessary functional skills are not available since it could be unsafe and cause the driver to lose control of the vehicle. An example would be an upper extremity that has a stereotypical flexor pattern with little isolated control. If the patient cannot use the affected arm safely, then various kinds of adaptive equipment and driving aids are available that can be used to aid one-handed steering or for reach of secondary control functions that the impaired extremity should operate. For example, the left hand generally operates the turn signals and the right hand generally operates the gear selector. Fig. 23-7 gives examples of adaptive equipment for driving that is recommended by the OT Specialist in Driving to assist with various vehicle controls. Some states require a spinner knob even if the person can

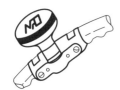

Spinner knob

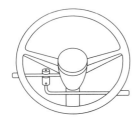

Left foot accelerator

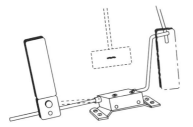

Turn signal crossover

Figure 23-7 Typical driving aids for a person recovering from stroke. (Courtesy Mobility Products and Design, Winamac, Ind.)

palm the wheel and control it well with the remaining good arm. Compensatory techniques with special equipment can assist only with physically controlling a vehicle and do not resolve the person's other potential problem area with cognitive and sensory-perceptual skills.

Regarding lower extremity function, if the patient does not have isolated control in the right lower extremity, then the person will require a left foot gas pedal (see Fig. 23-7). If the person has recovery in muscle strength, sensation, and coordination in the right leg, then the patient may be able to continue using this leg normally on the pedals. If the person wears a lightweight short leg brace and has some minimal movement in the ankle, and all other factors—such as strength, sensation, and coordination—are good, then this person still may be able to use the right leg for gas and brake operation or just gas operation. If movement to the brake pedal is slow with or without a brace, or the hip or knee fatigues quickly, then teaching a two-footed driving method may be possible if this is allowed in the state of residence and the person has plantarflexion and dorsiflexion in the affected ankle. Proprioception is necessary and should be evaluated carefully. The OT Specialist in Driving will determine if the stroke survivor has good foot placement, good pedal regulation, and acceptable reaction time using the affected leg. The in-vehicle and on-road evaluation will determine which method and what

equipment, if any, is viable and necessary. After the moving assessment, the therapist may determine that the person requires equipment when initially it was thought he or she could use the affected upper or lower limb.

For secondary controls that are operated in a stationary position, the stroke survivor may be able to use compensatory methods for these controls; for example, using the left hand for inserting and turning the ignition key or operating the gearshift lever. If this is difficult, adaptive aids such as a gear selector crossover and key extension may be appropriate. Special panoramic mirrors can be beneficial when neck range of motion is limited or to increase visual awareness to the rear, sides, and blind spots (Figs. 23-8 and 23-9). These mirrors do not compensate for loss of peripheral vision, so they are not useful for correction of homonymous hemianopsia.

Sensory-Perceptual Assessment

A visual assessment is crucial because driving depends so much on visual input. A visual assessment in regards to the task of driving is more than mere checking of a patient's visual acuity and depth perception. Scheiman,[32] a rehabilitation optometrist who works with patients with various diagnoses, stated that good vision is more than clear vision: "the individual must have the ability to use his eyes for extended periods of time without discomfort, be able to analyze and interpret the incoming

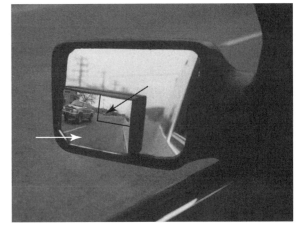

Figure 23-8 SmartView Mirror by Interactive Driving Systems. This mirror eliminates the confusion noted in the typical spot convex mirror and increases rear vision by dividing the mirror into two areas. The outside half of the SmartView mirror *(white arrow)* shows objects in the blind spot of the vehicle, or Danger Zone. If a car is detected in the Danger Zone, the driver must not move in front of it. In this photograph, the car shown is detected by the mirror to be in the driver's Danger Zone. The upper inside quadrant of the mirror *(black arrow)* is boxed and shows the Safe Zone. If a car is seen in the box—and stays in the box—the driver may move in front of it. (Courtesy Interactive Driving Systems, Cheshire, Conn.)

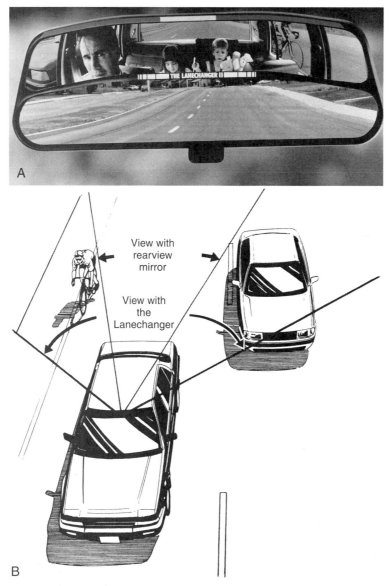

View with
rearview
mirror

View with
the
Lanechanger

Figure 23-9 **A,** The Lanechanger mirror combines a standard rearview mirror with a convex mirror. **B,** This convex mirror provides a wider angle of vision and increased safety. (Courtesy The Lanechanger, Quebec, Canada.)

information, and respond to what is being seen." His experience indicates that nearly half of the patients admitted to a rehabilitation center with stroke or traumatic brain injury have visual system deficits, primarily in the area of binocular vision and accommodation. Other commonly reported vision problems include reduced visual acuity, decreased contrast sensitivity, visual field deficits, visual neglect, strabismus, oculomotor dysfunction, and accommodative and stereopsis dysfunction. See Chapter 16.

The stroke survivor should be evaluated visually according to the vision requirements for licensing of the state. This usually includes visual acuity of 20/40 in at least one eye and a total field of vision of at least 130 to 140 degrees. Eye test charts can be used to ascertain visual acuity. A commercially available stereoscopic vision tester that is self-contained and often used by driver licensing agencies may be applicable to a clinical setting. In addition to visual acuity, these machines also screen for depth perception or stereopsis, contrast sensitivity, road sign recognition, phoria, fusion, and horizontal perimeter vision. These machines have limitations that the therapist must take into consideration when using them and interpreting the results. For example, stereoscopic vision testers rely on binocular vision. If a patient does not possess binocular vision for whatever reason, this machine can be used only on a limited basis. Box 23-4 lists vision testing resources. If any suspicions

Box 23-4

Resources for Vision Testing Equipment

Bernell Corporation
4016 North Home St.
Mishawaka, IN 46545
(800) 348–2225

Keystone View
www.keystoneview.com

Porto-Clinic
Driver Testing Equipment
1309 South Main Ave.
Scranton, PA 18504

Stereo Optical Company
www.stereooptical.com

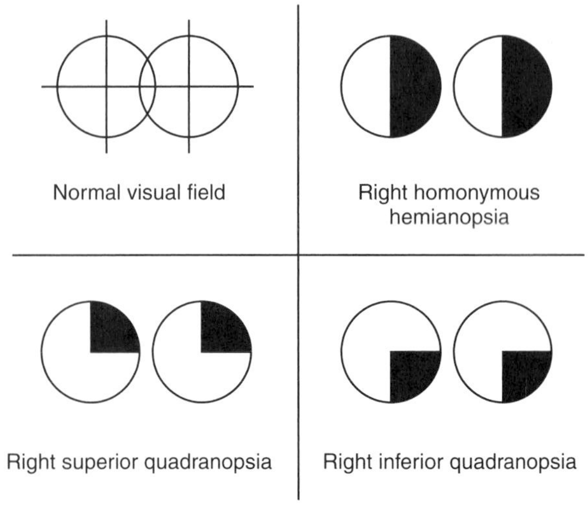

Figure 23-10 Representation of normal visual field in the eyes and typical visual field defects.

of problem areas arise, the stroke survivor should be referred to an eye care specialist. If the patient does not meet basic state requirements, an eye care specialist should see the patient before an on-road assessment. For example, if the stroke survivor does not meet the state's visual requirement for peripheral vision, then he or she and the family should be educated on this fact and never referred to the OT Specialist in Driving. This information should be reported to the state's medical review board with the Department of Driver Licensing, so the state can make a decision to suspend the person's driving privileges (see Box 23-4).

Some states allow a loss of vision in the upper quadrant as long as the lateral median in the superior quadrant is normal (Fig. 23-10). The exact degree of visual field available in each eye should be assessed quantitatively. Gianutsos and Suchoff[13] have suggested that perimetric and functional visual fields also are important to assess. A patient with complete homonymous hemianopsia may have only 110 degrees of total visual field. Whenever an occupational therapist suspects that a patient has any degree of peripheral vision loss, an objective test using machines such as the Goldman or Humphrey perimeter test should be used. An OT clinic generally cannot afford expensive, large objective perimeter machines that can quantitatively measure exact degrees of visual fields in all quadrants. The therapist can perform a finger confrontation test or use a horizontal perimeter tool, and while this will confirm a complete hemianopsia, the test is not inclusive or objective. Before concluding that the patient cannot drive with this impairment, the therapist must make a referral to a local eye care specialist that uses one of the machines noted previously to get an accurate report of the exact field of vision.

Aside from visual deficits that may occur because of the stroke, the occupational therapist also must consider the normal change in visual skills occurring due to the person's age. Testing eye range of motion, tracking, pursuits, and saccades can be done quickly with a few handheld sticks or a tracking ball. As does any organ in the body, the eye loses some of its capability with age. The pupil of the eye becomes less elastic and restricts the amount of light let into the retina. Many elderly patients complain of difficulty driving at night or during weather conditions when the illumination is poor, such as in rain, fog, or snow. Cataracts, glaucoma, and macular degeneration are common among elderly persons. Cataracts, a clouding of the lenses, also can affect night driving and can produce hazy vision during the day. Cataract surgery has a 90% success rate in a healthy older person who does not have comorbidities. Glaucoma, an increase in ocular pressure that damages the optic nerve and retinal nerve fibers, begins by affecting side vision first and eventually compromises central vision. It is a treatable condition, and a referral to the appropriate eye care specialist is important before performing the on-road assessment. The therapist should consider diabetic retinopathy for a person with a history of diabetes. When the degree of macular degeneration is so great that it affects the central vision to a point that the person cannot see anything in this visual area, then the patient needs to stop driving. Therapists can assess visual scanning, awareness, and attention in the clinic by using some of the subtests in the visual-perceptual and cognitive tests discussed later in this chapter.

Because speed and movement can influence visual and visual-perceptual skills, the therapist must make the final determination of the proficiency and effectiveness of these areas for driving in the vehicle and in the dynamic moving traffic environment. For example, the speed of a vehicle decreases visual acuity and side vision. If a person has 200 degrees of visual field, at 20 miles per hour, the field is reduced to 104 degrees; at 40 miles per hour, to 70 degrees; and at 60 miles per hour, to 40 degrees. Speed also decreases visual acuity; the faster the speed, the less time available to react to visual stimuli in the environment.[34] The Visual Attention Analyzer Model 2000 (Visual Resources, Chicago, Ill.) assesses the size of the useful field of view and comprises three subtests to evaluate processing speed, divided attention, and selective attention (see Chapter 19). This machine can be helpful to the OT Generalist in Driving as the machine evaluates and provides training modules that can be used in intervention to improve the person's visual attention and processing speed.

Visual-Perception and Cognitive Assessment

According to Toglia,[40] the limitation to the deficit-specific approach to perception is that "it equates difficulty in performance of a specific task with a deficit . . . [and] does not consider the underlying reasons for failure or the conditions that influence performance." For example, a patient may score low on a typical OT clinical test of visual-perceptual skills; nevertheless, the results may be a consequence of reduced visual acuity or accommodation and not necessarily a specific visual-perceptual deficit.

A stroke survivor who has serious visual-perceptual deficits will have difficulty throughout rehabilitation.[43] The occupational therapist will complete documentation and observations of deficits in these areas during routine evaluation and intervention. The stroke survivor should not be referred to the OT Specialist in Driving until the deficit areas no longer interfere with basic ADL. If the therapist understands the definition of each visual-perceptual category and the way deficits in each area affect a person's basic self-care skills, a further analysis of the activity demands of driving can show the way persistent problems in these areas can interfere with driving performance skills (see Chapter 18 and Chapter 19).

Driving requires a combination of perceptual skills in which cognitive performance plays a major role. Strong cognitive abilities are fundamental to attentiveness in the driving task, recognition of stimuli, and choice of the appropriate way to respond. A decline in cognitive abilities can significantly influence a person's ability to plan, judge, and act adequately. A cognitively impaired person may have difficulty maneuvering a vehicle through rapidly changing traffic with many unexpected actions and reactions from other drivers, passengers, pedestrians, and bicyclists. Cognitive impairment has been linked to higher motor vehicle crash rates in elderly individuals.[6] Problem areas may involve attention,

orientation, concentration, learning (short-term memory), and problem-solving. Diffuse cognitive deficits occur more frequently in patients with large frontal strokes, visuospatial deficits in right hemisphere strokes, and apraxia in left hemisphere strokes.[46] Unilateral neglect has been reported in half of the patients with right brain damage and in 20% to 25% with left brain damage.[38] Diller and Weinberg[7] reported that "patients with left hemiparesis often experience accidents that are related to difficulties in dealing with space, while accidents in patients with right hemiparesis are often related to slowness in processing information."

Patients are generally more aware of motor problems than they are of cognitive problems.[13] Gresham and colleagues[14] noted that "unawareness of the stroke (or its manifestations) is often found in patients with lesions in the nondominant hemisphere. It can lead to impulsive, unsafe behavior in a patient who may otherwise appear relatively normal with respect to physical functioning." Patients' poor insight into their own problem areas can be dangerous because patients may not be aware of serious driver errors and the potentially fatal consequences of their actions.

The occupational therapist can use common verbal and written tasks to assess the areas of visual perceptual functioning such as spatial relations, visual discrimination, form constancy, depth perception and visual memory, sequential memory, and visual closure. Two commonly used tests are the Gardner Test of Visual Perceptual Skills and the Motor-Free Visual Perception Test—3, which is standardized for adults age 70-years-old or older. The Motor-Free Visual Perception Test—Vertical is for those who have difficulty with horizontally presented stimuli such as stroke survivors.

Therapists can use a variety of cognitive tests to assess memory, language, orientation, attention, concentration, reasoning, and problem-solving. The Helm-Estabrooks Cognitive Linguistic Quick Test can be administered in 20 to 30 minutes; is standardized for adults with acquired neurological dysfunction, ages 18- to 89-years-old; and can be used to identify a person's cognitive strengths and weaknesses. This test gives a "snapshot" assessment of the status of these five cognitive domains: attention, memory, language, executive functions, and visuospatial skills (see Chapters 18 and 19).

During the administration of these clinical tests, one must remember that these tests are static and two-dimensional and do not begin to simulate the dynamics of the driving task. French and Hanson[10] stated "controversy continues about which cognitive-perceptual assessments are the best predictors of behind-the-wheel performance." The authors summarized studies performed by Galski, Bruno, and Elhe in 1992 that found a significant correlation between seven tests: "Part A of the Trailsmaking Test, the Rey-Osterreith Complex Figure Test, the Porteus Maze Test, the Visual Form Discrimination, the Double Letter Cancellation, the Wechsler Adult Intelligence Scale—Revised Block Design Test, and Raven's Progressive Matrices and the behind-the-wheel evaluation . . . . the [continued] research suggests that a combination of neuropsychological testing, visual screening, physical functioning, and actual driving (simulators and on-the-road evaluations) is necessary to predict driving performance."

Engum and colleagues[9] defined basic operational and behavioral skills as "attention, concentration, rapid decision-making, stimulus discrimination/response differentiation, sequencing, visual-motor speed and coordination, visual scanning, and acuity and attention shifting." Table 23-3 describes several performance areas and the way deficits in these areas can affect driving performance.

An appropriate end to the predrive clinical evaluation may involve several tests to assess procedural memory for driving, knowledge of road rules, and road sign and/or situational problem-solving, reasoning, and judgment. Several formal tests can be used. The Driver Performance Test, distributed by the Advanced Driving Skills Institute (Orlando, Fla.), is a video of simulated real-world driving scenes and provides insight into the patient's perceptual capabilities, psychomotor responses, and decision-making strategies. Using a driver education defensive driving technique of identifying, predicting, deciding, and executing, the Driver Performance Test requires the patient to search for hazardous situations or conditions, identify potential and immediate hazards, predict the effect of the hazard, decide the way to evade the hazard, and execute evasive driving actions.[44] The drawback to this test is that it takes about 45 minutes to administer. Additional time is then necessary to review the answer video with the patient, an essential step for any learning or understanding to take place for the patient or the therapist.

Because the Driver Performance Test has no statistical validity, the therapist should decide whether to use valuable time administering it during this phase or letting the driver rehabilitation therapist use it in the next phase of the process. An important consideration is that this rapidly timed test may produce stress in the stroke survivor because it requires quick problem-solving and decision-making, marking on an answer sheet while having attention divided, and retaining information. The test taker has only a few seconds to choose an answer and then must go on to the next traffic scene because the test has no built-in delay or pause. If the test taker gets behind, he or she may become disorganized or distracted and not be able to respond to the next scene. Although quick thinking and reaction are important for driving, the Driver Performance Test may be a better tool to use after the patient has passed all clinical tests and road tests, and may be a more effective tool to use when the therapist determines that the patient needs more practice, training, or review in the areas tested by the Driver Performance Test (Box 23-5).

Table 23-3

Effects of Various Deficits in a Stroke Survivor on Driving Performance

TYPE OF DEFICIT	EFFECT ON DRIVING PERFORMANCE
Higher cognitive functions, memory, ability to learn	Cannot remember route to take to location or loses way if makes wrong turn; may not remember road names but can remember the route; severe deficits in higher functions may impede safe driving; unless the patient recovering from stroke is a new driver, the inability to learn new tasks may not impede safe driving; may require directions to be repeated
Motor	Usually does not impede safe driving because compensatory driving techniques or adaptive driving aids can be used
Disturbances in balance and coordination	May impede car transfers or loading of mobility device (e.g., wheelchair or walker); steering device, left-foot accelerator, or turn signal adaptation may compensate for inability to use the upper or lower extremity
Somatosensory	Generally does not interfere with driving because a person does not use an extremity with lack of sensation or with limiting pain while driving
Vision disorders	Severe visual loss or ocular motility disturbances may impede safe driving; the deficit may lead to the patient not meeting driver licensing requirements; persons with homonymous hemianopsia are not allowed to drive in most states; other age-related deficits such as glaucoma, cataracts, and diabetic retinopathy may impede safe driving.
Unilateral neglect	A contraindication for safe driving
Speech and language	Expressive aphasia, dysarthria, or apraxias of speech are usually not problems in driving, although attempting to carry on a conversation while driving may cause distraction; receptive aphasia may impede the driver from understanding directions or conversation.
Pain	The unaffected extremities may be used to drive; does not impede driving unless it is so severe it causes a distraction.

Box 23-5

Resources for Assessment of Driving Knowledge and Judgment

Driver Performance Test and Safe Performance
   On-Road Test:
Advanced Driving Skills Institute
www.advdrivskills.com

Drivers Edge Rehabilitation Course:
InterActive Enterprises
852 Martin Drive
Palatine, IL 60067
1–847–358–9508 (fax)
interactiveenterprises@comcast.net

IMPORTANCE OF THE COMBINATION OF A CLINICAL EVALUATION AND AN ON-ROAD EVALUATION

A comprehensive driver evaluation should involve the two phases of a clinical evaluation and an on-road evaluation. A therapist's decision regarding the patient's motor, sensory-perceptual, and cognitive abilities for driving should not be based solely on a clinical test(s) or solely on an on-road test. In a 1994 review of driver assessment methods at the Jewish Rehabilitation Center in Montreal, Canada, the chief of research and her associates found that 95% of their patients were given on-road tests because no clear cutoff score based on typical clinical tests was reliable in predicting whether a person was unsafe to drive.[21] Earlier studies suggested that persons who pass tests for cognitive deficits do not require road tests.[25,33] Experienced certified driver rehabilitation specialists (CDRS) typically do not agree with this opinion, and other more recent studies have found that clinical testing alone is insufficient and recommend a mandatory driving test.[4,20,42]

A therapist should not deny a stroke survivor the opportunity to have the road test based on the clinical findings only unless the patient has obvious serious performance skill issues or does not meet the basic requirements given by the department of driver licensing. The therapist at this point can make only an assumption regarding significant deficits and the potential for them to interfere with driving performance. There is little correlation between typical clinical tests and real driving performance, so the therapist performing the formal driving test on the road should make the conclusion regarding the stroke survivor's driving abilities. Occupational therapists who are experienced driver rehabilitation therapists say that some patients who do well on clinical tests perform poorly in the car. However, they agree that some patients who do poorly in the clinic perform well in the familiar environ-

ment of the car. Again, the decision lies in the occupational therapist's skill to combine clinical observations and analysis with clinical reasoning and judgment of in-car performance.

DETERMINATION OF READINESS FOR THE ROAD TEST

Driving is one of the most complex activities a person may perform, requires integration of many performance areas, and should always be at the top of the ADL pyramid. Because of its complexity, driving should be one of the last ADL attempted following a stroke.[28] The stroke survivor must have reached all other ADL goals before being ready for the difficult ADL of driving. With abbreviated inpatient rehabilitation stays for stroke survivors becoming the norm, the driving evaluation should not take place until the patient has been discharged from the outpatient treatment program or has recovered to a maximal level of independence in the performance of other ADL. If the person is referred too early, he or she may not do well and may lose driving privileges. If the person is referred too late, then he or she may begin driving without an evaluation or the necessary medical approval and put other persons at risk.

Timeliness of the referral for the formal road test is important. Typically, the appropriate time for a referral to the driver rehabilitation therapist is not until two to four months after discharge from the inpatient facility. An exception to this timeline is if the person suffered a mild stroke or transient ischemic attack and recovered quickly with minimal residual deficits. This person may be evaluated as early as two to four weeks after discharge from the inpatient facility. The clinical occupational therapist is the best person to determine whether the stroke survivor is ready for the formal road test before discharge as an inpatient or to determine an estimation of time for readiness after discharge to include in the team's discharge planning and final recommendations to the patient and family. Input from all team members should be sought. The physician should provide only medical clearance when all parties agree that the stroke survivor is ready for the on-road evaluation.

A timely referral by the physician or other team members may reduce the likelihood that the patient may begin driving with no supervision from a family member or friend. The physician should communicate effectively to the stroke survivor that he or she should abstain from all driving until an evaluation has been completed. This recommendation should be documented and verbally communicated to the person's caregivers. For liability protection of the rehabilitation facility and team members, the patient should be required to sign a form demonstrating understanding of the recommendations given and indicating willingness to comply. Each team member that has verbally given the same recommendations to the patient should document in the progress notes or discharge summary when and what instructions were given to the patient. If it appears that the person will not comply with the recommendations, the rehabilitation team (doctor or therapists) should advise the department of driver licensing.

The therapist should caution the patient and the family against practicing a week or so before the appointment with the driver rehabilitation therapist. This strategy is unsafe and needless and puts the patient at risk to be sued by parties for driving while impaired, which can cause personal and property damage. In addition, insurance companies may be able to claim fraud and violation of their regulations, so that they are not monetarily responsible for any damages ordered by a court. The potential consequences are not worth the risk and associated liability, and family members should be informed.

OCCUPATIONAL THERAPIST AS A SPECIALIST IN DRIVING OR DRIVER REHABILITATION THERAPIST

The impact of persisting sensory, perceptual, motor, and cognitive deficits on driving risk levels must be addressed through an objective, formal evaluation on the road and in a specially adapted evaluation vehicle. The professional performing this part of the driving evaluation must have a medical background, knowledge of driver education principles, and special training and skill in in-vehicle techniques and methods. The allied health professional in this role is called the driver rehabilitation therapist to distinguish the therapist from a commercial driving school instructor.

According to the 2009 membership directory of the Association of Driver Rehabilitation Specialists, most therapists certified by this organization have an OT background. Since 2005 the AOTA created an Older Driver Initiative to coordinate multiple projects related to increasing the occupational therapist's awareness and professional training in addressing the occupation of driving and community mobility. The projects completed as of 2009 include an evidence-based literature review, publication of OT Practice Guidelines for Driving and Community Mobility for Older Adults (2006), Older Driver Microsite (www.aota.org/olderdriver), and a specialty certification in driver rehabilitation and community mobility. AOTA also has a variety of educational opportunities available at their annual conference or at their website for continuing education. The AOTA offers a professional certification designation (specialty certification in driving and community mobility [SCDCM] or driving and community mobility assistants [SCADCM]) through a portfolio and professional

development process that is available for application year round. Adaptive Mobility Services, based in Orlando, Florida, has offered since 1984 educational workshops for the allied health professional who need advanced knowledge and skill in the field of driver evaluation as a OT Generalist in Driving or an OT Specialist is Driving. It now offers in-person and online CE opportunities. Box 23-6 has contact information on these organizations.

After receiving a referral on a stroke survivor for a comprehensive driver evaluation, the first step for the OT Specialist in Driving or the driver rehabilitation therapist is to talk with the primary clinical occupational therapist in the inpatient or outpatient unit to obtain any pertinent information about the stroke survivor. If any questions arise about performance skill areas that the occupational therapist cannot answer, the driver rehabilitation therapist would talk with the person in the appropriate discipline, such as physical therapy, speech therapy, neuropsychology, or rehabilitation optometry.

Second, the driver rehabilitation therapist interviews the patient and the family and obtains a full medical

---

Box 23-6

Resources for Professional Education, Driver Education Materials, and Networking

AAA
Traffic Safety
1000 AAA Drive, Box 78
Heathrow, FL 32746–5080

Adaptive Mobility Services (AMS)
Department of Continuing Education
1000 Delaney Ave.
Orlando, FL 32806
(407) 426–8020
www.adaptivemobility.com

American Occupational Therapy Association (AOTA)
4720 Montgomery Lane
Bethesda, MD 20814–1220
(800) 877–1383
www.aota.org

Association of Driver Rehabilitation Specialists (ADED; formerly called Association of Driver Educators for the Disabled)
www.aded.net or www.driver-ed.org

Safety Industries
P.O. Box 1137
McGill, NV 89318
1–775–235–7766
www.safety-industries.com

history including any other medical or health issues in addition to the stroke that must be considered. The therapist should review the patient's progress in rehabilitation, discuss the unaccomplished goals in each discipline, and confirm all facts regarding the patient's occupation of driving including driving history, the role of driving for this person, and contextual and environmental factors. Driving abilities may be impaired because of adverse drug effects or age-related factors such as physiological changes and age-associated diseases and conditions including arthritis, cataracts, memory loss, and hearing loss. The therapist should explore the stroke survivor and family's knowledge and perspective of problems with other coexisting medical conditions in areas that may not necessarily be related to the stroke diagnosis to understand the whole person. For example, if the stroke survivor has a history of diabetes and has had the right leg amputated, the driver rehabilitation therapist would be prudent to explore the potential problems that may occur in the patient's left leg. This may affect equipment recommendations in terms of a left foot gas pedal versus a set of hand controls.

The therapist should check the status of the person's driver's license, ensure that it is still valid, and note any restrictions already placed on the license. A driver's license is considered public property, so the therapist can contact the appropriate office with the department of driver licensing to check on the license status. Most departments of driver licensing do not allow a person to drive if the license has been suspended or has expired. Most states have a Medical Advisory Board that with the appropriate medical approval may issue a temporary driving permit for evaluation purposes only. The stroke survivor and family must be told that this permit is not to be used to practice before the actual road test appointment with the driver rehabilitation therapist.

The on-road phase of the driver evaluation is crucial to the final decision about a person's driving abilities. The value of the in-vehicle and the in-traffic assessment cannot be underestimated. The professional performing this step must have knowledge of driver education principles, road rules, and state laws and must know how to assess all driving abilities in the car. This person must know the breakdown of performance components involved in specific driving tasks and must understand the purpose of planning a specific route for each person, what to look for, and what can be done to elicit underlying suspected behaviors. This professional is not a passive passenger sitting on the right side of the car simply giving directions. The person must have verbal, visual, and physical skills required to control the driver and the vehicle throughout the test.[31] The therapist must know how to approach the driver with constructive criticism and how to react and handle the emotional and psychological factors that come into play with this portion of the evaluation.

The occupational therapist's unique skill in analysis of activity and occupational performance is of great benefit in this role. The therapist's keen observation skills and knowledge of what to look for are also invaluable during the in-car work. Because the therapist understands the diagnosis and all implications, the therapist can plan a route specific to each client. The therapist should strive for ecological validity, which simply means that the (evaluation and) training takes into consideration the actual environment from which the client comes and will return. The environment includes home, neighborhood, and community where the person works, plays, and/or goes to school.[29]

The driver rehabilitation therapist must have a working knowledge of deficits associated with a stroke, age-related issues, medication implications, and the relationship of all to the driving task. The driver rehabilitation therapist must appreciate the importance of driving to the stroke survivor and work in the client's best interest while also considering the safety and well-being of the public. An allied health professional is most qualified by education and skill standards to perform the clinical evaluation based on professional licensure, ethical standards, and guidelines. Some hospitals and rehabilitation centers consider using a commercial driving school instructor or a retired driver educator from a school to complete the on-road assessment so they do not have to invest in an evaluation car. They may consider the liability cost reduced by using a driving school, but this is not always the case.

USE OF DRIVING SCHOOL INSTRUCTORS AND DRIVER EDUCATORS

The use of an individual without an allied health background in this role should be studied carefully and considered by the rehabilitation team, the employer, and legal counsel. This decision could result in an inadequate outcome if the person performing the road test does not understand diagnoses, disabilities, and the way to observe and assess each performance skill level in the car. The person's educational background, personal references, work history, and working knowledge of diagnoses should be considered carefully. State requirements for licensing as a commercial driving school instructor varies greatly, with no special training required to work with persons with disabilities. In many states, a person can obtain a commercial driving instructor (CDI) license by having a high school diploma, a good driving record with no criminal record, and proof of good health. Some states do require taking an in-depth driver education course to be licensed as a CDI; however, other states require less. Many driving schools exist to teach new drivers to pass a road test so that they can obtain driver's licenses; the focus is not on analyzing driving behavior.

In summary, a typical commercial driving school instructor is usually not a professional, has no understanding of disabilities, and tends to concentrate on teaching a person to pass a road test. The instructor's motivation is often to provide a revenue-generating service. A rehabilitation driving program would need to find a knowledgeable and experienced driving school instructor who has also obtained specialized training with disabilities. An instructor listed as a CDRS with the Association of Driver Rehabilitation Specialists will have met their criteria for this credential.

A person with a degree in education and a certification in driver education may have a more professional approach. This individual has a professional college degree in education with special study in driver education and is well-equipped to educate a person regarding the whole responsibility of driving. This person, although having the professional background, would not have the medical background for understanding all medical implications of a stroke survivor. The biggest limiting factor today to finding a driver educator is that many high school driver education programs are being closed because of funding and liability issues; therefore, fewer individuals opt for special study in this field, and consequently, fewer study programs exist for them.

Whether a CDI or a driver educator is used, the occupational therapist must work with and advise this person about the patient's strengths and weaknesses and probable behaviors that may be observed or expected based on the clinical evaluation and intervention. The therapist also can assist this person in handling particular problem areas and can provide recommendations for appropriate remedial training to see whether the driver can compensate for problems seen in the car.

If the driving instructor or driver educator has little or no experience working with stroke survivors, the therapist must remain closely involved with the road test to ensure proper and continued understanding of the driver's deficits and that the progress or lack of progress is observed correctly. The therapist may need to be in the evaluation vehicle only for the first and last session, but the therapist's collaboration with in-car person for the outcome is very important and should be documented. The OT Generalist in Driving or Specialist in Driving should remain as the supervisor of the person performing the road test and can be held responsible for any decisions or actions made by this person. The members of the "driving team," comprised of the driver rehabilitation therapist and the driving school instructor or driver educator, always should keep in mind that they must follow a standard of care, show reasonable judgment, and avoid negligent action in their work and decisions. Any accidents or collisions in an evaluation car or wrongly clearing a person for driving can produce potential litigation against all parties associated with the driver evaluation process. The liability is not passed completely onto the person just performing the road test. The therapist and/or rehabilitation team that referred the stroke survivor to a particular person for the road test may share liability if wrong decisions are made or poor conclusions are drawn and incompetence is proved.

VEHICLE AND EQUIPMENT ASSESSMENT

Before conducting the road test, the driver rehabilitation therapist must determine if any problem areas exist in the performance skills areas, client factors, contextual and environment factors that may have an impact on making the recommendations for adaptive equipment, setting the driving route, and drawing a conclusion regarding the entire picture of the occupation of driving and community mobility for this person. Final determination of adaptive driving equipment needs should be confirmed in a moving assessment in the evaluation vehicle; however, the patient's own vehicle must be considered at some point. The majority of adults, particularly elderly adults, typically own a vehicle with automatic transmission, which is required for the installation of most driving aids.

Usually the driving equipment needed by a person with left or right hemiplegia is minimal and not costly (between $100 and $1000); but additional costs exist for special instruction and training on the devices in a dual-controlled vehicle. For example, if a left foot gas pedal device is required, the stroke survivor must be instructed in its safe use and be given time for a cerebral transfer from using the right foot to the left foot to take place. This in-car training and practice with the driver rehabilitation therapist should help prevent any accidents and allow the stroke survivor to be safe in the vehicle operation with the new device and the new way of driving. Proper use of the equipment also should be ascertained in a dynamic situation; however, the driver should be given sufficient learning time before being taken into complex traffic situations. A driving range or neighborhood with light traffic and speeds of 15 to 25 miles per hour is a safe, undemanding, and nonthreatening environment in which to start. Even if the patient has no equipment needs, this environment provides time for the patient to become familiar with the evaluation vehicle and the verbal directions of the therapist or instructor.

ON-ROAD DRIVING EVALUATION

A driver must make multiple decisions constantly and interpret information correctly and quickly for safe driving (Fig. 23-11). Smith[35] stated the following: "Driving a modern passenger vehicle on a clear day in light traffic does not overtax any dimension of performance (perceptual, cognitive, or physical). However, in heavy traffic at high speed, at night on poorly marked roads, at a complex

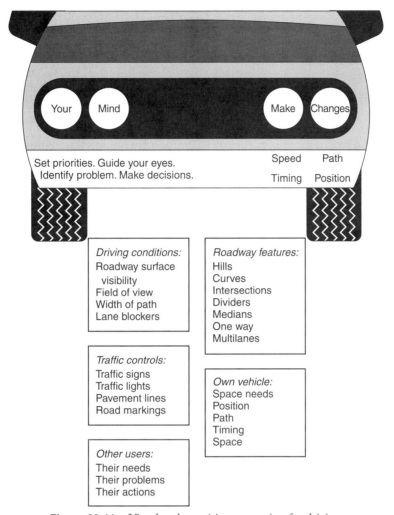

Figure 23-11   Visual and cognitive processing for driving.

intersection, or in a potential accident situation, the demands placed on drivers can exceed their abilities."

Smith[35] described a step procedure necessary for safe driving:

1. The driver must see or hear a situation developing (stimulus registered and sampled at the visual, auditory, or perceptual level).
2. The driver must recognize it (stimulus recognition at the cognitive level).
3. The driver must decide the way to respond (cognitive level).
4. The driver must execute the physical maneuver (motor level).

According to Gianutsos,[12] the New York State Vocational and Educational Services for Individuals with Disabilities committee that addressed this issue concluded in its report on August 13, 1993 that no candidate should be advanced to driving without a behind-the-wheel test. Numerous studies have investigated driving after a stroke or head injury. These patients can be most difficult to assess for driving because they may not only have physical disabilities

that are readily visible but also may have more subtle visual, visuoperceptual, or cognitive problems not easily apparent by observation.

More than half of all stroke survivors who drove cars before their strokes stop driving afterward.[23] Factors that are associated most commonly with driving cessation are older age at the time of stroke and the presence of cognitive deficits.[14] Wilson and Smith[46] investigated the driving performance of patients after stroke using two control groups on a planned driving course. The results indicated that the patients recovering from stroke performed more poorly than did the control subjects. Specific problems identified included difficulties entering and leaving an interstate, lack of awareness of other potential interacting vehicles, and difficulty in reacting to emergencies. Analyses of the more likely performance components causing the driving errors were concluded to be difficulty in visual scanning, lane positioning, appropriate speed, coordination of separate visual scans, interaction with same directional traffic, and maintaining a safe distance from other vehicles.

A simple five- to 10-minute road test given by a state driver's license examiner is not adequate to assess fully all areas that must be considered in driving after a stroke. The examiner primarily is evaluating physical control of the vehicle during basic skills tests such as perpendicular or parallel parking, backing up, three-point turns, and right and left turns. Many times drivers are not even tested in traffic, or if they are, traffic exposure is light and short. The panel of the U.S. Department of Health and Human Resources that determined poststroke rehabilitation guidelines reflected in their report that "stroke survivors may be able to pass a driving test despite having visual spatial deficits or problems with easy distractibility, impulsive behaviors, or slowed decision making that may impair their ability to drive safely under unpredictable road conditions."[14] In addition, the driver license examiner rarely has knowledge of all the adaptive equipment available for physical deficits to determine recommendations. The stroke survivor requires a medical-oriented evaluation and training in a dual-controlled vehicle, neither of which is available from driver license examiners. If adaptive equipment is required for continued safe driving, the stroke survivor generally requires a longer period of training because compensation or adaptation involves breaking old habits (e.g., using the left foot on a left side mounted gas pedal rather than the right foot).

Driving is an overlearned skill for the experienced elderly driver, so the on-road driving assessment phase generally does not require teaching the patient to drive. Many operational components come back naturally to the patient unless a problem associated with dementia, agnosia, or apraxia is evident. Patients' strategic skills may be impaired by any sensory-perceptual, or cognitive deficits that remain. Not to be overlooked is the increased anxiety and stress that this phase of the driver evaluation can invoke for the person being evaluated. The driver rehabilitation therapist can be a valuable asset in a supportive, therapeutic way during the first 15 minutes of the road test. The therapist should make every effort to relax the patient and to let the patient know what to expect and how the verbal directions will be given. The evaluation car may be different from the stroke survivor's, and this can affect his or her disposition. The evaluation vehicle may have many different types of adaptive equipment, and the therapist needs to know how to remove equipment that may get in the way of a driver. For example, if the brake or gas rod of a hand control interferes with a driver who uses his or her right foot moving on and off the factory gas pedal and brake, the therapist should know how to remove the rods for this patient.[30] By allowing time to let the person become familiar with the evaluation vehicle, the driver may be more relaxed for the rest of the test. The driver rehabilitation therapist always should keep in mind how important driving is to each person and how crucial the final decision is on the rest of the person's life.

This perspective aids the therapist in spending sufficient and quality time during the work in the car.

The therapist must understand and plan the goals, objectives, and structuring for the in-traffic evaluation. Every mile of road the patient is requested to drive should have a purpose. Ramsey,[31] a driver educator from West Virginia who has more than 30 years of experience working with persons with diverse disabilities, stated that if driver evaluators or educators go straight for more than a mile, they are "taking a joy ride" and are not assessing effectively a person's ability to drive. Driving straight is easier than making vehicle and speed adjustments for left and right turns and for merging. The visual and mental demands on the driver are greatly increased in executing multiple-step procedures with divided attention demands. The therapist can use a planned route by which to evaluate every patient. The route for a stroke survivor should focus on problem areas seen with the patient's particular deficit areas. Routes familiar and unfamiliar to the driver may have to be used to expose the person to many complex driving situations. If possible, the driver rehabilitation therapist should start or end the test in the driver's home environment, because the patient likely will perform better and be more relaxed on familiar roads. In this familiar context, the driver rehabilitation therapist can get an understanding of the traffic and roads that the stroke survivor normally encounters during driving and can get a picture of how well the driver plans his or her routes. If routes are dangerous, such as one that includes an unprotected left turn against heavy traffic, the driver rehabilitation therapist can counsel the driver about the danger of this maneuver and the high risk and accident potential of this situation and can assist in finding a safer route.

The therapist must be flexible during the road test, guiding the patient on and off the planned route as needed. For example, if a stroke survivor with poor insight and visual awareness starts to miss a stop sign or run through a yield sign without looking both ways or does not show any reaction to a lane ending sign, then this person should be taken off the planned route for instruction and practice to see whether improvement is possible. This driver should not be taken into more complex driving situations in which a hazard may be posed to other road users until the problem is corrected. A stroke survivor with expressive and receptive aphasia may be distracted from the driving scene while attempting to process the therapist's verbal directions during driving. In this case, the patient may benefit from being taken around the familiar home environment and allowed to self-direct in driving from one destination to another such as the bank, drugstore, or doctor's office.

Common driving errors committed by elderly drivers may be related to sensory-perceptual or cognitive dysfunction, or an overall decline (Box 23-7). The driver not only must see objects in the path of travel but also must

Box 23-7

Common Driving Errors in Older Drivers

- Difficulty backing up and making turns
- Not seeing traffic signs or other cars quickly enough
- Difficulty in locating and retrieving information from dashboard displays and traffic signs
- Delayed glare recovery when driving at night
- Not checking rearview mirrors and blind spots
- Bumping into curbs and objects
- Not yielding to oncoming traffic or right-of-way vehicles
- Irregular or slow vehicle speeds

Box 23-8

Examples of Driving Behaviors to be Observed during the In-Traffic Assessment

- Visually searching traffic environment (20 to 30 seconds ahead)
- Demonstrating safe physical control of the vehicle at all times
- Maintaining safe speeds
- Smooth braking
- Demonstrating good lane selection
- Maintaining a safe following distance
- Backing the vehicle
- Making turns
- Navigating curves
- Changing lanes and merging
- Judging gaps at intersections
- Making passing maneuvers
- Performing parallel and angle parking
- Interacting with traffic in a low-risk manner
- Entering and exiting expressways
- Using turn signals appropriately
- Demonstrating proper use of all mirrors
- Checking blind spots
- Finding and using turn lanes properly
- Observing and responding to road signs

understand their implications for safety to adjust driving accordingly. The most frequent citations for older drivers, noted by McKnight[24] in his report "Driver and Pedestrian Training," involved failure to heed stop signs, traffic lights, no left turn signs, and other signs and signals. Underwood[41] noted that "safe driving requires complex cognitive skills, including vigilance, rapid visual scanning with attention to environmental detail, rapid processing of multiple stimuli in several sensory modalities, adequate judgment, and rapid decision-making." Emotional and behavioral factors and characteristics also come into play many times.

There is synergistic performance of many skills and abilities for safe driving. Activity analysis is a valuable tool in which the occupational therapist is well-trained. Breaking the driving task down to its simple performance components can assist greatly with relevant analysis of the clinical test results and in starting a patient in the car in a nonthreatening and stress-reducing fashion (Box 23-8).

A well-planned road and traffic route for the on-road evaluation has the following purposes:

- To assess the driver's ability to enter and exit the vehicle safely and store any mobility aids efficiently
- To assess the driver's understanding and operation of all vehicle primary and secondary controls
- To assess the driver's need for adaptive devices or techniques for driving safely
- To assess the driver's operational and strategic abilities in various traffic, speed, and road conditions
- To assess the driver's memory for the roads and paths to various common locations
- To assess driving performance skills in the real dynamic driving environment

ADAPTIVE EQUIPMENT MOBILITY PRESCRIPTION

After the stroke survivor has been through the clinical evaluation, the vehicle and equipment evaluation and the on-road evaluation, the driver rehabilitation therapist makes a decision regarding the stroke survivor's ability to continue driving safely with or without restrictions. The occupational therapist's clinical reasoning and judgment skills are invaluable at this point to consider all observations, findings, and results from both the clinical and the on-road evaluation. Results from both phases and conversations with family members and other team members must be considered in drawing a conclusion.

If the therapist determines that the stroke survivor can continue to drive, then the driver rehabilitation therapist should write an evaluation summary supporting licensure and specifying vehicle and equipment recommendations as needed. The 2000 edition of the *American Heritage Dictionary of the English Language*, Fourth Edition, defined *prescription* as "a formula directing the preparation of something." In the context of driving, the term *mobility prescription* is used to direct the patient, the equipment installer, and possibly a funding source to the specific equipment needs of the patient.[30]

The document should be written specifically for the stroke survivor and his or her vehicle. The mobility prescription should be inclusive, considering every aspect of the vehicle, the driving task, and all related mobility factors such as the way the driver operates the steering column controls, loads or carries a manual wheelchair or quad cane, or opens the door or trunk of the vehicle.

The mobility prescription should not be guesswork or estimation but should be based on a thorough and objective assessment after the stroke survivor has been observed using each piece of equipment or device safely. Many stroke survivors often need several driving sessions until they are deemed safe drivers with new adaptive equipment. The mobility prescription should indicate to all appropriate parties that the patient has completed a comprehensive driving evaluation successfully, that the driver rehabilitation therapist has made an objective determination that the patient can drive safely, and that the equipment prescribed is necessary for the person to return to safe driving.[30]

Guiding the stroke survivor to a competent and qualified mobility equipment dealer or installer is important. The driver rehabilitation therapist should identify all of the appropriate dealers in the patient's community and communicate with the business by sending the mobility prescription to them. The dealer should be factory trained or certified by the equipment manufacturer to install the specific devices prescribed. The dealer should respect the therapist's expertise and role so as not to overstep boundaries and install equipment without a prescription or substitute, delete, change, or add items on the document.

FOLLOW-UP RECOMMENDATIONS

The final task for the driver rehabilitation therapist is to provide any necessary follow-up recommendations from the on-road assessment. These may include the following:

1. *Additional driver training:* for further practice with the adaptive equipment in a dual-controlled evaluation vehicle
2. *A final equipment inspection and fitting:* Inspection and fitting of equipment by the driver rehabilitation therapist should be done after the installation of the equipment and before the client is released to drive. The purposes for the inspection and fitting are: (1) to verify that all mobility prescription items have been installed, (2) to verify that the equipment is installed and working properly, and (3) to observe the client driving with the equipment to determine if any adjustments are needed. The dealer does not have the knowledge about the patient and may not know or understand the way to adjust equipment for a particular person's needs. Equipment may be installed properly and still not work optimally for the driver if it has not been adjusted for safe use. For example, the therapist may prescribe a spinner knob at the 5 o'clock position on the steering wheel, but the dealer may place the knob at 1 o'clock position. The stroke survivor has a weak right shoulder and fatigues quickly if the arm is held suspended against gravity for a long period. The lower position on the wheel allows the patient to maintain the arm in a resting position while steering straight. Another example is a patient who wears a large shoe size, and the dealer does not account for this fact when determining the location of the left foot gas pedal in relation to the brake. The therapist must check the position of both pedals to make sure that the patient does not inadvertently hit both pedals simultaneously.

3. *Driver licensing or relicensing:* The driver rehabilitation therapist should inform the client of the requirements of the department of driver licensing and provide assistance if necessary in obtaining a valid driver's license with the appropriate restrictions. The client may need to be taken for a road test in the evaluation vehicle or may require the driver rehabilitation therapist's guidance and assistance to communicate with the medical review board for having the driver's license reinstated after a suspension for medical reasons.

4. *Communication with the rehabilitation team:* Written and/or verbal communication, particularly with the physician and the family regarding the outcome of the driving evaluation, is important so that all parties understand and support the results and any follow-up services that have been recommended. If the client has a progressive condition such as the beginning of cataracts, macular degeneration, reflex sympathetic dystrophy or complex regional pain syndrome, Parkinson's disease, dementia, or Alzheimer's disease, the physician and medical review board should be notified of the need for periodic driver reevaluation.

5. *Client and family counseling:* Counseling is important if the stroke survivor can no longer drive safely. This outcome requires the therapist to gently inform the patient directly with compassion, support, and understanding and give the person time to express his or her emotions and feelings about retiring from driving. As hard as it is to complete this part of the job, this is an important aspect for the driver rehabilitation therapist to handle with respect of the person's dignity.

The loss of a driver's license changes a person's life dramatically. The person may no longer be able to live alone or remain in the house that has been home for decades. The person may become dependent on others for transportation and may have to cut out many social activities. The person may be forced to use a taxi or public bus to get to destinations important for purchasing services and goods for daily living. The person should be informed that taxis are expensive means of transportation but are still cheaper than owning a car and paying for maintenance, gas, and insurance.

The occupational therapist can use his or her psychological background and holistic thinking to counsel the stroke survivor and the family on community mobility choices after driver cessation. The therapist needs to give the client and family additional information and resources at this time and should discuss transportation choices available to the person. The following are suggestions to ease the psychological effects of learning about negative outcomes of a driving evaluation:

1. The therapist should give the person a frank and honest description of observable driving behaviors or problems areas that do not allow for safe driving. Discussion of the clinical results and the road test is helpful because time is needed for the information and consequences to be processed. The therapist should give the person an opportunity to discuss the results and ask questions.

2. A significant other should be present with the stroke survivor at this point for psychological support, for help in deciding the best way of securing other transportation choices, and perhaps for a discussion of selling a vehicle and turning in a driver's license for a state identification card.

3. Available counseling through the doctor, psychologist, or other senior health counselor should be sought to assist the person psychologically. The client likely will go through an expression of a variety of feelings and emotions such as denial, anger, resentment, and depression. Family members and friends should be available to check on the person in case depression becomes deep enough to require frequent counseling.

4. Community mobility must be resolved for the person who can no longer drive. The therapist should recruit family members or friends for personal errands and appointments. Information about optional transportation for senior citizens and persons with disabilities should be given in detail and in writing. If necessary, the person should be taken on a city bus route to an appointment and instructed in the way to use the route and bus map guide. The therapist may discuss the option of keeping the personal car and hiring a neighbor or friend to drive it several days of the week for any necessary trips. To continue community mobility goals to the end, it may be necessary for the occupational therapist to evaluate the stroke survivor's ability to use other transportation options by actually observing the person using the various options and determine which is best suited for the client.

LIABILITY CONSIDERATIONS

Because of the inherent nature of driving, all parties must address the degree of liability concerning the stroke survivor who drives, including the physician, the rehabilitation team, the clinical occupational therapist addressing driving as an IADL, the driver rehabilitation therapist, the client, and the family. The physician and other treating professionals of stroke survivors should be diligent in always recommending a thorough driving evaluation and supporting all aspects of the evaluation. Health care professionals working with stroke survivors must remember that protective privilege ends where public peril begins.[30] Every physician and rehabilitation staff member, if for no other reason than because of the liability, should consider the issue of driving after a stroke. If the facility does not have a driving program, a referral to a qualified program in the community should be made, and the referral should be documented in the chart. A discussion of the concept of shared liability in each party follows.

Patient's Liability

The driver has an ethical responsibility to avoid harming self or others. Each state department of motor vehicles grants a person the privilege of a driver's license based on criteria and regulations that vary from state to state. The driver must realize that the driving privilege can lead to potential disaster through injury to persons and destruction of property if residual functional deficits interfere with driving skills. Persons recovering from a stroke who cannot master the operational, tactical, and strategic skills necessary to operate a motor vehicle safely present a clear risk of injury to themselves, their passengers, pedestrians, and other operators of motor vehicles.[2]

The OT should address the liability issues for the family before discharge as an inpatient. The family should understand that following the rehabilitation team's recommendations for driving cessation until a driving assessment can be made will lessen their liability risk. Families are entrusted with ensuring compliance with the recommendations after discharge from the inpatient rehabilitation stay. They should be encouraged, if necessary, to take the stroke survivor driver's license and/or vehicle keys and even relocate any vehicle to which the person may have access before the person is discharged from the rehabilitation facility. The entire rehabilitation team must reinforce this information so the family is informed properly, prepared, and willing to take their role and responsibility seriously and to follow through with the recommendations.

The rehabilitation team or family member should never hesitate to report the stroke survivor to the department of driver licensing if the person does not comply with the team's recommendations and is deemed unsafe to self or the public while driving. If the physician hesitates to address driving to a patient or thinks liability may be avoided by not addressing the issue, another team member should contact the department of driver licensing if allowable in that state. Each state differs in the requirements for reporting a person, so the occupational therapist should investigate the procedure for the patient's resident state. Obtaining a copy of the state's statute is important, as is talking to the department of driver licensing or medical review board. By performing a an internet search using the letters "DMV," each state Division of Motor Vehicles website can be found.

The March 1993 AOTA physical disabilities special interest section newsletter discussed the legal considerations for driver rehabilitation programs in terms of the responsibility of the patient, physician, and occupational therapist.[30] To avoid any legal difficulties with the driver's insurance, the stroke survivor should notify his or her car insurance company about the stroke, the results of the driving evaluation, and the validation of the person's driving ability by the department of motor vehicles. Failure to notify the insurance company may result in a claim of fraud if the patient has an accident. As a result, the stroke survivor who is driving may be held completely or partially liable for costs rewarded in court judgments for property damage, bodily damage, pain, suffering, and loss of any parties involved in the accident because of contributory negligence.

Physician's Liability

In the past 20 years, court precedent has established that physicians have responsibility for protecting the public health even if it conflicts with the patient's right to privacy and confidentiality. This duty to warn society for the greater good has been upheld by the courts. Consequently, the physician's liability to inform third parties has increased. Few, if any, exceptions to this rule exist, so any person who has had a brain trauma or damage should be assessed objectively for safe driving skills. Failure to address these issues with the stroke survivor and concerned others may expose a health care provider to a charge of negligence.

Some states have mandatory reporting laws. A physician must report a new disability or diagnosis to the department of driver licensing. In states that lack this law, some physicians may overlook, ignore, or hesitate to report a patient for fear of losing a patient. The physician may feel a loyalty toward patients he or she has treated for many years. A patient may attempt to influence the physician's decision by indicating that he or she is the only driver in the family and driving is crucial to continued independent living. Although this may be true, the physician's first thought should be the safety and protection of the patient and the public. If the physician or others on the rehabilitation team are unsure the patient will comply with the recommendations as given regarding driving, the person should be reported to the department of driver licensing without hesitation.

The American Medical Association (AMA) now encourages physicians to make driver safety a routine part of geriatric medical services. The AMA in 2003 published the *Physician's Guide to Assessing and Counseling Older Drivers.* Information about this book and other resources is available through their website at www.ama-assn.org/go/olderdriver.

The physician's decision to report a patient should be based on the amount of risk involved in allowing the person to continue driving. The physician should protect patients from further harm or injury to themselves or others. States that have a mandatory reporting law also protect individuals by a state statute who report medical conditions from being sued for slander or character defamation by divulging personal information to the department of driver licensing. For further protection, the name of the reporting person is not revealed to the licensee.

A review of past court opinions and judgments reveals rulings for and against physicians. Jacobs,[17] in a 1978 article titled "Reporting the Handicapped Driver," cited several lawsuits against physicians. In a 1920 invasion of privacy lawsuit, *Simonsen v. Swenson*, the physician was vindicated of any wrongdoing by proving that the public welfare was being protected. In *Freese v. Lemmon*, 210 NW2d 576 (Iowa, 1973), a physician was found guilty of malpractice because he failed to warn and counsel a patient about the possible effects a medical condition might have on driving ability. In this case, the patient had been diagnosed with epilepsy. The physician did not advise the person to stop driving. The person had a seizure while driving and struck a pedestrian. In a 1986 lawsuit *Tarasoff v. Regents of the University of California* (551 p. 2d 334, at 344 [1986]), a psychologist working in the student health department on campus was held liable because of his failure to alert and advise campus authorities properly when a student reported to him an intention to murder his girlfriend. The court ruled the psychologist had a duty to break confidentiality and warn the potential victim. The court's opinion concluded that the "protective privilege ends where the public peril begins." The court also stated the following:[3] "The physician treating a mentally ill patient, just as a doctor treating a physical illness, bears a duty to use reasonable care to give threatened persons such warnings as are essential to avert foreseeable danger arising from his patient's condition or treatment."

Antrim and Engum,[2] in an article titled "The Driving Dilemma and the Law: Patients Striving for Independence Versus Public Safety," described other legal cases illustrating practitioner liability. In *Naidu v. Laird*, 539 A2d 1064 (Del. 1988), the court heard that Laird was killed in a car accident by a known psychotic person who had been involved in several similar accidents in which he drove his car deliberately into someone else's car. When taking his medication, the psychotic person was generally manageable, appropriate, and capable of living semi-independently. When not taking his medication, he had violent tendencies that presented a risk of harm to himself and others. Laird's widow sued the psychotic person and the treating physician, Dr. Naidu, for wrongful death. The court ruled in favor of the plaintiff. The court stated "a psychiatrist owes an affirmative duty to persons other than the patient to exercise reasonable care in the treatment and discharge of their patients." Antrim defined *reasonable care* as the degree of care, skill, and diligence that a reasonably prudent psychiatrist engaged in a similar practice and in similar conditions ordinarily would have exercised in like circumstances.

Antrim and Engum[2] further discussed the California case *Myers v. Quesenberry*, 144 Cal App 3d 888 (1983), which involved a car accident of a patient of Dr. Quesenberry who was being treated for diabetes and receiving prenatal care. The doctor knew that his patient had been seriously affected during two previous pregnancies that resulted in one stillbirth. During the third pregnancy, the patient's diabetes could not be stabilized. During an office examination, the physician discovered the fetus had died. Dr. Quesenberry advised the patient to have a dilation and curettage procedure. He instructed her to drive immediately to a hospital. Emotionally distraught, the patient suffered a diabetic attack in route and lost control of her car, striking a pedestrian, Myers. The court noted that a fundamental principle of tort law held physicians liable for injuries caused by their failure to exercise reasonable care. A physician must warn a patient if the patient's condition or medications renders certain conduct such as operating a motor vehicle dangerous to others.

A physician must appreciate the complexity and dangers of driving and understand that certain conditions or deficits may impair driving performance. A physician should recognize limitations in having the tools and abilities to evaluate a person's driving skills fully in the office or hospital. A physician should be informed about the expertise and role of the occupational therapist and the driver rehabilitation therapist to refer patients for a medical-oriented and comprehensive driving evaluation.

Occupational Therapist's Liability

The occupational therapist's responsibility can be as great and serious as the physician's is. The level of liability increases as the therapist's role and responsibility increase. The therapist seeing the patient in the acute care setting who addresses only driving from a factual standpoint has little liability, if any. However, if the inpatient or outpatient occupational therapist chooses not to inform the patient or the family of their responsibility with this issue, then the therapist may be liable for an act of omission.

The OT Specialist in Driving or the driver rehabilitation therapist has the greatest degree of vulnerability to liability lawsuits compared with an occupational therapist in the clinic or hospital. The nature of the job, in which the therapist takes a person in traffic, has inherent risks. A definitive legal case that eases the liability position of the driver rehabilitation therapist was *White v. Moss Rehab, et al.* (Philadelphia, 1995) when the court declined "to recognize a common-law third party cause of action for educational malpractice against a driving school." The

driver rehabilitation program was found not to be liable for the driving mistake of a former patient that resulted in a motor vehicle accident that caused the death of a passenger in another vehicle.

For risk management the driver rehabilitation therapist should follow safe, accepted practices (Box 23-9). The evaluation car must be viewed as an evaluation tool that must be adjusted to each client's use and maintained in proper working order just as any machine in the OT clinic. Proper training by qualified professionals in the field and practice with in-car skills prepares the therapist for the work in the car. An Adaptive Mobility Services workshop titled *Take the Wheel: A Driver Education Workshop for the Therapist* provides this type of knowledge, instruction, and practice in a real evaluation vehicle with mock patients.

An occupational therapist must be credentialed adequately to enhance the value of his or her professional opinion. The therapist must have a strong working knowledge of each step of a comprehensive driving evaluation and must use the accepted practices in the industry conscientiously. The therapist must follow any industry guidelines, standards of practice, and code of ethics that exist for the OT profession. Wendy Kaplan[19] in a 1999 AOTA physical disabilities special interest section quarterly newsletter article titled "The Occupation of Driving: Legal and Ethical Issues" stated that "Therapists should be aware of medical reporting requirements for impaired driving laws that exist in their state of practice. The AOTA Code of Ethics creates an obligation for administrative occupational

---

Box 23-9

Strategies for Risk Management

The driver rehabilitation therapist can reduce liability risk by the following:

- Have a medical background with knowledge in driver education principles.
- Have advanced and specialized education and skill in the field of driver evaluation.
- Have a working knowledge of each step of the comprehensive driving evaluation.
- Know and practice accepted standard of care in driver evaluations.
- Ensure that the evaluation vehicle is equipped with instructor's safety equipment.
- Set the vehicle for each client per the individual needs.
- Know how to control the vehicle from the right side, physically and verbally.
- Use sound judgment and good clinical reasoning.
- Use good observation and visual skills.
- Use good documentation and communication procedures.
- Carry professional liability insurance.

therapists to be aware of the laws related the health care practitioners and driving as well as to disseminate that knowledge. It is the role of the manager to create departmental policies consistent with those laws and provide the administrative support necessary for observance of those policies." For legal protection, all therapists, and especially those in this specialty area, should have their own professional liability insurance in addition to coverage from the employer. If the therapist is ever drawn into a lawsuit, he or she must have representation by a personal attorney and not a third-party interest.

The driver rehabilitation therapist should possess all necessary clinical and vehicle tools, tests, and skills used to pass judgment fairly and accurately on a person's driving future. The therapist should evaluate a client's driving ability fully, considering the safety of the client and the public at large. The therapist should avoid zealousness as an advocate for the client whose skills are in question. The occupational therapist's perspective of looking at the whole person is key to making the best decision. The contextual and environmental factors are very important to consider. The person may only need to drive within a 5 mile radius of his or her home and has lived at the same address for many years. If the patient will require a manual wheelchair permanently, then this may affect the vehicle and equipment recommendations. If the person will be moving to a different location to be close to family and is unfamiliar with the area, then memory, learning skills, and directionality may be greater factors than when a person will be returning to a familiar environment in which he or she has resided for many years.

Antrim[2] is a practicing attorney and a member of the board of reviewers of the journal *Cognitive Rehabilitation.* He strongly suggests that current legal authority appears ready to impose liability on health care professionals for negligence in failing to address their patients' abilities to drive. Antrim recommends that health care professionals use a standard of care in making these recommendations and that their evaluation process should include guidelines for making those decisions reasonably and responsibly. *The AOTA Practice Guidelines for Driving and Community Mobility for Older Adults* offers recommended practices for the occupational therapist.

In a 1986 article, Steich[37] explained that the law holds professionals to a higher standard than it does the public because professionals consider themselves more highly skilled in their particular fields of expertise. For example, the driver rehabilitation therapist owes a greater duty of care to a client and the public than does a parent teaching a child to drive. Steich goes on to explain that the occupational therapist must do something wrong or fail to do something that should have been done to be held liable. If the policies and procedures of a program define the steps that should be performed to complete a comprehensive driver evaluation but the therapist fails to use the tool or

procedure defined, the therapist may be held liable for omitting that portion of the test. Legal counsel should review the wording of the driving program policies and procedures.

The therapist is responsible for ensuring that all evaluative or testing equipment works when needed. For example, therapists can use several commercially available devices to test visual acuity and night vision. If the machine that measures night vision is not working when the therapist evaluates a patient with a diagnosis in which night vision could be a suspected problem (such as glaucoma), the therapist may be found negligent for not having the machine fully functioning when the patient was evaluated. The therapist may make a statement in the summary indicating that rendering an opinion on the issue was impossible; however, in making a conclusion regarding the person's driving ability, night vision should be tested appropriately.

Communication and Documentation

Communication and documentation are important keys to lessening everyone's liability throughout the entire process of addressing driving issues for the stroke survivor. The stroke survivor and the family need to be informed of the requirements of the state department of driver licensing. These requirements vary from state to state. In the rehabilitation phase, the stroke survivor and family should sign a document that becomes a permanent part of the medical record that describes the information, recommendations, and follow-up plans given by the rehabilitation team regarding driving and community mobility.

Documentation of addressing the IADL of driving and community mobility is crucial and necessary for several purposes. This documentation can be used to justify an adaptive equipment purchase for a third-party payer, inform the department of motor vehicles and a physician of the patient's driving performance, and help defend the therapist in a court of law or during a deposition in which professional judgment or expertise is deposed. The therapist should keep in mind that if something is not documented on paper, in the eyes of the court it was not done. This documentation is more vulnerable than usual because it is scrutinized far more than is the documentation of in-house therapy for ADL training. Because driving is an ADL that can kill,[28] the parties involved must maintain the highest degree of competence, thoroughness, and seriousness at all times. The documentation of a driving program is at greater risk to be subpoenaed by an attorney searching for liability for a lawsuit.

The OT notes should document all aspects of how the IADL of driving was addressed just as they would for any other ADL or IADL. For example, reports throughout the continuum of OT at the various levels of rehabilitation and recovery should include such things as interactions with the stroke survivor, the way the patient performed in each step, and the clinical reasoning inherent in the decision-making and final outcome regarding the person's ability to drive. Therapists should avoid statements such as "the patient has potential to be a safe driver." The therapist must have enough confidence with the patient's abilities and in his or her own professional judgment to document "the patient is a safe driver."

Another method of documentation is to say "today the patient drove safely in the following situations." The documentation should account for the time and days spent with a patient. The therapist should note positive and negative observations or scores. Incomplete, illegible, and poorly written documentation is hard to defend in court if an expert witness is used to judge the driver rehabilitation therapist's work and decisions. As with the physician cases noted previously, an expert witness with similar practice to the therapist's may be called to testify regarding standard procedure in similar conditions. This witness may not be able to testify that the driver rehabilitation therapist acted with a reasonable care of duty if the documentation cannot support conclusions with evidence. Evidence of professional continuing education is important to show that the therapist knowledge is updated with current standard of practice.

After a complete driving evaluation, the therapist should explain final recommendations thoroughly to the stroke survivor and family members. The referring physician should receive written notification of the outcome of the evaluation. The therapist should document the results, recommendations, and follow-up services to be done in the client's chart. The client should sign the written recommendations to demonstrate legal proof of explanation of the findings. If the results of the evaluation are negative, a team member may inform the proper driver licensing authority in the client's state of residency.

SUMMARY

Driving and community mobility must be included and addressed as an IADL in the OT evaluation and intervention for the stroke survivor. Driving after a stroke is possible for some persons, but addressing driving along the continuum of OT is necessary so that a driver evaluation with a qualified driver rehabilitation therapist is completed before the person returns to driving. The physician and other team members must educate stroke survivors and their families early in rehabilitation concerning the necessity and importance of the evaluation. The issues of liability and insurance arising from a stroke survivor driving without a valid license, without the doctor's approval, without necessary equipment, and/or without a documented formal driving evaluation should be explained carefully. Emphasis should be on the detrimental effects on the client and family's finances, assets, and security if an accident occurs.

Since driving and community mobility are in the domain of OT as an IADL, the occupational therapist must address and be involved in the evaluation, intervention, and outcome for determining safety to return to driving or to use other transportation choices. AOTA is the primary provider of information and education for the occupational therapist in addressing the IADL of driving and community mobility as an OT Generalist in Driving or as an OT Specialist in Driving. A stroke survivor presents unique problems that must be looked at individually. The outcome regarding the client's driving abilities must be made on reliable, objective information and with good clinical reasoning and judgment.

REVIEW QUESTIONS

1. Describe why the occupational therapist should include driving and community mobility as an IADL.
2. Describe at least five activities that illustrate the importance of community mobility to a patient who has had a stroke.
3. Describe the requirements for an occupational therapist to be an OT Specialist in Driving or a driver rehabilitation therapist.
4. What specific areas should be evaluated during the clinical evaluation portion of a comprehensive driver evaluation for a client with left hemiplegia from a stroke?
5. Describe the liability issues involved for the client, physician, therapist, and facility.
6. Identify four driving behaviors or errors that may be seen in a driver with left side neglect.
7. Identify specific performance skills (e.g., motor, sensory-perceptual, cognitive, and communication) used in the following steps of each driving task:
   - Lane change to the right
   - Rearview mirror check
   - Right outside mirror check
   - Right turn signal
   - Right head check
   - Gradual and small turn of wheel to right
   - Cancel turn signal
   - Accelerate as appropriate
8. List at least six factors influencing a successful driving evaluation process.
9. What is the purpose of the mobility prescription? List all its uses.
10. What adaptive driving equipment may be used for the following deficits?
    - Use of one hand only for steering
    - Nonuse of right lower extremity
    - Nonuse of left upper extremity
    - Lack of neck motion (particularly rotation)

11. List four purposes for the road test.
12. How can a therapist plan a driving route with ecological validity for the stroke survivor?
13. Describe why the occupational therapist is suited to perform the on-road assessment.

REFERENCES

1. American Occupational Therapy Association: Occupational Therapy practice framework: domain and process. *Am J Occup Ther* 62(6):625–683, 2008.
2. Antrim MJ, Engum ES: The driving dilemma and the law: patients striving for independence versus public safety. *Cognit Rehabil* 7(2):16–19, 1989.
3. Blum J: Keeping seniors on the move. *Columbus Monthly* 8:72, 1993.
4. Brooke MM, Questad KA, Patterson DR, et al: Driving evaluation after traumatic brain injury. *Am J Phys Med Rehabil* 71(3):177–182, 1992.
5. Carp FM: Significance of mobility for the well being of the elderly. *Transport Aging Soc* 2:1–20, 1988.
6. Committee for the Study on Improving Mobility and Safety for Older Persons. In *Transportation in an aging society*, vol 1, Washington, D.C., 1988, Transportation Research Board.
7. Diller L, Weinberg J: Evidence for accident-prone behavior in hemiplegic patients. *Arch Phys Med Rehabil* 51(6):358–363, 1970.
8. Engum ES: Criterion-related validity of the cognitive behavioral driver's inventory: brain-injured patients versus normal control. *Cognit Rehabil* 8(2):20, 1990.
9. Engum ES, Pendergras T, Cron L, et al: Cognitive behavioral driver's inventory. *Cognit Rehabil* 6(5):34–50, 1988.
10. French D, Hanson C: Survey of driver rehabilitation programs. *Am J Occup Ther* 53(4):344–7, 1999.
11. Gianutsos R: Driving advisement with the elemental driving simulator (EDS): when less suffices, behavior research methods. *Instrum Comput* 26:183, 1997.
12. Gianutsos R: Personal communications, Sept 1996 and July 2010. Refer to www.driverrehab.com and www.sites.google.com/site/elementaldrivingsimulator for more information.
13. Gianutsos R, Suchoff IB: Visual fields after brain injury: management issues for the occupational therapist. In Scheiman M, editor: *Vision: screening and intervention techniques for occupational therapists*, Thorofare, NJ, 1996, Slack.
14. Gresham GE, Duncan P, Stason W, et al: *Post-stroke rehabilitation: clinical practice guideline*, Rockville, MD, 1995, US Department of Health and Human Services, Public Health Service, Agency for Health Care Policy and Research, No 16, AHCPR Pub No 95–0662.
15. Hibbard MR, Gordon WA, Stein DN, et al: Awareness of disability in patients following stroke. *Rehabil Psychol* 37:103, 1992.
16. Hunt L, Pierce S: *Driving and Community Mobility for Older Adults: Occupational Therapy Roles.* AOTA online course, 2009, pg 35, lesson 1.
17. Jacobs S: Reporting the handicapped driver. *Arch Phys Med Rehabil* 59(8):387–390, 1978.
18. Johansson C: *Top 10 emerging practice areas to watch in the new millennium* (website). www.aota.org/members/area7/index.asp. Accessed March 12, 2002.
19. Kaplan W: The occupation of driving: legal and ethical issues. *AOTA Phys Disabil Spec Interest Section Newsletter* 22:3, 1999.
20. Katz RT, Golden RS, Butter J, et al: Driving safety after brain damage: follow-up of 22 patients with matched controls. *Arch Phys Med Rehabil* 71(2):133, 1990.
21. Korner-Bitensky N, Sofer S, Kaizer F, et al: Assessing ability to drive following an acute neurological event: are we on the right road? *Can J Occup Ther* 61(3):141–148, 1994.
22. Deleted.
23. Legh-Smith J, Wade DT, Hewer RL: Driving after a stroke. *J R Soc Med* 79(4):200–203, 1986.
24. McKnight JA: *Driver and pedestrian training*, vol II, Washington, D.C., 1988, Transportation Research Board.
25. Nouri FM, Tinson DJ, Lincoln NB: Cognitive ability and driving after stroke. *Int Disabil Stud* 9(3):110–115, 1987.
26. Eberhard J: On the road again. *AOTA OT Week* 5:16, 1998.
27. Persson D: The elderly driver: deciding when to stop. *Gerontologist* 33(1):88–91, 1993.
28. Pierce S: A roadmap for driver rehabilitation. *AOTA OT Pract* 10(1):30–38, 1996.
29. Pierce S: Restoring competence in mobility. In Trombly C, Radomski M, editors: *Occupational therapy for physical dysfunction*, ed 5, Philadelphia, 2002, Lippincott Williams & Wilkins.
30. Pierce S, Blackburn C: *Building blocks for becoming a driver rehabilitation therapist*, Orlando, FL, 2008, Adaptive Mobility Services.
31. Ramsey B: *Take the wheel: a driver education course for the therapist*, course notes, Orlando, FL, 1996, Adaptive Mobility Services.
32. Scheiman M: *Understanding and managing visual deficits: theory screening procedures, intervention techniques*, course notes, Atlanta, 1996, Vision Education Seminars.
33. Sivak M, Olson PL, Kewman DG, et al: Driving and perceptual/cognitive skills and behavioral consequences of brain damage. *Arch Phys Med Rehabil* 62(10):476–483, 1981.
34. Slavin S: Association of Driver Educators for the Disabled conference presentation, Keynote Speaker Address, Orlando, FL, 1987.
35. Smith EE: Choice reaction time: an analysis of the major theoretical positions. *Psychol Bull* 69:77, 1968.
36. Stav WB, Pierce S, Wheatley CJ, Davis ES: Driving and community mobility. *Am J Occup Ther* 59(6):666–670, 2005.
37. Steich T: Malpractice insurance important for occupational therapy personnel. *OT News* 40:7, 1986.
38. Stone SP, Wilson B, Wroot A, et al: The assessment of visuo-spatial neglect after acute stroke. *J Neurol Neurosurg Psychiatry* 54(4):345–350, 1991.
39. Stressel DL: American Occupational Therapy Association continuing education article: Driving issues of the older adult. *OT Practice* 5:CE1–CE8, 2000.
40. Toglia JP: Visual perception of objects: an approach to assessment and intervention. *Am J Occup Ther* 43(9):587, 1993.
41. Underwood M: The older driver: clinical assessment and injury prevention. *Arch Intern Med* 152(4):737, 1992.
42. Van Zomeran AH, Brouwer WH, Minderhoud JM: Acquired brain damage and driving: a review. *Arch Phys Med Rehabil* 68(10):697–705, 1987.
43. Warren M: A hierarchical model for evaluation and treatment of visual perceptual dysfunction in adult acquired brain injury, part 2. *Am J Occup Ther* 47(1):55–66, 1993.
44. Weaver J: In *Driver performance test*, Orlando, FL, 2009, Advanced Driving Skills Institute.
45. Wilson B, Cockburn J, Halligan P: Development of a behavioral test of visuospatial neglect. *Arch Phys Med Rehabil* 68(2):98–102, 1987.
46. Wilson T, Smith T: Driving after stroke. *Int Rehabil Med* 5(4):170–177, 1983.

wendy avery

chapter 24

Dysphagia Management

key terms

alternative nutrition
aspiration
bedside evaluation
bolus
cervical auscultation

dysphagia
feeding trials
fiberoptic endoscopic evaluation
of swallowing

laryngeal penetration
modified barium swallow
silent aspiration

chapter objectives

After completing this chapter, the reader will be able to accomplish the following:

1. Describe the normal anatomy and physiology of the swallowing mechanism.
2. Discuss the effects of stroke on the swallowing mechanism.
3. Describe clinical and instrumental assessment of dysphagia following stroke.
4. Describe various rehabilitative and compensatory techniques used to treat dysphagia after a stroke.
5. Discuss the efficacy of dysphagia intervention following stroke.

Dysphagia comes from the Greek prefix *dys*, meaning difficult, and the Greek term *phagein*, meaning to eat. The occurrence of dysphagia, or difficulty swallowing, immediately after stroke is common, with a reported incidence as high as 51%.[82] In patients with brainstem stroke, the incidence may be as high as 81%.[60] Intervention for dysphagia is a part of occupational therapy care for patients with stroke in a variety of settings. While initial evaluation and treatment for dysphagia is critical in the acute care setting, patients often require reassessment in postacute settings as well.[35] See Chapter 1.

NORMAL ANATOMY AND PHYSIOLOGY OF THE SWALLOWING MECHANISM

A prerequisite for successful intervention with patients with dysphagia is knowledge of the anatomy and physiology of the swallowing mechanism. Fig. 24-1 represents a midsagittal view of the anatomical landmarks of the head and neck important in swallowing. Fig. 24-2 represents anatomical landmarks of the oral cavity. The act of swallowing may be divided into five separate stages: preoral, oral-preparatory, oral, pharyngeal, and esophageal. Fig. 24-3 illustrates the anatomical division of the oral preparatory through esophageal stages.

Preoral Stage

During the preoral stage, the patient engages in tray or plate setup and preparation; visual, visual-perceptual, and olfactory awareness of the food; and transportation of the food to the mouth (feeding) using a utensil, cup, or fingers. Patients with stroke often have challenges with preoral stage activities that benefit from occupational therapy interventions, even in the absence of dysphagia.

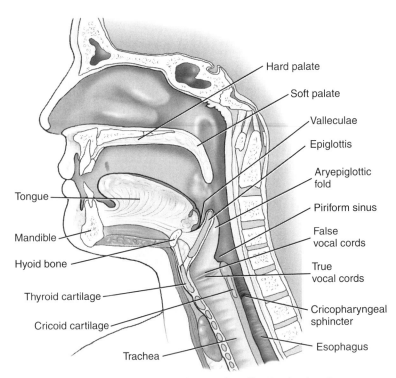

Figure 24-1   Midsagittal view of swallowing landmarks.

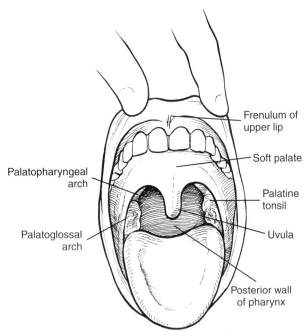

Figure 24-2   Landmarks of the oral cavity.

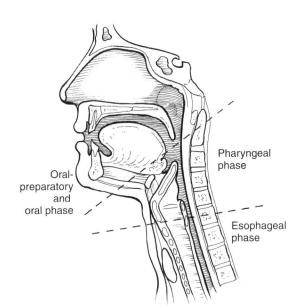

Figure 24-3   Stages of a normal swallow sagittal view.

Oral-Preparatory Stage

During the oral-preparatory stage (Fig. 24-4, *A*), the patient demonstrates adequate mouth opening, bolus reception, containment in the oral cavity, oral sensation for the bolus, and appreciation of the flavor and texture of the bolus. The muscles of mastication prepare the food, if solid, into a bolus of suitable texture for swallowing by manipulating the bolus using the muscles of mastication, the jaw, and the cheeks. During this stage, the soft palate rests on the back of the tongue to prevent food or fluid from trickling into the pharynx.

Oral Stage

During the oral stage of the swallow, the prepared bolus is propelled through the oral cavity toward the pharynx (see Fig. 24-4, *B*). The lips and buccal muscles contract and transport the bolus posteriorly as the tongue sequentially pushes the bolus posteriorly against the hard palate, propelling it through the oral cavity, to the base of the tongue.

Pharyngeal Stage

During this stage of the swallow, the following events occur in rapid sequence, producing a swallow response. The soft palate elevates, closing off the nasopharynx. Swallowing apnea, or cessation of breathing, occurs as the vocal folds close, protecting the airway from aspiration and laryngeal penetration. The epiglottis folds over the opening to the larynx (the laryngeal vestibule) (see Fig. 24-4, *C*), also preventing airway penetration into the larynx and directing the bolus toward the piriform sinuses. The larynx rises and tilts anteriorly, and pharyngeal peristalsis squeezes the bolus downward through the pharynx toward the cricopharyngeal sphincter (see Fig. 24-4, *D*). The cricopharyngeal sphincter, which is at the superior aspect of the esophagus, relaxes and allows the bolus to pass into the esophagus.

Esophageal Stage

The esophageal stage begins as the bolus passes through the cricopharyngeal sphincter (see Fig. 24-4, *E*). The bolus is propelled through the esophagus by a sequential peristaltic "stripping wave." The lower esophageal sphincter

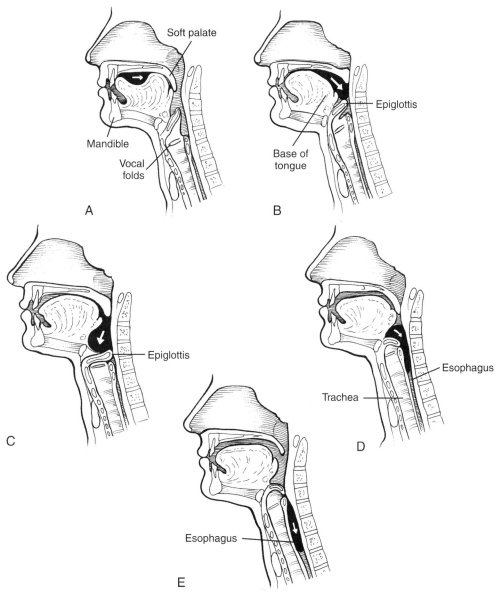

Figure 24-4 **A,** The oral-preparatory stage. **B,** The oral stage. **C** and **D,** The pharyngeal stage. **E,** The esophageal stage.

located at the base of the esophagus then relaxes, allowing the bolus to pass into the stomach.

Neural Control of Swallowing

Cortical and subcortical centers control the voluntary aspects of the swallow, particularly during the preoral, oral-preparatory, and oral stages. The swallow response, which can be initiated voluntarily or involuntarily, is controlled by cranial nerves and their nuclei in the medulla, with input from cortical and subcortical centers. Six cranial nerves are involved in the swallow process[50] (Box 24-1).

SIGNS OF DYSPHAGIA ASSOCIATED WITH STROKE

A variety of signs are observed directly or by videofluoroscopy during swallowing following stroke. Veis and Logemann[91] found that 75% of patients assessed by videofluoroscopy demonstrated more than one specific sign with their swallowing. Signs and symptoms vary with location and size of the lesion or lesions caused by stroke. Table 24-1 delineates specific impairments that one may observe. Fig. 24-5 illustrates some of these impairments. Patients with dysphagia and stroke may have a tracheostomy and may require mechanical ventilation. Although this chapter does not cover these topics, the suggested reading will provide the reader with more information. Studies have observed the differences between dysphagia in stroke patients by lesion location.

Hemispheric Stroke

In general, patients with hemispheric stroke have difficulty with voluntary triggering of the swallow.[6] Patients with right hemispheric middle cerebral artery stroke tend to have greater incidence of laryngeal penetration and aspiration than those with left hemispheric middle cerebral artery stroke. Patients with right hemispheric stroke take longer to initiate a swallow response than those with a left hemispheric stroke. Oral and pharyngeal bolus mobilization is slower in persons with right hemispheric stroke than in healthy individuals. Patients with left hemispheric stroke experience slower bolus mobilization through the pharynx compared with healthy individuals. Oral time transit time may also be delayed in those with left hemispheric stroke. Apraxia is present in those with left hemispheric stroke.[85] A study by Irie and Lu[42] suggested that, in general, patients with left hemispheric stroke tended to have primarily oral phase impairments and those with right strokes tended to have impairment of oral and pharyngeal phases. Patients with left hemispheric stroke tended to require fewer dysphagia interventions and to require alternative nutrition less than those with a right sided stroke did. Pharyngeal and laryngeal sensory loss may play a role in reduced ability to respond to the presence of a bolus in some stroke patients.[5]

Brainstem Stroke

Patients with brainstem stroke have greater occurrence of persistent dysphagia than those with hemispheric stroke.[6,59] With lateral medullary infarction (Wallenberg syndrome), oral control may be near intact, but the ability to trigger and achieve an effective swallow is weak bilaterally, despite a unilateral lesion.[6] Reduced laryngeal elevation, unilateral pharyngeal weakness, and reduced adduction of the vocal cords may be seen, resulting in aspiration.[91] A delayed or absent swallow response may be seen.[55,60] Recovery does occur in 88% of patients; however, it takes longer than in those with hemispheric stroke.[60]

Pseudobulbar or Suprabulbar Palsy

Pseudobulbar or suprabulbar palsy refers to stroke that causes dysphagia affecting the lower motor neuron. The corticospinal pathways are spared. Lesions may be located in the corona radiata, internal capsule, or lenticular hemorrhage.[12] Symptoms may disappear within several weeks.[12] Lacunar infarcts with suprabulbar palsy demonstrate delayed trigger, absent trigger, and/or slow swallow.[30]

Lacunar Infarcts

Lacunar infarcts, often occurring in the periventricular areas, are not always associated with specific dysphagic signs.

Multiple Strokes

Patients with multiple strokes may demonstrate slow oral movements and a delayed swallow response.[55] Often multiple deficits exist, resulting in a greater risk of aspiration. Patients with bilateral stroke are more likely to have sensory deficits in the pharynx and larynx.[5]

Box 24-1

Cranial Nerve Functions

STAGE

Oral	Cranial nerve V (trigeminal): tactile and proprioceptive sensation and motor
	Cranial nerve VII (facial): taste and motor
Pharyngeal	Cranial nerve IX (glossopharyngeal): taste, pharyngeal peristalsis, salivation, and taste
	Cranial nerve X (vagus): taste and motor, intrinsic laryngeal muscles, pharyngeal peristalsis, and swallow initiation
	Cranial nerve XI (accessory): pharyngeal peristalsis and head and neck stability
Oral and pharyngeal	Cranial nerve XII (hypoglossal): lingual movement and laryngeal and hyoid movement

Table 24-1

Dysphagia Signs and Symptoms in Stroke Associated with the Stages of Swallowing*

STAGE OF THE SWALLOW	BEDSIDE EVALUATION SYMPTOMS	MODIFIED BARIUM SWALLOW SIGNS	PHYSIOLOGICAL SYMPTOMS
Preoral	Poor sitting posture	Unable to view	Reduced trunk control
	Reduced orientation to food		Reduced cognition
	Inability to identify edibles from nonedibles or to recognize food		Visual-perceptual or sensory deficits
	Inability to open packages or to prepare and cut food on plate		Reduced upper extremity function, control, or coordination
	Inability to get bolus to mouth using utensils or hand		Apraxia
			Ataxia
Oral-preparatory	Reduced mouth closure	Loss of bolus onto lips, drooling	Reduced oral-motor strength, tone, range
	Reduced lip, tongue, and cheek control	Decreased ability to form bolus, incohesive bolus	Abnormal reflexes
	Perioral food residue (on lips and/or face), drooling	Barium observed on lips or cheeks	Reduced perioral sensation
	Tongue thrust	Anterior tongue movements	Reflexive tongue movements
	Disorganized tongue movements	Random tongue motions	Tongue tremors, weakness, reduced coordination
	Reduced mastication	Ineffective mastication, with unchewed bolus	Weakness, tone alterations
	Slow oral preparation time	Slow oral time observed	Weakness, poor sensory awareness
	Oral fatigue	Slow oral movements	Weakness, low muscle tone
	Lengthy mealtime	Unable to visualize length of meal	Slow or poorly coordinated overall movements
Oral	Use of fingers to manipulate the bolus posteriorly	Fingers observed at mouth	Reduced awareness of or ability to propel the bolus posteriorly
	Holding of food in the mouth	Slow oral transit time	
	Pocketing of food in oral sulci (pooling)	Oral residue on tongue and sulci, lips, or palate	Reduced/absent muscle control to direct bolus
	Drooling	Barium observed outside of mouth	Reduced or absent intraoral sensation
	Oral residue after attempts at swallowing	Barium residue in mouth	Difficulty collecting or propelling the entire bolus
	Reduced tongue elevation to propel the bolus posteriorly	Tongue pumping	Apraxia, ataxia, muscle tone alteration, discoordination
	Reduced anterior to posterior tongue movement/bolus propulsion, disorganized tongue movements	Random tongue motions	
	Slow oral transit time	Slow oral transit time observed	Fatigue, poor coordination
Pharyngeal	Coughing/choking	Premature loss of bolus into hypopharynx	Cranial nerves X and IX: reduced/absent swallow, weakness of swallow response
		Wet/gurgly breath and vocal quality	Delayed or absent swallow response
	Absent swallow response		
	Difficulty initiating a swallow		
	Weak cough	Repeated attempts at coughing/clearing	Reduced respiratory support/capacity
		Ineffective cough, cannot clear aspirated or penetrated material	Bilateral or unilateral vocal fold paralysis

*This table is not an exhaustive list of signs and symptoms but is meant to suggest some causative factors for swallowing dysfunction.

Continued

Table 24-1

Dysphagia Signs and Symptoms in Stroke Associated with the Stages of Swallowing—cont'd

STAGE OF THE SWALLOW	BEDSIDE EVALUATION SYMPTOMS	MODIFIED BARIUM SWALLOW SIGNS	PHYSIOLOGICAL SYMPTOMS
			Cranial nerves IX and X: reduced or absent sensation
	Complains of food sticking in throat	Pharyngeal wall residue	Cranial nerves IX and X: Reduced pharyngeal peristalsis
	Increased throat clearing	Valleculae and piriform sinus pooling	
	Multiple swallows (more than two)	Ineffective multiple swallows to clear residue	
	Nasal regurgitation	Penetration of bolus into nasopharynx	Incompetence of palatal seal of nasopharynx
		Penetration of bolus into trachea above level of vocal folds	Reduced epiglottal movement, reduced laryngeal elevation
		Aspiration of bolus into trachea below level of vocal folds	Reduced ability to prevent entry of food material into airway
	Lengthy mealtime		Delayed swallow
Esophageal	Regurgitation, sour taste, heartburn, awaking with a wet pillow	Reflux: reduced upper esophageal sphincter opening caused by reduced pharyngeal/laryngeal movement, reflux	Esophageal or gastric reflux
	Altered esophageal motility observed on instrumental testing		

Resolution of Dysphagia Following Stroke

Dysphagia clinicians and researchers have noted that difficulty with swallowing lessens in the seven days following acute stroke, although in one study 27% of patients still were considered to be at risk by the physician. After six months, only 8% retained dysphagia; however, 3% had developed new difficulty with swallowing.[82] Logemann noted that 95% of patients with a single, uncomplicated stroke returned to full oral intake after nine weeks, regardless of the location of the stroke.[55] However, among that 95%, pharyngeal function was not completely normal and possibly contributed to even more severe dysphagia with a subsequent stroke.[55]

MEDICAL COMPLICATIONS ASSOCIATED WITH DYSPHAGIA IN STROKE

Medical complications associated with dysphagia following stroke include aspiration pneumonia, dehydration, compromised nutrition, and death.[81]

Aspiration

Aspiration refers to the penetration of food or liquid into the airway, below the level of the vocal folds, before, during, or after the swallow. *Laryngeal penetration* refers to the entrance of food or liquid into the larynx, above the level of the vocal folds.[55] *Silent aspiration* is defined as the entrance of saliva, food, or liquid below the level of the true vocal folds without a cough or any clinical signs of difficulty.[38] Aspiration and laryngeal penetration occur when the ability of the swallowing mechanism to prevent material from entering the airway is impaired.

Aspiration is common in the acute phase following stroke, with a greater incidence in severe strokes and in patients with pharyngeal sensory loss.[33] Approximately 40% of stroke patients with dysphagia who aspirate do not exhibit symptoms of aspiration during the bedside evaluation (silent aspiration).[38] Of stroke patients selected for a videofluoroscopic study, 48% to 55% were shown actually to aspirate.[28] Veis and Logemann[91] found that 32% of the subjects assessed by videofluoroscopy aspirated from pharyngeal stage problems, which the bedside evaluation cannot detect. Mann and Hankey[58] found that aspiration was correlated with delayed oral transit and incomplete oral clearance of the bolus. Sensory deficits in the larynx and pharynx may be associated with aspiration.[5] Patients with brainstem, subcortical, or bilateral stroke are at greater risk for aspiration.[26]

Tolerance for aspiration appears to be individual and may depend on the frequency, volume, and content of what is aspirated. Tolerance may also depend on the

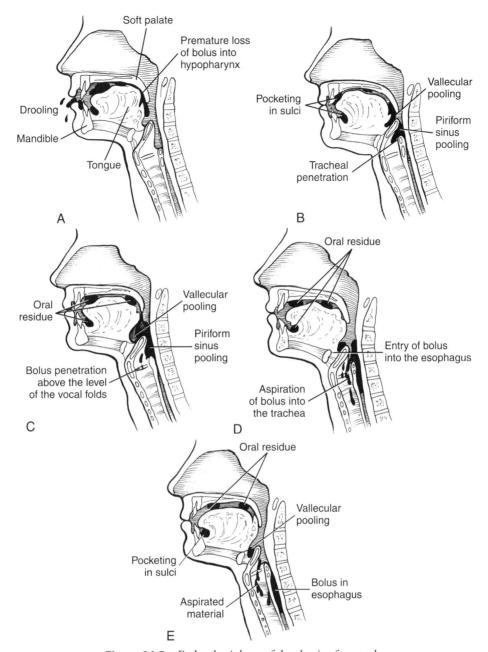

Figure 24-5 Pathophysiology of dysphagia after stroke.

overall health of the individual patient. Information regarding who may tolerate aspiration and in what parameters is scarce.

Aspiration Pneumonia

Aspiration can lead to aspiration pneumonia in patients with stroke,[56,59,63,76,81] which may lead to hospitalization or death.[63] Pneumonia is particularly common in stroke patients with multiple-location strokes, a history of airway disease, hypertension, diabetes, and aspiration during modified barium swallow (MBS).[26,59] As aspiration may occur with greater frequency in brainstem stroke, and it

may occur in 11% of those with brainstem stroke.[89] It occurs primarily the first few days after stroke.[27] Saliva contains pathogens that may be causative factors for pneumonia when saliva is aspirated.[44,45]

Dehydration and Compromised Nutrition

Dehydration is another possible consequence of dysphagia. Schmidt and colleagues[76] were unable to identify an increased risk of dehydration for patients with aspiration compared with those who did not aspirate. Dehydration may be caused by the use of dysphagia diets that provide only thickened liquids to avoid aspiration.[31,95] Dehydration also may be caused by the patient's inability to recognize thirst or to request a drink when thirsty. Nutritional status also may be compromised by stroke[81] for a variety of reasons, including dysphagia, loss of appetite, decreased mental status, depression and other psychosocial factors, and medication interactions.

Aspiration and Site of Lesion

Teasell, Bach, and McRae[88] reported that aspiration occurred in at least 9.9% of all patients who had unilateral right hemispheric strokes, 12.1% of those who had unilateral left hemispheric strokes, 24% of those who had bilateral hemispheric strokes, and 39.5% of those who had brainstem strokes. Horner, Massey, and Brazer[39] reported that aspiration occurred twice as often in those with bilateral stroke compared with those with unilateral stroke. Aspiration after bilateral stroke may be caused primarily by incomplete laryngeal elevation and closure, which encourages aspiration during the swallow and reduces pharyngeal peristalsis after the swallow, causing aspiration of residue. Alberts and colleagues[2] reported that patients with only small vessel infarcts had a decreased incidence of aspiration versus those with large and small vessel infarcts. Aspiration may be correlated with pharyngeal transit time, swallow response time, and duration of laryngeal closure.[69]

ROLE OF THE SWALLOWING TEAM

In inpatient settings, optimal management of dysphagia is performed by a multidisciplinary team. The team is responsible for identification, evaluation, diagnosis, treatment, and overall management of patients with dysphagia.

The multidisciplinary team includes a designated primary dysphagia therapist, usually the occupational therapist or speech-language pathologist, and the nurse, physician, respiratory therapist, dietitian, and the patient, who plays an active role in decision-making. For management of the dysphagic patient to be successful, *all* persons involved in the patient's care should understand the swallowing impairment and the management techniques used. Ongoing education and follow-up are often necessary.

EVALUATION OF SWALLOWING

Evaluation is the process of gathering and interpreting information needed for intervention.[37] *Assessment* refers to use of specific standardized tools or tests used as part of overall evaluation.[37] Dysphagia can be evaluated clinically and instrumentally. Clinical evaluation, which cannot rule out aspiration in those with stroke,[83] usually precedes instrumental evaluation. Instrumental evaluation is better at determining aspiration risk, and clinical evaluation helps to determine whether instrumental evaluation is needed.

Dysphagia screening tools identify patients in need of a complete clinical evaluation. Screening has been shown to reduce the incidence of pneumonia, regardless of severity of the stroke.[36] Several screenings are available in the literature, including the 3 ounce water test,[24] the Burke Dysphagia Screening Test,[25] and the Gugging Swallow Screen,[90] which was developed for those with acute stroke. Facilities may also develop their own screening tests. Screening is least likely to identify the presence of dysphagia following stroke, clinical assessment is more sensitive, and MBS is most sensitive.[59]

Identifying those at risk for aspiration and reducing possibility of severe medical consequences is a critical purpose of evaluation. However, a complete evaluation of swallowing addresses many other important issues for those with stroke. The swallow may be simply mildly impaired; however, that may lead to a more seriously decompensated swallow in the future as illness proceeds. Mild challenges with swallowing may lead to inadequate nutrition. Pleasure, enjoyment, and socialization at meals may be severely impacted by mild impairments and may gravely affect quality of life.

Clinical Evaluation and Assessment

When the physician suspects dysphagia, the physician orders a dysphagia evaluation. The physician, patient, nursing staff, and family also may identify the need for dysphagia evaluation. For patients who are NPO (not eating food by mouth), the physician must stipulate whether evaluation will include attempting trials of food by mouth with the patient. The evaluation examines factors that interfere with feeding and swallowing function, the patient's risk for aspiration, and factors that may contribute to a decrease in oral intake. The evaluation includes observational and direct examination components: chart review, patient and caregiver interview, functional status, oral motor examination, abnormal reflexes, pharyngeal examination, feeding trial, and a statement of impression and recommendations.

Specific assessment tools may be developed by facilities or a standardized assessment may be used. Appropriate dysphagia standardized assessments for patients with stroke include the Dysphagia Evaluation Protocol,[4] the Mann Assessment of Swallowing Ability,[57] and the Functional Oral Intake Scale.[21] The latter two were standardized on stroke populations. All of these assessments demonstrate a high degree of reliability.

Chart Review

The therapist first must review the patient's chart carefully to ascertain pertinent facts from the medical and feeding history. Pertinent information includes the following:

- Age[52]
- Previous evaluations and tests indicating current status (positive infiltrate on chest x-ray examination; ear, nose, and throat evaluation)

- Primary diagnosis and date of onset
- History of present illness, secondary diagnoses, and medical history, including history of dysphagia due to conditions other than stroke
- History of aspiration pneumonia
- History of weight loss, appetite, and nutrition, especially with current inpatient admission
- Reduced oral intake and its possible relation to depression, pain, feeding dependence, and food preferences or dislikes
- Aspiration precautions
- Dietitian, chest physical therapy, and/or respiratory therapy evaluations
- Current method of nutritional intake
- Current type of diet ordered
- Whether calorie counts are in place
- Length of time on current diet
- Dietary restrictions (diabetic: no concentrated sugars; cardiac: low sodium or low fat)
- Food allergies
- Current respiratory status

When reviewing the chart, the therapist must consider the patient's ability to participate in the evaluation, which contributes to the ability to feed and swallow safely. Factors to consider for mental status include primary language spoken, level of alertness, ability to follow directions, insight into swallowing difficulty, cognitive and perceptual status, and ability to communicate needs. Because eating requires a coordination of breathing and swallowing, respiratory problems may affect a person's ability to eat safely. The therapist should consider the following factors when evaluating the patient's ability to eat orally: excessive oral secretions, presence of tracheostomy, ventilator dependence and ability to wean, and frequency and route of suctioning.

Patient/Caregiver Interview

Initial contact begins with medical nursing staff and in the patient's room, where the occupational therapist may ask questions of the patient, family, and caregivers regarding the patient's past and present eating function. This information may expand on that obtained during the chart review.

Observation begins as soon as the practitioner enters the patient's room. The therapist should observe the room for any types of food that may indicate the patient's recent diet. Details to observe include the presence of an untouched meal tray; residual food on the patient's face, clothing, bed, or tray; and wet or hoarse breath sounds and abnormal vocal quality. The patient's positioning in the bed or chair is also relevant.

Functional Status

Functional status refers to the patient's ability to move in space and interact in the environment. Some functional interventions may be needed during evaluation to elicit optimal feeding and swallowing.

If a patient is unable to self-position to achieve an upright sitting position, this may interfere with feeding and swallowing. The occupational therapist should determine the amount of assistance required to position the patient in the bed or chair and whether the patient is able to maintain the position independently. Ideally the patient should sit upright in a chair with the pelvis in a slight anterior tilt, forearms weight-bearing on the tabletop, and the head and neck at midline and upright. The therapist also evaluates upper extremity and hand function as they relate to feeding.

Adaptive equipment or environmental adaptations may enable patients to feed themselves if possible. Adaptations for positioning include supporting feet that do not reach the floor with a telephone book or foot rest, using wheelchair cushions and other devices to improve upright posture, and adjusting the table height as needed. Wheelchairs with removable or swing-away armrests allow the patient to eat at the table. Alternatively, a full lap tray can be used with a wheelchair.

The therapist should assess the patient's ability to initiate and complete oral hygiene. A clean mouth is necessary for sensory appreciation of food, and good oral hygiene has been shown to reduce rates of pneumonia in an elderly populations.[97] One-handed techniques and equipment create independence with oral care. See Chapter 28.

For feeding, helpful items include Dycem to prevent the plate from slipping, a rocker knife and plate guard for one-handed eating, a covered cup or straw for bringing beverages to the mouth without spilling, and built-up utensils for weak or poorly controlled grasp to encourage use of a hemiplegic dominant arm. Bent spoons for using a non-dominant upper extremity to feed also may be helpful. Adapted cups with lids reduce spilling and provide handles for easy manipulation with a gross grasp; lids may have holes for straws, if appropriate. Specially angled dysphagia cups allow sipping without tilting the neck into extension.

Adaptations for reduced visual acuity, perception, and cognition may be useful at the table. The patient should wear eyeglasses if they usually are used at mealtime. A colorful piece of paper or "anchor" may be needed to draw the patient's attention or vision to the neglected side of the food array. A simplified presentation of one food item at a time can help to focus visual and general attention to the eating task. For stroke patients who are distractible, eating in a quiet, reduced-distraction setting promotes attention. Safety and pacing cues and supervision may be needed, especially for those with left hemiplegia. For right hemiplegic patients with aphasia and apraxia, minimal use of verbal directions and setup of the eating environment that makes the activity obvious are helpful.

Oral Examination

The therapist must administer an oral motor examination of the lips, cheeks, tongue, jaw, and palate before presenting food to the patient. The occupational therapist determines whether range of motion, muscle tone, and sensation (intraorally and extraorally) are decreased, increased, or within normal limits. Strength of oral structures is observed but may not be appropriate to assess because of the presence of abnormal muscle tone, which may invalidate strength testing.

Abnormal Reflexes

If present, abnormal "primitive" reflexes can interfere with feeding. Primitive reflexes include the bite reflex, rooting reflex, and the jaw jerk. The gag reflex may be hypersensitive, and hypersensitivity of internal and external oral structures also may be present.

Pharyngeal Examination

Although unseen, the therapist may assess aspects of pharyngeal function. Clinical features associated with dysphagia severity include dysphonia, dysarthria, abnormal volitional cough, abnormal gag reflex, coughing after swallowing, and voice change after swallowing.[22]

- *Dry swallow.* The ability to "dry" swallow (without food) provides information on the patient's ability to initiate a swallow response.
- *Vocal quality.* A wet, gurgly vocal quality can indicate pooling of secretions above the vocal cords, which normally are cleared by coughing or throat clearing. The patient may not perceive the presence of pooled secretions or may be unable to cough them up and clear the throat. Voice hoarseness or weakness may be due to unilateral or bilateral weakness of the vocal cords. Wet voice or a weak-hoarse voice suggests that weakness of the laryngeal structures may compromise the protection of the airway during swallow.[74]
- *Volitional or reflexive cough.* A volitional cough provides information about the strength of the vocal cords and breath support for coughing. Presence of reflexive cough indicates a lower risk of aspiration and pneumonia.[1]
- *The gag reflex.* In normal individuals, the presence or absence of a gag reflex can vary. Horner and Massey[38] noted that a poor gag reflex proved to be a poor indicator of prognosis for safer swallowing. Triggering of the gag reflex with a tongue depressor is different from triggering the gag reflex by a misdirected bolus. Food does not (normally) trigger a gag, because it is not a foreign substance or a noxious stimulus. The presence or absence of a gag reflex in patients with neurological impairments is not an accurate indicator of the patient's ability to swallow safely.[55] However, presence of a gag reflex does indicate some level of sensory and motor function of the tenth cranial nerve, which is responsible for innervating many structures that contribute to sensory and motor aspects of the swallow.

Feeding Trial

Feeding trials are appropriate for patients who are alert, able to follow commands, and medically stable. Factors that may contraindicate feeding trials include absence of or significantly reduced laryngeal elevation during dry swallows, moderate to severe dysarthria, lethargy or severely impaired mental status, and severe pulmonary compromise.[4,68]

Therapists may observe patients in a formal evaluation setting or informally at mealtime. Informal mealtime observation provides an efficient indication of the patient's eating ability and allows the evaluator to assess the patient's ability to concentrate despite distractions and interruptions. An informal evaluation allows for observation of the rate of intake and the patient's reaction to the presentation of the meal.[68] If the evaluation takes place in a formal setting, or if this is the patient's first attempt at eating following a stroke, trials should begin with foods that are less likely to be aspirated, such as thick purees, which do not require much oral manipulation, since thin liquids are more difficult to control in the oral cavity and pharynx. The evaluation then progresses to include foods of more difficult consistencies, depending on the patient's tolerance and medical status. Box 24-2 shows the usual progression of consistencies (from easiest to most difficult) as standardized in the National Dysphagia Diet (NDD). The NDD is the American Dietetic Association's recommended diet level hierarchy, developed in an attempt to standardize dysphagia diets offered in hospitals in the United States.[3]

The therapist may evaluate all the food and fluid consistencies shown in Box 24-2 or begin at the consistencies

---

Box 24-2

Bolus Consistency Progression: The National Dysphagia Diet

SOLID FOODS

Level 1: Dysphagia-Pureed: homogenous, cohesive, and puddinglike; little chewing required; examples: applesauce, pudding

Level 2: Dysphagia Mechanical-Altered: cohesive, moist, semisolid foods requiring some chewing; examples: soft macaroni and cheese, soft cooked vegetables

Level 3: Dysphagia-Advanced: Soft foods requiring more chewing

Regular: all foods allowed, including foods requiring chewing (meat) and mixed textures (cereal and milk; pills and water)

FLUIDS

Spoon-thick
Honeylike
Nectarlike
Thin

(ADA, 2002)

the patient currently tolerates. During the feeding trial, the occupational therapist should pay close attention to the nature and quality of oral manipulation of food and to the following indicators of laryngeal function.

An automatic cough occurs under many conditions, including a dry throat, or when secretions have accumulated around the vocal cords even before eating begins. To some extent, coughing occurs with normal breathing and at times when swallowing. Although an automatic cough may not be heard during a meal or feeding trial, its presence may signal that the patient is making efforts to clear the airway of food or secretions and that there is difficulty with airway protection or aspiration of a particular texture or textures. In normal swallowing, laryngeal penetration occurs occasionally; material that is penetrated is cleared from the larynx with throat clearing and reswallowing and often does not result in a cough. However, laryngeal reaction to aspirated material below the true vocal folds is normally a cough, which ideally expels the aspirated material.[80] A strong cough is necessary to protect the airway well. Horner, Massey, and Brazer[39] reported that a weak cough is more likely to occur in aspirating patients than in nonaspirating patients. As with the gag reflex, the presence of a reflexive cough indicates that the structures of the larynx and pharynx innervated by cranial nerve X have sensory and motor function to some extent and protect the airway during meals.[1]

Full laryngeal elevation and depression indicates that a swallow has occurred. Perlman and colleagues[68] concluded that reduced hyoid elevation impairs the pharyngeal stage of the swallow, thereby increasing the risk of vallecular residue and pharyngeal stasis. These factors may result in aspiration. Fig. 24-6 demonstrates the proper positioning of the examiner's hand and digits on

the patient's neck for palpation of the larynx to assess laryngeal elevation.

The therapist may assess breath and voice quality by the ear and by cervical auscultation with a stethoscope. Cervical auscultation is accomplished by placing the diaphragm of the stethoscope lateral to the trachea and inferior to the cricoid cartilage.[87] The therapist may adjust placement until hearing cervical breath sounds. The normal pharyngeal stage includes swallow initiation promptly after oral transit, an apneic period during the swallow, and exhalation immediately after the swallow, with clear breath sounds and vocal quality.[98] Breath and vocal quality differ in patients with dysphagia and often are characterized by gurgling sounds, increased throat clearing, and a "wet" vocal quality, which may indicate pooling. The therapist also may assess voice quality with the naked ear. Although cervical auscultation is an imprecise clinical method for the evaluation of aspiration, it has some correlation with aspiration found on an MBS,[98] and may be helpful in quickly identifying those at high risk for aspiration.[14]

Research of usefulness of pulse oximetry to detect aspiration has shown mixed results and may not be particularly useful.[93]

Common dysphagia signs and symptoms in stroke are compiled in Table 24-1. The therapist should make observations relating to these signs and symptoms for the oral-preparatory, oral, and pharyngeal stages for each food and fluid consistency presented. Recommendations and intervention goals are based on these observations, medical history, prognosis, and instrumental assessment results.

Instrumental Assessment of Dysphagia

Instrumental evaluation refers to diagnostic testing using instrumentation, the most important of which are MBS (sometimes referred to as *videofluoroscopy*) and fiberoptic endoscopic evaluation of swallowing (FEES) examinations.[11,21,48] These evaluations use diagnostic imaging techniques and provide information about the anatomy and physiology of the swallow, including aspiration, which cannot be determined during a clinical assessment.[70] They also may be rehabilitative procedures to assess efficacy and progress of compensatory techniques. The MBS and FEES provide information regarding the oral stage and the unseen pharyngeal stage of the swallow and can provide information about the patient's ability to protect the airway during swallow, which clinical evaluation cannot. Other instrumental evaluations commonly used to assess dysphagic patients with stroke include ultrasound and electromyography.

Modified Barium Swallow

The MBS or videofluoroscopic evaluation of swallowing allows the clinician to directly view the oral, pharyngeal, and esophageal aspects of the swallow. The MBS also allows the clinician to observe aspiration before, during, and

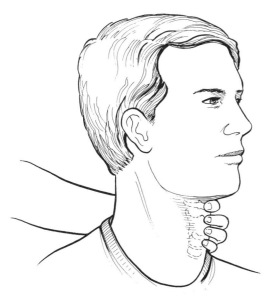

Figure 24-6 Palpation during the swallowing evaluation.

after the swallow.[51] MBS allows for greater accuracy in identifying dysphagia in stroke patients compared with clinical evaluation or screening.[59] The MBS ideally is performed jointly by the radiologist and the occupational therapist. Food and liquid boluses are mixed with barium, which is radiopaque. Alternatively, plain barium may be used, which is available in different thicknesses. The patient must be positioned in an upright position and preferably feeds himself or herself. The swallows are noted by a fluoroscopy unit and are recorded onto videotape or DVD. Thus, each stage of the swallow may be viewed during the assessment and reviewed later. The MBS not only allows the clinician to view swallow function and rule out aspiration but also provides useful information regarding compensatory swallowing strategies, discussed later in this chapter, and provides a determination of the amount, frequency, and quality of aspiration. The MBS also can assess how well the patient is able to deal with aspirated or penetrated material (e.g., his or her ability to clear aspirated material back into the pharynx). One study indicated that three specific observable aspects are related to aspiration in those with stroke: pharyngeal transit time, swallow response time, and duration of closure of the larynx.[69]

The MBS does expose the patient to some levels of radiation, and the ability of the patient to cooperate and follow directions is important for the success of information gathering and for minimizing radiation exposure. The MBS is difficult to achieve with patients who are in the intensive care unit, are difficult to position, and/or are difficult to transport to a radiology suite, although newer technology available at some medical centers permits MBS at the bedside. Naturally, MBS presents function at a specific moment in time, and reliability with real world swallowing function is not guaranteed, which therapists who use MBS results must consider. Additionally, interrater reliability of MBS performance assessment may vary.[86]

Fiberoptic Endoscopic Evaluation of Swallowing

FEES involves passing an endoscope with a light and camera through one of the patient's nares, down to the level of the valleculae. Before the assessment, lidocaine spray is used to numb the nares. Liquid and solid boluses are dyed with green food coloring for easy visualization. Images of the pharynx and larynx then are visualized and can be videotaped. This assessment is performed by an otolaryngologist, a trained occupational therapist, or a speech-language pathologist. The FEES allows the examiner to evaluate pharyngeal and laryngeal function and to assess the amount of residue present on the vocal cords or pooled in the valleculae or pyriform sinuses after a swallow. Thus, one can assess aspiration and competence in protecting the airway. One study suggested that FEES may be more sensitive in detecting aspiration than MBS.[46] However, FEES cannot always explain the reason that aspiration occurs, and the presence of the endoscopy tube

inhibits a completely normal swallow. The FEES is minimally invasive, and the patient must be able to tolerate the procedure. This procedure is contraindicated for patients with cardiac dysrhythmias, respiratory distress, bleeding disorders, anatomical deviations (narrow nasal passage), agitated or hostile patients, or patients with movement disorders.[84] The FEES is particularly useful for patients who cannot undergo a MBS for the foregoing reasons or who require frequent reassessment. Clinical benefits of FEES include assessment of airway protection when vocal cord involvement or impaired adduction is suspected, assessment of laryngeal/pharyngeal sensation, and direct visualization of anatomy when it is believed to be a contributing factor in dysphagia.

Ultrasound

Ultrasound is the method of choice if only oral function is to be assessed. Ultrasound is a noninvasive, dynamical evaluation of swallowing that shows the anatomy. This procedure uses normal foods and liquids and is safe to use with patients who are unable to follow directions.[84] The disadvantage of ultrasound is that it can visualize only the oral preparatory and oral stages of the swallow.

Electromyography

Surface electromyography measures myoelectrical impulses resulting from the firing of motor units. Surface electrodes are applied to the skin over specific muscles or muscle groups, producing a line tracing representing amplitude or strength of a contraction. Targeting of one muscle or the pharyngeal constrictor muscles is not possible. Placement of electrodes under the chin is used to detect motion of the suprahyoid muscles to assess whether a swallow has occurred.[40]

OUTCOME SCALES

Outcome scales are useful in categorizing dysphagia once evaluation is completed. The Dysphagia Outcome and Severity Scale is a seven category scale;[66] the Functional Outcome Swallowing Scale is a five point scale.[75] The Functional Oral Intake Scale, a seven point scale, was developed for patients with stroke.[21]

EVALUATION IMPRESSIONS AND RECOMMENDATIONS

After gathering information from all aspects of the clinical assessment and instrumental evaluations, the therapist must determine whether further instrumental evaluation of swallowing, discussed subsequently, is warranted. Often concerns about unseen pharyngeal function determine whether a referral for instrumental assessment is appropriate, important since pharyngeal stage deficits are common in acute stroke. Whether feeding should be oral or nonoral is a decision to be made by the team.[32] If, following a compete assessment, a patient clearly is aspirating or is at high risk for aspiration, NPO is recommended.

In acute care settings, NPO is often a short-term situation for stroke patients until swallowing improves, which it often does. For patients with complex medical conditions including stroke and resulting long-term dysphagia, for whom NPO may be a longer situation, the team should consider the impact of such a decision on the patient and family.[47] The caregivers and patient provide information about the patient's quality of life and preferences regarding medical intervention. If oral feeding is initiated against medical advice, mealtime management guidelines should be provided to optimize safety and emphasize food consistencies least likely to be aspirated.

ALTERNATIVE MEANS OF NUTRITION

Following evaluation, some patients may not be deemed candidates for oral feeding. They require alternative means of nutrition[19] unless they or their designated surrogate have made a purposeful choice not be given artificial feedings. The medical team must determine the length of time the patient will be NPO and the optimal nutritional route. One study has suggested that stroke patients who are not tolerating spoon-fed thick fluids or purees by 14 days following their stroke will need an alternative nutritional route such as a percutaneous endoscopic gastrostomy, defined later.[96] Two primary feeding routes generally are used: enteral, which uses a gastrointestinal route, and parenteral, which uses an intravenous route. Table 24-2 summarizes the risks and benefits of alternative feeding routes.

Enteral Feedings

Noninvasive Tube Feedings
Noninvasive tube feedings are most appropriate for short periods. A nasogastric tube is placed through the nose. Food in the form of an enteric feeding formula and water pass through the tube into the stomach (Fig. 24-7). Feedings may be given intermittently via boluses with a large syringe or constantly using a pump. Nasogastric tubes do not prevent pneumonia, however.[27]

Table 24-2

Risks and Benefits Associated with Oral, Enteral, and Parenteral Nutritional Support

TYPE OF NUTRITIONAL SUPPORT	POSSIBLE RISKS AND DRAWBACKS	BENEFITS
Oral	Possible tracheal aspiration	Psychologically pleasurable
	Possible inability to ingest sufficient calories	Allows occupational performance of eating and feeding
	Poor patient satisfaction (with limited dysphagia diet)	Provides socialization experience
		Promotes normal digestion
Nasogastric	Ulceration	Routine procedure
	Bleeding	Affordable
	Fistula	Begins immediately
	Gastroesophageal reflux, aspiration	Easily reversible
	Oropharyngeal discomfort	
	Poor patient satisfaction and compliance	
Surgical gastrostomy	Requires general anesthesia	Common procedure
	Bleeding	Good for long-term care if gastrointestinal tract is inaccessible
	Gastroesophageal reflux, aspiration	Easily replaceable
	Diarrhea	Removes tube from head/neck region
	Stomal irritation	Nonsurgical placement available (PEG)
Jejunostomy	Peritonitis	Minimizes gastroesophageal reflux
	Diarrhea	Can be used when stomach cannot tolerate diet
	Difficult to replace	Nonsurgical placement available (PEJ)
TPN	Sepsis	Fewer complications in patients with dysphagia and malnutrition
	Infection at site	For use in nonfunctioning gastrointestinal tract
	Short-term alimentation	Minimizes risk of aspirating stomach contents
	Pneumothorax	
	Expensive	

Adapted from Groher ME: Formulating feeding decisions for acute dysphagic patients, *Occup Ther Pract* 3:27, 1992.
PEG, Percutaneous endoscopic gastrostomy; *PEJ,* percutaneous endoscopic jejunostomy; *TPN,* total parenteral nutrition.

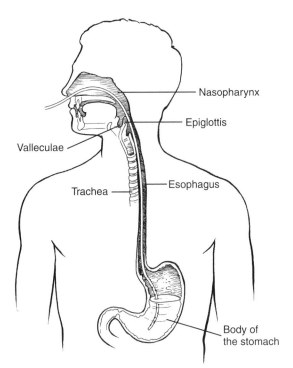

Figure 24-7   Placement of a nasogastric tube.

Invasive Feeding Methods

Invasive feeding methods are used when a patient is activity aspirating, for whom prolonged and severe dysphagia is expected. Tube feeding may be considered a rehabilitative technique when recovery is anticipated.[43] Percutaneous gastrostomy tubes are most often used and are placed with the patient under local anesthesia. The surgeon inserts an endoscope through the mouth into the stomach, makes a small incision in the stomach, and then threads a tube through the endoscope out through the abdominal wall. Special enteric formulas and water are administered for tube feeding. A percutaneous endoscopic gastrostomy may be "advanced" into the jejunum, creating a percutaneous endoscopic jejunostomy to help avoid reflux.

Occasionally, a patient will require a surgical gastrostomy. Often this is the case if there is a history of gastric disease and/or scarring. With the patient under general anesthesia, a surgeon makes an incision in the abdomen and then places a gastrostomy tube directly into the stomach. Occasionally, a tube is placed into the jejunum to reduce the reflux of stomach material into the esophagus, which gastrostomy tubes may cause. Food passes through the tube into the stomach.

Parenteral Feedings

Total parenteral nutrition administers a complete metabolic diet through a central vein, whereas peripheral parenteral nutrition administers the diet through a peripheral vein.

DYSPHAGIA INTERVENTION IN STROKE

Following evaluation, the patient and occupational therapist jointly determine specific swallowing goals. Family members and other caregivers may be involved in this process. For some patients, an initial goal is developing insight into their dysphagia, lack of which is commonly seen in patients with stroke.[67] Development of insight is associated with better swallowing outcomes as patients understand and follow intervention strategies.[67]

Interventions for dysphagia caused by stroke may be remedial (rehabilitative), compensatory, or a combination of both. Whether remedial or compensatory, the goals of intervention include reduction of aspiration risk, improving the quality of the swallow, and developing independence in feedings skills and behaviors at mealtime. In the acute phase after a stroke, patients may require daily reevaluation and adjustment in the intervention plan because their status may change daily.

Intervention Techniques

Treatments for dysphagia include positioning, feeding techniques, improvement of oral responses, facilitation of pharyngeal and laryngeal movements, facilitation of swallowing, therapeutic swallowing techniques, and diet modification. Assuring good nutrition and hydration, maintenance of eating by mouth, oral hygiene programs, and use of oral, pharyngeal and laryngeal structures in conversation are critical.

Positioning

An upright seated position allows optimal function of the muscles of swallowing, maximizes alertness for the fatigued or somewhat lethargic patient, and minimizes reflux. It aids in optimizing expiration during cough,[28] which is an important safety reflex. An upright seated position can be achieved in a chair or wheelchair, at the edge of the bed if balance allows, or in bed if necessary.

Feeding

Feeding oneself allows the optimal coordination of upper extremity and oral motor responses and the best awareness of bolus approach. Awareness of the bolus, via visual and olfactory appreciation, provides oral readiness for the bolus.[54] Manual guiding for stroke survivors with partial dominant upper extremity movement, particularly those with left cerebrovascular accident and apraxia, is a useful way to facilitate feeding in concert with upper extremity functional goals. Constraint induced therapy may encourage use of the affected dominant arm for eating. See Chapter 10.

Improving Oral Responses

Interventions begin with symmetrical body position and then are directed toward the affected side of the face to try to create symmetrical movement. When increased skeletal muscle activity (hypertonicity) is present, passive stretching of tight musculature such as a tight cheek with the back of a spoon or gloved finger is useful. When patients present with hypotonicity or low-toned motion in the oral structures, the therapist encourages movement using functional speech and eating tasks; for example, using oral exercises such as blowing or sucking tasks to elicit movement. Overflow motions or increased activity of undesired motions should be discouraged. The therapist can provide sensory stimulation for reduced sensation using a gloved hand inside and outside the mouth. Having the patient accomplish regular oral hygiene helps to establish sensory awareness and motor responses. For abnormally heightened sensation, graded sensory stimulation programs help the patient tolerate stimulation of the face and oral cavity to accept food and utensils. The therapist addresses abnormal reflexes with positioning and avoiding the stimuli that trigger the response.[23]

Weakness (as opposed to hypotonicity) of oral structures may be an issue with the debilitated stroke patient with reduced endurance. Some dysphagia therapists find that direct oral range of motion exercises are useful and often progress patients to gentle oral progressive resistive exercises. Tongue exercises have been shown to improve swallow pressure and airway safety in patients with both acute and chronic stroke.[72] Lip exercises have been found to improve lip force for eating in stroke patients.[34] A new study suggests that strength training does not exacerbate spasticity, as previously thought.[7]

While the patient eats, alteration in bolus qualities may help to trigger oral responses to food and thus improve the ensuing pharyngeal responses. Pushing down slightly with the spoon on the tongue as the bolus is introduced into the mouth can help with sensory awareness. Presentation of a cold bolus[13] or a sour bolus[53] can facilitate oral and also pharyngeal responses. Alternating food textures with each mouthful—for example, alternating fluids with solids—is a way of altering sensory input with each bite.[55]

Facilitation of Pharyngeal and Laryngeal Movements

Exercises involving pulling the tongue back, yawning, and gargling with saliva serve to strengthen retraction of the base of the tongue,[92] which is necessary to execute a swallow. Shaker exercises strengthen laryngeal elevation.[79] To accomplish Shaker exercises, the therapist has the patient perform repetitive tucking of the chin to the chest while supine. Shaker exercises have been shown to help patients with chronic dysphagia who are fed by tube to return to eating food by mouth.[78] Encouraging the patient to talk, cough, and clear the throat intermittently provides functional exercise for motions of the pharynx and larynx.

As with facilitation of oral motions, pharyngeal and laryngeal, strength training may assist in improving the force with which motions can be accomplished.[16]

Facilitation of Swallowing

Different methods are available to facilitate a swallow when its initiation is weak or delayed:

- *Thermal-tactile stimulation* consists of stroking the faucial arches with a chilled laryngeal mirror before eating and has been shown to speed the onset of the swallow response and the total swallow time in stroke patients.[73] A study indicated that the use of citrus flavored cold stimulus was optimal; however, the effect lasted for only one swallow.[77]
- *Surface electromyography* has been used to retrain brainstem stroke patients with chronic dysphagia to eat safely by mouth[20] and also has been demonstrated to be useful in providing biofeedback for relaxing high tone in laryngeal musculature, which allows an improved swallow response.[40]
- *Electrical stimulation.* Neuromuscular electrical stimulation therapy is used to target specific muscle groups to strengthen the swallow response. The VitalStim unit was developed by the Chattanooga group specifically for swallowing therapy. Practitioners must be certified to perform this therapy. One metaanalysis has demonstrated that this modality is effective for strengthening the swallow.[18]
- *Improving quality of the swallow.* Different techniques to improve the bolus direction during the swallow have been attempted with dysphagia patients. Patients with stroke often have residue in the affected cheek; using the tongue to clear the bolus or massaging the cheek with the hand are helpful to route the bolus back to the center of the tongue. Holding the affected lip closed with a finger to allow oral containment of the bolus may be necessary. Having the patient chew with the hemiparetic side of the jaw stimulates movement and function and helps the patient to practice transfer of the bolus between the two molar surfaces.

Using a chin tuck position during the swallow may be beneficial in decreasing aspiration in persons who experience a delayed pharyngeal swallow and reduced airway closure if the source of aspiration is material pooled in the valleculae.[80] The study by Shanahan and colleagues[80] did not find a decrease in the risk of aspiration with pooling in the piriform sinus with chin tuck. Chin tuck causes the structures of the pharynx to move posteriorly, reducing the size of the opening to the larynx.[94]

Full rotation of the head causes the bolus to move away from the direction of rotation and can be used to direct the bolus down the intact side of the pharynx.[65]

The "effortful swallow" is done by contracting the muscles of the throat hard during the swallow; this moves the base of the tongue posteriorly and helps to clear bolus from the valleculae.

The Mendelson maneuver, accomplished by pushing the tongue into the hard palate while swallowing, has been demonstrated to open the cricopharyngeal sphincter better and for a longer period, allowing the bolus to pass.[10]

Throat clearing and reswallowing may be useful in clearing pooled residue and can be done with other swallowing techniques.

Diet Modification

Research demonstrates that stroke patients aspirate less on pureed textures compared with liquids and soft solids.[28] The American Dietetic Association has standardized levels of a dysphagia diet, called the National Dysphagia Diet, which is appropriate for many diagnoses, including stroke.[3] Box 24-2 presents levels of diet based on the NDD. Naturally, patients will require an individual approach to determining safe and manageable textures to swallow. For example, carbonated liquids, not noted on the NDD, have been found to reduce incidence of aspiration compared with noncarbonated thin fluids.[15]

Follow-Up Care

Follow-up dysphagia care is advised for determining whether caregivers and patients understand and are complying with recommendations; outpatient visits after acute and rehabilitative inpatient care may be needed. Diets may need to be upgraded as improvements occur, and the patient and caregiver should be reminded about safe swallowing strategies and food textures.

Patient and Caregiver Education

The education process begins with initial contact with the patient and caregivers and continues with follow-up visits, informational pamphlets, and referrals to other health care professionals. Patients and caregivers must understand the concept of dysphagia, including the causes and consequences of aspiration, because they cannot follow recommended treatment without knowledge of the problem and its possible consequences. Anatomical pictures, handouts, and verbal explanations are useful educational tools. Precautionary signs placed by the bed also may be helpful in reinforcing the need to follow mealtime management guidelines.

Types and Efficacy of Dysphagia Intervention

Recovery of swallowing function is likely due to a combination of natural recovery and therapeutic effects. These effects include *facilitation* of available motions where structures and functions have been lost due to reduced sensation and altered muscle tone, and volitional strengthening of weak structures. Neuroplasticity is facilitated by these interventions[9] in ways that rehabilitation science has yet to fully understand.[71]

While swallowing compensations are used initially to encourage function in early stroke recovery, the goal for many is recovery of premorbid function. In those for whom recovery of lost function cannot be achieved, compensatory strategies may be permanent.

Regardless of whether it is rehabilitative or compensatory in nature, dysphagia intervention has been shown to improve aspects of oral and pharyngeal function[61] and nutritional status in patients with stroke.[29] Dysphagia intervention is associated with the ultimate ability to eat by mouth in those with neurological diagnoses.[17,62] Intervention has been shown in one small study to enable those with chronic dysphagia requiring alternative nutrition sources to return to eating by mouth with the use of surface electromyography biofeedback.[41] Dysphagia intervention for patients with stroke has been shown to reduce the risk of aspiration pneumonia[62] and thus is cost-effective.[64]

CASE STUDY 1

Swallowing After Right Hemispheric Stroke

Mrs. Jones was admitted to the hospital with a right middle cerebral artery stroke, resulting in a left hemiplegia with dysphagia. She had a nasogastric tube and was not referred for dysphagia evaluation until she was medically stable, a week after her admission. On evaluation, she demonstrated a left facial droop involving reduced muscle tone in the lip, cheek, and tongue. Drooling from the left side of her mouth was a problem because of reduced sensation. The gag reflex was reduced on the left side of the pharynx, although she could elicit a dry swallow with difficulty. Once her dentures were inserted and the nasogastric tube was removed, a feeding trial was done. During the feeding trial, Mrs. Jones demonstrated pocketing of food in her left cheek and in the sulcus between her lower jaw and cheek. She was able to swallow soft purees and honey-thick fluids, although thin fluids extracted a cough. An MBS further revealed pooling in the pyriform sinuses and occasional laryngeal penetration with honey-thick fluids, which was alleviated with a chin tuck and by intermittent throat clearing. At this time, she still had an intravenous line, so hydration was not a concern. She was able to feed herself with her dominant right hand once her tray was set up, with frequent cues to regard the left side of her plate because of left neglect. She also needed cues to swallow each mouthful and eat slowly because of reduced judgment and impulsivity. Mrs. Jones massaged her left cheek with tactile cues to move pocketed food back onto her tongue. Within a week, Mrs. Jones progressed to soft solids and nectar-thick fluids, and her intravenous line was discontinued. The following week, she proceeded to thin fluids and ground solids and was able to prepare her tray independently. She still needed occasional safety cues to eat slowly, to take single sips, and to look at the left side of her plate.

CASE STUDY 2

Swallowing after Left Hemispheric Stroke

Mr. Smith was admitted to the hospital with a left middle cerebral artery stroke and was referred for dysphagia evaluation the day after admission. His oral movements and ability to follow commands were difficult to assess formally because of aphasia. Active and symmetrical motion of his lips, cheeks, and tongue were observed on attempts to speak. Mr. Smith's dentition was intact. His gag reflex was intact, although palatal movement was not observed because of inability to phonate on command; he was unable to produce an automatic cough. On the feeding trial, he initially demonstrated slow initiation of oral and hand-to-mouth movement characteristic of apraxia, but once he had eaten several bites, he was able to manipulate foods more efficiently during the preoral and oral-preparatory stages of the swallow. Mr. Smith was able to manage soufflé textures and soft chewable solids and to drink thin fluids using a dysphagia cup to prevent tipping his head back to swallow. He required some tactile guiding to self-feed with his dominant right upper extremity, which had exhibited isolated but weak movements. Within the week, he was able to chew and swallow food with regular textures. Upper extremity function improved as well, and he could prepare his tray independently and cut solid foods using his right hand in dominant fashion.

REVIEW QUESTIONS

1. Define aspiration.
2. Define laryngeal penetration.
3. Describe the five stages of swallowing. Indicate three signs or symptoms of dysphagia at each stage.
4. Name the cranial nerves and identify their functions in swallowing.
5. Name 10 items important for chart review.
6. Describe the elements of a dysphagia intervention program for a stroke patient.
7. Describe two advantages of FEES.
8. Describe two advantages of an MBS.

REFERENCES

1. Addington WR, Stephens RE, Gilliland KA: Assessing the laryngeal cough reflex and the risk of developing pneumonia after stroke. *Stroke* 30(6):1203–1207, 1999.
2. Alberts MJ, Horner J, Gray L, et al: Aspiration after stroke: lesion analysis by brain MRI. *Dysphagia* 7(3):170–173, 1992.
3. American Dietetic Association: *National Dysphagia Diet: Standardization for Optimal Care*, Chicago, 2002, American Dietetic Association.
4. Avery-Smith W, Rosen AB, Dellarosa DM: *Dysphagia evaluation protocol*, San Antonio, TX, 1997, Therapy Skill Builders.
5. Aviv JE, Martin JH, Sacco RL, et al: Supraglottic and pharyngeal sensory abnormalities in stroke patients with dysphagia. *Ann Otol Rhinol Laryngol* 105(2):92–97, 1996.
6. Aydogdu I, Ertekin C, Sultan T, et al: Dysphagia in lateral medullary Infarctions (Wallenberg's Syndrome). *Stroke* 32(9):2081–87, 2001.
7. Badics E, Wittmann A, Rupp M, et al: Systematic muscle building exercises in the rehabilitation of stroke patients. *Neurorehabilitation* 17(3):211–4, 2002.
8. Badr C, Ekins MR, Ellis ER: The effect of body position on maximal expiratory pressure and flow. *Aust J Physiother* 48(2):95–102, 2002.
9. Barrett AW, Smithard DG: Role of cerebral cortex plasticity in the recovery of swallowing function following dysphagia stroke. *Dysphagia* 24(1):83–90, 2009.
10. Bartolome G, Neumann S: Swallowing therapy in clients with neurological disorders causing cricopharyngeal dysfunction. *Dysphagia* 8(2):146, 1993.
11. Bastian RW: The videoendoscopic swallowing study: an alternative and partner to the videofluoroscopic swallowing study. *Dysphagia* 8(4):359–367, 1993.
12. Besson G, Bogousslavsky J, Regli F, Maeder P: Acute pseudobulbar or suprabulbar palsy. *Arch Neurol* 8(5):501–507, 1991.
13. Bisch EM, Logemann JA, Rademaker AW, et al: Pharyngeal effects of bolus volume, viscosity, and temperature in clients with dysphagia resulting from neurologic impairment and in normal subjects. *J Speech Hear Res* 37(5):1041, 1994.
14. Borr C, Hielscher-Fastabend M, Lucking A: Reliability and validity of cervical auscultation. *Dysphagia* 2(3):225–34, 2007.
15. Bulow M, Olsson R, Ekberg O: Videoradiographic analysis of how carbonated thin liquids and thickened liquids affect the physiology of swallowing in subjects with aspiration on thin liquids. *Acta Radiologica* 44(4):366–372, 2003.
16. Burkhead LM, Sapienza CM, Rosenbek JC: Strength training in dysphagia rehabilitation: principles, procedures, and directions for future research. *Dysphagia* 22(3):251–65, 2007.
17. Carnaby G, Hankey GJ, Pizzi J: Behavioural intervention for dysphagia in acute stroke: a randomized controlled trial. *Lancet Neurol* 5(1):31–7, 2007.
18. Carnaby-Mann GD, Crary MA: Examining the evidence on neuromuscular electrical stimulation for swallowing: a meta-analysis. *Arch Otol Head Neck Surg* 133(6):564–571, 2007.
19. Ciocon JO: Indications for tube feedings in elderly patients. *Dysphagia* 5(1):1–5, 1990.
20. Crary MA: A direct intervention program for chronic neurogenic dysphagia secondary to brainstem stroke. *Dysphagia* 10(1):6–18, 1995.
21. Crary MA, Carnaby Mann GD, Groher ME: Initial psychometric assessment of a functional oral intake scale for dysphagia in stroke patients. *Arch Phys Med Rehabil* 86(8):1516–20, 2005.
22. Daniels SK, McAdam CP, Braily K, Foundas AL: Clinical assessment of swallowing and prediction of dysphagia severity. *Am J Speech Lang Path* 6:17–24, 1997.
23. Davies PM: *Starting again*, Berlin, 1994, Springer-Verlag.
24. DePippo KL, Hosas MA, Reding MJ: Validation of the 3–oz water swallow test for aspiration following stroke. *Arch Neurol* 49(12):1259–1261, 1992.
25. DePippo KL, Hosas MA, Reding MJ: The Burke dysphagia screening test: validation of its use in patients with stroke. *Arch Phys Med Rehabil* 75(12):1284–1286, 1994.
26. Ding R, Logemann JA: Pneumonia in stroke patients: a retrospective study. *Dysphagia* 15(2):51–57, 2000.
27. Dziewas R, Ritter M, Schilling M, et al: Pneumonia in acute stroke patients fed by nasogastric tubes. *J Neurol Neurosurg Psychiatry* 5(6):852–856, 2004.
28. Dziewas R, Warnecke T, Olenberg S, et al: Towards a basic endoscopic assessment of swallowing in acute stroke-development and evaluation of a simple dysphagia score. *Cerebrovascular Dis* 6(1):41–47, 2008.

29. Elmstahl S, Bulow M, Ekberg O, et al: Treatment of dysphagia improves nutritional conditions in stroke patients. *Dysphagia* 14(2):61–66, 1999.

30. Ertekin C, Aydogdu I, Tarlaci S, et al: Mechanisms of dysphagia in suprabulbar palsy with lacunar infarct. *Stroke* 1(6):1370–1376, 2000.

31. Finestone HM, Foley NC, Woodbury MG, et al: Quantifying fluid intake in dysphagia stroke patients: a preliminary comparison of oral and nonoral strategies. *Arch Phys Med Rehabil* 82(12):1744–1746, 2001.

32. Groher ME: Determination for the risks and benefits of oral feeding. *Dysphagia* 9(4):233–235, 1994.

33. Groher ME, Bukatman R: The prevalence of swallowing disorders in two teaching hospitals. *Dysphagia* 1(1):3, 1986.

34. Hagg M, Anniko M: Lip muscle training in stroke patients with dysphagia. *Acta Otolaryngologica* 128(9):1027–1033, 2008.

35. Heckert KD, Komaroff E, Adler U, Barrett AM: Postacute re-evaluation may prevent dysphagia-associated morbidity. *Stroke* 40(4):1381–85, 2009.

36. Hinchey JA, Shephard T, Furie K, et al: Formal dysphagia screening protocols prevent pneumonia. *Stroke* 36(9):1972–1976, 2005.

37. Hinojosa J, Kramer P, Crist P, Evaluation P: *Obtaining and interpreting data*, 2nd ed, Bethesda, MD, 2005, AOTA Press.

38. Horner J, Massey EW: Silent aspiration following stroke. *Neurology* 38(2):317–319, 1988.

39. Horner J, Massey EW, Brazer SR: Aspiration in bilateral stroke patients. *Neurology* 40(11):1686–1688, 1990.

40. Huckabee ML: Maximizing rehabilitation efforts for dysphagia recovery: SEMG biofeedback monitoring. Lincoln Park, NJ, 1997, Kay Elemetrics Corp. Application Note.

41. Huckabee ML, Cannito MP: Outcomes of swallowing rehabilitation in chronic brainstem dysphagia: a retrospective evaluation. *Dysphagia* 14(2):93–109, 1999.

42. Irie H, Lu CC: Dynamic evaluation of swallowing in patients with cerebrovascular accident. *Clin Imaging* 19(4):240–243, 1995.

43. James R, Gines D, Menlove A, et al: Nutrition support (tube feeding) as a rehabilitation intervention. *Arch Phys Med Rehabil* 86(12): 82–92, 2005.

44. Johnson ER, McKenzie SW, Sievers A: Aspiration pneumonia in stroke. *Arch Phys Med Rehabil* 74(9):973–976, 1993.

45. Kalra L, Yu G, Wilson K, et al: Medical complications during stroke rehabilitation. *Stroke* 26(6):990–994, 1995.

46. Kelly AM, Drinnan MJ, Leslie P: Assessing penetration and aspiration: how do videofluoroscopy and fiberoptic endoscopic evaluation of swallowing compare? *Laryngoscope* 117(10):1723–7, 2007.

47. Kidd D, Lawson J, Nesbitt R, et al: The natural history and clinical consequences of aspiration in acute stroke. *Q J Med* 88(6):409–413, 1995.

48. Kidder TM, Langmore SE, Martin BJW: Indications and techniques of endoscopy in evaluation of cervical dysphagia: comparison with radiographic techniques. *Dysphagia* 9(4):256–261, 1994.

49. Deleted.

50. Linden-Castelli P: Treatment strategies for adult neurogenic dysphagia. *Semin Speech Lang* 12(3):255, 1991.

51. Logemann JA: Criteria for studies of the treatment for oral-pharyngeal dysphagia. *Dysphagia* 1(4):193, 1987.

52. Logemann JA: Effects of aging on the swallowing mechanism. *Otolaryngol Clin North Am* 23(6):1045–1056, 1990.

53. Logemann JA, Pauloski BR, Colangelo L, et al: Effects of a sour bolus on oropharyngeal swallowing measures in clients with neurogenic dysphagia. *J Speech Hear Res* 38(3):556–563, 1995.

54. Logemann JA: Preswallow sensory input: its potential importance to dysphagic patients and normal individuals. *Dysphagia* 11(1):9–10, 1996.

55. Logemann JA: *Evaluation and treatment of swallowing disorders*, Austin, TX, 1997, Pro-Ed.

56. Lorish TR, Sandin KJ, Roth EJ, et al: Stroke rehabilitation evaluation and management. *Arch Phys Med Rehabil* 75(5 Spec No): S47–S51, 1994.

57. Mann G: MASA: *The Mann assessment of swallowing ability*, Clifton Park, NY, 2000, Singular.

58. Mann G, Hankey GJ: Initial clinical and demographic predictors of swallowing impairment following acute stroke. *Dysphagia* 16(3): 208–215, 2001.

59. Martino R, Foley N, Bhogal S, et al: Dysphagia after stroke: incidence, diagnosis, and pulmonary complications. *Stroke* 36(12): 2756–63, 2005.

60. Meng NH, Wang TG, Lien IN: Dysphagia in patients with brainstem stroke: incidence and outcome. *Am J Phys Med Rehabil* 79(2):170–175, 2000.

61. Neumann S: Swallowing therapy with neurologic patients: results of direct and indirect therapy methods in 66 patients suffering from neurologic disorders. *Dysphagia* 8(2):150–153, 1993.

62. Neumann S, Bartolome G, Buchholz D, et al: Swallowing therapy of neurologic patients: correlation of outcome with pretreatment variables and therapeutic methods. *Dysphagia* 10(1):1–5, 1995.

63. Noll SF, Roth EJ: Stroke rehabilitation. I. Epidemiologic aspects and acute management. *Arch Phys Med Rehabil* 75(5 Spec No): S38–S41, 1994.

64. Odderson IR, Keaton JC, McKenna BS: Swallow management in patients on an acute stroke pathway: quality is cost effective. *Arch Phys Med Rehabil* 76(12):1130–1133, 1995.

65. Ohmae Y, Ogura M, Kitahara S, et al: Effects of head rotation on pharyngeal function during normal swallow. *Ann Otol Rhinol, Laryngol* 107(4):344–8, 1998.

66. O'Neil, KH, Purdy M, Falk J, Gallo L: The Dysphagia Outcome and Severity Scale. *Dysphagia* 14(3):139, 1999.

67. Parker C, Power ML, Hamdy S, et al: Awareness of dysphagia by patients following stroke predicts swallowing performance. *Dysphagia* 19(1):28–35, 2004.

68. Perlman AL, Langmore SE, Milianti FJ, et al: Comprehensive clinical examination of oropharyngeal swallowing function: Veteran's Administration procedure. *Semin Speech Lang* 12(3):246, 1991.

69. Power ML, Hamdy S, Goulermas JY, et al: Predicting aspiration after hemispheric stroke from timing measures of oropharyngeal bolus flow and laryngeal closure. *Dysphagia* 4(3):257–264, 2009.

70. Ramsey DJC, Smithard DG, Kalra L: Early assessments of dysphagia and aspiration risk in acute stroke patients. *Stroke* 34(5):1252–1257, 2003.

71. Robbins J, Butler SG, Daniels SK, et al: Swallowing and dysphagia rehabilitation: translating principles of neural plasticity into clinically oriented evidence. *J Speech Lang Hear Res* 51(1):S276–S300, 2008.

72. Robbins J, Kays SA, Gangnon RE, et al: The effects of lingual exercise in stroke patients with dysphagia. *Arch Phys Med Rehabil* 88(2):150–8, 2007.

73. Rosenbek JC, Roecker EB, Wood JL, et al: Thermal application reduces the duration of stage transition in dysphagia after stroke. *Dysphagia* 11(4):225–233, 1996.

74. Ryu JY, Park SR, Choi KH: Prediction of laryngeal aspiration using voice analysis. *Am J Phys Med Rehabil* 83(10):753–7, 2004.

75. Salassa J: A Functional Outcome Swallowing Scale for staging oropharyngeal dysphagia. *Dig Dis* 7(4), 230–234, 1999.

76. Schmidt J, Holas M, Halvorson K, et al: Videofluoroscopic evidence of aspiration predicts pneumonia and death but not dehydration following stroke. *Dysphagia* 9(1):7, 1994.

77. Sciortino KF, Liss JM, Case JL, et al: Effect of mechanical, cold, gustatory, and combined stimulation to the human anterior faucial pillars. *Dysphagia* 18(1):16–26, 2003.

78. Shaker R, Easterling C, Kern M, et al: Rehabilitation of swallowing by exercise in tube-fed clients with pharyngeal dysphagia secondary to abnormal UES opening. *Gastroenterology* 122(5):1314–1321, 2002.

79. Shaker R, Kern M, Bardan E, et al: Augmentation of deglutitive upper esophageal sphincter opening in the elderly by exercise. Am J Physiol 272(6 pt 1):G1518–G1522, 1997.

80. Shanahan TK, Logemann JA, Rademaker AW, et al: Chin-down posture effect on aspiration in dysphagic patients. *Arch Phys Med Rehabil* 74(7), 1993, 736–9.

81. Smithard DG, O'Neill PA, Parks C, et al: Complications and outcome after acute stroke: does dysphagia matter? *Stroke* 27(7):1200–1204, 1996.

82. Smithard DG, O'Neill PA, England RE, et al: The natural history of dysphagia following stroke. *Dysphagia* 12(4):188–193, 1997.

83. Smithard DG, O'Neill PA, Park C, et al: Can bedside assessment reliably exclude aspiration following acute stroke? *Age Ageing* 27(2):99–106, 1998.

84. Sonies BC: Instrumental procedures for dysphagia diagnosis. *Semin Speech Lang* 12(3):186, 1991.

85. Steinhagen V, Grossmann A, Benecke R, Walter U: Swallowing disturbance pattern relates to brain lesion location in acute stroke patients. *Stroke* 40(5):1903–1906, 2009.

86. Stoeckli S, Huisman TA, Seifert B, et al: Interrater reliability of videofluoroscopic swallow evaluation. *Dysphagia* 18(1):53–57, 1991.

87. Takahashi K, Groher ME, Michi K: Methodology for detecting swallowing sounds. *Dysphagia* 9(1):54–62, 1994.

88. Teasell RW, Bach DB, McRae M: Prevalence and recovery of aspiration poststroke: a retrospective analysis. *Dysphagia* 9(1):35–39, 1994.

89. Teasell RW, Foley N, Doherty T, et al: Clinical characteristics of patients with brainstem stroke admitted to a rehabilitation unit. *Arch Phys Med Rehabil* 83(7):1013–1016, 2002.

90. Trapl M, Enderle P, Nowotny M, et al: Dysphagia bedside screening for acute-stroke patients: The Gugging Swallowing Screen. *Stroke* 38(11):2948–2952, 2007.

91. Veis SL, Logemann JA: Swallowing disorders in persons with cerebrovascular accident. *Arch Phys Med Rehabil* 66(6):372–375, 1985.

92. Veis SL, Logemann JA, Colangelo L: Effects of three techniques on maximum posterior movement of the tongue base. *Dysphagia* 15(3):142–145, 2002.

93. Wang T-G, Chang Y-C, Chen S-Y, Hsiao T-Y: Pulse oximetry does not reliably detect aspiration on videofluoroscopic swallowing study. *Arch Phys Med Rehabil* 86(4):730–734, 2005.

94. Welch MV, Logemann JA, Rademaker AW, et al: Changes in pharyngeal dimensions effected by chin tuck. *Arch Phys Med Rehabil* 74(2):178–181, 1993.

95. Whelan K: Inadequate fluid intakes in dysphagic acute stroke. *Clin Nutr* 20(5):423–428, 2001.

96. Wilkinson TJ, Thomas K, MacGregor S, et al: Tolerance of early diet textures as indicators of recovery from dysphagia after stroke. *Dysphagia* 17(3):227–232, 2002.

97. Yoneyama T, Yoshida M, Ohrui T, et al: Oral care reduces pneumonia in older patients in nursing homes. *J Am Geriatr Soc* 50(3): 430–433, 2002.

98. Zenner PM, Losinski DS, Mills RH: Using cervical auscultation in the clinical dysphagia examination in long-term care. *Dysphagia* 10(1):27–31, 1995.

SUGGESTED READINGS

Carnaby-Mann G, Lenius K, Crary MA: Update on assessment and management of dysphagia post stroke. *Northeast Florida Medicine* 58(2):31–34, 2007.

Clark HM: Neuromuscular treatments for speech and swallowing: A tutorial. *Am J Speech Lang Pathol* 12(4):400–415, 2003.

Clark HM: Clinical decision making and oral motor treatments. *ASHA Leader*, June 8-9, 2005.

Crary MA, Groher ME: *Adult swallowing disorders*, Philadelphia, 2003, Elsevier.

Davies P: The neglected face. In *Steps to follow*, New York, 2000, Springer-Verlag.

Fornataro-Clerici L, Roop TA: *Clinical management of adults requiring tracheostomy tubes and ventilators*, Gaylord, MI, 1997, Northern Speech Services.

Groher ME: *Dysphagia: diagnosis and management*, Boston, 1997, Butterworth-Heinemann.

Ramsey DJC, Smithard DG, Kalra L: Early assessments of dysphagia and aspiration risk in acute stroke patients. *Stroke* 34(5):1252–1257, 2003.

jessica farman
judith dicker friedman

chapter 25

Sexual Function and Intimacy

key terms

aging	sexual function	sexuality counseling
disability	sexual rehabilitation	
sexual dysfunction	sexuality	

chapter objectives

After completing this chapter, the reader will be able to accomplish the following:

1. Identify and describe the normal human sexual response cycle and the changes that occur during the aging process.
2. Understand the effects of stroke on sexual function.
3. Identify the occupational therapist's role in sexuality intervention.
4. Understand and apply the levels of the PLISSIT model that are appropriate for occupational therapists.
5. Identify sexual impairments and how they affect function.
6. Plan treatment interventions for impairments affecting sexual function.

A discussion of sexuality includes not only specific sexual practices but also the attitudes, behaviors, thoughts, and feelings associated with sex and sexuality. These include an individual's perception of self as a sexual being, body image, self-esteem, participation and roles in relationships (sexual and other), sexual orientation, and beliefs and attitudes toward a wide range of sexual behaviors, including masturbation, coitus, oral-genital sex, cuddling, and sensuality. Romano[66] defined sexuality expertly: "Sexuality is more than the art of sexual intercourse. It involves for most . . . the whole business of relating to another person; the tenderness, the desire to give as well as take, the compliments, casual caresses,

reciprocal concerns, tolerance, the forms of communication that both include and go beyond words . . . sexuality includes a range of behavior from smiling through orgasm; it is not just what happens between two people in bed."

Everyone can enjoy sex. Health care professionals must be aware of their own attitudes toward sexuality. Our patients may be different from ourselves: they may be older, may be of a different sexual orientation, or may have permanent or temporary disabilities. Just as differences among human beings are inherent, therapists must consider and respect the variances in sexual behaviors, preferences, and beliefs among individuals.

NORMAL HUMAN SEXUAL RESPONSE

One must have an understanding of the normal human sexual response cycle before one can explore the relationship between sexuality and disability. Masters and Johnson[48] divided the human sexual response cycle into four segments: (1) excitement, (2) plateau, (3) orgasm, and (4) resolution. In each phase, definite physical changes occur in both sexes. During the excitement phase, physiological reactions occur because of somatosensory or psychogenic stimulation. In females, the nipples become erect, the vagina swells and becomes lubricated, the clitoris and the labia minora and majora swell, and the uterus and cervix retract. In males, the penis grows erect and the testes rise. In both sexes, blood pressure and heart rate increase.

During the plateau phase, respiration increases and blood pressure and heart rate escalate further. In females, the areola surrounding the nipple swells, the orgasmic platform forms (vasocongestion of the outer two thirds of the vagina), and the color of the labia minora deepens from pink to red. In males, a full erection is achieved as the testes elevate further and the Cowper gland secretes preejaculatory fluid.

Orgasms differ between the sexes; some women can achieve multiple orgasms. In both sexes, peak pulse rate, blood pressure, and respiration increase, as does muscle tone. Rhythmic contractions of the orgasmic platform and the uterus occur in women, and rhythmic contractions of the penis project semen forward in males.

Masters and Johnson[48] recorded cardiac response and found peak heart rates of 110 to 180 beats per minute during orgasm. However, the mean maximum heart rate during sexual activity was 117.4 beats per minute in a study of middle-aged men with postcoronary disease.[34] During sexual activity, systolic and diastolic pressure increase (from 30 to 80 and 20 to 40 mm Hg, respectively). Respiration rates of up to 40 breaths per minute have been recorded, depending on the level of intensity and duration of sexual activity.[48]

The resolution phase is characterized by the return to preexcitement status, including reductions in blood pressure, heart rate, and respiration. The genitals and breasts return to preexcitement size.

Aging and the Human Sexual Response Cycle

In normal human development, changes occur during the aging process. Such changes affect sexuality[61] in males and females and already may affect patients who have sustained cerebrovascular accidents.

Women

Generally women experience menopause between the ages of 40- and 50-years old; the cessation of menstruation is caused by a lack of production of estrogen that occurs over a period of several months to a few years.[43] The major effects of menopause are as follows:

- Vasomotor syndrome (hot flashes)[43]
- Atrophic vaginitis (thinning of the vaginal walls)[43]
- Osteoporosis[43]
- A decrease in the rate, amount, and type of vaginal fluid, which can cause pain during intercourse and may lead to infection[74]
- Loss of contractility of vaginal muscles, which can cause shorter orgasms[74]
- Decreased size of the uterus and clitoris and atrophy of the clitoral hood[43]
- Loss of elasticity in breast tissue, causing sagging

According to Laflin,[43] regular muscle contractions help maintain the integrity of vaginal muscle tone, and "contact with the penis helps preserve the shape and size of the vaginal space." Therefore, an active sex life can have a positive effect on genital function.

Men

As men grow older, the following changes occur:

- Erections are often less full, take longer to achieve, and may require direct stimulation.[74]
- Ejaculatory control increases, ejaculation may only occur every third sexual episode and is less forceful, and loss of erection after orgasm may occur faster.[43,74]
- The man may not be able to achieve another erection for 12 to 24 hours after orgasm.[39]
- Sperm volume decreases and the ejaculation may be less intense, which may affect the intensity of orgasm.[43,74]
- The size and firmness of the testes diminish.
- The testosterone level decreases.

Many elderly persons continue to enjoy sexual activity; however, a decline in sexual activity among elderly persons is common. Older persons do not necessarily lose their desire for sex, but circumstances can make it difficult for them to engage in active sexual relationships. Leading causes of altered sexual activity in the older adult include difficulty finding partners, illness, medication effects, widowhood, divorce, biases about masturbation, societal attitudes about sex and the elderly, and even their own biases and prejudices toward sexuality.[65] Elderly persons may view sex as something that only young, attractive persons do.

SEXUALITY AND NEUROLOGICAL FUNCTION

Sexual function is controlled by the brain, spinal cord, and peripheral nerves, whereas control of libido and sexual pleasure are mediated by several areas in the cortex, midbrain, and brainstem.[56] Men experience reflexogenic and psychogenic erections. Reflexogenic erections are caused by direct stimulation to the penis and may occur without conscious awareness, even in the absence of penile sensation. Psychogenic erections originate from mental activity such as sexual fantasies and stimulating visual input and do not require direct penile stimulation. Reflexogenic erections are controlled by the nervous system through the sacral roots, and psychogenic erections involve the sympathetic nerves between T11 and L2. Female sexual function is similar to that of males regarding nerve innervation.[77] The parasympathetic nerves S2 to S4 influence the clitoris and vaginal lubrication. "Contraction of the vaginal sphincter and pelvic floor occur with stimulation of the somatic aspect of the pudendal nerves (S2-S4)," according to Zasler.[77] Neurological disability can cause organic impotence by altering the blood flow needed for penile erection and can cause problems with emission and ejaculation in males and with lubrication, clitoral engorgement, and orgasm in females. Some of the subcortical structures theorized to be involved in the neurology of sexuality are the reticular activating system and the hippocampus, amygdala, and hypothalamus. According to Zasler,[77] the thalamus and basal ganglia are hypothesized to be involved with the mediation of sexual function. Some of the cortical areas involved are the frontal lobes and the nondominant temporal lobe. "Lesions in the dominant hemisphere may produce aphasia or apraxia, both of which could impede sexual activity. Nondominant hemisphere injury may result in . . . visuoperceptual deficits, denial, and impulsiveness, all of which could impede expression of sexuality," according to Zasler.[77] Sexual stimulation is caused by stimulation of the brain or peripheral nerves, the former of which results from thoughts and psychological processes and the latter of which results from direct physical stimulation.[54,72]

EFFECTS OF STROKE ON SEXUAL FUNCTION

The literature shows that common effects of stroke on sexual function are decreased libido, impaired erectile and ejaculatory function, decreased vaginal lubrication, impaired ego and self-esteem, and depression. The motor, sensory, cognitive, and physiological effects of stroke have been shown to affect the desire and ability to engage in sexual activities in many ways. Some research has been focused on relating sexual dysfunction to the location of the lesion. Some of the scientific literature recommends counseling for patients following stroke but does not provide specific interventions.* As a result, therapists are left with insufficient information to treat sexual dysfunction adequately.

Numerous studies have found that among men and women who had sustained strokes, libido was decreased,

abilities to achieve erection and vaginal lubrication were impaired, and the frequency of intercourse was diminished.[11,38,40,41,53,73] In contrast, at least one study documented that a small group of stroke survivors (19 of 192 patients studied) indicated an increase in libido following stroke.[41] Isolated cases of hypersexuality and abnormal sexual behavior have been found to occur in individuals with temporal lobe lesions and concurrent histories of poststroke seizure activity.[28,54] In a study of 13 female stroke survivors, the most common complaint was found to be a decreased desire for sexual activity after the stroke; only 5% of the women reported actual impairment in the production of vaginal secretions after the stroke.[2] Most of the women reported no changes in their abilities to achieve orgasm or in their menstrual periods. In addition, although the stroke impaired sexual desire, physiological function remained unimpaired. The authors concluded that nondominant hemispheric stroke is related to decreased desire; five of seven patients with decreased desire had right brain involvement.

The authors of several studies have attempted to determine cerebral hemisphere dominance related to sexual function. Although some investigators found a greater decline in sexual function with left-sided cerebrovascular accident, others found little or no difference between right and left cerebral hemisphere strokes.* One study of 109 men poststroke revealed that lesions in the right hemisphere resulted in a significant decline in sexuality functioning poststroke, including desire and frequency.[36] Garden[25] concluded, "There seems to be an overall consensus that stroke patients maintain prestroke sexual desire but commonly experience sexual dysfunction including erectile and libido problems. Changes in coital frequency and libido are also common. As a result there can be great potential for depression and loss of self esteem."

The individual's prestroke sexual activity is usually a better indicator of poststroke activity.[7,26,29,33,42,73] If the individual was leading an active sex life before a stroke, the likelihood of returning to sexual activities is good. Younger age is also a predictor of resumption of sexual activity, although less so.[33] Individuals who were without a partner before a stroke have less opportunity to develop new partnerships and resume sexual activity after a stroke. This decreased opportunity has to do with the effects of stroke itself and an individual's impaired social contact, possible placement in a nursing home or other long-term setting, depression, altered self-image, and the multitude of psychological effects caused by stroke. In a study of 192 stroke survivors and 94 spouses, the decline in sexual activity after stroke was associated largely with individuals' attitude toward sexuality, fears including erectile dysfunction, and the inability to discuss sexuality issues.[41]

---

*References 6, 11, 13, 14, 24, 26 28, 29, 36, 41, 68-70, 73

*References 6, 11, 14, 26, 28, 38, 42, 57, 73

Erectile dysfunction may occur as a direct result of stroke* and also may occur in men whose sexual partners have sustained strokes because of fear of causing another stroke or hurting the partner or averse feelings toward the disabled partner.[26,28,29,30] In women, vaginal lubrication may be insufficient, causing painful intercourse.[2,11,25,26,40,73]

The presence of nocturnal erections indicates psychological versus organic reasons for erectile dysfunction. In a study by Korpelainen, Nieminen, and Myllyla,[41] all of the male subjects did experience nocturnal erections after stroke, although 55% had impaired nocturnal erections. Individuals with a history of taking cardiovascular medications and those who had diabetes mellitus exhibited a greater frequency of erectile dysfunction after stroke than those without. Bener and colleagues[5] found similar results in a study of 605 men following stroke; the likelihood of erectile dysfunction increased with cardiovascular medications and comorbities including hypertension, hypercholestermia, and diabetes. Similarly, impaired vaginal lubrication was more common in women who had taken cardiovascular medications prestroke.[41]

Initiation of sexual activity after discharge from the hospital may be difficult. A couple may delay sexual activity because each partner waits for the other to initiate sex.[29,30] In a study by Goddess, Wagner, and Silverman,[29] one couple put off sexual activity for 15 months after the husband's stroke. The man was unsure whether his wife would find him attractive or a suitable partner, and the wife was concerned that sexual play for her husband may be unsafe.

Sensory impairment is common after stroke. Considering the significant role of touch in sexual expression, its dysfunction also may contribute to sexual dysfunction.[24,40] In subjective reports of 50 stroke survivors, 19% of the subjects reported sensory deficits as the reason for diminished sexual activity.[40] However, the research is inconclusive; a study by Aloni and colleagues[1] of 15 male stroke patients showed that disturbed superficial and deep sensation were not correlated with decreased desire.

Motor impairment can affect sexual function. Decreased range of motion, strength, endurance, balance, abnormal skeletal muscle activity, impaired coordination, and oral motor dysfunction may interfere with intercourse or other sexual activities. However, some research suggests that the degree of hemiplegic impairment is not a major factor in sexual dysfunction.[24,26]

Cognitive deficits also may affect the stroke survivor's social and sexual function. Fundamental cognitive abilities such as attention and concentration are prerequisites for social and sexual activities; distractibility and overstimulation may cause anxiety and agitation, which prevent interaction.

Decreased initiation, impulsivity, poor memory, decreased speed of processing, and impaired executive functions are possible effects of neurological dysfunction and clearly can affect sexual relations.[71]

McCormick, Riffer, and Thompson[51] noted that sexual activity is itself a form of human communication. When verbal or nonverbal communication is impaired, sexual activity may be affected.[77] One study found that sexual adjustment was easiest for physically intact individuals with aphasia with spared comprehension and nonverbal communication.[76] However, in one study involving 110 subjects, no correlation between aphasia and poststroke sexual activity was found.[70] Lemieux, Cohen-Schneider, and Holzapfel[44] reported that individuals with moderate and severe aphasia are not included in most studies because they are difficult to interview, so little is known about their sexuality after stroke. In their small study of aphasia and sexuality in six couples, the researchers developed pictograms to facilitate communication with aphasic respondents. Although the effects of stroke on sexuality in this study were similar to those of previous studies, almost all the aphasic persons and their partners reported that aphasia had a negative effect on their sex lives.

The effect of stroke on psychological function is enormous[11,28,36,42] (see Chapter 2). Studies by Giaquinto and colleagues[28] and Korpelainen and colleagues[40] found that the psychological impact of stroke was a greater factor in sexual function after stroke than associated neurological deficits. The loss of function, including hemiparesis, sensory and balance disorders, pain, and cognitive, perceptual, and impaired communication skills may have an enormous negative effect on an individual's self-image. As Strauss[71] noted, the formulation of relationships, sexual or other, requires some level of self-esteem. An impaired image of one's body and appearance can affect the ability to make new relationships or maintain existing ones. Loss of confidence and decreased self-esteem may result from the following:

- Changes in appearance, including facial asymmetries and diminished facial expression
- Changes in clothing style (inability to don pantyhose or walk in high heels due to required ankle-foot orthosis)
- Need for adaptive equipment or assistive devices such as a splint, wheelchair, or cane
- Dependence in activities of daily living (ADL), such as the need to have food cut and to have assistance with toileting

In addition to changes in self-perception, the stroke survivor suddenly may find a new role in relationships. For instance, a wife may discover that she is no longer able to carry out the functions related to her role as wife because of the effects of a stroke. The stroke survivor may depend more on other family members. Role changes could affect the quality of an existing relationship.[9,65] Such changes may be confusing and

---

*References 5, 11, 28, 33, 36, 40, 42, 69, 73

stressful for the patient and the partner, particularly if the stroke survivor requires assistance with self-care activities such as toileting or bathing. Dependence in ADL is a major predictor of decreased sexual activity level after a stroke. In a study by Kimura and colleagues,[38] subjects who demonstrated ADL impairments also exhibited a decline in sexual activity. Sjogren and Fugl-Meyer reported similar findings as early as 1982.[70]

Impaired bladder function also may affect sexual activity. Stroke often occurs in the elderly who may have underlying genitourinary dysfunction (prostatic hypertrophy, stress incontinence). Proper evaluation by a urologist is indicated.[47,62] Marinkovic and Badlani[47] recommended treatment of incontinence before addressing sexual dysfunction. Medications used to treat incontinence have side effects such as dry mouth, which can make kissing or other oral activities unpleasant. If the individual takes additional medication for other reasons (for example, diuretic agents), urine output may be increased. For the individual with mobility impairments, quick and frequent access to the bathroom may be difficult, resulting in episodes of incontinence. Incontinence may affect self-esteem and may be a source of embarrassment.[37] Bowel incontinence is less common after cerebrovascular accident because stroke patients typically are constipated because of immobility, inactivity, and poor food and fluid intake, which can cause bloating and discomfort.[75]

Hypertension is a major risk factor for stroke, and research indicates that hypertension is associated with sexual dysfunction in men and women. Burchardt and colleagues[8] reported a higher incidence and greater severity of erectile dysfunction in men with hypertension compared with an age-matched population without hypertension. The study also suggested that the erectile dysfunction was linked to the hypertension and not to side effects of antihypertensive medications. Grimm and colleagues[31] also found that "sexual dysfunction in hypertensive individuals may be related more to hypertension level than to drug treatment." Hypertensive women also report decreased lubrication, less frequent orgasm, and more frequent pain with sexual activity than women without hypertension; again, the effects were not related to the type of treatment.[19]

Individuals who have had strokes often have a history of other medical problems, including heart disease, which alone can cause functional impairments related to sexual activities. Often individuals with a history of myocardial infarction or bypass surgery fear the resumption of sexual activities.[31,45,55] Muller and colleagues[55] studied 858 patients who were sexually active in the year preceding myocardial infarction and found that although the risk of myocardial infarction increases in the two hours following sexual activity, the risk is almost equivalent in patients with and without heart disease. The research indicated that the risk of myocardial infarction caused by sexual activity is two in one million for a person with heart disease and that individuals who experience periods of anger or heavy exertion have a greater increase in actual risk because these behaviors occur with more frequency than sexual activity. However, the overall risk of myocardial infarction is lower for patients who engage in regular exercise, which has been shown to decrease the amount of cardiac work required during sexual activity.

"At its peak, sexual activity is about as physically strenuous as walking two to four miles per hour. The greatest levels of 'exertion' actually occur during orgasm, which lasts only a brief amount of time."[67] Studies to determine cardiac expenditure are often performed on treadmills. Palmeri and colleagues[60] compared cardiac response during sexual activity to treadmill testing; results indicated that the amount of "work" during sexual activity was half the maximal found on treadmill testing and that there are different physiological responses to upright (i.e., treadmill testing) versus supine activity (i.e., sexual activity). Average heart rates ranged from 108 to 128 beats per minute. From a cardiac rehabilitation perspective, a patient is "safe" to resume sexual activity when the person can climb two flights of stairs or walk the length of a city block or its equivalent at a brisk pace with no discomfort.[34,45] This parameter may be difficult to assess in some stroke patients because of mobility deficits, and alternative activities may have to be explored (for example, propelling a wheelchair at a brisk pace with the use of unaffected arms and legs). The effect of stroke on sexual function is difficult to assess without examining the types of medications patients are taking. Antihypertensive agents have been found to cause erectile dysfunction, impede ejaculation, and decrease libido.[10,13,23,24,26] Some β-blockers are known to affect erectile function and cause depression. One antihypertensive diuretic medication, spironolactone, is known to cause breast tenderness, galactorrhea (excessive secretion of the mammary glands), and gynecomastia (overdevelopment of the mammary glands), which is not always reversible in men.[13] In a study by Aloni, Schwartz, and Ring,[2] six of the seven women who reported decreased sexual desire were taking anticoagulant drugs, suggesting that the medications may affect sexual function. Medications other than those prescribed for stroke management or hypertension may have additional side effects such as rashes and feelings of fatigue that may affect a patient's desire to participate in sexual activities. Considering the potential side effects of various medications on sexual function and informing patients as necessary is the rehabilitation team's responsibility.

SOCIETAL ATTITUDES

Attitudes on the part of the public or the patient's family members also may affect the patient emotionally or psychologically. Although the Americans with Disabilities Act has resulted in some improvement in public attitude, the fact remains that many persons still harshly judge individuals who appear "different" from the rest of society and regard disabled individuals with fear and shame. Stroke survivors and persons with other disabilities perceive these attitudes and, as a result, avoid social or public situations. The media seldom depict persons with disabilities as full partners in sexual relationships. The stroke patient and partner, family members, and others may share the view that persons with disabilities are sexless, "different," and undeserving of social and sexual fulfillment. These attitudes can affect patients' existing relationships and their willingness to pursue new relationships.

ROLE OF OCCUPATIONAL THERAPY

When persons experience changes in sexual function, they may require professional intervention to cope with these changes in sexual function and sexuality. What is the role of occupational therapy in sexuality intervention for these patients, and what is required to fulfill this role?

Sexuality long has been considered an appropriate area for occupational therapy intervention. Andamo[3] stated that "sexual function should be included in the occupational therapy evaluation as it relates to the identification of the patient's abilities and limitations in his daily living necessary for the resumption of his various roles." Neistadt[56] noted that as "holistic caregivers, dedicated to facilitating quality lives, occupational therapists should be prepared to address sexuality issues with their adolescent and adult patients." Couldrick[15] argued that "with awareness and skill development, occupational therapists can affirm sexual identity, they can listen, and, with sometimes simple measures, they an address issues that fall within their professional roles." The American Occupational Therapy Association has continued to confirm the role of occupational therapy by including sexual activity as an ADL within the areas of occupation in the Occupational Therapy Practice Framework.[59]

Occupational therapists are well-prepared to address sexuality problems in stroke patients; the sensory, motor, cognitive, and psychosocial impairments that interfere with sexual function are the same ones that affect other performance areas addressed by occupational therapy, including other ADL and work and leisure activities. Occupational therapists' skills of activity analysis and adaptation, holistic orientation, and knowledge of biological and behavioral sciences help them deal effectively with patients' sexual difficulties.[21] Research indicates that dependence in ADL is a major factor in decreased sexual activity after stroke,[38,70] further supporting the role of occupational therapists in sexual rehabilitation by restoring patients to the highest possible level of independence and role function.

Most occupational therapists receive some training in sexuality intervention. Even before the American Occupational Therapy Association listed sexual activity as an ADL, the authors of a 1988 study reported that 88% of 50 occupational therapy programs included formal classroom training about sexual function, with an average of three and a half hours of class time devoted to this subject.[63]

TEAM APPROACH

Although occupational therapists must be involved in sexual health care, effective sexual rehabilitation, like all rehabilitation, requires a team approach. The rehabilitation team must address all the individual's problems in a holistic way, and all team members should be knowledgeable about sexual issues and treatment options.[46,77] If each member of the treatment team is educated and skilled in this area, the patient can choose the team member with whom he or she is most comfortable to address sexual issues. In addition, each team member has different expertise from which the patient may benefit. The physician may best address problems related to erectile dysfunction, relationship changes may require social work intervention, and the speech and language pathologist may best address communication difficulties.

In reality, the health care team often ignores sexuality issues, especially for the stroke population. A support group of 37 wives of stroke patients at a Veterans Administration center reported that no one had spoken to them about poststroke sexuality.[51] In a 1988 study of sexuality counseling in an inpatient rehabilitation program, only 20% of non–spinal cord injured patients (55% of whom had a diagnosis of stroke) had received written materials on sex. Sexuality information was given voluntarily to 32%.[16] Rehabilitation professionals cite various reasons for not addressing sexuality with their patients, with the most common responses being that another team member is responsible for this intervention and that their knowledge is inadequate.[51,57] In a pilot study of health care professionals who treat stroke patients, including occupational and physical therapists, lack of training and experience were cited as reasons to not address sexuality. Over half felt that they would be inhibited by either potentially offending or embarrassing the patient. Perceptions of which team member is responsible for addressing sexual function varied.[51] The physician, social worker, and psychologist most often are cited as responsible for sexuality intervention.

In yet another study on sexuality counseling following spinal cord injury, patients indicated a preference to speak with their occupational or physical therapist or nurse about their sexual concerns. Participants reported a positive response to therapists who used an open and direct style of communicating and otherwise were frustrated, embarrassed, or intimidated by therapists who did not. Although many of the subjects were not ready to discuss sexuality early in their rehabilitation, they concurred that knowing resources were available when they needed them was vital.[49]

Besides being neglected in the clinic, sexual rehabilitation has received little attention in research. However, a general positive correlation has been found between successful sexual rehabilitation and positive adjustment to disability. The literature shows that patients with disabilities are interested in the inclusion of sexuality in rehabilitation and give sexuality a high priority.[27] Studies confirm that stroke survivors and their partners are interested in information and/or counseling about sexuality after stroke.[20,41]

In clinical rehabilitation, "a job title does not always define competencies," and "no job title . . . excludes discussion of sexuality," according to Chipouras and colleagues.[12] The qualities necessary in a competent sexuality counselor for persons with disabilities have been described variously. Chipouras and colleagues[12] emphasize comfort with sexuality, including one's own, comfort with disability, empathy, nonprojection of one's own morals onto the patient, awareness of available resources, basic knowledge of human sexuality, and awareness of one's own competency and willingness to refer to others as necessary. The foundation of sexuality counseling consists of awareness and knowledge, which one can gain through reading, in-service education, coursework, and workshops. Therapists must develop skill in sexuality counseling through practice, as for all clinical skills. Discomfort in dealing with sexuality need be no different from discomfort with other difficult disability issues. Occupational therapists address many personal and sometimes painful issues with their patients. Increased competency, skill, and comfort comes with practice. Practice of sexuality interventions through role play with other staff members may be helpful in achieving greater comfort in conducting sexuality interventions.

PERMISSION, LIMITED INFORMATION, SPECIFIC SUGGESTIONS, AND INTENSIVE THERAPY

The therapist may use various frameworks and models to address sexuality issues in health care. Among the earliest and most prevalent is the PLISSIT model, developed by psychologist Annon.[4] *PLISSIT* is an acronym for four levels of intervention: Permission, Limited Information, Specific Suggestions, and Intensive Therapy (Fig. 25-1). Using this model, the practitioner can determine the type and extent of sexuality intervention needed, whether he or she has the skills to perform the intervention, and whether to refer to a more qualified counselor.

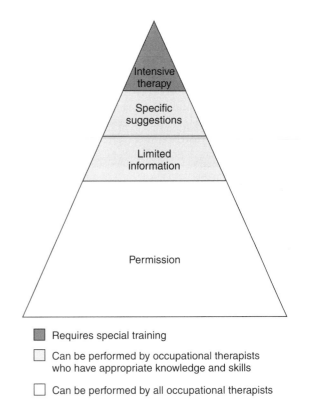

Figure 25-1   The PLISSIT model. PLISSIT, *P*ermission, *Lim*ited *I*nformation, *S*pecific *S*uggestions, and *I*ntensive *T*herapy.

Permission

Permission is the most basic and most frequently required intervention. Permission consists of reassuring patients that their actions and feelings are normal and acceptable. All occupational therapists should strive to perform permission-level sexuality interventions. Recognizing that sexual behavior varies widely and not projecting one's own values or morals onto the patient is most important.

The practitioner must be proactive to provide patients with permission. Waiting for the patient to bring up sexual issues is not enough; the therapist must let the patient know that expressing sexual concerns is acceptable. The simplest way to do this is to ask, "People who have had strokes sometimes have concerns or questions about how they will be affected sexually. Do you have any concerns or questions in this area?" This line of questioning serves to normalize the concerns and gives patients the opportunity to say "no" if they are not comfortable discussing sexuality with that person at that time. Asking also lets patients know that sexual concerns are considered legitimate and gives them permission to bring up sexual issues again if their needs change. The therapist should ask questions in a language appropriate for the patient's understanding, including the use of slang terms if necessary.

The best time to bring up sexuality is usually at the initial evaluation, when other ADL issues also are being addressed. If this is not feasible because of time constraints or because the evaluating therapist will not be treating the patient, sexuality should be brought up as soon as is comfortable. Sexual concerns should be explored before home visits and in the formulation of discharge plans because the patient's needs and concerns change throughout rehabilitation.

Opportunities to give patients permission to express themselves as sexual beings often occur spontaneously. On one rehabilitation unit, a 38-year-old Hispanic man with a diagnosis of right cerebrovascular accident was playing a getting-to-know-you game with the other patients, all of whom were older women. As part of the activity, each member of the group was asked to name something he or she liked. The women named things such as chocolate, flowers, and pets. The man said, "I like women." After a few seconds of silence, the occupational therapist running the group said, "Of course you do; what could be more natural?" The group members all nodded, and the activity continued.

Limited Information

Sometimes simply reassuring patients about sexuality is not enough. If patients do have concerns or questions, they may require specific information related to their stated concerns. Most occupational therapists are qualified to provide patients with limited information. This level of intervention often is concerned with dispelling myths or misconceptions about sexuality. Limited information may be related to facts about the effect of disability on sexuality and sexual function. Handouts, pamphlets, and group education programs are good ways to provide limited information. The patients may read and absorb information on their own and ask the practitioner for clarification as needed. The important issue is to limit the information to the patient's specific concerns. The accuracy of the information is also paramount. If the therapist does not have the information, he or she should help the patient get it before making a referral to another practitioner. For example, a patient with a recent stroke and complex cardiac history asks whether it is safe to have sex. Although the patient's physician can provide the answer, it is not enough for the therapist to say, "Ask your physician." By bringing up the concern to the therapist, the patient has chosen that person as an advocate. The therapist might respond, "Your physician is best equipped to answer that question. Would you feel comfortable asking him or her yourself, or would you like me to contact him or her for you?"

Specific Suggestions

If a patient is experiencing a sexual problem, limited information may not be enough to solve it. The next level of intervention is specific suggestions aimed at solving the specific problem. This type of intervention requires more knowledge, time, and skill from the therapist but is appropriate for some occupational therapists (Box 25-1). The therapist should meet with the patient (and partner, if appropriate) in a comfortable, private setting and obtain a sexual problem history. This history should include the following:

- The patient's assessment of the problem and its cause, onset, and course
- The patient's attempts to solve the problem
- The patient's goals

Box 25-1

Competencies for Sexuality Interventions at Each PLISSIT Level

PERMISSION

To perform this level of sexuality intervention, the therapist should do the following:
- Acknowledge the sexuality of all persons.
- Be comfortable with his or her own sexuality.
- Believe that interest in sexuality is appropriate for everyone.
- Be comfortable speaking directly about sexual issues (or be willing to overcome discomfort).
- Refrain from projecting personal sexual morals and values onto others.

LIMITED INFORMATION

To provide this level of intervention, the therapist should fulfill the criteria listed for Permission and do the following:
- Have a basic understanding of human sexuality and its many variations.
- Understand the physiology of human sexual response.
- Be able to analyze the effects of physical disability on various sexual activities.
- Be willing to seek and provide accurate sexual information.
- Be aware of the limitations of his or her own knowledge base.

SPECIFIC SUGGESTIONS

To perform this level of intervention, the therapist should fulfill the criteria for Permission and Limited Information and do the following:
- Be familiar with various sexual activities.
- Be comfortable discussing specific sexual activities.
- Be able to conduct a sexual problem history.
- Be able to adapt various sexual activities to accommodate functional limitations.

INTENSIVE THERAPY

To perform this level of sexuality intervention, the therapist should fulfill the criteria for Permission, Limited Information, and Specific Suggestions and do the following:
- Have formal training in sex therapy, sexuality counseling, or psychotherapy.

Just as the occupational therapist would not initiate treatment of other problems without a full evaluation, the therapist must understand the sexual problem fully before making specific suggestions. After obtaining the sexual problem history, the therapist should develop treatment goals in collaboration with the patient. These goals may address learning the effects of stroke on sexual function; adapting to changes in sensory, motor, or cognitive function; adapting to psychosocial and role changes; and improving sexual communication.

One male stroke patient reported sexual problems after a weekend visit home. A sexual problem history revealed that he had always preferred the male-superior position for intercourse. Since his cerebrovascular accident, increased leg extensor skeletal muscle activity and weakness had prevented adequate pelvic thrusting in this position. With his occupational therapist, the patient discussed various new positions to increase mobility: lying on the affected side with knees bent or sitting in a chair with his partner seated facing him.

Intensive Therapy

If the patient's problems are beyond the scope of goal-oriented specific suggestions, he or she may require intensive therapy. This level of intervention is based on specialized treatment skills and is beyond the scope of most occupational therapists. Finding an appropriate referral for such patients, such as a psychologist, social worker, or sex therapist, is advisable. If the sexual problems predate or are not related to the onset of disability, the patient may require referral.

The PLISSIT model enables the health care professional to adapt a sexuality program to the needs of the setting and the population served. Although permission to express sexual concern is universal, the need for limited information and specific suggestions varies. The best way to assess the need for sexuality intervention is to ask patients about their concerns. Occupational therapist Andamo's treatment model[3] uses a written problem checklist in which the patient is asked to identify problems in whatever role he or she fills, including that of sexual partner. By addressing sexuality in a multiproblem context, this model helps normalize sexual concerns. The checklist includes two items related to sexual problems and concerns about sexual activity. Patients who check either item receive further intervention as needed, including problem clarification, sexual history taking, and the development of treatment goals and planning. Therapists can adapt any evaluation to include verbal questions about sexual concerns and can repeat questions before home visits or as discharge approaches because patients' concerns change over time.

Underlying some health care workers' reluctance to address sexuality may be a fear of opening a Pandora's box of issues too difficult or intimate for them to handle. This is seldom the case. Most persons do not wish to disclose their sexual problems or to include strangers in their intimate relationships. They want and benefit from the least intervention possible to help them solve their sexual problems and deal with their concerns. Other therapists fear that providing permission to discuss sexual concerns will facilitate inappropriate patient sexual behavior. Recent literature indicates that many health care workers are exposed to inappropriate sexual behavior on the part of patients during their careers, and they often lack training in dealing with these behaviors. Less experienced therapists and students tend to ignore the behaviors even when they are severe, which may result in high stress and difficult working conditions.[35,50] Of course, any therapist who is exposed to sexual or other inappropriate behavior by anyone should address the problem immediately. Patient behaviors should be documented in the medical records; other staff members also may be affected. All new therapists and students should be encouraged to report harassment and seek help with difficult situations.

Providing permission to patients to address sexual issues directly actually decreases inappropriate behaviors. Flirting, sexual jokes, and innuendos are often a patient's way of indirectly expressing doubts and concerns about sexuality after disability. One stroke patient, M.G., overheard his occupational therapist inviting some coworkers to her home and asked, "When are you going to invite me over?" The therapist replied, "You know, M.G., that I am your therapist, and although you're a really nice person, it would be unethical for us to have a social relationship. But tell me, are you interested in developing new social relationships?" This question led to a lively discussion about M.G.'s returning interest in women and sex. The therapist was understanding and supportive. The patient made no further advances to her. By refocusing attention on the patient, the therapist deflected the unwanted attention and responded to the patient's real need for permission to acknowledge his returning sexual feelings.

DEVELOPING COMPETENCY

Competency in sexuality intervention comprises three elements (see Box 25-1): comfort, knowledge, and skill. These elements are interrelated; individuals are more comfortable with things they know well (knowledge) and do well (skill). Suggestions for improving these competencies follow.

- Comfort
  - Reading (See resources and references at end of chapter.)
  - Films (Be aware that many are related to spinal cord injuries.)
  - Disability literature
- Knowledge
  - Readings (See resources and references at end of chapter.)

- Lectures
- In-service education
- Skill
  - Role playing with other staff members
  - Acquiring skill through practice
  - Seeking a mentor for private supervision who specializes in sexuality

SPECIFIC SUGGESTIONS FOR TREATMENT

Many impairments that occur after cerebrovascular accident may affect sexual function and sexuality. These deficits include sensorimotor, cognitive, communication, and psychosocial changes. With sexuality, as with other ADL, determining the underlying causes of the performance problem can be challenging. The following section comprises a list of suggestions one may use during treatment.

Hemiparesis/Sensory Loss

Patients with hemiparesis or sensory loss and their partners may try the following suggestions:

- Having the hemiplegic partner lie on the affected side frees the uninvolved side for touching; this position also provides support, permits active movement, and focuses attention on the intact side. Early treatment by the rehabilitation team (occupational and physical therapy) should include instructing the patient to lie comfortably on the affected side (Fig. 25-2).
- Impaired motor control (limb and trunk) may require a change in coital positioning because the hemiplegic partner may find it difficult to assume certain positions. Alternatively, the unaffected partner may assume the superior position in bed or on a chair or lying on his or her side (Figs. 25-3 to 25-5).
- Positioning for comfort with the use of pillows can be incorporated into foreplay.

- Partners should discuss sensory loss beforehand; in hemiplegia, there may be absent or diminished light touch, impaired proprioception, kinesthesia, or loss of stereognosis. Stimulation on areas of intact sensation and incorporation of stimuli to intact senses (e.g., using scents, keeping lights on for visual stimulation, music, and stimulating language) may help improve sensory abilities.
- Individuals with severe sensory deficits must consider skin protection during sexual activity to prevent skin breakdown.
- In the case of impaired hand function, a vibrator can be attached with the use of Velcro to enable stimulation.
- Treatment of weakened muscles of facial expression to improve body image and facial expression and strengthening of oral-motor muscles may enhance oral sexual activities such as kissing and oral-genital sex.

Cognitive/Perceptual/Neurobehavorial Impairments

Patients with cognitive/perceptual/neurobehavioral impairments and their partners may try the following suggestions:

- Simple positions are recommended (see Figs. 25-4 and 25-5). Achieving a routine of sexual activity may be helpful if the person has difficulty moving spontaneously. When the brain becomes used to a routine, it does not have to work as hard to plan movements and the patient does not have to concentrate on how he or she is moving.[57]
- Hemianopsia or unilateral neglect may cause a person to ignore parts of the partner's body or not respond when approached from the affected side. The unaffected partner must be sensitive to these deficits.

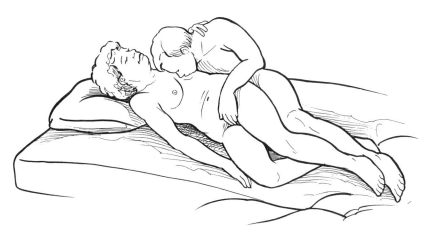

Figure 25-2 This position allows for genital fondling during rear entry vaginal or anal penetration and is appropriate for opposite or same-sex couples. Either partner can participate fully if lying on the hemiplegic side.

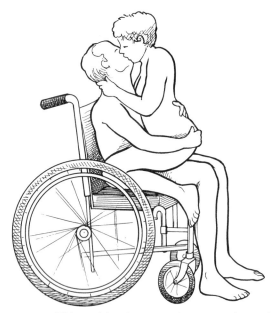

Figure 25-3 This position is appropriate as an alternative to lying on a bed or other surface; it is a nice alternative for wheelchair use and may break the barrier of the wheelchair being used only for transport.

- Nonverbal communication such as touching and gesturing are encouraged with partners who may have speech or language disorders.[57]
- Distractions such as loud music should be kept to a minimum.[57]
- Individuals with memory impairment should keep a log of daily activities, including sexual activities, in an effort to remain oriented.[57]
- Sexual role changes such as increased sexual initiation by the nondisabled partner can help minimize the effects of cognitive changes on sexual function.
- Partners may share fantasies or intimate thoughts in writing or by using augmentative communication devices before and after sexual activity.[57]
- A team approach may be helpful. Speech and language pathologists can help the patient improve or compensate for verbal and nonverbal communication deficits.

Decreased Endurance

Patients with decreased endurance and their partners may try the following suggestions:
- Sexual activities should be planned. The patient should wait three hours after meals before engaging in activities and avoid sex when fatigued. Instead, this may be a good time for intimate cuddling, hugging, or participating in massage.
- Partners can deemphasize intercourse through exploration of other sexual activities such as mutual masturbation and oral-genital sex.
- Partners should consider sexual positions that use less energy (see Figs. 25-4 and 25-5).
- Sexual activities may be easier to do in the morning, when energy may be greater, instead of the evening.

Inadequate Vaginal Lubrication

Patients with inadequate vaginal lubrication and their partners may try the following suggestions:
- A water-based lubricant should be used.
- Foreplay should be extended to ensure adequate lubrication of the vagina before intercourse.
- Lubricated condoms may be helpful.
- Both partners should keep in mind that impaired vaginal lubrication also might be a normal age-related change.
- A consultation with a gynecologist may be warranted.

Erectile Dysfunction

Patients with erectile dysfunction and their partners may try the following suggestions:
- Medications for erectile dysfunction may be indicated, which include Sildenafil citrate (Viagra), Vardenafil (Levitra), and Tadalafil (Cialis).[67] They are considered safe in combination with most cardiac medications and can be "safely recommended in all patients with stable cardiac conditions."[67] However, they all come with warnings about use in patients with history of stroke.[64] Although inconclusive, sildenafil citrate has been reported to have potentially

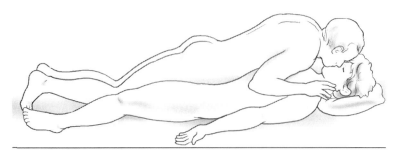

Figure 25-4 This position is recommended if the female partner sustained motor or cognitive impairment and requires less endurance for the partner on the bottom.

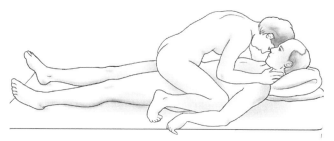

Figure 25-5 This position is recommended if the male partner sustained motor or cognitive impairment and requires less endurance for the partner on the bottom.

positive effects in the treatment of neurological disease, including stroke.[22] For any person with stroke and/or cardiovascular disease, a physician should assess the safety of sexual activity and use of these medications.

- Certain medications may have an effect on erection in addition to the stroke itself. The patient and physician should discuss this possibility.
- The patient and partner should consider alternatives to intercourse.
- If erectile dysfunction is related to depression or another psychological issue, the therapist should suggest that the patient discuss it with the appropriate team member, such as the psychologist or psychiatrist.
- A ring placed on the base of the penis may help maintain blood flow into the penis and help the patient maintain an erection.
- Other treatment options for erectile dysfunction require consultation with a urologist. These include vacuum constrictor devices, injection of vasoactive agents, and penile prosthesis implantation.[32] Use of these therapies has not been studied in stroke survivors[52] and has decreased greatly since the advent of sildenafil.[18]

Incontinence

Patients with incontinence and their partners may try the following suggestions:

- The patient should avoid fluids before engaging in sexual activity.[40]
- Men may wear a condom to prevent leakage onto the partner.
- Patients on a voiding schedule should be encouraged to adhere to the schedule to prevent accidents.
- Towels should be available in case of accidents, and the patient should discuss his or her situation before engaging in sexual activity to prevent embarrassment.
- The patient should empty his or her bladder before engaging in sexual activity.

- Pelvic muscle reeducation (with or without biofeedback) to improve strength and control of pelvic floor muscles may be indicated.[58]

Contraception and Safer Sex

Most stroke patients are past the childbearing years; however, contraception remains an issue for those who are still fertile. Menses may be affected after a stroke, although studies are inconclusive.[48] However, the exploration of contraceptive methods may be necessary, depending on the patient's impairments. The functional abilities needed to use condoms, a diaphragm, or a cervical cap include fine motor abilities, motor praxis, and intact cognitive and perceptual function.[57] However, in some cases, the nondisabled partner can assist with contraception and work it into the sexual repertoire. For example, if a woman had a stroke and her contraception of choice is the diaphragm but she cannot insert the device because of hemiplegia, her partner might do this for her. If the couple prefers, they can explore alternative methods of contraception. A review of other methods may be warranted, particularly if the patient previously used the pill or other contraceptive hormones, which have side effects, some of which affect circulation.[72]

Latex condoms are preferred for safer sexual practices against sexually transmitted diseases; however, an erect penis is required. If the male has difficulty maintaining or achieving an erection, it may not be possible for him to use condoms effectively. Female condoms or alternative sexual practices minimizing contact with body fluids may be explored, and individuals and couples should be educated on options such as mutual masturbation and oral sex with the use of a dental dam, which is a latex sheet placed over the vulva during cunnilingus. The therapist is responsible for staying updated on current guidelines related to safer sex practices if education on safer sex will be included in treatment.

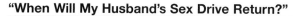

CASE STUDY 1

"When Will My Husband's Sex Drive Return?"

P.R. is a 52-year-old married man who previously suffered a hemorrhagic left basal ganglia stroke. He was admitted to a subacute rehabilitation center with right hemiplegia and language and short-term memory deficits. His right upper and lower extremity sensation was absent for tactile stimulation. He demonstrated increased flexor activity and had no active arm movement. P.R. required maximal assistance with all transfers and ADL, and his activity tolerance was poor. Before admission he had lived with his wife of 1½ years and ran a business requiring frequent travel. P.R.'s wife also worked full-time and taught women's exercise classes in her free time.

By his 18-day team conference, P.R. had made substantial gains. He was independent in stand-pivot

Continued

CASE STUDY 1

"When Will My Husband's Sex Drive Return?"—cont'd

transfers and required minimal assistance in dressing. He demonstrated emerging sensation and motor control in his right arm and lower extremities. He was able to walk during physical therapy with a cane and assistance from a therapist. His language function had improved, with only some word-finding deficits remaining. He and his wife attended the team meeting. Her last question to the team was, "When will his sex drive return?" P.R. said, "Don't worry, Honey, it will come back like everything else." The staff recommended discussing this issue with the new neurologist, with whom the couple had an appointment the following day.

On return from his neurologist, P.R. reported to his speech therapist that he and his wife had "forgotten" to bring up sexuality. He reported achieving only partial erections. The therapist offered him a consultation with an occupational therapist on staff who was knowledgeable about sexuality and disability, and he agreed. The speech therapist had received no training or information about sexuality and had no experience in this area. P.R.'s treating occupational therapist, who was not present at the team meeting, was willing to use part of P.R.'s scheduled treatment time for the sexuality intervention.

The occupational therapist who specialized in sexuality issues introduced herself to P.R. and made an appointment to meet with him the next week in his private room. She asked whether he had any specific questions or concerns so she could prepare information for their meeting. He said the concerns were mostly his wife's and that he was confident his sex drive would "return just like use of my arm and leg are going to return." The occupational therapist suggested including P.R.'s wife in the meeting, but P.R. said she was unavailable during the daytime so the occupational therapist might as well speak to him alone.

A brief sexual history revealed that P.R. had been single for 11 years before this second marriage and that he had been sexually active with a variety of women during that time. He and his wife considered sex an extremely important part of their relationship. "People can be very sexy even though they don't look it," he explained. P.R. volunteered that he and his wife would not need help with sexual positioning for intercourse because they preferred the female-superior position. P.R. admitted to decreased sexual desire, which he attributed to fatigue, separation, and the nonconducive environment. He reported having erections that he estimated at "three quarters of normal hardness," which was an improvement. He reiterated that he was sure everything would come back.

The intervention included three levels of the PLISSIT model.

Permission
The therapist assured P.R. that concern about sexuality was common among stroke survivors and their sex partners and that, after a life-threatening event, sexual concerns are a sign of returning health. They discussed the myth that middle-aged persons are not attractive and society's insistence in portraying only young, thin, beautiful persons as "sexy." The therapist explained that although health care workers are sometimes reluctant to bring up sexuality, P.R. had the right to be assertive in getting any assistance he needed in this area.

Limited Information
P.R. was provided a verbal summary of the research on stroke and sex. He was informed that some persons experience sexual dysfunction after stroke and that desire, libido, erection, ejaculation, and orgasm might be affected. The therapist emphasized the lack of correlation of sexual dysfunction to motor or sensory deficits and the high correlation between prestroke and poststroke sexual function. The therapist and P.R. discussed the effect of antihypertensive medications on sexual function. P.R. reported telling his physician that he would not take any medication that had side effects on sexual function. The physician prescribed a medication without sexual side effects.

Specific Suggestions
Although P.R. reported no need for ideas to improve his sexual function, a level of denial was evident in his assurances that "everything would come back." The occupational therapist said, "Just as you're participating in therapy to improve your arm, leg, and speech, your sexual function will improve faster if you don't just sit around waiting for its return." P.R. agreed that he felt as if he had a new, different body and that he would find it helpful to explore and learn the responses of the new body. They discussed including his wife in the sexual explorations, but she was uncomfortable with the lack of privacy in the facility.

Because P.R. would be unlikely to have sexual relations with his wife before discharge, strategies were discussed for initiating sexual activity in a positive, nonthreatening way because early problems with erectile function are not necessarily predictive of continuing problems. Alternative sexual activities also are considered "real sex."

Because of their prestroke sexual function, motivation, interest, maturity, and willingness to communicate, P.R. and his wife were likely to make a good sexual adjustment to the effects of stroke. However, the therapist did offer information on treatment of erectile or other sexual dysfunction, for in the future, if problems arose, she would not be available to P.R. after discharge. She also reported the latest medical interventions for erectile dysfunction, which would be familiar to any urologist. Although he felt he would not need it, P.R. seemed glad to know that treatment was readily available.

At this facility, sexual concerns were not addressed by any rehabilitation discipline. While treating P.R., the therapist had provided written information on the sexual effects of cerebrovascular accident and the role of speech and language therapists in sexuality counseling to the speech therapist who referred him and summarized the results of the counseling session. Staff members became aware that other patients might have sexual concerns but lacked the comfort level or assertiveness to initiate the communication. The therapist was asked to provide an in-service on sexuality, which was well-attended by members of the occupational therapy department and other interested staff.

CASE STUDY 2

"I Want to Get Out of the Wheelchair So I Can Chase a Man"

W.A. is a 62-year-old woman who previously suffered a right middle cerebral artery stroke with resulting left hemiparesis. After her initial and rehabilitation hospitalizations, she was discharged home for continued occupational and physical therapy. She lived in a senior housing development, which had a social room on the premises. W.A. had been widowed for more than 15 years and reported that her husband had been an alcoholic and a "terrible man." During W.A.'s initial evaluation at home, the occupational therapist asked what her goals for rehabilitation were. W.A. was quick to reply, "I want to be able to get out of the wheelchair so I can chase a man." Sexuality had not been addressed until this point in the evaluation. The therapist took the opportunity to ask W.A. whether she had a significant man in her life, to which W.A. replied "no." The therapist asked W.A. whether she had any concerns about resuming sexual activities after the stroke; again W.A. replied "no." She explained that she was not looking to marry again and simply wanted to be exposed to others so she could flirt. During this conservation, the therapist realized that further exploration of sexual function was geared toward getting W.A. out into the community again. W.A. had been limited in this endeavor because of poor mobility and wheelchair dependency.

In this example, the therapist used the permission level of the PLISSIT model. The patient brought up the topic herself, and it was discovered through further questioning that W.A. was really referring to a need to socialize, not so much as to act on her sexual desires. In subsequent conversations, W.A.'s occupational therapist reassessed this situation, particularly as W.A. made progress with ADL and functional mobility. After six months of treatment, W.A. was getting back out into the community, attending an adult day care center, and participating in bingo games in her building. She was taught how to transfer on and off the furniture in the social room to allow greater independence and a sense of normalcy. All areas of function, including sexuality, were reevaluated periodically during W.A.'s treatment program, and her goals remained unchanged from her initial evaluation.

In this example, the issue of sexuality was related less directly to actual sexual activities than to socialization and flirting. Had the therapist neglected to pursue W.A.'s early statement about wanting to "chase a man," the patient's needs might never have been met.

CASE STUDY 3

"Will I Ever Have Sex Again?"

L.E. was a 57-year-old woman with an unknown social history who was admitted to a rehabilitation hospital and who previously suffered a right cerebrovascular accident with left hemiplegia and perceptual deficits. At the initial evaluation, the occupational therapist asked whether L.E. had any sexual concerns. "Yes, I want to know whether I'll ever have sex again," she said tearfully. The occupational therapist realized that such a question could not be answered and that the patient's concerns needed clarification. Was L.E. concerned about being able to find a partner? About "performing" sexually? The therapist helped L.E. clarify her question with some probing, "What are you concerned about specifically? What do you think might get in the way of your having sex again?" L.E. reported having a male friend with whom she had an active sex life. Her major concerns were whether she would regain enough function to return home and whether sexual activity would provoke further strokes. The occupational therapist reassured L.E. that most persons can resume sexual activity safely after a stroke and offered to help her consult her physician for medical clearance. The therapist provided the limited information L.E. was looking for through reassurance and by obtaining medical clearance through another team member (that is, the physician). The therapist was able to tie in all the rehabilitation goals with the patient's desire to return to her home and previous lifestyle, which strengthened the collaboration between L.E. and the rehabilitation staff.

PROGRAM DEVELOPMENT

The therapist should have support, resources, and referrals available when addressing sexual issues. The therapist should inform supervisors and others on the rehabilitation staff of activities. Resources and referral services should be identified in other departments and outside the facility, if appropriate. The therapist should check the existing policies on sexuality (if any) at the facility and strive to be in compliance. The therapist should report experiences and provide education to others. If possible, an interdisciplinary committee should be formed to address sexual issues and develop appropriate programs.

DOCUMENTATION AND BILLING

Sexuality interventions may be billed and documented in various ways, depending on the billing system and the issues discussed. Appropriate categories include ADL training, patient and family education, discharge planning, and psychosocial training.

As in treatment, sexuality is best addressed in a multiproblem context. Patient privacy and confidentiality must be maintained. Examples of goals include the following:

1. Patient will independently identify proper bed positioning for sleep and sexual activity.
2. Patient's spouse will accurately assess patient's safety to engage in physical and sexual activities.

SUMMARY

All persons are sexual, and sexual activity is important to most persons throughout their lives. Interest in or desire for sexual activity does not necessarily diminish as persons grow older. Stroke may interfere with sexual expression by affecting the survivor's desire, libido, erectile or lubrication response, orgasm or ejaculation, and sensorimotor, cognitive, psychosocial, ADL, and role function. Stroke also may affect the partner's response or the patient's ability to find a sexual partner. Research has shown that sexual desire most often is affected; however, prestroke sexual activity is the strongest predictor of poststroke sexual activity. Occupational therapists can use a holistic approach and training in activity analysis and adaptation to assist persons who have had strokes to regain their desired sexual function. A team model is best for sexual rehabilitation, with each team member knowledgeable about sexuality and providing special expertise. The PLISSIT model helps the practitioner identify the type of sexuality intervention required. All occupational therapists should be able to provide patients with permission, limited information, and specific suggestions and should be able to make appropriate referrals for sexual concerns related to stroke. Therapists must be sensitive to the multiple components of sex.

REVIEW QUESTIONS

1. What are the stages of the sexual response cycle and the associated physiological changes in males and females?
2. What are some of the normal changes in sexual function in aging men and women?
3. Why does sexual activity decline among older persons?
4. What are the four levels of sexuality intervention in the PLISSIT model? Which may be performed by occupational therapists?
5. What skills are needed to provide sexuality counseling to patients who have had strokes?
6. What common effects of stroke interfere with sexual function and sexuality? What are the best predictors of poststroke sexual function?

REFERENCES

1. Aloni R, Ring H, Rosenthal N, et al: Sexual function in male patients after stroke a follow up study. *Sex Disabil* 11(2):121, 1993.
2. Aloni R, Schwartz J, Ring J: Sexual function in post-stroke female patients. *Sex Disabil* 12(3):3, 1994.
3. Andamo EM: Treatment model: occupational therapy for sexual dysfunction. *Sex Disabil* 3(1):26, 1980.
4. Annon JS: The PLISSIT model: a proposed conceptual scheme for the behavioral treatment of sexual problems. *J Sex Educ Ther* 2(1):1–15, 1976.
5. Bener A, Al-Hamaq A O A A, Kamran S, Al-Ansari A: Prevalence of erectile dysfunction in male stroke patients, and associated comorbidities and risk factors. *Int Urol Nephrol* 40(3):701–708, 2008.
6. Boldrini P, Basaglia N, Calanca MC: Sexual changes in hemiparetic patients. *Arch Phys Med Rehabil* 72(3):202–207, 1991.
7. Bray GP, DeFrank RS, Wolfe TL: Sexual functioning in stroke survivors. *Arch Phys Med Rehabil* 62(6):286–288, 1981.
8. Burchardt M, Burchardt T, Baer L, et al: Hypertension is associated with severe erectile dysfunction. *J Urol* 164(4):1188–1191, 2000.
9. Burgener S, Logan G: Sexuality concerns of the post-stroke patient. *Rehabil Nurs* 14(4):178–181, 1989.
10. Chen K, Chiou CF, Plauschinat CA, et al: Patient satisfaction with antihypertensive therapy. *J Hum Hypertens* 19(10):793–799, 2005.
11. Cheung RTF: Sexual functioning in Chinese stroke patients with mild or no disability. *Cerebrovasc Dis* 14(2):122–128, 2002.
12. Chipouras S, Cornelius DA, Makas E, et al: *Who cares? A handbook on sex education and counseling services for disabled people*, ed 2, Baltimore, MD, 1982, University Park Press.
13. Cole TM, Cole SS: Rehabilitation of problems of sexuality in physical disability. In Kottke FJ, Lehman JF, editors: *Krusen's handbook of physical medicine and rehabilitation*, ed 4, Philadelphia, 1990, Saunders.
14. Coslett HB, Heilman KM: Male sexual function: impairment after right hemisphere stroke. *Arch Neurol* 43(10):1036–1039, 1986.
15. Couldrick L: Sexual expression and occupational therapy. *British Journal of occupational Therapy* 68(7):315–318, 2005.
16. Cushman LA: Sexual counseling in a rehabilitation program: a patient perspective. *J Rehabil* 54(2):65–69, 1988.
17. DeBusk R, Drory Y, Goldstein I, et al: Management of sexual dysfunction in patients with cardiovascular disease: recommendations of the Princeton Consensus Panel. *Am J Cardiol* 86(2):175–181, 2000.
18. Ducharme S: From the editor. *Sex Disabil* 20(2):105–107, 2002.

19. Duncan LE, Lewis C, Jenkins P, et al: Does hypertension and its pharmacotherapy affect the quality of sexual function in women? *Am J Hypertens* 13(6 pt 1):640–647, 2000.

20. Edmans J: An investigation of stroke patients resuming sexual activity. *Br J Occup Ther* 61(1):36–8, 2002.

21. Evans J: Sexual consequences of disability: activity analysis and performance adaptation. *Occup Ther Health Care* 4(1):1, 1987.

22. Farooq MU, Naravetla B, Moore PW et al: Role of sildenafil in neurological disorders. *Clin Neuropharmacol* 31(6):353–362, 2008.

23. Francis ME, Kusek JW, Nyberg LM, Eggers PW: The contribution of common medical conditions and drug exposures to erectile dysfunction in adult males. *J Urol* 178(2):591–596, 2007.

24. Fugl-Meyer AR, Jaasko L: Post-stroke hemiplegia and sexual intercourse. *Scand J Rehabil Med* 7:158–166, 1980.

25. Garden FH: Incidence of sexual dysfunction in neurologic disability. *Sex Disabil* 9(1):1, 1991.

26. Garden FH, Smith BS: Sexual function after cerebrovascular accident. *Curr Concepts Rehabil Med* 5:2, 1990.

27. Gatens C: Sexuality and disability. In Woods NF, editor: *Human sexuality in health and illness*, ed 3, St Louis, 1984, Mosby.

28. Giaquinto S, Buzelli S, DiFrancesco L, et al: Evaluation of sexual changes after stroke. *J Clin Psychiatry* 64(3):302–307, 2003.

29. Goddess ED, Wagner NN, Silverman DR: Poststroke sexual activity of CVA patients. *Med Aspects Hum Sex* 13:16, 1979.

30. Goldberg RL: Sexual counseling for the stroke patient. *Med Aspects Hum Sex* 21(6)86–92, 1987.

31. Grimm RH, Grandits GA, Prineas RJ, et al: Long-term effects of sexual function of five antihypertensive drugs and nutritional hygienic treatment in hypertensive men and women. *Hypertension* 29(1 pt 1):8–14, 1997.

32. Hatzichristou DG, Bertero EB, Goldstein I: Decision making in the evaluation of impotence: the patient profile-oriented algorithm. *Sex Disabil* 12(1):29, 1994.

33. Hawton K: Sexual adjustment of men who have had strokes. *J Psychosom Res* 28(3):243–249, 1984.

34. Hellerstein HK, Friedman EH: Sexual activity and the postcoronary patient. *Arch Intern Med* 125(6):987–999, 1970.

35. Jones MK, Weerakoon P, Pynor RA: Survey of occupational therapy students' attitudes towards sexual issues in clinical practice. *Occup Ther Int* 12(2):95–106, 2005.

36. Jung JH, Kam SC, Choi SM, et al: Sexual dysfunction in male stroke patients: correlation between brain lesions and sexual function. *Urology* 71(1):99–103, 2008.

37. Kaplan SA, Brown WC, Blaivas JG: When stroke patients suffer urologic dysfunction. *Contemp Urol* January 1990.

38. Kimura M, Murata Y, Shimoda K, et al: Sexual dysfunction following stroke. *Compr Psychiatry* 42(3):217–222, 2001.

39. Kloner RA, Brown M, Prisant LM, et al: Effect of sildenafil in patients with erectile dysfunction taking antihypertensive therapy. *Am J Hypertens* 14(1):70–73, 2001.

40. Korpelainen JT, Kauhanen ML, Kemola H, et al: Sexual dysfunction in stroke patients. *Acta Neurol Scand* 98(6):400–405, 1998.

41. Korpelainen JT, Nieminen P, Myllyla VV: Sexual functioning among stroke patients and their spouses. *Stroke* 30(4):715–719, 1999.

42. Kwon SC, Kim JS: Poststroke emotional incontinence and decreased sexual activity. *Cerebrovasc Dis* 13(1):31–37, 2002.

43. Laflin M: Sexuality and the elderly. In Lewis CB, editor: *Aging: the health care challenge—an interdisciplinary approach to assessment and rehabilitative management*, ed 2, Philadelphia, 1990, FA Davis.

44. Lemieux L, Cohen-Schneider R, Holzapfel S: Aphasia and sexuality. *Sex Disabil* 19(4):253, 2001.

45. Mackey FG: Sexuality in coronary artery disease. *Postgrad Med* 80(1):58–60, 1986.

46. MacLaughlin J, Cregan A: Sexuality in stroke care: a neglected quality of life issue in stroke rehabilitation? A pilot study. *Sex Disabil* 23(4):213–226, 2005.

47. Marinkovic SP, Badlani G: Voiding and sexual dysfunction after cerebral vascular accidents. *J Urol* 165(2):359, 2001.

48. Masters WH, Johnson VE: *Human sexual response*, Boston, 1966, Little, Brown.

49. McAlonan S: Improving sexual rehabilitation services: the patient's perspective. *Am J Occup Ther* 50(10):826–834, 1996.

50. McComas J, Hebert C, Giacomin C, et al: Experiences of student and practicing physical therapists with inappropriate patient sexual behavior. *Phys Ther* 73(11):762–769, 1993.

51. McCormick GP, Riffer DJ, Thompson MM: Coital positioning for stroke afflicted couples. *Rehabil Nurs* 11(2):17–19, 1986.

52. Monga TN, Kerrigan AJ: Cerebrovascular accidents. In Sipski ML, Alexander CJ, editors: *Sexual function in people with disability and chronic illness: a health professional's guide*, Gaitherburg, MD, 1997, Aspen.

53. Monga TN, Lawson JS, Inglis J: Sexual dysfunction in stroke patients. *Arch Phys Med Rehabil* 67(1):19–22, 1986.

54. Monga TN, Monga M, Raina MS, et al: Hypersexuality in stroke. *Arch Phys Med Rehabil* 67(6):415–417, 1986.

55. Muller FE, Mittleman MA, Maclure M, et al: Triggering myocardial infarction by sexual activity. *JAMA* 275(18):1405–1409, 1996.

56. Neistadt M: Human sexuality and counseling. In Hopkins HL, Smith HD, editors: *Willard and Spackman's occupational therapy*, ed 8, Philadelphia, 1993, Lippincott.

57. Neistadt ME, Frieda M: *Choices: a guide to sex counseling with physically disabled adults*, Malabar, FL, 1987, Robert E Krieger.

58. Neuman B: Using behavioral treatment for urinary incontinence. *OT Pract* September:10–16,2002.

59. Roley SS, Delany JV, Borrow, CJ et al: Occupational therapy practice framework domain and process. *Am J Occup Ther* 62(6):625–683, 2008.

60. Palmeri ST, Kostis, JB, Casazza L, et al: Heart rate and blood pressure response in adult men and women during exercise and sexual activity. *Am J Cardiol* 100(12):1795–1801, 2007.

61. Parke F: Sexuality in later life. *Nurs Times* 87(50):40–42, 1991.

62. Patel M, Coshall C, Lawrence E, et al: Recovery from poststroke urinary incontinence: associated factors and impact on outcome. *J Am Geriatr Soc* 49(9):1229–1233, 2001.

63. Payne MS, Greer DL, Corbin DE: Sexual functioning as a topic in occupational therapy training, a survey of programs. *Am J Occup Ther* 42(4):227, 1988.

64. *Physicians Desk Reference*, ed 63, Montvale NJ, 2009, PDR Network.

65. Purk JK, Richardson RA: Older adult stroke patients and their spousal caregivers. *J Contemp Hum Serv* 75(10):608–615, 1994.

66. Romano MD: Sexuality and the disabled female. *Accent Living* winter, 1973.

67. Schwarz ER, Rodriguez J: Sex and the heart. *Int J Impot Res* 17 suppl 1:S4–S6, 2005.

68. Sjogren K: Sexuality after stroke with hemiplegia. II. With special regard to partnership adjustment and to fulfillment. *Scand J Rehabil Med* 15(2):63–69, 1983.

69. Sjogren K, Damber JE, Liliequist B: Sexuality after stroke with hemiplegia. I. Aspects of sexual function. *Scand J Rehabil Med* 15(2):55–61, 1983.

70. Sjogren K, Fugl-Meyer AR: Adjustment to life after stroke with special reference to sexual intercourse and leisure. *J Psychosom Res* 26(4):409–417, 1982.

71. Strauss D: Biopsychosocial issues in sexuality with the neurologically impaired patient. *Sex Disabil* 9(1):1, 1991.

72. Szasz G, Miller S, Anderson L: Guide to birth control counseling of the physically handicapped. *Can Med Assoc J* 120(11):1353, 1979.

73. Tamam Y, Tamam L, Akil E, et al: Post-stroke sexual functioning in first stroke patients. *European Journal of Neurology*, 15(7):660–666, 2008.

74. Thienhaus OJ: Practical overview of sexual function and advancing age. *Geriatrics* 43(8):63–67, 1988.
75. US Department of Health and Human Services: *Post-stroke rehabilitation*, Rockville, Md, 1995, Public Health Service Agency for Health Care Policy and Research, Clinical practice guideline 16, AHCPR Pub No 95–0662.
76. Wigg EH: Counseling the adult aphasic for sexual readjustment. *Rehab Couns Bull* Dec:10–119, 1973.
77. Zasler ND: Sexuality in neurologic disability: an overview. *Sex Disabil* 9(1):1, 1991.

SUGGESTED READINGS

Finger WW: Prevention, assessment and treatment of sexual dysfunction following stroke. *Sex Disabil* 11(1):1, 1993.
Kroll K, Levy Klein E: *Enabling romance*, Bethesda, MD, 1995, Woodbine House.
Novak PP, Mitchell MM: Professional involvement in sexuality counseling for patients with spinal cord injuries. *Am J Occup Ther* 42(2): 105–112, 1988.

SEXUALITY RESOURCES

American Association of Sex Education Counselors and Therapists
435 North Michigan Ave., Suite 1717
Chicago, IL 60611
(312) 644–0828
www.aasect.org

American Congress of Rehabilitation Medicine
6801 Lake Plaza Drive, Suite B-205
Indianapolis, IN 46220
(317) 915–2250
www.acrm.org

American Stroke Association
National Center
7272 Greenville Ave.
Dallas, TX 52231
1–888–4–STROKE
www.strokeassociation.org

Hazel K. Goddess Fund for Stroke Research
785 Park Ave.
New York, NY 10021–3552
(212) 734–8067
www.thegoddessfund.org

National Stroke Association
9707 East Easter Lane
Englewood, CO 80112–5112
1–800–STROKES
www.stroke.org

Planned Parenthood Federation of America
www.plannedparenthood.org
SIECUS (Sex Information and Education Council of the United States)
90 John St., Suite 704
New York, NY 10038
(212) 819–9770
www.siecus.org

Sexuality and Disability Training Center
Boston University Medical Center
88 East Newton St.
Boston, MA 02118
(617) 638–7358
www.stanleyducharme.com

The Stroke Association
www.stroke.org.uk

Stroke Clubs International
805 Twelfth St.
Galveston, TX 77550
(409) 762–1022
www.strokeclubs@earthlink.net

Specific Websites:

Disability resources: www.menstuff.org
National Institute of Aging: www.nia.nih.gov
Sexual Health Network: www.sexualhealth.com
Institute on Independent Living: www.independentliving.org
Stroke Survivors without Partners: www.dateable.org

mary shea
christine m. johann

chapter 26

Seating and Wheeled Mobility Prescription

key terms

client education	mat evaluation	seating system
deformity	pressure distribution	symmetrical postural alignment
functional mobility	product trial	team approach
functional positioning	seated posture	wheelchair

chapter objectives

After completing this chapter, the reader will be able to accomplish the following:

1. Understand the seating system and mobility system evaluation process.
2. Appreciate the difference between seating for rest and seating for activity performance.
3. Implement a treatment plan and identify the goals of the mobility device and seating and positioning system.
4. Appreciate the pros and cons of different mobility bases and seating system components.
5. Understand the influence of the seating system on carryover of treatment goals.
6. Appreciate the importance of the team process throughout the evaluation and fitting/ delivery process.
7. Understand the importance of fitting and training with the recommended seating system and mobility device.

The statistics from the National Stroke Association indicate that stroke is the leading cause of serious adult disability in the United States.[12] Despite advances in rehabilitation and treatment approaches, many individuals have difficulty with mobility and performance of activities of daily living (ADL). An appropriate seating system and mobility base is essential to maximize each client's potential to achieve the upmost independence and safety with ADL. Consequently, it is important for a therapist to develop a working knowledge of assistive technology. *Assistive technology* is an umbrella term that includes seating and wheeled mobility, including manual and power wheelchairs, electronic aids to daily living (formerly known as environmental control units), computer access including workstation setup, and augmentative and alternative communication devices.

This chapter provides a general introduction and then focuses on the basic principles of seating and positioning, the evaluation process, the fitting/delivery and training process, and the features of various seating system products and mobility devices. Although the emphasis is on the seating and wheeled mobility process specific to persons with a stroke, many of these principles are appropriate for use with all individuals with disabilities who have impaired functioning and disability.

The terms *client* and *individual with disability* are used interchangeably throughout the chapter for appropriate semantics. These terms consistently refer to the same person.

The wheelchair and seating system provision process is a collaborative process that begins with a client interview and ends with fitting, training, and follow-up with the recommended wheelchair and seating system. A team approach throughout this process is essential to ensure achievement of safety and the client's goals. The ideal wheelchair and seating system team consists of the client; health care practitioners such as a medical doctor, an occupational and/or physical therapist, and a speech pathologist (as needed); the caregiver and/or significant other; and an assistive technology supplier. The client is the central person in the wheelchair and seating system process, and the client's goals are given the highest priority.

If a client can communicate his or her needs and has the cognitive functioning to participate in decision-making, then the therapist's role is to empower him or her, through education, to be more active in the decision-making process. If a client has cognitive changes that limit his or her ability to function and be involved in the decision-making process, then he or she is still central; however, increased attention may be given to the caregiver's needs and goals.

In the past 35 years, numerous changes have occurred in the health care industry. These changes were primarily at the environment level and include societal attitudes and expectations of persons with disabilities, rehabilitation service provision, manufacturer production of durable medical equipment, reimbursement policies, and system changes that include the development of authorities and organizations to organize, control, and monitor assistive technology services. Due to these changes in the wheelchair industry, increased emphasis is on the client taking a more active role in medical care, increased expectations of returning to a previous level of activity and function, minimization of deformities and secondary complications, actual evaluation of trial equipment, and the certification of a group of therapists and suppliers with a basic wide-range knowledge base

of seating system and mobility device evaluation and provision.

SOCIETAL ATTITUDES AND EXPECTATIONS OF PERSONS WITH DISABILITIES

For the past 35 years, individuals with disabilities have been lobbying for their needs and rights and have been relatively successful with the passage of several laws. The Americans with Disabilities Act has played a major role at the International Classification of Functioning, Disability and Health (ICF)[6] activities and participation level to increase access to transportation and public places. This increase in environmental accessibility has enabled many individuals with disabilities to pursue their education, employment, and leisure interests to become more active, productive members of society. These changes have fueled the wheelchair manufacturing industry to develop and provide appropriate equipment to meet these more active lifestyles.

REHABILITATION SERVICES

The provision of rehabilitation services has changed drastically regarding length of stay on rehabilitation units and knowledge required to appreciate the variety of wheelchair and seating system options. Initially, clients had sufficient time in rehabilitation programs to adjust to the changes in their bodies and reach their full potential before they received a wheelchair and integrated into their discharge environment, preferably home. Today, because of the influence of traditional insurance funding limitations, clients are discharged from rehabilitation units once they are medically stable, have demonstrated restoration gains, and have a support system in place to enable them to be relatively safe with their basic ADL. As a result, therapists are forced to look at a permanent seating system early to ensure that it will facilitate functional restoration and minimize the risk for increased deformity and secondary complications.

Years ago an overall one-size-fits-all philosophy prevailed and a limited number of wheelchair and seating system options were available for individuals with disabilities. Because of changes in the manufacturing industry, a multitude of product options now are available to facilitate optimal positioning for individuals with a wide variety of needs. The knowledge base of therapists and the increased number of seating systems and accessories now available can help decrease the progression of deformities, pain, and other secondary problems. An individual who is seated appropriately can access available motor function, perform ADL with increased sense of security, and can lead a healthier, more enriching life. Specific product options are addressed later in this chapter.

MANUFACTURER PRODUCTION OF DURABLE MEDICAL EQUIPMENT

The durable medical equipment industry has grown tremendously in the past 35 years to meet the increasing population of persons with disabilities and the increasing demand for more versatile, lighter-weight products. The increase in product options and advancement to lighter-weight materials such as aluminum and titanium has resulted in a vast selection of off-the-shelf products that have the potential to meet a wide array of needs. Manufacturers understand the need for persons with disabilities to try specific products to ensure they will meet their needs. Accordingly, they often provide evaluation equipment for clients to try.

REIMBURSEMENT POLICIES

Insurance companies are the funding source for the majority of durable medical equipment provided for individuals with disabilities. Unfortunately, as a result, the funding source often influences the decision-making process. This discussion will focus primarily on Medicare guidelines because many private insurance companies follow these guidelines, and Medicare is the primary funding source for individuals who are older than 65-years-old and have had a stroke. Medicare has specific codes and reimbursement guidelines for durable medical equipment. It is concerned primarily about mobility within the home and will consider payment for a device only after an individual has received it. As a result, durable medical equipment suppliers have to take the risk and supply equipment without receiving any guarantee of payment from Medicare. Consequently, differences exist between individual supplier policies and what wheelchair and seating system products suppliers are willing to provide. As one can imagine, some suppliers hesitate to provide more complex, expensive equipment for individuals with more involved needs. It is essential for the team to work together to ensure that each individual has access to the best product to meet his or her needs. If this is not possible under Medicare guidelines, the client should notify the local congressional representative, and the team should consider other funding sources.

SYSTEM AND POLICY CHANGES: DEVELOPMENT OF STANDARDS AND ORGANIZATIONS TO MONITOR ASSISTIVE TECHNOLOGY SERVICES

System changes have evolved over the past three decades and include the development of authorities and organizations to organize, control, and monitor assistive technology services. The Rehabilitation Engineers Society of North America (RESNA), the National Registry of Rehabilitation Technology Suppliers (NRRTS), the American Academy of Physical Medicine and Rehabilitation, and the Foundation for Physical Medicine and Rehabilitation have been created to develop or have been active in developing standards to ensure a higher standard of practice with wheelchair service provision. A monumental accomplishment was the American National Standards Institute/RESNA Wheelchair Standards. These standards provided the industry with increased consistency for wheelchair performance characteristics and measurements that are widely used by manufacturers to categorize and test wheelchairs. Consequently, these standards provide the wheelchair team with the ability to compare similar products from different manufacturers.

Another major accomplishment has been the development of credentialing programs. The RESNA awards therapists and suppliers credentials for an assistive technology professional and a seating and mobility specialist. The NRRTS awards a certified rehabilitation technology supplier credential. These credentials increase the likelihood that the professional members of the treatment team have a certain knowledge base of client's needs and assistive technology products.

Numerous outcome studies have been performed and are being performed at a multitude of levels to determine the efficacy of wheelchairs, seating system products, and wheelchair service provisions. Specific topics studied include long-term wheelchair use, wheelchair design, repetitive stress injuries, propulsion methods, pressure relief techniques, and community integration. Many of these studies have focused on the individuals with spinal cord injury; however, the results are meaningful for all individuals who use wheelchairs as their primary means of mobility. The results from these studies have influenced manufacturing focuses and current practice with wheelchair prescription trends. This has translated into higher-quality products that minimize an individual's risk of injury and increase their efficiency with mobility for increased integration into society. Continued involvement of health care practitioners in education, research, and product development is essential to ensure that all individuals with disabilities receive the best possible equipment to minimize their risk for secondary complications and maximize their ability to function indoors and outdoors.

BIOMECHANICS OF SITTING

To appreciate and evaluate postural alignment, it is important to have an understanding of biomechanics. A therapist should understand basic anatomy of skeletal structures and their relationship to one another. The pelvis is the foundation for sitting; consequently, knowledge of the anatomy and biomechanical features of the pelvis and its relationship with the musculature and fascia of the spine and lower extremities is essential to understand how changes in lower-extremity positioning influence the pelvis and subsequently the spine.

The pelvis moves anteriorly and posteriorly in the sagittal plane around a coronal axis, laterally tilting in a frontal plane around an anteroposterior axis and rotationally in a transverse plane around a vertical axis. A stable neutral position of the pelvis must be attained to provide the optimal postural alignment of the spine (Fig. 26-1). In a neutral pelvic position, the anterior superior iliac spine (ASIS) is level in a frontal plane and level with or slightly lower than the posterior superior iliac spine (PSIS) in the sagittal plane. A pelvis is also positioned in neutral when both ischial tuberosities bear weight equally (Fig. 26-2). Palpating the ASIS and PSIS and then both right and left anterior superior iliac spine can help the therapist to determine the position of the pelvis. Fig. 26-3 shows optimal sitting posture with a stable neutral pelvic position and symmetrical positioning of the lower extremities and trunk.

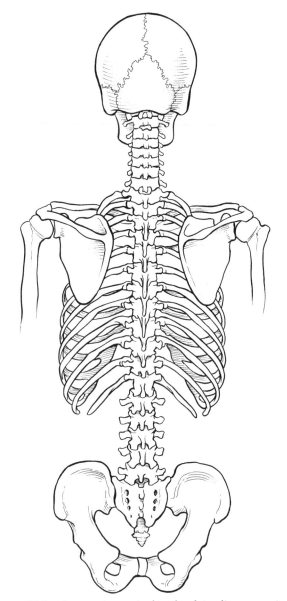

Figure 26-2 Appropriate spinal and pelvic alignment viewed posteriorly.

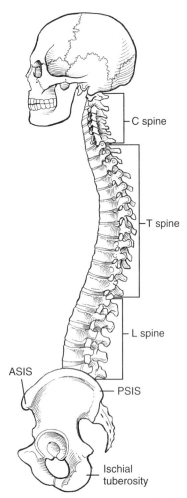

Figure 26-1 Lateral view of the spine and pelvis with appropriate alignment and spinal curvatures. *C,* Cervical; *T,* thoracic; *L,* lumbar; *ASIS,* anterior superior iliac spine; *PSIS,* posterior superior iliac spine.

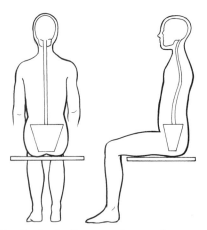

Figure 26-3 Optimal alignment in seated posture. Note the symmetrical pelvis and spinal alignment.

ASSYMMETRICAL PELVIC POSITIONS, CONCERNS, AND COMMON CAUSES

Fig. 26-4, *A*, *B*, and *C*, shows changes in pelvic alignment. Part *A* demonstrates lateral tilting of the pelvis, in which one ASIS is higher than the other is. This pelvic obliquity results in unequal weight distribution through the ischial tuberosities and a C- or an S-shaped spinal curve. This posture places an individual at a high risk for developing a pressure sore under the lower, weight-bearing ischial tuberosity and secondary shoulder and neck discomfort. This problem is seen commonly in individuals with asymmetrical muscular strength, asymmetrical muscle tone, limited hip joint mobility, lower extremity hip flexion or internal/external rotation range of motion limitations, asymmetrical lower extremity muscle strength, and midline orientation deficits.

Fig. 26-4, *B* demonstrates a posterior pelvic tilt. A posterior pelvic tilt occurs when the ASIS is higher than the PSIS. This abnormal pelvic position results in a kyphotic spinal posture. A posterior pelvis with lumbar and thoracic spinal kyphosis results in changed weight distribution, with increased pressures on the sacrum and coccyx, and a compensatory cervical hyperextension. This posture can lead to pressure sores on the sacrum and coccyx, neck and back pain, limited neck range of motion, and a decreased visual field. Posterior pelvic tilt is commonly seen in individuals with trunk weakness, muscle imbalance, limited pelvic mobility, limited hip joint mobility, limited lower extremity hip flexion, and/or limited hamstring muscle length.

With anterior pelvic tilt, the ASIS is lower than the PSIS. This pelvic position usually results in a more pronounced lordotic curve in the spine. This posture is typically seen in individuals with decreased muscle recruitment and overall muscle weakness.

A pelvic rotation is present when one ASIS is farther forward than the other (see Fig. 26-4, *C*). The posture can present as unequal leg length posturing when an individual is seated. This abnormal pelvic rotation influences the spine to move into a rotated position and predisposes an individual to a scoliotic curvature of the spine. Pelvic rotation can create unequal weight distribution between the ischial tuberosities, which can lead to pressure sores. This posture is commonly seen in individuals with asymmetrical muscle strength, asymmetrical muscle tone, limited hip joint mobility, lower extremity abduction, or adduction limitations.

WHEELCHAIR AND SEATING SYSTEM ASSESSMENT

Basic Principles

Although accessibility and wheelchair technology have changed drastically over the past 30 years, Judai's study[7] is a reminder that the process still is evolving. Judai used the Psychosocial Impact of Assist Device Scale to assess the psychosocial impact of assistive devices on individuals one and three months following the stroke. His findings for individuals who used wheelchairs indicated that some individuals reported a negative effect on their self-esteem, competence, and adaptability. This is a reminder to be attentive to the social and attitudinal environment that includes the stigma associated with using a wheelchair. Approaching each treatment session with a positive tone and educating individuals about the benefits of increased comfort and the potential ability to function independently indoors and outdoors are important.[7] It is also helpful if the team has a working knowledge of community resources (i.e., support groups, transportation, and general accessibility) by which to educate the client about strategies for increased integration in the community.

Unfortunately, no specific formula exists to choosing the "right" seating system and mobility base. However, the set of guidelines discussed next can help the team achieve the best combination of mobility base and seating system with each client. The wheelchair and seating system decision is the result of an intricate interplay among an individual's postural seated needs, personal preferences and goals, home and community environment, financial situation, and method of transportation. It is important to remember that the one-size-fits-all philosophy has no place in seating system and mobility device prescription.

The wheelchair and seating system assessment is specific to each individual's needs. After obtaining demographic data, the assessment process generally begins at the ICF activities and participation level and progresses to the body functions and structures level. Initially, an indepth comprehensive interview with the wheelchair team

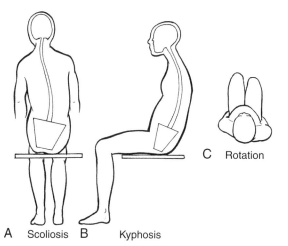

Figure 26-4 Common posturing following a stroke. **A**, Lateral tilting of the pelvis in a client with right-sided weakness. **B**, Posterior pelvic tilt with kyphosis. **C**, Trunk and pelvic rotation (superior view).

takes place to develop an understanding of an individual's functional goals, environments he needs to function in, ability to participate in ADL, and knowledge base of wheelchair and seating system needs. The assessment then continues to screen numerous body functions such as muscle strength, balance, and cognition. This includes a mat evaluation, client education regarding postural needs and pros/cons of various seating and mobility base options, seating product and mobility product trial, and specifications of the wheelchair and seating system products. It is extremely important to take the time to perform a thorough assessment to avoid compromising the result and to minimize time spent fixing mistakes.[2]

Step 1: Conduct a Comprehensive Interview

The therapist should lead the team and conduct a comprehensive interview that includes the client's diagnosis; medical and surgical history; skin history; future medical and surgical considerations; allergies; precautions; pain; funding sources; social support network; use of splints or orthotics; previous and current level of functioning; likes and dislikes with current equipment; equipment fit in home environment, work environment, and community; transportation method(s) (car, van, taxi, or bus); and the client's goals for the new or modified equipment. The interview should include psychosocial issues with respect to roles and lifestyle preferences; basic and instrumental ADL performance, including indoor and outdoor mobility; and transfer status. A physical status screening should take place to ascertain passive and active range of motion, available movement patterns, muscle strength, sensation, endurance, balance, visual-perception, and cognition. If the client has moderate to severe oral-motor control issues, a speech pathologist should be a member of the treatment team to ensure that the client's communication and/or augmentative communication needs are addressed thoroughly. See Chapter 20.

If this is a client's first wheelchair, a home evaluation form is generally provided and additional education is necessary to ensure that the client and significant others understand the environments that wheelchair maneuverability will have impact on.

Step 2: Perform a Supine and Seated Mat Assessment

A mat assessment is an intimate evaluation that can be intimidating and confusing to the client and significant others. The assessment involves therapeutic handling, palpation, and range of motion. The results of the mat assessment are essential to determine the amount of support an individual requires for upright sitting, the goals and overall setup of the seating system, and the mobility base options needed to accommodate the recommended seating system. The therapist must take the time to articulate the purpose and importance of the mat evaluation to ensure that everyone "understands what you are looking for, how you will be going about it, and why this information is important to reach a good end result."[2]

Before beginning a mat assessment, it is important for the therapist to understand some basic biomechanical and seating principles. One of the main concepts is the distinction between flexible, difficult to correct, and fixed postural deformities. These concepts clarify skeletal positions in the supine and seated mat assessment.

The initial focus with a mat evaluation is to determine whether neutral pelvic and trunk alignment can be achieved. If the pelvis is in an oblique position and lower extremity influence has been accommodated for or ruled out, the therapist should attempt to correct the pelvis manually.

If the pelvis stays in the corrected position, without handling, the deformity is considered flexible.[19] If the pelvis goes back into the oblique position but is repositioned easily to neutral and requires gentle therapeutic handling to stay in neutral, the deformity is considered difficult to correct.[19] If the pelvis cannot be repositioned manually into a neutral position, the deformity is considered fixed.[19] A pelvic obliquity is measured by the height difference between each ASIS and is named for the side that is lower.[19] A subsequent section discusses seating considerations for flexible, difficult to correct, and fixed body structures.

A thorough mat assessment can require two to four persons and consists of four major components:

1. Observation of the client in the clinic with the current or loaned equipment; the therapist assesses postural positioning in the wheelchair and screens muscle tone and strength. The specific focus should include the influence of tone on movement, influence of movement on tone, and influence of tone on postural control.

2. For a supine mat assessment, the client is positioned on a mat. This is essential to determine the bony structure, muscle flexibility (including muscle tone), and range of motion of the client to achieve optimal spinal-pelvic alignment. The assessment provides the therapist with a "true" picture of each individual's potential to be seated with optimal spinal-pelvic alignment. The results from the supine assessment are essential to guide how an individual is positioned or supported for the seated mat evaluation

3. A seated mat assessment is essential to determine the influence of gravity on the individual's ability to sit upright. The therapist can usually perform the seated assessment with the client seated on the edge of the mat with therapeutic handling by the therapist and other members of the treatment team. At this time, muscle tone may be increased as the individual attempts to hold his or her body up against gravity. If a client has moderate to significant

postural needs, a positioning simulator can be helpful to support the client in the upright position. A more detailed description follows.

4. Once an individual is positioned with maximum aligned posture on the mat or in the simulator, the time and location are ideal to take accurate measurements of the client's body. The five basic measurements for an active individual are seat width, seat depth, knee to heel (with shoe), elbow height, and distance from the seating surface to inferior angle of the scapula. All measurements can be documented in half-inch or one inch increments (e.g., 17.5-inch seat width). Chest width, axilla, top of shoulder, and occiput measurements are important to obtain if an individual requires more aggressive support (Fig. 26-5).

A simulator is a tool that permits the team to evaluate a sitting client more easily with various angles and amounts of support. This simulator is composed of planar surfaces that can be adjusted to different depths, and recline, and tilt to provide appropriate support. In addition, it consists of easily adjusted components (headrest, lateral support, hip support, armrest, and footrest) that can be placed in numerous positions and are adjustable through knobs. The simulator permits therapists to evaluate the seated position with an individual, evaluate the level of function with different positions, educate the client on the potential to achieve the best possible resting posture, take more accurate measurements, visually document potential for increased alignment via pictures to funding sources, and save an enormous amount of time with evaluating different products. The simulator can help narrow the product options necessary for evaluation to provide optimal support (Fig. 26-6).

Step 3: Provide Client and Team Education

Educating the client about the mat evaluation findings and their effect on postural alignment in a seated position is important. At that time, the therapist can review a client's goals, and each team member should articulate their goals to ensure that all are headed in the same direction. Education is essential to enable an individual to participate actively in the wheelchair and seating system trial and decide what compromises he or she is willing to make to maximize the ability to function in a wheelchair. Although the client is the primary decision-maker, the therapist and assistive technology supplier should freely discuss their professional opinions. Part of the educational process is to help a client prioritize what is most important, especially when future health, skin integrity, and secondary complications are a concern. There is no one wheelchair and seating system that is perfect for individuals with stroke; the solution is perfect only when a client makes informed decisions about what various components will work best for his or her lifestyle.

It is helpful to discuss wheelchair and seating system needs in a general way and then to select products so that a client can choose from two or three options. Using the mat evaluation results and understanding product features and benefits is essential and described in detail later in this chapter. The therapist and assistive technology supplier have the responsibility to clearly articulate the features, benefits, and pros and cons of various options to empower the clients to select products to best meet their needs. Providing this information empowers the client and significant others to be educated, reinforces their confidence in the decision of the team, and increases their satisfaction with the final product.

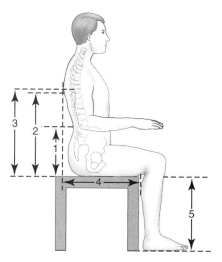
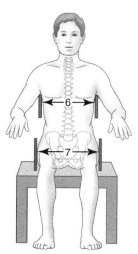

Figure 26-5 Measurements during the mat assessment. *1*, Elbow height; *2*, seat to inferior angle of scapula; *3*, axilla; *4*, seat depth; *5*, knee to heel; *6*, chest width; *7*, hip width.

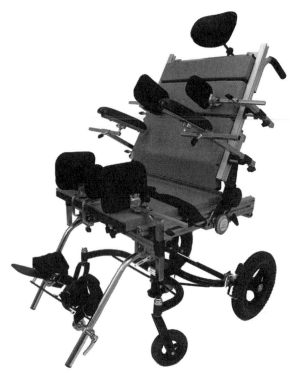

Figure 26-6   Planar Simulator. (Courtesy of Prairie Seating Corporation.)

Step 4: Equipment Trial

Actual trial of seating system and wheelchair options is the best case scenario; however, this is not always possible. If a manufacturer is unable to provide the team members with the equipment they are considering, simulating the type of seating design and components is important for the team to ensure that the product is accomplishing what they had hoped to achieve.

Actual trial of more complex, expensive equipment is highly recommended to minimize unseen compatibility and fit problems and ensure that the full system can meet the client's needs and goals.

Once the ideal wheelchair and seating system is decided upon, the team gathers around the client in the "evaluation" wheelchair and seating system. At this point, the team decides the measurements of the product, specifies wheelchair and seating system features with order forms, and provides additional education about the pros and cons of specific features (such as pneumatic versus solid tires). In an ideal situation, this is truly a collaborative team process.

Step 5: Documentation

At this point, the therapist has gathered all the information needed to write a letter of medical necessity. This letter is a concise summary of the client's activities and participation status, mat evaluation findings, problems with existing equipment, wheelchair and seating needs to maximize activity and participation, and medical and functional justification for the wheelchair, wheelchair features, and seating system recommendations. This is the letter that the medical doctor reviews and signs once the final additions are completed.

As the medical professionals are generating the letter of medical necessity and organizing the medical chart notes and prescriptions, the assistive technology supplier contacts each of the manufacturers for price quotes and generates a product description form. The doctor reviews and signs this form. It is sent with the letter of medical necessity and other insurance documentation to the assistive technology supplier for funding approval.

Step 6: Fitting, Training, and Delivery

After the team has recommended and documented the person's equipment needs, the job is only half over. It is common for funding sources to question the team's recommendation. It is important to respond as promptly as possible to these inquiries and clearly communicate the team's goals.

Once the assistive technology supplier feels secure that the equipment will be funded and in some cases "approved" by the funding source, the equipment is ordered. All team members who were involved in steps 1 to 5 should be available for steps 6 and 7. During fitting, training, and delivery, the wheelchair and seating system is set up and adjusted to specifically meet each client's needs. At this time, the therapist and assistive technology supplier educate the client and significant others regarding wheelchair and seating system parts management, care, and general maintenance, including whom to contact if problems arise. For example, if a client needs replacement parts, he or she is advised to contact the assistive technology supplier; if a client experiences physical changes and is no longer comfortable, he or she is advised to contact the medical doctor and the therapist.

Mobility skills training is essential to provide clients with strategies and techniques for maximum safety and independence with mobility. This includes training for manual wheelchair operation using the traditional ipsilateral arm-foot propulsion technique,[3] a one-arm drive wheelchair, or a power mobility product. Rudman and colleagues[16] concluded that training was needed beyond the prescription of the wheelchair. This training is essential to provide clients with the ability to reach their full functional potential with activities and participation.

This fitting and delivery step is essential to ensure that the end product accomplishes the team's goals and minimizes an individual's risk for deformity and secondary problems. Another benefit to this step is that it significantly reduces the potential for product abandonment.

Step 7: Functional Outcome Measurement and Follow-Up

The ideal situation would be for an individual to attend a follow-up treatment session three months after the fitting and delivery or at least to participate in a phone interview with the therapist to determine the success of the wheelchair and seating system intervention. This step is a true test to ensure achievement of the team's goals. Follow-up should focus on issues such as whether the equipment is holding up to the individual's specific needs and has made a difference on pain, quality of life, and independent functioning.

Barker and colleagues[1] reported that wheelchairs were an enabler of community participation. Pettersson and colleagues[13] used the Psychosocial Impact of Assistive Devices Scale and found that wheelchairs increased quality of life for individuals after stroke.

MATCHING EQUIPMENT TO CLIENT FUNCTION: SEATING SYSTEM PRINCIPLES

Translating the Mat Evaluation into the Seating System

Once the mat assessment is completed, the therapist must translate the measurements and ranges into the set-up of the seating system and wheelchair. For example, if Mr. S. has only 80 degrees of hip flexion range, the seat-to-back angle must be set up to accommodate this 10-degree limitation. Most back canes have an 8-degree bend rearward, and therefore a back support with some adjustability is provided with an additional 2 to 7 degrees of open seat-to-back angle. The extra 5 degrees is necessary to allow for some adjustment for comfort. It is important not to position an individual at the maximum range available. Likewise, if Mr. S. has hamstring tightness (−70 degrees of knee extension with his hip at 80 degrees of flexion), the therapist must be cautious about using an elevating leg rest, because it generally positions the lower extremity in −65 degrees of knee extension and would overstretch his tight hamstring musculature. Because Mr. S.'s hamstring muscle cannot sufficiently elongate to tolerate this open knee angle, his body will automatically compensate for this, which would result in Mr. S sitting with a posterior pelvic tilt. In this situation the team can order a 70-degree standard footrest and use a longer heel loop for foot position rearward for a −70- to −75-degree knee angle, being mindful of caster (front wheel) clearance. This is essential to adequately accommodate his hamstring muscle tightness and allow for optimal pelvic and spine positioning.

Flexible, Difficult to Correct, and Fixed Deformities

Once a therapist establishes what type of deformity is present, he or she must figure out how to support the client to minimize his or her risk for increased deformity. If an individual has a flexible or difficult to correct deformity, the seating system should be set up to imitate the therapeutic handling to "correct" the deformity. At this time, client education regarding repositioning strategies is helpful to ensure the client is aligned properly and to facilitate neuromuscular reeducation. It is important to carefully monitor each client's tolerance for correction and adjust the seating system accordingly to maximize success. The process may require incremental steps to achieve increased alignment or may involve backing down from an aggressive start. If a deformity is fixed, as much aggressive support as possible is important to assist the client around his deformity to decrease progression and to minimize his or her risk for increased deformity.

With more aggressive seating systems, a mobile person can be "locked" up by the aggressive supports used to achieve optimal spinal-pelvic alignment. Unfortunately, this often limits an individual's ability to function. With positioning for function, a compromise occurs to provide as much support as possible for the resting body position without affecting or limiting an individual's ability to function. Consequently, wheelchair seating is a continuum with safety and maximum postural support on one end and mobility for activity and participation on the other end. An ideal seating system should have some flexibility to provide optimal spinal-pelvic alignment and facilitate function. It is important to maximize the potential movement options of individuals who use wheelchairs as their primary means of mobility. Individuals with good motor control may choose to sit on a chair or stool for more active functioning. For individuals who do not have as many mobility options available, the wheelchair must have the ability to accommodate both active and resting seated postures.

Although online resources for wheelchair and seating system products are an excellent source of information and education, online purchase of these products is not recommended because a client does not receive any of the benefits that an assistive technology supplier provides (i.e., assistance with set-up and assembly, on-site adjustments, and personalized modifications).[9] In addition, an individual purchasing equipment online misses the opportunity for the team evaluation and product trial and may not be in-tune to mild physical changes that have occurred since last receiving a wheelchair and seating system.

GENERAL SEATING SYSTEM PRINCIPLES FOR INDIVIDUALS WITH STROKE

Therapeutic intervention for individuals with brain damage caused by a stroke depends on the severity of the infarct and the amount of functional change that has occurred, including physical, visual-perceptual, and cognitive changes. Accordingly, wheelchair and seating system intervention also depends on the level of functional changes and confounding variables, including the environment in which the individual is functioning and the presence of other diagnoses such as diabetes, hypertension, and coronary artery disease. Seating systems for individuals with more involved needs may be more supportive because of decreased plasticity in the central nervous system and permanent brain damage.[5]

Individuals with hemiplegia resulting from stroke often have difficulty controlling posture, balance reactions, and smooth movement patterns that enable the performance of functional tasks. Davies[5] described the typical patterns of adult hemiplegia (Table 26-1).

For individuals who use a wheelchair as their primary means of mobility, seating and mobility recommendations should address these typical patterns of adult hemiplegia. The following are typical seating system goals and seating principles specific to individuals with stroke.

Goals of the Seating System

The primary goals of seating and positioning at the ICF body functions and structures level are as follows:

Provide adequate postural support

- To prevent deformity or minimize the risk of increased deformity
- To balance skeletal muscle activity
- To minimize compensatory postures
- To maximize pressure distribution and minimize the risk of pressure ulcers
- To enhance distal extremity control
- For adequate comfort to maximize sitting tolerance
- For autonomic nervous system functioning

The primary goals of seating and positioning at the ICF[6] activities and participation level are as follows:

Provide adequate postural support

- To maximize ability to perform functional activities
- Aesthetically to enhance dignity and self-esteem and quality of life
- To increase comfort for increased social interaction and participation in community activities

Postural Stability and Control. Abnormal skeletal muscle activity and pathological reflexes often influence the postural alignment of an individual with neurological insult. A seating system should provide a stable foundation for maximum postural alignment to reestablish the length tension relationship of the muscles, balance muscle activity, normalize muscle tone, and decrease compensatory posturing. Improved postural stability provides individuals with the freedom to interact, move their extremities, and hold their heads in the midline position.[2] Secondary benefits of improved stability and control are increased ability to attend to what is happening in the environment, increased interaction with the environment, improved ability to assist in or perform ADL, and increased independence with mobility.

Proximal Muscle Stability to Enhance Distal Muscular Control. A stable base of support for the pelvis provides individuals with the opportunity to develop control and balance of their trunk musculature. When the pelvis is stable, an individual's center of gravity passes through the base of support, which helps promote stability. This central stability allows for distal extremity control. The client is better able to access muscles for arm or leg movement, head control, or oral motor control to perform functional tasks (i.e., hand function for dressing, leg movement for wheelchair propulsion, midline head orientation for improved visual tracking of objects, and oral motor control for speech articulation or swallowing).

Decrease Development of Muscle Contracture and Skeletal Deformity. Decreased pelvic control, muscle weakness, and muscle imbalance contribute to asymmetrical posturing. Asymmetrical postures can result in shortening or tightening of muscle groups, which can lead to a decreased range of motion in joints, increased tone, muscle contractures, and skeletal deformity. Asymmetrical posture must be corrected in a resting seated position

Table 26-1

Typical Patterns of Adult Hemiplegia

BODY PART	COMMON POSTURE
Head	Flexion toward hemiplegic side, neck rotation toward unaffected side
Upper extremity (flexion pattern)	Scapula retraction, shoulder girdle depression, humeral adduction and internal rotation
	Elbow flexion, forearm primarily in pronation; occasionally supination dominates
	Wrist flexion and ulnar deviation
	Thumb and finger flexion and adduction
Trunk	Trunk rotation backward on hemiplegic side with lateral trunk flexion
Pelvis	Posterior tilt with obliquity (lower on unaffected side)
Lower extremity	Hip extension, adduction, and internal rotation
	Knee extension
	Foot plantar flexion and inversion
	Toe flexion and adduction

to minimize an individual's risk for development of a fixed deformity. If soft tissue and skeletal flexibility is preserved, an individual can be encouraged successfully to sit with improved spinal-pelvic alignment through seating and seating system accessories. This positioning serves as a guide that eventually can promote the development of more balanced muscle control in that desired position. If muscle control cannot be improved, good positioning provides adequate support.

Enhance Comfort and Appearance. With optimal postural support in the seated position, individuals feel and look better. However, the process is not always a one-time event; seating system modifications can be introduced gradually to facilitate neuromuscular reeducation. Once an individual can tolerate increased postural alignment, the benefits are tenfold. Individuals who feel comfortable and feel good about themselves are much more productive and functional. This can lead to increased social interaction, communication, and an improved quality of life.

Minimize Development of Pressure Ulcers. When impaired sensation, motor control, or judgment affect an individual's ability to shift body weight, the client is usually at risk for developing pressure ulcers. Essential aspects of seating are to focus on pressure-redistributing cushions to maximize seating surface pressure dissemination and to consider a method of pressure relief (power tilt or recline) that the client can operate independently or a tilt-in space or recliner wheelchair in which a caregiver can perform the pressure-relief technique. Performance of regular (i.e., every half hour) pressure relief technique is essential to minimize risk of pressure ulcers.

Improve Function of the Autonomic Nervous System. Abnormal posturing, muscle shortening, and the inability to shift weight can increase pressure on internal organs and other structures. When an individual is leaning forward or to the side because of poor pelvic or spinal muscle control, a strain on circulation, digestion, and cardiopulmonary function can result. Postural supports can facilitate optimal pelvic, spinal, and trunk alignment, which in turn can provide improved physiological functioning of the autonomic nervous system. Sufficient head and neck support can decrease the potential for aspiration when swallowing problems exist.[2]

Increase Sitting Tolerance and Energy Level. If an individual is well-supported and can function from the wheelchair, sitting tolerance increases along with the ability to participate in therapy programs and functional activities. Individuals who receive adequate postural support experience less fatigue and pain than those who fix and stabilize continually with a higher level of abnormal muscle activity

and reflexes to support the body upright against gravity. The increased energy level associated with a more symmetrical posture increases sitting tolerance and an individual's ability to participate in functional activities within the home and the community.

Functional Positioning: An Active Seating System. Although the primary focus for seating intervention thus far has been on symmetry and alignment, a therapist must remember that functional movement is asymmetrical and dynamic. As a result, it is essential to consider seating systems that allow for function and activity performance and yet provide individuals with as much postural support as necessary to minimize their risk for increased deformity. It is important to remember that "body control is interpreted and performed when the body understands its relationship to gravity, primarily through activation of the vestibular system."[8]

The pelvis is the foundation for seated posture. With this in mind, it is important to consider Kangas' perspective on pelvic stability. Kangas[8] stated, "pelvic stability is not simply a musculoskeletal posture but rather is a movement of the body that includes an ongoing interaction of numerous systems, including the musculoskeletal, neuromuscular, circulatory, respiratory, gastrointestinal, and endocrinological systems." Pelvic stability is "not simply a musculoskeletal posture." It involves a position of actively holding still rather than being passively restricted. For individuals with a stroke, an active seating system generally provides as much seating surface as possible, a slightly anterior tilted seat, mild contour for upper leg positioning, and weight-bearing of the feet on the floor to enable the individual to position them as he or she chooses. This base of support can provide the body with sufficient pelvic stability, and this position of active weight-bearing allows an individual to assume an active task performance position for eating, writing a check, or working at a computer.[8]

An active seating system can be attained easily with minor adjustments to the wheelchair and seating system that is set-up slightly higher on the continuum for increased safety and adequate support. This is beneficial for times when an individual is more active (i.e., meal preparation in the kitchen). A seat wedge can be placed under the cushion and the footrests and positioning straps removed to allow an individual to achieve a more active position. As with all intervention recommendations, the therapist and client should evaluate this intervention together to ensure that it provides adequate stability for maximum safety with functioning. The art with mobility and seating system prescription is to achieve a balance between positioning for functional activity performance and symmetrical postural alignment for more sedentary activities (i.e., watching television) and to minimize an individual's risk for increased deformity and secondary complications.

MATCHING EQUIPMENT TO CLIENT FUNCTION: SEATING SYSTEMS

Seating and positioning is a continuum that encompasses all of the foregoing goals and principles. It is important for clients to understand that the *wheelchair* is not uncomfortable; usually the *seating system* is. The seating system is the primary unit that influences body posture because it is the direct interface between the client and the wheelchair and provides the client with the foundation for adequate postural support to rest and function. The mobility base is a frame that has some seating components such as footrests and armrests; however, its primary focus is mobility indoors and outdoors. It is essential to have a seating system that provides sufficient postural support interfaced with a wheelchair frame set at the appropriate angles to facilitate optimal spinal-pelvic alignment. Without appropriate postural support, an individual may be able to move about the environment; however, the risk for further deformity and pain is a major concern. A good rule of thumb for optimal positioning is to start with the pelvis and then proceed to the trunk and extremities. This approach follows the "support proximal to distal philosophy" inherent in numerous treatment approaches for individuals with neurological dysfunction.

The importance of seating, goals, and assessment of biomechanics and posture were reviewed previously. This section describes the types of seating systems available and their various features. Three basic styles of seating exist: linear, contoured, and custom contoured. Each of these provides different levels of support to promote postural alignment and pressure distribution. The definition of each with their respective benefits and concerns follows.

Linear Seating Systems

Linear seating systems (Table 26-2) are flat, noncontoured planes of support. Linear seat cushions or backs can be custom-made or ordered from the factory in various sizes, densities, and with different fabric covers.

Linear seating provides a firm, rigid seating base that can be beneficial for active individuals. Individuals with minimal musculoskeletal involvement typically benefit the most from linear seating. This seating is generally a lower cost option, and because of the flat surface, independent transfers are easy to achieve. Linear seating systems provide the least amount of postural support; however, because the human body is contoured, lack of support can result in higher peak pressures and pressure ulcers for individuals with prominent bony structures.

Contoured Seating Options

Contoured seating system options (see Table 26-2) are designed to support the body ergonomically. They are generally available in predetermined shapes of varying contours in a wide range of sizes.

Contoured seating options provide a range of contours from mild to aggressive. This type of seating system provides an excellent surface area for support that can enhance postural alignment and pressure relief. Individuals with minimal neuromuscular or central nervous system insults can benefit from the gentle cues that the slight contours of this seating system provide. Individuals can also achieve independent transfers with the mild contour options.

Individuals with moderate impairments benefit more from moderately contoured seating systems. These individuals are less likely to perform independent transfers, and the increased contours can meet their more involved postural support and pressure distribution needs. An advantage to an off-the-shelf contoured seating system is that it can be modified as an individual's needs change. It is important to remember that more aggressive contoured supports really hold and support an individual, which is ideal for postural alignment but can make transfers more difficult.

Custom Seating Options

Custom seat cushions and backs provide adapted support to meet an individual's specific needs. Customized seating systems are essential to provide maximum support, accommodation, and comfort for individuals with moderate to severe deformities. The concerns with custom-molded seating systems is the lack of flexibility for changing postural support needs, the high cost, and the amount of labor to create a customized seating system. An experienced therapist and assistive technology supplier is essential to achieve a successful end product with this level of seating system.

In addition to the primary support surface contours, the angles and degree of postural support from gravity are major considerations. Two dynamic seating system options available are recline and tilt-in-space seating systems. Both of these systems can position a person posterior from the upright, 90-degree sitting for postural support from gravity. A recline seating system is one in which the back support can be shifted backward or forward for varying levels of support and upright posture (Fig. 26-7). A tilt-in-space seating system is one in which the whole seating system (cushion and back support) tilts backward for increased postural support from gravity. Both of these systems can provide individuals with increased postural support and a method of pressure distribution through movement of the seating system. A recliner or a tilt-in-space wheelchair is often beneficial for individuals who need moderate to maximal support for upright sitting. These seating system options are available in both manual and power wheelchairs. With a manual seating system, a caregiver is essential to perform the movement. A power-operated seating system can provide an individual in the wheelchair with the ability to shift

Text continued on p.683

Table 26-2

Seating Systems

SEATING COMPONENT		INDICATIONS FOR USE	POSTURAL AND FUNCTIONAL CONSIDERATIONS
Solid insert	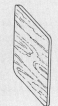	Insert can provide a level base of support on the sling wheelchair seat. Slide insert inside the cover, under the cushion, and secure to cushion base with Velcro. The cushion cover usually has Velcro to attach the cushion securely to sling upholstery of the wheelchair.	A sling wheelchair seat encourages a posterior pelvic tilt with hip adduction and internal rotation. This sets an individual up for a "slumped" posture. A solid insert is necessary to provide a firm and level base of support on the sling wheelchair seat. This facilitates more neutral pelvic positioning for upright posture and upper body movement for functional activities.
1.5–inch seat wedge		Wedge slides inside the cushion cover, under the cushion. Wedge can provide an anterior or posterior seat tilt.	Wedge is a lightweight, easy to remove component to use for an anterior-sloped seat or a posterior-sloped seat. An anterior tilt would facilitate upright positioning for an individual who is working at a workstation or propelling with one arm and one foot. A posterior tilt can assist with decreasing extensor spasticity or creating a set, slight tilt for increased postural support in a standard wheelchair.
Solid seat	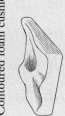	Remove wheelchair upholstery to install. To mount, solid seat hooks lock down on seat rails of wheelchair. The adjustable hooks on the solid seat can be positioned to provide an anterior or posterior tilt of solid seat and subsequently the cushion on the wheelchair frame.	Seat also encourages neutral pelvic alignment and lower extremity alignment. One concern is that it adds a significant amount of weight to the wheelchair. Unless necessary to achieve a low seat-to-floor height that cannot be achieved with a super low wheelchair, the weight disadvantage outweighs the positioning advantages.
Foam cushion	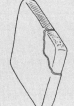	Foam linear cushions provide a stable base of support for individuals with mild postural support needs. The foam comes in varying densities and can be layered in different densities to provide support, comfort, and some pressure relief.	Cushions can enhance sitting posture, pressure distribution, and increase comfort.
Contoured foam cushion	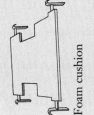	Contoured foam cushion provides an increased surface area of support and pressure relief for individuals with mild to moderate support and pressure distribution needs. A variety of foam densities are available.	The combination of stability and pressure relief is a major advantage to this cushion. The weight is a consideration; however, the advantage of a stable and pressure-distributing base of support minimizes the need for external supports.

Continued

Table 26-2

Seating Systems—cont'd

SEATING COMPONENT	INDICATIONS FOR USE	POSTURAL AND FUNCTIONAL CONSIDERATIONS
"Pressure-relieving" cushion (fluid medium) 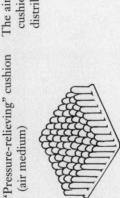	A firm, contoured cushion base with pressure-distributing gel fluid pad on top provides stability and a high level of pressure relief appropriate for all individuals who need moderate to significant postural support and pressure distribution. The gel bladder allows the pelvis to sink into it for full contact support for adequate pressure distribution to minimize the risk of pressure sores.	These off-the-shelf cushions provide a superior level of pressure distribution and good pelvic stability. This stability is important for improved balance and for adequate support. It can improve function at a wheelchair level and minimize compensatory posturing.
"Pressure-relieving" cushion (air medium) 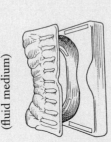	The air medium allows the seated individual to sink into this cushion for contoured support and a high degree of pressure distribution to minimize the risk of pressure ulcers.	The pressure distribution and lightweight qualities of this cushion are unsurpassed. However, this cushion does not provide any stability, and additional postural supports such as hip guides and adductors are essential for optimal alignment. These supports increase weight of the whole wheelchair system. Another concern is the continual air maintenance required with this cushion.
Lumbar-sacral back support	This component can provide support to the lumbar-sacral region to support the pelvis in neutral pelvic alignment. A more secure attachment method is recommended to keep it in position.	This support is a low-cost method to provide minimal postural support for increased spinal-pelvic alignment. The support is easy to remove, which is an advantage for car transport but a disadvantage because the support is not stable and can shift out of place easily.
Solid back support 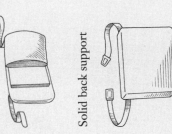	The solid back insert provides firm support to facilitate improved postural alignment for individuals with good pelvic and trunk control. The support is easy to remove for transportability of the wheelchair and usually is attached to the wheelchair back canes with Velcro straps.	This support is a low-cost method to provide minimal postural support for increased spinal-pelvic alignment. The support is easy to remove, which is an advantage for car transport but a disadvantage because the support is not stable and can shift out of place easily.

Pita back

This solid back insert provides a firm support to facilitate improved postural alignment for individuals with good pelvic and trunk control. The support is easy to remove for transportability of the wheelchair and slides into and out of a pocket in the back support upholstery.

This simple, low-cost back support can provide minimal postural support for increased spinal-pelvic alignment. The lack of foam makes the support easy to use; however, lack of sufficient padding is a concern for individuals using the wheelchair as a primary means of mobility.

Linear back support

This solid back insert provides a more durable back support for increased spinal-pelvic alignment. It is beneficial for individuals with good postural control, is attached to the wheelchair frame with quick-release hardware, and usually is linear with a solid posterior base with foam in front. The support may be covered in vinyl or other materials.

This is a planar back support to enhance upright sitting. The adjustable mounting brackets makes it possible to open up seat-to-back angle to accommodate a hip range of motion limitation or for increased postural support and balance via gravity. This hardware is durable. One concern is the weight added to the wheelchair.

Adjustable-angle off-the-shelf back support

This back support can be attached to the wheelchair with quick-release hardware. The support has generic, gentle contours that provide a guide for increased postural alignment for individuals with mild to moderate positioning needs and can be used in its original configuration or can accommodate a contoured foam in-place back support.

This back support provides mild contour to facilitate neutral trunk posturing and increased spinal-pelvic alignment. The angle can be adjusted to open up seat-to-back angle to accommodate a hip range of motion limitation or for increased postural support and balance via gravity. This support is a lightweight option that provides good support. One concern is that more durable hardware may be necessary for individuals with significant spasticity.

Adjustable-angle custom back support

This rigid back support can be attached to the wheelchair with quick-release or stationary hardware. The support often is positioned at an angle with a custom-contoured amount of support. The shell can be reused if the foam insert needs to be modified. This support benefits individuals with moderate to significant trunk weaknesses and/or flexible or fixed postural deformities.

This back support can provide moderate to significant support for individuals with flexible and fixed deformities. The hardware can open up the seat-to-back angle for the foregoing reasons. The contoured support provides maximum surface area contact to maximize alignment, accommodate deformities, and maximize pressure distribution to minimize the risk for increased deformities and pressure sores.

Pelvic positioning belt

Pelvic belts are designed to maintain optimal pelvic alignment and minimize an individual's risk for sliding out of the wheelchair. They are mounted to the seat frame via screws or straps and are available with various angles of pull and various buckles such as auto and airline style.

This support can be positioned at various angles depending on the individual's needs and functional level. A pelvic belt at the traditional 45 degrees can limit pelvic mobility for an anterior weight shift for forward reach and functioning at a table. Padded belts are available to minimize pressure concerns, and various buckles are available for maximum independence with opening/closing.

Continued

Table 26-2

Seating Systems—cont'd

SEATING COMPONENT	INDICATIONS FOR USE	POSTURAL AND FUNCTIONAL CONSIDERATIONS
Leg adductors 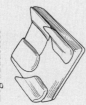	A leg adductor can be attached to the wheelchair cushion base, under the seat, or on the footrest hanger and is designed to maximize lower extremity alignment and prevent the legs from rolling into abduction or external hip rotation. This is an example of an adductor added to the front of the cushion.	Adductors can facilitate increased lower extremity alignment to minimize an individual's risk of increased deformity and pain. The height of the adductor can limit side-to-side transfers; a removable one can provide adequate support and increased safety with side transfers.
Hip guides	Hip guides provide support to maximize pelvic alignment, can be contoured or linear, and usually are made of different density foams with a solid back. Hip guides can be mounted onto the wheelchair armrests, seat pan, or back canes. The hardware can be fixed or removable. This is an example of hip guides that are attached to the rear of the cushion.	In addition to the lateral supports, hip guides can provide a third point of control for individuals with fixed or flexible spinal curves or individuals who have a pelvic obliquity. Removable hardware is often necessary for individuals who perform side-to-side transfers.
Medial knee block (pommel) with flip-down hardware 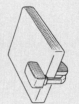	Medial knee blocks or pommels can maximize lower extremity alignment. They are designed to minimize leg adduction and internal hip rotation. For optimal support the medial knee blocks are custom-made in a variety of shapes and sizes. This contour is essential for adequate contour and fit for increased pelvic and lower extremity alignment. The knee blocks and pommels typically are constructed of a variety of foams with a solid inner component and are attached to the wheelchair with various types of hardware.	Medial knee blocks are often necessary for individuals with severe adductor spasticity. They are most successful when used with the other postural supports to maximize overall postural alignment. They can promote increased lower extremity alignment. Small medial knee blocks are helpful as a guide for more neutral lower extremity posturing.
Pelvic obliquity build-up 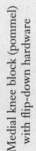	This component is usually mounted under the gel pad or created with foam; it can be a gel or foam medium and can provide increased support under the lower ischium to "correct" a deformity, under the weaker side to accommodate for muscle atrophy, or under the higher ischium to accommodate a deformity. This component may be used with hip guides to minimize lateral tilting of the pelvis for increased spinal-pelvic alignment.	Foam or gel inserts are helpful for individuals with asymmetrical muscle strength. They can compensate for the decreased muscle bulk to facilitate a more level pelvic position. When used with hip guides, inserts can support optimal pelvic alignment in individuals who have a flexible pelvis. One concern is the amount of pressure the inserts place on the ipsilateral ischial tuberosity.[17] Monitoring of pressure with this treatment approach is important. If a pelvic obliquity is fixed, positioning an insert under the higher side is necessary. This will accommodate and support the fixed pelvic obliquity, increase pressure distribution, and minimize the risk of increased deformity.

Continued

Lateral trunk supports, straight and curved

These supports usually are mounted off the back support or back canes and are available in various sizes in planar or contoured levels of support. They are beneficial for individuals with trunk weakness or a tendency to lean to one side. Another point of control, usually via hip guides, is necessary for adequate trunk support to correct a flexible deformity or accommodate a fixed deformity.

The hardware to mount to the wheelchair can be stationary or quick release.

Individuals who have decreased trunk support often hold themselves upright with their upper extremities. Lateral supports can provide increased trunk support to these individuals so that they can use their extremities for bilateral upper extremity tasks. Lateral supports also can provide the upper two points of control to correct or accommodate a lateral spinal curve for increased midline positioning of the torso in the wheelchair. The swing-away hardware is helpful to position the lateral support out of the way for transfers, dressing, and initial positioning in the wheelchair. Lateral support hardware that aggressively contours to the back support contour is necessary to keep the hardware profile minimal to allow for adequate upper extremity mobility. Curved lateral support pads provide improved contour and support over planar lateral support pads.

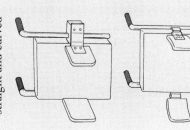

Harness/anterior chest support

Anterior chest supports are mounted to the wheelchair via four points of attachment, usually to each side of the back support and the seat rails. They are available in a variety of styles and are beneficial for individuals with severe trunk weakness. These supports often are used with a tilt or recline seating system to maximize postural support when an individual is more upright against gravity.

This component can provide anterior trunk support to allow an individual with poor trunk control to be more upright against gravity. This is helpful for more dynamic, engaging activities (i.e., working at a desk). Therapists should consider this component after evaluating a recline or tilt-in-space seating system for increased postural support in a more sedentary, posterior position. The component can be helpful for maximum trunk support for increased safety and stability when negotiating varying terrain (i.e., ramps and door saddles).

Head/neck support

Head/neck supports can be mounted to the back support via quick-release or flip down hardware. A headrest and/or neck support is essential to provide adequate head support for individuals with poor head or neck control. The quick release and flip down hardware is necessary to maneuver the headrest out of the way for positioning the client in the wheelchair, hair washing, etc.

This component is necessary for individuals with fair head control and for head and neck support when an individual tilts back for pressure relief or improved postural support. Additional pads and head bands are available for individuals with significant head positioning needs. The head and neck supports should be adjusted to support the head in as neutral alignment as possible for optimal functioning (i.e., respiration and feeding) and speech.

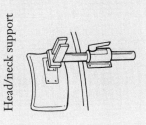

Table 26-2

Seating Systems—cont'd

SEATING COMPONENT	INDICATIONS FOR USE	POSTURAL AND FUNCTIONAL CONSIDERATIONS
Wheel lock extension	Wheel lock extensions can be mounted over the existing wheel lock handle. They are available in various sizes. Wheel lock extensions provide a longer lever arm to make it possible to access and lock/unlock the wheel locks if an individual cannot negotiate the standard wheel lock.	Extensions are important for maximum independence and to stabilize the wheelchair for functioning and safety with transfers to and from the wheelchair. For individuals with stroke, a wheel lock extension on the wheel on the client's weaker side is often very helpful for independent use with either the weaker or the stronger upper extremity.
Upper extremity support, full and half lap trays	Lap trays can be mounted over the armpad with "slide" hardware with an additional strap for stability, if necessary. They come in full or half tray models in various sizes. They can provide individuals with a support surface for their paretic upper extremity.	Adequate upper extremity support is essential to minimize an individual's risk for increased shoulder pain and deformity. A lap tray can provide a work surface for functional activities such as writing and feeding. The clear version can also provide an individual with a clear view of the feet for maximum safety with wheelchair propulsion. Upper extremity edema is often present in individuals who are unable to move their upper extremity functionally. A lap tray can facilitate increased awareness of this extremity for edema management, weight-bearing, and positioning to minimize upper extremity edema.
Arm trough	An arm trough can be mounted on the standard armrest in place of the armpad. The trough can provide more aggressive support for adequate upper extremity joint protection. Full length armrests are often necessary to provide sufficient stability for an arm trough.	An arm trough provides optimal support for individuals with absent to poor upper extremity control. Support is important to minimize the risk for pain, subluxation, and edema. An arm trough can provide an individual with a surface for upper extremity weight-bearing for functional reaching activities or for repositioning his/her body in the wheelchair.

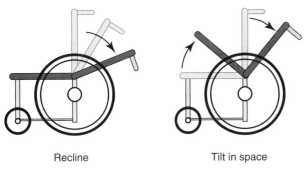

Recline   Tilt in space

Figure 26-7 Recline versus tilt options.

position independently for pressure distribution, increase postural support due to fatigue, decrease postural support for more upright seated functioning (i.e., feeding), or meet varying environmental demands (i.e., increased recline for improved support when descending a ramp).

The concept of reclining the back of the seating system or slightly tilting the seating system can be performed in 5- to 15-degree ranges in a standard wheelchair through add-on back supports and/or seat wedges. This is often necessary to accommodate hip range limitations or provide an individual with improved postural support and balance to function upright against gravity. One consideration is that this is a fixed, stationary position in a standard wheelchair. The stability of a recliner or tilt-in-space wheelchair that is specifically designed for tilt or recline is essential for this position to be a dynamic seating function.

Table 26-2 describes a variety of seating system products and secondary support products for seating systems and depicts the seating component, its indications for use, considerations for use, and the functional benefit.

FITTING THE PERSON BASED ON FUNCTIONAL STATUS

The following list addresses body structures and the seating components that can be used for individuals with hemiplegia and flexible deformities. This list encompasses individuals who have a wide range of functional abilities. One concept that is present throughout neurological rehabilitation and seating and positioning is to always provide proximal support first and then support distally. An example of this concept with an upper extremity support is to provide sufficient trunk support first, before supporting the upper extremity on a half-lap tray. This is essential to minimize the risk of injury to the shoulder girdle.

- Pelvic positioning: Wheelchair upholstery stretches over time; consequently, the sling facilitates poor postural alignment with a posterior pelvic tilt, a pelvic obliquity, and lower extremity adduction and internal rotation. A cushion with a solid base of support (such as a wood insert) is highly recommended

to provide a firm and level base of support for the pelvis on the sling wheelchair seat. This is essential for all individuals at various stages of the rehabilitation process. Initially, the support can facilitate carryover of rehabilitation restoration goals and later can provide a seating surface for upright functioning at a wheelchair level.

- Lower extremity positioning: The affected side is typically postured in a position of hip adduction and internal rotation.[2] This posture can be decreased significantly with a mild contoured cushion and a solid insert. For individuals with more significant spasticity and lower extremity adduction, postural support via gravity through tilt, a padded pelvic belt, hip guides, and a medial knee support should be considered. For individuals with severe adduction and internal rotation, medial knee blocks are necessary to minimize the risk for hip dislocation.

- Trunk: The affected hemiplegic side typically postures with lateral trunk flexion.[5] The lateral trunk flexion is often a consequence of decreased pelvic alignment. Optimal pelvic positioning with a good cushion and sacral support with a mild contoured back support can significantly decrease or fully correct the lateral trunk flexion. For individuals with severe weakness, hip guides and a build-up in the cushion can compensate for asymmetrical muscle loss and provide optimal pelvic alignment. In addition, lateral trunk supports can be added as needed to support the body in alignment. Three points of control are essential for optimal trunk support. Fig. 26-8 shows placement of these supports. It is important to remember that a fixed

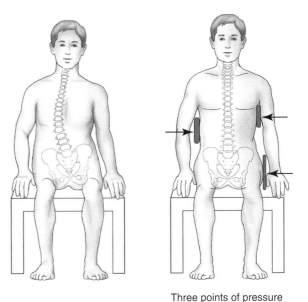

Three points of pressure

Figure 26-8 Three points of support for a lateral spinal curve.

deformity is supported to minimize the risk of increased deformity. A flexible deformity can be "corrected"; however; the therapist should monitor an individual's tolerance of this correction.

- Upper extremity: If a client has mild limitations, active use is encouraged. If an individual has significant weakness, the affected upper extremity requires adequate scapula and glenohumeral support and thus stability from a lap tray or arm trough to minimize the risk for increased pain and subluxation. Appropriate positioning is essential to facilitate optimal upper extremity alignment and motor return, and to maximize function. For a paretic upper extremity, optimal upper extremity alignment is with the shoulder in 5 degrees of abduction and flexion with neutral rotation, the elbow in 90 degrees of flexion and positioned slightly forward of the shoulder joint, the forearm in a neutral or pronated position, and the hand in a functional resting position. Functional hand splints are often integrated into the seating system for optimal wrist and hand support with the forearm supported on a lap tray. More aggressive supports and straps may be used for individuals with more severe spasticity.

- Head/neck: Typically, if an individual is seated with a stable base of support at the pelvis and lower extremities and has adequate trunk control or support, the asymmetrical neck posture decreases or disappears. For individuals with moderate to severe involvement who require hip guides and lateral supports, a headrest can be placed on the chair to ensure proper support of the cervical spine and head. After stroke, head support is generally recommended for clients with head/neck weakness, reflex activity, and/or to optimize head positioning to address visual field neglect or other visual-perceptual challenges.

- Feet: Foot support typically is determined by the person's functional level. Most individuals with hemiplegia who propel wheelchairs have the best success with propulsion using the unaffected arm and leg. Consequently, the top of the cushion to floor (seat-to-floor height) is a crucial measurement. The seat-to-floor height must allow the person's heel to access the ground for a successful heel strike to propel the wheelchair effectively. It is also important to consider the depth of the seat cushion. This should be slightly shorter than a client's seat depth or have an undercut/beveled base of the cushion for adequate freedom of movement. A leg rest or footrest should support the affected lower extremity. In general, individuals with stroke do not benefit from elevating leg rests. Elevating leg rests tend to cause overstretching of the hamstring muscles and facilitate posturing with a posterior pelvic tilt when muscle imbalance or spasticity is present.

MOBILITY BASE CONSIDERATIONS

The primary goals are to increase safety and independence with mobility and to provide an efficient method of mobility. The primary goal of the mobility base at the ICF[6] activities and participation level is to maximize an individual's ability to function and interact with the environment. An example of this would be the ability to access a closet for clothing to dress.

Unilateral Neglect

Depending on the stroke, some clients present with unilateral neglect at the body structures and function level. This leads to significant challenges with activities and participation. Several studies investigated unilateral neglect and mobility including wheelchair mobility. Qiang and colleagues[15] used a wheelchair collision test to assess behavioral unilateral neglect. Their investigation found high test-retest reliability with this as a simple screening test for unilateral neglect.

In addition to the test, several studies investigated the effect of unilateral neglect on mobility. Turton and colleagues[18] found that differences in environmental navigation were dependant on their mobility product use. They found that subjects with left side neglect tended to drift to the left with wheelchair use. However, two of the same clients consistently drifted to the opposite side, the right side, when they ambulated. Punt and colleagues[14] found that differences in subject's mobility tendencies with drifting to the ipsilesional versus contralesional side were dependant on the environment. In open spaces, the clients with neglect tended to drift toward the ipsilesional side, and in tighter spaces. clients with neglect tended to drift toward the contralesional side. Both of these studies[14,18] have implications in training individuals with neglect for safe mobility using both manual and power wheelchairs. See Chapters 18 and 19.

Manual Wheelchair Frame Styles

Two basic types of manual wheelchair frame styles are available: rigid and folding. Rigid wheelchairs tend to be lighter weight and more maneuverable than their folding counterparts. This is because of fewer moving parts and a shorter base length resulting from the integrated footrest design. Folding wheelchairs are designed with a cross brace that allows the chair to fold in half for transport and storage. The wheelchair style commonly recommended for individuals with stroke is the folding style, which is because the style is traditional and most familiar to medical professionals, can be folded up to store in the corner, fits into certain reimbursement codes, and is recognized easily by the general public.

An individual's medical condition, functional status, seating system support needs, home environment, method of community mobility, and funding source are important variables that influence the style of wheelchair frame recommended. Wheelchair frames are made of different materials to meet various chair weight requirements. The weight of the wheelchair is important if the person's strength, endurance, and propulsion abilities are in question. A basic wheelchair is constructed of aluminum, is relatively heavy, and is appropriate for persons who are not active and do not use a wheelchair as their primary means of mobility. These wheelchairs are durable enough for light everyday use and are reasonably priced. Ultra-lightweight wheelchair frames typically are constructed with aircraft aluminum or titanium and are durable but more costly than standard wheelchairs. In general, these wheelchairs are not typically recommended for individuals with stroke, even for individuals who will use a wheelchair for their primary means of mobility. There are many thoughts on why this better quality wheelchair is not recommended, which include the wheelchair code that the principal funding source Medicare has for this level wheelchair and the documentation necessary for this level of wheelchair.

Because of the increased incidence of repetitive stress injuries in individuals who use wheelchairs as their primary method of mobility, a strong case can be made for justification of an ultra-lightweight wheelchair for individuals who have sustained a stroke. For individuals with hemiplegia, trunk weakness and use of one upper extremity for all mobility, transfers, and ADL performance is of great concern. A study by Cowan and colleagues[4] focused on novice older adults and found that a more anterior axle position decreased the forces necessary to propel the wheelchair, especially on everyday surfaces such as carpets and ramps. This author feels these results support the use of an ultra-lightweight wheelchair for mobility. Ultra-lightweight wheelchairs typically have an adjustable axle that can be adjusted lower for increased trunk balance and slightly forward for a different center of gravity and an optimal hand-to-wheel relationship. This adjustment can decrease the mechanical forces required for wheelchair propulsion and is essential for energy conservation and adequate joint protection of the upper extremity. For the same reasons, power mobility can be considered as a viable option to preserve upper extremity function and maximize overall functioning and community mobility for individuals who have sustained a stroke.

Fig. 26-9 shows the basic wheelchair frame style. Consideration of frame style, wheelchair accessories, and the seating system is crucial to ensure adequate postural support and maximum function at a wheelchair level.

The following are wheelchair and wheelchair frame features that are important to consider when recommending a folding manual wheelchair.

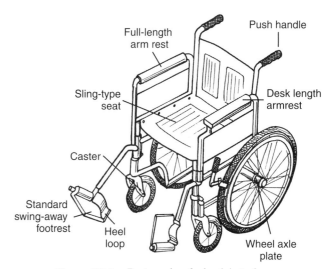

Figure 26-9   Basic style of wheelchair frame.

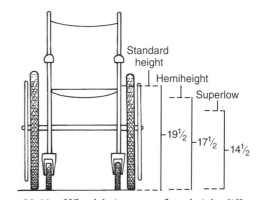

Figure 26-10   Wheelchair seat-to-floor height differences.

Wheelchair Frame Seat-to-Floor Height

Three common seat-to-floor heights are these (Fig. 26-10):
- Standard: 19.5 inches from seat to floor
- Hemi height: 17.5 inches from seat to floor
- Super low: 14.5 inches from seat to floor

The seat-to-floor height is the height from the floor to the sling seat of the wheelchair. It is important to remember that the height of the cushion chosen also influences the seat-to-floor height. The wheelchair frame height decision is based on the individual's lower extremity knee-to-heel measurement and what type of wheelchair propulsion the client uses.

If an individual pushes the wheelchair with both arms or is not independently propelling the wheelchair, the footrest clearance is a major concern. After the client is positioned with good femoral support on the wheelchair cushion, approximately 3 inches of clearance should be between the footplate and the ground. This is essential so that the client can negotiate ramps and uneven surfaces without scraping the footplates on the ground. This seat-to-floor height is often compromised to

2 inches of clearance to allow for improved table and desk access.

If an individual is negotiating the wheelchair with one arm and one foot, then the seat-to-floor height is crucial for comfort of the hemiparetic lower extremity on the foot rest and adequate heel access for propulsion of the wheelchair with one or both lower extremities.[3] The individual's knee-to-heel measurement (taken with shoe on) is generally the exact measurement from the top of the wheelchair cushion to the floor. The wheelchair should not be too high because the client will slide into a posterior pelvic tilt to obtain improved heel contact for efficient mobility.[3]

Wheel Style. Several styles of inner wheel support structure are available. For the purpose of this chapter, discussion is limited to mag wheels and spoke wheels. Wheel style is chosen based on an individual's ability to care for and maintain the wheelchair.

The team should consider the following:

- The advantage of mag wheels is that they do not require maintenance. However, they do not have as much shock absorption as spoke wheels and can be slightly heavier.
- Spoke wheels are lighter than mag wheels; however, they require periodic tightening of the individual spokes. A local bicycle shop can perform this adjustment.

Rear Wheel Size. Wheelchair wheels are measured from the ground to the top of the wheel. They are available in 12-, 20-, 22-, 24-, 25-, and 26-inch diameters. For individuals with stroke, the seat-to-floor height needs of the individual primarily determines the size of the rear wheel.

The team should consider the following:

- The standard wheel size is 24 inches.
- If an individual requires a super low wheelchair height to fit a petite frame and/or for foot propulsion, the size of the rear wheel can be 20 inches.

Tire Style. Numerous tire options are available; however, for simplicity this section focuses on the types of tires available for standard, folding wheelchairs: pneumatic, pneumatic with flat-free inserts, and polyurethane.

The team should consider the following options:

- Pneumatic tires provide a smoother ride because of good shock absorption ability. The traction of the tires provides good wheelchair stabilization for safety with transfers, and the tires handle varying terrain better than the other two options. The disadvantages are maintenance of air pressure and the risk of a flat tire.
- Pneumatic tires with flat-free inserts are pneumatic tires with an insert to replace the air. This eliminates the need for air pressure maintenance and the possibility of flats. The benefit of this combination is the traction of the tire that results in increased stability of the wheelchair for safe transfers. Unfortunately, the flat-free inserts decrease the shock absorption potential and add weight to the tire.
- Polyurethane tires are the least expensive and are durable; however, they are heavier than pneumatic tires, provide no shock absorption, and handle varying terrain poorly. In addition, the smoothness of the tire does not provide any traction of the wheelchair wheel on smooth flooring. Often these tires are the reason wheelchairs slide when persons transfer to and from them.

Wheel Handrims and One-Arm Drive Wheelchairs. Handrims are the circumferential rim on the outside of the tire to allow stroking and propulsion of the wheel. Hand rims are available in aluminum, plastic-coated, or projection styles. One-arm drive wheelchairs have two hand rims on one wheel only (Fig. 26-11).

The team should consider the following options:

- Aluminum or composite hand rims are standard on most wheelchairs. Aluminum hand rims can become slippery or cold in different weather conditions. As a result, most active wheelchair users wear specific gloves to compensate for this.
- Plastic-coated hand rims are beneficial for individuals with decreased grasp. The plastic coating provides traction against an individual's hand or a Dycem glove. The one disadvantage is that individuals cannot let the rim run through their hands as they descend hills and ramps because the friction will burn the skin on their hands.
- Projection handrims are occasionally used for individuals with decreased grasp. The disadvantages are that they can increase the overall width of the wheelchair if they are not vertical and the propulsion method is more labor intensive because one has to look continually at the handrim to hit the projection.

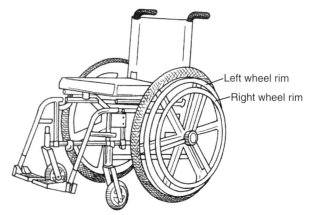

Figure 26-11 One-arm drive wheelchairs have two hand rims on one wheel only.

One-arm drive wheelchairs have right- and left-hand rims on the same side. This wheelchair was designed for individuals with only one functional upper extremity (see Fig. 26-11). The double hand rim allows one upper extremity to control the wheelchair in all directions. Use of these wheelchairs takes much strength and a high degree of coordination to move straight. In addition, this propulsion method has a longer learning curve because the concept is difficult to master. Mandy and colleagues[11] documented the inefficiency of mobility using a one-arm drive wheelchair and investigated an ankle controlled prototype product to increased efficiency with manual wheelchair use. This product demonstrated promising potential for increased efficiency with mobility in a manual wheelchair. However, it is still in the prototype phase and not readily available for purchase at this time. Unfortunately, unilateral hand-foot propulsion or a one-arm drive propulsion style are the only options available for individuals with hemiplegia at this time. Asking an individual to use his or her one functional upper extremity for wheelchair propulsion is an excessive request if one considers that the client also uses this one extremity for all other ADL. The study by Barker colleagues[1] study supports this and found the effort to mobilize a manual wheelchair was a contextual barrier for activities and participation. This study supports the concept that a power wheelchair should be strongly considered for independent mobility along with adequate upper extremity joint protection and energy conservation. The increased community participation with power mobility is supported in studies performed by Barker and colleagues[1] and Pettersson and colleagues.[13]

Wheel Axle Positioning. Standard wheelchairs allow minimal or no axle adjustment. If a standard wheelchair allows for axle positioning, it only allows the wheel to go up and down in proportion to the front caster to create a hemi- or standard-height wheelchair. On ultra-lightweight wheelchairs, an adjustable wheel axle plate allows for wheel positioning up and down and back and forth.

An adjustable axle position allows the chair to be fine-tuned by adjustment of the wheel to the best position for propulsion. This is essential for optimal wheel set-up for an energy-efficient propulsion stroke[4] and for minimizing an individual's risk for upper extremity repetitive strain injuries. As the wheel is shifted slightly into a forward position, wheel access is improved and propulsion is easier for an individual. This adjustment should be performed with caution as it affects the balance of the wheelchair. One concern is for individuals who have had a lower extremity amputation (because of a compounding diagnosis such as diabetes); the axle is better placed in a rear position to stabilize the wheelchair adequately.

Casters. Casters are the front wheels of the wheelchair (see Fig. 26-9). They are available in several diameters

(3, 4, 5, 6, and 8 inches) and two thicknesses (1 and 1.5 inches).

The team should consider the following:

- Large casters handle uneven terrain and door saddles well; however, they increase the turning radius of the wheelchair and provide higher rolling resistance to the user.
- Small casters are typical in super low and ultra-lightweight, rigid wheelchairs. They provide the client with a lower front seat-to-floor height and improved maneuverability in small areas. The disadvantage of small casters is that they become stuck in cracks and bumps on sidewalks and streets.
- Narrow-width casters handle smooth surfaces well but can become stuck easily in uneven terrain.
- The 1.5-inch width is available on the 5- and 6-inch diameter casters. This option balances maneuverability and performance over uneven surfaces; the smaller diameter provides improved maneuverability in tight areas and the increased width facilitates transitioning over different surfaces such as door saddles and prevents the casters from getting stuck in sidewalk cracks.

Elevating Leg Rests and Footrests. Elevating leg rests can raise or lower the lower extremities if an individual requires this because of a medical condition (Fig. 26-12). Footrests have a fixed knee angle and support the lower extremity in sitting.

The team should consider the following:

- Elevating leg rests typically are recommended for individuals with limited knee angles (because of arthritis or other orthopedic diagnosis), poor circulation in the lower extremities, or edema. These leg rests typically are overprescribed and should be considered carefully. An elevating leg rest usually protrudes out farther than a footrest. This increases the overall length of the wheelchair and compromises

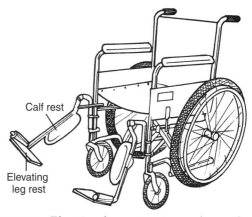

Calf rest

Elevating leg rest

Figure 26-12 Elevating leg rests raise or lower the lower extremities.

maneuverability. If an individual does not have adequate hamstring muscle elongation to tolerate this large knee angle change, he or she will sit with a posterior pelvic tilt to compensate for the lack of muscle flexibility (Fig. 26-13).[9]

- The circulation benefits of these leg rests are questionable, since they do not raise the lower extremity above the heart in a standard wheelchair.
- A major disadvantage to elevating leg rests is the significant amount of weight they add to the wheelchair.
- Footrests are available in different knee angles, typically 60, 70, and 75 degrees. The angle recommended should be based on the individual's knee range and hamstring range from the mat evaluation. Proper adjustment of the footrest length is important to ensure lower extremity stability and support in sitting. Swing-away removable footrests enable the footrests to be shifted out of the way for increased safety with transfers and improved table accessibility.
- A 70-degree angle is usually a standard option and provides a shorter turning radius than a wheelchair with the 60-degree angle footrest.

Footplates. Footplates are available in different materials such as composite and aluminum and are available in different sizes with different angle options: angle adjustable or standard.

The team should consider the following:
- The aluminum option is heavier and more durable than a composite footplate.
- An angle-adjustable footplate is essential to accommodate ankle range of motion limitations and can be helpful in accommodating hamstring muscle limitations.

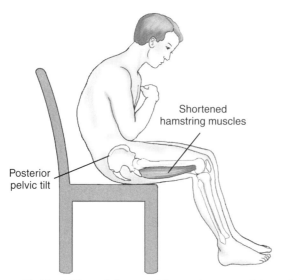

Posterior pelvic tilt

Shortened hamstring muscles

Figure 26-13   Effect of shortened hamstrings on pelvic positioning.

Armrests. Depending on the level of wheelchair, armrests (see Fig. 26-9) are available in different styles: (1) fixed or removable with different height options: fixed and adjustable height, and (2) with two different length options: full and desk length.

The team should consider the following:
- Fixed armrests are welded to the frame and set at a standard height; they cannot be adjusted. This is good for an individual who stands from the wheelchair; however, this design does not work for an individual who needs to transfer sideways to and from the wheelchair.
- Removable armrests can be positioned out of the way to allow an individual to transfer sideways into and out of the wheelchair. The armrests also can be removed from the wheelchair frame for more compact storage locations such as the trunk of a car.
- Adjustable-height armrests allow for height adjustment to provide sufficient glenohumeral support. This is important for individuals with hemiparesis and shoulder subluxation.
- Full-length arms provide full arm support at rest and upper extremity support during sit to stand and stand-pivot transfers.
- Desk-length armrests are shorter. This can provide an individual with the ability to maneuver close to desks and tables for functional activities such as feeding or writing.

Power Mobility Products

Barker and colleagues[1] studied stroke survivors and wheelchair use. They found that a manual wheelchair was actually a contextual barrier for individuals with stroke and power wheelchair use enabled community participation. Studies by Makino and colleagues[10] and Mandy and colleagues[11] also documented the inefficiency of mobility using current techniques and products (a one-arm drive wheelchair and ipsilateral hand/foot propulsion technique) and investigated different prototype products to increased efficiency with manual wheelchair use. There have been several products developed that show promising potential for increased efficiency with mobility in a manual wheelchair.[10,11] However, these products are in the prototype phase, are not necessarily practical for daily use, and are not readily available for purchase at this time. As a result, power mobility appears to be an enabling option for individuals with denser hemiplegia.

Power mobility products frequently are recommended for individuals who do not have the strength, endurance, or coordination to negotiate a wheelchair manually. Power mobility can provide individuals with increased independent and safe mobility within the home and the community. This mobility is essential to provide individuals with increased ability to perform ADL and to perform their life roles. At this time, it is important to note that clients need to present with a basic level of visual-perceptual and cognitive functioning and be available for power wheelchair mobility skills training for a power wheelchair to be a safe method of mobility. The wheelchair industry has progressed significantly in the past 20 years; consequently, a wide array of products now exist to meet the most challenging physical needs. This section gives an overview of power mobility products with a general list of considerations for each option.

Power Scooters

Scooters provide individuals who have good balance and upper extremity control with a means of power mobility. They are available in three- or four-wheel bases (Fig. 26-14). Scooters have a long and narrow base, and as a result, they are great for open areas and general outdoor community mobility. They can be disassembled for car transport; however, this is an awkward task to perform and may present an injury risk for the caregiver.

The team should consider the following:

- Scooters generally have mildly contoured seating systems. They are similar to car seats, with a limited number of options. As a result, they cannot provide sufficient postural support for individuals who need a moderate level of trunk support.
- In general, scooters are long and narrow. As a result, they have a large turning radius and often do not fit and maneuver in well in most apartments and homes.
- Four-wheeled scooters handle outdoor terrain better but are less maneuverable in smaller areas. In addition, they are heavier and therefore are more difficult for a caregiver to break down for car transport.

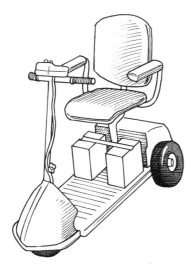

Figure 26-14 Clients are appropriate for power scooters if they have good functional control of their upper extremities, trunk control, and appropriate visual, perceptual, and cognitive skills.

Power Wheelchairs

Power wheelchairs are available with a folding frame or a power-base frame with the drive wheel in the front, middle, or rear position. For ease of discussion, power wheelchairs are divided into the front-, center-, and rear-wheel drive bases with the understanding that each of these models can be classified further into a basic-level wheelchair and a power-base wheelchair.

After the therapist determines that an individual has the range of motion to sit in most wheelchair styles and the sufficient visual-perceptual and cognitive level abilities to move safely, the next important consideration is fit of the wheelchair into and within an individual's home environment. This fit is critical and often influences the type of drive-wheel base selected.

Front-Wheel Drive Wheelchairs. A front-wheel drive wheelchair is a base with the large drive wheel in the front. This style of wheelchair is a very stable base and is beneficial for individuals with significant hamstring muscle limitations. Accommodation of hamstring tightness in a rear-wheel drive base either places excessive weight on the casters and compromises driving or an individual often has to be positioned high up to keep his feet above the caster wheels. A front wheel drive base is the only base that can accommodate positioning the feet as far back as possible without compromising the seat height and interfering with casters or motors. The team should consider the following:

- A front-wheel drive wheelchair is an excellent option for individuals who have certain environmental limitations. This style of wheelchair is excellent for tight turns into doorways at the end of a hall and maneuvering at a desk, counter, or table.
- A portable ramp is necessary for individuals to negotiate curbs or one-step entrances more than 3 inches high.
- Because of the design of this base, turning occurs in the rear, outside of the driver's visual field. Consequently, an individual requires excellent proprioception to know where the wheelchair is for safe mobility. This wheelchair base generally is not recommended if an individual has visual or cognitive limitations.

Mid-Wheel Drive Wheelchairs. For the purpose of this chapter, the term *mid-wheel drive wheelchair* includes center-wheel drive wheelchairs. A mid-wheel drive wheelchair is a wheelchair base that has the drive wheel in the center of the wheelchair with smaller wheels in the front and the rear. This base requires wheels in the front and the back for maximum stability of the wheelchair base. Because the drive wheel is in the middle, this wheelchair usually has the smallest turning radius and is the most maneuverable in tight areas.

The team should consider the following:

- Because of the design of this base, turning occurs at the center, which is the same axis on which the body turns. As a result, some individuals feel that this is an easier drive method to learn; however, one concern is that some of the turning occurs in the rear, outside of the driver's visual field. Consequently, an individual requires good proprioception to know where the wheelchair is for safe mobility. This wheelchair base generally is not recommended if an individual has more involved visual or cognitive limitations.
- A portable ramp is necessary for individuals to negotiate curbs or one-step entrances more than 3 inches high.

Rear-Wheel Drive Wheelchairs. A rear-wheel drive wheelchair is the original style of power wheelchair in the United States. Because the drive wheel is in the rear position, most of the weight of the wheelchair is in the rear. As a result, this style of wheelchair has small "anti-tipper" wheels in the back for maximum safety ascending inclines.

The team should consider the following:

- This wheelchair base maneuvers similar to a car, and consequently, many individuals find the drive familiar and, as a result, the wheelchair easy to operate.
- This wheelchair base is easier to control at higher speeds than the comparable front-wheel drive and mid-wheel drive models.
- Because of the design of this wheelchair base, the turning wheels are in front of the driver. As a result, all turns happen within the driver's visual field. This is the optimal situation for individuals with sensory (auditory), visual, or cognitive limitations because this base provides the driver with the maximum amount of visual input about the environment they are negotiating.
- Because of the design of this wheelchair base, the footrests have to be positioned in front to allow the casters to turn. This increases the overall length of the wheelchair and results in a larger turning radius. Consequently, a rear-wheel drive base is not as maneuverable in tight areas as a mid-wheel drive base.
- This wheelchair base can be assisted up an 8-inch step and curbs, if necessary. If a rear-wheel drive wheelchair is tipped back onto the tippers, the amount of caster clearance determines the actual height one can negotiate with assistance of another person. This is important for one-step entrances and curbs that are 6 to 8 inches in height. This feature is not a luxury but a necessity for individuals to access their favorite restaurants and stores without a ramp. This is an advanced skill and should only be performed with a skilled therapist or supplier.

Basic Power Wheelchair

A basic power wheelchair is durable and can handle relatively level terrain. Most basic power wheelchairs operate by joystick. The joystick controls the speed and direction of the wheelchair. Some basic power wheelchairs can even be folded for car transport.

The team should consider the following:

- Basic power wheelchairs have basic electronics with little programmability. Consequently, if an individual requires a higher degree of electronics adjustments because of tremors, spasticity, or ataxia, a power base with more flexible electronics may be indicated.
- If an individual requires a moderate or aggressive level of postural support, including a tilt or recline seating system, this wheelchair base would not meet that person's needs.
- Because of its folding crossbar and flexible frame, a power folding frame does not handle terrain as well as a power base. However, for basic power mobility, the model is an efficient and reasonably priced alternative.
- Power folding frames are practical in theory but not in reality. Although the frame can be folded by pulling out the batteries and battery tray, the wheelchair components are still heavy and awkward. Two strong adults can lift the folded power frame in and out of a van or car; however, daily use with one person assisting the individual with a stroke is difficult and unrealistic.

Power Wheelchair Bases. Power wheelchair bases are much more durable than basic power wheelchair frames. The frame style is more rigid, which translates into increased durability, increased ability to handle uneven terrain, and a smoother ride. In addition, the base style wheelchairs are often available with the option for more advanced, higher-level electronics and the option for a more supportive seating system such as a tilt or recline seating system.

The team must consider that power bases cannot be disassembled for car transport. As a result, these individuals would need access to transportation by a bus, ambulette, or accessible van.

Power Wheelchair Options. For most power wheelchairs, a wide array of joystick handle and joystick mounting options are available to position the joystick in the best location for an individual with a stroke. These include larger ball joystick handles, built-up cylindrical-type joystick handles, swing-away joystick mounts, and midline joystick mounting brackets.

On power wheelchairs with more advanced electronics, alternative drive methods such as a single-switch scanner, a head array, or a pneumatic controller can be easily set up. These options can enable individuals who do not have the upper extremity control to operate a joystick or modified joystick to maneuver the wheelchair safely and independently.

REVIEW QUESTIONS

1. What are the most important considerations when recommending a wheelchair and seating system?
2. Why is a mat evaluation an important first step before considering a wheelchair and seating system?
3. What is the treatment approach difference for a fixed versus a flexible deformity?
4. What is a wheelchair contributing factor to sitting with a posterior pelvic tilt?
5. What are the basic differences between a rigid and a folding wheelchair?
6. In addition to the mat evaluation, what are important areas to screen when considering power mobility?
7. What are the differences between a front-wheel drive, mid-wheel drive, and rear-wheel drive power wheelchair?

REFERENCES

1. Barker DJ, Reid D, Cott C: The experience of senior stroke survivors: factors in community participation among wheelchair users. *Can J Occup Ther* 73(1):18–25, 2006.
2. Bergen A: Assessment for seating and wheeled mobility systems. *Team Rehab Rep.* April 1998, 16.
3. Buck S: Wheelchair propulsion by foot: assessment considerations. *Top Stroke Rehabil* 11(4):68–71, 2004.
4. Cowan RE, Nash MS, Collinger JL, et al: Impact of surface type, wheelchair weight, and axle position on wheelchair propulsion by novice older adults. *Arch Phys Med Rehabil* 90(7):1076–1083, 2009.
5. Davies PM: *Steps to follow: a guide to the treatment of adult hemiplegia*, Heidelberg, Germany, 1985, Springer-Verlag.
6. *International classification of functioning, disability and health: ICF short version*, Geneva, 2001, World Health Organization.
7. Judai JW: Psychosocial impact of assistive devices in stroke. *Proceedings of the twenty-sixth International RESNA Conference on Technology and Disability: Research, Design, Practice, and Policy*, Atlanta, June 2003.
8. Kangas KM: The task performance position: providing seating for accurate access to assistive technology. *Physical Disabilities Special Interest Section Quarterly* 23(3), 2000.
9. Lipka DD: BuyerBeware.com. *Physical Disabilities Special Interest Section Quarterly* 23(3):3, 2000.
10. Makino K, Wada F, Hachisuka K, et al: Speed and physiological cost index of hemiplegic patients pedaling a wheelchair with both legs. *J Rehabil Med* 37(2):83–86, 2005.
11. Mandy A, Lesley S: Measures of energy expenditure and comfort in an ESP wheelchair: a controlled trial using hemiplegic users. *Disabil Rehabil Assist Technol* 4(3):137–142, 2009.
12. National Stroke Association: *What is stroke?* (website). www.stroke.org/site/DocServer/STROKE_101_Fact_Sheet.pdf?docID=4541. Accessed April 11, 2009.
13. Pettersson I, Ahlstrom G, Tornquiat K: The value of an outdoor powered wheelchair with regard to the quality of life of persons with stroke: a follow up study. *Asst Technol* 19(3):143–153, 2007.
14. Punt TD, Kitadono K, Hulleman J, et al: From both sides now: crossover effects influence navigation in patients with unilateral neglect. *J* et al: 79(4):464–466, 2008.
15. Qiang W, Sonoda S, Suzuki M, et al: Reliability and validity of a wheelchair collision test for screening behavior assessment of unilateral neglect after stroke. *Am J Phys Med Rehabil* 84(3):161–166, 2005.
16. Rudman DL, Heber D, Reid D: Living in a restricted occupational world: The occupational experiences of stroke survivors who are wheelchair users and their caregivers. *CJOT* 73(3):141–152, 2006.
17. Shea M: A wheelchair cushion insert and its effect on pelvic pressure distribution. *Proceedings of the twenty-third International RESNA Conference: Technology for the New Millennium*, Orlando, FL, June 2000.
18. Turton AJ, Dewar SJ, Lievesley A, et al: Walking and wheelchair navigation in patients with left visual neglect. *Neuropsych Rehabil* 19(2), 274–290, 2009.
19. Zollars JA: *Special seating: an illustrated guide*, Minneapolis, MN, 1996, Otto Back Orthopedic Industry.

SUGGESTED READINGS

Angelo J: *Assistive technology for rehabilitation therapists*, 1997, Philadelphia, FA Davis.
Axleton P, Chesney D, Minkel, J, et al: *The manual wheelchair training guide*, Santa Cruz, CA, 1998, Pax Press.
Axleton P, Minkel J, Chesney D: *A guide to wheelchair selection: how to use the ANSI/RESNA wheelchair standards to buy a wheelchair*, Washington, DC., 1994, Paralyzed Veterans of America.
Bergen AF: *Positioning for function*, Valhalla, NY, 1990, Valhalla Rehabilitation.
Carr EK: Positioning of the stroke person: a review of the literature. *Int J Nurs Stud* 29(4):355, 1992.
Ferido T: Spasticity in head trauma and CVA persons: etiology and management. *J Neurosci Nurs* 20(1):17, 1988.
Lange ML: Positioning the upper extremities. *OT Practice* May 1999.
Lange ML: Power wheelchair access methods. *OT Practice* July/Aug 1999.
Lange ML: Tilt in space versus recline: new trends in an old debate. *Tech Spec Interest Section Q* 10(2): 1–3, 2000.
Minkel JL: *Sitting solutions: principles of wheelchair positioning and mobility devices*, New Windsor, NY, 1996, Minkel Consulting.
Ramsey C: Power mobility access methods. *Tech Spec Interest Section Q* 9(3):1–3, 1999.
Sparacio J: The effects of seating on upper-extremity function. *Tech Spec Interest Section Q* 9(2):1–2, 1999.
Sweet-Michaels B: Alternative methods for power wheelchair control: then and now. *Tech Spec Interest Section Q* 9(3):1–4, 1999.
Taylor SJ: The head control dilemma. *Tech Spec Interest Section Q* 9(2): 1–3, 1999.
Trefler E: Then and now: simulators have evolved from simple positioning chairs into devices with multiple uses and benefits. Is it time your facility purchased one? *Team Rehab Rep* Feb:32, 1999.
US Department of Health and Human Services: In *Pressure ulcers in adults: prediction and prevention*, Rockville MD, 1992, US Department of Health and Human Services, AHCPR Pub No 92–0050.
Vogel B: Maintaining your chair. *New Mobility* June:25, 2003.

RESOURCES

Clinician websites

www.gatech.edu
www.iss.pitt.edu
www.resna.org
www.pva.org

Manufacturer websites

www.aelseating.com
www.artgrouprehab.com
www.bodypoint.com
www.invacare.com
www.pdgmobility.com
www.permobilus.com
www.pridemobility.com
www.sunrisemedical.com
www.supracor.com
www.therohogroup.com
www.varilite.com

Consumer websites

www.rolli-moden.com
www.spinlife.com
www.sportaid.com
www.stroke.org

Accessibility websites

www.access-board.gov – US Access Board

catherine a. duffy

chapter 27

Home Evaluation
and Modifications

key terms

accessibility
adaptations
architectural barriers

durable medical equipment
home environment

mobility
safety

chapter objectives

After completing this chapter, the reader will be able to accomplish the following:

1. Apply methods of assessing the home environment for barriers.
2. Understand architectural guidelines as established by the American National Standards Institute.
3. Implement methods for modifying the home environment and increase safety and mobility independence for patients recovering from stroke.

A barrier-free environment in the home and community is essential to successful independent living for individuals who are elderly or physically disabled and particularly for individuals who have suffered stroke.[2] Throughout the rehabilitation process, therapists work with patients toward the goal of achieving independence in mobility and self-care. However, this process usually occurs in an institutionalized setting that is relatively free of architectural barriers.[1] *Architectural barriers* are defined as architectural features (e.g., stairs and doors) in the home and community that make negotiating at will difficult or impossible for an individual.

Most individuals with disabilities wish to return to their own homes. For many, some type of durable medical equipment and home modifications are necessary to achieve easy access.[3]

Understanding the patient's home environment is an integral part of treatment and discharge planning. A home visit with the patient should occur well before the discharge date to provide recommendations to facilitate safety and independence. The therapist uses information gained from this home visit to modify the existing treatment plan and establish appropriate therapy goals. This chapter focuses on architectural barriers commonly found in the home, ways to eliminate them, basic wheelchair information, and a general overview of methods for assessment appropriate for patients who have had a stroke. This chapter—with its bulleted, quick-reference format—is intended to be used as a resource for practical suggestions that will assist the occupational therapist's clinical reasoning process when evaluating the homes of stroke survivors.

BASIC GUIDELINES AND WHEELCHAIR INFORMATION

The wheelchairs shown in Figs. 27-1 to 27-6 are based on a standard adult-size chair. Dimensions vary with the size of the patient using the chair. See Chapter 26 for information regarding specific wheelchair adaptations. The therapist must know the specific size and type of wheelchair being prescribed for the patient before making recommendations for home modifications.

EVALUATING THE HOME

Evaluation for architectural barriers usually is organized by room. In this approach, the therapist considers the following information during a home evaluation:

Exterior

Suggestions include the following:
- Assess type of residence: Note whether dwelling is a house or apartment building; determine whether dwelling has elevator or staircase access; examine steps (their number, height, width, and depth); note walkway railings and width; and assess distance and grade between the dwelling entrance and the curb or driveway.

- Note protection from the weather: Examine the condition of surfaces over which the wheelchair must travel (e.g., grass that becomes mud, concrete with cracks, shaded bricks covered with moss, and asphalt that softens in the hot summer sun).
- Examine driveway: Note size and ability to accommodate a wheelchair van; assess composition (solid or boulevard style with a strip of dirt in the middle); and determine whether surface is paved or gravel.
- Survey surrounding area: Look for trees that drop nuts, branches, leaves, and pine cones; note location of mailbox.

Entrances

Suggestions include the following:
- Consider all entrances to evaluate accessibility; note any entrances inaccessible to the patient.
- Measure steps and landings and note the presence and height of railings.
- Measure all doorway widths and heights, including interior doors to closets and between rooms.
- Note the direction of each door swing, the presence and height of any sills, and the height of any installed locks; determine whether screen doors open outward and solid doors open inward, and assess the

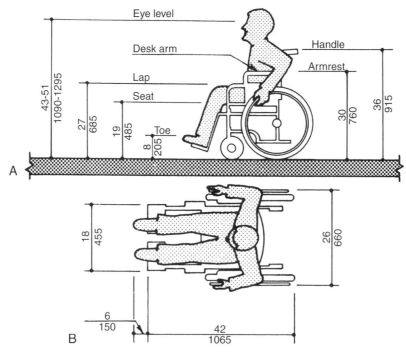

Figure 27-1 Dimensions of standard adult manual wheelchair (metric measurements are in millimeters). Width: 24 to 26 inches from rim to rim. Length: 42 to 43 inches. Height to push handles from floor: 36 inches. Height to seat from floor: 19 to 19½ inches (excluding cushion). Height to armrest from floor: 29 to 30 inches. NOTE: Footrests may extend farther for very large persons. (From American National Standards Institute: *Accessible and usable buildings and facilities*, New York, 1992, The Institute.)

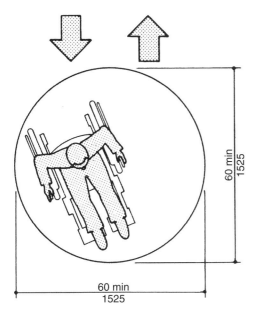

Figure 27-2 Wheelchair turning space of 360 degrees (metric measurements are in millimeters). A 360-degree turn requires a clear space of 60 by 60 inches. This space enables the individual to turn without scraping the feet or maneuvering multiple times to accomplish a full turn. *min,* Minimum. (From American National Standards Institute: *Accessible and usable buildings and facilities,* New York, 1992, The Institute.)

weight of the doors and whether they can be moved from a wheelchair.

■ If the patient lives in a building with an elevator, note whether the chair can be maneuvered into the elevator; assess whether the elevator stops flush with the landing; and consider whether the patient can reach the buttons.

Interior

Suggestions include the following:

■ Assess the number of levels and whether the bedrooms are located upstairs or downstairs; consider relocating a bedroom downstairs for improved mobility.

■ Count and measure all steps (their height, width, and landing), and note whether handrails exist on both sides.

■ Measure the dimensions of the staircase; note the stair height, width, and depth.

Living Room and Hallways

Suggestions include the following:

■ Consider phone accessibility; height of light switches, thermostats, and electrical sockets; furniture arrangement; floor covering; and doorway width and thresholds. Note the width of the hallway and number of turns.

■ Determine whether the patient will be able to open and close windows; note whether the windows slide up and down or swing outward; and measure the height of the latches.

Bedroom

Suggestions include the following:

■ Measure doorway width, threshold height, and mattress height.

■ Consider space for hospital bed and bedside commode; note floor space and covering (i.e., carpet, wood, tile, or linoleum) because these may have an effect on walking and wheelchair mobility.

■ Note whether the bed is stable for transfer.

■ Assess the accessibility of dressers and closets.

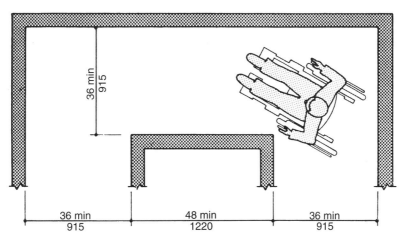

Figure 27-3 Wheelchair turning space of 90 degrees (metric measurements are in millimeters). A 90-degree turn requires a minimum of 36 inches for the wheelchair user to have clear space for the feet and prevent scraping the hands on the wall. *min,* Minimum. (From American National Standards Institute: *Accessible and usable buildings and facilities,* New York, 1992, The Institute.)

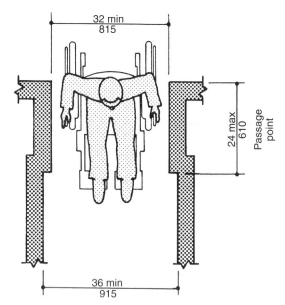

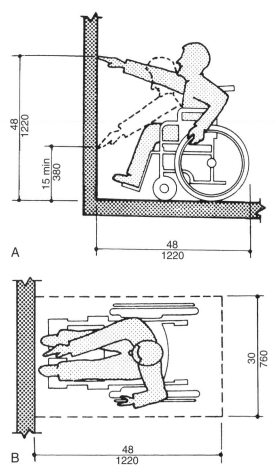

Figure 27-4 Minimum clear width for doorways and halls (metric measurements are in millimeters). A minimum of 32 inches of doorway width is required; the ideal is 36 inches. Hallways should be a minimum of 36 inches wide to provide sufficient clearance for wheelchair passage and allow the user to propel the chair without scraping the hands. *max*, Maximum; *min*, minimum. (From American National Standards Institute: *Accessible and usable buildings and facilities*, New York, 1992, The Institute.)

Figure 27-5 Forward reach (metric measurements are in millimeters). The maximal height an individual can reach from a seated position is 48 inches. Height should be at least 15 inches to prevent the wheelchair from tipping forward. *min*, Minimum. (From American National Standards Institute: *Accessible and usable buildings and facilities*, New York, 1992, The Institute.)

■ If a mechanical lift is being prescribed, ensure enough room is available to maneuver it around the bed.

Bathroom

Suggestions include the following:
■ Measure the door width and threshold height, and note the direction of the door swing (inward or outward).
■ Measure the entry width and note the type of entry of the shower or bathtub; determine the inside and outside sill height and sill width; measure the length, width (inside top and bottom), and height of the faucet; and note the type of shower head.
■ Note whether the wall is plasterboard, tile, or fiberglass; the type of wall affects the installation of grab bars.
■ Measure the height of the toilet, the available space on the left and right, and the space in front of it; check whether the toilet paper roll is within easy reach; and consider the sink height and counter distances to the left and right.
■ Determine the presence of any nonslip treatment in the tub; note whether the patient has a shower curtain or a glass door.

Kitchen

Suggestions include the following:
■ Measure the height and depth of the basin of the sink, the distance to the faucet knobs, cabinet and counter heights, and refrigerator door heights.
■ Consider table height in relation to wheelchair fit.
■ Note outlet height and location, type of controls and location on the stove and microwave, and height and accessibility of light switches.

Laundry

Suggestions include the following:
■ Note the location and measurements of the washer and dryer if relevant.
■ Determine whether the washer and dryer are front loading or top loading.

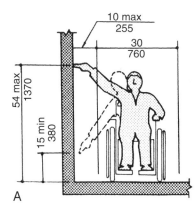

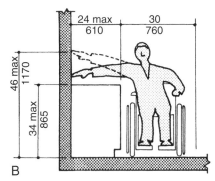

Figure 27-6 Side reach (metric measurements are in millimeters). The maximal height for reaching from the side position without an obstruction is 54 inches. If an obstruction such as a countertop or shelf is present, the maximal height for side reach is 46 inches. *max*, Maximum; *min*, minimum. (From American National Standards Institute: *Accessible and usable buildings and facilities*, New York, 1992, The Institute.)

■ Assess whether the washer and dryer are installed permanently or must be moved into place and set up each time for use.

Basement

The therapist should examine the staircase, railings, windows, furnace controls, fuse box, and lighting.

Sketches of each room with notations of problematic areas are useful for the therapist attempting home simulation during treatment sessions. The therapist should provide a brief summary of findings with recommendations for modifications and safety to the family.

HOME EVALUATION FORMS

Evaluation formats range from simple to complex, depending on the therapist's and patient's needs. Figs. 27-7 to 27-10 show samples of home assessments.

MODIFICATIONS

The therapist's recommendations should meet the patient's need to function with the greatest level of independence and safety. The therapist must consider the patient's

budget and the extent of the structural changes necessary to attain the patient's goals. The therapist should consult building contractors and obtain bids for extensive reconstruction needs and to assist with determining the feasibility of structural modifications. Generally, modifications should be made in accordance with the guidelines established by the American National Standards Institute.[1]

The American National Standards Institute publishes the document American *National Standards for Buildings and Facilities,*[1] which provides specifications to make buildings and other facilities accessible and usable for individuals with physical disabilities. The examples provided are reprinted to increase occupational therapists' understanding of specifications needed for patients who are recovering from a stroke and who rely on wheelchairs for independent mobility.

Exterior

A parking space with a 4-foot aisle adjacent to it allows an individual to maneuver a wheelchair alongside the car. Pathways and walkways should be a minimum of 48 inches wide and have smooth surfaces to prevent tipping and difficult wheelchair mobility. Motion-sensitive or automatically timed lighting along walkways provides safety. At least one entrance to the home should have easy access. If all entrances are reached by stairs, the number of steps influences the solution to creating a no-step entrance. Options include ramps, stair gliders, or porch lifts.

General Comments on Ramps
The therapist should consider the following:
■ Ramps should be a minimum of 36 inches wide and have nonskid surfaces.
■ The ideal ratio of slope to rise is 1:12—every inch of vertical rise requires 12 inches of ramp (Fig. 27-11).
■ Ramps should have level landings at the top and bottom of each run; the landing should be at least as wide as the ramp; and to allow unobstructed ability to open the door, a 24-inch area is needed.
■ Handrails should be waist high for individuals who can walk (a minimum of 34 to 38 inches) and should extend a minimum of 12 inches beyond the top and bottom runs.
■ Ramps require railings or curbs at least 4 inches high to prevent individuals from slipping off the ramp

General Comments on Stairs
The therapist should consider the following:
■ According to American National Standards Institute, all steps on a flight of stairs should have uniform riser heights (a maximum of 7 inches) and tread depth (a minimum of 11 inches)
■ All stairs should have handrails; the handrail grasping surface should be ½ inch to 2 inches in diameter

Text continued on p.708

OCCUPATIONAL THERAPY
HOME ASSESSMENT WORKSHEET

Address visited_____

Date of assessment_____

Exterior:

Type of residence:

☐ House   ☐ Own   ☐ Rent

☐ Apartment   ☐ Care home

Distance from parked car to home:_____

Distance from home to curb:_____

Ramping space: 1 foot of ramp to 1 inch of elevation

Maximum length: 30 ft

Level platform: 5 square ft

Platform at door: 5 square ft

Railings

Type of terrain:

☐ Incline   ☐ Concrete/asphalt

☐ Smooth   ☐ Rough

Walkway width: _____inches wide

AREA	IDEAL	ACTUAL	COMMENTS/DIAGRAM
Entrance:			
Most accessible entry:			
Front Rear Side		Front Rear Side	
Steps (ground to porch)	7 inches high with nonskid stripes	Number_____ Height_____ Width_____ Depth_____ Carpet Nonskid strip_____ Artificial turf_____	
Landing		Number_____ Width_____ Depth_____	
Railings (ascending steps)	32 inches high– extends 1½ ft beyond top and bottom step	Left _____ Right _____ Height_____	
Porch size	4 or 5 square ft	Width_____ Depth_____	
Height of step from porch to house level	7 inches high		
Doorway width	36 inches wide		
Swing of door		In _____ Out _____	
Screen door swing		In _____ Out _____	
Threshold	Level with floor		

Staff   Date   Time

Figure 27-7   Occupational therapy home assessment worksheet. (Courtesy K. Hatae, V. Tully, N. Wade; Honolulu, Hawaii.)

AREA	IDEAL	ACTUAL	COMMENTS/DIAGRAM
Interior:			
Number of levels within the house			
Number of steps			
Steps	7 inches high with nonskid stripes	Number _____ Height _____ Width _____ Depth _____	
Railings (ascending steps)		Left _____ Right _____	
Landing		Height _____ Number _____ Width _____ Depth _____	
Living Room:			
Threshold	Level with floor		
Doorway width	36 inches wide		
Floor covering	Wood/tile		
Furniture arrangement	5 square feet turning space		
Favorite chair	Wheelchair height		
Density	Firm	Height _____	
Armrest	Both sides		
Phone accessibility	No long wire Cordless		
Television accessibility	Remote control		
Outlets	18 inches from floor		
Light switches	36 inches from floor		
Hallways:			
Width	36-48 inches wide	Turns _____ Straight	
Turns	Straight		
Floor covering	Wood/tile		
Bedroom:			
Doorway width	36 inches wide		
Door swing		In _____ Out _____	
Threshold height	Level with floor		
Floor covering	Wood/tile		
Telephone accessibility	Next to bed		
Bed size	Single, double, queen, king		
Mattress height	Wheelchair height		
Mattress density	Firm		
Space for hospital bed	36 inches x 88 inches		
Space for bedside commode	24 inches x 24 inches		
Night light	Next to bed		

Staff   Date   Time

Figure 27-7, cont'd

Continued

AREA	IDEAL	ACTUAL	COMMENTS/DIAGRAM
Bell	Next to bed		
Outlets	18 inches from floor		
Light switches	36 inches from floor		
Wheelchair turning space	5 square ft × 5 square ft		
Dresser accessibility	Toe space below		
Closets:			
Accessibility	Bifold, curtain		
Rod height	No higher than 48 inches		
Bathroom:			
Threshold	Level with floor		
Door width			
Door width (with door)	36 inches wide		
Door swing		In _____ Out _____	
Shower/tub:			
Entry width		Entry width _____	
Type of entry	Curtain	Curtain, glass door	
Sill height (outside)			
Sill height (inside)			
Sill width			
Sill width–wall			
Width (inside top)			
Width (inside bottom)			
Length (inside top)			
Length (inside bottom)			
Faucet height			
Shower head (type)	Removable for hose		
Wall type (e.g., tile, fiberglass)		Tile, fiberglass	
Toilet			
Height			
Distance on left (sitting on toilet)	3-9 inches minimum		
Distance on right	3-9 inches minimum		
Distance in front	30 inches		
Lavatory			
Height	26-30 inches		
Distance on left			
Distance on right			
Distance in front			
Accessibility below			

Staff   Date   Time

Figure 27-7, cont'd

AREA	IDEAL	ACTUAL	COMMENTS/DIAGRAM
Electric outlets	Open for knee space	Yes ——— No ———	
Wall surface	Wood		
Floor covering	No scatter rugs Tile/linoleum		
Wheelchair turning space	5 square ft		
Kitchen:			
Door width			
Sink			
Height			
Knee space			
Basin depth	$6^1/_2$ inches deep		
Type		Double/single	
Faucet control		Double/single	
Distance to faucet			
Cabinets			
Stove		Gas/electric	
Height			
Controls	Front	Front/back/top	
Oven-handle height			
Type		Wall/integral	
Refrigerator			
Door height			
Door hinge		Left/right	
Freezer			
Door height			
Door hinge		Left/right/side	
Outlets			
Light switches	36 inches from floor		
Table height			
Chair height			
Counter height	30 inches high		
Telephone accessibility			
Appliances:			

Staff   Date   Time

Figure 27-7, cont'd

Continued

AREA	IDEAL	ACTUAL	COMMENTS/DIAGRAM
Laundry:			
Location			
Doorway width	36 inches		
Number of steps		Number _____	
		Height _____	
		Width _____	
		Depth _____	
Railings (ascending steps)		Left ____ Right ____	
		Height _____	
Washer door	Front opening		
Controls	Front panel	Front/back	
Dryer door	Front opening		
Controls	Front panel	Front/back	
Clothes line location		Height _____	
Patio:			
Doorway width	36 inches		
Type of door		Sliding/hinged	
Threshold	Level with floor		
Steps		Number _____	
		Height _____	
		Width _____	
		Depth _____	
Railings (ascending steps)		Left ____ Right ____	
		Height _____	

_____
Staff   Date   Time

Figure 27-7, cont'd

HOME VISIT EVALUATION

Name of patient: _____ M/F _____ Age: _____

Address: _____ Phone number: _____

Diagnosis and disability: _____

_____

_____

Status of patient on discharge:

Ambulatory Status

Is patient ambulating independently?   Yes _____ No _____

Does patient use assistive device? If yes, what type? _____

Wheelchair?   If yes: Standard _____ Motorized _____

Cognitive Status

Is patient alert and oriented?   Yes _____ No _____

Does patient have memory deficits?   Yes _____ No _____

Judgement and safety awareness: Intact _____ Impaired _____

Vision: _____

Hearing: _____

- -

Who will be home to assist patient?

   Family member _____ Home attendant _____ hours per day

In what capacity?

   Self-care _____ Domestic _____ Total _____

For whom will patient be responsible?

   Self _____ Spouse _____ Children (number) _____

For which activities of home management was patient formerly responsible?

   Cooking _____ Laundry _____ Cleaning _____

   Shopping _____ Child care _____

For which activities of home management will patient now be responsible?

   Cooking _____ Laundry _____ Cleaning _____

   Shopping _____ Child care _____

Actual home visit

Type of residence patient lives in:

   House _____ Apartment _____

                    What floor? _____

                    Is there an elevator?   Yes _____ No _____

                    Width of elevator (for w/c) _____

Are there stairs to enter house/apartment?   Yes _____ No _____

   How many? _____

Are structural alterations allowed in residence?   Yes _____ No _____

How many rooms in house/apartment? _____

Can patient get to all rooms?

   Bedroom _____ Kitchen _____ Bathroom _____ Living room _____

   (If patient is in a wheelchair, width of doorway must be at least 30-32 inches.)

If private house:

   Can patient sleep on ground floor?   Yes _____ No _____

   Are there bathrooms on every floor?   Yes _____ No _____

Figure 27-8   Home visit evaluation. (Courtesy K. Hatae, V. Tully, N. Wade; Honolulu, Hawaii.)

Continued

Bedroom

Width of doorway: _____

Height of bed: _____

Is there room for bedside commode?   Yes _____ No _____

Kitchen

Width of doorway: _____

Height of: Sink _____ Stove _____ Cabinets _____ Table _____ Chair _____

Where are meals eaten?   Kitchen _____ Dining room _____

How far is table from cooking area? _____ From refrigerator? _____

Living Room

Width of doorway: _____

Height of: Sofa _____ Chair _____

Do chairs have armrests?   Yes _____ No _____

Bathroom

Width of doorway: _____

Toilet

Height: _____

Width of space to nearest surface (e.g., wall, sink):   Right _____ Left _____

Are walls sturdy enough for grab bars?   Yes _____ No _____

Is there a shower stall? _____ Bathtub? _____ Bathtub with shower? _____

Does patient shower? _____ Bathe? _____ Shower in tub? _____

Shower stall

Glass doors _____ Shower curtain _____

Is there a step up or down? _____ Height _____

Are there grab bars?   Yes _____ No _____

Height of faucets: _____

Width of shower stall: _____

Length of shower stall: _____

Bathtub

Glass doors _____ Shower curtain _____

Facing tub—where are faucets?   Right _____ Left _____ Straight ahead _____

Height of faucets: _____

Height of bathtub: _____

Width of bathtub: _____

Length of bathtub: _____

Miscellaneous

Carpeting? _____ Area rugs? _____

How many telephones does patient have? _____ Wall phones _____ Desk phones _____

Does patient currently own any adaptive equipment? What type? _____

Figure 27-8, cont'd

Equipment recommendations

Home adaptation recommendations

Follow-up

Equipment ordered from _____ , _____
(Vendor)   (Phone number)

on _____ .
(Date)

Equipment to be delivered to _____ on _____ .
(Date)

Date of home visit: _____

Did patient go on home visit? _____

_____   _____
(Name of occupational therapist)   (Phone number)

Figure 27-8, cont'd

To: _____

Address: _____

From: _____

Date: _____

Purpose:

**RECOMMENDATIONS FOR PREVENTING FALLS
AND/OR INCREASING ACCESSIBILITY WITHIN THE HOME**

Exterior

☐ Entrance: Use   ☐ Front   ☐ Back   ☐ Side   ☐ Other

☐ Stairs: ☐ Use nonskid stripes on step edges.

    ☐ Reinforce stairs.   ☐ Remove: _____

☐ Handrails: ☐ Install: Right/left   ☐ Secure handrails.

☐ Walkway: ☐ Cover with nonslip material.   ☐ Remove: _____

    ☐ Repair broken walkway.

☐ Door: ☐ Assist with door.

    ☐ Install door-closing mechanism.

    ☐ Add hook to door and _____

Notes:

Living Room

☐ Entrance: ☐ Locate lamp close to entry of room.

☐ Floor: ☐ Remove throw rugs.   ☐ Tape or tack down carpet.

    ☐ Clear walking path of electrical/phone cords.

☐ Space: ☐ Clear room of furniture and other obstacles.

☐ Furniture: ☐ Ensure that tables and chairs can provide support if leaned on.

    ☐ Remove furniture with wheels or unsteady bases.

    ☐ Remove low-lying objects (e.g., coffee tables).

Notes:

Hallway/Stairwell

☐ Lighting: ☐ Install light.   ☐ Change light bulb.

☐ Handrails: ☐ Install: Right/left   ☐ Secure for sturdiness.

☐ Other: ☐ Remove obstacles: _____

Notes:

Bedroom

☐ Lighting: ☐ Install nightlight and/or bedside lamp.

☐ Path from bed

    to bathroom: ☐ Remove obstacles: _____

☐ Bed: ☐ Rearrange: _____

    ☐ Lower/elevate bed: _____

☐ Clothes: ☐ Arrange closet: _____

☐ Other: ☐ Install bell/intercom.

Notes:

Figure 27-9   Recommendations for preventing falls and/or increasing accessibility within the home. (Courtesy K. Hatae, V. Tully, N. Wade; Honolulu, Hawaii.)

OCCUPATIONAL THERAPY
RECOMMENDATIONS FOR HOME MODIFICATIONS
FOR SAFETY AND ACCESSIBILITY

Patient name: _____

AREA OF CONCERN	PROBLEM	RECOMMENDATIONS	RESPONSIBLE PERSON
Bathroom entrance	☐ Doorway is too narrow. ☐ Tub/shower entrance is too narrow: _____ inches wide. ☐ Towel rack is unsteady as support. ☐ Throw rugs pose a trip hazard.	☐ Remove/widen door. ☐ Remove tub/shower door and replace with curtain. ☐ Remove and replace with grab bars. ☐ Remove rugs.	
Bathing	☐ Balance is unsteady. ☐ Rinsing is difficult. ☐ Tub/shower floor is slippery when wet.	☐ Sit to bathe. ☐ Use a bath bench. ☐ Use grab bars. ☐ Use a flexible shower hose. ☐ Use a nonskid bath mat.	
Dressing	☐ Balance is unsteady.	☐ Dress on _____ .	
Using toilet	☐ Getting on/off toilet is difficult. ☐ Toilet is too low.	☐ Keep toilet seat raised. ☐ Use right/left toilet guard rails. ☐ Use grab bars on _____ .	
Kitchen			
Laundry			
Comments			

Occupational Therapist   Date

Figure 27-10 Occupational therapy recommendations for home modifications for safety and accessibility. (Courtesy K. Hatae, V. Tully, N. Wade; Honolulu, Hawaii.)

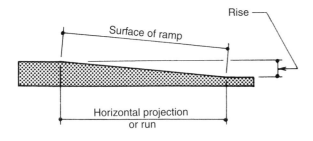

Figure 27-11 Slope and rise of ramps. This diagram provides the components of a single ramp run and a sample of ramp dimensions. The slope ratio is an important consideration when designing a ramp; slope creates hazardous wheelchair propulsion conditions if it is too steep. (From American National Standards Institute: *Accessible and usable buildings and facilities,* New York, 1992, The Institute.)

	Maximum rise		Maximum horizontal projection	
Slope	in	mm	ft	m
1:12 to 1:15	30	760	30	9
1:16 to 1:19	30	760	40	12
1:20	30	760	50	15

and have a nonslip surface; and handrails should be mounted approximately 1½ inches away from the wall to allow for adequate grasping space.

General Comments about Doors and Landings

Standard door width should be a minimum of 32 inches. Several solutions to narrow door problems do not require replacing the entire frame and door with a wider doorway. Existing hinges may be replaced with swing-clear hinges. Thus the clear opening of the door may be enlarged by 1½ to 2 inches. Doorstops may be removed, adding an additional ¾ inch to the clear opening width of the doorway. Removal of existing doors can provide an additional 1½ to 2 inches. Removing doors and doorstops can increase door width 2¼ to 2¾ inches.

Small landings on either side of the door present problems for a wheelchair or walker user because pulling a swinging door open is difficult if the assistive device already is occupying the landing area over which the door must swing. A minimum of 18 inches for walkers and 26 inches for wheelchairs is needed outside the door swing area (Fig. 27-12). Rather than enlarging a landing by removing walls and partitions, three options are available. The door can be removed, an automatic door opener can be installed, or a door pull loop with Velcro-type attachments can be devised. The latter can assist individuals

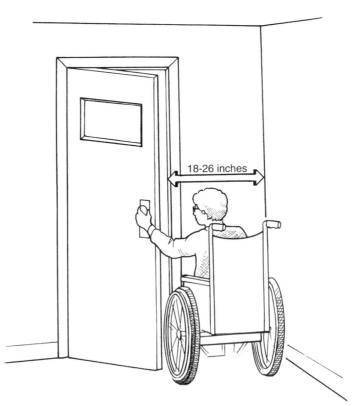

Figure 27-12 Door swing area. A minimum of 18 inches for walkers and 26 inches for wheelchairs is needed outside the swing area.

with closing a swing-in door. The loop can be constructed from 2-inch wide webbing material and should be at least 30 inches in length. A loop sewn at one end assists patients with weak grasps. The other end can be fastened to the door lever or knob using 1-inch wide Velcro-type loops and hooks.

If doors are to be replaced, several options are available. If space is a limiting factor, sliding doors are useful (Fig. 27-13). However, their weight and lateral movement can make maneuvering difficult. Moreover, some sliding doors require floor tracks, which are obstacles for wheelchairs and persons who have difficulty walking. Pocket doors are effective if only occasional privacy is necessary (Fig. 27-14). Folding doors require lateral movement but

are lighter in weight (Fig. 27-15). Door thresholds higher than ¼ inch should be removed or beveled to prevent tripping hazards and to remove barriers for wheelchair users.

Hardware

Lever door handles or doorknob adapters are preferable to round twist doorknobs. Slide bolts, which can be reached from a seated position, may replace dead bolt locks. Kick plates can be installed on doors to prevent gouging and scratches from wheelchairs and walking aids. They should be as thin as possible to allow clear door width opening. They should extend from the bottom of the door to a height of 10 to 16 inches.

Interior

Hallways, Living Room, and Dining Area

Hallways should be a minimum of 36 to 48 inches wide. They should be free of protruding objects such as low tables, coat racks, and planters. Thresholds should be eliminated. Nonslip and low-friction surfaces are recommended. Scatter rugs should be removed. Carpeting should be removed or tacked or taped down to eliminate trip hazards. Furniture should be rearranged to accommodate a wheelchair turning area of 5 square feet. Coffee tables, ottomans, and other trip hazards should be eliminated for patients who walk with assistive devices. A favorite chair can be increased in seat height by adding medium-density foam cushions. Telephone and appliance wires should be taped or tacked down. Easy access to light fixtures and outlets is recommended. Appropriate height

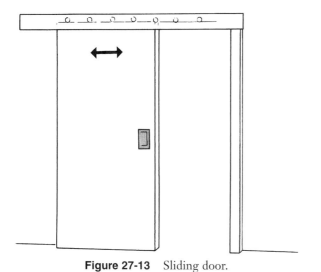

Figure 27-13 Sliding door.

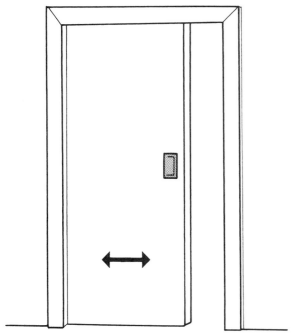

Figure 27-14 Pocket door.

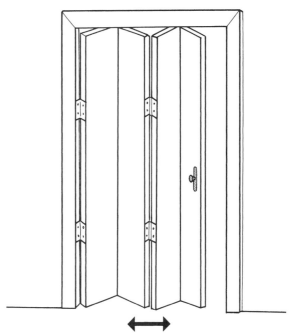

Figure 27-15 Folding door.

for wall switches is 36 to 48 inches. Outlets should be a minimum of 18 inches above the floorboard. Rocker switches and dimmer switches can reduce the fine manipulation required for operating light switches, or automatic timer lights can be installed. Inexpensive environmental control units can aid in independent operation of television sets, radios, and other appliances.

Bedroom

The bedroom should be free of clutter and scatter rugs. A minimum of 3 feet should be available on the side of the bed to allow for wheelchair transfers. The height of the bed should be equal to the height of the wheelchair for safe transfers. If the bed is too low, it may be elevated on blocks or a platform. Raising the bed also increases ease for sit-to-stand transitions if the patient is ambulatory. A firm mattress is recommended to improve bed mobility. A trapeze can assist with mobility in bed if necessary. Side rails provide safety from falls and also can be used as assistive devices for rolling in bed. Dressers should have toe space underneath and easy-glide drawers. Stackable baskets may be a substitute for clothing storage. Closet doors should be removed or replaced with folding doors or a curtain. The height of the clothing rod should be a maximum of 48 inches.

Bathroom

Doorway width may preclude bathroom access for the wheelchair user. Removing the door, installing a pocket or sliding door, or using a narrow rolling commode chair are options for entry to the bathroom for nonambulatory individuals. The optimal toilet seat height should be 17 to 19 inches, which allows for level transfers from a wheelchair and decreases the amount of bending required to get up and down for those who can stand. Options for raising the height of the toilet include a raised toilet seat, an over-toilet commode, a drop-arm commode, or a Toilevator (Fig. 27-16). For individuals who have greater weakness in their lower extremities than in their upper extremities, a toilet safety frame may assist with sit-to-stand transitions. Grab bars should be installed throughout the bathroom because surfaces become slippery and falls are more likely. The height of horizontal bars should range from 33 to 36 inches above the floor. The width of the bar should be 1¼ to 1½ inches to accommodate grasp efficiently. When bars are mounted adjacent to the wall, the distance between the wall and the bar should be 1½ inches so that the patient's fingers can reach around the bar but the arm cannot slip through. Walls around the tub or shower stall should be reinforced. Bars should be mounted securely into the wall studs. Towel racks should be removed if they are likely to be used for support.

Glass doors on tub and shower stalls should be removed and replaced with a curtain. Glass doors can detach from tracks and fall on the person. This renovation

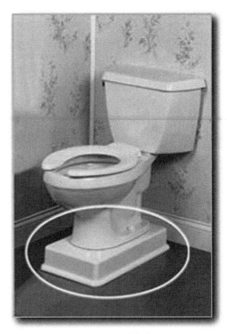

Figure 27-16 Toilevator.

increases accessibility for transfers and improves safety conditions. The recommended height for tub rims is 17 to 19 inches. Shower stall thresholds should be ½ inch high. A roll-in shower may be recommended for nonambulatory individuals and should be a minimum of 30 by 60 inches. Some tubs have rounded bottoms. This can present stability problems if a stationary leg of a tub bench is supposed to be positioned inside. A clamp-on tub bench is more suitable for such tubs. Regardless of the type of tub, the therapist should evaluate the individual's balance and transfer method and architectural constraints carefully to determine the most appropriate and safest type of seat. A flexible shower spray unit assists with rinsing; the hose should be a minimum of 60 inches long. The handle can be adapted for individuals with limited hand dexterity. Nonskid tub strips or a rubber bath mat should be applied to the floor of the tub or shower stall and outside the tub to prevent falls. Fig. 27-17 gives samples of shower stall and shower seat dimensions.

Sink and Lavatories

The height of the sink should be a maximum of 34 inches above the floor. Wheelchair users need a minimum of 29 inches of height underneath the sink to enable them to have close access to the faucets and basin. Access problems may be eliminated by removing cabinets or doors. The mirror above the sink should be angled ¼ to ½ inch for individuals who are seated. Water pipes should be insulated to prevent contact burns. Hot and cold water should mix and empty through a single faucet to mix water of variable temperatures. Water temperature controls

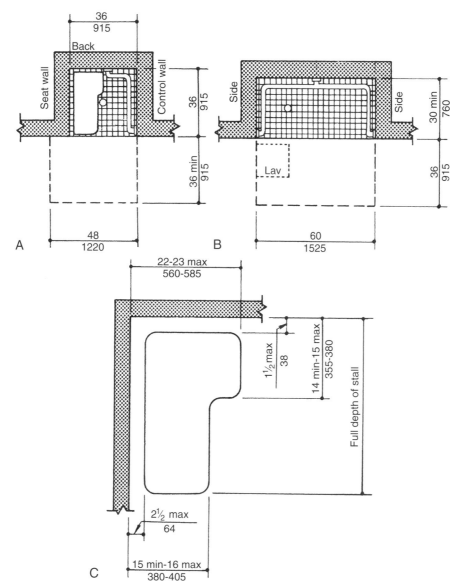

Figure 27-17 Transfer-type shower stall, roll-in shower stall, and shower seat design (metric measurements are in millimeters). *Lav*, Lavatory; *max*, maximum, *min*, minimum. (From American National Standards Institute: *Accessible and usable buildings and facilities*, New York, 1992, The Institute.)

should be set no higher than 115 degrees F. Ordinances in some cities mandate a fixed maximum temperature for hot water for safety. Single-lever faucet controls are recommended because they provide visual indication of water temperature and do not require fine motor dexterity to operate.

Kitchens

The three most common kitchen layouts are L-shaped, aisle, and U-shaped. The L- or U-shaped configuration can improve efficiency (Fig. 27-18). Work surfaces should be free of clutter, and small appliances that are used frequently should be placed within reach.

Countertops are generally 36 inches high, making accessibility difficult for wheelchair users. Alternate counter or work surfaces can be adapted by adding pullout cutting boards or placing a cutting board on top of a drawer that has been opened partially. Height-adjustable countertops and cabinets provide easy access for individuals with limited reach; however, this option is expensive. The countertop should have a maximum depth of 24 inches. The corners and edges should be rounded. Base cabinets should have enough toe space at the bottom to accommodate wheelchair footplates. Retractable doors and lazy Susans increase accessibility to stored items. Adapted knobs or D-loop handles assist individuals with decreased

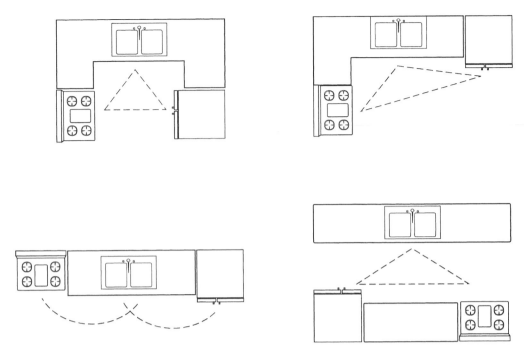

Figure 27-18   Common kitchen layouts.

coordination and grasp strength. Easy-glide drawers and pullout shelves may decrease energy expenditure.

The therapist also must take appliances into account. A side-by-side refrigerator is recommended for increased access to the refrigerator and freezer. Shelves should be adjustable; lazy Susans may provide easier access to stored food items. A wall-mounted oven and range top with staggered burners are recommended for wheelchair users. A mirror placed above the stove allows seated individuals to see the cooking process. Transparent pots are another alternative. Range controls should be located at the front or side to eliminate the need to reach over hot elements. Controls can be adapted for individuals with limited hand dexterity. Tactile or audible cues can assist individuals with limited vision. For wall-mounted ovens, the controls should be no higher than 40 inches above the floor for wheelchair user access. Microwave and toaster ovens may be convenient and safe alternatives for cooking.

Sink basins should be a maximum of 6½ inches deep. A plastic or wooden rack can be used to raise the working level. A retractable hose can increase the ease of rinsing dishes. Single-lever faucet controls are recommended and should be positioned no farther than 21 inches from the edge of the counter.

Moving Around the Obstacles

General mobility and transfers will be difficult for the individual who has severe motor deficits. After a discussion of prognosis for motor return, it may be appropriate to recommend a safe mechanical transfer system for the primary caregiver to use within the home.

From a historical perspective, standard lift systems were difficult to use because they generally required more than one person to operate and were difficult to maneuver in limited spaces. Modern advances in technology have resulted in effective, safe, and more affordable equipment available to mobilize the more physically involved individual.

An example of one system is the Barrier Free Lift. With this system, tracks usually are custom installed on the ceilings in patients' homes. They allow the caregiver or home attendant to stay close to the patient during the transfer process but do not require physical exertion from the caregiver. Several benefits to using a Barrier Free track system include prevention of caregiver injuries and ensuring that furniture, carpets, and other equipment do not get in the way of the lift (Fig. 27-19).

FALL PREVENTION

The checklist in Fig. 27-20 is an adaptation from the fall prevention checklist used at the Rehabilitation Hospital of the Pacific located in Honolulu, Hawaii. This checklist originally was used as a tool to provide education to family members and caregivers after the home evaluation process. The adjustments incorporate options for durable medical equipment. See Chapter 14.

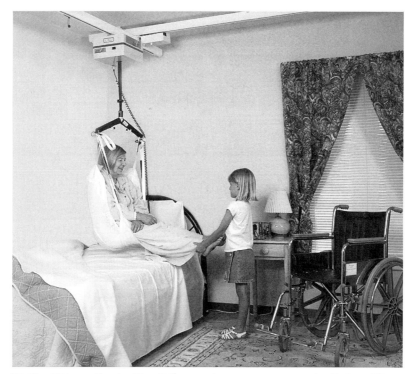

Figure 27-19   Using a Barrier Free Lift, caregivers can now come in all sizes. (Courtesy Ted Hensley, Barrier Free Lifts.)

Exterior
__ Walkways have a smooth surface and are clear of objects.
__ Outdoor lighting is sufficient for safe ambulation and wheelchair maneuvering at night.
__ Step surfaces are nonslip and edges are clearly marked to prevent tripping.
__ Steps are sturdy and handrails are secure.

Living Room
__ Entryway and room are free of clutter to allow safe walking or wheelchair mobility.
__ Stepstools, ottomans, coffee tables, and other low-lying objects are out of the way to prevent trip hazards.
__ Chairs have armrests and are sturdy.
__ Telephone and lighting are accessible; cords are tucked down.
__ Environmental controls are accessible.

Hallway
__ Doors that open into halls are removed.
__ Floor is clear of objects.
__ Carpet borders and runners are secured.

Bathroom
__ Door width is wide enough to permit wheelchair access.
__ No thresholds are trip hazards.
__ Scatter rugs are removed.
__ Grab bars are installed near toilet, tub, and entryway.
__ Toilet is proper height.
__ Nonskid bath mat or strips are installed on floor of tub or shower.
__ Tub or shower seat is available for bathing.

Bedroom
__ Doorway entry is proper width.
__ Bed is proper height and firmness.
__ Night lights are present.
__ Hospital bed is available.
__ Side rails are installed.
__ Bedside commode is available.

Kitchen
__ Table is sturdy.
__ Frequently used items are located at waist level.
__ Use of range top is avoided.
__ Microwave or toaster oven is available.
__ Throw rugs are removed.
__ Electrical cords are tied up or taped down.

Figure 27-20   Fall prevention checklist.

CASE STUDY

Returning Home Safely and Independently after Stroke

J.J. is a 72-year-old woman who was admitted to the hospital with a diagnosis of right hemispheric stroke. Her hospital course was uncomplicated, and she was transferred to the rehabilitation unit four days later.

An occupational therapy evaluation was performed and clinical findings were reported. Passive range of motion was within functional limits throughout all joints in the upper extremities bilaterally. Strength was good in the right upper extremity. Minimal active movement was present in the left shoulder, and one-finger subluxation was noted. Sensation was intact for light touch, pain, and temperature. Functional abilities were impaired moderately because of decreased ability to bear weight on the left upper and lower extremities. Sitting balance was fair. Standing balance was poor. J.J. required moderate assistance for bed mobility. Sit-to-stand required maximal assistance of one person, and transfers required moderate to maximal assistance depending on the surface. She was unable to walk at the time of evaluation, and wheelchair mobility skills required moderate assist. In self-care, a left neglect was noted during all activities. J.J. required set-up assistance for eating and grooming. Dressing and bathing required moderate to maximal assistance.

J.J. was treated in occupational and physical therapy for six weeks. During her fourth week of treatment, a home evaluation was scheduled. The therapy team felt that having the patient present during the visit would be useful because she lived alone and still required the use of a wheelchair. She lived in a two-bedroom rental apartment in a building with a no-step entry and elevator. The apartment had large rooms, but wheelchair accessibility was limited because of excessive furniture and thick carpeting. The hallway was narrow. Her bedroom and bathroom were located off to the right of the hallway, and the second bedroom was located at the end of the hallway. She was unable to negotiate the turn into her bedroom with the wheelchair because of the hall and door width. The therapist suggested that she switch bedrooms and use the second bedroom as her own. The bed was low with a soft mattress and the closet was not accessible because of narrow paths and excessive furnishings. The bathroom was spacious and easily could accommodate a wheelchair; however, the door was only 19 inches wide, preventing wheelchair access. The bathroom had a combination tub and shower with sliding glass doors. The toilet was located behind the door. The sink had round fixtures that were difficult to turn. The kitchen was wheelchair accessible.

The refrigerator door opened to the right, and the stove had controls at the back of the range top. The cabinets were high and not accessible from a seated position. The following recommendations were made:

Living room
1. Remove one couch and coffee table.
2. Remove the area carpet and scatter rugs.
3. Relocate the lamps for easier access.

Bedroom
1. Elevate the bed 4 inches on cinder blocks to equal the height of the wheelchair.
2. Place a plywood board beneath the mattress to increase firmness.
3. Remove the closet door and one dresser.
4. Lower the height of the closet rod to 40 inches above the floor.
5. Place a drop-arm commode chair next to the bed.
6. Place a night-light in the wall socket.

Bathroom
1. Remove the sliding glass doors and replace with a shower curtain.
2. Use a tub transfer bench and flexible shower hose for bathing.
3. Place a 24-inch grab bar on the wall of the tub 33 inches from the floor.
4. Park the wheelchair in front of the bathroom door and walk with assistance.
5. Place a chair in the bathroom in front of the sink to perform grooming and dressing tasks.
6. Tilt the mirror ½ inch.

Kitchen
1. Reverse the door swing on the refrigerator.
2. Relocate frequently used items to the counter.
3. Relocate the toaster oven to the kitchen table.

Communication
1. Purchase a portable cordless phone.
2. Consider registration with an emergency call service.

J.J. agreed with the foregoing recommendations and requested permission from the landlord to install the grab bar. During the rest of her inpatient rehabilitation stay, the focus of treatment was placed on achieving independence in bed-to-commode transfers, short-distance walking, light meal preparation, and kitchen tasks from wheelchair level in a home-simulating environment. At the time of discharge, J.J. was independent in all self-care, transfers, and meal preparation. She required contact guard for short distance ambulation with a hemiwalker and was independent with wheelchair mobility. She was recommended for home care services for follow-up therapy and assistance from a home health aide.

REVIEW QUESTIONS

1. What options can an occupational therapist consider if existing doorways are too narrow for a wheelchair?
2. What issues does an occupational therapist need to address for a wheelchair-dependent patient recovering from stroke who is returning home?
3. What modifications should be considered to make bathrooms safe and accessible?
4. What are architectural barriers?

REFERENCES

1. American National Standards Institute: *Accessible and usable buildings and facilities*, New York, 2003, The Institute.
2. AOTA: *AOTA's societal statement on livable communities*, Bethesda, MD, 2008, AOTA.
3. Sabata DB, Shamber S, Williams M: Optimizing access to home, community, and in workplace. In Radomski MV, Latham CAT, editors: *Occupational therapy for physical dysfunction*, ed 6, Baltimore, 2008, Williams & Wilkins.

patricia a. ryan
jennie w. sullivan

chapter 28

Activities of Daily Living Adaptations: Managing the Environment with One-Handed Techniques

key terms

adaptive devices	energy conservation	instrumental activities of daily living
adaptive techniques	environmental modifications	
basic activities of daily living		work simplification

chapter objectives

After completing this chapter, the reader will be able to accomplish the following:

1. Explore a variety of adaptive techniques and assistive devices to allow for completion of activities of daily living.
2. Enhance performance of activities of daily living using principles of energy conservation and work simplification.
3. Explore environmental modifications to enhance safety and ease of mobility in the performance of activities of daily living.

Occupational therapy intervention for stroke survivors is geared toward ameliorating deficits resulting from stroke and varies tremendously from one patient to another. For certain individuals, limited return of functional use of the involved extremity makes performance of self-care and instrumental activities of daily living (IADL) uniquely challenging. According to the study described in "Compensation in Recovery of Upper Extremity Function After Stroke,"[1a] the emphasis of intervention during rehabilitation for patients with extensive upper extremity paralysis should be on teaching one-handed compensatory techniques. The occupational therapist is called to use creative problem-solving abilities to enhance independence in a wide range of activities, helping the patient achieve meaningful, realistic goals. Indeed recent evidence strongly suggests that focused occupational therapy makes a substantial impact in this area of activities limitations (Box 28-1). (See Chapter 21 for a comprehensive overview of IADL.)

BASIC ENVIRONMENTAL CONSIDERATIONS

Before initiating basic activity of daily living (BADL) training, the therapist should address the variety of environments in which the patient is required to perform. While surveying the patient's environment, the therapist should consider the following criteria:

1. Safety factors
2. Ease of mobility and performance of activities of daily living (ADL)

Box 28-1

Evidence Briefs: ADL Retraining after Stroke

■ A recent systematic review and metaanalysis aimed to determine whether occupational therapy focused specifically on personal ADL improves recovery for patients after stroke. Nine randomized controlled trials including 1258 participants met the inclusion criteria. The authors concluded, "Occupational therapy focused on improving personal activities of daily living after stroke can improve performance and reduce the risk of deterioration in these abilities. Focused occupational therapy should be available to everyone who has had a stroke." (Legg, et al, 2007)

■ Steultjens and colleagues conducted a systematic review to determine from the available literature whether occupational therapy interventions improve outcomes for stroke patients. The authors identified and included 32 studies (18 were randomized controlled trials). They documented significant effect sizes for the efficacy of comprehensive occupational therapy on primary ADL, extended ADL, and social participation.

■ Trombly and Ma examined 15 studies involving 895 participants (mean age = 70.3-years-old). Of these studies, 11 (7 randomized controlled trials) "found that role participation and instrumental and basic activities of daily living performance improved significantly more with training than with the control conditions." The authors concluded that "occupational therapy effectively improves participation and activity after stroke and recommend that therapists use structured instruction in specific, client-identified activities, appropriate adaptations to enable performance, practice within a familiar context, and feedback to improve client performance."

Safety

Helping patients negotiate the bedroom environment safely is a priority because this is an area in which many self-care activities are performed. The height of the bed should allow the patient to sit comfortably with both feet flat on the floor to provide a good base of support. If the bed is too high or too low, the therapist can consider the following adaptations. Several inches can be sawed off or added to the bedposts of a wooden bed to adjust the bed height. Leg extensions are commercially available from a variety of rehabilitation catalogs. Another alternative is to remove the bed frame entirely and use only the box spring and mattress. Ideally, a double mattress should be used to improve ease of mobility and provide an increased sense of security. The mattress should be firm to allow for increased postural stability and improved balance. The bed should be placed within the room to allow access from both sides. Use of a transfer handle positioned on the patient's noninvolved side improves safety and ease of mobility in and out of the bed (Fig. 28-1).

Bedroom furniture should be rearranged to eliminate obstacles hindering the patient from negotiating a path to the bathroom or room exit. If possible, changes in the floor surface should be avoided. Bare floor surface changing to raised carpeting, for example, may increase the risk of falls.

The sensory environment is another component to consider. Factors such as sufficient lighting and a comfortable room temperature must be ensured. If inadequate,

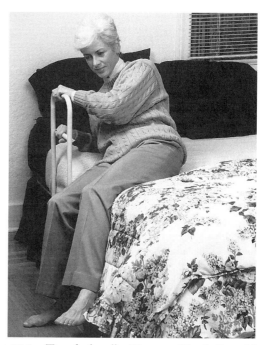

Figure 28-1   Transfer handle. (Courtesy North Coast Medical, San Jose, Calif.)

both conditions present safety obstacles. For example, if the room temperature is too cold, the patient may experience an increase in muscle activity, possibly decreasing postural stability and the ability to perform self-care tasks successfully. (See Chapter 27 for a detailed review of home modifications.)

Ease of Mobility and Performance of Activities of Daily Living

In addition to the safety of the environment, the therapist also must consider arrangement of the bedroom to increase ease of mobility and performance of ADL. The therapist may use energy conservation and work simplification techniques to teach the patient ways to prioritize, organize, and limit work to save time and energy and to enhance the successful outcome of task performance. The following techniques should be considered:

1. Eliminate excess space. Enough space must be available for ease of mobility without excess. Excess space forces a patient to travel greater distances, draining personal energy resources. For example, the bathroom ideally should be directly off the bedroom rather than down the hall. If this arrangement is not possible, a bedside commode and sitting table with a mirror that can be set up to allow for performance of toileting and grooming are useful modifications. A living room can be used to replace an out-of-the-way bedroom.
2. Arrange the room so that sequential tasks can be performed with minimal travel time in between.
3. Place appliances and controls where they can be accessed easily. Lamps, alarm clocks, and telephones should be placed where they are needed most often and are most convenient for the patient. The use of environmental control units should be considered.
4. Eliminate clutter. Thorough cleaning and organization is essential to allow for easy retrieval of commonly needed items.
5. Arrange for easy access of clothing and toileting supplies by eliminating excess reaching and bending. Shelves are easier to access than drawers are. If drawers are used, they are easier to open with a central knob rather than handles. Also, closet rods can be lowered to eliminate excess reaching. An alternative solution includes use of a reacher.

Therapists must be aware of the neurobehavioral deficits that affect BADL and IADL. These deficits influence equipment choices and training techniques (see Chapters 17 and 18).

FUNCTIONAL ASSESSMENT

The World Health Organization's 2001 International Classification of Functioning, Disability and Health[4] provides a useful conceptual framework while considering using functional assessment instruments in stroke rehabilitation. Many instruments have been used in research and clinical practice to assess functional outcomes in patients who have survived a stroke (Table 28-1). See Chapter 21 for a review of standardized tools to assess IADL.

BASIC ACTIVITIES OF DAILY LIVING

Grooming and Hygiene

When performing hygiene and grooming, assistive devices and alternative methods often provide increased independence and safety and decreased energy expenditure.

Toileting. A toilet tissue dispenser should be mounted within easy reach of the unaffected side and allow for easy, one-handed retrieval of tissue sheets. Two possibilities include a tissue box dispenser mounted on the bathroom wall or an easy-load toilet paper holder, which eliminates excessive paper roll waste. This alternative gives a more aesthetic appearance, possibly improving acceptance by the patient (Fig. 28-2). Moist towelettes can be used in place of toilet paper and are a viable alternative for patients with urgency or impaired sphincter control.

Two devices that are available and recommended to increase independence in bladder care for women who have survived a stroke include the Asta-Cath and the Feminal. Both products are available from A+ Products. The Asta-Cath female catheter guide is a simple device that assists women in locating their urinary meatus. As the Asta-Cath is inserted into the vagina, it spreads the labia, and one hole aligns with the urinary meatus. The patient then can pass a No. 14 French or smaller catheter into the bladder for emptying. The three alignment holes allow for most anatomical differences (Fig. 28-3). The Feminal is designed so that a woman can urinate in a reclined, seated, or standing position. When gently pressed against the body, the unique shape creates a leak-proof seal (Fig. 28-4).

Showering and Bathing. Transferring from a slippery tub, controlling water temperature, and washing adequately in a slippery tub are safety factors to consider during bathing. Nonslip mats should be placed inside and outside the tub. All toiletries should be placed where they can be reached easily. Articles should be moved close together if the individual is sitting on a tub bench to ensure safe reaching. To ensure safety of water temperature and ease of bathing, a handheld shower hose with control of water flow may be used to prevent scalding. This device can be purchased through a variety of catalogs.

Long-handled scrub sponges and bath brushes are excellent assistive devices for washing. A flex sponge is able to bend in any direction to wash all of the body, including the nonaffected arm, axilla, and shoulder,

Table 28-1

Examples of Functional Assessments for Stroke Survivors

INSTRUMENT	BRIEF DESCRIPTION
American Heart Association Stroke Outcome Classification (Kelly-Hayes and colleagues, 1998)	The purpose of this instrument is to serve as a standardized and comprehensive classification system to document the impairments and disability resulting from a stroke. The scale considers the number of neurological domains involved, severity of impairment, and level of function.
A-ONE (Arnadottir, this volume)	Documents level of functional independence in basic ADL and mobility and underlying neurobehavioral impairments. See Chapter 18.
Barthel ADL Index (Mahoney, 1965)	Scores for activities are weighted so that the final item scores range from 0 for dependent performance to 15 for independent performance. Total score ranges from 0 to 100. Activities include feeding, bathing, grooming, transfers, dressing, bowel, bladder, toileting, walking, wheelchair use, and stair climbing.
Canadian Occupational Performance Measure (Law and colleagues, 2005)	Measures clients' perceptions about performance and satisfaction with self-care, productivity, and leisure. After identifying occupational performance issues, the clients rate their perception of performance and satisfaction with performance on a 1 to 10 scale. The same scale is used for reassessment.
Functional Independence Measure (FIM) (Keith and colleagues, 1987)	Administered by members of the rehabilitation team by direct observation. A detailed scoring system is used, and therapists are trained to administer the FIM in a standardized manner. Items scored on a 1 to 7 scale include self-care, sphincter control, mobility, locomotion, communication, social skill, and cognition.
Modified Rankin Scale (van Swieten and colleagues, 1988)	A 5 point scale used to rate disability and need for assistance.

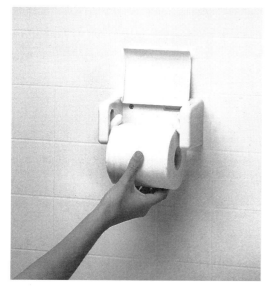

Figure 28-2 Easy-Load toilet paper holder. (Courtesy Sammons Preston, a BISSELL Company.)

which may be difficult to reach (Fig. 28-5). Soap on a rope or a suction soap holder may be used to prevent soap from slipping about or getting lost in the water. The soap on the rope is hung around the neck or hung within easy reach. Another alternative is to use liquid soap in a pump container. A soaper sponge also may be used to wash without having to hold a slippery bar of soap. If grasp is limited, the patient can use a terry cloth wash mitt with a pocket to hold the bar of soap. The aforementioned devices may be purchased through a variety of rehabilitation catalogs. For those who must rely on another to bathe them, a mechanical lift positions the person in a body sling. This lifting device has a swing arm to allow a person to be suspended in a shower or over a tub.

Shampooing. Shampoo in a pump spray bottle helps avoid waste and reaches a broader area of the scalp. A full-spray handheld shower is convenient for rinsing.

Drying. To decrease energy expenditure while drying, an extra large towel or terry wraparound robe can be worn to absorb most of the water. The back and nonaffected arm are the most difficult areas to dry. The following procedure can be incorporated:

1. Place the towel over one shoulder.
2. Reach behind and grasp the other end, pulling the towel down across the back.
3. Repeat the same procedure over the opposite shoulder.

An alternative method is to toss the towel over the top of a doorway and shut the door as much as possible to hold the towel in place. The patient then can pull the towel across the back and shoulder with the nonaffected extremity.

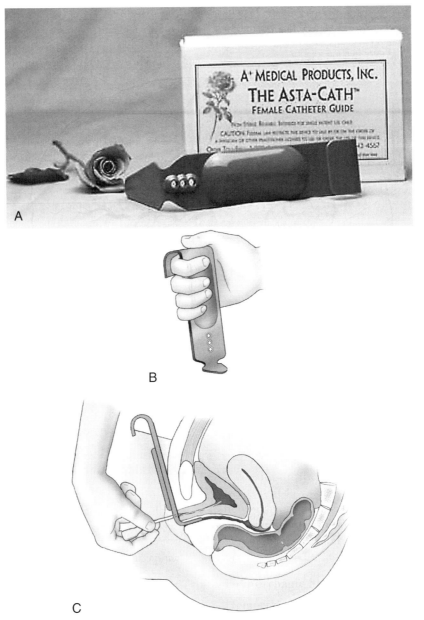

Figure 28-3 The Asta-Cath. (Available from A⁺ Products, www.aplusproducts.biz, [888] 843–3334.)

Washing at the Sink. Some individuals may have difficulty showering or bathing for a variety of reasons. An alternative method is to have body washes at the sink. The easiest position in which to wash the affected arm is to place the arm and axilla in the sink basin. To wash the unaffected arm, the individual steadies the soapy washcloth over the edge of the sink and rubs the arm and hand over it. The patient then washes the rest of the body with one hand. Again, a flex sponge is useful to wash all of the body, including the nonaffected extremity. A supplement to washing at the sink is the use of a bidet. The Hygenique Plus Bidet/Sitz Bath System is designed specifically for personal hygiene needs. This system combines a spray wand for bidet cleansing and a sitz bath (Fig. 28-6).

For individuals with low endurance who are unable to shower or bathe at the sink, a total-body, pH-balanced cleanser may be used for shampooing, bathing, and incontinence care. This product is available through a variety of rehabilitation catalogs. Drying techniques are the same as previously described.

Performing Oral Hygiene. Oral hygiene care can be done easily with one hand. A toothpaste dispenser can dispense the correct amount of toothpaste on the brush

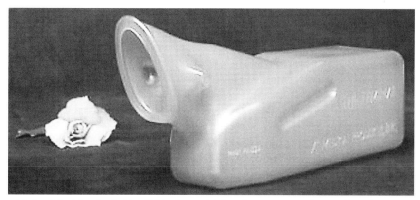

Figure 28-4   The Feminal. (Available from A+ Products, www.aplusproducts.biz, [888] 843–3334.)

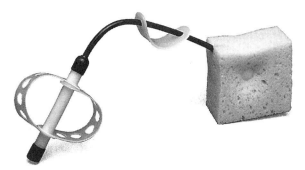

Figure 28-5   Flex sponge. (Courtesy Sammons Preston, a BISSELL Company.)

for individuals with limited hand function (Fig. 28-7). The method of brushing (electrical or manual) is a personal choice. The use of an electrical toothbrush may decrease energy expenditure because the brush vibrates up and down, and the patient holds the arm in one position. A Waterpik attachment is excellent for massaging the gums and rinsing between the teeth. Suction toothbrushes may be attached to a suction unit to prevent dysphagia-related aspiration in individuals who cannot tolerate thin liquids.

The simplest method for denture care is to soak the dentures overnight in a commercial denture cleanser. If additional cleansing of dentures is needed, the patient can use a suction denture brush.

Flossing teeth with one hand can be performed easily and effectively with a commercially available dental floss holder.

Applying Deodorant. Aerosol sprays are easier to apply to the unaffected arm unless the individual has sufficient function to reach the axilla with a roll-on or stick applicator. The affected axilla must be placed passively away from the body to apply deodorant. This can be accomplished by bending forward at the hips and allowing gravity to assist the arm away from the body.

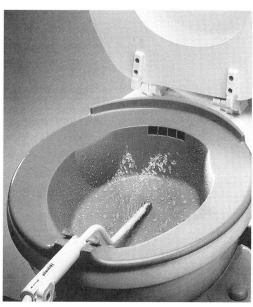

Figure 28-6   Hygenique Plus Bidet/Sitz Bath System. (Courtesy North Coast Medical, San Jose, Calif.)

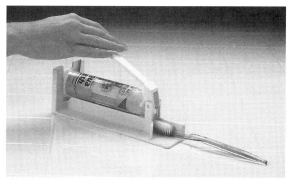

Figure 28-7   Toothpaste dispenser. (Courtesy Sammons Preston, a BISSELL Company.)

Caring for Fingernails. Nail care of the affected hand can be done easily with the noninvolved hand. Cleaning, cutting, and filing the nails of the unaffected hand are more difficult.

The following strategies may be used to ease nail management:

1. To clean the unaffected hand, a nailbrush with suction cups for cleaning fingernails can be used.
2. To cut the nails of the unaffected hand, the patient may use a one-hand fingernail clipper. When the patient presses down on the board, the jaws of the clipper close (Fig. 28-8).
3. Filing the nails of the unaffected hand can be done in a variety of ways. A suction emery board is useful. Other individuals may choose to use a homemade device such as an emery board or sandpaper glued to a piece of wood, a nail file secured to a table with masking tape, or a file wedged in a drawer.
4. Applying nail polish to the unaffected hand can be done by mounting a clothespin on a piece of wood with a C-clamp to hold the polish brush. The polish is applied when the person moves the nail in relation to the brush.

Caring for Toenails. Cleansing toes can be accomplished with the use of a footbrush or Footmate System (Fig. 28-9). Clipping toenails is easier if the feet are soaked in warm water first. A pistol-grip remote toenail clipper is one of several devices designed for one-handed use to clip toenails; it allows one to reach the foot with less bending (Fig. 28-10).

Hairstyling. Simple, short hairstyles are the easiest to manage with one hand. Combing or styling long hair may be easier using adjustable, long-handled grooming accessories, available through various rehabilitation catalogs.

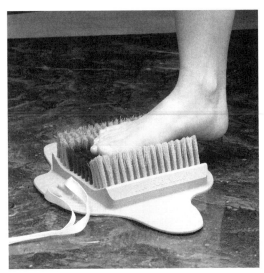

Figure 28-9   Footmate System. (Courtesy North Coast Medical, San Jose, Calif.)

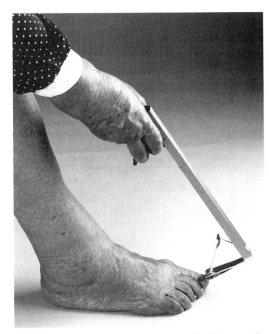

Figure 28-10   Pistol-grip remote toenail clipper. (Courtesy Maddack, Pequannock, NJ.)

Lightweight splinting material also may be used to extend the handles of an individual's favorite grooming tools.

Blow-drying hair can be made easier by using a commercial product called the Hands-Free Hair Dryer Holder, which allows the unaffected hand free operation to style hair (Fig. 28-11). An alternative method is a home-devised product such as a position-adjustable hair dryer. A lightweight blow-dryer, a desk lamp with spring-balanced arms, a tension control knob at each joint, and a mounting

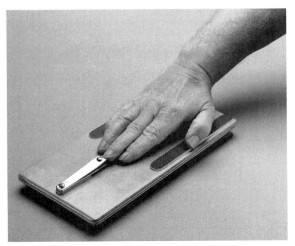

Figure 28-8   One-hand fingernail clipper. (Courtesy Maddak, Pequannock, NJ.)

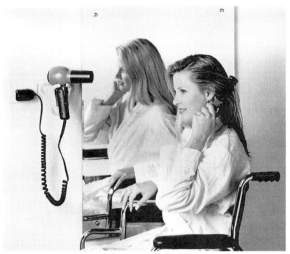

Figure 28-11 Hands-free hair dryer holder. (Courtesy Sammons Preston, a BISSELL Company.)

bracket are the only materials needed to fabricate the device. The position-adjustable hair dryer requires limited body movement because the dryer can be positioned in any plane desired.[1]

Brush attachments to the hair dryer also can be used for blow-drying styles. A hot brush curling system can be used for setting hair in simple hairstyles.

Shaving. Shaving can be done one-handed with any type of razor. If a patient is unsteady with the motor skills, a Silk Effects razor reduces the risks of nicking the skin. An electric razor is easy to manage with one hand and is recommended for safety to prevent nicks.

Applying Makeup. The patient may apply makeup one-handed with practice. Grip and bottle makeup holders are useful to stabilize supplies; suction cups and rubber mats also help stabilize grooming items.

Dressing

Retraining an individual with hemiplegia who is limited to the use of one hand to dress presents challenges to the patient and the therapist. Specific deficits that the therapist must address include the following:
1. Impaired postural stability and balance
2. Decreased dexterity and work speed
3. Impaired ability to stabilize clothing articles and body parts
4. Decreased endurance accompanied by increased energy demands on the body
5. Impaired sensory capabilities
6. Possible cognitive and perceptual limitations

When retraining the patient in dressing techniques, the therapist should incorporate adequate time and allowances for rest breaks into the session. The patient should be able to achieve success without undue effort. Loose-fitting clothes should be selected. Roomy clothes with limited fasteners allow for increased ease of movement and easier donning and doffing.

Dressing and undressing invariably involve awkward movement patterns and a certain amount of sitting down and standing up. Care must be taken to ensure that the danger of falling is minimized. Management of clothes is always difficult at first; the occupational therapist should reinforce to the individual that independence and efficiency are achieved through practice.

Fasteners
Many individuals with hemiplegia can learn to manage fasteners if the following requirements are met:
- Garments fit loosely.
- Buttons and hooks are of a larger size.
- Fasteners are positioned in front of or on the nonaffected side of the garment and are within sight.

Buttons. If the patient is unable to manage fasteners, the therapist can use the following adaptation:
1. Remove the buttons from the garment and then sew them back on over the buttonholes.
2. Using Velcro squares, sew the loop side of the Velcro over the original button side of the garment.
3. Sew the hook side of the Velcro under the buttonholes.

The patient then simply uses hand pressure to close the garment. A standard collar extender also can be used. With this item, collars and cuffs are increased by ½ inch, increasing ease of management.

Zippers. Zippers may be easier to manage if a ring or loop is added to the zipper tab. Patients should avoid open-ended zips. Patients can leave the zip fastened at the bottom and don the garment by pulling it on over the head. A large safety pin left fastened can prevent the zipper from sliding all the way down and detaching during overhead donning.

Adaptive Dressing Techniques. Before initiating dressing training, the therapist should ensure the patient is seated on a stable, supportive surface, preferably a sturdy armchair. Both of the patient's feet should be securely positioned on the floor to establish a solid base of support and increase postural stability. Clothing should be placed within easy reach and in the order in which each item is required. This helps maximize energy preservation.

A wide variety of dressing techniques are described in the literature, depending on the particular treatment theory incorporated by the therapist. Some general principles that facilitate ease of one-handed dressing are described in the following sections.

Upper Extremity Dressing

Donning Garments with Front Fasteners. The patient should follow these instructions for donning garments with front fasteners (Fig. 28-12):

1. Pull the shirtsleeve onto the affected arm.
2. Pull the shirtsleeve over the affected shoulder.
3. Swing the garment around until the other sleeve hangs down the back or pull the sleeve over the head and around the neck. The patient may even anchor it by biting the sleeve.
4. Reach to the back with the nonaffected arm and place it into the opening of the remaining sleeve.
5. Use a shrugging motion with the nonaffected arm, and straighten the sleeve into place.

Shirtsleeves may need to be expanded or loose fitting to be pulled over the noninvolved hand. This can be achieved by sewing a piece of elastic into the sleeve cuff to allow for easy passage over the hand[2] and to eliminate the difficulty of managing a cuff button.

The top button of a shirt collar is often difficult to fasten. The button is usually small, and the collar fits snugly around the neck. The problem can be eliminated by replacing the button with a Velcro fastener.[2]

Donning Ties. Ties are difficult to manipulate single-handedly. The simplest solution is to use a conventional, already-tied tie. A piece of elastic may be inserted into the back of the tie to replace a small part of the fabric. This allows for easy passage of the tie over the head. Clip-on ties also are convenient to use.

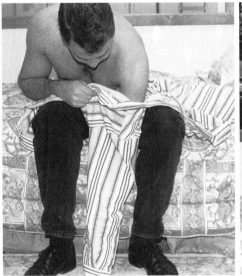
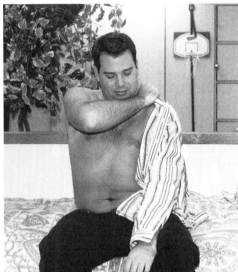
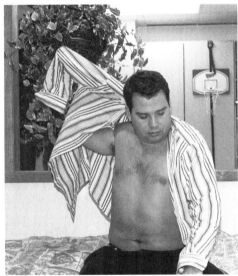

Figure 28-12   Sequence for upper extremity dressing for a patient with left hemiplegia.

Donning Pullover Shirts

The patient should follow these instructions for donning pullover shirts:

1. Use shirt tags or labels to identify the front and back sides of the garment.
2. Pull the correct sleeve onto the affected arm, and pull the garment onto the affected shoulder.
3. Bend the head forward through the neck opening.
4. Put the unaffected arm into the other sleeve.
5. Straighten the sleeve by rubbing the arm against the leg.
6. Pull the garment over the torso.

Donning Brassieres. Front-fastening bras are easier to manage than bras that fasten in back. The bra should be donned by putting the affected arm in first. Another method is to fasten the bra first and then put the bra on by donning it over the head. Larger hooks can be substituted for smaller hooks, or a Velcro strap and D ring may be sewn in as substitutions for the fastener. A bra extender can be purchased and interchanged between bras; increasing the girth accommodation can ease donning.

Patients may manage back-closure bras in the following way:[2]

1. Align the bra around the waist so that the cups face backward. The strap can be held in place by hugging it with the affected arm, by tucking it into the elasticized panty waist, or by using a clothespin to hold it onto the pants.
2. Fasten the hooks in front.
3. Swivel the bra around so that the cups are in front.
4. Pull the strap over the affected shoulder.
5. Using the thumb of the unaffected hand, pull the strap over the unaffected shoulder.

The easiest solution, although not necessarily the most aesthetic, is a fully elasticized bra such as a sports bra, which can be slipped on over the head. A hook-and-eye bra can be adapted by sewing the back fasteners together.

Lower Extremity Dressing

Donning Pants and Underwear While Lying in Bed

The patient should follow this procedure for donning underwear and pants in bed:

1. Bend the affected leg until the foot is within reach. The patient may use the unaffected leg to assist with this.
2. Place the pants over the affected foot and allow the leg to straighten into the pant leg.
3. Put the unaffected leg into the pants and pull the pants up as far as possible.
4. Using the unaffected leg, or if possible both legs, lift the pelvis off the bed. Wriggle the pants up to the waist.
5. Fasten the pants. (Velcro may be used in place of buttons.)

Donning Pants and Underwear While Sitting Up

The patient should follow this procedure for donning underwear and pants while sitting up (Fig. 28-13):

1. While sitting (preferably on a firm surface), cross the affected leg over the unaffected leg. Use clasped hands to lift the leg.
2. Put the correct pant leg over the affected foot and pull it onto the leg.
3. Dress the unaffected leg.
4. Pull the pants up as far as possible while sitting; shift weight over each buttock.
5. Stand up to pull the pants up around the waist. If balance is impaired, lean against a wall or sturdy piece of furniture to provide support and minimize the risk of falling. The patient also can use a pant clip. The pant clip attaches to the pants and an upper body garment, and the clip holds the pants up while the patient transitions to standing, thereby improving safety and function.

Donning Skirts

The patient should follow this procedure for donning skirts:

1. Put the skirt over the head and then pull it down.
2. Make sure to maneuver the fasteners to the front or the unaffected side for increased ease of fastening.
3. Twist the skirt around to the correct position.

A skirt with an elasticized waist that expands to pass over the head may be simpler.

Donning Socks

The patient should follow this procedure for donning socks (Fig. 28-14):

1. Cross the affected leg over the other leg, using clasped hands to lift the leg.
2. With the leg in place, open the sock using the thumb and index finger of the unaffected hand. Roll the sock down to the heel before slipping it on for greater ease in donning.
3. Bend forward at the hips to assist in reaching the foot. Pull the sock over the foot.
4. Don the sock on the unaffected foot in the same fashion.

Donning Shoes

The patient should follow this procedure for donning shoes (Fig. 28-15):

1. Choose shoes that provide good support. A broad heel can provide better stability if balance is poor. Men's standard dress shoes have a toe spring built into the front. For a patient recovering from stroke, the toe spring may assist with toe clearance during the swing phase of gait.
2. Bring the affected foot closer to the body by crossing it over the unaffected leg or by using a small footstool.

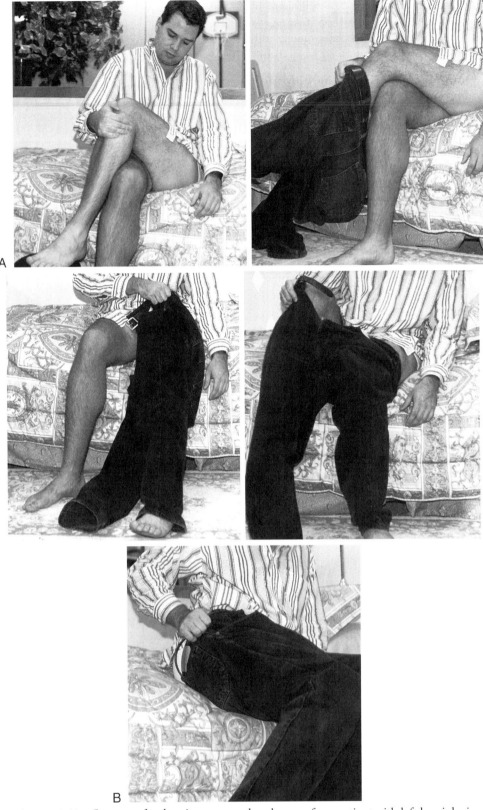

Figure 28-13   Sequence for donning pants and underwear for a patient with left hemiplegia.

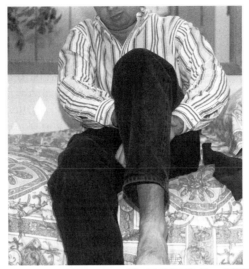

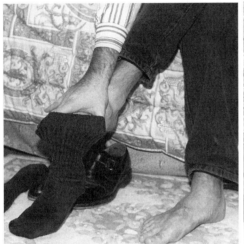

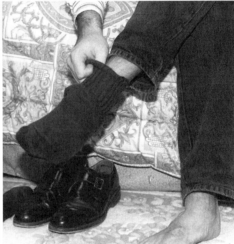

Figure 28-14   Sequence for donning socks for a patient with left hemiplegia.

3. With the leg in place, open the shoe as much as possible before attempting to put it on.
4. Bend forward at the hips to reach the foot. Place the shoe over the ball of the foot and pull it on. A helpful technique to aid with getting the shoe over the foot is to mold a small piece of splinting material onto the shoe heel and allow it to harden. This helps to keep the heel rigid, preventing it from buckling under as the foot slides in.
5. Shoes with Velcro closures are easy to manage with one hand. Shoelaces can be substituted with elastic laces or coilers that do not require tying.

Donning Lower Extremity Orthotics. Lower extremity orthotics can be difficult for patients to manage one-handed, and patients may require assistance. In general, the donning of orthotics is easier if placed into the shoe first. An adaptation to the pant leg that may be helpful in donning the orthotic is to open the inseam of the pant cuff to the desired length. Stitch the loop side of a Velcro strip underneath the top of the seam and the hook side to the front of the seam. The pant leg then can be opened up, allowing for easier manipulation of the orthotic over the calf.

Adaptive Devices

The therapist should introduce adaptive dressing devices only if the patient cannot otherwise perform dressing safely or efficiently. Dressing devices to consider might include the following:

- A reacher, particularly if a patient has poor trunk control
- A dressing stick, which can be useful to extend reach if trunk balance is impaired and to push garments off the affected side
- A long-handled shoehorn, which may assist the patient in slipping on shoes

All of the aforementioned devices are available from a variety of rehabilitation catalogs.

Walker, Drummond, and Lincoln[3] completed a randomized crossover study. One group ($n = 15$) received

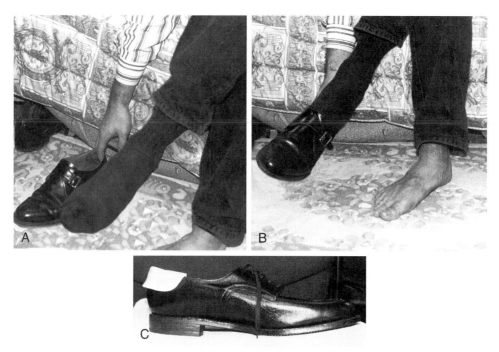

Figure 28-15 **A** and **B**, Sequence for donning shoes for a patient with left hemiplegia. **C**, Heel support fabricated from low-temperature plastic.

three months of no intervention followed by three months of treatment; the other group (*n* = 15) received three months of treatment followed by three months of no treatment. Treatment was provided by an occupational therapist and focused on dressing training for the subjects and their families. The subjects were assessed by an independent evaluator using the Nottingham Stroke Dressing Assessment; the Rivermead ADL Assessment, self-care section; and the Nottingham Health Profile. Both groups showed statistically improved performance during the treatment phase, neither group showed a change during the nontreatment phase, and subjects who received treatment in the first three months maintained their improvement.

Feeding Techniques

Positioning at the Table. The affected extremity should be supported in a good weight-bearing position on the table. This position promotes appropriate upper extremity alignment, visual awareness of the extremity, and trunk symmetry.

Use of Adaptive Devices. To avoid embarrassment while dining with others and to reach full independence with feeding, the patient often uses compensatory strategies and adaptive equipment. The following equipment is recommended:

- Nonskid mats should be used to prevent slippage of plates and bowls and to hold them steady during meals.

- Plate guards and scoop dishes are recommended to eliminate food getting pushed off the plate while scooping or when buttering bread.
- A rocker knife or knife with serrated and curved edges is easy to use with one hand if safety awareness is intact.
- Combined implements such as knife and fork or knife, fork, and spoon are available for purchase. Safety in using these combined instruments is a concern if loss of sensation or weakness in oral-motor structures is present. Utensils with built-up handles also may be used to assist a weak grasp.

INSTRUMENTAL ACTIVITIES OF DAILY LIVING

Kitchen Activities

An individual with hemiplegia can accomplish kitchen tasks safely with adequate activity pacing; properly placed, secured equipment; and provision of adaptive devices.

Energy Conservation and Work Simplification. A consequence of weakness and impaired upper extremity function is that the individual with hemiplegia tires more quickly and thus needs to work at a slower pace. The following energy conservation guidelines should be included in treatment plans focusing on increasing IADL:

- Allow increased time for task completion.
- Take frequent, short rest breaks.
- Sit when working, when possible.

- Avoid complicated procedures.
- Use ready-prepared foods when possible.
- Use labor-saving equipment. (Electrical equipment such as microwaves and food processors with easy-to-control on-off switches and self-cleaning ovens and self-defrosting freezers reduce manual labor requirements.) A variety of cookbooks are available for use with microwave ovens. Recipes tend to be simpler and require less preparation and shorter cooking times.
- Arrange work surfaces at a height that allows for maximal efficiency.
- Avoid excessive reaching and bending.
- Reduce clutter.

To allow for easy access to supplies, items needed most often should be kept on convenient shelves at the front of the most accessible cupboards and drawers or at the back of the work surface.

Storage

A variety of storage devices can be purchased that enhance easy equipment access:

- Plastic-covered racks slide under or clip to the underside of shelves, increasing visible storage space. They can be purchased at hardware stores.
- Peg-Boards can be hung on the wall and used to hang small pots, strainers, kitchen tongs, and spatulas.
- Magnetic knife racks can be placed over a counter top and can be used to store knives, peelers, and kitchen scissors.
- Lazy Susans, which can be placed in easy-to-reach cupboards or at the back of a counter, are useful for persons who have trouble bending or reaching beyond the front of the cabinet; they allow for convenient storage of jars, cans, and bottles.

Transport. Moving supplies safely about the kitchen is another significant challenge for the person with hemiplegia. To avoid lifting and carrying, the patient can use a rolling cart for transporting items from one side of the kitchen to the other. Ideally, the cart should have a handle at one end to provide support while walking. Dycem can be used to help secure items on the cart shelves. A clip secured to the side of the cart with glue can be used to hold a cane or walking device while the person pushes the cart with the noninvolved hand.

Stabilization. Patients can accomplish cooking activities successfully single-handedly with adequate stabilization of items. Tasks such as opening packages and containers, peeling, slicing, making sandwiches, stirring, and mixing create problems that usually can be solved by a variety of self-help devices. The following paragraphs describe commonly used and readily accessible items for self-help.

The Zim jar opener is mounted easily to the wall or underside of a cabinet and allows for one-handed screw cap removal of lids measuring from ½ to 3½ inches in diameter (Fig. 28-16).

A jar opener combined with a Belliclamp allows for easy opening of jar lids for individuals with weak grasps or use of only one hand. The Belliclamp holds jars and bottles securely during use of the jar opener. The Spill Not Jar and Bottle Opener has a plastic nonskid base with three rubber-lined openings to accommodate jars from 1 to 3 inches in diameter. A rubber lid opener provides a firm grip for easy opening of jar tops. Lightweight electrical or cordless can openers are easy to use with one hand and are available from a variety of product catalogs and appliance stores. An example is the E-Z Squeeze One Handed Can Opener (Sammons-Preston).

Patients can open cardboard boxes containing cereals, rice, and instant potatoes one-handed by stabilizing them firmly in a kitchen drawer and then carefully using scissors or the point of a knife to slit the boxtop open. Box toppers are inexpensive devices that easily slide open box tops and are ideal for one-handed use (Fig. 28-17).

Pan holders keep pots and pans stabilized on a range top while the individual stirs or sautés one-handed and are important to prevent spillage of hot food (Fig. 28-18).

A common device for stabilizing equipment and food items during food preparation is Dycem. The product is made from gelatinous material, is nonslip on both sides, and is an easy, inexpensive alternative to help secure items such as pans and mixing bowls in place during cooking. The Stay Put Suction Disc provides another means of securing bowls and plates to any smooth surface using vacuum pressure (Fig. 28-19). Mixing bowls with suction

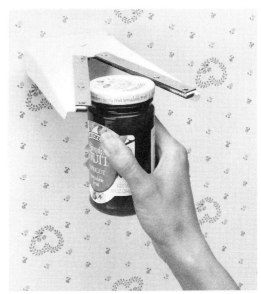

Figure 28-16 Zim jar opener. (Courtesy North Coast Medical, San Jose, Calif.)

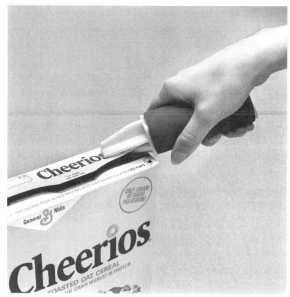

Figure 28-17 Boxtopper. (Courtesy North Coast Medical, San Jose, Calif.)

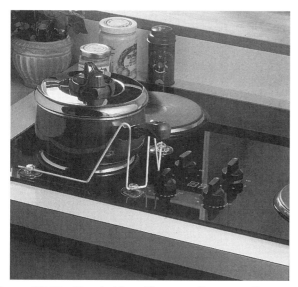

Figure 28-18 Pan holder. (Courtesy Sammons Preston, a BISSELL Company.)

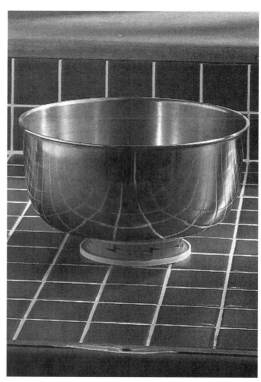

Figure 28-19 Stay Put Suction Disc. (Courtesy Sammons Preston, a BISSELL Company.)

Stainless steel nails hold food in place for cutting and chopping. Food guards keep food from sliding while the individual spreads butter or sandwich spreads. Cutting boards can be fabricated easily using 2-inch thick wood and nails.

Food Storage. Rigid plastic containers with overlapping lids usually are easy to open and seal with one hand.[2] Plastic containers with screw-top lids are ideal for storing rice, sugar, flour, and other items that pour. Aluminum foil molds easily with one hand and is useful for covering containers and wrapping food that requires refrigeration.

Dish Washing. Nonstick cooking utensils are easy to clean and make the cleanup process go quicker. Oven-to-table cookware cuts down on the number of supplies used. Pots and pans can be stabilized for scrubbing by positioning them on a wet dishcloth positioned in the corner of the sink. For washing cups and glasses, the patient can use a brush suctioned to the inside of the sink, such as a suction bottle brush (Fig. 28-20).

Home Maintenance

Work simplification methods should be applied in the performance of household tasks. Housework requires a great deal of mobility and necessitates getting into awkward

bases are available from a variety of product catalogs and allow for more vigorous one-handed stirring without sliding or tipping. Similarly, the Little Octopus Suction Holders are inexpensive and provide double acting grip to anchor glasses, dishes, bowls, and other common objects during meal preparation. Other items such as suction bottom nail brushes can useful during meal preparation to clean fruits and vegetables.

Cutting boards designed for one-handed use and designed from wood, Formica, or plastic come equipped with rubber suction feet to secure the board in place.

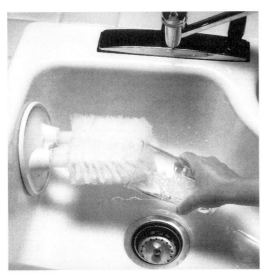

Figure 28-20 Suction bottle brush. (Courtesy North Coast Medical, San Jose, Calif.)

positions. Housework can be made easier by removing clutter from the house. Time spent dusting is cut in half without added clutter. To conserve personal energy and ensure ease of performance, adaptive devices such as lightweight, long-handled, and electronic tools may serve as useful supplements.

Caring for the Floor. Long-handled, freestanding dustpans; self-wringing sponge mops; electrical floor scrubbers; light upright vacuum cleaners with helping hand attachments; and no-wax floors can ease the maintenance of floor care. While mopping the floor, the individual should use a rectangular bucket. This allows the sponge mop to be soaked fully with water in a half-filled bucket as opposed to partial soaking in a round bucket. The bucket should be filled and emptied on the floor with a plastic jug to avoid heavy lifting.

Cleaning the Bathroom. The patient should use a long-handled reach sponge mop to clean the bathroom. This product is available through a variety of rehabilitation catalogs. The risk of falling is great, and kneeling or sitting should be considered in the performance of this household task.

Extra cleaning materials should be kept upstairs and downstairs to avoid unnecessary journeys. Items can be transported in an apron with large pockets, a shoulder bag, or a wheeled cart.

Bed Making. Bed making can be difficult with only one hand. Beds should be positioned so that access to both sides is easy. To conserve energy, the patient can make the bed by completing each corner of one side from the undersheet to bedspread before moving to the other side to repeat the operation.

Changing Sheets. Patients can manage sheets easily if they are folded or unfolded in position on the bed. Pillows should be kept on the bed during changing of the pillowcases so that the bed takes the weight of the pillow.

Laundry

Machine Washing Clothes. The patient should select fabric and garment designs that are completely machine washable and dryable and should use automatic machines.

Hand Washing Clothes. Soaking articles overnight in soap or detergent can minimize the effort to remove dirt with one hand. A washboard can be useful for scrubbing out dirt and stubborn stains.

Wringing Clothes. Small articles can be rolled in a towel and squeezed to remove excess water. Clothes can be wrung out with one hand. Drip-dry clothes should be placed on a hanger before they are removed from the sink.

Ironing

The patient should use a lightweight iron. Steam irons are efficient at removing creases from many materials.

Most ironing boards are height adjustable so that the individual can sit or stand when using them. Ironing boards can be difficult and heavy to manage with one hand. The board may be left permanently standing if space permits. Ironing also can be done on the kitchen table or a counter covered with a folded towel or sheet.

Sewing

Threading Needles. A patient can thread a needle easily with one hand if the needle is held in a pincushion, padded armchair, or bar of soap. Self-threading needles and automatic needle threaders also are available at most major department stores.

Cutting. A patient can cut material if it is stabilized by weight to prevent slipping. Although most scissors are for right-handed use, scissors and shears for left-handed use are available.

Hand Sewing. The patient can perform hemming and sewing seams easily by placing material over a curved object such as an armchair and holding it down with weights.

Machine Sewing. A patient can use a sewing machine with one hand with practice according to safety guidelines.

Communication

Writing. Individuals whose strokes have affected their dominant sides need to consider dominance retraining to learn to write with the noninvolved hand. An important goal for such individuals is to be able to sign their names legibly.

Writing practice begins with exercises consisting of continuous circles and connected up and down strokes. Patients practice large strokes first and progress to smaller ones. With increasing proficiency, patients practice alphabet letters. At the initiation of training, patients should use a larger-size pencil, crayon, or rubber pencil grip attached to a standard pencil. The paper may be stabilized with Dycem or a clamp or by weighting the paper down.

Except for meeting the requirement of a functional signature, individuals may prefer to use another method of written communication. Individuals with hemiplegia can access equipment such as personal computers, tape recorders, and word processors easily.

Using the Telephone. Providing for easy access to the telephone is not a significant problem. Use of a speakerphone can facilitate telephone use. Another product, the commercially available phone holder, frees the noninvolved hand for dialing or taking messages. This device consists of a flexible arm clamped to a table, which holds the telephone receiver in a stationary position; the device is available through product catalogs.

COMMUNITY-BASED ACTIVITIES

Marketing and Grocery Shopping

Energy conservation should be applied in marketing and grocery shopping. The individual should make a list of necessary items and anticipate weekly expenses to minimize trips to the cash machine. The patient should categorize items according to aisles, thus limiting excess walking around the store. The patient can use a lightweight pushcart to carry items around the store and home if a car is not available. Individuals using wheelchairs require assistance with shopping trips. The patient should place money in an easily accessible pocket or purse to ensure easy retrieval at the checkout line. An alternative is mail, phone, or online shopping.

Banking

Banking has become easier during the past decade. Individuals can go the bank, access money through automatic teller machines, and bank by phone or online. If the patient's signature has been altered because of loss of function in the dominant hand, the bank must be notified. Banks have varying policies regarding this situation. For the most part, the new signature can be placed on file easily. Some banks, however, require a written and notarized letter from a physician before a new signature can be authorized.

CASE STUDY

One-Handed Training after Stroke

E.B. is a 74-year-old male recovering from a left stroke with right hemiplegia and a medical history of significant hypertension. E.B. worked as an engineer for 50 years but has been retired for the past two years. He currently is married, and his wife works full-time. E.B. resides in a ground-floor apartment with three steps up to enter the building.

E.B. was referred for home care services on discharge from the hospital. Initial occupational therapy evaluation revealed the following: He was alert and oriented to person, place, situation, and time. His cognitive perceptual status was intact. Before his stroke, E.B. was right-hand dominant. On evaluation, his right upper extremity was flaccid. His left upper extremity had functional range of motion and strength. Sensation was intact throughout. Static and dynamic sitting balance was good. When standing, however, he was unsteady while performing challenging tasks. His endurance for light activity was poor. E.B. required assistance with the following ADL tasks: bathing, grooming, feeding, dressing, simple meal preparation, writing, and community-based activities.

The therapist established a number of treatment goals with the patient:

Long-Term Goals

1. E.B. will be independent in managing BADL using adaptive techniques and assistive devices as required.
2. E.B. will be independent with simple meal preparation.
3. E.B. will be independent in shopping and banking.

Short-Term Goals

1. E.B. will independently bathe himself using assistive devices.
2. E.B. will independently clean and floss his teeth with use of assistive devices.
3. E.B. will be able to cut and butter food independently with a rocker knife.
4. E.B. will independently dress himself using adaptive techniques and devices.
5. E.B. will independently prepare himself lunch.
6. E.B. will independently perform home-based financial responsibilities.

Adaptations

Before initiating basic ADL training, the therapist surveyed the environment to ensure safety and ease of mobility. The following changes were recommended and implemented:

1. Excess clutter was removed from the bedroom, bathroom, kitchen shelves, and drawers to ensure

easier access of needed supplies. Closet rods were lowered to allow for easier access of clothing.

2. The bathroom floor rug was replaced with nonslip mats inside and outside the tub. A tub transfer bench with handheld shower attachment was provided.

3. A board was placed under the mattress to increase firmness, and a bedrail was placed on E.B.'s uninvolved side to increase safe transfers in and out of bed.

4. A lamp was placed on a bedside table next to E.B. to ensure sufficient lighting.

ADL training was initiated with implementation of several adaptations:

Bathing

1. Soap on a rope was used to stabilize the soap.
2. A flex sponge enabled E.B. to reach all body parts successfully.
3. A pump spray shampoo bottle was used to avoid excess waste and keep shampoo from getting into eyes.
4. E.B. reviewed one-handed drying techniques.

Oral Hygiene

1. A toothpaste dispenser allowed for easy one-handed access.
2. The Floss Aid dental floss holder allowed E.B. to floss his teeth.

Nail Management

1. A one-handed home device was fabricated from a nail clipper secured to a piece of plywood with suction feet attached.
2. A pistol-grip toenail clipper enabled E.B. to cut his toenails with less bending.

Dressing

1. Energy conservation techniques were reviewed because of E.B.'s poor endurance.
2. E.B. was able to don and doff shirts but unable to manipulate fasteners. Velcro was substituted for buttons.
3. E.B. was able to don his pants successfully with the support of a sturdy dresser placed next to the bed, which he leaned against to pull up his pants safely while standing.
4. E.B. was able to don his shoes after a piece of splinting material was molded into the shoe heel. Elastic laces allowed for easy fastening.

Feeding and Simple Meal Preparation

A rocker knife, nonskid mat, and plate guard allowed E.B. to cut and butter his food successfully and without spillage.

E.B. also was required to make lunch for himself while his wife was at work. His favorite lunch was a ham and cheese sandwich with lettuce and tomato and a glass of apple juice.

The following kitchen adaptations were made:

1. E.B. used a rolling cart to gather necessary supplies at one time and maneuver them to the kitchen table, where he could sit to complete the task.
2. A cutting board was fabricated using 2-inch thick wood, nails, and a plastic food guard glued to the side of the board. Using the board, E.B. was able to cut tomato slices successfully, stabilize lettuce, and spread mayonnaise on a slice of bread while stabilizing it against the food guard.
3. Presliced ham and cheese were stored in a plastic zipper bag that E.B. could access easily and seal using the zipper bag sealer.
4. Using a Zim jar opener, E.B. was able to open the apple juice bottle top.

Dominance Retraining and Financial Management

E.B. was initially right-hand dominant. An important goal for him was to be able to sign his name legibly on legal documents. He was put on a program of writing practice exercises. After obtaining a legible signature, E.B. contacted the bank and was required to submit a copy of his new signature to be placed on file.

Marketing and Grocery Shopping

As E.B.'s endurance improved, shopping outings with his wife were encouraged. The following energy conservation guidelines were incorporated:

1. E.B. made a list of necessary items and grouped them according to aisles to limit excess walking.
2. A lightweight pushcart was purchased to carry items around the store and into the home.
3. Before leaving home, E.B. would place his money in an easily accessible pocket from which he could retrieve it quickly at the checkout line.

SUMMARY

This chapter describes equipment recommendations and practical and creative solutions that the occupational therapist can incorporate to assist patients in becoming more independent in performing BADL and IADL. For individuals with limited functional return of the involved upper extremity, compensatory techniques are crucial during the rehabilitation process and maximize the potential for reaching meaningful goals. As always, the therapist should concentrate on activities the patient finds most meaningful and curtail activities the individual does not want to perform. For individuals with extensive paralysis resulting from stroke, family members or hired outside help may be required to assist with ADL.

REVIEW QUESTIONS

1. When is use of compensatory strategies most advantageous as part of the rehabilitation process?
2. What environmental considerations need to be taken into account before the initiation of ADL training?
3. Where can specific information regarding the reliability and validity of BADL evaluation instruments be obtained?
4. What are some compensatory techniques and adaptive devices an individual may use during grooming and hygiene to compensate for loss of one upper extremity?
5. Which specific deficits need to be considered before the initiation of dressing training?
6. What energy conservation and work simplification techniques should be considered during IADL training?
7. Which compensatory techniques and adaptive devices should be considered to compensate during kitchen-based activities for loss of one upper extremity?
8. What types of adaptive devices should be considered for easier performance of home-maintenance activities?
9. If a signature has been altered because of loss of function in the dominant hand, what issues need to be addressed before the patient resumes financial responsibilities?

REFERENCES

1. Feldmeier DM, Poole JL: The position-adjustable hair dryer. *Am J Occup Ther* 41(4):246–247, 1987.
1a. Nakayama H, Jorgensen HS, Raaschou HO, et al: Compensation in recovery of upper extremity function after stroke: the Copenhagen stroke study. *Arch Phys Med Rehabil* 75(8):852–857, 1994.
2. U. S. Department of Health and Human Services: *Clinical practice guidelines #16: post stroke rehabilitation*, Rockville, MD, Agency for Healthcare Policy and Research 1995.
3. Walker MF, Drummond AER, Lincoln NB: Evaluation of dressing practice for stroke patients after discharge from hospital: a crossover design study. *Clin Rehabil* 10(1):23, 1996.
4. World Health Organization: *International classification of function*, Geneva, 2001, The Organization.

SUGGESTED READINGS

Berger PE, Mensh S, Whitaker J: *How to conquer the world with one hand . . . and an attitude*, ed 2, Merrifield, VA, 2002, Positive Power Publishing.

Keith RA, Granger CV, Hamilton BB, et al: The functional independence measure: a new tool for rehabilitation. In Eisenberg MG, Grzesiak RC, editors: *Advances in clinical rehabilitation*, vol 1, New York, 1987, Springer-Verlag.

Kelly-Hayes M, Robertson JT, Broderick JP, et al: The American Heart Association Stroke Outcome Classification: executive summary. *Circulation* 97(24):2474–8, 1998.

Law M: *The Canadian occupational performance measure*, ed 4, Ottawa, 2005, CAOT Publications ACE.

Legg L, Drummond A, Leonardi-Bee J, et al: Occupational therapy for patients with problems in personal activities of daily living after stroke: systematic review of randomised trials. *BMJ* 335(7626):922, 2007.

Mahoney FI, Barthel D. Functional evaluation: the Barthel Index. *Md State Med J* 14:56–61, 1965.

Mayer TK: *One-handed in a two-handed world*, ed 2, Boston, 2000, Prince-Gallison Press.

Nakayama H, Jorgensen HS, Raaschou HO, et al: Compensation in recovery of upper extremity function after stroke: the Copenhagen stroke study. *Arch Phys Med Rehabil* 75(8):852–857, 1994.

Steultjens EMJ, Dekker J, Bouter LM, et al: Occupational therapy for stroke patients: a systematic review. *Stroke* 34(3):676–687, 2003.

Trombly CA, Ma HI: A synthesis of the effects of occupational therapy for persons with stroke, Part I: Restoration of roles, tasks, and activities. *Am J Occup Ther* 56(3):250–9, 2002.

van Swieten J, Koudstaal P, Visser M, et al: Interobserver agreement for the assessment of handicap in stroke patients. *Stroke* 19(5):604–607, 1988.

Leisure Participation
after Stroke

key terms

adaptive equipment   leisure   leisure satisfaction

extrinsic barriers   leisure attitudes   types of leisure

intrinsic barriers   leisure roles

chapter objectives

After completing this chapter, the reader will be able to accomplish the following:

1. Define leisure, types of leisure, and functions of leisure activities.
2. Discuss the changes in an individual's ability to engage in leisure tasks after a stroke.
3. Describe problems that may interfere with a patient's participation in leisure tasks.
4. Present possible solutions to these problems.
5. Discuss research addressing leisure participation and occupational therapy interventions after stroke.
6. Outline ways occupational therapists can adapt leisure tasks to allow partial or full participation by someone with a disability caused by a stroke.

Comprehensive stroke rehabilitation must include the consideration of leisure. This is particularly true as there is a renewed focus on decreasing activity limitations and participation restrictions and on improving quality of life as a critical outcome to measure after stroke. Rehabilitation professionals are obligated professionally to address changes in patients' leisure roles and to use patients' leisure interests to plan treatment sessions. This area of functioning is critical in the assessment of patients' motivation, quality of life, and self-esteem. Effective approaches to improving leisure skills and participation usually requires a team approach to meet the complex needs of stroke survivors.

This chapter provides a conceptual framework to help therapists evaluate the leisure skills and improve the leisure participation of patients who have survived a stroke. It focuses on increasing the ability of occupational therapists to improve the leisure skills and the quality of life of this population. Readers are encouraged to review Chapter 3 with this chapter.

DEFINITION OF LEISURE

The Practice Framework[1] of the American Occupational Therapy Association includes leisure under the heading Performance in Areas of Occupation. *Leisure* is described as being "nonobligatory behavior, intrinsically motivated, and engaged in during discretionary time, that is, time not committed to obligatory occupations such as work, self-care, or sleep."[32] The Practice Framework includes the following two subcategories:

1. Leisure exploration: identifying interests, skills, opportunities, and appropriate leisure activities
2. Leisure participation: planning and participating in appropriate leisure activities, maintaining a balance of leisure activities with other areas of occupation, and obtaining, using, and maintaining equipment and supplies as appropriate

The Practice Framework also includes the following related definitions:

- Play: "any spontaneous or organized activity that provides enjoyment, entertainment, amusement, or diversion."[32] Play is further broken down into play exploration (identifying appropriate play activities), and play participation defined as "participating in play; maintaining a balance of play with other areas of occupation; and obtaining, using, and maintaining toys, equipment and supplies appropriately."

- Social participation: "organized patterns of behavior that are characteristic and expected of an individual or a given position within a social system."[30] Social participation can include community (engaging in activities that result in successful interaction at the community level), family (engaging in required or desired family roles), and peer/friend (engaging in activities at different levels of intimacy including engaging in sexual activity). See Chapter 25.

Leisure attitude is defined as the expressed amount of affect toward a given leisure-related object. According to Feibel and Springer,[14] "this attitude is a multiplicative function of a person's beliefs that an object has certain characteristics and a personal evaluation of these characteristics." Many factors affect an individual's leisure attitudes. These factors include social influences, personality, past experiences, and motivation. Leisure attitudes play an important role in the choice and pursuit of leisure activities. A positive experience during an activity usually results in the person continuing to engage in this pursuit.

A *leisure role* is defined as a perceived identity associated with a leisure task. Changes in a person's roles throughout life are accompanied by shifts in leisure participation. Role changes resulting from disability may cause role strain and role conflict: "Role strain refers to the difficulty an individual experiences when attempting to meet role obligations. Role conflict occurs when the occupant of a position perceives that he or she is unable to meet role expectations."[20]

Use of time is an important factor in leisure participation. It is well-documented that individuals have impoverished time use after stroke including leisure and social participation. The therapist should analyze the person's schedule to determine whether intervention is necessary. In an inpatient rehabilitation unit, those with stroke spend more time inactive and alone as compared to those without stroke.[6] Additionally, at one month post-discharge, survivors struggle with establishing routines in their day and coping with an increased amount of idle time. Subjects' strategies for managing increased idle time include "passing time," "waiting on time," and "killing time." [37]

LEISURE, STROKE, AND OCCUPATIONAL THERAPY

In their review of the literature regarding the role of occupational therapy and leisure after stroke, Parker, Gladman, and Drummond[33] summarized the following:

- Stroke survivors often fail to resume full lives, regardless of whether they make a good physical recovery.
- Participation restrictions such as a decline in social and leisure pursuits are prevalent.
- Customary goals of rehabilitation are focused on mobility and independence in self-care, but recovery in a broader sense may not be maximized if health professionals concentrate exclusively on these goals.
- Leisure has been shown to be associated closely with life satisfaction and is a worthwhile goal of rehabilitation.
- Elderly persons show a decline in leisure activity, which has been well-studied. This information may provide a useful model for the more rapid decline seen in stroke patients.
- Further research is needed to confirm the finding that specialized occupational therapy can be effective in raising leisure activity and to show whether this translates into improved psychological well-being.

Widen-Holmqvist and colleagues[42] studied a community-based sample of 20 patients living at home one to three years after hospitalization for stroke and who perceived that they were in need of rehabilitation services. Their results included the following:

- Most of the subjects reported a change in activity and interest patterns after stroke.
- Subjects had high motivation for current activities.
- Cognitive functions were within normal limits for all tested subjects.
- Motor abilities and verbal performances frequently were affected and varied considerably.

- Social and leisure activities outside the home were identified as the most promising goals for community-based rehabilitation programs and that by focusing on such activities, improvement in quality of life for this population could possibly be achieved by individually planned rehabilitation programs.

Amarshi, Artero, and Reid[2] published a qualitative study of 12 stroke survivors and aimed to investigate the types of social/leisure activities engaged in pre/poststroke, the meaning attributed to leisure pursuits, and the process involved in social/leisure participation following stroke. The authors identified four themes from their data:

- Life has changed when characterized by reduced social/leisure activity, giving up favored leisure occupations, and having to rely on others.
- Limitations to participation include physical impairments, cognitive impairments, transportation issues, and cost.
- Requirements for participation include social supports and interactions with others, fitting in with others, accommodations related to transportation, and organization support such as structured groups and programs.
- Moving on with life and reengaging in leisure and social participation including initiate new activities, adapting activities, and maintaining a meaning life.

FACTORS AFFECTING LEISURE PERFORMANCE

Many factors affect leisure participation, including the following:

- Patterns of underlying impairments (i.e, cognitive, motor, psychological, or combinations)
- Types of leisure tasks available
- Stage of life
- Social and cultural environments
- Leisure attitudes, roles, and satisfaction
- Use of time as discussed previously
- Barriers to leisure participation

A strong, well-coordinated person may prefer physical leisure activities such as baseball, soccer, and basketball. Persons with less developed physical skills may be interested in more intellectual leisure tasks such as reading, playing chess, and working puzzles. They also may be interested in creative leisure pursuits such as painting, photography, and quilting.

Geographic location also may affect participation in leisure activities. If a person lives in a rural environment, leisure activities may include hiking, horseback riding, swimming, and fishing. Someone in an urban environment may go shopping or to theaters, lectures, and museums.

Leisure assumes various forms throughout life. The amount and type of leisure activities depend on the person's developmental stage.[18] During adulthood, leisure pursuits are important for establishing and maintaining social networks. A balance between work and play is important. Factors that influence participation in active leisure activities include financial constraints, decreases in functional skills, and decreases in social supports. Many older individuals replace active leisure tasks with more passive ones after experiencing decreases in physical and cognitive abilities.

LEISURE ACTIVITIES DURING OCCUPATIONAL THERAPY

Occupational therapists working with patients who have had a stroke are concerned with the way these individuals spend their time. Often leisure and play interventions are considered secondary during the rehabilitation process as therapists focus on self-care and instrumental activities of daily living (ADL). However, leisure activities can be equally meaningful to patients as they redefine their life roles.[2,39] Occupational therapists can integrate leisure activities into the rehabilitation process in two ways: *occupation-as-end* and *occupation-as-means*.[40]

Occupation-as-end[40] refers to activities and/or tasks that comprise a role. The patient chooses the occupation as a meaningful activity he or she wants to perform, needs to perform, or has to perform. Therapists may become aware of these activities (e.g., bowling, crossword puzzles, and making jewelry) via an interview process or a semistructured interview such as the Canadian Occupational Performance Measure (COPM).[25] When a (leisure) activity is defined by the patient, the therapist collaborates with the patient to accomplish the goal through a variety of interventions including adaptation (e.g., enlarged print on books), education (e.g., providing information regarding transportation methods to and from a local pool), using remaining abilities, and/or remediation. Trombly[40] pointed out that when a therapist uses occupation-as-ends, the therapist is not focused on using leisure activities to make a change at the impairment level (e.g., improve scanning ability), although this may occur as a secondary gain. Trombly suggested that the therapist use the following principles to implement occupation-as-end:

- Organize the subtasks to be learned so the patient will succeed.
- Give clear instructions.
- Use feedback to promote success (see Chapter 5).
- Structure the practice to ensure learning (see Chapter 5).
- Make adaptations when needed (see Chapter 28).

Occupation-as-means[40] may be described as using (leisure) occupations as a treatment to improve body system and body structure impairments. The (leisure) activity is the change agent. The therapist may use leisure activities like the Nintendo Wii to remediate impairments such as weakness, postural dyscontrol, and neglect. Valued leisure activities may be incorporated into the treatment plan to improve other functional areas. For example, the patient may achieve postural and motor goals in a standing position while engaging in a game of air hockey. See Chapter 10 for examples of using occupation-as-means to remediate upper extremity motor control dysfunction and Chapter 19 for examples to improve cognitive-perceptual dysfunction (Box 29-1). Therapists should be cautious about relying too much on using occupation-as-means during treatment sessions; patients should be given a clear explanation related to why the activity was chosen. For example, when a patient has mild neglect, the therapist might say, "As we've both discovered, you are forgetting to look for items on your left, such as not finding your tooth brush on the left side of the sink or the juice in the left side of the refrigerator. We are going to try to get you to look left more often. We are going to play dominoes, and I will put all of your dominoes on the left side. Try to look left as often as possible, and I will remind you as needed." After the activity, processing should occur related to whether the patient met the goals of the session (see Chapter 19). If patients are not given this information, they will not be able to make the connection between the therapeutic activity and their functional goals.

Evaluation of Leisure Skills

When evaluating the leisure roles of patients, therapists must consider seven factors that can affect leisure performance:

1. Evaluation findings related to impairments and performance in areas of occupation
2. Types of leisure activities that interest the patient
3. Patient's stage in the life cycle
4. Physical, social, and cultural environments
5. Patient's previous leisure attitudes, roles, and satisfaction
6. Patient's past and present use of time
7. Premorbid barriers

These factors can guide therapists in identifying leisure activities that must be modified and in assisting patients with leisure exploration. A checklist (Fig. 29-1) can assist

Box 29-1

Role of the Occupational Therapist

- Evaluate patient's physical, cognitive, and perceptual skills and environmental factors (social and cultural) that affect leisure participation.
- Provide treatment to improve patient's limitations.
- Provide adaptive equipment and adapt techniques to improve leisure participation.
- Provide education about various community resources and alternative transportation methods to increase participation.

therapists in determining the type of leisure tasks patients enjoyed before their stroke.[17,28]

Other usual and customary assessments can assist therapists in making decisions regarding leisure interventions. For example, information regarding range of motion, skeletal muscle activity, strength, endurance, postural control and alignment, motor control, praxis, fine motor coordination, and visual-motor integration is critical. The complete cognitive and perceptual assessment provides necessary information regarding the level of arousal, orientation, recognition, attention span, initiation and termination of activities, memory, sequencing, categorization, concept formation, spatial operations, problem-solving, learning, and generalization.

Therapists should review the type of leisure activities the patient performed before the stroke. For instance, someone who mostly participated in individual leisure tasks may have been content with little social contact. If the person enjoyed relational leisure tasks, social interactions may be important.

The therapist must consider the patient's stage in the life cycle because participation in leisure changes during the aging process. During adulthood, an individual's participation in leisure activities decreases because of demands such as work, household maintenance, and childcare. The importance and meaning of leisure also change as a person matures.

The physical, social, and cultural environments are critical in the development of leisure practices and the pursuit of leisure activities during adulthood. Information on the patient's social and cultural networks helps the therapist focus the treatment plan.

The patient's leisure attitudes, roles, and satisfaction before the stroke are important factors to consider after the stroke. The therapist should identify the importance of the selected leisure tasks and the patient's level of satisfaction with them. Identifying the specific aspects of the activity the patient finds enjoyable is helpful. The therapist also should document the patient's leisure roles by discussing topics such as family expectations.

The therapist can address past and present use of time by asking patients to describe the way they spent their time before the stroke, whether they achieved a balance between work and play, and whether they now require additional time for nonleisure activities.

The therapist must address premorbid barriers to leisure participation, which are obstacles that kept patients from participating in the full scope of leisure activities before their stroke and include intrinsic, environmental, and communication barriers (Box 29-2).

Many ways are available to assess an individual's leisure interests, such as a leisure interest checklist (see Fig. 29-1), a structured interview form, and a time log (Fig. 29-2) that requires the patient to record previous and current use of time. Therapists should strive to use standardized assessments.

Examples of assessments the therapist can use to assess leisure skills and participation in stroke survivors include the following:

■ Nottingham Leisure Questionnaire:[11,12,35] This assessment was developed to measure the leisure activity of stroke patients. The results of the interrater reliability study were "excellent," and the results for the test-retest reliability study were "excellent" or "good." Recently, the Nottingham Leisure Questionnaire has been shortened (from 37 to 30 items) and the response categories have been collapsed (from five to three categories) to make it suitable for mail use.[11] Higher Nottingham Leisure Questionnaire scores were associated with higher subscores on the Nottingham Extended Activities of Daily Living Scale, and lower Nottingham Leisure Questionnaire scores were associated with living alone and worse emotional health.

■ Activity Card Sort:[4] The card sort is used to measure an individual's participation or lack of participation in instrumental, leisure, and social activities. See Chapter 3 for a full description.

■ Canadian Occupational Performance Measure:[25] This semistructured interview covers three areas: leisure, self-care, and productivity. The patient identifies and ranks areas of meaningful occupational performance and rates the level of performance and satisfaction.

Date _____   Occupation_____

Name _____   Marital status _____

Age _____   Onset of stroke _____

Cultural background _____   Children's ages _____

Favorite leisure task _____   Male _____   Female _____

Please answer the following questions to enable your therapist to assist you in resuming/persuing your leisure interests:

1. When do you perform leisure activities?

_____ Morning   _____ Afternoon   _____ Evening   _____ Weekdays

_____ Weekends   _____ Holidays   _____ Vacations

2. What type of leisure activities do you enjoy?

_____ Physical   _____ Intellectual   _____ Arts   _____ Social

_____ Solitary   _____ Structured   _____ Unstructured

3. Place a check mark next to the people who are involved in your leisure activities.

_____ Significant other   _____ Spouse   _____ Children   _____ Parent

_____ Sibling   _____ Friend   _____ Co-worker   _____ Pets

_____ Relatives   _____ Grandparents _____ Grandchildren

4. Do you want to resume your past leisure activities?

_____ Yes   _____ No   _____ Do not know

5. If you do not want to resume past leisure activities, please place a check mark next to the reasons.

_____ Loss of skills   _____ No time   _____ Depressed   _____ Resources not available

_____ Afraid   _____ No transportation _____ Decreased leisure performance

_____ Decreased communciation skills   _____ No interest

_____ Other—Please state the reason. _____

_____

6. Are you satisfied with your present leisure activites?

_____ Yes   _____ No—why? _____   _____ Do not know

Figure 29-1 Leisure interest checklist.   *Continued*

Please check the types of leisure activities you enjoy:

Music
_____ Attending concerts
_____ Singing
_____ Playing instruments
_____ Conducting
_____ Watching concerts on television
_____ Listening to the radio

Dance
_____ Tap
_____ Ballet
_____ Folk
_____ Jazz
_____ Ballroom
_____ Modern
_____ Other

Arts and Crafts
_____ Carpentry
_____ Sewing
_____ Knitting
_____ Needlepoint
_____ Painting
_____ Quilting
_____ Ceramics
_____ Model making
_____ Drawing
_____ Sculpture
_____ Photography
_____ Other

Community
_____ Volunteering
_____ Travel
_____ Church
_____ Temple
_____ Other

Sports
_____ Skiing
_____ Softball
_____ Baseball
_____ Football
_____ Running
_____ Jogging
_____ Biking
_____ Hockey
_____ Basketball
_____ Skating
_____ Sailing
_____ Other

Table Games
_____ Table tennis
_____ Cards
_____ Scrabble
_____ Dominoes
_____ Puzzles
_____ Chinese checkers
_____ Checkers
_____ Othello
_____ Chess
_____ Monopoly
_____ Backgammon
_____ Trivial Pursuit
_____ Other

Relaxation
_____ Meditation
_____ Yoga
_____ T'ai chi
_____ Horticulture
_____ Pet care

Figure 29-1, cont'd

- Leisure Competence Measure:[22,23] This measure provides information about leisure functioning and measures change in leisure function over time. The tool includes nine areas: social contact, community participation, leisure awareness, leisure attitude, social behaviors, cultural behaviors, leisure skills, interpersonal skills, and community integration skills. Items are rated on the 7-point Likert scale.
- Leisure Satisfaction Scale:[5,36] This scale measures the degree to which people's personal needs are met through their leisure activities (24 items scored from 1 to 5; higher scores indicate greater satisfaction).
- Leisure Diagnostic Battery:[7] The original version includes 95 items, whereas the newer, shorter version includes 25 items. Items are rated on 3-point scale. Assessment areas include playfulness, competence, barriers, and knowledge.
- Frenchay Activities Index:[41] This tool is used for assessing general (i.e, other than personal care) activities of stroke survivors. The tool comprises 15 individual activities summed to give an overall score from 0 (low) to 45 (high).

Interventions to Improve Leisure Skills

The intervention process begins with obtaining the patient's leisure history. The therapist then reviews the results of the evaluation and determines the patient's strengths and limitations in relation to the performance components.

Box 29-2

Factors Affecting Leisure Performance after Stroke

Type of leisure tasks	Unconditional
	Compensatory or recuperative
	Relational
	Role-determined
Stage in the life cycle	Childhood
	Young adult
	Middle age
	Later life
Social and cultural	Support system (i.e, family
environments	and friends)
	Nationality
	Religion
Leisure attitudes, roles,	Attitudes
and satisfaction	Roles
	Satisfaction
Use of time	Present
	Past
Barriers to leisure	Internal barriers
participation	Lack of knowledge
	Decreased skills
	Decreased opportunities
	Environmental barriers
	Attitudes
	Architectural
	Transportation
	Rules and regulations
	Barriers of omission
	Economic
	Communication barriers
	Social skills
	Ability to speak
	Ability to listen

Leisure tasks may be used to achieve the goals of occupational therapy treatment. Leisure activities may be used during treatment sessions to remediate impairments, enhance the skill itself, or adapt the leisure activity itself. Therapists must identify the skills necessary to perform the tasks and modify them according to each patient's ability. The occupational therapist may provide treatment for neuromuscular, psychological, and cognitive deficits that will enable the patient to engage in the leisure activity.

The National Therapeutic Recreation Society proposes a continuum model of leisure service delivery. According to one description, "the 'Leisure Ability Model' serves as a guide for community recreation professionals to facilitate the movement of individuals with disabilities from more intrusive, specialized recreation services into integrated leisure environments."[38] This model consists of a continuum with four levels:

1. Noninvolvement
2. Segregated

3. Integrated
4. Accessible

At the first level noninvolvement, the person who has the disability does not participate in any leisure tasks. At the second level segregated, the patient participates in structured activities developed for group members with the same disability group. Examples include community activities through local stroke organizations, stroke support groups, and specialized sports programs (aquatics).

The third level integrated "provides persons with disabilities the opportunity to be mainstreamed into regular community recreation programs and to participate alongside nondisabled participants. This approach appears to go a long way toward helping to change the negative attitudes, stereotypes, stigmas, and myths associated with persons with disabilities and the systems that serve them."[38] The occupational therapist can instruct patients in the use of adaptive equipment and methods to pursue leisure activities successfully in the community.

The fourth level accessible occurs when the individual with a disability "is able to select and access preferred recreation programs with no more effort than his or her counterpart who is not disabled.... The participant is able to realize his or her ultimate goal of achieving a satisfying leisure lifestyle, free of any significant individual and external constraints."[38]

The therapist can use these levels to improve an individual's involvement gradually. For instance, if a patient enjoys bowling and wants to return to this activity, the therapist may locate or form a specialized bowling program. When the patient develops skills, he or she may join an integrated bowling program and eventually an accessible bowling program. This model can serve as a guide for occupational therapists when introducing resources for leisure services. Occupational therapists can assist patients in exploring alternative types of leisure tasks that fulfill their needs. This may include expanding their leisure activity repertoires to improve the quality of their lives. Occupational therapists educate patients on available services.

Treatment also can focus on helping patients and family members overcome barriers to leisure participation. Common barriers are intrinsic, environmental, and communication-related.

Intrinsic barriers are the results of the disability. These barriers may include lack of knowledge about leisure activities and programs, decreased educational activities, health problems related to the disability, psychological and physical dependence, and decreased skills.[21]

Occupational therapists can address intrinsic barriers in a variety of ways. Remaining informed about current community resources, support groups in the area, and professional leisure organizations designed to serve individuals

Time	Activity	Environment	Physical assistance	Cognitive skills required	Feelings
6:30 AM					
7:00					
7:30					
8:00					
8:30					
9:00					
9:30					
10:00					
10:30					
11:00					
11:30					
12:00 PM					
12:30					
1:00					
1:30					
2:00					
2:30					
3:00					
3:30					
4:00					
4:30					
5:00					
5:30					
6:00					
6:30					
7:00					
7:30					
8:00					
8:30					
9:00					
9:30					
10:00					
10:30					
11:00					

Figure 29-2   Patients can use a time log to record their previous and current use of time.

who have a physical disability is essential.[8] These organizations include stroke support groups, wheelchair sport leagues, and the American Heart Association.

Environmental barriers include attitudes, architectural and ecological obstacles, transportation, rules and regulations, and barriers of omission.[21] The attitudes of others are a serious problem for persons who have disabilities. Attitudinal barriers result in negative behaviors, stigmas, and decreased acceptance and participation in leisure tasks. Occupational therapists can suggest strategies that patients can use to address social prejudices.

Architectural barriers prevent individuals who have physical disabilities from participating in leisure activities. The main problem is accessibility as many buildings and sport facilities are not wheelchair accessible.

Occupational therapists can consult with architects, builders, and contractors to determine necessary modifications, such as installing a lift for a swimming pool. See Chapter 27.

Transportation barriers are another issue. Many persons with disabilities cannot drive or take public transportation independently. Public transportation is not always wheelchair-accessible and when it is accessible, it does not always foster independence because a driver may be required to operate the lift for the person to enter. The Americans with Disabilities Act is correcting this problem gradually by requiring wheelchair-accessible transportation. Occupational therapists can educate patients about the Americans with Disabilities Act and alternate methods of transportation. See Chapter 23.

Economic barriers also play a role in preventing individuals with disabilities from performing leisure activities. For example, gym memberships are too costly even for many able-bodied persons. Disabled individuals often live on a fixed income and have many medical and living expenses. Occupational therapists can educate their patients about available resources and community groups and encourage participation.

The final barrier involves communication. Disabilities that affect the ability to speak, listen, or respond lead to poor social interaction during the leisure task. By training patients in the use of assistive technology to improve communication skills, occupational therapists can play an active role in correcting this environmental barrier (see Chapter 20).

LEISURE INTERVENTIONS FOR STROKE SURVIVORS: EVIDENCE-BASED PRACTICE

A number of research studies address the issue of leisure activities after stroke. This literature can provide occupational therapists with valuable information about assessment and adaptation of leisure skills for stroke patients.[10,24,26,31] Research has demonstrated that many individuals who sustained a stroke do not resume many of their favorite social and leisure activities.[19,29] Factors that affect leisure participation after stroke include the following:

- Time
- Meaningfulness of activities
- Personal standards
- Internal/external control
- Range of interests
- Performance
- Transportation
- Social relations

Other studies have found the following:

- Individuals who sustained strokes do not resume leisure tasks because they do not have time. Their days usually are filled with exercises and self-care tasks. In addition, subjects reported that time passed slowly and they were bored.[19,29]
- Disabilities resulting from stroke can lead to changes in family roles and social relationships, which may result in role strain or role conflict.[20]
- Depression after stroke is related strongly to a decrease in social activities.[14]
- Stroke survivors do not resume normal social activities after stroke. Factors include social and environmental issues, emotional difficulties, and organic brain dysfunction. Activities outside the home appear more difficult to resume than activities in the home.
- Factors that affect life satisfaction after stroke include depression, poor ADL performance, and decreased social activity outside the home.[3]

Occupational therapists need to document what types of intervention are most successful in improving engagement in leisure activities after a stroke. At this point, clinical trials focused on this issue had conflicting results.

Desrosiers and colleagues[9] evaluated the effect of a leisure education program on participation in and satisfaction with leisure activities (leisure-related outcomes), and well-being, depressive symptoms, and quality of life (primary outcomes) after stroke via a randomized controlled trial. Experimental participants received the leisure education program at home once a week for eight to 12 weeks. Control participants were visited at home at a similar frequency. Participants were evaluated before and after the program by a blinded assessor. The leisure education program was carried out by an occupational and recreational therapist for a maximum of 12 sessions. The program was divided into three components, as defined by Desrosiers and colleagues:

- Leisure awareness (i.e, the perception and knowledge people have of their leisure activities and how important they consider them)
- Self-awareness (i.e, people's perception of themselves, and their values, attitudes, and capacities in regard to leisure activities)
- Competency development that encompassed the perceived and real constraints identified by the person and knowledge of alternatives to achieve autonomy in leisure activities (Fig. 29-3)

The authors found that the leisure education program was effective for improving participation in leisure activities, improving satisfaction with leisure, and reducing depression in people with stroke. There were no differences between the groups on the General Well-Being Schedule or the Stroke-Adapted Sickness Impact Profile.

Drummond and Walker[13] carried out a randomized, controlled trial to evaluate the effectiveness of a leisure rehabilitation program on functional performance and mood. Subjects were allocated randomly to three groups: a leisure rehabilitation group, a conventional occupational therapy group, and a control group. The subjects assigned to the leisure and conventional occupational therapy group received individual treatment at home after discharge from hospital. Baseline assessments were carried out on admission to the study and at three and six months after discharge from hospital by an evaluator blind to the trial. The results showed an increase only in the leisure scores for the leisure rehabilitation group, despite an age imbalance in the study. The authors also concluded that subjects receiving leisure rehabilitation performed significantly better in mobility and psychological well-being than the subjects in the other two groups.

Parker and colleagues[34] evaluated the effects of leisure therapy and conventional occupational therapy via a randomized controlled trial (multicenter) using the outcomes of mood, leisure participation, and independence

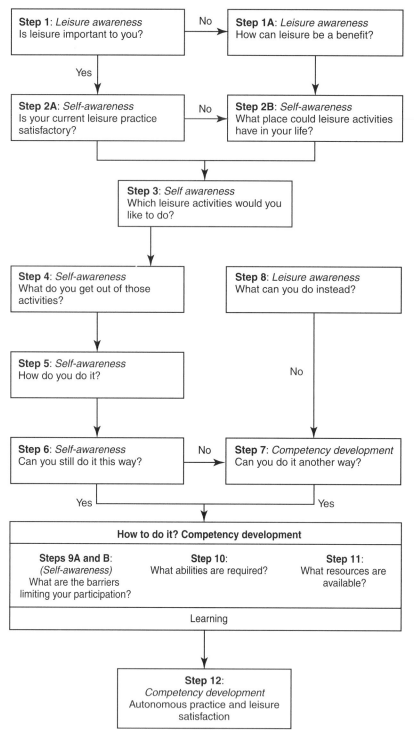

Figure 29-3   Summary of the leisure education program. (From Desrosiers J, Noreau L, Rochette A, et al: Effect of a home leisure education program after stroke: a randomized controlled trial. *Arch Phys Med Rehabil* 88(9):1095–1100, 2007.)

in ADL. Subjects included stroke survivors six and 12 months after hospital discharge. In total, the study included 466 patients from five centers in the United Kingdom. The standardized assessments used in the trial included the General Health Questionnaire (12 items), the Nottingham Extended ADL Scale, and the Nottingham Leisure Questionnaire, assessed by mail and with telephone follow-up for clarification. Eighty-five percent of survivors and 78% of survivors responded at six- and 12-month follow-up, respectively. At six months and compared with the control group, those allocated to leisure therapy did not have significantly better General

Health Questionnaire scores, leisure scores, and extended ADL scores. The group assigned to ADL did not have significantly better General Health Questionnaire scores and extended ADL scores and did not have significantly worse leisure scores. The results at 12 months were similar. The authors concluded that in contrast to the findings of previous smaller trials, neither of the additional occupational therapy treatments showed a clear beneficial effect on mood, leisure activity, or independence in ADL measured at six or 12 months.

A post hoc analysis by Logan and colleagues[27] of the previously mentioned study by Parker and colleagues[34] further examined the ADL and leisure groups. The ADL group received significantly more mobility training, transfer training, cleaning, dressing, cooking, and bathing training, while sport, creative activities, games, hobbies, gardening, entertainment, and shopping were used significantly more in the leisure group. Fifteen items from the outcome measures were identified as specific to these interventions. The authors found no evidence that specific ADL or leisure interventions led to improvements in specific relevant outcomes.

Gilbertson and Langhorne[15] evaluated a short post-discharge home-based occupational therapy service for stroke patients, including an assessment of the patients' satisfaction with occupational performance and service provision using a single-site, blind, randomized, controlled trial. One hundred thirty-eight patients were assigned randomly to a conventional outpatient follow-up or conventional services plus six weeks of home-based occupational therapy. The data were collected before discharge and at seven weeks and six months after discharge using the COPM, the Dartmouth Cooperative (COOP) Charts, the London Handicap Scale, and a patient satisfaction questionnaire. At seven weeks, the intervention group reported significantly greater changes in performance and satisfaction (COPM), better emotional scores (Dartmouth COOP Charts), and improved work and leisure activity scores (London Handicap Scale). The authors concluded that a six-week postdischarge home-based occupational therapy service could improve patients' perceptions of their occupational performance and satisfaction with services but may not have a long-term effect on subjective health outcomes.

Gladman and Lincoln[16] reported findings of the Domiciliary Stroke Rehabilitation (DOMINO) study that compared home-based and hospital-based rehabilitation services for stroke patients via a randomized, controlled trial, with 327 subjects enrolled after discharge from the hospital. No difference between the services had been found at six months, but home therapy was better than outpatient therapy related to improving household ability and leisure activity in the subjects who originally were discharged from a stroke unit.

Jongbloed and Morgan[19] designed a study to determine the efficacy of occupational therapy intervention related to the leisure activities of stroke survivors. The study included 40 discharged stroke patients who were assigned randomly to an experimental group, which received occupational therapy intervention related to leisure activities, or to a control group. An independent evaluator assessed the patients' involvement in activities and satisfaction with that involvement on three separate occasions. The authors found no statistically significant differences between the experimental and control groups in activity involvement or satisfaction with that involvement. The authors point out that the lack of significant differences may be due to the intervention being limited in scope (five therapist visits) and the observation that many environmental factors strongly influence activity participation and satisfaction.

ADAPTING THE LEISURE TASK

Reintroducing leisure activities to patients who have sustained a stroke is important. If the patient does not regain the skills needed to perform these leisure tasks, many adaptive devices are on the market to enable full participation in these tasks. To select the most effective adaptive aid, the occupational therapist analyzes the skill components necessary to perform the chosen activity. After identifying the components that limit performance, the therapist selects and introduces an appropriate adaptive device. Occupational therapists provide patients with information about various organizations, adaptive methods, and adaptive equipment that enhance and promote participation in leisure activities. Use of these resources enables patients to lead meaningful and productive lives.

Many types of adaptive equipment enable patients who have use of one hand to participate in leisure tasks (e.g, card holders, knitting-needle holders, fishing-pole holders, and needlepoint holders). These products are available from the Internet, catalogs, occupational therapists, and specialized organizations and stores.

SUMMARY

Leisure is a complex phenomenon. A review of the literature reveals that leisure may be defined in various ways. Many factors influence an individual's participation in leisure activities, such as roles, attitudes, satisfaction, stage in the life cycle, and intrinsic and extrinsic barriers. The role of the occupational therapist is multifaceted, including assessment, intervention through techniques and adaptive equipment, and patient and family education, with an emphasis on community resources. Leisure activities may be used to improve a patient's motivation, quality of life, and self-esteem.

CASE STUDY

Leisure Skills after Stroke

R.S. is a 74-year-old woman who sustained a right-sided stroke four months ago. After completion of the central nervous system assessment, interest checklist, time log, and activity analysis form, the occupational therapist established goals with R.S.

Briefly, the results of the central nervous system assessment were as follows. Right upper extremity function was within normal limits. Left upper extremity function revealed poor motor control with stereotypical patterns present and impaired sensation throughout. Ability to shift weight anteriorly and laterally while in a seated position was fair. Sustained attention skills were limited. She had a minimal left-sided inattention to self and environment and minimal impairments with spatial relations.

R.S. has been widowed for five years and reported feeling lonely, depressed, and fearful of falling. Her three adult children live out of state, and her social network consists of supportive neighbors, church members, and her dog.

Currently a home health aide assists R.S. with self-care and home management tasks. R.S. requires activity set-up for grooming and upper body hygiene, minimal assistance with upper body dressing and bathing, moderate assistance with lower body dressing and bathing, moderate assistance for stand-pivot transfers, minimal assistance for bed mobility, and moderate assistance with meal preparation from a seated level. She is not performing her favorite leisure task of knitting. How can an occupational therapist assist R.S.?

ACKNOWLEDGMENTS

The author would like to thank early contributors Denise A. Supon and Nancy C. Whyte.

REVIEW QUESTIONS

1. List and define the types and purposes of leisure tasks.
2. What are the factors the therapist must address when evaluating an individual's leisure participation and performance after sustaining a stroke? Describe how these factors affect leisure participation and performance.
3. What are leisure attitudes, roles, and satisfaction?
4. List and describe the environmental barriers that affect leisure participation.
5. What is the role of the occupational therapist in assessing and improving a patient's leisure participation after a stroke?
6. How would the occupational therapist assist a patient and family members in resuming leisure activities in their community?

REFERENCES

1. Amarshi F, Artero L, Reid D: Exploring social and leisure participation among stroke survivors: Part two. *Int J Ther Rehabil* 13(5):199–208, 2006.
2. American Occupational Therapy Association (AOTA): Occupational therapy practice framework: Domain and process, 2nd ed. *Am J Occup Ther* 62(6):625–683, 2008.
3. Astrom M, Asplund K, Astrom T: Psychosocial function and life satisfaction after stroke. *Stroke* 23(4):527–531, 1992.
4. Baum CM, Edwards DF: *Activity Card Sort*, 2nd ed. Bethesda, MD, 2008, AOTA Press.
5. Beard JG, Ragheb MG: The leisure satisfaction measure. *J Leis Res* 12(1):20–33, 1980.
6. Bear-Lehman J, Bassile CC, Gillen G: A comparison of time use on an acute rehabilitation unit: Subjects with and without a stroke. *Phys Occup Ther Geriatr* 20(1):17–27, 2001.
7. Chang Y, Card JA: The reliability of the leisure diagnostic battery short form version B in assessing healthy, older individuals: a preliminary study. *Ther Recreation J* 28(3):163, 1994.
8. Dattilo J: *Inclusive leisure services: responding to the rights of people with disabilities*, State College, PA, 1994, Venture Publishing.
9. Desrosiers J, Noreau L, Rochette A, et al: Effect of a home leisure education program after stroke: a randomized controlled trial. *Arch Phys Med Rehabil* 88(9):1095–1100, 2007.
10. Drummond AE: Leisure activity after stroke. *Int Disabil Stud* 12(4):157–160, 1990.
11. Drummond AE, Parker CJ, Gladman JR, et al: Development and validation of the Nottingham leisure questionnaire (NLQ). *Clin Rehabil* 15(6):647–656, 2001.
12. Drummond AE, Walker M: The Nottingham leisure questionnaire for stroke patients. *Br J Occup Ther* 57:414–418, 1994.
13. Drummond AE, Walker MF: A randomized controlled trial of leisure rehabilitation after stroke. *Clin Rehabil* 9(4):283, 1995.
14. Feibel JH, Springer CJ: Depression and failure to resume social activities after stroke. *Arch Phys Med Rehabil* 63(6):276–277, 1982.
15. Gilbertson L, Langhorne P: Home-based occupational therapy: stroke patients' satisfaction with occupational performance and service provision. *Br J Occup Ther* 63(10):464, 2000.
16. Gladman JR, Lincoln NB: Follow-up of a controlled trial of domiciliary stroke rehabilitation (DOMINO Study). *Age Ageing* 23(1):9–13, 1994.
17. Holbrook M, Skilbeck CE: An activities index for use with stroke patients. *Age Ageing* 12(2):166–170, 1983.
18. Iso-Ahola S, Jackson E, Dunn E: Starting, ceasing and replacing leisure activities over the life span. *J Leisure Res* 26(3):227–249, 1994.
19. Jongbloed L, Morgan D: An investigation of involvement in leisure activities after a stroke. *Am J Occup Ther* 45(5):420–427, 1991.
20. Jongbloed L, Stanton S, Fousek B: Family adaptation to altered roles following a stroke. *Can J Occup Ther* 60(2):70, 1993.
21. Kennedy D, Austin D, Smith R: *Special recreation opportunities for persons with disabilities*, Dubuque, IA, 1987, WC Brown.
22. Kloseck M, Crilly RG: *Leisure competence measure: adult version I*, London, Ontario, 1997, Data System.
23. Kloseck M, Crilly RG, Hutchinson-Troyer, L: Measuring therapeutic recreation outcomes in rehabilitation: Further testing of the Leisure Competence Measure. *Ther Recreation J* 35(1):31–42, 2001.
24. Krefting L, Krefting D: Leisure activities after a stroke: an ethnographic approach. *Am J Occup Ther* 45(5):429–436, 1991.
25. Law M, Baptiste S, Carswell A, et al: *Canadian occupational performance measure manual*, ed 3, Ottawa, 1998, CAOT Publications ACE.

26. Lawrence L, Christie D: Quality of life after stroke: a three year follow-up. *Age Ageing* 8(3):167–172, 1979.

27. Logan PA, Gladman JR, Drummond AE, Radford KA: A study of interventions and related outcomes in a randomized controlled trial of occupational therapy and leisure therapy for community stroke patients. *Clin Rehabil* 17(3):249–255, 2003.

28. Matsutsuyu J: The interest checklist. *Am J Occup Ther* 23(4):323–328, 1969.

29. Morgan D, Jongbloed L: Factors influencing leisure activities following a stroke: an exploratory study. *Can J Occup Ther* 57(4):223, 1990.

30. Mosey AC: *Applied scientific inquiry in the health professions: An epistemological orientation*, 2nd ed, Bethesda, MD, 1996, American Occupational Therapy Association.

31. Niemi M, Laaksonen R, Kotila M, et al: Quality of life 4 years after stroke. *Stroke* 19(9): 1101–1107, 1988.

32. Parham D, Fazio L, editors: *Play in occupational therapy for children*, St. Louis, MO, 1997, Mosby.

33. Parker CJ, Gladman JR, Drummond AE: The role of leisure in stroke rehabilitation. *Disabil Rehabil* 19(1):1–5, 1997.

34. Parker CJ, Gladman JR, Drummond AE, et al: A multicentre randomized controlled trial of leisure therapy and conventional occupational therapy after stroke, TOTAL Study Group, trial of occupational therapy and leisure. *Clin Rehabil* 15(1):42–52, 2001.

35. Parker CJ, Logan PA, Gladman JRF, Drummond AER: A shortened version of the Nottingham Leisure Questionnaire. *Clin Rehab* 11(3):267–68, 1997.

36. Raghed, M, Griffith, C: The contribution of leisure participation and leisure satisfaction to life satisfaction of older persons. *J Leis Res* 14(4):295–306, 1982.

37. Rittman M, Faircloth C, Boylstein C, et al: The experience of time in the transition from hospital to home following stroke. *J Rehabil Res Devel* 41(3A):259–68, 2004.

38. Schlelen S, Ray M: *Community recreation and persons with disabilities: strategies for integration*, Baltimore, 1988, Paul B Brookes.

39. Soderback I, Ekholm J, Caneman G: Impairment/function and disability/activity 3 years after cerebrovascular incident or brain trauma: a rehabilitation and occupational therapy view. *Int Disabil Stud* 13(3):67–73, 1991.

40. Trombly CA: Occupation. In Trombly CA, Radomski MV, editors: *Occupational therapy for physical dysfunction*, ed 5, New York, 2002, Lippincott Williams & Wilkins.

41. Wade DT, Legh-Smith J, Langton Hewer R: Social activities after stroke: measurement and natural history using Frenchay activities index. *Int Rehabil Med* 7(4):176–181, 1985.

42. Widen-Holmqvist L, de Pedro-Cuesta J, Holm M, et al: Stroke rehabilitation in Stockholm: basis for late intervention in patients living at home. *Scand J Rehabil Med* 25(4):173–181, 1993.

salvatore dimauro*

chapter 30

A Survivor's Perspective

THE EVENT

It happened during breakfast, on a bright December morning, unannounced, almost gently, and absolutely painlessly. I was wearing a thick terry cloth robe, which buffered my slumping to the floor and gave it (at least in my visual memory) a slow-motion appearance.

I ended up on my left side on the parquet floor, rejecting my father-in-law's offers of help, thrashing my right leg, holding onto the seat of my chair with my right hand, a little embarrassed and miffed that I did not seem able to stand up. I also remember distinctly my irritation at my mother-in-law's plaintive demands that her husband remove a piece of bread I was chewing on when the stroke hit. She, a keen observer with an artist's eye for detail, had noticed that chewing motions had ceased on the left side of my mouth and food was stuck under the cheek.

Because I was recuperating from open heart surgery—a mitral valve repair that had been performed two weeks earlier—little diagnostic acumen, especially for a neurologist, was required to conclude that I had suffered a stroke. Lying on my dining room floor waiting for the ambulance, I ruminated about the inappropriateness of the word *stroke* to describe what had happened to me, which had been more like the gentle snuffing of a candle than a violent hit. Nevertheless, the term *stroke* (from the Latin *ictus*, which is still widely used in medical jargon) is universally accepted and has equivalent words in most Western languages. I concluded one of two things: either stroke referred to the suddenness of the event rather than to its outward manifestations or I had had an unusual stroke. Now I know both things are probably true.

The fact that I was musing about words minutes after my stroke illustrates the most important "lucky" feature of this unfortunate event: it had spared mentation and speech. Although at times I suspect that my friends and relatives may have welcomed a little aphasia on my part, talking, reading, and, soon enough, working have been vital parts of my recovery, and I am certainly grateful for whatever forces, natural or supernatural, pushed the blood clot into the right rather than into the left carotid artery.

Finding myself totally incapacitated in a hospital bed was not as traumatic an experience as it would be now, maybe because it occurred so shortly after a similar post-operative intensive care experience. Or else, unbeknown to me, I was in a slightly stuporous state that blessedly quenched the emotional reactions to what was happening. Although I seemed to remember every detail of those first days after the stroke, later I discovered some curious gaps. For example, I have no memory of having received a Doppler scan. Months later, when a repeat scan was performed and I was shown the results of the first examination, I had to admit to myself that I must have been in that same laboratory, which I did not remember, subjected to the same procedure, which seemed new to me, by the same technician, who greeted me cordially but whom I did not recognize.

The question most often asked, especially by other neurologists, is "What does it feel like to be hemiplegic?" I had asked myself the same question when seeing patients who had lost various degrees of motor control. The answer, again, at least in my case, is disappointingly simple: it really felt like nothing, like I had never been able to use my left limbs; no exasperating feeling of formulating a mental command and getting no action occurred. Nor do I think that this was because of loss or diminution of left-body awareness (asomatoagnosia) or sensation, because I had neither to any detectable extent. Peculiarly, the frustration and anger with the sluggish and clumsy left limbs, especially in the hand, came later

---

*This chapter is dedicated to Maria Laura, Beppe, Giorgio, and Alessandra. My recovery would have been a lot slower without their loving assistance and support.

as I was gradually regaining function and continue to this day. I do not remember how many times I have cursed and actually punched my left hand for not performing adequately, knocking things over, being in the way, or simply being ridiculously (and embarrassingly) tremulous in reaching for objects.

However, at the time of admission to neurology, my only frustration was related to being totally dependent on others for everything, from turning in bed to performing bodily functions. As an intensely (maybe a bit neurotically) private person, as I had been all of my life, the loss of privacy that comes with major illness was initially a big problem for me. The "silver lining" has been, in fact, the acceptance of my physical frailty as a matter of fact.

How does a neurologist live with a neurological disease? I cannot answer this question appropriately because I lived my stroke as a patient, not as a neuroscientist. I asked few neurological questions and never wanted to see my magnetic resonance imaging films. As I had done at the time of my heart operation, I had full trust in the skill of my physicians and colleagues first and my physical and occupational therapists later and took a passive though cooperative attitude throughout the healing process. I think this consciously ignorant and trusting position may have done me more good than a critical, controlling approach.

Of course, seeing my own left toe go up in a classical Babinski sign, witnessing my own excessive knee jerk, and feeling odd paresthesias in the left side of my body and "pins and needles" in my left hand were strangely interesting experiences. Some peculiar phenomena may have escaped an untrained observer; for example, I noticed at some point (perhaps two months after the stroke) that a spontaneous Babinski sign occurred whenever I initiated urination. This happened without exception and consisted of two or three jerky dorsiflexions of the left toe that promptly subsided as the stream of urine became steady. This "urinary Babinski" persisted throughout the first year after the stroke and continues to occur sporadically to this day. My colleagues in the stroke unit swear they have never heard of a similar phenomenon, but physicians and therapists may find inquiring about this systematically with patients recovering from stroke a worthwhile task. Who knows, perhaps the "urinary Babinski" (DiMauro sign?) will be added to the spontaneous Babinski sign observed by H. Houston Merritt on removing a patient's slippers.

As every patient does, I worried about the extent of recovery I could expect. I was encouraged by the fact that I could bend my leg from the very beginning. I would show this proudly to visitors and colleagues with the expectation of rosy prognostic pronouncements. I was concerned by the total lack of movement in my left arm, but I learned later from a good friend, a pediatric neurologist, that he had felt optimistic about my future recovery because from the first day I could flex my fingers. Wisely,

however, he kept his own council about his positive prognosis until much later, when my arm had in fact regained a good deal of function.

Another weird aspect of my stroke (and as it turned out a positive one) has been the complete lack of spasticity, which has greatly facilitated the rehabilitation process. The only hint of spasticity appeared during automatic reactions such as stretching and yawning, when both left limbs would spontaneously and uncontrollably go into extreme flexion.

THERAPY

When the editor of this book, who had been my occupational therapist, asked me to write about my experiences as a patient recovering from stroke and suggested the title "Notes of a Survivor," I asked him whether he meant survivor of the stroke or survivor of physical and occupational therapy. Lest my later comments sound too enthusiastic or be considered self-serving on the part of the editor, let me start with a few negatives.

Both physical and occupational therapy are boring, consisting as they must of highly repetitive exercises and activities: the patient soon learns to count "reps," longing to reach the magic number (usually 10—do therapists have a functional rationale for this quota?) requested by the therapist. And no cheating is tolerated; therapists have mastered a secret way of keeping track of reps automatically and privately even as they keep up a conversation with you, and they will not be defrauded of even a few reps.

Another thing—therapists have a bit of a sadistic trait that may be innate and predisposing to the job or else part of their professional training. As soon as you feel comfortable doing the required number of reps for any given exercise, the number of reps usually goes up by five. The idea, I think, is to keep you challenged, and you are. Furthermore, consider pain; did you know that therapists distinguish between "good" pain and "bad" pain? Good pain is the muscle soreness that comes from those five cycles of ten reps, a guarantee for the therapist that you are doing your exercises and using the proper muscles. Bad pain is classified in imaginative ways; my occupational therapist, a man, used a scale of severity that ranged from "paper cut pain" to "labor pain," at which point the secretary on the occupational therapy floor, a woman, invariably reminded us that we men did not know what we were talking about.

One other piece of good news and bad news—exercise works, but only as long as you keep exercising. The moment you stop, you start losing ground, so that you are in fact condemned to exercising for life, which to a Mediterranean soul such as I is a pretty harsh sentence. My way of surviving this torture is to make exercise part of a highly routinized wake-up ritual, something I do almost automatically, like brushing my teeth. This way I feel slightly guilty when I skip the routine and, conversely, when I do exercise, I enjoy that little heady virtuous feeling I remember from my jogging days.

So much for the negatives. The positive side of the ledger is much larger. As a neurologist and a student of neuromuscular diseases, I am ashamed to confess that I had virtually ignored physical therapy and occupational therapy—a never-never land where patients usually ended up after the physicians concluded their brilliant diagnostic workups—and I had a vague notion of physical and occupational therapists as robotlike technicians. A few sessions of occupational therapy and physical therapy sufficed to change my views drastically. The first thing that impressed me was their knowledge of muscle anatomy and physiology; I thought I knew muscles! Throughout the rehabilitation process, I was amazed at their understanding of movement and lack thereof, muscle coordination, and compensatory mechanisms. Thus, I had at all times the comforting notion that all exercises and activities were rationally planned on the basis of my specific deficits and needs and were not part of a "canned" program. Another encouraging sign was the therapists' obvious satisfaction at every sign of improvement; far from being automata, these people clearly loved their profession and took pleasure in a job well done. In fact, I came to admire both the dedication and the professionalism of my therapists so much that I developed the conviction—which I expressed to the chairman of our Department of Neurology—that all neurology residents ought to spend at least a few weeks observing occupational and physical therapists at work. All too often we neurologists are content with our diagnostic workup of stroke patients and our intervention in the acute phase, only to lose sight of patients' progress.

I developed a pain syndrome in my left shoulder that not only gave me sleepless nights (partly because of pain, partly because of an exaggerated fear of dislocating my arm by sleeping on the left side) but also resulted in a "frozen shoulder," a very painful condition that interfered with my occupational therapy. Again, I was impressed by the variety of approaches used by my therapists not just to alleviate the pain but also to resolve the problem, including slinging, supporting my arm on an over-the-shoulder bag, and taping my shoulder in conjunction with passive mobilization and massage. On that occasion, I found myself in another situation I usually experience from the other side; I volunteered to be the subject of a teaching conference for occupational therapy trainees. Although I derived some satisfaction from being materially useful to the medical profession (something akin to but fortunately short of donating your body to the Department of Anatomy) at our clinical conferences, I am now much more aware of the discomfort caused to the patient by being an object of study.

GOING HOME

Falling is, of course, the big fear. I had fallen once in my hospital room, and I fell once again a few days after my return home. Finding myself on both occasions next to a wall, I went through the steps my therapists had so carefully rehearsed with me in the hospital gym, and on both occasions I got up on my own. However, after my relatives left, I had nightmares about falling in the middle of a room and not being able to get up and reach the phone or the intercom. The problem was solved by the acquisition of a portable phone, which I slipped into my pocket every night as soon as I entered my house. I never had to use it, but it served its purpose as a "security blanket."

Showering and getting dressed in the morning also took some adjusting, but I soon learned that what had appeared in the hospital as slightly ridiculous procedures (left sleeve and pants leg first; hook the sock on your big toe first, then slip in the other toes) were in fact precious clues to a highly routinized and reasonably rapid process. I took several months to remaster the tie knot, but I remember with joy the pride of my occupational therapist when I appeared at a clinic appointment wearing shirt and tie instead of the usual turtleneck.

Lest all this appear an exceedingly smooth return to normal life, let me dwell for a moment on the frustrations to which I alluded in my opening paragraphs. Even a mild residual hemiparesis is an endless source of frustration in just about every aspect of daily life. I find dropping objects especially irritating and often remember with new empathy my son's frequent outbursts as a clumsy adolescent—"I hate gravity!" Buttoning shirts, especially cuffs, can be a trying experience, and I have more than a few shirts with ripped-off buttons to prove it. Frustration at times turns to rage, and I have occasionally punched my sluggish left hand with my agile right one; even worse, I have punched a table, with the only result of having still a sluggish left hand and a painful right one. One less disruptive way to deal with frustrating experiences is to curse; I have invented a peculiar English/Italian hybrid curse (unprintable in either language) that I use as a mantra many times a day. Naturally, the level of frustration and the threshold for the "tantrums" vary considerably from day to day and are influenced by mood; on some "bad days," I notice that I am almost looking for a frustrating experience so I have an excuse to explode, thus using the stroke as a scapegoat for my bad mood.

Although I have never been a sportsman (library mouse would be a more fitting definition), as my rehabilitation progressed, I have repeatedly had vivid dreams in which I ran; I just ran for the sake of running, and it felt both exhilarating and as easy as it had been before the stroke. I actually tried the motions of running while holding onto a shopping cart in the hallway of my apartment building, but somehow the exhilaration of the dream wasn't there.

CONCLUDING REMARKS

Although I cannot run, I can walk without a cane, I am independent in my daily activities, I have been able to resume my (fortunately sedentary) job, and I travel around the world. To be sure, this is not the typical outcome of stroke. Every patient is different, and I have been unusually lucky in that I was spared speech impediments and spasticity. This in turn has made my rehabilitation easier and more effective.

However, my left side was totally paralyzed only two and a half years ago (at age 54), and I am now enjoying a nearly normal life. Much of my progress has been because of the patient, steady, intelligent, and compassionate work of my physical and occupational therapists. The punchline of these "Notes of a Survivor" has to be that not only can one survive a stroke, but brain plasticity does exist, and good physical and occupational therapy does improve the condition of every patient recovering from stroke to a remarkable degree. Some improvement continues to occur (if you exercise, that is!) for a long time, although at a reduced pace. So, who knows, maybe I will be able to run again before I turn 60.

P.S. Just as Alexandre Dumas père felt obliged to write "Twenty Years Later," a follow-up to *The Three Musketeers*, so 10 years after my stroke I also feel obliged to offer a follow-up. The good news is that I still walk independently, work full-time, and travel extensively. The bad news is that I never ran again—although running remains a recurrent subject of my dreams—and I still have paresthesia in the left side of my body, mostly in the hand. Additional problems are due to two situations, one of which is totally outside my will, while for the other I have to take full responsibility. The first has to do with aging and related troubles (still preferable to the alternative, to quote Woody Allen). Thus, generalized arthritis has necessitated a total left hip replacement, adding insult to the injury of the stroke and accentuating my limp. The second has to do with my physical laziness and my weakness for the Mediterranean diet (which is the opposite of the Atkins diet): lack of exercise and excessive weight are not what my physical therapist recommended. And I hear about it about every day because my physical therapist and I have developed a wonderful personal relationship. You can call this development a positive side effect of the stroke for me, and an occupational hazard for her. But it is a happy ending for both, and who does not like a happy ending?

chapter 31

A Survivor's Perspective II: Stroke

Somehow, I thought it would never happen; cancer, yes, but not this. My right arm lay lifeless at my side, and my right leg was too weak to lift from the sheet. For the second time in a week, I was in a hospital bed. My left arm was hooked up to a plastic bottle suspended from an intravenous (IV) pole, and a slender tube was relaying medication via my veins to the rest of my system. At least my body was someone else's problem now, and I did not have to pretend any longer that everything was all right. But rather than feeling relaxed, my mind was racing, replaying the events of the past six days.

"I've had a TIA [transient ischemic attack]." On Monday morning, I finally had to admit this to myself. It was the third day of gradually increasing weakness of my entire right side, and I knew I had a transient ischemic attack, which temporarily interrupts the flow of blood to the brain but then generally resolves itself within 24 hours. It is often the first warning of a stroke.

I was strangely calm—nonfeeling—but then, the topic of stroke was no stranger to me; for over 40 years I had been an occupational therapist and was familiar with neurological problems. It was ironic—too ironic even for my ability to find humor in the darker side of life. I had worked with men and women who themselves were the survivors of strokes and other serious illnesses, and I had found great satisfaction as I showed them how to manage daily life during their recovery. I had listened to the stories men and women told me of their strokes, recalling exactly where they were and what they were doing when they were struck. Most stories included a dramatic part of losing consciousness and falling. These stories and many like them formed the content of the teaching that was the natural progression of my career from practice to education. Until retiring, I had been a professor at Columbia University, and patient vignettes that helped to illustrate a particular point punctuated many of my classes.

It took getting used to the new experience as a patient. It differed from other patient stories in many ways. I never lost consciousness, nor did I suddenly collapse. I watched for three days and went about my business while my right side got weaker. It was a busy time for me, since I was anticipating a vacation trip to Europe with my brother and sister-in-law, and we exchanged frequent phone calls to discuss plans. I felt I had no time to pay attention to the annoying weakness that hardly interfered with my ability. On Sunday night a friend came to dinner. The symptoms were still not fully in my consciousness, and I was able to prepare the meal by compensating with my left side. On the return from walking my friend to the bus, I felt a strange urgency to get home to do the dishes before I got weaker. When I finally got to bed, I fell into a fitful, uneasy sleep. The next morning I couldn't ignore that I had had what the textbook refers to as a transient ischemic attack.

I had to repeat the hated phrase, "I think I've had a TIA," two more times; first, to the doctor's receptionist to get an appointment, then to my brother in New Jersey, asking him to take me to the doctor, since I knew I couldn't maneuver the car.

I tried to keep myself busy until my brother's arrival. Although I was still trying to deny the reality, I packed an overnight bag just in case I had to stay in the hospital. An added unpleasantness was the slurring of my speech that I couldn't control.

Much to my satisfaction, once we had arrived in his office, the doctor confirmed my diagnosis and made an appointment for me right away to see a neurologist who specializes in stroke. This was truly weird; just two months before, in my role as a retired adjunct professor, I had been coordinating a course for student occupational and physical therapists covering neurological problems, and this doctor had been our guest lecturer on the topic of stroke. I had liked his calm, confident manner and the clarity with which he sketched out to the students the various areas of the brain that might be affected. I had even remarked to a colleague that he was definitely someone I would consult if I ever needed a neurologist. All of this played back to me now as I sat in his waiting room, anxiously anticipating my turn.

Luckily, I was in familiar territory. The neurologist's office was only three stories below where my own office had been. I felt a slight twinge of embarrassment as he came out to greet me.

"I'm wearing a different hat today," I slurred and forced a weak smile. His smile was warm and reassuring. His neurological examination further established that I had had a stroke, and he confirmed the need to be hospitalized for further tests.

While the doctor made the necessary phone calls to admit me, my brother and sister-in-law took me to the fifth floor of the adjoining hospital building where a single room overlooking the Hudson was waiting for me. When my family was satisfied that I was in capable hands, I urged them to leave. I needed some time to myself and yet, when the door closed behind them, I felt like a little girl on the first day at camp after the parents have gone home.

It was difficult for me to grasp the seriousness of my condition, although a slow dread began to hover in the back of my mind. I had no pain and did not feel really sick, so the idea of getting into an ill-fitting hospital gown in the middle of the afternoon seemed ridiculous. What was this going to do to my plans for the trip? Before I had much time for reflection, a very young resident stood at my bedside, poised to take blood from my arm; her deft handling of the needle belied her youthful appearance. She was the first of a long line of men and women who entered my room at all hours of the day and night to perform some service that was much more useful to them than it was to me. The idea of using the hours around midnight for sleeping was not part of their thinking.

Sometime during the next several hours, I was roused from a restless sleep by something metallic banging into my bed. It was a stretcher on wheels.

"Your doctor ordered a CT [computed tomography] scan," the orderly said with false cheeriness.

"Now?" It was hard to believe that my neurologist would suddenly awaken with one thought in his mind—to order a CT scan to be carried out during the next hour. Obediently I slid from my mattress to the stretcher that was parked alongside the bed. The orderly covered me with a blanket and without another word, whisked me rapidly down numerous corridors and elevators to another section of the hospital. We were now clearly in the basement approaching the double doors of the CT scan suite where two technicians were waiting for me. Without interrupting the flow of their conversation, each of them grabbed one end of the sheet on which I was lying, and similar to the motion used to move sacks of meal to a waiting truck, transferred me onto the cold, hard surface of a narrow table. With two swift movements, the technician wrapped the sheet around me in mummy fashion.

"Let me have your glasses." His outstretched hand was close to my face, and I surrendered my last link with a world I could see. "First, you'll hear the motor start, and then the scan will start to turn. Don't move until I tell you." With that, he and his companion left the room.

I tried to dredge up all the things I had read about CT scans, but all I could focus on was the cold and my temporary blindness. The machine had started to whir at a considerable volume. A lighted circle above my head began to rotate and then gathered speed as the entire halo moved slowly back and forth. I shivered with cold and felt terribly vulnerable and alone. If I called for help, no one would hear me above the din of the machine.

After what seemed like an interminable time, the motor slowed down and stopped. The door was flung open, and the technician returned. It was only after the noise had stopped that I became aware of its unnerving effect. An unparalleled fatigue took over my body.

"Here are your glasses. I've called for a pickup," were the last words the technician spoke before he vanished again, this time for good. The silence in the room now became as frightening as the noise had been before. I closed my eyes and must have dozed off. When the orderly arrived, he seized the stretcher silently and retraced the circuitous route until I was back in my room.

Although my body felt exhausted, I could not get comfortable in the bed. Each time I awoke from what seemed hours of sleep, the large clock on the wall indicated that only a single hour had passed since I last checked. Now I had ample time to study the view from the large window by my bed. I looked out on the majestic Hudson, a coal-black ribbon bordered by the blinking lights of the Jersey edge. Finally, the first hues of the morning began to lighten the sky, and the hospital came to life. Someone entered my room and switched on the bright overhead lights.

"I've come to take your blood pressure." The speaker in white slacks and a pink T-shirt could have been anyone. Through my years as a therapist I was familiar with the subtle signs of hospital dress and behavior code; a stethoscope loosely slung around the neck meant that you were a nurse.

"Can you wash yourself?"

"I think so."

"Someone will bring you the basin in a few minutes."

"Can I go to the bathroom first?"

"When the aide comes to wash you, she'll give you a bed pan. We don't have time to take you to the bathroom now. All the patients have to be washed before the shift ends at seven." With that, she left the room. It was the first example of hospital rules, made for the convenience of the staff, without consideration of patients' needs. A feeling of utter powerlessness swept over me, and I knew that, like thousands of others before me, I had now entered the world of the patient, aptly named for the quality that is the keystone for survival in the hospital setting.

The day was punctuated by more tests and the visit of a hierarchy of doctors who represented all the developmental steps in a physician's career. Each of them questioned and probed. All of them wanted to feel my extremities, to see the amount of movement I could demonstrate, and to ask about my medical history. For all of them, I was the cheerful, cooperative patient, an approach that came to haunt me in the days that followed.

Evaluations by the physical therapist, occupational therapist, and speech and hearing therapists were part of the day's schedule. The physical therapist that I recognized from sight as a sweet, gentle young woman went over most of the leg motions I had performed for the various doctors, but then she asked me to move back and forth in the bed and to sit on the edge. It was clear that my right side hardly took part in carrying out all the requested movements, but the years of keeping fit were paying off; I could support myself on my left side and even hobbled around the room, firmly hanging on to Kathy, the physical therapist.

I had never met the speech pathologist before. Her manner was cheerful and matter-of-fact. Her role was not only to listen to the formation of sounds and words but also to test my comprehension and memory. I was appalled when I listened to myself; no matter how much I tried to enunciate clearly, certain words came out slurred. I fared better with the comprehension and memory tests. Thank goodness, that part of me seemed to be intact.

When I returned from more tests in another part of the hospital, the occupational therapist entered the room. I was very familiar with most of the occupational therapists in the rehabilitation department; 12 of them had been research subjects in a study I had conducted and published, and I was currently gathering information from their patients for a study that I was conducting with one of them. Fortunately, I was not acquainted with the two who worked with the patients on the stroke service but knew that a former student was doing her internship there. My patient role was still too new for me, and I was not ready for the exchange that would inevitably result from seeing a colleague-in-becoming.

As soon as I saw the occupational therapist, I knew I was in good hands. She was in her mid-20s, short, with Asian features. She spoke with a slight accent, but I could not identify her country of origin. She moved and talked with an air of competence. Directly behind her was the student.

"I'm Romana, the occupational therapist, and I've brought a friend of yours to do the evaluation with me."

I hoped that my discomfort at seeing Yaffa was not too obvious; I remembered her well from my class. I was certain that she felt an equal degree of unease. Romana checked me over carefully, noting on her clipboard all the areas of function that I could or could not do. Occasionally, she asked a question of the student. She left me some therapy putty and a piece of theraband, both familiar parts of the beginning exercise program for the hand and arm.

"You know what to do with these," she laughed somewhat apologetically; I returned the laugh.

"You want me to squeeze the putty?" She nodded and then watched my efforts to close my fingers around the apple-green mass. Although I squeezed as hard as I could, I had not even dented the putty and felt utterly defeated. Our eyes met briefly, and Romana said the thing that I had offered lamely a hundred times when I had overestimated a patient's ability, "Try using the putty every day; you'll see that it will get easier each time you try."

After Romana and Yaffa had left, I had little time to take stock of my situation before a new round of people stood in my doorway. This time it was Dr. Mitchell, the neurologist, with seven residents in tow. I recognized some of them from the interviews and blood tests of the day before. Dr. Mitchell greeted me with a question, "May we come in and talk to you for a few minutes?" I appreciated his consideration and was eager to cooperate. Between asking me to move my right side, he addressed the young doctors, asking them questions and sharing information about my condition. Then he turned to me. "The CT scan shows a very small lesion deep in the brain. The weakness should resolve itself in a few days, and you can go for outpatient therapy. You may call your brother now to take you home. I'll sign the necessary discharge papers." With a cheery wave, he and his entourage walked out. I was left with a million unanswered questions.

Although I should have been ecstatic about the verdict, the news left me stunned. Nothing had changed in my condition since I had arrived yesterday. The fingers on my right hand could hardly move, my leg could barely support me, and I had to hold on to furniture to move around the room. I had expected more improvement than this before being allowed to go home. But hadn't the doctor said that I would get my strength back? The most important thing now was to share the good news with my brother and sister-in-law before the staff members changed their minds.

My family's delight made me feel a tinge of guilt at my own lack of enthusiasm. They offered to take me to their spacious house for a few days, a prospect I always enjoyed. Why wasn't I glad to be going home? Aside from a loss of appetite, I did not feel ill, but I could not shake a vague uneasiness that dampened my spirits. But as I waited, once again, for their arrival, I passed the time getting into my clothes as best I could. I recalled the hours of sitting with a patient, giving him or her advice on how to put a paralyzed arm into a sleeve, putting on slacks while supported by the bed. Fastenings like shoelaces I left for my sister-in-law to do; we were on such good terms that I did not hesitate to broach this subject with her.

The genuine pleasure at seeing my family pushed aside the uncomfortable feeling that was gnawing at the back of my mind. I was grateful for the wheelchair that was required by the hospital to take me to the front door. Was it really only 24 hours since I had entered? Aside from the numerous black-and-blue marks left from the blood tests on both forearms I was certainly no worse, but was I better? Again, I reminded myself that I needed more time to get stronger.

Once we were in the car, Jeff and Helen told me that they had made numerous phone calls in the morning to cancel our European trip.

"But why shouldn't you go? I'll surely be able to take care of myself by next Sunday," I protested. "You were so much looking forward to seeing our cousins and your friend. Why should you give it all up on my account?"

"We wouldn't go without you." Their reply was almost in unison. "Anyway, we can go next year." For the first time in 24 hours, I was near to tears, perhaps because it was the first moment when I had dared to think about my feelings. All I could mutter was a bland, "Thank you; I know I've spoiled the trip for all of us, and I'm truly sorry." Helen reached over from the driver's seat and squeezed my hand.

As we headed toward their home in New Jersey, I knew I would be well cared for, and I began to feel better. Our conversation turned to everyday matters and to the things we might do together now that the pressure of the trip was off. Having an unexpected guest presented no problems to Helen and Jeff. As the parents of five children and grandparents to four, life was a never-ending chain of filled and empty beds and the feeding that was a part of this. I knew I was welcome in every family activity, but in spite of our intimate relationship, each of us had maintained separate lives with a different set of friends and daily responsibilities.

"Do you know, this is the first time I will be staying overnight at a time other than Christmas," I volunteered as we approached their house. I had always loved the canopy of old trees that joined branches over the street; they were an important part of keeping the summer heat from their large old house. It sat at the top of a hill with a steep driveway that had been the bane of my existence on many winter nights after a family gathering.

"Oh, yes!" Helen was genuinely excited by the prospect of being together for several days.

The walk from the car was supported by Jeff; it seemed doable. When I got into the house, I found refuge in the first available chair and stayed there for most of the evening. Not until it was time to go to bed did I realize that the stairs would create a real obstacle, especially since the banister was only on the right side and my right hand was too weak to hold on to pull my body from stair to stair. The only sensible, but thoroughly undignified, way was to go up on all fours, getting little help from the right side. I saw myself as a lame wolf I had recently seen in a nature film; my heart had gone out to the wolf that kept collapsing onto his weak side and was no longer able to keep up with the pack.

By the time I got into a bed where I had slept many times before, I was totally exhausted. I had not realized that every move involved a carefully strategized plan that required the mental layout of the room and each piece of furniture in relation to and its distance from its nearest neighbor. As long as I did not have to traverse any wide-open spaces, I would be all right. With that thought in mind, I fell asleep.

For the next two days, we spent the hours with all the routines that kept us close to the house. Knowing that I was safe, Helen and Jeff went for their usual swim in their large backyard pool while I stayed at the kitchen table or in a comfortable chair, reading. The canceled trip was still preying heavily on my mind, and it was hard to keep my attention focused on a printed page. My usual nonflagging energy had not returned, and I was most content to stay in one place. In the afternoon, Helen suggested that the two of us might drive to the two stores from which we had purchased gifts for the cousins in Germany and Switzerland. Now we were taking the gifts back to the stores where we had spent such a pleasant afternoon choosing items that were suited to the temperaments of our friends and relatives.

I was grateful to Helen for suggesting this outing, since she and I always enjoyed doing things together. I knew that she would understand when I declined the chance to go into the stores with her; I just did not have the energy to walk from the car. While I waited for Helen to return to the car, I tried to move my fingers and my leg and had to admit that I could not voluntarily move them any better than the day before. Why was it taking so long to get my strength back? Actually, in my 11 years of practice, I had never worked with anyone who had only a temporary stroke; by the time patients were referred to therapy, they were recovering from much more serious conditions, but I could not shake the knowledge that I was not getting better.

That evening, we decided that since it would be easier for me to manage in my apartment, Jeff and Helen would take me home and stay with me there for a few days. After all, the cancellation of the trip had left us with lots of free time. An overnight visit by Jeff and Helen was a real novelty; the thought of it buoyed up my spirits immediately. They could sleep in my room, while I would be comfortable on the couch in my study. What I failed to remember at the time of making these plans was that a major repair of the outside of my apartment building was underway, and all tenants had been asked to move all terrace furniture and plants inside. Since I thought that I would be away for several weeks anyway, I had piled most of the planters on the floor in the study, with just enough room to move to the desk and the bed.

We retired at a reasonable hour, and I was glad not to have to climb stairs tonight. Sometime in the night I got up to go the bathroom. Apparently, my right leg had become even weaker and when I tried to stand next to the couch I lost my balance and fell backwards into one of the planters. I was conscious of a cracking sound, fortunately not of a bone but the branch of a flowering geranium plant that had cushioned my fall and now held me captive. The ridiculousness of the situation made me laugh in spite of myself, and for a moment I simply enjoyed the humor without having to figure out a way to return to my bed. Then I saw that I could not rely on my body only to get me out of this predicament. I reached for a solid piece of furniture, pulled myself up with my left arm, and stood firmly on my left leg. Thank goodness, it supported me well.

Once back on the couch, I could not get to sleep. My mind was racing almost as fast as my heart. I knew that I wasn't getting better, and somehow I was not prepared for this. Would I just keep getting weaker and weaker? So far, my sensation was intact; I could feel everything that touched my right side, but was it only a matter of time before that too disappeared?

My bodily needs became all too clear for me. I again had to leave the couch to go to the bathroom. In almost a Xerox copy of my previous escapade into the flowerpot, I fell again into one of the plants. This time I did not laugh, but again, unhurt, I was able to extricate myself quickly. At this rate, I would not have any flowers left. I was becoming a hazard to myself and to the environment.

When I had returned from the bathroom a second time by holding onto all the pieces of furniture along the way, I tried in vain to find some rest. I stared at the ceiling, contemplating what lay ahead. I dared not face up to the reality of what my body had imposed on me. Like a worn-down music box that is ready to stop, the same tune played over and over again, "You know you're getting worse and worse. Why did you leave the hospital?" Finally the first pink stripes along the visible sky told me that another hot day had started. I couldn't bear lying there any longer, and I got up to take a shower; the warmth of the water had often cleared my head after sleepless nights and always made me feel better.

Although there was nothing to hold on to around the tub, at least it wasn't dark. Probably that was why I had fallen during the night. The water felt soothing to my skin, and for a moment I felt cleansed of the demons that had become a part of my thinking. I turned off the water and approached the edge of the tub to get out. I would have to sit down on the edge and then lift my legs out one by one. Somehow I lost my footing and came crashing down. When I finally came to rest on the floor of the empty tub I noticed with relief that my head was about three inches from the wall while I was lying on my back. Once again I was unhurt, but, like a beetle that had been turned on its back, I felt utterly helpless for fight or flight. If I called loudly enough, Helen or Jeff would no doubt hear me. Considering that option for a moment, I decided I was not ready to capitulate to that extent; the thought of being pulled out of the bathtub stark naked by my brother did not appeal to me, even in my helpless state. "Calm down!" I firmly told myself. "You're supposed to be a problem-solver." I was able to call on the dormant forces that are part of our emergency system, and they did not desert me. I turned over and with my left arm and leg, got myself first to a kneeling position with the left side holding all my weight and then to sitting on the edge of the tub. Holding onto the sink, I pulled myself to standing next to the tub. I found that I was shaking, totally exhausted by the ordeal. Somehow I got myself dressed and returned to the study where I had spent the night.

By now Helen was up and came to look for me.

"I've got to go back to the hospital," were my words of greeting. I then relayed the details of the three falls to her.

"I'm so glad you've decided to go back; we were thinking the same thing as we watched you last night." She seemed as relieved as I was that the decision had been made.

When I called Dr. Mitchell, his secretary told me he was on rounds but would call me as soon as he got back to his office. If he was at all surprised by my call, his voice certainly did not reflect this when he called back. Instead, he said calmly we should come right over.

Our departure from the house this time did not go unnoticed by my fellow tenants who were just leaving for work. It was not so easy to flash a cheery "Hi!" to neighbors from the compromised position of being held up by Jeff and Helen while we made our way through the lobby out to the car. This time we drove right up to the busy front door of the hospital.

"There are always wheelchairs there," I told Jeff, grateful that I could give in to my inability to walk the long corridors to Dr. Mitchell's office. As an automatic gesture on approaching the hospital doors, I slipped the chain with my ID over my head; "This will give us much faster entree to the different buildings," I told Jeff and Helen. What I did not tell them was that the simple act of wearing the ID firmly established my role as faculty member rather than having to yield completely to the patient role.

For the second time in four days, Dr. Mitchell confirmed my diagnosis following the neurological examination. "I thought I was supposed to be getting stronger, not weaker." My voice did not hide the indignation I felt.

"You're experiencing a progressive stroke, which can go on over several days," he said. In my long experience I had not heard of this, and I questioned him further about the length of time it would continue. "Usually it is finished by the fifth day," he replied. Silently I counted back to the day I had felt the first signs of weakness; that was six days ago. By the time I figured it out, Dr. Mitchell had left the room to ask his assistant to make the necessary calls to get me readmitted to the hospital.

When Dr. Mitchell returned, he stayed just long enough to tell me to go to the admitting office where they would tell us when the room was ready. "I'll stop in to see you later on," was all he said as a sign that the session was over.

I was very grateful for the wheelchair that Jeff now pushed through the many corridors that took us back to the hospital. At the admitting office, they already had papers for me that I now had to sign. I had not expected that I would be totally unable to sign my name. After several futile attempts at guiding the pen, I had to admit that this was impossible for me.

"Just do the best you can; you can even put an X if you want."

The humiliation was almost more than I could stand; I choked back the tears as best I could. We were told to wait until the bed was ready, and we sat in the waiting room along with other patients. At first it was rather interesting to watch and listen to the different snatches of life stories unfolding around us. I was comfortable in the wheelchair with two good friends at my side; I had made all needed decisions for the moment and was ready to relinquish my body to the wonders of the healing sciences.

It was hard to sustain my interest in the fate of other people when my own had a much higher priority. Repeated inquiries of the clerk at the desk about the readiness of my bed resulted in the same answer: "They should be calling from the floor any minute now." It was the first of a chain of broken promises that I came to recognize as one of the hallmarks of patient treatment. No one wants to give a straight answer when they know how unpleasant the truth may be to the patient; it is far easier to promise a fulfillment of the patient's request than to be in the role of the bad guy. And so the minutes turned into hours. Finally, three hours after we had entered the waiting area, we were told that the bed was indeed ready, and I could report to the fifth floor of the hospital. My room—with only one bed—was again on the river side. After another wait to get the necessary hospital paraphernalia, I was able to convince Jeff and Helen that I was in good hands, and they left for home. It was then that I became aware of the enormous fatigue in my body, but even more so, the seriousness of my condition now faced me squarely. I had to admit to myself I had lost the exhausting battle with denial, and I gave full expression to the overriding despair that gripped me. My body shook with sobs that I did not try to control.

After a few moments of this, when I had begun to collect myself, the door burst open and the first of the ever-present residents came in, sporting the now familiar blood-taking kit.

"We'll be checking your blood every few hours." Her manner was friendly but businesslike. Hardly had she left when a nurse entered, carrying the floppy plastic bag filled with clear fluid; this meant that I was to have an infusion. Without a word she hung the sack of liquid on an arm of the pole that she wheeled from the corner of the room to my bedside. With a minimum of wasted motion, she inserted the needle in my left forearm and held it in place by a strip of adhesive tape. She fitted the slender tube that extended from the bag of liquid into the needle and turned the valve, and the liquid began to drip slowly into my veins. In response to my inquiry, she told me that I was to receive an infusion of heparin, which I recognized as a so-called blood thinner. I let out a long sigh of relief; at last someone was doing something that seemed vaguely helpful, and for a moment I relaxed. Then I realized that I was not only tethered to the IV pole, but that this virtually made my left arm as useless as my right. Before I allowed myself to go into a full-blown panic, I tested the slack in the tube and how far I could reach with my arm before a tweak reminded me that I had reached the limit of my arm motion. I had to admit that this wasn't too bad; after all, I could reach as far as the top of my head, and if I sat up, I could reach my knees. These were the limits of my world for now; I let out a sigh of resignation and fell into an exhausted sleep.

After what seemed to be only moments later, I woke up to the cheery sound of a man's deep bass voice humming a tune as he entered my room.

"Hi, I'm Malcolm, your night nurse," he smiled broadly, and his rich Caribbean accent was undeniable. "I've come to check your pulse and blood pressure."

"Could you also call someone to help me to the bathroom? I need help with walking. Besides, I don't know how I can manage with the IV pole."

"Sure. I can take you."

This was not exactly what I had bargained for. The idea of a man taking me into the bathroom was not very appealing, but since I could not think of a graceful way of getting around this, I moved myself to the edge of the bed in anticipation of getting up.

Malcolm turned out to be a great help. He held me up effortlessly with his right arm while wheeling the pole with the other hand. In spite of my sorry condition, I smiled inwardly. We were indeed an odd couple as we headed toward the bathroom door. Once inside the bathroom, I had to face another hurdle. Could I balance my body by standing solely on my left leg and use my left hand to pull down my pants? I decided to risk it, rather than ask Malcolm to perform this task for me. There was a limit to how much I was willing to ask for assistance, and I needed to prove to myself that I was not totally helpless.

"I'll be all right now, Malcolm. Thanks a lot for your help," I managed a smile.

"Just pull this cord when you're finished." Malcolm handed me a slender cord that was attached to the switch for the bell. A fleeting thought crossed my mind; whatever needs my body or soul now had had to be carried out with the help of other people or exclusively by my less skilled left hand. This, like everything else that was happening to my independent lifestyle, would take some adjustment on my part.

The three days that followed were filled with the dull hospital routine; frequent visits by doctors in all stages of their development, always physically probing and asking for more information; and the change in nursing shifts and the actions performed by each, depending on where they found themselves on the hierarchy of professionals and helpers. Some were extremely cheerful and encouraging; some showed the strain of severe staff shortages.

There were also the small annoyances like a stuck window that took five days to get fixed. Of greater consequence to me were the details of my care that suddenly loomed larger than reality and reminded me at every moment just how helpless I really was. Perhaps in an effort to be kind or perhaps in a moment of absentmindedness, someone had shut my door at night, thereby leaving me at the mercy of my left hand to call the nurse. The first time the beeper announced that the heparin bag was empty, I rang the bell, and the remote voice at the end of the intercom told me that a nurse would come right away. The beeper screeched unceasingly, without the appearance of the promised nurse. I began to feel my heart pounding fiercely, certain that I would have another stroke because my blood was not getting the required dose of heparin. I tried feebly to call for help, but I had to admit that my voice barely reached to the door. At last the nurse arrived with the new bag, totally unmoved by my near-panic state.

"A short interruption like this doesn't make any difference." Her matter-of-fact response to my concern made me realize that I was losing my cool and had become just like all the frightened patients whom I had tried to reassure during my professional life.

I had struggled to view the whole experience with an objective clinical gaze, but I found myself forced into the role of docile sufferer, lacking the necessary willpower to do otherwise. Nothing seemed to be happening that was changing my condition; I began to feel very sorry for myself.

I was aroused from this "blue funk" by the arrival of an exquisitely blooming exotic plant sent by my colleagues at the University. How had they learned of my whereabouts? According to the calendar, I was supposed to be on my way to Europe! I thought that since no one was expecting me back for three weeks, my secret was safe. But there were enough people in the hospital that knew me, and the news soon leaked out. From then on, during the weeks of my stay in the hospital, the wide windowsill of my room was always filled with fresh flowers or potted plants, thanks to the dozens of people whose good wishes were expressed in this touching way. I felt ashamed of the feelings of self-pity that I had allowed to take over.

Soon after the flowers, the first of a steady flow of visitors from the University arrived. They managed to squeeze in friendly calls before, during, and after their work hours in the University. Now I had to face my deficits head-on, and I experienced a sense of shame, especially at my slurred speech. It was also exhausting to answer "How did it happen?" again and again. Still, the visitors were bright spots in the monotony of the hospital days. The ones I anticipated with the greatest pleasure were Helen and Jeff, my sister-in-law and brother. They always brought fresh news of their family and also delivered my mail. I could count on them for all the support and understanding I needed. Jeff had taken over the management of my finances; Helen took the bag of dirty clothes from the floor of my closet, and when I started to object, she silenced me. I surrendered a further aspect of my independence, this part more willingly.

Another break in the routine was the daily visits of the therapists. I was concerned that nothing was being done for my arm. I had seen too many tight, painful shoulders and permanently weak wrists to risk similar complications, frequently the result of lengthy disuse. When I voiced this to Romana, she brought me two wrist splints to try. I also began to exercise my arm with my other hand. It was the first action toward resuming charge of my life, and it felt good.

Now the next hurdle to overcome was the decision by the doctors and therapists of if and when I could be moved to the rehabilitation floor. Of course, I was still receiving the heparin infusion; the needle would have to be removed before I could begin a strenuous rehabilitation program. Finally, six days after my second admission, the order came from the doctors; my blood had been thinned to the required level, and I was to be moved to the eighth floor.

As promised, the two needles were removed from my arm, and I was liberated from my tether. In spite of my relief at the prospect of starting the rehabilitation program, I felt the slightest twinge of sadness, much as I felt in grade school when I advanced to the next grade. I had begun to think of the familiar routine of the fifth floor as more or less safe, and I had become used to the staff. I knew that on the rehabilitation floor, patients were in double rooms; there were also much higher expectations for helping oneself placed on the patients; would I be able to measure up? As always, there was a long wait ahead until finally, an attendant with a stretcher announced that he was moving me. But why the stretcher?

"Oh that," he explained, "That's not for you. That's for all your plants and stuff. I'll come back for you in a little while with a wheelchair." Then he left me sitting in bed, once again feeling abandoned. There was nothing to do but wait; to amuse myself, I looked out at the river, which was changing to its evening glow in preparation for the sunset. Most of my life I had lived within sight of a river; first, during my early childhood, it was the Danube with its rushing brown current in spring, and during many of my adult years, it was the Hudson. Now the steady flow had become a source of comfort and assurance of the continuity of life. The lights on the side of the river were already starting to blink when the door was flung open by the returning orderly, this time pushing a wheelchair. He lifted me nimbly into the chair and whisked me toward the elevator to the eighth floor. Halfway down the hall he pushed me into a large double room with a similar picture window facing the Hudson. My new roommate approached me, pushing a walker.

"Hi, I'm Virginia," she extended her hand in a confident way, and I shook it with my left. Virginia was a tall, black woman with a matter-of-fact manner and a smile that hovered just behind her eyes. I liked her immediately.

"Why are you here? Did you have a stroke?" I knew that I bore all the signs of patients with whom I shared this diagnosis, but Virginia's direct query caught me off guard. For the first time in days, I burst into tears.

"No sense feeling sorry for yourself." Virginia was right, and her words became my special mantra during the weeks that followed. But for now I was content to let Virginia talk; it was obvious that she knew the routine of the floor. When we said good night, I felt relieved that there was a person on the other side of the curtain that was drawn during sleeping hours.

I woke frequently during the night; each time I awoke, the big clock on the wall showed that only an hour and a half had passed. Now that I was free to move in the bed, I realized that I couldn't change my position much more than I had when my left arm was held in place by the tubes. Besides, my right side kept getting in my way and I needed to move both the arm and the leg with the other side. I was once again grateful that at least I knew the technique, but that didn't make the situation more palatable nor me more comfortable. I watched the sky for the first signs of summer dawn that arrived at the same time as the noise in the corridor that announced that the rehabilitation floor was coming to life. Shortly thereafter, a hand reached for the light switch that changed night into day.

"Time to get up," the raspy voice of the nurse called loudly; I noticed that the clock confirmed that it was only 5:30.

"Do you want to bathe yourself in bed or sit by the sink in the bathroom?" the nurse asked. I had noticed with satisfaction that each of us had a private bath.

"The sink," I responded, eager to have the chance to fend for myself.

"Do you have slacks and a shirt to wear? Here we expect people to wear their own clothes." To be able to shed the hospital gown after a week! Suddenly I realized how much I wanted to be restored to my former self and to leave the patient role behind.

The nurse brought a wheelchair into our large room and parked it next to my bed.

"Can you transfer into this?" Her voice sounded friendlier than before, and although I hadn't attempted to move from the bed to the wheelchair by myself, I had worked with dozens of patients to teach them this skill. I sat on the edge of my bed, slid down to stand on my left leg, pivoted around and grasped the left armrest before letting myself down in the chair. I had to gather each garment I wanted to wear from the drawers of the nightstand and the closet and wheel myself to the bathroom door. Moving the wheelchair with only my left foot and arm took a lot more skill than I remembered, but after several attempts to stop myself from merely going in a circle, I got the knack. The nurse moved an armchair into the bathroom to the small space between the wall and the sink. "Once you're in the bathroom, I'll help you transfer to the chair and then take the wheelchair out. Otherwise, you won't be able to close the door." I welcomed the privacy that this would give me; how I would get back the wheelchair when I had finished was too far in the future to consider.

Now began the long, arduous process of washing and dressing myself, but the idea of doing all of this by myself behind a closed door seemed like the best thing that had happened to me in a week! For the next 50 minutes, I was fully occupied in breaking down each task into tiny steps and then, mostly by trial and error, carrying out each step with my left arm and leg and with my teeth and any working part of my body that I could involve in completing a given task. I had never thought of myself as even remotely ambidextrous, and my left hand had only complemented my right for any task that naturally called for bilateral skill. Now I not only had to resort to being one-handed but also confining all hand use to the left.

One of the first challenges was putting toothpaste on the toothbrush before I brushed my teeth. Like all of the activities of daily living, I had worked with patients on this, so there was no mystery connected to it, but the frustration I experienced before I even had toothpaste on the brush was enormous. Flipping up the top of the tube presented no problem, although it meant grasping the tube without my thumb, since I needed the thumb free to push open the top. Obviously, I was out of practice; otherwise, I would have remembered that the toothbrush has to be laid flat and braced against an object to keep it from moving while the toothpaste was squeezed onto the bristles. Now I had to put the toothpaste down; why wasn't there at least a ledge on the edge of the sink on which to place the tooth-brush? When I put down the toothpaste to pick up the brush, the heavy tube fell into the sink where I left it momentarily; at least it couldn't fall on the floor. Once I had wedged the toothbrush against the left faucet in hopes that it would stay there, I was ready to retrieve the toothpaste and squeeze it onto the waiting toothbrush. Then, finding a place for the toothpaste, I picked up the toothbrush with my left hand. However, before it reached my teeth, the toothpaste had fallen off the brush and was clinging in a soggy mess to the edge of the sink. The second time I repeated the whole routine, I was successful and began to brush my teeth rather clumsily with my left hand. When I had at last advanced to my socks, I was already so tired that the thought of the struggle was almost more than I could face. Then the "achiever half" of me chided the "flagging half"; I picked up the first of two socks that were the only remaining garments on the arm of the chair in which I was sitting. Surely I could do this last step. Happily, I had not lost the agility that has always allowed me to squeeze through narrow spaces and bring my knees close to my chest! At least I could bring my left foot up to rest it on my right knee. I decided to tackle the left sock first and found that my left foot cooperated nicely in the task by extending the big toe so I could hook the sock over it. Then it was just a question of pulling the sock first over the rest of the toes and the heel.

It was a different story with the right sock. I lifted the right foot up to the left knee but without the muscle power to hold it, it slid down to the floor. I remembered that I could expect no help from my right side. I leaned over and brought my body closer to the foot, but I was afraid that if I leaned over too far I would tip over. I sat back as far as I could in the chair and leaned forward again, but when I was ready to hook the sock over the toe, the foot stayed flat on the floor. No sooner was the sock on the toe than I would pull it off accidentally in attempting to move the sock over the foot. After several more tries, I succeeded in getting the sock over the toe and gradually working it over the static foot. In my delight at seeing socks on both feet, I was glad to overlook that the right sock was completely stretched out and hung limply at the ankle.

"Oh, well," I sighed to myself with resignation. I realized that I would have to lower my standards for achieving anything. I would have to settle for just doing a task without looking for quality. And I had to muster all the patience I had slowly learned in the socialization process of becoming a therapist; only now it was not a question of sitting on my hands in order not to give in to my desire to help a struggling patient. I had to serve as my own cheerleader, goading myself on and applauding when I was done.

When the nurse came back to check on my progress, I reported triumphantly that I needed help only with fastening my bra and putting on the sneakers that were still in the closet. It was then I felt my exhaustion; I had used up every ounce of energy of my body before the day had even officially started.

Virginia was already seated in her chair fully dressed, her walker at her side.

"I'm supposed to graduate to a cane today," she announced, "I'll be going home when I can walk by myself." How I envied her! She seemed so competent with everything. A funny thought crossed my mind; I had often told my students how patients compared their own progress to that of other patients even when they had quite different diagnoses, "You should have seen me two weeks ago; I couldn't do anything." Invariably, the second patient would gather hope from seeing that progress. Now I had reached that stage of using Virginia as a role model, even though she had undergone thigh surgery only and her arms and hands were totally intact. In spite of everything, this type of black humor never ceased to amuse me!

Three hours after our untimely reveille, breakfast arrived. I realized that I was also weak from hunger and fell on the food for the first time since leaving home. Just as we finished, one of the physical therapists came to introduce herself as the person who would be working with me. I recognized her immediately as a graduate of the physical therapy program whose students shared many science classes with our occupational therapy students. She had been working several years and had fortunately lost some of the tentativeness of novice therapists. After we had talked for a few minutes and she had given me a quick once-over, she promised to return later with my total therapy schedule; the rest of the day I could relax! I was terribly disappointed and had to keep myself from crying again. For this I had gotten out of bed at 5:30!

Thank goodness the day's visitors and several phone calls took my mind off the letdown. Virginia returned from therapy sporting her new cane and was mighty proud of herself. Would I ever get to use a cane? It was hard to think beyond today, and I was not ready to create a new image of myself as anything other than my former self. In the effort to get used to so many new things, time had ceased to exist for me. I lived from moment to moment, and the outlandishness of my current existence enveloped me totally. Once again, I was grateful that all responsibilities had been taken from me, and no one was expecting anything more from me than being a good patient for my caretakers, a role that I had described at great length to my students. Although never expressed, the message was, "Be compliant, don't complain, don't ask too many questions, get well, and go home!" Here I was, very quickly behaving just like every good patient in the hospital.

Now that I was on the rehabilitation floor, life had a peculiar déjà vu feel; just a week before I became ill, I was interviewing patients in many of the rooms on this floor for a research project I was conducting with the occupational therapy department. Before I had time to dwell on this, Dr. Mitchell appeared, cheerful and energetic as always and seemingly very interested in my condition.

"I'd like to get an MRI [magnetic resonance imaging] on you. You're not claustrophobic, are you?" he asked. The question was almost rhetorical, but it hit me hard. For years I had heard reports of this procedure and had seen videotapes of patients' heads encased by the confining cagelike structure; I had often remarked that I would die of fright—how easily we speak of death when it is not imminent—if I ever had to have an MRI.

"Yes, I'm terribly claustrophobic," I said and remembered the time I thought I was suffocating when I woke in the upper bunk at camp with the ceiling ostensibly only inches from my face. "Do I have to have an MRI?" I felt ashamed of my childish, almost petulant question.

"I think you'd better, so we can tell the exact place of the lesion. I'm conducting a research project on brain function during hand movement at various points of recovery after stroke, and I'll be there with you." The dual possibility of contributing to research in an area that had always fascinated me and having Dr. Mitchell close by quickly convinced me, and I gave my consent. Besides, it was to be scheduled for next week and that seemed far in the future.

Meanwhile, I had to face the weekend without having started any therapy. My disappointment was mixed with the fear that I would begin to see in myself many of the complications that were the result of disuse. At night, during several sleepless hours, I suddenly discovered that I could slide my arm and leg across the sheet. That meant that a small amount of strength was returning to my limbs! I was so excited that I had to fight my urge to wake Virginia, who was sleeping soundly. After that, each time I awoke after a period of sleep, I had to move first my leg and then my arm to make sure that it had not been a dream. As I knew, the slight movement did not have any functional value, but the feeling that resulted from it gave me a boost that got me through the rest of the weekend. I had hoped that perhaps we would be allowed to sleep longer on Saturday and Sunday, but the routine was unchanged, since the only purpose of the early rising was the schedule of the night nurses; their duty ended at 7 AM, by which time all the patients had to be washed and dressed. "Patient-centered care," one of the buzzwords of the 1990s, this was not. Like much of hospital practice, it served the staff and the administration long before the wishes of the patients were taken into consideration.

Finally, it was Monday, and today therapy was to begin for me. As promised, Ilsa, the physical therapist, stopped in our room before she started working and had attached my therapy schedule to the back of my wheelchair in order to let the staff know where I was to be at any time during the day. Until I became familiar with the routine,

Ilsa had told me, the therapists would come for me at the appointed hour. I was to start with physical therapy at 9:30, then on to occupational therapy at 10:10, and followed by speech therapy until 11:30. Luckily for me, Romana was to remain as my occupational therapist, although she usually worked with the acute patients only. I felt that it was better to have someone who was new to me, rather than any of the 12 occupational therapists who had served as subjects for a study I had conducted and which meanwhile had been published in a professional journal. As a patient, I had been stripped of all the professional trappings that one is bound to accumulate, but after 15 years of serving as director of a university program, I was afraid that my history would serve to intimidate the young therapists. It was quite different with the physical therapists, most of whom I did not know and from whom I could expect ordinary patient treatment. When it came time to meet the speech therapist, we recognized each other immediately as colleagues who had shared the same monthly administrative department meetings for many years. Anne-Marie was nearer my own age than some of the others, and I felt we understood each other right away. And yet I felt the stigma of being a disabled patient more acutely in speech than I did in either of the other two therapies.

As expected, the first morning in therapy was taken up by a detailed assessment by each of the therapists. I was glad to show off the movement in my arm and leg and was pleased that these were not the only things that were recognized as strengths. Rather than experiencing the depression that was common when patients realized how much they couldn't do, I felt a surge of the need to excel that had driven me from my earliest years. As a child I had responded to the desire to please a very critical father whom I adored; now I wanted to be the "best" rehabilitation patient.

From frequent visits to the rehabilitation floor, I knew that both occupational therapy and physical therapy were extremely lively places. The large, airy physical therapy gym had mats in several places where patients with diverse problems were working with their therapists on strengthening exercises or resting between the different parts of their program. While I sat in my wheelchair waiting for Ilsa to finish with her first patient of the morning, I had a chance to survey the other patients with whom I would be sharing rehabilitation. I knew that in coming to this floor, I had become part of a distinct society who were bound together only by the fact that each of them had incurred a temporary and not-so-temporary loss of function, of self-image, and of role. I knew nothing of my new associates except that they were patients; they, in turn, knew nothing of me. Once again, I was reminded of one of the topics I had chosen for lectures: "People in the Patient Role." Was it part of a self-fulfilling prophecy? I decided that here I had an opportunity to fashion a totally new personality, but the thought seemed entirely too fatiguing. True to my old self, curiosity took over; I made up my mind to experience the new role as a fully participating member rather than an inquisitive spectator. Besides, I thought ruefully, I actually had little choice. The realization of this made me feel teary. I turned my attention to the bustling environment; I did not want to start my first physical therapy session as an emotional disaster.

Approximately eight other patients were engaged in some type of exercise or walking practice with their own therapist. Laughter and jokes resounded everywhere; it was obvious that therapists and patients enjoyed working together. One woman with a newly fitted artificial leg was practicing walking in the parallel bars; she was perspiring with the effort of lifting the heavy prosthesis in preparation for each step, but she wanted us all to know that she was there. A man, who seemed younger than the rest of us, was learning to step up and down simulated curbs using a cane. A very old and frail-looking lady was objecting strenuously that she couldn't stand on her operated side; the therapist firmly but gently insisted that she try in spite of the pain, and in a few minutes the patient was on her feet, tightly clenching the walker in front of her. Then it was my turn to begin.

Ilsa approached me with a broad smile and told me to wheel myself to one of the mats that was raised about 18 inches from the floor. I was told to transfer from the wheelchair to the mat pivoting on my left leg. It was an activity I had performed countless times with patients of all sizes and in need of varying degrees of help; I remembered how I was filled with dread at the sight of patients who were taller and heavier than myself and needing a great deal of assistance. Thank goodness I was well-schooled in this task and needed no help to get to the mat. Ilsa then checked every muscle for active and passive motion and pain. I was glad to be able to show the slight motion I had in both arm and leg; Ilsa told me that was a very good sign. Before the session ended, she let me try one of the walkers in the gym, but since I couldn't hold on with my right hand, this was still too difficult for me to attempt. It became a goal for a future session, something that seemed a distinct possibility. I had concluded my first session in physical therapy; Romana now pushed my wheelchair to occupational therapy.

This place was extremely familiar to me; first, from my years as a clinician in similar departments, and more recently, as the place where I had been coming to gather information on the patients who were the subjects in my current study. Conducting research in occupational therapy was one of the retirement projects I had promised myself, and since this department had accepted my offer with enthusiasm, I had been a weekly visitor on this floor, interviewing patients about their perceptions of occupational therapy. I had chosen the supervisor of occupational therapy as a research partner; Glen and I had known each other for many years and knew that we could work well together. He was also a favorite clinical instructor of our students. Glen and one of his colleagues were editing a book on stroke rehabilitation, and several months before, much to my surprise, had asked me to write the foreword. I had told Glen that I was no longer as well-versed with the topic as I had been when I was teaching clinical courses, but when he asked a second time, I agreed. The book was to appear on the market in several weeks. I thought of this when Romana and I entered the occupational therapy clinic and I spotted Glen working with a young man.

This was the place where I felt at home. In one of the momentary flashbacks that catch one unaware, I recalled the reason for my becoming an occupational therapist over 40 years ago. I was still in high school searching for a career in medicine without blood when I heard about occupational therapy. It allowed for direct work with people using my hands and a great deal of creativity of a special sort; assisting patients with the kinds of day-to-day physical, cognitive, and emotional problems that were preventing them from living ordinary lives. All of the patients here, like myself, were learning to live with what they had left after injury or disease had robbed them of a part of their function. In occupational therapy, they found a place and people who allowed them to mourn their losses and then to move ahead to learning new ways of accomplishing tasks. The aspect of my clinical work that I found most satisfying was literally to get into patients' heads, to discover which tasks had the most meaning for them, and then to elicit each patient's readiness to work on those tasks together until a satisfactory solution had been found. This had allowed me to glimpse deeply into other people's lives and to discover what kinds of activities were most important to people at different points in their lives. It had also given me a chance to be a partner in the roller coaster experience of recovery with men and women from all walks of life. Now I was acutely aware that a long process of moving through all the emotions from despair to exhilaration that probably lay ahead for me as well.

The occupational therapy clinic was a room with two distinct parts. There were also two large raised mats where people were practicing all sorts of movements in preparation for carrying out some functional activity. The other part was the "Easy Street" unit that had arrived only several months before. "Easy Street" had received much publicity in professional journals, and one of its features was that, depending on the needs of the particular rehabilitation center, it could include one or more daily life units such as a model apartment, a supermarket, a street with curbs and a traffic light, a factory setup, a golf driving range, or a stationary car. I remembered the discussions we had as a faculty, wondering whether this highly touted and equally highly priced equipment would really be worth the price and the large amount of space that was needed to house the various components. But even before I arrived as a patient, I had my answer. The majority of subjects in my recent study had all remembered some aspect of their occupational therapy that they practiced with their therapist in "Easy Street." I had never dreamed that I would be a candidate for validation of the equipment.

But clearly there was much I had to do before I got to that point. Romana first asked me to demonstrate all the motion I had and also checked strength and coordination in both arms. Then she asked me to describe a typical day, making sure that I mentioned not only major tasks and responsibilities, but also what I did for pleasure, where, and with whom. At the end I felt she had quite a complete picture of who I was and the types of skills, manual, cognitive, and social, I needed to approach my previous lifestyle. We ended the session with setting long-range and more immediate short-term goals. If the whole procedure would not have been so familiar and right to me, I suppose I would have been more bewildered and overwhelmed than I was; I knew what I had to do to get where I was going, but would I find the strength to do the work that would get me there?

Across the hall from occupational therapy was Anne-Marie's office, where I was to go for speech therapy. We talked about old times, especially the monthly meeting both of us had attended; Anne-Marie filled me in on details of the current politics in the department, and I responded to her news. This gave her the opportunity to listen to my thick, slurred speech and also to assess the extent of the breathlessness that had plagued me since the stroke. The deficient speech was of far greater concern to me than the paralyzed arm and leg, perhaps because speech and intellect are so closely linked on the social measurement scale. It was good that Anne-Marie and I could laugh together when I bungled sounds; otherwise, the situation would have been even harder to face.

At 11:30, when I was totally exhausted, I was told that during the hour before lunch, each patient was assigned to a group for further physical activity, depending on one's needs. I was sent to the strengthening group, which on that day consisted of about 10 other people. Seated in a circle in our wheelchairs, we were an odd cross-section of New York City demographics: black, white, and Hispanic men and women, dressed in sweat suits or shorts, shirts, and sneakers, we vaguely resembled a crowd at Yankee Stadium on a Saturday afternoon, although the average age was certainly above 50-years-old. Most of us were recovering from strokes, with varying degrees of disability on either the right or the left side. Some people were obviously seasoned members and knew the routine, which was not difficult to understand. Far more difficult for all of us was to carry out the commands issued by one of the therapists in charge. The purpose of the group was to encourage use of our limbs in sport or recreational activities that

were simplified to make it possible for all of us to participate in games like beanbag toss with a laundry basket as the target or modified soccer with the goal of kicking a big but light ball to each other. A very important aspect of the group was clearly socialization, and most of us got into that component effortlessly. It was amazing to see the inventiveness and enthusiasm of our leaders; I was quickly caught up in the laughter and the chance to be utterly ridiculous. During moments of waiting for my turn, I was reminded once again of my own incapacity; the newly regained motion in my arm and leg was of little help to me, and I had to confront the reality that I was one of thousands of people who were hemiplegic—"hemis," as we affectionately used to call them as therapists. I recalled the group traits that characterized the "hemis," depending on the side of the brain where the lesion was located; thank goodness, I thought once again, I'm a right hemi whose dominant side was affected but who was not expected to have problems in thinking or behavior. My experience as a therapist had borne out much of the textbook information, and I had always enjoyed working with right hemis, many of whom had aphasia, a language problem, or, like myself, dysarthria, which is a problem involving the clarity but not the content of speech. I had liked the challenge of developing a partnership with a patient with aphasia and together discovering a new mode of communication, something like a secret language between us at first. But I was awakened from this reverie by a large balloon being tossed my way and the struggle to catch it with my left hand before it hit me squarely in the face. "Go, Barbara, go!" the therapist encouraged; no one seemed to mind that I dropped the ball. So ended my first morning in therapy. I was too drained by the morning's activity to acknowledge the fact that in an hour and a half, the therapy routine would begin again.

In the middle of the week, my roommate Virginia went home, feeling satisfied that the recovery from the surgery had progressed to the extent that she could carry on alone at home. For one night, I had the room all to myself, and I welcomed the solitude between the steady pace of visitors—professional and friends and family—that continued. I longed for a chance to be left alone, at least long enough to appraise where I was, not fully two weeks since the onset of the stroke. I also wished for an opportunity to take off the cheerful mask that I was wearing, but the anticipated depression still had not come. I was just glad to be alive, and aside from the obvious paralysis of my right limbs and the breathless exhaustion, I felt perfectly well. This came as a total surprise to me. In all the conversations I had with patients who were recovering from a stroke, it always seemed they had pain or other discomfort. The movement in my arm and leg was definitely returning; I could not yet move even against gravity. I still wore the splint on my right wrist to keep that joint from tightening up in a contracted position.

Before I got too used to the luxury of having the large sunny room all to myself, my new roommate arrived. My first impression of her was quite favorable; in a few sentences, Mrs. Gold told me not only her medical history, but also enough details about her life that I knew she lived near me, "in a very good section" of the neighborhood as she emphasized, that she liked good quality and always bought the best, and that she had a daughter in California, whose marriage to a penniless college professor—at least 20 years ago—of which she still did not approve. Her daughter had come East to transfer her mother from another hospital, "a regular hellhole" she noted, where she had been taken after being hit by a van while crossing the street. Now her only remaining injury was a small tear in her bladder. She also needed to practice walking, since she was off her feet a number of weeks. She was greatly relieved when, in response to one of her first questions, I told her that yes, I was Jewish, too. She then asked for my marital status and many other details about my personal life that I had not expected to divulge within the first half-hour of our meeting.

When Mrs. Gold had been put to bed for the night, she began to rummage in her pocketbook for her checkbook, declaring it stolen after a few moments. I urged her to look again and then suggested that it might be in her night table. Sure enough, there it was! She began to flip through the check register and announced that her daughter, who now had power of attorney over Mrs. Gold's finances, was squandering her money on God knows what.

"Why, here is a check for one hundred dollars to Channel Thirteen! I never told her to do that."

For the rest of the evening she repeated the action of getting the checkbook from the drawer and narrative of the check. I tried to reassure her by saying that she could ask her daughter about the money the next day. This resulted in a new cascade of accusations against her daughter. Finally, after both of us were exhausted, Mrs. Gold fell asleep. For the next three and a half weeks, Mrs. Gold and I shared the room, and she became both the much-needed scapegoat on whom to vent my anger and the equally needed comic relief. How much of her confusion was her normal state and how much could be attributed to the accident I never found out, but although she had moments of complete clarity, she also was beset by feelings of persecutions and paranoia that made ordinary conversation almost impossible. Luckily, we spent many hours attending our respective therapies, and thus I did not encounter Mrs. Gold for most of every day.

When Dr. Mitchell next came to see me, he told me that the MRI had been scheduled for the following day. While he spoke very reassuring words, I could feel the familiar cold dread spreading over me that was part of a childhood fear of suffocating. To my knowledge, the closest I had ever come to that state was in third grade when we were rehearsing for a play. As a prank, one of the boys

in my class decided to wrap me in the dark red velvet curtains that hung open at the edge of the stage. Before I could object, I felt myself being spun around as the heavy material enveloped me. I can still smell the thick dust that saturated the curtain; I felt trapped and unable to breathe. I let out a piercing shriek, and the boy released the curtain. While I sobbed hysterically, the curtain fell away from me and I stood free, feeling utterly humiliated in front of my laughing classmates. That image stayed with me all these years and became particularly vivid while Dr. Mitchell spoke further about the procedure.

"I'll be with you in the room; you'll be able to see me through a mirror, and I'll tell you exactly what to do, first with your left hand and then with your right." Since I had already told him about my anxiety, I decided that my telling him again would change nothing. If the procedure were really life-threatening, I decided, I would have read about the consequences by now. "I'll meet you down there tomorrow," with a breezy wave of his hand, Dr. Mitchell was gone, and I was left alone with my irrational fear.

At least I would have a respite for an hour tomorrow from the twice-daily therapy that consumed six hours of every day. With that small bit of comfort, I fell asleep. The next morning, an orderly arrived with the now-familiar stretcher that took patients to special services in other parts of the huge hospital. We arrived in one of the basement corridors clearly marked with a large sign that announced that we were approaching the MRI suite. "Caution— Electromagnetic Equipment—No Unauthorized Personnel beyond this point!" a second sign heralded ominously. In response to a special bell pressed by the orderly, the double doors swung open and closed behind us as soon as we were inside.

Contrary to the CT scan room where I had been alone with the machine, this room was a lively place, mostly occupied by outpatients and a variety of technicians. After a long wait where no one seemed aware of my presence, a man in shirtsleeves greeted me.

"You're Doctor Mitchell's patient, aren't you? I'm Doctor Timoshenko, his assistant, and will prepare you for the actual procedure. Please remove everything metallic you are wearing, like your watch and your rings."

A nurse holding a little plastic box was standing next to me, her hand outstretched in anticipation.

"I can only remove the ring on my left hand," I volunteered, "my other hand is paralyzed." Didn't she realize that herself? Without a word she slipped the ring from my right finger, removed my watch, and proceeded to tackle my earrings. I wanted to scream! I was systematically being stripped of my identity, and felt the last vestige of myself disappearing into the little white box.

"I need to take your glasses, too." Reluctantly, I relinquished my remaining hold on reality. Anything could happen to me now, and I couldn't even see my aggressors!

Dr. Timoshenko wheeled me into another room where I could dimly see several people in lab coats seated before computers. Beyond this outer room was the actual chamber with the large white machine into which I would be placed during the test. Now Dr. Timoshenko and another man seized the sheet on which I was lying on both sides and at the familiar count of three hoisted my body onto the platform of the machine. I felt the hard, cold surface against my spine and hoped that I would not have to remain in this position very long. With deft hands, the two men strapped me down to the table, first making sure that I was covered by a flannel sheet. Then a strip of adhesive tape across my forehead tethered my head to the platform and gave the finishing touch to my immobilized, mummy-like state.

"Here are earplugs to block out the noise made by the machine," Dr. Timoshenko said. What else was part of the preparation? I was beginning to feel utterly dehumanized, and this was only the preparation! With their work apparently completed, the two men left me alone. A dull, whirring sound came from somewhere in the machine; I could vaguely hear voices on the other side of the window that looked into the next room. Just then the door was flung open, and Dr. Mitchell entered with a technician. His usual cordial greeting sounded oddly remote through the rubber earplugs that a moment later, when the machine was turned on, did little to drown out the penetrating noise like a jackhammer all around my head. Before I was fully aware what was happening, the entire platform on which I was lying slid soundlessly into the machine that now encased my head. I could only make out that the top of the enclosure was just inches from my face. This was the moment I had been dreading, and I sensed raw panic flooding over me. I could feel my breath coming in short gasps, and in spite of the chilly air that had bothered me moments before, I felt that I was burning up and had to get out of this place. But before I could act on this impulse, I told myself that I was not the third grader wrapped in a curtain and that there was plenty of air inside the box enclosing my head so that I would not suffocate. I closed my eyes, took several deep breaths and slowly felt my equilibrium returning. I then surrendered myself to the state of imprisonment and waited for whatever was ahead.

After what seemed to be hours, I saw Dr. Mitchell's striped shirt through the small overhead mirror. "How are you doing?" he asked. I could hardly distinguish his voice over the clanging knock of the jackhammer. "Are you ready to begin? First, with your left hand and then with your right, open and close your fist as quickly as you can for thirty seconds. Wait until I say 'go.'" He glanced at his watch and then signaled with his hand and voice that I was to begin. The left hand was easy, but when the procedure was repeated with the right hand, I could not make the fingers move, no matter how hard I tried. The sheer effort of racing against the clock with nothing to show for it was

overwhelming, but I remembered my discussion of this with Dr. Mitchell before the test.

"I'm only looking for brain activity while you attempt the movement." His response had been reassuring, at least for the moment. This got me through the second half of the test, touching each of my fingers to the thumb with equal lack of success on the right side.

At the end of this trial, Dr. Mitchell patted my hand approvingly. "You did very well." He gave me a broad smile. "In about 10 minutes you'll be finished." He left the test chamber, and I was once again by myself. The clanging abated slightly. At least, I could expect an end to the ordeal.

I wondered why, after Dr. Mitchell had completed his experiment, I had to remain in the machine, but all signs of human staffing of the machine had vanished on the other side of the window, and I was once again all alone. Time seemed at a standstill; I recalled a story from the *New Yorker* that my father had told me when I was a little girl. An elderly lady lived alone with her servants in a brownstone house with an elevator. On a Friday night, after the butler and cook had gone off for the weekend, the woman got stuck in the elevator. She knew she could not expect anyone to find her until the servants returned on Sunday night, and to maintain both her mental and physical health until that time, she fashioned a totally rational plan for spending the next 48 hours in the elevator. When her servants found her on Sunday night, she was not only quite composed, but aside from feeling parched and empty, was in good condition. Although I had long since forgotten the details of the woman's ordeal, her resourcefulness and self-control remained as a metaphor for survival under adverse conditions. I now invented a plan for an eventual escape if no one came back to liberate me within a reasonable time. But what was reasonable? I asked myself. And how would I know how much time had elapsed? Before I could ponder these questions, one of the technicians entered, removed the adhesive tape and the other fetters, and placed me back on the mattress of the stretcher that was a welcome relief from the granite-like surface of the machine platform.

The nurse with the little white box was no longer in the outside room. Who would return my belongings to me? An attendant with a Herculean build approached my stretcher.

"Do you know where my glasses and other belongings are?" I asked.

"Yes, I have them." He handed me my glasses and one by one brought out my rings, earrings, and watch.

"I need help with putting on everything except my glasses and one ring. I don't suppose you've ever put a pair of earrings on a woman?" I teased him, secretly hoping that he would become flustered at my question.

"Oh, sure, I have a wife and two daughters." Undaunted, with deft fingers, he replaced my earrings. Once again, as he leaned over me with his big hulk, I felt my private space invaded, but he sensed nothing of this and, after completing his task, wheeled me outside the MRI suite to a "holding station," where other patients on stretchers and in wheelchairs were also waiting to be returned to their floors. We were not a happy group; on the stretcher next to me, a tiny, shriveled old woman was weeping quietly to herself, while a heavyset middle-aged man on the other side moaned loudly in pain. In the far corner of the room, a seemingly disoriented figure in a hospital gown swore loudly and effusively at no one in particular. Yet no one at the desk paid the slightest attention to any of us. The laughter and teasing of the orderlies and nurses at the desk continued. I recalled an illustration of the powerlessness of the individual patient I had frequently used in my teaching: a ladderlike hierarchy of the hospital staff with a small, nondescript patient on the bottom rung. I was struck again by the feeling of powerlessness not only in terms of myself, but more importantly, in any of the other patients to whom the hospital was a strange, bewildering place where no one was willing to listen, much less understand their fear, pain, or loneliness. And I, a supposed helper, was just as vulnerable as they were. I was relieved when a female attendant, without a word, took hold of my stretcher and wheeled me back to the eighth floor.

By the end of the first week in therapy, I was standing upright with a walker and with one of the therapists at my side, taking the first halting steps. From the sheer social acceptance of devices, the wheelchair had always seemed preferable to a walker, but I was glad to be able to move forward from a standing position. At first, my grip was still so weak that I needed an auxiliary upright grab bar for my right hand, but at least I was putting my right side to some good use. Ilsa had built up the handle with ace bandages to make the grasping surface thicker, but unless I concentrated on my hand, it would slip off inadvertently and would need to be replaced in the required position. Within days I was walking all over the rehabilitation floor and felt elated when I was able to see my visitors to the elevator.

With Romana, occupational therapy was also taking on a more functional note, albeit with simulated tasks. My least favorite activity—I groaned at the mere sight of the plastic milk crate that held plastic bottles and containers of various sizes and weights—was picking up these items one by one and placing them on the raised mat on which I was sitting. As I remembered from my clinical practice days, grasping an object was far easier than letting it go, unless the item was so heavy that I would drop it before I had a decent grip on it. This activity was clearly the most tiring I attempted, and there was a noticeable point of no return, when all of Romana's encouraging remarks could not restore the required strength to pick up another object, no matter how small or light. After the first few times

of hating myself for being a quitter, I was glad that Romana recognized my readiness to work on something else until my strength had returned.

Romana had provided me with elastic shoelaces that stayed laced up and knotted in place and did not require tying. Now there were just two dressing items with which I needed help: my bra and the strap of my watch. I remembered trying to teach a one-handed bra technique to patients and usually decided with the patient that it was not worth the enormous strain nor the equally great frustration that this entailed. I had not been part of the bra-burning generation, and therefore never understood the symbolism of going without a bra. Getting into the bra was high on my priority list, and I was willing to spend the time it took to learn this elusive skill. The idea was to fasten the bra first, then slip the involved arm and the head into the opening as if putting on a tee shirt, and finally pushing the healthy arm into the other armhole. Theoretically, this works, but the reality was, at least with me, that I was left with the bra hanging on my right shoulder and around the neck. It was the closest I had come to screaming, but before I uttered a sound, I began to see the ridiculousness of the situation, and I laughed instead. I decided to put on the bra without fastening it and dressing the rest of my body; sooner or later some female would appear in the room, and I could ask her to fasten my bra.

I enjoyed speech therapy simply because Anne-Marie and I were definitely on a compatible wavelength, but I saw little progress in the clarity of my speaking. We spent much time working on silly word exercises, and I even practiced these in my room, but certain consonants like "d" and "p" were slurred and ugly sounding. When any of my colleagues or former students came to see me, I felt very self-conscious about my speech, but no one ever mentioned it, although my family often commented on the low volume of my voice during our conversations.

Although I was very grateful for the good wishes and cheerful conversation they brought, the many visitors from the University were becoming a real burden, mainly for their unpredictability. I had always found that the ID card that allowed university employees carte blanche access to the hospital to be a great help when we needed some clinical information or even for using one of the corridors as a short cut. Now the privilege of going into the hospital at any time came back to haunt me; at any hour of the day, I could expect visitors in my room, and I felt I had to be "on stage." When I told Anne-Marie that these visits were even more fatiguing than five to six hours of therapy, she suggested that I tell my drop-in guests that I had to rest my voice during mealtimes, a measure I accepted and applied gratefully.

Far better were the announced or mutually arranged visits that I anticipated with pleasure. Such a visit was from Marie, a colleague and friend who telephoned one

Saturday and announced that she was bringing dinner. Marie, of Italian descent and a marvelous cook, was certain that I wasn't eating enough and needed some home cooking. She came bearing not only a delicately prepared dinner but also a bright tablecloth, real silver, cloth napkins, and pottery plates! At one of the round tables, Marie spread out her wealth, and we proceeded to have a gourmet meal while the other patients ate the usual hospital fare nearby, casting envious glances in my direction. For a moment I almost forgot that I still couldn't cut meat and had to eat everything except finger food with an awkward left hand.

After my first days on the rehabilitation floor, I decided that eating a meal alone or with a roommate in the same room that served as a bedroom was not conducive to stimulating my still lagging appetite, and so I chose to take my meals in the day room, a large open space that served as a recreation or meeting room for both patients and staff. A folding wall could be closed off to divide the space in half, thereby allowing it to be used for several purposes simultaneously. The last activity of the morning—the "upright" group—was held on one side of the wall at the same time as members of the staff met on the other to discuss the progress and eventual discharge of patients. At mealtimes, the large round tables were pulled into the center of the room and patients who wished could take their meals there. Some of us chose this setting, while others preferred the privacy of their own rooms. Since most of the staff were in the day room with the majority of the patients, it was easier there to get assistance with any aspect of a meal. Perhaps if I had not been used to watching people with chewing and swallowing difficulty eat, I too would have preferred to stay in my room during mealtimes, but after working with both children and adults who experienced these problems, I knew the atmosphere would not be as unpleasant for me as it appeared to be for patients who did not return to the day room after their first meal there. Besides, I knew that my own eating was not up to the aesthetic standards I had been taught as a child. For a strongly right-handed person like me, it was awkward to eat with the left hand, and I often ended with much of the meal in my lap.

Although the quality and the quantity of most meals were quite adequate, and those of us who had no dietary restrictions could ask for as many dishes as we wished, the plastic wrapping of the utensils and much of the food was a daily source of frustration to those of us who did not have use of two hands. Certain wrappings could be removed only by helping with the teeth or developing other questionable methods for tearing the plastic. When one of us had devised a technique that seemed particularly effective, we quickly shared it with the others. To me, this teaching aspect was particularly important; it was the first small sign that I was reclaiming a part of my former self.

Mealtimes were also useful for seeing the similarities and differences among patients in response to their disability. I marveled at the way that premorbid personality surfaced and either aided or impeded progress in different patients. A tiny, very old lady whose strong accent I recognized as Viennese complained and demanded things in a penetrating voice throughout each meal. She was quite deaf and could not hear when one of the nurses told her she would come right away and so continued calling for help. I soon found out that the only way to calm her down was to sit next to her and engage her in conversation close to her ear. She then cheered up instantly and listened to my shouted explanations that help was on its way. Mrs. Siegel told me repeatedly about many aspects of her life, particularly her age—she was 93-years-old—and the fact that she was now cut off from her sister in California because she could not hear her on the telephone. At home she had a special phone; in fact, since she had no family here, she had to rely on a friend who was not really a friend. Her repertoire of conversation topics remained constant from meal to meal, and I soon became familiar with her litany of complaints. She frequently whimpered that the physical therapists made her work too hard by forcing her to stand with her walker and take steps. Looking at the tiny, frail, and unhappy woman, I almost agreed with her, but I was pleasantly surprised when several days after our first encounter, I saw her slowly taking steps pushing the walker, still complaining about working too hard.

Seating arrangements for meals in the day room were up to us—one of the few choices we had. I usually sat with the same crowd who was by nature, and as a circumstance of their diagnoses, most communicative. Mrs. Gold, who at first could not find her way anywhere on the rehabilitation floor, was my steady companion as we dragged our walkers along the hall to the dayroom for meals. Once there, we would sit together because that seemed to be the simplest way to deal with her. According to Mrs. Gold, she never got the dishes she had ordered, but when I looked at the menu on her tray that she herself had completed the day before, she usually had not circled the missing items on her order, and I had to listen to her complaints during the whole meal. When I could not seem to satisfy her demands, she called whatever staff person whom she could see in the day room, addressing them with a loud, "Mi-iss!" no matter who they were. The residents often visited their patients at meals, when the doctors knew that the patients were not in one of the therapies. They were frequently the only staff in sight, but Mrs. Gold did not discriminate in the persons selected to carry out her demands; generally, the young doctors chuckled at these requests for help and good-naturedly said they would call one of the aides. Mrs. Gold and I then agreed that it would be more reasonable if I helped her fill out the menu for the following day to assure that she would get the dishes she had selected. Filling out the menu then became part of our daily ritual; I would read aloud the choices to Mrs. Gold who said that she could not see enough to read the menu. When she had made her selection, I held the pencil and circled the items with my very awkward left hand much as I did when I completed my own menu. I marveled that the helpers in the kitchen could decipher which dishes I had actually circled since my scribbles on the page hardly resembled circles. But I knew that handwriting difficulties were a rather common-place deficit among most of the patients on the rehabilitation floor.

Almost every one of us was eager to take advantage of the therapies. Although we each had at least two 30-minute sessions of individual treatment of each type of therapy daily, there were always other people around who were simultaneously working with their therapists. Only speech therapy was private, a fact that made it much easier for me. As a result of spending so much time with the rehabilitation patients, I became very familiar with the rate or degree of progress of other people and they with mine. Pretty much everything we did in therapy was public knowledge, and for me, this served as a strong motivation to try to succeed at everything I was asked to do. Both Ilsa and Romana expected more of us each day, and in spite of being naturally fearful and in a constant state of fatigue, I tried to rise to the challenges of their demands. When I was successful, my flickering battery of self-esteem felt recharged. But at the end of each day of therapy, in spite of steady progress, I was so drained of energy that I dragged myself back to my room just to sit and relax a few moments before it was time to walk back to the day-room for dinner. Usually there were already visitors waiting for me, and I was forced to muster a new round of power for conversation and answers to the well-meaning inquiries about my progress.

After three weeks in rehabilitation, my life had settled into a routine that served as a stable background for the changes in my body and, I suppose, my soul. I became aware that I was living only in the present; I did not dwell much on the past because that could be painful, but I also did not think ahead about my future. As long as I was in rehab, I must still be moving ahead, and so I really did not think of myself as a fixed being, but rather as a work in progress. Since I was still sleeping fitfully, I often found myself at night in a state of semiconsciousness, when I envisioned the same image of myself. I was a paper doll folded at the waist because the upper half of my body was not strong enough to allow me to stand upright. By morning this had faded back into my subconscious, but every night it returned. During the day, there were many opportunities to prove to myself that I could indeed do more than stand upright. My activities with both Ilsa and Romana had taken on a more practical tone; in occupational therapy, we practiced getting in and out of the

bathtub, and I actually went to the grocery store of Easy Street to do some "shopping." There was a small shopping cart in the store, the kind found in New York City neighborhood grocery stores. My task was to pick up various items from the shelf, place them in the shopping cart, and walk to the cash register. Each of the plastic fruits and vegetables and the empty boxes of cereal or containers of detergent were filled with a substance that calibrated its approximate real weight. I was expected to use my right hand for all one-handed tasks and could use my left hand only to assist with normally bilateral activities. After picking up a simulated tomato, a cucumber, and a banana out of the vegetable bin, my arm was totally worn out. Letting go of the objects was almost harder than picking them up; my right hand hovered over the basket until I was able to release whatever I held in my hand. Although I had done similar tasks with patients for many years, I had never imagined that fatigue was the constant companion of even the simplest tasks.

Although I still tired quickly with any type of physical activity, I experienced the massive fatigue more totally when using my right hand. When I reached the end of my muscle power, I felt literally like a windup toy that had run down and needed a new boost, one that was not immediately available to me. I was surprised how long it took before I felt ready to use the hand or arm again for a task requiring lifting of any but the lightest items. This was one of the few areas where I felt that the therapists did not fully understand that when a patient states unequivocally, as I did on several occasions, "I can't do it again; I'm exhausted!" that a two-minute rest period won't restore the expended energy. I began to wonder whether, as a practicing therapist, I had been as sensitive to each patient's fatigue as I should have been; I sent a silent apology to the many patients I had treated years ago.

I had never experienced the kind of massive exhaustion that now held my body in its grip. It was probably apparent to others in the breathlessness I experienced many times during the day, especially when I was walking and talking at the same time. This brought to mind the old dare we tried on one another as children: "Try rubbing your stomach and patting the top of the head at the same time!" I did not succeed even as a child, and the memory of that made me smile somewhat ruefully each time I had another breathless episode. When I mentioned these to Anne-Marie, she suggested I try to slow down my speech in normal conversation and continue to practice in my room the breathing exercise I did with her twice every day—blowing as hard as I could into a thick tube that was connected to a plastic bottle with a calibrated gauge that registered the volume of my lung capacity. The gauge was useful in measuring my progress, but I never advanced beyond a certain point, in spite of Anne-Marie's motivating cheers. For the rest of my body, there did not seem to be an immediate remedy. I always knew I had reached the end of my energy supply when I began to experience actual nausea and a strong desire to lie down and shut off the world. I never acted on the impulse, however; instead, I simply sat down on whatever surface was available and waited for my equilibrium to be restored. Generally, that did not take longer than five minutes, and no one ever questioned my "time out."

My days took on another dimension when a patient called Ben became more visible on the rehabilitation floor and took his meals with the rest of us. He was younger than I was by about 10 years, but like me, he had survived a stroke that affected his right arm and leg; he also had considerable slurring in his speech and, because the paralysis affected his chewing and swallowing muscles, he was on a special pureed diet. As a result, his tray always included many small dishes of unappetizing-looking pureed food of varying colors and several soft desserts. At first, he preferred to eat alone in his room or at a table by himself in a corner of the large day room, but one day I asked him to move to our table, mainly because I sensed he would be a better communicator than were some of the other people.

I recognized him from the various therapies, especially the movement group where his attempts at kickball or ring toss were as unsuccessful as mine most of the time. He caught my immediate attention by his unfailing sense of humor that resounded readily with me. I had decided that among other sequelae of the stroke, the slow, awkward way of carrying out most everyday activities would appear utterly ridiculous if compared to my past life; I could tolerate my present lack of speed only if I looked upon my performance as being a caricature of myself. Many of the quips that Ben tossed out to the group in general indicated to me that he operated on an equal wavelength with me. When we were not sitting at the table with the others, we sat in other parts of the day-room, from where he and I could joke or make sarcastic comments about the food, the routine, and the other patients without our being heard. Our favorite topic was, of course, Mrs. Gold, who gave us ample material for a new script each day. She felt that most therapy was a waste of time and was quite vocal about this, especially in the "upright group," individually adapted to meet the needs of every member of the group. A staff person carefully monitored each of us, since most were unsteady at best in an upright position. During one of our particularly lively games that must have looked grotesque to the uninitiated, Mrs. Gold announced in a loud voice, "I think this is a big waste of time!" Thereafter, from our corner Ben and I invented situations where we would tell Mrs. Gold that the doctors and therapists had selected her as captain of all team sports or other similar crazy ideas. Ben grew so enamored with his ideas that at times I felt I had to restrain him from carrying out the pranks. Although this was surely not my proudest hour, it helped

to diminish the reality of our condition that confronted us every waking moment of each day. With Ben I could count on being amused, and our shared laughter had a beneficial effect on both of us. Every afternoon just before dinner, Ben's wife Charlotte appeared and stayed with him until visiting hours had ended. From what I learned, they had married less than 10 years ago, and she appeared to be a housewife, free to spend many hours of each day at the hospital. The couple readily accepted me in their hospital dinners, and I was grateful to have one meal daily away from the complainers.

I knew that I was progressing well, but I was still walking with a walker and using my right hand only to assist my left. The walker was light to move about, but it was wider than I was and required enough space to get into the places that were part of my present environment. As a result, I missed most of my phone calls, because the phone was on the nightstand on the right side of my bed and meant walking around the bed to answer it. Maneuvering the walker and myself into the narrow space between the window and the bed took me much longer than most callers were willing to wait. No matter how quickly I tried to move—and my quickest pace still resembled that of a sloth—I never reached the phone before the caller had hung up. Much as I tried to tell my callers that they should let the phone ring at least a dozen times, anyone who called for the first time did not reach me. At first, this was a source of frustration and disappointment, but after a while I realized that I was not in control of this, and I accepted the missed calls as a matter of course.

I had now reached the third week in rehab. One of the most dramatic physical challenges was climbing the set of four or five practice steps in the gym. Even with the aid of the banister on the left, going up was bad enough, but when I arrived at the platform on the top and faced forward, the sight of the steps below me was a daunting prospect that made my heart beat madly. How would I get down? I was suddenly transported back to my childhood to the Sunday hikes in the German evergreen forest that frequently ended with a climb of the deserted observation tower for hunters and forest rangers. My father deemed that this activity would be a healthy challenge to my brother and me. Although Jeff was quite unathletic and much preferred reading to sports, he did have the advantage of being older by a year and a half and thereby having longer legs. Outwardly, at least, he showed no fear. Scaling the ladder meant going up the rickety rungs that were much too far apart for my short legs, but I was expected to follow my brother. Under loud protestations I actually reached the top. My immediate expression of victory was clouded by the dreaded moment when I would have to descend. As a simultaneously ambitious and compliant child, I never thought of refusing the climb up, especially when my older brother accomplished this without difficulty, but when I saw how far I had come and realized that the tiny man below with the smiling upturned face was really my father, I froze and sobbed that I couldn't come down. Eventually, my father's encouraging words and explicit directions on placement of each foot guided me down, but it spoiled the hike for me for that day and many days to come when I realized the performance had to be repeated. Now I could feel the same terror, but Ilsa was less than six feet below; the sight of her brought me back to the present and to the entirely achievable task of descending the steps, again holding on to the banister on the left side.

When I saw how difficult it was to accommodate to the early bedtime routine of the hospital—if I went to sleep at 9 PM, as many of the patients did, I woke at 2 AM and lay awake waiting for dawn and the 5:30 reveille without ever falling asleep again—after a week of this, I decided to go into the deserted day room and read. No one objected to my being there, since by now all the nurses knew that I did not need help getting myself ready for bed. I soon discovered that this was the hour and place for the aides' dinner, but they tolerated my presence on the other side of the room with cheerful indifference. Instead of reading—I still found it difficult to concentrate for an extended period of time—I watched whatever "drama" the aides had selected as their dinner accompaniment on the large-screen television and listened to their high-spirited banter in the Caribbean patois I had come to love after many visits to the islands. The performances on the screen fascinated me by their sheer novelty; in my white, middle-class culture I had never tuned in to an all black channel. Now I watched the screenplays and commercials in which all black stars were featured, accompanied by the comments of the aides. A favorite topic of conversation was the Caribbean food that some of them brought from their homes. Although I was extremely interested to see what they were eating, I did not want to spoil my coveted role of silent participant-observer in their mealtimes. At the end of an hour, with a collective sigh as someone glanced at her watch, the dinner break ended, and they quickly cleaned up the remains of their meal before returning to their posts. One of them always passed close to my chair to hand me the remote control. Now I was truly on my own, sitting in the semidark with only the huge screen of the television coming between me and the drowsiness that overcame me shortly after I was left alone. I don't think I ever saw the end of a program that I had selected. With my last bit of energy, I pushed my walker through the silent corridor to my room, where I soon joined Mrs. Gold in sleep.

Whether it was part of the denial that carried me through the first few days following the onset of the stroke or another part of my psyche, I found myself on several occasions using the "magical thinking" that many of my patients employed to escape a painful reality. More than once, when I arrived in my room after a particularly exhausting day, I found myself wishing for a miracle. A soundless voice from a part of myself that I rarely used would say to me, "For just five minutes, I would like to feel normal again so I could move with ease!" I never considered what would happen when those five minutes were up; that was part of the magical thinking, of course. Once I had uttered that wish and cried for a moment with the certainty of knowing I was asking for the impossible, I somehow felt empowered again to carry on.

I was really so much better than I had been; I no longer wore the splint during the day and began to use my right hand more spontaneously. At night, as a precaution, I put the splint on for several additional days, and then developed the habit of putting my hand under the pillow so that the weight of my head would keep the fingers from curling up and the wrist supported. In occupational therapy, Romana and I were working on my handwriting; at this point, we were still unsure whether I should switch to using the left hand. As children we had all practiced writing with the left hand, as many of my classmates did, but I never perfected this skill and now found it awkward and fatiguing. With the right hand, at first, the pen or pencil often fell from my grasp. Romana had a large selection of adapted pens, all of which I tried with limited success.

Whenever I practiced writing, I was reminded of a visit by one of the rehabilitation physicians who, after reading my chart, quipped in an almost jovial way, "You should do very well, but you'll never get your handwriting back." With that, he left the room. I was furious and hurt. How could he predict my recovery merely from reading my medical chart? Since I never saw him again, I did not even have the satisfaction of asking him to explain the basis of his prognosis. Nevertheless, Romana and I continued in our efforts to find a writing utensil that was really useful for me. I was given sheets of writing exercises (large script on wide lines not unlike the ones that I remembered from elementary school when learning to write for the first time). I traced over the sample letters and then completed the sheet on my own with varying results. Like with everything else, I tired rapidly; I also found this activity to be terribly boring, and I had to force myself to do it in the rare moments without prescribed activity or visitors.

At the end of the fourth week, the entire rehab team discussed my case as reported to me by Dr. Stuart, who had been my attending physician and in charge of all the patients on our floor. She and I related easily to one another, first, because we had attended the same department meetings for several years, and second, because as women, we had a similar perspective on many aspects of life. Now she reported that the team had agreed that I should be ready for discharge in seven days, exactly five weeks from the date of my second admission. This would give me time to work on additional tasks that were important for my particular lifestyle—living alone in an apartment on the northern fringes of New York City. My initial reaction was neither surprise nor alarm. I was familiar with the regulations that medical insurance dictated the maximum length of stay by diagnosis, not status. I knew that by the date that Dr. Stuart mentioned, I would have received the maximum number of days of inpatient treatment covered for a stroke.

Until that moment I had not allowed myself to think a great deal about discharge; now I had to face the outside world with the residual changes wrought by the stroke. The first thing that came to mind was that I really was ashamed to be seen in my community with a walker that to me signified a far greater degree of dependency than I was willing to accept. It also would place me in a large group of elderly people who, for one reason or another, used walkers to get around our community, usually accompanied by another person. I hated the thought of joining that group at this point in my life, and again I realized the importance for me to get on the cane as quickly as possible. The cane had become a metaphor for an older but independent person.

My three therapists, Romana, Ilsa, and Anne-Marie, all talked to me about the discharge date and the goals I wanted to attain before leaving the hospital. Clearly, I had to be able to prepare meals for myself and to increase my endurance, not only for speaking without getting out of breath but also for tackling the five-block walk to the grocery store. Before we could put into practice any of these plans, I was faced by another weekend without therapy, and this time I really resented the forced idleness imposed by the five-day treatment schedule. On Saturdays the two recreation therapists were in charge of keeping our minds and bodies stimulated, and since I had seen for three weeks that attendance at the morning current events group and the afternoon cooking group was sparse, I decided to join the groups once more in a show of collegial solidarity. I felt much closer to the other patients during therapy and meals where our disabilities formed a common bond. It was much harder to feel the same connection when we had a somewhat artificial conversation about sports or the latest scandal from the daily news. Still, I gave the two young therapists a great deal of credit for their enthusiasm and inventiveness week after week.

On Monday, my rehabilitation took on a new note of immediacy; there were only four days of therapy before leaving the hospital! Both Ilsa and Romana had prepared a list of very practical activities they wanted me to perform before Friday, which included preparing my habitual lunch from a shopping list prepared by myself and walking outside and taking a ride on a city bus with Ilsa along in the event that I needed assistance. Ilsa and Romana had also planned a home visit with me to see if any changes were needed in the set-up of my apartment. It seemed to be an awful lot for me to accomplish in the short time, but the therapists assured me that we could get everything done. After this afternoon's walk outside on the street, Ilsa

would be able to judge if I could exchange the walker for a cane.

Wisely, Ilsa had decided that I needed to save my energy for the actual walk in the street; I could therefore use the wheelchair until we were outside. Our first stop on this venture was the elevator that would take us down to the lobby. I realized that there were many hurdles along the way that six weeks before would have been just routine parts of dealing mindlessly with the interaction of human beings and technology. Suppose I could not wheel myself through the open doors of the elevators before they closed again automatically? Was I strong enough to manage the various doors that led to the busy hospital lobby? Thank goodness Ilsa was there to ward off any real danger. I could feel the fierce beating of my heart as the elevator stopped on our floor. I rolled over the threshold into the narrow space left by the other passengers before the doors closed behind us and then rolled out again at the lobby level. One hurdle had been conquered. I exhaled gratefully and approached the entrance to the lobby feeling somewhat less anxious.

As we left the hospital building, I realized that this was the first fresh air I had breathed in five weeks. I had missed most of July and within the air-conditioned rooms of the hospital had forgotten how oppressive the August heat could be in New York. Now it hit me as I stood up and took hold of the walker. Before I took the first steps on the sidewalk, Ilsa bent toward me and said, "There's a good chance that you'll meet up with some of the people you know around here; do you think that will that bother you?"

I was touched by her sensitivity. In the same way that I had felt when the first colleague had approached my bed when the news of my stroke reached the university, I decided that only the first encounter would be difficult. Before I had a chance to ponder this, I saw a colleague crossing the street and approaching me.

"Hi, how are you? It's good to see you again!" He treated me quite normally, and I knew I would have little difficulty relating to other colleagues in the same way. Not until I left the hospital environment would I have to deal with the questions I expected from my neighbors. At this moment, I was much more concerned with managing the uneven pavement and the hazards of crossing the street that Ilsa had included in the itinerary.

For the last 25 years of my professional life, this had been one of the most familiar corners; it was the intersection where the university and the hospital met. How many times in all seasons had I crossed here, running to and from classes, going to my office and the administration building? It was a bustling, unruly place, teeming with students, medical personnel, and ambulatory patients, some patiently waiting for the light and others, perennially rushed and darting between the traffic to make it quickly to the other side. Gypsy cabs, unmindful of either traffic lights or the people, were everywhere, adding to the noise and confusion by blasting their horns at the slightest provocation. Did Ilsa really expect me to get into the midst of this?

"I don't think I can make it across before the light changes." I hoped that she would agree with me, and we could call the whole thing off.

"Of course you can! Just don't stop walking. Besides, I'll be right next to you."

I knew that I could trust Ilsa not to set a challenge beyond my ability to meet it, and so, when the light turned the next time, I stepped off the curb and met the onrushing pedestrian traffic. Again I could hardly breathe for the wild beating of my heart. Was this going to be my partner in every new situation facing me? This time I felt almost overwhelmed; Ilsa's presence served both as a protective and as an empowering mantle whenever a menacing task was ahead, and now, too, I made it safely to the other side. But I was not yet free to gloat over my victory.

"Now let's go back. Cars will stop when they see the walker," Ilsa said, as confident as ever, and I could not disappoint her. I held my breath and dragged myself back across the street. The waiting wheelchair was a welcome haven, and I sank back into it, too exhausted to speak. Would every outing require that much courage and energy? Where would I find an endless supply of both? Once again I was reminded how much the stroke had taken from me. Could I really reclaim the missing parts of my former self?

Ilsa's cheerful voice roused me. "You made it, you see! You also showed me that tomorrow we can start with the cane." I immediately cheered up and could hardly wait to tell my family about my accomplishments.

Helen then told me of her decision to stay with me at my apartment for at least a week, thereby eliminating the need for home care from a stranger. This piece of news cheered me enormously, since the thought of having a stranger stay with me was thoroughly unappealing and had caused me a great deal of concern. After my outing with the walker, there were only four days of hospitalization left. As promised, Ilsa had a cane waiting for me in physical therapy the next morning. I took my first steps rather unsteadily, with Ilsa holding the back of my slacks for support. It was difficult to think of all the parts of walking simultaneously and sequentially. Compared to the walker, the cane had a much narrower base of support. I was grateful that I was not totally on my own as I walked along the long corridor. To give me additional practice, a young male therapy aide was given the job of walking with me twice each day around the extended quadrangle that covered the entire eighth floor.

I had done my homework for Romana for the next day: making a list of all the items I would need for the salad I was to prepare in the occupational therapy kitchen. It had taken me almost half an hour to print out the names of six vegetables! And they were barely legible. At least I had found a built-up pencil that I could grasp, and Romana had given it to me to take home. However, for today I was to remove and replace the sheets on the bed in the Easy Street apartment. This was a task I remembered well from my days of being a clinician: one-handed bed-making is a slow, arduous procedure; the help that my right hand could offer at this point reduced neither the effort nor the length of time that elapsed until the bedspread was safely back on the bed. Changing the pillowcase was especially hard; all the two-handed steps that turn this into an efficient, easily done task now became mostly unilateral. Since I was still too unsteady with the cane, I had to use the walker. I circled the bed a dozen times to tuck in sheets and the blanket, but I proved to Romana and myself that I was capable of performing this task by myself; once I got home, only I would need to know how much time and energy it cost!

I had progressed sufficiently to eating most of each meal with my right hand in an awkward manner. At first, my hand often overshot its mark, and the food dropped back on the plate or in my lap. I was plagued more by the lack of coordination now than by the weakness. Also, I had discovered another annoying aspect of hand function over which I had no control; whenever I coughed or was surprised by an unexpected noise, my hand shot up and I dropped whatever I was holding. Worst of all, if I was startled while I held a cup of juice or coffee, I would spill the liquid all over the table. The first time this happened was during lunch at our large round table. I was holding a roll in my right hand and was ready to take a bite when an uncontrollable cough shook my body. My hand shot up and flung the roll across the room in what must have looked like very crazy behavior. I looked around quickly to see if anyone had noticed, but luckily, everyone was too absorbed with his or her own meals. Though I was initially amused at my action, it was a painful reminder of the extent of neurological damage I had incurred. How many years I had explained to my students that "a brain injury can actually 'undo' the learning that has occurred in the neurological system in the course of normal development of an infant. All of us are born with a 'startle' reflex that makes an infant raise its arms in response to a loud noise or sudden striking of the surface on which the baby lies. This reflex is suppressed as part of normal development. A stroke will undo the suppression, and the reflex operates as in early infancy." Now as I lay awake in the early hours of the following day, I recognized that this had actually happened to me as part of the larger picture of irreversible neurological loss. All of my recovery thus far was probably due to the fact that the brain is such a versatile organ with spare neurological pathways that can take over lost functions. This was powerful stuff, and while I accepted it as theoretical information, I was not ready to accept it as inevitable fact. When I next saw Dr. Mitchell, I asked him whether I would ever lose the startle reflex. His answer was terse but friendly, "Probably not."

As planned, Ilsa and Romana met me at 10 AM the next morning to do the home visit at my apartment. At the front door of the hospital, one of them hailed a cab. Since neither of them knew the way to my house, I felt totally in charge of this outing. I gave the driver instructions of the route that had brought me home every day—not seated in the back of a taxi, to be sure—but relishing the short, pleasant drive along the Hudson in back of the wheel of my own car. Now as I watched the trees and the sky flash by, I wondered whether I would ever be capable of enjoying the degree of independence that both night and day driving of my car had allowed. Thank goodness that was not one of my immediate concerns.

I was surprised at the amount of anticipation that I now felt as the taxi turned the last corner and swung into the driveway of the apartment building. Except for one brief visit by Helen to fetch me more shirts and slacks, no one had entered the apartment since I had left it almost five weeks ago. A quick composite of Sleeping Beauty and Rip van Winkle flashed across my mind; would the rooms be covered by cobwebs?

The doorman rushed from the building when the cab pulled up; his face lit up with a huge smile as he opened the door.

"Welcome back! How are you?" He extended his arm and helped me out of the car, flanked by the two therapists. Before we could enter the building, however, I had to mount the single step that led up to the front door. In more than 10 years of living in this place, I had never noticed that there was no railing and was genuinely surprised to see that oversight now.

"Yipes!" was the only word I could utter. In her usual calm manner, Ilsa called out, "Just use the technique you used on the practice curbs in the gym." I was very glad that she was standing next to me as I mounted the step.

Everything looked pleasantly familiar as I crossed the lobby and went up the three steps to the elevator, this time firmly holding on to the banister. Even taking stairs with the cane presented few problems now that I could carry the cane in my right hand while the left grasped the railing.

I felt as if I were welcoming new friends to my home as I unlocked the door. My absence from the familiar rooms suddenly seemed much longer than the actual five weeks. I could recall coming home from college after a semester away from home; there was always a comfortable recognition of the furnishings, but I was no longer the same person who had left. This time I was returning from a journey to unexplored terrain, and my physical relationship to the objects was changed as well.

Romana's voice brought me back to reality. "Is it OK if we just look around?" I knew the considerations of a routine home visit, and I pointed out to Romana all the features of accessibility and safety they would be looking for: no scatter rugs to trip on, the placement of kitchen utensils and dishes that I had to use every day, the location of the telephone, and the layout of the bathroom.

"You'll need a bench for the shower, and we'll order that in the hospital today. Otherwise, the apartment looks good and you should be able to manage everything."

"Did you really think that an occupational therapist's apartment would be full of hazards?" I couldn't resist the chance to tease the therapists.

Leaving the apartment after such a brief visit was less difficult than I had thought it would be. There were several things I needed to practice while I was still in rehabilitation, such as the cooking experience and the ride on the city bus. Besides, Mrs. Gold was going home today, and I actually looked forward to the next two days alone.

That evening for the first time I allowed myself to think about what it would be like at home. I realized how much I had employed denial as a useful method of dealing with an unpleasant or unacceptable reality. I could make the problem disappear temporarily by just not thinking about it; when it next confronted me, as it inevitably did, I was more ready to face it and work on a solution. Although I would not recommend this style of problem-solving to anyone else, it had certainly worked for me until now. Therefore, I was finally ready to concentrate on life at home, fully aware that there were hazards and hurdles that would have to be surmounted, and I would somehow manage them as I had all the previous ones during my rehabilitation. Thank goodness I had learned long ago to hide my fears quite well and thereby keep face. I recognized once again how unacceptable it was to me to lose face. With these thoughts I finally drifted off to sleep.

Practicing the various curbs while using the cane was my assignment in physical therapy the next morning. At one point, Ilsa made a seemingly innocent comment about doing this alone once I was home. Suddenly, all the emotions that I had kept to myself for five weeks broke the thin shell that held them in check; I was caught completely off guard and burst into uncontrollable tears. Ilsa, seeing my state, quickly ushered me into an empty back room, where I spent the next 20 minutes sobbing noisily in a way that was completely foreign to me. Try as I might, I could not stop crying. Ilsa tactfully left me alone and even brought me moist paper towels for my red eyes when the torrent seemed to be abating. The enormity of what had happened had finally dawned on me. I was totally overcome by the thought of leaving the safe haven of the rehabilitation floor where we all had problems and had been completely sheltered from the outside world. No explanation about one's condition was necessary, and if anyone needed medical or psychological help, it was always available. Now I would have to cut through all the red tape that stood between the health care system and me. And then the dreaded "S" word flashed through my mind; suppose I would have a second stroke! I knew that the threat of a second stroke was much greater than that for the first time; the only preventable factor in my own case was keeping the blood pressure under control. The twice-daily reading of blood pressure had made me painfully aware that it fluctuated considerably from day to day. Before this episode, I had never been concerned about my blood pressure, which, as I was repeatedly told by my doctor at my annual checkup, was within normal limits for my age. In the hospital I was on the verge of panic when it seemed particularly high one day. I asked to see Dr. Mitchell since I was sure I was having a second stroke. He reassured me that this was not the case and to be prepared for the frequent ups and downs. After his visit I felt ashamed about my hysterical reaction, but it was a fear that did not leave me. Who would respond to my cries for help from home? As always, I calmed myself by calling on my reasoning system. At last I felt that my equilibrium was at least partially restored. Although I was drained by the experience, it was a necessary part of the healing process.

I realized how long I had been in the back room when I saw Romana searching for me; she was ready to take me through the salad-making experience that would give her a chance to observe my performance in the kitchen. I hoped that my red eyes were not too obvious as I followed her into the occupational therapy kitchen where a bag with the salad ingredients on my shopping list was waiting for me.

"I know I don't have to show you any of the equipment or the techniques," she laughed, "You probably know them better than I do. I'll just observe you from here. I'd like to try out a new test on you; it includes such aspects of your performance as safety, sequencing, and time. Please use your right or both hands whenever you can, especially for removing dishes from the cabinets."

Romana was right; I had been through countless cooking experiences with patients. In fact, cooking and baking had been among the most successful therapy sessions I had with many types of patients who needed not only to reacquire the physical skill but also to restore their self-concept and self-confidence. While I was washing lettuce and peeling the cucumber, I felt vaguely like the schoolmaster Mr. Chips, who in his dreams recalled dozens of his former pupils marching in front of him.

Romana watched me wordlessly from a corner of the large table at which I worked, sometimes standing, sometimes sitting, while the salad slowly took shape. The sequential steps were in and of themselves not difficult for me to do, mostly one-handed. I was appalled to realize how long the simple process of washing, peeling, and cutting six vegetables took—45 minutes—and all my remaining energy went into the process. Walking from the sink or counter to the table meant holding the cane in my left hand. This left the weak right hand to carry objects. After the first attempt I found that this was still too difficult for me. Romana had pointed out the teacart on which I placed all the objects that ordinarily I would have carried in both hands. This, too, was familiar, but nevertheless it struck me as totally wrong that now I was the patient rather than the teacher who showed patients how to carry objects on the cart that also served as a support while walking. My reward for completing the activity was the finished salad that Romana carried to the dining room for me. Although I knew, theoretically, that walking and carrying objects would be a problem at home, the cooking experience reminded me that I still had a lot of work to do at home.

I found it difficult to believe that this had been my last full session in occupational therapy, since the afternoon's therapy would be cut short as a result of the planned bus trip to Fort Tryon Park, and, after getting off the bus and crossing the street, taking the bus back to the hospital. This was an outing I did not anticipate with pleasure. Even with Ilsa's guidance, I could not see myself being able to hold the rail with my left hand while mounting the bus step in the time New York bus drivers usually allow before starting up the bus again.

The ride on the elevator and walk to the front of the hospital were almost routine for me. I was glad that I did not need many repetitions of a procedure to overcome my greatest fears. However, when the bus approached our corner, I would gladly have told Ilsa that I was not ready for this challenge. This was my last chance to practice this skill with supervision, and once more, reason took charge. I noticed that there were several other men and women of my vintage with canes waiting for the bus. I would let some of them precede me and try to watch the technique they employed. But then it was my turn. With Ilsa following close behind, I moved the cane to my right hand, grasped the handrail with my left hand, and pulled myself up. Ilsa managed the tokens for us while I walked to one of the seats in front that had been vacated by a younger rider when he saw me coming. Gratefully, I fell into one of the places designated "For elderly and disabled," a seat that only five weeks before I would gladly have left for the people who fit one of these groups. Now, involuntarily, I had joined their ranks. I was so totally preoccupied with these thoughts that I paid no attention to the passing scene or my fellow passengers, which would have been unthinkable for me before the stroke. Ilsa stood in front of me and reminded me that the next corner was the last stop, and once the bus had come to a stop, we would be getting out. Again, I feared that I would not be able to get out in time and slid to the edge of my seat to be ready as soon as the bus came to a halt. Ilsa preceded me on the way out so she could supervise my getting down the bus steps. In my eagerness to descend the steps, I stumbled and would have landed on the sidewalk had Ilsa not caught me. By now I was trembling all over.

"The bus drivers will always wait until you are well outside." Ilsa's voice was reassuring, but I could tell she was not pleased by my performance. "Let's cross the street since the bus is coming." I was still completely rattled when I remounted the bus steps, but both the ascent and descent were accomplished without further incident. Still, I did not think I could ever find the courage again to ride a city bus.

I was too excited to sleep more than a few hours that night, anticipating all the good things connected to life in my own apartment. One of the most annoying things of sleeping in the hospital bed had been the rubber covering of the mattress that was stiff, hot, and noisy each time I changed my position. The thing I hated most, though, were the light blue hospital gowns, most of them too big for me, so that they resulted in a rakish, off-the shoulder look that gave me at the same time a waiflike appearance not helpful to my sagging self-confidence. Worst of all, in spite of daily washings in the hospital laundry, was the acrid smell of having been worn by too many bodies, each with its personal odor. Tomorrow I could return to my own bed and wear my own nightgown!

When dawn finally came, I relished the sight of the Hudson whose steady, relentless flow had had such a calming influence on me during the past five weeks. It had been a source of silent, steady support that spoke of the continuity of life even in the face of changing seasons and circumstances. It was comforting to know that it would always be there, whether I regarded it or not. The view of the river had served me well, and I wished that the sight of it would be equally calming to future inhabitants of this bed.

Even the early reveille and the sponge bath at the sink were easier to bear today, knowing that a few hours hence I would be able to put hospital life behind me. But every small part of the morning routine was tinged with a bit of sadness, nevertheless. Would I ever have that much guidance and support again from the people around me?

The head nurse breezed into my room. "I've come to give you the prescriptions for all the medications Dr. Mitchell wants you to take. Get these filled as soon as you get home." She handed me several prescriptions in an envelope. Her visit started a procession of various staff members, each with his or her written orders for my new life. Dr. Stuart, who had checked on me almost daily, left me a prescription for another rehabilitation center where I was to take a driving evaluation when I felt ready. At this point, that seemed like a distant goal, but I was pleased that she considered me a future candidate for resuming driving. Even the social worker that I had hardly ever seen told me that a visiting nurse would evaluate my need for a home health aide. For the moment, Helen would be my helper, and I was relieved that I would not need other assistance.

I had been told that I would not have therapy this morning, but my three therapists were available for final questions and instructions. It was hard to say good-bye to all three: Anne-Marie and I had laughed together over the small successes and rough going as the slurring slowly left my speech; Romana, kindness personified, yet nevertheless very businesslike when it came to all of the activities of living; and Ilsa, to whom I had formed a deep relationship based on her understanding and unfailing confidence in my ability; all three had guided my progress in a way that far exceeded my expectations. I knew I would be back for occasional visits, since I still had the unfinished research project that I was hoping to complete, and this made it easier to leave them behind. I felt I owed the therapists so much; I could never adequately express my feelings to them without breaking down.

When I returned to my room, Helen was already waiting, and I was eager to go. The obligatory wheelchair was brought by an orderly who took me down to the front door, where I happily exchanged the wheelchair for my cane and the front seat of Helen's car. At last I was free and could put life in the hospital behind me!

I felt the same kind of euphoria that always signaled the end of an examination in college. Suddenly I could understand patients with whom I had worked who relied on magical thinking that "everything will be all right once I get home." It was a way of avoiding unpleasant challenges in the hospital or confronting realities that seemed too awful to face. In my case, it was somewhat different; I was tired of practicing in simulated situations and wanted to try what is was really like to have to solve a particular problem.

On the drive home, Helen and I talked about the way we would spend the days together; her goal was to make sure I could manage taking care of myself and preparing meals with minimal help from a home care worker, whose salary for a few hours each day was covered by my insurance. We would practice walking as much as I could to build up my endurance. It seemed like a practical plan, and I was eager to get started.

My arrival at home was similar to my visit, except for one important difference; since it was later in the day, many of my neighbors were passing through the lobby on their way in or out, and I was warmly greeted by several people. "We heard about your illness from Carlos." Leave it to the doorman to inform the entire building population! I was touched by so much concern and offers of all kinds of help by tenants I hardly knew.

When we reached my apartment, I was overcome by exhaustion and sank into an easy chair where I stayed for several hours, grateful that no one was expecting me to be anywhere or do anything. Helen plied me with food and drink, after which I felt a new surge of energy. I was surprised that the visiting nurse that was scheduled to look in on me called to announce her house call in an hour. When the doorbell rang, I picked up my cane and walked to the door to let in the visitor.

"Hello, I'm Donna Vasquez. Are you the patient?" When I nodded my head, she continued, "I expected you to be in bed! I've never had a patient greet me at the door before; you made my day!" With that she began her interview and evaluation, reviewed my medications, and said she would call me the next day, but since I was already so independent and had Helen for the present, she felt that her services were not required. Besides, the home therapists were to evaluate me the next day to determine what type of physical therapy and occupational therapy were to be ordered.

Her assessment increased my confidence to the extent that, almost giddily, I suggested to Helen that we celebrate by going out to dinner, since we had no food in the house.

"Are you sure you're up to it?" Her query was prompted by genuine concern, but when I answered in the affirmative, she was ready to take me up on the suggestion. I thought it would be a good idea to face the public while I was feeling so high.

People did not even look up from their dinners when we entered. I became aware of the number of diners using canes, crutches, and wheelchairs who passed our table; I felt I was in good company. It was the last time I ever worried about the cane in public. Far more worrisome was my tortoiselike gait; everyone on the sidewalk easily passed me. In the hospital this was the normal speed with which patients progressed. Now obviously I had to compete primarily with able-bodied individuals, and the match was not a good one. Nevertheless, Helen and I enjoyed our first outing; I was beginning to shed my patient skin.

It was heavenly to sleep in my own bed again, and I slept soundly. Next morning I stepped into the tub gingerly, holding on to the sink for support, and was glad to sit on the shower bench that Romana had ordered for me. The fall in the shower five weeks before was still fresh in my memory, and I did not want to repeat it. On the other hand, a nurse had given me a shower only twice during more than a month in the hospital, and I was ready for the experience of feeling really clean and refreshed.

As expected, the physical therapist came to assess my strength and gait. She was very young but appeared competent in checking my status. When she was finished, she gave me some exercises to do on my own but said I was too advanced for the home therapy to which I was entitled. Shortly after she had left, the occupational therapist arrived, and like Romana on the home visit, she wanted to inspect the apartment for safety hazards, after she had determined my functional status. She was older than the

physical therapist, and experience had seasoned her to be more thorough. We enjoyed talking shoptalk for a few minutes before she rose to leave.

"You're really doing very well, and I don't believe you need any home therapy. Just do the exercises on the staircase that I'll show you." With that she took me to the apartment house staircase where she demonstrated a number of exercises for strengthening my ankle. Then she, too, took the elevator down, leaving me in the questionable position of having lost all eligibility for further therapy because I was too well! Instead of feeling elated that all three health professionals independently of each other had pronounced me in such good condition, I felt rather abandoned and let down. Helen considered the therapists' verdict as good news, and so I agreed with her.

Now we were really on our own, rejoicing in the fact that we could schedule the time together in any way that suited our fancy. It was delightful to be free of the rigid hospital schedule!

We filled the next days with short walks and frequent rests to build up my endurance. During a trip to the supermarket by car, I found that I could use the grocery cart almost like a walker, and so could look forward to shopping by myself. I was aware that the store made deliveries, and I decided to investigate the possibility at a future time.

With every day we added another block to my destination, and although I was completely exhausted each time I reached my house, I saw that an increased distance was well within the realm of possibility. Helen allowed me to try everything in the kitchen; she knew that I would not risk doing the impossible. Finally, seven days after I came home, I was able to walk to the supermarket and back—the goal I had set for myself. Helen and I agreed that I could carry on by myself.

As she packed her bag, we talked about the fact that my illness had brought us even closer together. Difficult though it was to say good-bye, I was eager to try to fend for myself as the new person I had become during the last six weeks. Seven weeks ago, the chance of my having a stroke at this time was not even in my realm of possibilities. I was anticipating many years of the good health that I enjoyed and that I considered my responsibility. Six weeks ago, when I first took my place among the seriously ill men and women in the hospital, I did not remotely envision that exactly 42 days later I would be well enough to resume my former life with only a few adjustments. But would I ever get back my prior self? Perhaps not, but as I had learned, I had been blessed with a rich dose of the resilience that allows both body and spirit to seize the second chance.

Index

Page numbers followed by *f* indicate figures; *t*, tables; *b*, boxes.

A

Abdominal wall muscles
  obliques, 159-160
  rectus abdominis, 159
  transversus abdominis, 160
Abducens nerve, 213-215f
ABILHAND questionnaire, 221
Absorption, venous and lymphatic, 308-309
  manual stimulation methods, 313-317
Accommodation, 418t, 420, 423
Acquisitional occupation, 569f, 571, 580
Acquisition stage of learning, 106
Action
  ecological approach to, 81
  ineffective, compensation for, 580-581
Action Research Arm Test, 222
Active robot systems, 282
Active seating system, 675
Activities of daily living (ADL). *See also specific activities*
  AMPS for, 88
  apraxia and, 512-514, 513b
  and clinical reasoning with A-ONE, 489-490
  definitions of, 457
  driving and community mobility as crucial ADL,
    600-601
  dysfunction of area of occupation, 469-486
  effect of spatial impairments, 432-434f
  enhancement
    in assisted living setting, 555-573
    for elderly client living at home, 573-575
  grading, during acute stroke rehabilitation, 41b
  instrumental. *See* Instrumental activities of daily
    living (IADL)
  neurobehavioral deficit effects, 462-467
    assessment methods, 490-494
  one-handed techniques
    adaptive devices, 727-728
    dressing, 723, 724-727
    feeding techniques, 728
    grooming and hygiene, 718-728
  performance of, 458
  processing during, 467-469
  for regaining trunk control, 186
  retraining after stroke, 717b, 750
  and systems model of motor behavior, 83-84
  taxonomy, 559-561f
  trunk control during, 176-180
  weight-bearing during, 232f
Activities-Specific Balance Confidence Scale, 199, 382t
Activity-based intervention
  amount of practice, 106
  background concepts, 101-102
  constraint-induced movement therapy, 103
  expectation for goal achievement, 111
  foundational strategies for task performance, 104-105
  freedom from mechanical constraints to movement,
    110
  goals of training and learning, 104
  neuroscience studies of brain plasticity, 102-103
  occupational therapy practice
    framework, 101-102
    guidelines for adults, 102
  prerequisites to engaging in activity-based practice,
    109-110
  promoting generalization of learning, 106-109
  self-monitoring skills, 110-111
  structuring activity demands, 112-114
  task analysis and problem-solving skills, 111
  types of learning, 105-106
Activity Card Sort, 70f, 72t, 739
Activity processing, in cognitive rehabilitation, 508
Activity synthesis, 114

Acute care
  functional assessments in, 74
  goal setting in, 42b
  issues of driving addressed during, 603
  team approach in, 754
Acute stroke rehabilitation
  assessments used in, 31
  CIMT during, 236
  communication, 37
  discharge planning, 42
  dysphagia screening, 37
  early cognitive management, 36
  early intervention, 26
  edema management, 35
  family training, 39-42
  goal setting in acute care, 42
  increasing spatial awareness, 36
  interventions for, 31-35
  monitoring, 27-31
    basic ICU monitor, 28
    feeding tubes, 30
    ventilator, 30-31
  positioning, 31-35
    functional activity during acute phase, 33-34
    weight-bearing for function, 34-35
  self-care training, 37-39
  shoulder management, 35-36
  skin protection, 36-37
  team approach, 26-27
Adaptation(s)
  baby care, 584-585
  dimension of OTIPM, 562, 576
  to doors in home, 709
  of environment, 92-93, 186-187, 503, 518
  motor, 163
  one-handed techniques
    basic ADL, 718-728
    basic environmental considerations, 717-718
    community-based activities, 732-734
    IADL, 728-732
  of performance, 566f
  as treatment approach, 502t
Adaptive equipment
  for baby care
    bedtime, 588-589
    childproofing, 589
    diapering, 589
  dressing devices, 727-728
  eating/dining devices, 728
  mobility prescription, 621-622
Adaptive occupation, 569f, 570, 580-581
Adelaide Activities Profile, 556-558t
Adhesive changes, in hemiplegic shoulder, 261
Adjustable inflatable hand splint, 33b
Adjustment, to role and task performance limitations,
  90-91
Age effects
  on driving, 603-605
  on functional mobility, 351
  on sexual response cycle, 649
Agnosia, 460
  treatment for, 521
Air splint, 331
  for hand edema, 317-318
Alcohol, heavy consumption of, 26
Alexia, 522
Alignment
  biomechanical
    loss of, 264-268
    and splinting distal extremity, 339-340
  normal, and malalignments after stroke, 170t
  ocular, 427

Alignment *(Continued)*
  of scapulothoracic and glenohumeral joints, 254f
  spinal, 668f
  trunk, observations of, 169-170
Alternate Cover Test, 428
Alternating attention impairment, 527
Ambulation
  intervention advancements, 397
  speed, 391, 392-393
Ambulatory patients, treatment activities and goals for,
  202b
American Association of Motor Vehicle Administrators
  (AAMVA), 606
American Heart Association Stroke Outcome
  Classification, 719t
Amnesia
  anterograde, 524-525t
  retrograde, 524-525t
AMPS, 88, 221, 381, 430-431, 505-506t, 555
  evaluation of ADL performance in assisted living
    setting, 564-568
  graphic report, 561-562, 567f
  items observed and evaluated in, 559b
  performance skill summary, 561, 565f, 566f
Ampullar nerves, 211f
Anarthria, 538-539
Anatomy
  of shoulder, 269f
  of swallowing, 629-632
  of trunk
    muscular system, 159-161
    skeletal system, 157-159
Aneurysm, saccular, 9-10
Anger, and stroke risk, 50
Angular motion, system of naming, 390f
Ankle-foot orthoses (AFOs), 403, 404f, 405f
Ankle strategy, 191, 195, 205
Anomic aphasia, 546, 547t
Anosognosia, 471, 482-484
Anterior lobe of cerebellum, 399
Anterograde amnesia, 524-525t
Antibiotics, for aspiration, 23
Anticlaw splint, 341f
Anticoagulation agents, 16, 19
Antiplatelet agents, 16, 18-19
Antiseizure medication, signs of excess of, 21b
Antithrombotic therapy, 16
Anxiety
  after stroke event, 21
  coupled with depression, 53
  in MRI machine, 765
  PTSD in stroke survivors, 53-54
Anxiety disorders, 55t
A-ONE, 430-431, 457, 458-461t, 476, 489-494,
  491-493t, 495-497f, 505-506t, 719t
Apathy, 52, 55t, 471
Aphasia, 536, 539
  Broca, 540-542, 543t
  fluent types of, 544
  transcortical motor, 542-544, 544t
Apraxia
  assessing, 505-506t
  functional deficits secondary to, 515b
  ideational, 464f, 472, 479-481f
  interventions
    direct training of whole activity, 514
    errorless completion, 512-514
    strategy training, 511-512
    task-specific training, 514-516
  motor, 473, 476-478, 484
  of speech, 542, 543t
  treatment for, 510-516